the calorie carb and fat bible 2009

Juliette Kellow BSc RD, Lyndel Costain BSc RD & Rebecca Walton

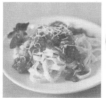 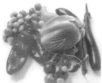 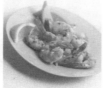 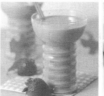 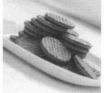 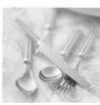

The UK's Most Comprehensive Calorie Counter

The Calorie, Carb & Fat Bible 2009

Published by:
Weight Loss Resources Ltd
29 Metro Centre
Woodston,
Peterborough
PE2 7UH.

Tel: 01733 345592
www.weightlossresources.co.uk

Companies and other organisations wishing to make bulk purchases of the Calorie, Carb and Fat Bible should contact their local bookstore or Weight Loss Resources direct.

ISBN 978 1 904512 07 3

Authors: Lyndel Costain BSc RD
Juliette Kellow BSc RD
Rebecca Walton, Weight Loss Resources

Database Editor: Laura Meads

Design & Layout: Jonathan Lansdown

Printed and bound in Finland by:
WS Bookwell Oy

Contents

Losing Weight - the Easy Way 5

Getting Ready for Weight Loss Success 13

Coping with Common Slimming Saboteurs.............. 21

Your Step-by-Step Guide to Using this Book
and Shifting Those Pounds 26

Healthy Eating Made Easy 32

Useful Tools 36

Food Information 44

Weights, Measures & Abbreviations 47

General Foods and Drinks A-Z 49

Eating Out Brands A-Z.. 442

Useful Resources... 506

Losing weight – the easy way

Juliette Kellow BSc RD

CHINESE TAKEAWAYS, curries, chocolate, chips and a glass of wine! Imagine being told the best diet to help you lose weight includes all these foods and more. It sounds too good to be true, doesn't it? But the truth is, these are exactly the types of foods you can still enjoy if you opt to lose weight by counting calories.

But you'd be forgiven for not knowing you can still eat all your favourite foods *and* lose weight. In recent years, endless trendy diets that cut carbs, boost protein intake or skip entire groups of foods, have helped to make dieting a complicated business. Added to this, an increasing number of celebrities and so-called nutrition experts have helped mislead us into thinking that dieting is all about restriction and denial. Is it any wonder then that most of us have been left feeling downright confused and miserable about what we should and shouldn't be eating to shift those pounds?

Dieting doesn't have to be complicated or an unhappy experience. In fact, there's really only one word you need to remember if you want to shift those pounds healthily and still eat all your favourite foods. And that's CALORIE!

It's calories that count

When it comes to losing weight, there's no getting away from the fact that it's calories that count. Ask any qualified nutrition expert or dietitian for advice on how to fight the flab and you'll receive the same reply: quite simply you need to create a calorie deficit or shortfall. In other words, you need to take in fewer calories than you use up so that your body has to draw on its fat stores to provide it with the energy it needs to function properly. The result: you start losing fat and the pounds start to drop off!

Fortunately, it couldn't be easier to create this calorie deficit. Regardless of your age, weight, sex, genetic make up, lifestyle or eating habits, losing weight is as simple as reducing your daily calorie intake slightly by modifying your diet and using up a few more calories by being slightly more active each day.

Better still, it's a complete myth that you need to change your eating and exercise habits dramatically. You'll notice I've said you need to reduce your calorie intake 'slightly' and be 'slightly' more active. It really is just LITTLE differences between the amount of calories we take in and the amount we use up that make BIG differences to our waistline over time. For example, you only need to consume one can of cola more than you need each day to gain a stone in a year. It's no wonder then that people say excess weight tends to 'creep up on them'.

10 simple food swaps you can make every day (and won't even notice!)

Make these simple swaps every day and in just 4 weeks you'll lose 7lb!

SWAP THIS...	FOR THIS...	SAVE...
300ml full-fat milk (195 calories)	300ml skimmed milk (100 calories)	95 calories
1tsp butter (35 calories)	1tsp low-fat spread (20 calories)	15 calories
1tbsp vegetable oil (100 calories)	10 sprays of a spray oil (10 calories)	90 calories
1tsp sugar (16 calories)	Artificial sweetener (2 calories)	14 calories
1tbsp mayonnaise (105 calories)	1tbsp fat-free dressing (10 calories)	95 calories
Regular sandwich (600 calories)	Low-fat sandwich (350 calories)	250 calories
Can of cola (135 calories)	Can of diet cola (0.5 calories)	12.5 calories
Large (50g) packet of crisps (250 calories)	Small (25g) packet of crisps (125 calories)	125 calories
1 chocolate digestive (85 calories)	1 small chocolate chip cookie (55 calories)	30 calories
1 slice thick-cut wholemeal bread (95 calories)	1 slice medium-cut wholemeal bread (75 calories)	20 calories
	TOTAL CALORIE SAVING:	**858.5 calories**

The good news is the reverse is also true. You only need to swap that daily can of cola for the diet version or a glass of sparking water and you'll lose a stone in a year – it really is as easy as that!

Of course, most people don't want to wait a year to shift a stone. But there's more good news. To lose 1lb of fat each week you need to create a calorie deficit of just 500 calories a day. That might sound like a lot, but you can achieve this by simply swapping a croissant for a wholemeal fruit scone, a regular sandwich for a low-fat variety, a glass of dry white wine for a gin and slimline tonic and using low-fat spread on two slices of toast instead of butter. It is also important to become more active and increase your level of exercise. Losing 1lb a week, amounts to a stone in 14 weeks, or just under 4 stone in a year!

Taking control of calories

By now you've seen it really is calories that count when it comes to shifting those pounds. So it should be no surprise that a calorie-controlled diet is the only guaranteed way to help you shift those pounds – and that's a scientific fact! But better still, a calorie-controlled diet is one of the few that allows you to include anything, whether it's pizza, wine or chocolate. A healthy diet means including a wide range of foods (see 'Healthy Eating Made Easy' page 32).

And that's where this book can really help. Gone are the days when it was virtually impossible to obtain information about the calorie contents of foods. This book provides calorie information for more than 22,000 different branded and unbranded foods so that counting calories has never been easier.

The benefits of counting calories

✓ *It's guaranteed to help you lose weight providing you stick to your daily calorie allowance*

✓ *You can include favourite foods*

✓ *No foods are banned*

✓ *It's a great way to lose weight slowly and steadily*

✓ *Nutrition experts agree that it's a proven way to lose weight*

Calorie counting made easy

Forget weird and wacky science, complicated diet rules and endless lists of foods to fill up on or avoid every day! Counting calories to lose weight couldn't be easier. Quite simply, you set yourself a daily calorie allowance to help you lose between ½-2lb (¼-1kg) a week and then add up the calories of everything you eat and drink each day, making sure you don't go over your limit.

To prevent hunger from kicking in, it's best to spread your daily calorie allowance evenly throughout the day, allowing a certain amount of calories for breakfast, lunch, dinner and one or two snacks. For example, if you are allowed 1,500 calories a day, you could have 300 calories for breakfast, 400 calories for lunch, 500 calories for dinner and two snacks or treats of 150 calories each. You'll find more detailed information on p26-31 (Your step-by-step guide to using this book and shifting those pounds).

QUESTION
What affects the calorie content of a food?

ANSWER:
Fat, protein, carbohydrate and alcohol all provide the body with calories, but in varying amounts:

- *1g fat provides 9 calories*

- *1g alcohol provides 7 calories*

- *1g protein provides 4 calories*

- *1g carbohydrate provides 3.75 calories*

The calorie content of a food depends on the amount of fat, protein and carbohydrate it contains. Because fat provides more than twice as many calories as an equal quantity of protein or carbohydrate, in general, foods that are high in fat tend to contain more calories. This explains why 100g of chips (189 calories) contains more than twice as many calories as 100g of boiled potato (72 calories).

DIET MYTH:
Food eaten late at night stops you losing weight

DIET FACT:

It's not eating in the evening that stops you losing weight. It's consuming too many calories throughout the day that will be your dieting downfall! Providing you stick to your daily calorie allowance you'll lose weight, regardless of when you consume those calories. Nevertheless, it's a good idea to spread your calorie allowance throughout the day to prevent hunger from kicking in, which leaves you reaching for high-calorie snack foods.

Eat for good health

While calories might be the buzz word when it comes to shifting those pounds, it's nevertheless important to make sure your diet is healthy, balanced and contains all the nutrients you need for good health. Yes, you can still lose weight by eating nothing but, for example, chocolate, crisps and biscuits providing you stick to your calorie allowance. But you'll never find a nutrition expert or dietitian recommending this. And there are plenty of good reasons why.

To start with, an unbalanced diet is likely to be lacking in essential nutrients such as protein, vitamins, minerals and fibre, in the long term putting you at risk of nutritional deficiencies. Secondly, research proves that filling up on foods that are high in fat and/or salt and sugar can lead to many different health problems. But most importantly, when it comes to losing weight, it's almost impossible to stick to a daily calorie allowance if you're only eating high-calorie foods.

Filling up on lower-calorie foods also means you'll be able to eat far more with the result that you're not constantly left feeling unsatisfied. For example, six chocolates from a selection box contain around 300 calories, a lot of fat and sugar, few nutrients – and are eaten in just six mouthfuls! For 300 calories, you could have a grilled skinless chicken breast (packed with protein and zinc), a large salad with fat-free dressing (a great source of fibre, vitamins and minerals), a slice of wholemeal bread with low-fat spread (rich in fibre and B vitamins) and a satsuma (an excellent source of vitamin C). That's a lot more food that will take you a lot more time to eat! Not convinced? Then put six chocolates on one plate, and the chicken, salad, bread and fruit on another!

Bottom line: while slightly reducing your calorie intake is the key to losing weight, you'll be healthier and far more likely to keep those pounds off if you do it by eating a healthy diet *(see 'Healthy Eating Made Easy' page 32).*

Eight steps to a healthy diet

1 *Base your meals on starchy foods.*

2 *Eat lots of fruit and vegetables.*

3 *Eat more fish.*

4 *Cut down on saturated fat and sugar.*

5 *Try to eat less salt - no more than 6g a day.*

6 *Get active and try to be a healthy weight.*

7 *Drink plenty of water.*

8 *Don't skip breakfast.*   SOURCE: FSA www.eatwell.gov.uk

Fat facts

Generally speaking, opting for foods that are low in fat can help slash your calorie intake considerably, for example, swapping full-fat milk for skimmed, switching from butter to a low-fat spread, not frying food in oil and chopping the fat off meat and poultry. But don't be fooled into believing that all foods described as 'low-fat' or 'fat-free' are automatically low in calories or calorie-free. In fact, some low-fat products may actually be higher in calories than standard products, thanks to them containing extra sugars and thickeners to boost the flavour and texture. The solution: always check the calorie content of low-fat foods, especially for things like cakes, biscuits, crisps, ice creams and ready meals. You might be surprised to find there's little difference in the calorie content when compared to the standard product.

Uncovering fat claims on food labels

Many products may lure you into believing they're a great choice if you're trying to cut fat, but you need to read between the lines on the labels if you want to be sure you're making the best choice. Here's the lowdown on what to look for:

LOW FAT	by law the food must contain less than 3g of fat per 100g for solids. These foods are generally a good choice if you're trying to lose weight.
REDUCED FAT	by law the food must contain 25 percent less fat than a similar standard product. This doesn't mean the product is low-fat (or low-calorie) though! For example, reduced-fat cheese may still contain 14g fat per 100g.
FAT FREE	the food must contain no more than 0.5g of fat per 100g or 100ml. Foods labelled as Virtually Fat Free must contain less than 0.3g fat per 100g. These foods are generally a good choice if you're trying to lose weight.
LESS THAN 8% FAT	this means the product contains less than 8g fat per 100g. It's only foods labelled 'less than 3% fat' that are a true low-fat choice.
X% FAT FREE	claims expressed as X% Fat Free shall be prohibited.
LIGHT OR LITE	claims stating a product is 'light' or 'lite' follows the same conditions as those set for the term 'reduced'.

10 easy ways to slash fat (and calories)

1   Eat fewer fried foods – grill, boil, bake, poach, steam, roast without added fat or microwave instead.

2   Don't add butter, lard, margarine or oil to food during preparation or cooking.

3   Use spreads sparingly. Butter and margarine contain the same amount of calories and fat – only low fat spreads contain less.

4   Choose boiled or jacket potatoes instead of chips or roast potatoes.

5   Cut off all visible fat from meat and remove the skin from chicken before cooking.

6   Don't eat too many fatty meat products such as sausages, burgers, pies and pastry products.

7   Use semi-skimmed or skimmed milk instead of full-fat milk.

8   Try low-fat or reduced-fat varieties of cheese such as reduced-fat Cheddar, low-fat soft cheese or cottage cheese.

9   Eat fewer high-fat foods such as crisps, chocolates, cakes, pastries and biscuits.

10   Don't add cream to puddings, sauces or coffee.

Getting Ready for Weight Loss Success

Lyndel Costain BSc RD

THIS BOOK not only provides tools to help you understand more about what you eat and how active you are, but guidance on how to use this information to develop a weight loss plan to suit your needs. Getting in the right frame of mind will also be a key part of your weight control journey, especially if you've lost weight before, only to watch the pounds pile back on.

The fact is that most people who want to lose weight know what to do. But often there is something that keeps stopping them from keeping up healthier habits. The same may be true for you. So what's going on? For many it's a lack of readiness. When the next diet comes along with its tempting promises it's so easy to just jump on board. But if you have struggled with your weight for a while, will that diet actually help you to recognise and change the thoughts and actions that have stopped you shifting the pounds for good?

Check out your attitude to weight loss programmes

Before starting any new weight loss programme, including the Weight Loss Resources approach, ask yourself:

Am I starting out thinking that I like myself as a person right now?	(YES or NO)
OR I feel I can only like myself once I lose weight?	(YES or NO)
Do I want to stop overeating, but at the same time find myself justifying it – in other words I want to be able to eat what I want, but with no consequences?	(YES or NO)
Do I believe that I need to take long-term responsibility for my weight?	(YES or NO)
OR Am I relying on 'it' (the diet) to do it for me?	(YES or NO)

Keep these questions, and your replies, in mind as you read through this chapter.

Next Steps

You may have already assessed the healthiness of your weight using the BMI guide on page 37. If not, why not do it now, remembering that the tools are a guide only. The important thing is to consider a weight at which you are healthy and comfortable – and which is realistic for the life you lead *(see opposite - What is a healthy weight?)*.

The next step is to have a long hard think about why you want to lose weight. Consider all the possible benefits, not just those related to how you look. Psychologists have found that if we focus only on appearance we are less likely to succeed in the long-term. This is because it so often reflects low self-esteem or self-worth – which can sabotage success – as it saps confidence and keeps us stuck in destructive thought patterns. Identifying key motivations other than simply how you look - such as health and other aspects of physical and emotional well being - is like saying that you're an OK person right now, and worth making changes for. Making healthy lifestyle choices also has the knock on effect of boosting self-esteem further.

Write down your reasons for wanting to lose weight in your Personal Plan *(see page 42)* – so you can refer back to them. This can be especially helpful when the going gets tough. It may help to think of it in terms of what your weight is stopping you from doing now. Here's some examples: to feel more confident; so I can play more comfortably with my kids; my healthier diet will give me more energy; to improve my fertility.

What is a Healthy Weight?

With all the 'thin is beautiful' messages in the media it can be easy to get a distorted view about whether your weight is healthy or not. However, as the BMI charts suggest, there is no single 'ideal' weight for anybody. Research also shows that modest amounts of weight loss can be very beneficial to health and are easier to keep off. Therefore, health professionals now encourage us to aim for a weight loss of 5-10%. The ideal rate of weight loss is no more than 1-2 pounds (0.5-1kg) per week – so averaging a pound a week is great, and realistic progress.

The health benefits of modest weight loss include:

✓ *Reduced risk of developing heart disease, stroke and certain cancers*

✓ *Reduced risk of developing diabetes and helping to manage diabetes*

✓ *Improvements in blood pressure*

✓ *Improvements in mobility, back pain and joint pain*

✓ *Improvements with fertility problems and polycystic ovarian syndrome*

✓ *Less breathlessness and sleep/snoring problems*

✓ *Increased self esteem and control over eating*

✓ *Feeling fitter and have more energy*

Are You Really Ready to Lose Weight?

When you think of losing weight, it's easy just to think of what weight you'd like to get to. But weight loss only happens as a result of making changes to your usual eating and activity patterns – which allow you to consume fewer calories than you burn *(see 'It's calories that count' page 5)*.

So here comes the next big question. Are you really ready to do it? Have you thought about the implications of your decision? If you have lost weight in the past, and put it all back on - have you thought about why that was? And how confident do you feel about being successful this time?

To help you answer these questions, try these short exercises.

Where would you place yourself on the following scales?

Importance

How important is it to you, to make the changes that will allow you to lose weight?

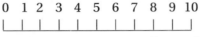

0 1 2 3 4 5 6 7 8 9 10

Not at all important   *Extremely important*

If you ranked yourself over half way along the scale then move on to the next question. If you were half way or less along the scale, you may not be mentally ready to make the required changes to lose weight. To further explore this, go to *'The Pros and Cons of Weight Loss' (page 17).*

Confidence

How confident are you in your ability to make the changes that will allow you to lose weight?

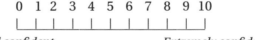

0 1 2 3 4 5 6 7 8 9 10

Not at all confident   *Extremely confident*

Now ask yourself (regarding your confidence ratings):

1. Why did I place myself here?

2. What is stopping me moving further up the scale (if anything)?

3. What things, information, support would help me move further up the scale? (if not near 10)

If you aren't sure about answers to question 3, then keep reading for some pointers.

The Pros and Cons of Weight Loss

Making lifestyle changes to lose weight is simpler if there are lots of clear benefits or pros, for example, clothes fit again, more energy, helps back pain - but there will also be associated downsides or cons. For example, some may feel it interferes with their social life, or don't have the time to plan meals or check food labels. Or overeating can help, if only temporarily, as a way of coping with unwanted feelings. Being overweight allows some people to feel strong and assertive, or to control their partner's jealousy. So in these cases there are downsides to losing weight, even if the person says they are desperate to do it.

If you are aware of the possible downsides, as well as the pros, you will be better prepared to deal with potential conflicts. Understanding what could be (or were with past weight loss efforts) barriers to success gives you the chance to address them. This boosts confidence in your ability to succeed this time, which in turn maintains your motivation.

Have a go at weighing up the pros and cons using the charts below and on page 18. Some examples are included. If you decide that the pros outweigh the cons, then great. You can also use the cons as potential barriers to plan strategies for *(see Personal Plan)*. If you find it's the other way around, this may not be the best time to actively lose weight. Try the exercise again in a month or so.

Making Lifestyle Changes to Lose Weight Now

CONS *e.g. Must limit eating out, take aways*	PROS *e.g. Feel more energetic, slimmer*

Not Making Changes Now – how would I feel in 6 months time?

PROS *e.g. Haven't had to worry about failing;* *Still able to eat take aways a lot*	CONS *e.g. Probably gained more weight;* *Back pain may be worse*

To change your weight, first change your mind

To lose weight you may already have a list of things to change, such as eating more fruit and veg, calculating your daily calorie intake, going for a walk each morning or buying low fat options. Others could also give you tips to try. But knowing what to do isn't the same as feeling motivated or able to do it. To be effective, you have to believe the changes are relevant, do-able and worth it.

What you think, affects how you feel, and in turn the actions you take.

Self-efficacy

In fact, research is telling us that one of the most important factors that influences weight loss success are your feelings of 'self-efficacy'. Self-efficacy is a term used in psychology to describe a person's belief that any action they take will have an effect on the outcome. It reflects our inner expectation that what we do will lead to the results we want. Not surprisingly, high levels of self-efficacy can enhance motivation, and allow us to deal better with uncertainty and conflict, and recovery from setbacks. But low levels, can reduce our motivation. We fear that whatever we do will not bring about our desired goal. This can lead self-defeating thoughts or 'self-talk', which make it hard to deal with set-backs, meaning we are more likely to give up. Here's some examples.

Examples: Low self-efficacy
' No matter how carefully I diet, I don't lose weight . . . '
' I have eaten that chocolate and as usual blown my diet, so I may as well give up now. '
' I had a rich dessert – I have no willpower to say no. I can't stand not being able to eat what I want. '

If you have a strong sense of self-efficacy, your mindset and 'self-talk' will be more like:

Examples: High self-efficacy
' I know from previous weight loss programmes, that if I stay focussed on what I am doing I do lose weight. I have always expected to lose too much too quickly which frustrates me. I know that I will lose weight if I keep making the right changes, and this time it is important to me. '
' The chocolate bar won't ruin my diet, but if I think it has and keep on eating, then my negative self-talk will. So I will get back on track. '
*' I don't like having to eat differently from others, but losing weight is very important to me, so I **can** stand it. After all, the world won't stop if I say no to dessert, and I will feel great afterwards. If I think about it, I am not hungry so would just feel bloated and guilty if I ate it. '*

Willpower is a Skill

Many people feel that they just need plenty of willpower or a good telling off to lose weight. But willpower isn't something you have or you don't have. Willpower is a skill. Like the dessert example on page 19, it's a sign that you've made a conscious choice to do something, because you believe the benefits outweigh any downsides. In reality everything we do is preceded by a thought. This includes everything we eat. It just may not seem like it because our actions often feel automatic *(see 'Look out for trigger eating' page 21)*.

When it comes to weight loss, developing a range of skills – including choosing a lower calorie diet, coping with negative self-talk and managing things that don't go to plan - will boost your sense of self-efficacy to make the changes you want. This is especially important because we live in such a weight-promoting environment.

Our weight-promoting environment

We are constantly surrounded by tempting food, stresses that can trigger comfort eating and labour-saving devices that make it easy not to be physically active. In other words, the environment we live in makes it easy to gain weight, unless we stop and think about the food choices we make and how much exercise we do. In fact, to stay a healthy weight/maintain our weight, just about all of us need to make conscious lifestyle choices everyday. This isn't 'dieting' but just part of taking care of ourselves in the environment we live in.

It is also true that some people find it more of a challenge than others to manage their weight, thanks to genetic differences in factors such as appetite control, spontaneous activity level and emotional responses to food – rather than metabolic rate, as is often believed. The good news is that with a healthy diet and active lifestyle a healthier weight can still be achieved. But do talk to your doctor if you feel you need additional support.

Coping with Common Slimming Saboteurs

Lyndel Costain BSc RD

Look out for 'trigger' eating

Much of the overeating we do or cravings we have are actually down to unconscious, habitual, responses to a variety of triggers. These triggers can be external, such as the sight or smell of food, or internal and emotion-led, such as a response to stress, anger, boredom or emptiness. Your food diary (see page 43) helps you to recognise 'trigger' or 'non-hungry' eating which gives you the chance to think twice before you eat (see below).

Get some support

A big part of your success will be having someone to support you. It could be a friend, partner, health professional, health club or website. Let them know how they can help you most.

Make lapses your ally

Don't let a lapse throw you off course. You can't be, nor need to be perfect all the time. Doing well 80-90% of the time is great progress. Lapses are a normal part of change. Rather than feel you have failed and give up, look at what you can learn from a difficult day or week and use it to find helpful solutions for the future.

Understand why you eat

When I ask people what prompts them to eat, hunger usually comes down near the bottom of their list of reasons. Some people struggle to remember or appreciate what true hunger feels like. We are lucky that we have plenty of food to eat in our society. But its constant presence makes it harder to control what we eat, especially if it brings us comfort or joy.

If you ever find yourself in the fridge even though you've recently eaten, then you know hunger isn't the reason but some other trigger. The urge to eat can be so automatic that you feel you lack willpower or are out of control. But it is in fact a learned or conditioned response. A bit like Pavlov's dogs. He rang a bell every time he fed them, and from then on, whenever they heard the bell ring they were 'conditioned' to salivate in anticipation of food.

Because this 'non-hungry' eating is learned, you can reprogramme your response to the situations or feelings that trigger it. The first step is to identify when these urges strike. When you find yourself eating when you aren't hungry ask yourself 'why do I want to eat, what am I feeling?' If you aren't sure think back to what was happening before you ate. Then ask yourself if there is another way you can feel better without food. Or you could chat to your urge to eat in a friendly way, telling it that you don't want to give into it, you have a planned meal coming soon, and it's merely a learned response. Whatever strategy you choose, the more often you break into your urges to eat, the weaker their hold becomes.

Practise positive self-talk

Self-talk may be positive and constructive (like your guardian angel) or negative and irrational (like having a destructive devil on your shoulder).

If you've had on-off battles with your weight over the years, it's highly likely that the 'devil' is there more often. 'All or nothing' self-talk for example, 'I ate a "bad food" so have broken my diet', can make you feel like a failure which, can then trigger you into the action of overeating and/or totally giving up *(see 'Diet-binge cycle' page 23)*. One of the most powerful things about it is that the last thoughts we have are what stays in our mind. So if we think 'I still look fat' or 'I will never be slim', these feelings stay with us.

To change your self-talk for the better, the trick is to first recognise it's happening (keeping a diary really helps, *see Keep a Food Diary, page 29*). Then turn it around into a positive version of the same events *(see Self-efficacy, page 18)* where the resulting action was to feel good and stay on track. Reshaping negative self-talk helps you to boost your self-esteem and feelings of self-efficacy, and with it change your self-definition - from someone who can't 'lose weight' or 'do this or that', to someone 'who can'. And when you believe you can…

The Diet – Binge Cycle

If this cycle looks familiar, use positive self-talk, and a more flexible dietary approach, to help you break free.

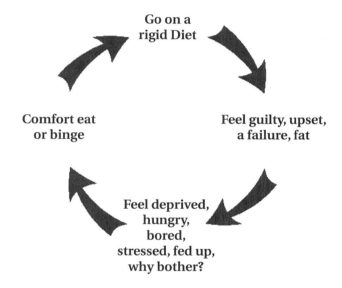

Go on a rigid Diet

Feel guilty, upset, a failure, fat

Feel deprived, hungry, bored, stressed, fed up, why bother?

Comfort eat or binge

Really choose what you want to eat

This skill is like your personal brake. It also helps you to manage 'trigger/non-hungry' eating and weaken its hold. It legalises food and stops you feeling deprived. It helps you to regularly remind yourself why you are making changes to your eating habits, which keeps motivation high. But it doesn't just happen. Like all skills it requires practise. Sometimes it will work well for you, other times it won't – but overall it will help. Basically, ask yourself if you really want to eat that food in front of you. This becomes the prompt for you to make a conscious choice, weighing up the pros and cons or consequences of making that choice, and feeling free to have it, reject it or just eat some. Remembering all the while that you can eat this food another time if you want to.

Action Planning

Successful people don't just wait for things to happen. They believe in themselves, plan ahead, take action and then refine their plan until it gets, and keeps on getting the results they want. Successful slimmers use a very similar approach. They don't rely on quick-fixes or magic formulas, but glean information from reliable sources to develop a plan or approach that suits their needs, tastes and lifestyle. Thinking of weight management as a lifelong project, which has a weight loss phase and a weight maintenance phase, is also a route to success.

When the Going Gets Tough - Staying on Track

If things start to go off track, don't panic. Learning new habits takes time. And life is never straightforward so there will be times when it all seems too much, or negative 'self- talk' creeps in to try and drag you back into old ways. So if the going gets tough:

- Value what you've achieved so far, rather than only focus on what you plan to do.
- Look back at your reasons to lose weight and refer to the list often .
- Don't expect to change too much, too quickly. Take things a step at a time.
- Accept difficulties as part of the learning and skill building process.
- Enjoy a non-food reward for achieving your goals (including maintaining your weight).
- Use recipes and meal ideas to keep things interesting.
- Talk to your supporters and get plenty of encouragement. This is really vital!

Strategies of Successful Slimmers

Thanks to research conducted by large studies such as the US National Weight Control Registry and the German Lean Habits Study, we now know more about what works best for people who have lost weight and successfully kept it off. So be inspired!

The key elements of success are to:

- Believe that you can control your weight and the changes involved are really worth it.
- Stay realistic and value what you have achieved rather than dwell on a weight you 'dream' of being.
- Be more active – plan ways to fit activity into your daily life – aim for 1 hour of walking daily.
- Plan ahead for regular meals and snacks, starting with breakfast.
- Choose a balanced, low-fat diet with plenty of fruit and vegetables (*see Healthy Eating Made Easy, page 32).*
- Watch portion size and limit fast food.
- Sit down to eat and take time over meals, paying attention to what you are eating.
- Have a flexible approach – plan in and enjoy some favourite foods without guilt.
- Recognise and address 'all or nothing' thinking and other negative 'self-talk'.
- Keep making conscious choices.
- Learn to confront problems rather than eat, drink, sleep or wish they would go away.
- Enlist ongoing help and support from family, friends, professionals or websites.
- Regularly (at least once a week but not more than once daily) check your weight.
- Take action before your weight increases by more than 4-5lb (2kg).
- Accept that your weight management skills need to be kept up long-term.
- Take heart from successful slimmers, who say that it gets easier over time.

Your step-by-step guide to using this book and shifting those pounds

Juliette Kellow BSc RD and Rebecca Walton

1. Find your healthy weight

Use the weight charts, body mass index table and information on pages 36-43 to determine the right weight for you. Then set yourself a weight to aim for. Research shows it really helps if you make losing 10% of your weight your first overall target. It also brings important health benefits too *(see 'What is a Healthy Weight?' page 15)*. You can break this down into smaller manageable steps, for example, 3kg/6.5lbs at a time. If 10% is too much, then go for a 5% loss – this has important health benefits too. In fact, just keeping your weight stable is a great achievement these days, because of our weight-promoting environment *(see page 20)*.

Waist Management

In addition to BMI, another important way to assess your weight is by measuring your waist just above belly button level. It is especially useful for men as they tend to carry more excess weight around their bellies, but women should test it out too. Having excess weight around your middle (known as being 'apple-shaped') increases your risk of heart disease and type 2 diabetes. A simple way to stay aware of your waist is according to how well, or otherwise, skirts and trousers fit. Talk to your doctor about any weight and health concerns.

WAIST MEASUREMENT

	Increased Health Risk	High Risk to Health
Women	32-35in (81-88cm)	more than 35in (88cm)
Men	37-40in (94-102cm)	more than 40in (102cm)

---

2. Set a realistic time scale

With today's hectic lifestyles, everything tends to happen at breakneck speed, so it's no wonder that when it comes to losing weight, most of us want to shift those pounds in an instant. But it's probably taken years to accumulate that extra weight, with the result that it's unrealistic to expect to lose the excess in just a few weeks! Instead, prepare yourself to lose weight slowly and steadily. It's far healthier to lose weight like this. But better still, research shows you'll be far more likely to maintain your new, lower weight.

If you only have a small amount of weight to lose, aim for a weight loss of around 1lb (½kg) a week. But if you have more than 2 stone (28kg) to lose, you may prefer to aim for 2lb (1kg) each week. Remember though, it's better to keep going at 1lb (½kg) a week than to give up because trying to lose 2lb (1kg) a week is making you miserable! The following words may help you to keep your goal in perspective:

'Never give up on a goal because of the time it will take to achieve it – the time will pass anyway.'

Weight Fluctuations

Weight typically fluctuates on a day to day basis. You know that shock/horror feeling when you weigh yourself in the morning then later in the day, or after a meal out, and it looks like youve gained pounds in hours! But this is due to fluid not fat changes. Real changes in body fat can only happen more gradually (remember, to gain 1lb you need to eat 3500 calories more than you usually do). Don't be confused either by seemingly very rapid weight loss in the first week or so.

When calorie intake is initially cut back, the bodys carbohydrate stores in the liver and muscles (known as glycogen) are used up. Glycogen is stored with three times its weight in water, meaning that rapid losses of 4.5- 6.6lb (2 -3 kg) are possible. These stores can be just as rapidly refilled if normal eating is resumed. True weight loss happens more gradually and this book helps you to lose weight at the steady and healthy rate of no more than 1-2 lbs per week.

3. Calculate your calorie allowance

Use the calorie tables on pages 39-40 to find out how many calories you need each day to maintain your current weight. Then use the table below to discover the amount of calories you need to subtract from this amount every day to lose weight at your chosen rate. For example, a 35 year-old woman who is moderately active and weighs 12 stone (76kg) needs 2,188 calories a day to keep her weight steady. If she wants to lose ½lb (¼kg) a week, she needs 250 calories less each day, giving her a daily calorie allowance of 1,938 calories. If she wants to lose 1lb (½kg) a week, she needs 500 calories less each day, giving her a daily calorie allowance of 1,688 calories, and so on.

TO LOSE...	Cut your daily calorie intake by	In three months you could lose...	In six months you could lose...	In one year you could lose...
½lb a week	250	6.5lb	13lb	1st 12lb
1lb a week	500	13lb	1st 12lb	3st 10lb
1½lb a week	750	1st 5.5lb	2st 11lb	5st 8lb
2lb a week	1,000	1st 12lb	3st 10lb	7st 6lb

TO LOSE...	Cut your daily calorie intake by	In three months you could lose...	In six months you could lose...	In one year you could lose...
¼kg a week	250	3.25kg	6.5kg	13kg
½kg a week	500	6.5kg	13kg	26kg
¾kg a week	750	9.75kg	19.5kg	39kg
1kg a week	1,000	13kg	26kg	52kg

4. Keep a food diary

Writing down what you eat and drink and any thoughts linked to that eating helps you become more aware of your eating habits. Recognising what is going on helps you feel in control and is a powerful way to start planning change. Keeping a food diary before you start to change your eating habits will also help you identify opportunities for cutting calories by substituting one food for another, cutting portion sizes of high-calorie foods or eating certain foods less often. Simply write down every single item you eat or drink during the day and use this book to calculate the calories of each item. Then after a few days of eating normally, introduce some changes to your diet to achieve your daily calorie allowance. Remember to spread your daily calorie allowance fairly evenly throughout the day to prevent hunger. You'll find a template for a daily food and exercise diary on page 43. Try to use it as carefully as you can as research shows that people who do, do best.

Top Tip

If you only fill in your main food diary once a day, keep a pen and notepad with you to write down all those little extras you eat or drink during the day – that chocolate you ate in the office, the sliver of cheese you had while cooking dinner and the few chips you pinched from your husband's plate, for example! It's easy to forget the little things if they're not written down, but they can make the difference between success and failure.

QUESTION: Why are heavier people allowed more calories than those who have smaller amounts of weight to lose?

ANSWER: This confuses a lot of people but is easily explained. Someone who is 3 stone overweight, for example, is carrying the equivalent of 42 small packets of butter with them everywhere they go – up and down the stairs, to the local shops, into the kitchen. Obviously, it takes a lot more energy simply to move around when you're carrying that extra weight. As a consequence, the heavier you are, the more calories you need just to keep your weight steady. In turn, this means you'll lose weight on a higher calorie allowance. However, as you lose weight, you'll need to lower your calorie allowance slightly as you have less weight to carry around.

5. Control your portions

As well as making some smart food swaps to cut calories, it's likely you'll also need to reduce your serving sizes for some foods to help shift those pounds. Even 'healthy' foods such as brown rice, wholemeal bread, chicken, fish and low-fat dairy products contain calories so you may need to limit the amount you eat. When you first start out, weigh portions of foods like rice, pasta, cereal, cheese, butter, oil, meat, fish, and chicken rather than completing your food diary with a 'guesstimated' weight! That way you can calculate the calorie content accurately. Don't forget that drinks contain calories too, alcohol, milk, juices and sugary drinks all count.

6. Measure your success

Research has found that regular weight checks do help. Weighing yourself helps you assess how your eating and exercise habits affect your body weight. The important thing is to use the information in a positive way – to assess your progress - rather than as a stick to beat yourself up with. Remember that weight can fluctuate by a kilogram in a day, for example, due to fluid changes, premenstrually, after a big meal out, so weigh yourself at the same time of day and look at the trend over a week or two.

People who successfully lose weight and keep it off, also tend to continue weighing themselves at least once a week, and often daily (but not in an obsessive way), because they say it helps them stay 'on track'. Probably because they use it as an early warning system. People who weigh themselves regularly (or regularly try on a tight fitting item of clothing) will notice quickly if they have gained a couple of kilograms and can take action to stop gaining more. Checking your weight less often can mean that you might discover one day that you gained 6kg. That can be pretty discouraging, and it might trigger you to just give up.

Top Tip

Don't just focus on what the bathroom scales say either – keep a record of your vital statistics, too. Many people find it doubly encouraging to see the inches dropping off, as well as the pounds!

7. Stay motivated

Each time you lose half a stone, or reach your own small goal – celebrate! Treat yourself to a little luxury – something new to wear, a little pampering or some other (non-food) treat. It also helps replace the comfort you once got from food and allows you to take care of yourself in other ways. Trying on an item of clothing that used to be tight can also help to keep you feeling motivated. Make sure you keep in touch with your supporters, and if the going gets tough take another look at the 'Coping with Slimming Saboteurs' section. Once you've reviewed how well you've done, use this book to set yourself a new daily calorie allowance based on your new weight to help you lose the next half stone *(see point 3 - page 28 - Calculate your calorie allowance).*

8. Keep it off

What you do to stay slim is just as important as what you did to get slim. Quite simply, if you return to your old ways, you are likely to return to your old weight. The great thing about calorie counting is that you will learn so much about what you eat, and make so many important changes to your eating and drinking habits, that you'll probably find it difficult to go back to your old ways – and won't want to anyway. It's still a good idea to weigh yourself at least once a week to keep a check on your weight. The key is to deal with any extra pounds immediately, rather than waiting until you have a stone to lose (see page 30). Simply go back to counting calories for as long as it takes to shift those pounds and enjoy the new slim you. Page 25 has more information about how successful slimmers keep it off.

QUESTION: Do I need to stick to exactly the same number of calories each day or is it OK to have a lower calorie intake during the week and slightly more at the weekend?

ANSWER: The key to losing weight is to take in fewer calories than you need for as long as it takes to reach your target, aiming for a loss of no more than 2lb (1kg) a week. In general, most nutrition experts recommend a daily calorie allowance. However, it's just as valid to use other periods of time such as weeks. If you prefer, simply multiply your daily allowance by seven to work out a weekly calorie allowance and then allocate more calories to some days than others. For example, a daily allowance of 1,500 calories is equivalent to 10,500 calories a week. This means you could have 1,300 calories a day during the week and 2,000 calories a day on Saturday and Sunday.

Healthy Eating Made Easy

Juliette Kellow BSc RD

GONE ARE THE DAYS when a healthy diet meant surviving on bird seed, rabbit food and carrot juice! The new approach to eating healthily means we're positively encouraged to eat a wide range of foods, including some of our favourites – it's just a question of making sure we don't eat high fat, high sugar or highly processed foods too often.

Eating a healthy diet, together with taking regular exercise and not smoking, has huge benefits to our health, both in the short and long term. As well as helping us to lose or maintain our weight, a healthy diet can boost energy levels, keep our immune system strong and give us healthy skin, nails and hair. Meanwhile, eating well throughout life also means we're far less likely to suffer from health problems such as constipation, anaemia and tooth decay or set ourselves up for serious conditions in later life such as obesity, heart disease, stroke, diabetes, cancer or osteoporosis.

Fortunately, it couldn't be easier to eat a balanced diet. To start with, no single food provides all the calories and nutrients we need to stay healthy, so it's important to eat a variety of foods. Meanwhile, most nutrition experts also agree that mealtimes should be a pleasure rather than a penance. This means it's fine to eat small amounts of our favourite treats from time to time.

To help people eat healthily, the Food Standards Agency recommends eating plenty of different foods from four main groups of foods and limiting the amount we eat from a smaller fifth group. Ultimately, we should eat more fruit, vegetables, starchy, fibre-rich foods and fresh products, and fewer fatty, sugary, salty and processed foods.

The following guidelines are all based on the healthy eating guidelines recommended by the Food Standards Agency.

Bread, other cereals and potatoes

Eat these foods at each meal. They also make good snacks.

Foods in this group include bread, breakfast cereals, potatoes, rice, pasta, noodles, yams, oats and grains. Go for high-fibre varieties where available, such as wholegrain cereals, wholemeal bread and brown rice. These foods should fill roughly a third of your plate at mealtimes.

TYPICAL SERVING SIZES

- *2 slices bread in a sandwich or with a meal*
- *a tennis ball sized serving of pasta, potato, rice, noodles or couscous*
- *a bowl of porridge*
- *around 40g of breakfast cereal*

Fruit and vegetables

Eat at least five portions every day.

Foods in this group include all fruits and vegetables, including fresh, frozen, canned and dried products, and unsweetened fruit juice. Choose canned fruit in juice rather than syrup and go for veg canned in water without added salt or sugar.

TYPICAL PORTION SIZES

- *a piece of fruit eg apple, banana, pear*
- *2 small fruits eg satsumas, plums, apricots*
- *a bowl of fruit salad, canned or stewed fruit*
- *a small glass of unsweetened fruit juice*
- *a cereal bowl of salad*
- *3tbsp vegetables*

Milk and dairy foods

Eat two or three servings a day.

Foods in this group include milk, cheese, yoghurt and fromage frais. Choose low-fat varieties where available such as skimmed milk, reduced-fat cheese and fat-free yoghurt.

TYPICAL SERVING SIZES

* *200ml milk*

* *a small pot of yoghurt or fromage frais*

* *a small matchbox-sized piece of cheese*

Meat, fish and alternatives

Eat two servings a day

Foods in this group include meat, poultry, fish, eggs, beans, nuts and seeds. Choose low-fat varieties where available such as extra-lean minced beef and skinless chicken and don't add extra fat or salt.

TYPICAL SERVING SIZES

* *a piece of meat, chicken or fish the size of a deck of cards*

* *1-2 eggs*

* *3 heaped tablespoons of beans*

* *a small handful of nuts or seeds*

Healthy Eating on a plate

A simple way to serve up both balance and healthy proportions is to fill one half of your plate with salad or vegetables and divide the other half between protein-rich meat, chicken, fish, eggs or beans, and healthy carbs (potatoes, rice, pasta, pulses, bread or noodles).

Fatty and sugary foods

Eat only small amounts of these foods

Foods in this group include oils, spreading fats, cream, mayonnaise, oily salad dressings, cakes, biscuits, puddings, crisps, savoury snacks, sugar, preserves, confectionery and sugary soft drinks.

TYPICAL SERVING SIZES:

- *a small packet of sweets or a small bar of chocolate*

- *a small slice of cake*

- *a couple of small biscuits*

- *1 level tbsp mayo, salad dressing or olive oil*

- *a small packet of crisps*

Useful Tools

Body Mass Index

The Body Mass Index (BMI) is the internationally accepted way of assessing how healthy our weight is. It is calculated using an individual's height and weight. Use the Body Mass Index Chart to look up your BMI, and use the table below to see what range you fall into.

BMI Under 18.5	Underweight
BMI 18.5-25	Healthy
BMI 25-30	Overweight
BMI 30-40	Obese
BMI Over 40	Severely Obese

This is what different BMI ranges mean.

- **Underweight:** you probably need to gain weight for your health's sake. Talk to your doctor if you have any concerns, or if you feel frightened about gaining weight.

- **Healthy weight:** you are a healthy weight, so aim to stay in this range (note that most people in this range tend to have a BMI between 20-25).

- **Overweight:** aim to lose some weight for your health's sake, or at least prevent further weight gain.

- **Obese:** your health is at risk and losing weight will benefit your health.

- **Severely obese:** your health is definitely at risk. You should visit your doctor for a health check. Losing weight will improve your health.

Please note that BMI is not as accurate for athletes or very muscular people (muscle weighs more than fat), as it can push them into a higher BMI category despite having a healthy level of body fat. It is also not accurate for women who are pregnant or breastfeeding, or people who are frail.

Body Mass Index Table

HEIGHT IN FEET / INCHES

	4'6	4'8	4'10	5'0	5'2	5'4	5'6	5'8	5'10	6'0	6'2	6'4	6'6	6'8	6'10
6st 7	22.0	20.5	19.1	17.8	16.7	15.7	14.7	13.9	13.1	12.4	11.7	11.1	10.6	10.0	9.5
7st 0	23.7	22.1	20.6	19.2	18.0	16.9	15.9	15.0	14.1	13.3	12.6	12.0	11.4	10.8	10.3
7st 7	25.4	23.6	22.0	20.6	19.3	18.1	17.0	16.0	15.1	14.3	13.5	12.8	12.2	11.6	11.0
8st 0	27.1	25.2	23.5	22.0	20.6	19.3	18.1	17.1	16.1	15.2	14.4	13.7	13.0	12.3	11.8
8st 7	28.8	26.8	25.0	23.3	21.8	20.5	19.3	18.2	17.1	16.2	15.3	14.5	13.8	13.1	12.5
9st 0	30.5	28.4	26.4	24.7	23.1	21.7	20.4	19.2	18.1	17.2	16.2	15.4	14.6	13.9	13.2
9st 7	32.2	29.9	27.9	26.1	24.4	22.9	21.5	20.3	19.2	18.1	17.1	16.2	15.4	14.7	14.0
10st 0	33.9	31.5	29.4	27.4	25.7	24.1	22.7	21.4	20.2	19.1	18.0	17.1	16.2	15.4	14.7
10st 7	35.6	33.1	30.8	28.8	27.0	25.3	23.8	22.4	21.2	20.0	18.9	18.0	17.0	16.2	15.4
11st 0	37.3	34.7	32.3	30.2	28.3	26.5	24.9	23.5	22.2	21.0	19.8	18.8	17.9	17.0	16.2
11st 7	39.0	36.2	33.8	31.6	29.6	27.7	26.1	24.6	23.2	21.9	20.7	19.7	18.7	17.8	16.9
12st 0	40.7	37.8	35.2	32.9	30.8	28.9	27.2	25.6	24.2	22.9	21.6	20.5	19.5	18.5	17.6
12st 7	42.3	39.4	36.7	34.3	32.1	30.1	28.3	26.7	25.2	23.8	22.5	21.4	20.3	19.3	18.4
13st 0	44.0	41.0	38.2	35.7	33.4	31.4	29.5	27.8	26.2	24.8	23.5	22.2	21.1	20.1	19.1
13st 7	45.7	42.5	39.6	37.0	34.7	32.6	30.6	28.8	27.2	25.7	24.4	23.1	21.9	20.8	19.8
14st 0	47.4	44.1	41.1	38.4	36.0	33.8	31.7	29.9	28.2	26.7	25.3	23.9	22.7	21.6	20.6
14st 7	49.1	45.7	42.6	39.8	37.3	35.0	32.9	31.0	29.2	27.6	26.2	24.8	23.5	22.4	21.3
15st 0	50.8	47.3	44.0	41.2	38.5	36.2	34.0	32.0	30.2	28.6	27.1	25.7	24.4	23.2	22.0
15st 7	52.5	48.8	45.5	42.5	39.8	37.4	35.2	33.1	31.2	29.5	28.0	26.5	25.2	23.9	22.8
16st 0	54.2	50.4	47.0	43.9	41.1	38.6	36.3	34.2	32.3	30.5	28.9	27.4	26.0	24.7	23.5
16st 7	55.9	52.0	48.5	45.3	42.4	39.8	37.4	35.2	33.3	31.4	29.8	28.2	26.8	25.5	24.2
17st 0	57.6	53.6	49.9	46.6	43.7	41.0	38.6	36.3	34.3	32.4	30.7	29.1	27.6	26.2	25.0
17st 7	59.3	55.1	51.4	48.0	45.0	42.2	39.7	37.4	35.3	33.3	31.6	29.9	28.4	27.0	25.7
18st 0	61.0	56.7	52.9	49.4	46.3	43.4	40.8	38.5	36.3	34.3	32.5	30.8	29.2	27.8	26.4
18st 7	62.7	58.3	54.3	50.8	47.5	44.6	42.0	39.5	37.3	35.3	33.4	31.6	30.0	28.6	27.2
19st 0	64.4	59.9	55.8	52.1	48.8	45.8	43.1	40.6	38.3	36.2	34.3	32.5	30.8	29.3	27.9
19st 7	66.1	61.4	57.3	53.5	50.1	47.0	44.2	41.7	39.3	37.2	35.2	33.3	31.7	30.1	28.6
20st 0	67.8	63.0	58.7	54.9	51.4	48.2	45.4	42.7	40.3	38.1	36.1	34.2	32.5	30.9	29.4
20st 7	69.4	64.6	60.2	56.3	52.7	49.4	46.5	43.8	41.3	39.1	37.0	35.1	33.3	31.6	30.1
21st 0	71.1	66.2	61.7	57.6	54.0	50.6	47.6	44.9	42.3	40.0	37.9	35.9	34.1	32.4	30.9
21st 7	72.8	67.7	63.1	59.0	55.3	51.9	48.8	45.9	43.3	41.0	38.8	36.8	34.9	33.2	31.6
22st 0	74.5	69.3	64.6	60.4	56.5	53.1	49.9	47.0	44.4	41.9	39.7	37.6	35.7	34.0	32.3
22st 7	76.2	70.9	66.1	61.7	57.8	54.3	51.0	48.1	45.4	42.9	40.6	38.5	36.5	34.7	33.1
23st 0	77.9	72.5	67.5	63.1	59.1	55.5	52.2	49.1	46.4	43.8	41.5	39.3	37.3	35.5	33.8
23st 7	79.6	74.0	69.0	64.5	60.4	56.7	53.3	50.2	47.4	44.8	42.4	40.2	38.2	36.3	34.5
24st 0	81.3	75.6	70.5	65.9	61.7	57.9	54.4	51.3	48.4	45.7	43.3	41.0	39.0	37.0	35.3
24st 7	83.0	77.2	71.9	67.2	63.0	59.1	55.6	52.3	49.4	46.7	44.2	41.9	39.8	37.8	36.0
25st 0	84.7	78.8	73.4	68.6	64.2	60.3	56.7	53.4	50.4	47.6	45.1	42.8	40.6	38.6	36.7
25st 7	86.4	80.3	74.9	70.0	65.5	61.5	57.8	54.5	51.4	48.6	46.0	43.6	41.4	39.4	37.5
26st 0	88.1	81.9	76.3	71.3	66.8	62.7	59.0	55.5	52.4	49.5	46.9	44.5	42.2	40.1	38.2
26st 7	89.8	83.5	77.8	72.7	68.1	63.9	60.1	56.6	53.4	50.5	47.8	45.3	43.0	40.9	38.9
27st 0	91.5	85.1	79.3	74.1	69.4	65.1	61.2	57.7	54.4	51.5	48.7	46.2	43.8	41.7	39.7
27st 7	93.2	86.6	80.8	75.5	70.7	66.3	62.4	58.7	55.4	52.4	49.6	47.0	44.7	42.4	40.4
28st 0	94.9	88.2	82.2	76.8	72.0	67.5	63.5	59.8	56.4	53.4	50.5	47.9	45.5	43.2	41.1
28st 7	96.5	89.8	83.7	78.2	73.2	68.7	64.6	60.9	57.5	54.3	51.4	48.7	46.3	44.0	41.9
29st 0	98.2	91.4	85.2	79.6	74.5	69.9	65.8	62.0	58.5	55.3	52.3	49.6	47.1	44.8	42.6
29st 7	99.9	92.9	86.6	80.9	75.8	71.1	66.9	63.0	59.5	56.2	53.2	50.5	47.9	45.5	43.3

WEIGHT IN STONES / LBS

Weight Chart

Underweight BMI less than 18.5

HEALTHY WEIGHT BMI 18.5-25

Overweight BMI 25-30

Obese BMI 30-40

Severely Obese BMI 40 or more

BMI: 10 11 12 13 14 15 16 17 18 19 20 21 22 23 24 25 26 27 28 29 30 31 32 33 34 35 36 37 38

Height:
6ft 6" / 197.5cm
6ft 5" / 195cm
6ft 4" / 192.5cm
6ft 3" / 190cm
6ft 2" / 187.5cm
6ft 1" / 185cm
6ft 0" / 182.5cm
5ft 11" / 180cm
5ft 10" / 177.5cm
5ft 9" / 175cm
5ft 8" / 172.5cm
5ft 7" / 170cm
5ft 6" / 167.5cm
5ft 5" / 165cm
5ft 4" / 162.5cm
5ft 3" / 160cm
5ft 2" / 157.5cm
5ft 1" / 155cm
5ft 0" / 152.5cm
4ft 11" / 150cm
4ft 10" / 147.5cm
4ft 9" / 145cm
4ft 8" / 142.5cm
4ft 7" / 140cm
4ft 6" / 137.5cm

Weight:
4st 7lb / 29kg
5st 0lb / 32kg
5st 7lb / 35kg
6st 0lb / 38kg
6st 7lb / 41kg
7st 0lb / 45kg
7st 7lb / 48kg
8st 0lb / 51kg
8st 7lb / 54kg
9st 0lb / 57kg
9st 7lb / 60kg
10st 0lb / 64kg
10st 7lb / 67kg
11st 0lb / 70kg
11st 7lb / 73kg
12st 0lb / 76kg
12st 7lb / 79kg
13st 0lb / 83kg
13st 7lb / 86kg
14st 0lb / 89kg
14st 7lb / 92kg
15st 0lb / 95kg
15st 7lb / 98kg
16st 0lb / 102kg
16st 7lb / 105kg
17st 0lb / 108kg
17st 7lb / 111kg
18st 0lb / 114kg
18st 7lb / 118kg
19st 0lb / 121kg
19st 7lb / 124kg
20st 0lb / 127kg
20st 7lb / 130kg
21st 0lb / 133kg
21st 7lb / 137kg
22st 0lb / 140kg
22st 7lb / 143kg
23st 0lb / 146kg
23st 7lb / 149kg

Calories Required to Maintain Weight
Adult Females

ACTIVITY LEVEL / AGE

WEIGHT IN STONES / LBS	VERY SEDENTARY			MODERATELY SEDENTARY			MODERATELY ACTIVE			VERY ACTIVE		
	<30	30-60	60+	<30	30-60	60+	<30	30-60	60+	<30	30-60	60+
7st 7	1425	1473	1304	1544	1596	1412	1781	1841	1630	2138	2210	1956
8st 0	1481	1504	1338	1605	1629	1450	1852	1880	1673	2222	2256	2008
8st 7	1537	1535	1373	1666	1663	1487	1922	1919	1716	2306	2302	2059
9st 0	1594	1566	1407	1726	1696	1524	1992	1957	1759	2391	2349	2111
9st 7	1650	1596	1442	1787	1729	1562	2062	1996	1802	2475	2395	2163
10st 0	1706	1627	1476	1848	1763	1599	2133	2034	1845	2559	2441	2214
10st 7	1762	1658	1511	1909	1796	1637	2203	2073	1888	2644	2487	2266
11st 0	1819	1689	1545	1970	1830	1674	2273	2111	1931	2728	2534	2318
11st 7	1875	1720	1580	2031	1863	1711	2344	2150	1975	2813	2580	2370
12st 0	1931	1751	1614	2092	1897	1749	2414	2188	2018	2897	2626	2421
12st 7	1987	1781	1648	2153	1930	1786	2484	2227	2061	2981	2672	2473
13st 0	2044	1812	1683	2214	1963	1823	2555	2266	2104	3066	2719	2525
13st 7	2100	1843	1717	2275	1997	1861	2625	2304	2147	3150	2765	2576
14st 0	2156	1874	1752	2336	2030	1898	2695	2343	2190	3234	2811	2628
14st 7	2212	1905	1786	2397	2064	1935	2766	2381	2233	3319	2858	2680
15st 0	2269	1936	1821	2458	2097	1973	2836	2420	2276	3403	2904	2732
15st 7	2325	1967	1855	2519	2130	2010	2906	2458	2319	3488	2950	2783
16st 0	2381	1997	1890	2580	2164	2047	2976	2497	2362	3572	2996	2835
16st 7	2437	2028	1924	2640	2197	2085	3047	2535	2405	3656	3043	2887
17st 0	2494	2059	1959	2701	2231	2122	3117	2574	2449	3741	3089	2938
17st 7	2550	2090	1993	2762	2264	2159	3187	2613	2492	3825	3135	2990
18st 0	2606	2121	2028	2823	2298	2197	3258	2651	2535	3909	3181	3042
18st 7	2662	2152	2062	2884	2331	2234	3328	2690	2578	3994	3228	3093
19st 0	2719	2182	2097	2945	2364	2271	3398	2728	2621	4078	3274	3145
19st 7	2775	2213	2131	3006	2398	2309	3469	2767	2664	4162	3320	3197
20st 0	2831	2244	2166	3067	2431	2346	3539	2805	2707	4247	3366	3249
20st 7	2887	2275	2200	3128	2465	2383	3609	2844	2750	4331	3413	3300
21st 0	2944	2306	2235	3189	2498	2421	3680	2882	2793	4416	3459	3352
21st 7	3000	2337	2269	3250	2531	2458	3750	2921	2836	4500	3505	3404
22st 0	3056	2368	2303	3311	2565	2495	3820	2960	2879	4584	3552	3455
22st 7	3112	2398	2338	3372	2598	2533	3890	2998	2923	4669	3598	3507
23st 0	3169	2429	2372	3433	2632	2570	3961	3037	2966	4753	3644	3559
23st 7	3225	2460	2407	3494	2665	2608	4031	3075	3009	4837	3690	3611
24st 0	3281	2491	2441	3554	2699	2645	4101	3114	3052	4922	3737	3662
24st 7	3337	2522	2476	3615	2732	2682	4172	3152	3095	5006	3783	3714
25st 0	3394	2553	2510	3676	2765	2720	4242	3191	3138	5091	3829	3766
25st 7	3450	2583	2545	3737	2799	2757	4312	3229	3181	5175	3875	3817
26st 0	3506	2614	2579	3798	2832	2794	4383	3268	3224	5259	3922	3869
26st 7	3562	2645	2614	3859	2866	2832	4453	3307	3267	5344	3968	3921
27st 0	3618	2676	2648	3920	2899	2869	4523	3345	3310	5428	4014	3973
27st 7	3675	2707	2683	3981	2932	2906	4594	3384	3353	5512	4060	4024
28st 0	3731	2738	2717	4042	2966	2944	4664	3422	3397	5597	4107	4076
28st 7	3787	2768	2752	4103	2999	2981	4734	3461	3440	5681	4153	4128

Calories Required to Maintain Weight
Adult Males

ACTIVITY LEVEL / AGE

WEIGHT IN STONES / LBS	VERY SEDENTARY			MODERATELY SEDENTARY			MODERATELY ACTIVE			VERY ACTIVE		
	<30	30-60	60+	<30	30-60	60+	<30	30-60	60+	<30	30-60	60+
9st 0	1856	1827	1502	2010	1979	1627	2320	2284	1878	2784	2741	2254
9st 7	1913	1871	1547	2072	2026	1676	2391	2338	1933	2870	2806	2320
10st 0	1970	1914	1591	2134	2074	1724	2463	2393	1989	2955	2871	2387
10st 7	2027	1958	1636	2196	2121	1772	2534	2447	2045	3041	2937	2454
11st 0	2084	2001	1680	2258	2168	1820	2605	2502	2100	3127	3002	2520
11st 7	2141	2045	1724	2320	2215	1868	2677	2556	2156	3212	3067	2587
12st 0	2199	2088	1769	2382	2262	1916	2748	2611	2211	3298	3133	2654
12st 7	2256	2132	1813	2444	2310	1965	2820	2665	2267	3384	3198	2720
13st 0	2313	2175	1858	2506	2357	2013	2891	2719	2322	3470	3263	2787
13st 7	2370	2219	1902	2568	2404	2061	2963	2774	2378	3555	3329	2854
14st 0	2427	2262	1947	2630	2451	2109	3034	2828	2434	3641	3394	2920
14st 7	2484	2306	1991	2691	2498	2157	3106	2883	2489	3727	3459	2987
15st 0	2542	2350	2036	2753	2545	2205	3177	2937	2545	3813	3525	3054
15st 7	2599	2393	2080	2815	2593	2253	3248	2992	2600	3898	3590	3120
16st 0	2656	2437	2125	2877	2640	2302	3320	3046	2656	3984	3655	3187
16st 7	2713	2480	2169	2939	2687	2350	3391	3100	2711	4070	3721	3254
17st 0	2770	2524	2213	3001	2734	2398	3463	3155	2767	4155	3786	3320
17st 7	2827	2567	2258	3063	2781	2446	3534	3209	2823	4241	3851	3387
18st 0	2884	2611	2302	3125	2828	2494	3606	3264	2878	4327	3917	3454
18st 7	2942	2654	2347	3187	2876	2542	3677	3318	2934	4413	3982	3520
19st 0	2999	2698	2391	3249	2923	2591	3749	3373	2989	4498	4047	3587
19st 7	3056	2741	2436	3311	2970	2639	3820	3427	3045	4584	4112	3654
20st 0	3113	2785	2480	3373	3017	2687	3891	3481	3100	4670	4178	3721
20st 7	3170	2829	2525	3434	3064	2735	3963	3536	3156	4756	4243	3787
21st 0	3227	2872	2569	3496	3112	2783	4034	3590	3211	4841	4308	3854
21st 7	3285	2916	2614	3558	3159	2831	4106	3645	3267	4927	4374	3921
22st 0	3342	2959	2658	3620	3206	2880	4177	3699	3323	5013	4439	3987
22st 7	3399	3003	2702	3682	3253	2928	4249	3754	3378	5098	4504	4054
23st 0	3456	3046	2747	3744	3300	2976	4320	3808	3434	5184	4570	4121
23st 7	3513	3090	2791	3806	3347	3024	4392	3862	3489	5270	4635	4187
24st 0	3570	3133	2836	3868	3395	3072	4463	3917	3545	5356	4700	4254
24st 7	3627	3177	2880	3930	3442	3120	4534	3971	3600	5441	4766	4321
25st 0	3685	3220	2925	3992	3489	3168	4606	4026	3656	5527	4831	4387
25st 7	3742	3264	2969	4054	3536	3217	4677	4080	3712	5613	4896	4454
26st 0	3799	3308	3014	4116	3583	3265	4749	4135	3767	5699	4962	4521
26st 7	3856	3351	3058	4177	3630	3313	4820	4189	3823	5784	5027	4587
27st 0	3913	3395	3103	4239	3678	3361	4892	4243	3878	5870	5092	4654
27st 7	3970	3438	3147	4301	3725	3409	4963	4298	3934	5956	5158	4721
28st 0	4028	3482	3191	4363	3772	3457	5035	4352	3989	6042	5223	4787
28st 7	4085	3525	3236	4425	3819	3506	5106	4407	4045	6127	5288	4854
29st 0	4142	3569	3280	4487	3866	3554	5177	4461	4101	6213	5354	4921
29st 7	4199	3612	3325	4549	3913	3602	5249	4516	4156	6299	5419	4987
30st 0	4256	3656	3369	4611	3961	3650	5320	4570	4212	6384	5484	5054

Calories Burned in Exercise

This table shows the approximate number of extra* calories that would be burned in a five minute period of exercise activity.

ACTIVITY	CALORIES BURNED IN 5 MINUTES	ACTIVITY	CALORIES BURNED IN 5 MINUTES
Aerobics, Low Impact	25	Situps, Continuous	17
Badminton, Recreational	17	Skiing, Moderate	30
Cross Trainer	30	Skipping, Moderate	30
Cycling, Recreational, 5mph	17	Squash Playing	39
Dancing, Modern, Moderate	13	Tennis Playing, Recreational	26
Fencing	24	Toning Exercises	17
Gardening, Weeding	19	Trampolining	17
Hill Walking, Up and Down, Recreational	22	Volleyball, Recreational	10
Jogging	30	Walking, Uphill, 15% Gradient, Moderate	43
Kick Boxing	30	Walking Up and Down Stairs, Moderate	34
Netball Playing	23	Walking, 4mph	24
Rebounding	18	Weight Training, Moderate	12
Roller Skating	30	Yoga	13
Rowing Machine, Moderate	30		
Running, 7.5mph	48		

*Extra calories are those in addition to your normal daily calorie needs.

My Personal Plan

Date: _____

Body Mass Index: _____

Weight: _____

Waist Measurement: _____

Height: _____

Body Fat % (if known) _____

10% Weight Loss Goal:

Current weight	16stone (224lb)	100kg
- 10% weight	1stone 8½lb (22½lb)	10kg
= 10% loss goal	14stone 5½lb (201½lb)	90kg

My smaller weight targets on the way to achieving my 10% goal will be:

_____ _____ _____ _____

Reasons why I want to lose weight:

_____

Changes I will make to help me lose weight:

Diet: _____

Activity: _____

_____

_____

Potential saboteurs or barriers will be:

_____

Ways I will overcome these:

_____

_____

_____

My supporters will be:

_____

I will monitor my progress by:

_____

_____

I will reward my progress with:

In the short term:

_____

In the long term:

_____

_____

Food and Exercise Diary

Date:

| / / |

Daily Calorie Allowance: 1534 **(A)** ~~1284~~

Food/Drink Consumed	Serving Size	Calories
B. Porridge + Blueberrys.	-	200
D. 2 Chicken Pieces with Mayo + Salad.		649.
2 Slices Bread.		
Yoghurt		118.
Apple		74.
T. Fish, Corn, Peas Wedges		497.

You are aiming for your Calorie Balance (Box D) to be as close to zero as possible - ie. you consume the number of calories you need.

Your Daily Calorie Allowance (Box A) should be set to lose ½-2lb (¼-1kg) a week, or maintain weight, depending on your goals.

Total calories consumed 1538 **(B)**

Exercise/Activity	No. mins	Calories

Daily Calorie Allowance (A) *plus* Extra Calories used in Exercise (C) *minus* Total Calories Consumed (B) *equals* Calorie Balance (D)

Calories used in exercise **(C)**

$A + C - B = D$

Calorie balance **(D)**

You can also write down any comments or thoughts related to your eating if you want to.

Food Information

Nutritional Information

CALORIE AND FAT values are given per serving, plus calorie and nutrition values per 100g of product. This makes it easy to compare the proportions of fat, protein, carbohydrate and fibre in each food.

The values given are for uncooked, unprepared foods unless otherwise stated. Values are also for only the edible portion of the food unless otherwise stated. ie - weighed with bone.

Finding Foods

The Calorie, Carb & Fat Bible has an Eating Out section which is arranged alphabetically by brand. In the General Foods and Drinks A-Z most foods are grouped together by type, and then put in to alphabetical order. This makes it easy to compare different brands, and will help you to find lower calorie and/or fat alternatives where they are available.

This format also makes it easier to locate foods. Foods are categorised by their main characteristics so, for example, if it is bread, ciabatta or white sliced, you'll find it under "Bread".

There are, however, some foods which are not so easy to categorise, especially combination foods like ready meals. The following pointers will help you to find your way around the book until you get to know it a little better.

FILLED ROLLS AND SANDWICHES - Bagels, baguettes, etc which are filled are listed as "Bagels (filled)" etc. Sandwiches are under "Sandwiches".

CURRIES - Popular types of curry, like Balti or Jalfrezi, are listed under their individual types. Unspecified or lesser known types are listed under their main ingredient.

BURGERS - All burgers, including chicken-type sandwiches from fast-food outlets, are listed under "Burgers".

CHIPS & FRIES - Are listed separately, depending on the name of the particular brand. All other types of potato are listed under "Potatoes".

SWEETS & CHOCOLATES - Well-known brands, eg. Aero, Mars Bar, are listed under their brand names. Others are listed under "Chocolate" (for bars) and "Chocolates" (for individual sweets).

READY MEALS - Popular types of dishes are listed under their type, eg. "Chow Mein", "Casserole", "Hot Pot", etc. Others are listed by their main ingredient, eg. "Chicken With", "Chicken In", etc.

EATING OUT & FAST FOODS - By popular demand this edition has the major eating out and fast food brands listed separately, at the back of the book. They are alphabetised first by brand, then follow using the same format as the rest of the book.

Serving Sizes

Many ready-meal type foods are given with calories for the full pack size, so that an individual serving can be worked out by estimating the proportion of the pack that has been consumed. For example, if you have eaten a quarter of a packaged pasta dish, divide the calorie value given for the whole pack by 4 to determine the number of calories you have consumed. Where serving sizes are not appropriate, or unknown, values are given per 1oz/28g. Serving sizes vary greatly from person to person and, if you are trying to lose weight, it's very important to be accurate – especially with foods that are very high in calories such as those that contain a fair amount of fat, sugar, cream, cheese, alcohol etc.

Food Data

Nutrition information for basic average foods has been compiled by the Weight Loss Resources food data team using many sources of information to calculate the most accurate values possible. Some nutrition information for non-branded food records is from The Composition of Foods 5th Edition (1991). Reproduced under licence from The Controller of Her Majesty's Stationary Office. Where basic data is present for ordinary foodstuffs such as 'raw carrots'; branded records are not included.

Nutrition information for branded goods is from details supplied by retailers and manufacturers, and researched by Weight Loss Resources staff. The Calorie Carb & Fat Bible contains data for over 900 UK brands, including major supermarkets and fast food outlets.

The publishers gratefully acknowledge all the manufacturers and retailers who have provided information on their products. All product names, trademarks or registered trademarks belong to their respective owners and are used only for the purpose of identifying products.

Calorie & nutrition data for all food and drink items are typical values.

Caution	
The information in The Calorie, Carb and Fat Bible is intended as an aid to weight loss and weight maintenance, and is not medical advice. If you suffer from, or think you may suffer from a medical condition you should consult your doctor before starting a	weight loss and/or exercise regime, If you start exercising after a period of relative inactivity, you should start slowly and consult your doctor if you experience pain, distress or other symptons.

Weights, Measures and Abbreviations

ABBREVIATIONS

kcal	*kilocalories / calories*
prot	*protein*
carb	*carbohydrate*
sm	*small*
med	*medium*
lge	*large*
tsp	*teaspoon*
tbsp	*tablespoon*
dtsp	*dessertspoon*

BRAND ABBREVIATIONS USED

ASDA

Good for You	*GFY*

MARKS & SPENCER *M & S*

Count on Us	*COU*

MORRISONS

Better For You	*BFY*

NEW COVENT GARDEN FOOD CO. *NCGF CO*

SAINSBURY'S

Be Good to Yourself	*BGTY*
Way to Five	*WTF*
Taste the Difference	*TTD*

TESCO

Healthy Eating	*HE*
Healthy Living	*HL*

WAITROSE

Perfectly Balanced	*PB*

	Measure INFO/WEIGHT	per Measure KCAL	FAT	Nutrition Values per 100g / 100ml KCAL	PROT	CARB	FAT	FIBRE
ABSINTHE								
Average	1 Pub Shot/35ml	127	0.0	363	0.0	38.8	0.0	0.0
ACKEE								
Canned, Drained, Average	1oz/28g	42	4.3	151	2.9	0.8	15.2	0.0
ADVOCAAT								
Average	1 Pub Shot/35ml	91	2.2	260	4.7	28.4	6.3	0.0
AERO								
Creamy White Centre, Nestle*	1 Bar/46g	244	13.8	530	7.6	57.4	30.0	0.0
Minis, Nestle*	1 Bar/11g	57	3.2	518	6.8	58.1	28.7	0.8
Mint, Nestle*	1 Bar/48g	256	14.3	533	4.9	61.2	29.8	0.4
Nestle*	1 Bar/46g	247	14.2	536	5.0	59.8	30.8	0.8
ALFALFA SPROUTS								
Raw, Average	1oz/28g	7	0.2	24	4.0	0.4	0.7	1.7
ALMONDS								
Blanched, Average	1oz/28g	171	15.0	610	25.0	7.2	53.5	8.5
Chocolate Covered, Bonneterre*	15 Almonds/45g	257	18.0	570	11.0	43.0	40.0	0.0
Chopped, Sainsbury's*	1 Serving/10g	61	5.6	614	25.4	6.5	55.8	7.4
Cocoa Dusted, Organic, Green & Black's*	1 Pack/110g	585	40.4	532	7.8	42.8	36.7	7.6
Flaked, Tesco*	1 Tbsp/7g	43	3.9	614	21.1	6.9	55.8	7.4
Ground, Average	1 Serving/10g	62	5.6	625	24.0	6.6	55.8	7.4
Smoked, Sainsbury's*	1 Serving/40g	264	23.1	660	26.0	9.0	57.8	7.5
Sugared, Co-Op*	1 Almond/5.5g	27	0.8	455	7.0	74.0	14.0	2.0
Toasted, Average	1oz/28g	178	15.8	634	25.0	6.6	56.5	6.6
Whole, Average	1 Portion/20g	122	11.0	612	23.4	8.1	54.8	8.4
Yoghurt Coated, Holland & Barrett*	1 Pack/100g	536	37.0	536	10.9	45.3	37.0	2.8
ALOO TIKKI								
Budgens*	1 Serving/25.2g	51	1.9	202	5.9	27.8	7.5	4.1
Mini, Indian Selection, Somerfield*	1 Serving/25g	49	1.6	199	4.5	30.3	6.6	0.2
ANCHOVIES								
Fillets, Flat, John West*	1 Can/50g	113	7.0	226	25.0	0.1	14.0	0.0
Fillets, Tesco*	1 Serving/15g	34	2.1	226	25.0	0.0	14.0	0.0
in Oil, Canned, Drained, Average	1 Serving/30g	58	3.4	194	22.9	0.0	11.3	0.0
Marinated, Sainsbury's*	¼ Pot/44.1g	78	4.0	177	22.0	2.0	9.0	0.1
Salted, Finest, Tesco*	1 Serving/10g	9	0.2	93	18.2	0.0	2.2	0.0
with Olives, Marinated, H Forman & Son*	1 Pack/200g	320	17.4	160	20.2	0.2	8.7	0.0
ANGEL DELIGHT								
Banana Flavour, Kraft*	1 Sachet/59g	289	12.4	490	2.5	72.0	21.0	0.0
Butterscotch Flavour, Kraft*	1 Sachet/59g	280	11.2	475	2.4	73.5	19.0	0.0
Chocolate Flavour, Kraft*	1 Sachet/67g	305	12.1	455	3.7	69.5	18.0	0.4
Strawberry Flavour, Kraft*	1 Sachet/59g	286	12.4	485	2.5	71.0	21.0	0.0
Strawberry Flavour, No Added Sugar, Kraft*	1 Sachet/47g	230	12.5	490	4.8	59.0	26.5	0.0
Strawberry Flavour with Topples, Kraft*	1 Sachet/59g	266	8.3	450	2.8	74.5	14.0	0.0
Vanilla Ice Cream Flavour, Kraft*	1 Sachet/59g	289	12.7	490	2.5	71.5	21.5	0.0
ANGEL HAIR								
Pasta, Sainsbury's*	1 Serving/100g	357	1.7	357	12.3	73.1	1.7	2.5
ANTIPASTO								
Artichoke, Sainsbury's*	1 Serving/50g	68	6.3	135	2.0	3.6	12.5	2.3
Mixed, Misto Cotto, Arrosto Erbe, Waitrose*	1 Slice/9g	11	0.4	129	22.2	0.0	4.4	0.0
Mixed Mushroom, Sainsbury's*	¼ Jar/72g	70	6.5	97	2.7	1.4	9.0	3.7
Mixed Pepper, Sainsbury's*	¼ Jar/68g	23	0.9	34	1.3	4.2	1.3	3.5
Seafood, Drained, Sainsbury's*	½ Jar/84g	150	9.7	178	14.3	4.1	11.6	1.4
Sun Dried Tomato, Sainsbury's*	¼ Jar/70g	275	25.0	393	4.5	13.4	35.7	6.2
APPETISERS								
Salmon, Smoked, Tesco*	1/3 Pack/33.3g	80	6.2	240	16.3	1.1	18.5	0.0

	Measure INFO/WEIGHT	per Measure KCAL	FAT	Nutrition Values per 100g / 100ml KCAL	PROT	CARB	FAT	FIBRE
APPLE & GRAPES								
Fresh, Morrisons*	1 Pack/90g	46	0.1	51	0.4	12.1	0.1	2.3
APPLES								
Bites, Average	1 Pack/118g	58	0.1	49	0.3	11.7	0.1	2.2
Braeburn, Average	1 Apple/165g	79	0.2	48	0.4	11.3	0.1	1.8
Cape, Tesco*	1 Apple/100g	50	0.1	50	0.4	11.8	0.1	1.8
Cooking, Baked with Sugar, Flesh Only, Average	1 Serving/140g	109	0.1	78	0.5	20.1	0.1	1.7
Cooking, Raw, Peeled, Average	1oz/28g	10	0.0	35	0.3	8.9	0.1	1.6
Cooking, Stewed with Sugar, Average	1 Serving/140g	104	0.1	74	0.3	19.1	0.1	1.2
Cooking, Stewed without Sugar, Average	1 Serving/140g	46	0.1	33	0.3	8.1	0.1	1.5
Cox, English, Average	1 Apple/108g	53	0.1	49	0.4	11.6	0.1	2.2
Dried, Average	1 Pack/250g	554	0.8	222	1.1	57.3	0.3	6.7
Empire, Tesco*	1 Apple/100g	50	0.1	50	0.4	11.8	0.1	1.8
Fuji, Organic, Sainsbury's*	1 Apple/130g	61	0.1	47	0.4	11.8	0.1	1.8
Gala, Average	1 Apple/152g	74	0.2	49	0.4	11.5	0.1	1.4
Golden Delicious, Average	1 Apple/102g	49	0.1	48	0.4	11.5	0.1	1.7
Granny Smith, Average	1 Apple/125g	62	0.1	50	0.4	11.9	0.1	2.0
Mackintosh, Red, Average	1 Apple/165g	81	0.5	49	0.2	12.8	0.3	1.8
Pink Lady, Average	1 Apple/125g	62	0.1	50	0.4	11.7	0.1	1.8
Sliced, Average	1oz/28g	14	0.0	49	0.4	11.6	0.1	1.8
Snack Pack, Garden Gang, Asda*	1 Pack/80g	42	0.1	53	0.3	12.5	0.1	2.8
Stewed, Sainsbury's*	¼ Can/100g	71	0.0	71	0.2	17.4	0.0	1.2
APPLETISE								
Schweppes*	1 Glass/200ml	98	0.0	49	0.0	11.8	0.0	0.0
APRICOTS								
& Prunes, in Fruit Juice, Breakfast, Sainsbury's*	1 Pot/150g	134	0.2	89	1.1	21.2	0.1	0.7
Canned, in Syrup, Average	1oz/28g	18	0.0	63	0.4	16.1	0.1	0.9
Dried, Average	1 Apricot/10g	17	0.1	171	3.6	37.4	0.5	6.3
Dried Fruit, Ultimate, Mariani Premium*	6 Apricots/48g	130	0.0	270	2.5	65.0	0.0	5.0
Halves, in Fruit Juice, Average	1 Sm Can/221g	87	0.1	40	0.5	9.2	0.1	1.0
Raw, Flesh Only, Average	1 Apricot/37g	19	0.2	52	1.5	12.0	0.4	2.2
Raw, Weighed with Stone, Average	1 Apricot/40g	19	0.2	48	1.4	11.1	0.4	2.0
Soft, Asda*	1 Bag/75g	124	0.5	165	3.9	36.0	0.6	6.3
Soft, Dried, So Organic, Sainsbury's*	1/3 Pack/83.3g	166	0.6	199	4.8	43.4	0.7	7.7
ARCHERS*								
Aqua, Peach, Archers*	1 Bottle/275ml	206	0.0	75	0.3	5.1	0.0	0.0
Peach (Calculated Estimate), Archers*	1 Shot/35ml	91	0.0	260	0.0	0.0	0.0	0.0
Vea, Wildberry, Schnapps, Archers*	1 Bottle/275ml	124	0.0	45	0.0	5.8	0.0	0.0
ARROWROOT								
Fresh, Average	1 Root/33g	21	0.0	64	4.2	13.3	0.0	1.2
ARTICHOKE								
Hearts, Canned, Drained, Average	½ Can/117g	35	0.1	30	1.9	5.5	0.1	2.2
Hearts, Chargrilled in Olive Oil, TTD, Sainsbury's*	¼ Jar/73g	150	15.2	205	1.0	3.4	20.8	0.0
Hearts, Marinated & Grilled, Waitrose*	1 Serving/50g	57	5.0	114	3.0	3.0	10.0	3.0
Marinated, Roasted, M & S*	1 Pack/200g	300	26.6	150	1.9	5.0	13.3	2.3
Raw, Fresh, Average	1oz/28g	13	0.0	47	3.3	10.5	0.2	5.4
ASPARAGUS								
Boiled, in Salted Water, Average	5 Spears/125g	33	1.0	26	3.4	1.4	0.8	1.4
Canned, Average	1 Can/250g	48	0.5	19	2.3	2.0	0.2	1.6
Raw, Average	1 Serving/80g	20	0.5	25	3.1	1.8	0.7	1.8
AUBERGINE								
Baked Topped, M & S*	1 Serving/150g	165	11.6	110	2.4	7.4	7.7	0.9
Fried, Average	1oz/28g	85	8.9	302	1.2	2.8	31.9	2.3
in Hot Sauce, Yarden*	1 Serving/35g	96	9.0	273	1.5	8.8	25.8	0.0

	Measure INFO/WEIGHT	per Measure KCAL	FAT	Nutrition Values per 100g / 100ml KCAL	PROT	CARB	FAT	FIBRE
AUBERGINE								
Marinated & Grilled, Waitrose*	½ Pack/100g	106	10.0	106	1.0	3.0	10.0	2.0
Parmigiana, M & S*	1 Pack/350g	333	18.6	95	4.6	7.6	5.3	1.1
Raw, Fresh, Average	1 Serving/120g	18	0.5	15	0.9	2.2	0.4	2.0
AVOCADO								
Flesh Only, Average	1 Med/145g	276	28.3	190	1.9	1.9	19.5	3.4

A

B

	Measure INFO/WEIGHT	per Measure KCAL	per Measure FAT	Nutrition Values per 100g / 100ml KCAL	PROT	CARB	FAT	FIBRE
BACARDI*								
37.5% Volume, Bacardi*	1 Shot/25ml	52	0.0	207	0.0	0.0	0.0	0.0
40% Volume, Bacardi*	1 Pub Shot/35ml	78	0.0	222	0.0	0.0	0.0	0.0
Bacardi & Diet Cola, Bacardi*	1 Bottle/275ml	85	0.0	31	0.0	1.0	0.0	0.0
Breezer, Apple, Half Sugar, Crisp, Bacardi*	1 Bottle/275ml	121	0.0	44	0.0	3.7	0.0	0.0
Breezer, Half Sugar, Bacardi*	1 Bottle/275ml	122	0.0	44	0.0	0.0	0.0	0.0
Breezer, Lemon, Diet, Bacardi*	1 Bottle/275ml	96	0.0	35	0.0	1.2	0.0	0.0
Breezer, Lime, Bacardi*	1 Bottle/275ml	182	0.0	66	0.0	9.1	0.0	0.0
Breezer, Orange, Bacardi*	1 Bottle/275ml	179	0.0	65	0.0	8.2	0.0	0.0
Breezer, Pineapple, Bacardi*	1 Bottle/275ml	171	0.0	62	0.0	8.6	0.0	0.0
Breezer, Raspberry, Half Sugar, Bacardi*	1 Bottle/275ml	122	0.0	44	0.0	3.7	0.0	0.0
Breezer, Watermelon, Bacardi*	1 Bottle/275ml	151	0.0	55	0.0	6.8	0.0	0.0
BACON								
Back, Dry Cured, Average	1 Rasher/31g	77	4.7	250	28.1	0.3	15.1	0.3
Back, Dry Fried Or Grilled, Average	1 Rasher/25g	76	5.5	304	26.5	0.1	21.9	0.0
Back, Lean, Average	1 Rasher/33g	57	4.0	174	16.3	0.1	12.0	0.5
Back, Smoked, Average	1 Rasher/25g	66	5.0	265	20.9	0.0	19.9	0.0
Back, Smoked, Lean, Average	1 Rasher/25g	41	1.2	163	28.2	1.1	5.0	0.2
Back, Smoked, Rindless, Average	1 Rasher/25g	60	4.3	241	21.0	0.1	17.4	0.0
Back, Tendersweet, Average	1 Rasher/25g	63	3.6	251	29.8	0.5	14.4	0.1
Back, Unsmoked, Average	1 Rasher/32g	78	5.5	243	21.3	0.4	17.3	0.0
Back, Unsmoked, Rindless, Average	1 Rasher/23g	56	3.9	241	22.5	0.0	16.9	0.0
Chops, Average	1oz/28g	62	4.2	222	22.3	0.0	14.8	0.0
Chops, Coated in American Style BBQ Glaze, Tesco*	1 Serving/200g	480	36.2	240	16.1	2.1	18.1	0.0
Chops, in Cheese Sauce, Tesco*	1 Serving/185g	405	26.5	219	12.6	10.0	14.3	1.1
Collar Joint, Lean & Fat, Boiled	1oz/28g	91	7.6	325	20.4	0.0	27.0	0.0
Collar Joint, Lean & Fat, Raw	1oz/28g	89	8.1	319	14.6	0.0	28.9	0.0
Collar Joint, Lean Only, Boiled	1oz/28g	53	2.7	191	26.0	0.0	9.7	0.0
Fat Only, Cooked, Average	1oz/28g	194	20.4	692	9.3	0.0	72.8	0.0
Fat Only, Raw, Average	1oz/28g	209	22.7	747	4.8	0.0	80.9	0.0
Gammon Rasher, Lean Only, Grilled	1oz/28g	48	1.5	172	31.4	0.0	5.2	0.0
Lardons, Smoked, Sainsbury's*	1 Serving/200g	476	30.8	238	21.4	0.1	15.4	0.1
Lean, Average	1oz/28g	40	1.9	142	19.6	0.9	6.7	0.2
Lean Only, Fried, Average	1 Rasher/25g	83	5.6	332	32.8	0.0	22.3	0.0
Lean Only, Grilled, Average	1 Rasher/25g	73	4.7	292	30.5	0.0	18.9	0.0
Loin Steaks, Grilled, Average	1 Serving/120g	229	11.6	191	25.9	0.0	9.7	0.0
Medallion, Steaks, Unsmoked, Grilled, HL, Tesco*	1 Medallion/50g	100	3.3	200	33.2	0.0	6.6	0.0
Medallions, Average	1 Rasher/18g	27	0.6	151	29.4	0.9	3.3	0.1
Middle, Fried	1 Rasher/40g	140	11.4	350	23.4	0.0	28.5	0.0
Middle, Grilled	1 Rasher/40g	123	9.2	307	24.8	0.0	23.1	0.0
Middle, Raw	1 Rasher/43g	104	8.6	241	15.2	0.0	20.0	0.0
Rindless, Average	1 Rasher/20g	30	1.7	151	18.5	0.0	8.5	0.0
Smoked, Average	1 Rasher/28g	46	2.1	166	24.8	0.3	7.4	0.0
Smoked, Crispy, Cooked, Average	1 Serving/10g	46	2.7	460	53.0	2.1	26.9	0.0
Smoked, Rindless, Average	1 Rasher/20g	21	0.6	106	19.8	0.0	3.0	0.0
Streaky, Average	1 Rasher/20g	54	4.2	270	20.0	0.0	21.0	0.0
Streaky, Cooked, Average	1 Rasher/20g	68	5.6	342	22.4	0.3	27.8	0.0
BACON BITS								
Average	1oz/28g	66	4.9	235	19.6	0.0	17.4	0.0
Flavoured Soya Pieces, Salad Topping, Schwartz*	1 Tbsp/6.5g	26	1.0	397	37.0	27.7	15.3	0.0
BACON VEGETARIAN								
Cheatin' Rashers, Redwood*	1 Rasher/16.3g	32	1.2	196	25.9	6.5	7.3	0.5
Realeat*	1 Rasher/18.75g	49	1.1	260	27.0	25.0	5.8	1.6
Streaky Style Rashers, Tesco*	1 Rasher/20g	43	2.1	215	23.7	5.0	10.6	2.2

	Measure INFO/WEIGHT	per Measure KCAL	FAT	Nutrition Values per 100g / 100ml KCAL	PROT	CARB	FAT	FIBRE
BAGEL								
Bacon, & Soft Cheese, Boots*	1 Serving/148g	481	25.2	325	12.0	31.0	17.0	2.2
Chicken, Lemon & Watercress, Safeway*	1 Pack/153g	329	6.3	215	12.8	28.2	4.1	0.0
Cream Cheese, & Salmon, Smoked, M & S*	1 Bagel/23g	64	2.8	280	10.9	31.7	12.2	2.9
Cream Cheese, M & S*	1 Bagel/22.5g	81	5.0	352	7.8	31.0	21.8	1.8
Ham, & Pesto, COU, M & S*	1 Pack/173g	260	2.4	150	11.1	23.5	1.4	1.7
Soft Cheese, & Salmon, Smoked, Finest, Tesco*	1 Pack/173g	396	10.0	229	13.1	31.2	5.8	1.7
Tuna, & Salad, BGTY, Sainsbury's*	1 Bagel/170g	325	7.1	191	10.4	26.0	4.2	1.0
Tuna, & Sweetcorn Relish, Safeway*	1 Bagel/162g	284	4.4	175	11.5	26.2	2.7	0.0
BAGEL CHIPS								
Sea Salt & Vinegar, Shapers, Boots*	1 Pack/25g	95	0.7	378	11.0	77.0	2.9	3.1
Smokey Ham Flavour, COU, M & S*	1 Pack/25g	91	0.6	365	10.5	75.6	2.5	5.2
Sour Cream & Chive, Shapers, Boots*	1 Bag/25g	94	0.7	377	9.7	78.0	2.9	1.9
BAGUETTE								
Cheese, & Ham, Snack 'n' Go, Sainsbury's*	1 Baguette/178g	381	9.0	215	12.6	29.6	5.1	1.9
Cheese, & Pickle, Fullfillers*	1 Baguette/280g	767	31.1	274	11.9	35.5	11.1	0.0
Cheese, Mixed, & Spring Onion, Asda*	1 Pack/190g	629	34.8	331	9.5	32.1	18.3	1.3
Cheese, Tomato, & Basil, Asda*	¼ Bread/42g	138	5.9	329	10.0	40.8	14.0	1.3
Chicken, & Mayonnaise, Asda*	1 Pack/190g	407	16.5	214	9.7	30.5	8.7	1.3
Chicken, & Salad, Asda*	1 Serving/158.3g	325	9.5	206	9.0	29.0	6.0	2.1
Chicken, & Salad, Boots*	1 Baguette/132g	202	2.4	153	11.0	23.0	1.8	2.0
Chicken, & Salad, Shapers, Boots*	1 Pack/132.1g	222	2.6	168	11.0	27.0	2.0	1.5
Chicken, & Stuffing, Hot, Sainsbury's*	1 Baguette/227g	543	16.3	239	13.7	29.6	7.2	0.0
Chicken, Honey & Mustard, BGTY, Sainsbury's*	1 Pack/186.8g	340	3.7	182	11.0	30.0	2.0	0.0
Chicken, Tikka, Asda*	1 Pack/190g	439	17.9	231	10.4	32.8	9.4	1.3
Chicken, Tikka, Hot, Sainsbury's*	1 Pack/190g	386	11.6	203	8.5	28.4	6.1	0.0
Egg, & Tomato, Oldfields*	1 Pack/198g	416	15.0	210	8.7	27.0	7.6	0.0
Egg Mayonnaise, & Cress, Cafe, Sainsbury's*	1 Pack/100g	480	20.4	480	13.8	60.2	20.4	0.0
Ham, & Turkey, Asda*	1 Baguette/360g	774	18.4	215	11.6	30.7	5.1	1.3
Mozzarella, Tomato, & Pesto, Darwins Deli*	1 Serving/210g	531	20.4	253	11.7	29.7	9.7	0.0
Prawn, French, Shell*	1 Baguette/63g	171	7.2	272	9.7	32.4	11.5	0.0
Prawn Mayonnaise, Asda*	1 Pack/190g	399	9.3	210	9.1	32.5	4.9	1.3
Steak, & Onion, Snack 'n' Go, Sainsbury's*	1 Baguette/177g	396	8.8	225	14.3	30.6	5.0	2.2
Tuna, Crunch, Shapers, Boots*	1 Serving/43.9g	100	1.5	228	14.0	35.0	3.5	3.1
Tuna, Melt, Sainsbury's*	1 Serving/204g	373	8.0	183	11.3	25.8	3.9	0.0
BAILEYS*								
Glide, Baileys*	1 Serving/200ml	212	2.4	106	0.0	18.0	1.2	0.0
Irish Cream, Original, Baileys*	1 Glass/37ml	121	4.8	327	3.0	25.0	13.0	0.0
BAKE								
Aubergine & Mozzarella Cheese, BGTY, Sainsbury's*	1 Pack/360g	194	7.2	54	3.0	6.0	2.0	1.3
Aubergine & Spinach, BGTY, Sainsbury's*	1 Pack/360g	148	6.5	41	2.2	4.0	1.8	1.3
Bean & Pasta, Asda*	1 Pack/450g	599	22.5	133	5.0	17.0	5.0	1.7
Bolognese, Mini Classics, Co-Op*	1 Pack/300g	405	15.0	135	9.0	13.0	5.0	1.0
Broccoli & Cheese, M & S*	1 Pack/400g	380	22.8	95	4.8	5.6	5.7	1.1
Cauliflower & Broccoli Bake, Tesco*	½ Pack/250g	178	10.3	71	2.8	5.8	4.1	1.0
Cheese & Spinach, Tesco*	1 Bake/140g	269	10.9	192	4.5	26.0	7.8	1.4
Chicken, Bacon & Potato, British Classics, Tesco*	½ Pack/375g	435	16.5	116	7.0	12.2	4.4	1.4
Chicken, Broccoli & Mushroom, Safeway*	1 Serving/175g	425	22.9	243	8.9	22.4	13.1	3.0
Chicken, Tomato, & Mascarpone, HL, Tesco*	1 Serving/400g	468	10.8	117	7.6	15.5	2.7	0.8
Chicken & Mushroom, COU, M & S*	1 Serving/360g	324	8.3	90	7.3	10.3	2.3	1.1
Chicken & Pasta, BGTY, Sainsbury's*	1 Pack/400g	394	10.0	99	9.0	10.0	2.5	2.5
Chicken Arrabbbiata, M & S*	1 Pack/450g	540	13.5	120	7.6	16.0	3.0	2.0
Chicken Spiralli, M & S*	1 Serving/400g	400	15.2	100	7.9	9.1	3.8	1.1
Cod & Prawn, COU, M & S*	1 Pack/400g	320	8.0	80	6.5	8.8	2.0	1.0

	Measure INFO/WEIGHT	per Measure KCAL	per Measure FAT	Nutrition Values per 100g / 100ml KCAL	PROT	CARB	FAT	FIBRE
BAKE								
Courgette & Tomato, Cauldron*	½ Pack/200g	416	26.0	208	10.0	17.0	13.0	6.4
Creamy Peppercorn, Vegetarian, Tesco*	1 Serving/140g	322	16.8	230	3.6	27.0	12.0	1.2
Fish & Vegetable, Youngs*	1 Serving/374.8g	446	23.6	119	5.6	10.0	6.3	1.3
Mediterranean Vegetable Bistro, Cauldron*	1 Bake/100g	190	10.0	190	4.0	21.0	10.0	3.0
Mushroom, Leek & Spinach, Cumberland, Sainsbury's*	1 Pack/450g	518	24.3	115	3.6	12.9	5.4	1.2
Penne Bolognese, BGTY, Sainsbury's*	1 Pack/450g	446	11.3	99	6.0	13.0	2.5	2.0
Potato, Cheese, & Bacon, Homepride*	1 Serving/210g	277	26.3	132	1.6	3.2	12.5	0.0
Potato, Cheese, & Onion, Tesco*	1 Pack/400g	376	19.6	94	2.4	10.0	4.9	1.0
Potato, Mushroom & Leek, M & S*	1 Serving/225g	225	13.3	100	3.5	10.0	5.9	2.0
Potato, Tomato & Mozzarella, M & S*	1 Bake/450g	585	34.2	130	5.2	9.8	7.6	1.8
Potato, with Cheese & Leek, Aunt Bessie's*	½ Pack/275g	300	13.8	109	3.4	12.7	5.0	2.7
Potato & Brie, Finest, Tesco*	½ Pack/200g	304	21.2	152	4.1	10.2	10.6	1.5
Potato & Vegetable, Co-Op*	1 Bake/340g	425	27.2	125	4.0	11.0	8.0	1.0
Roast Onion & Potato, COU, M & S*	1 Pack/450g	338	5.9	75	1.9	13.6	1.3	1.5
Roast Potato, Cheese & Onion, Asda*	½ Pack/200g	288	16.0	144	4.2	14.0	8.0	1.1
Salmon & Broccoli, Youngs*	1 Bake/375g	409	19.1	109	6.3	9.6	5.1	1.3
Salmon & Prawn, M & S*	1 Bake/328.6g	461	31.3	140	7.4	6.6	9.5	0.7
Smoked Haddock & Prawn, BGTY, Sainsbury's*	1 Pack/350g	319	2.5	91	7.5	13.6	0.7	1.1
Spicy Bean & Potato, Safeway*	1 Pack/385.7g	405	12.4	105	3.9	14.2	3.2	2.1
Spicy Chickpea & Apricot, Safeway*	1 Pack/400g	340	11.5	85	2.2	12.5	2.9	3.2
Tuna & Pasta, HL, Tesco*	1 Pack/400g	360	6.0	90	8.3	10.7	1.5	0.9
Vegetable & Lentil, Somerfield*	1 Pack/350g	319	6.3	91	4.9	13.8	1.8	2.5
BAKE MIX								
Potato, Creamy Cheddar Cheese, Colman's*	1 Pack/45g	189	11.7	420	11.5	34.8	26.0	9.6
Potato, Ham & Leek, Colman's*	1 Pack/44g	181	10.6	412	9.9	40.4	24.0	2.1
Quick Quisine, Atkins*	1 Serving/100g	286	2.7	286	44.0	16.0	2.7	19.8
Tuna & Pasta, Colman's*	1 Pack/45g	149	2.4	331	10.4	60.5	5.3	4.4
BAKING POWDER								
Average	1 Tsp/2g	3	0.0	163	5.2	37.8	0.0	0.0
BAKLAVA								
Assortment, TTD, Sainsbury's*	1 Pastry/23.9g	105	7.0	439	10.6	33.4	29.2	4.2
Average	1 Serving/100g	393	21.0	393	5.0	46.0	21.0	0.0
BALTI								
Chick Pea & Spinach, Cauldron*	1 Pack/400g	356	8.0	89	2.3	15.5	2.0	1.0
Chicken, From Indian Meal for One, Sainsbury's*	1 Pack/300g	384	20.4	128	12.9	3.7	6.8	2.1
Chicken, Indian Takeaway, Iceland*	1 Pack/402.2g	362	19.3	90	7.8	4.0	4.8	0.7
Chicken, M & S*	½ Pack/175g	245	15.2	140	13.0	2.0	8.7	1.7
Chicken, Morrisons*	1 Pack/350g	441	26.6	126	12.1	2.3	7.6	1.5
Chicken, Sainsbury's*	½ Pack/200g	222	11.2	111	11.6	3.6	5.6	1.3
Chicken, Takeaway, Sainsbury's*	1 Pack/400g	404	18.0	101	10.4	4.8	4.5	1.4
Chicken, Tesco*	1 Pack/460g	662	25.8	144	6.1	17.4	5.6	1.6
Chicken, Tin, Sainsbury's*	1 Serving/200g	168	6.8	84	9.4	4.0	3.4	1.0
Chicken, with Garlic & Coriander Naan, Frozen, Patak's*	1 Pack/375g	431	18.8	115	6.3	11.1	5.0	1.1
Chicken, with Garlic & Coriander Naan, Patak's*	1 Pack/375g	431	18.8	115	6.3	11.1	5.0	1.1
Chicken, with Naan Bread, PB, Waitrose*	1 Pack/375g	450	13.5	120	12.1	9.7	3.6	2.8
Chicken, with Naan Bread, Sharwood's*	1 Pack/375g	529	23.3	141	7.3	14.1	6.2	2.2
Chicken, with Pilau Rice, Asda*	1 Pack/504g	625	24.7	124	5.0	15.0	4.9	1.2
Chicken, with Potato Wedges, HL, Tesco*	1 Pack/450g	387	9.5	86	6.0	10.8	2.1	1.1
Chicken, with Rice, COU, M & S*	1 Pack/400g	380	6.0	95	6.9	14.1	1.5	1.2
Chicken, with Rice, Curry Break, Patak's*	1 Pack/220g	198	6.2	90	4.7	11.6	2.8	0.0
Chicken, with Rice, Patak's*	1 Pack/370g	440	13.0	119	6.1	16.7	3.5	1.7
Chicken, with Rice, Weight Watchers*	1 Pack/329g	253	5.6	77	4.8	10.7	1.7	0.5
Chicken & Mushroom, Tesco*	1 Serving/350g	326	10.5	93	12.3	4.2	3.0	0.7

	Measure INFO/WEIGHT	per Measure KCAL	FAT	Nutrition Values per 100g / 100ml KCAL	PROT	CARB	FAT	FIBRE
BALTI								
Chicken & Naan Bread, Somerfield*	1 Pack/335g	489	16.8	146	10.0	16.0	5.0	0.0
Chicken & Rice, M & S*	1 Pack/400g	380	6.0	95	6.9	14.1	1.5	1.2
Chicken Ceylon, Finest, Tesco*	1 Pack/400g	588	38.0	147	14.4	0.9	9.5	5.0
Chicken Tikka, Finest, Tesco*	½ Pack/200g	280	17.2	140	15.8	1.1	8.6	3.2
Chicken Tikka, Tesco*	1 Pack/400g	389	17.8	97	8.5	5.8	4.5	1.1
Chicken Tikka & Wedges, HL, Tesco*	1 Pack/450g	392	9.9	87	6.0	10.7	2.2	1.1
Lamb, Bhuna, Tesco*	1 Pack/400g	360	14.8	90	9.2	4.8	3.7	1.1
Prawn, Budgens*	1 Pack/350g	375	24.9	107	5.6	5.2	7.1	1.3
Vegetable, Asda*	½ Can/200g	206	12.0	103	2.2	10.0	6.0	2.5
Vegetable, GFY, Asda*	1 Pack/450g	324	4.1	72	1.9	14.0	0.9	1.5
Vegetable, Indian Meal for 2, Finest, Tesco*	½ Pack/150g	144	10.8	96	1.6	6.1	7.2	2.9
Vegetable, Naan Bread & Raita, Eat Smart, Safeway*	1 Pack/371g	315	7.0	85	3.8	12.5	1.9	3.1
Vegetable & Rice, Tesco*	1 Pack/450g	378	7.2	84	2.0	15.6	1.6	1.3
BAMBOO SHOOTS								
Canned, Average	1 Sm Can/120g	11	0.2	9	1.1	0.9	0.1	0.9
BANANA								
Raw, Flesh Only, Average	1 Sm/95g	90	0.3	95	1.2	20.9	0.3	4.2
Raw, Weighed with Skin, Average	1 Lge/185g	176	0.6	95	1.2	20.9	0.3	4.2
BANANA SPLIT								
Fresh Cream, Tesco*	1 Serving/240g	463	31.2	193	1.7	17.2	13.0	0.3
BANGERS & MASH								
& Beans, Blue Parrot Cafe, Sainsbury's*	1 Pack/300g	354	12.6	118	5.3	14.8	4.2	2.1
Asda*	1 Pack/400g	636	28.0	159	9.0	15.0	7.0	1.6
Bitesize, Birds Eye*	1 Pack/316.7g	285	9.2	90	2.7	13.3	2.9	1.5
Co-Op*	1 Pack/300g	375	18.0	125	4.0	13.0	6.0	0.8
Loved By Kids, M & S*	1 Pack/225g	191	7.4	85	5.4	8.1	3.3	1.2
Meal for One, M & S*	1 Pack/430.8g	560	34.0	130	4.7	9.5	7.9	1.1
Morrisons*	1 Pack/300g	306	14.7	102	3.0	12.3	4.9	0.8
Sausage, & Cabbage Mash, Eat Smart, Safeway*	1 Pack/400g	340	10.0	85	6.4	9.0	2.5	1.3
BARS								
All Bran, Apple, Kellogg's*	1 Bar/40g	158	7.6	395	8.0	48.0	19.0	5.0
All Bran, Honey & Oat, Kellogg's*	1 Bar/27g	99	2.2	366	6.0	67.0	8.0	12.0
All Day Breakfast, Weight Watchers*	1 Bar/50g	179	2.3	358	6.8	72.2	4.6	3.2
All Fruit, Frusli, Passion Fruit, Jordans*	1 Bar/30g	92	0.2	307	1.3	74.0	0.7	5.0
All Fruit, Frusli, Strawberry, Jordans*	1 Bar/30g	94	0.1	313	2.3	81.3	0.3	5.0
Almond, Apricot, & Mango, M & S*	1 Bar/50g	205	7.4	410	9.0	60.2	14.8	5.0
Am, Breakfast Muffin, Apple & Sultana, McVitie's*	1 Bar/45g	168	7.5	373	4.4	54.9	16.7	1.6
Am, Cereal, Apricot, McVitie's*	1 Bar/30g	146	6.2	486	6.5	68.8	20.5	0.5
Am, Cereal, Fruit & Nut, McVitie's*	1 Bar/35g	167	7.5	477	6.6	64.9	21.4	3.4
Am, Cereal, Orange Marmalade, McVitie's*	1 Bar/40g	151	7.2	378	4.5	53.3	18.0	1.8
Am, Granola, Almond, Raisin & Cranberry, McVitie's*	1 Bar/35g	133	4.0	380	7.1	62.9	11.4	4.0
Am, Muesli Fingers, McVitie's*	1 Bar/35g	154	6.9	440	6.0	59.8	19.6	3.1
Apple, Granola, McVitie's*	1 Bar/35g	128	3.4	366	6.6	63.1	9.7	4.3
Apple, Pear & Berry, Shapers, Boots*	1 Bar/30g	78	0.0	261	1.2	64.0	0.1	10.0
Apple & Cinnamon, Breakfast Snack, Tesco*	1 Bar/37.5g	139	4.8	365	4.3	58.8	12.5	2.0
Apple & Cinnamon, Chewy, GFY, Asda*	1 Bar/27g	95	0.7	351	6.0	76.0	2.6	3.5
Apple & Custard, Danish, Tesco*	1 Serving/100g	268	15.1	268	3.6	29.5	15.1	5.6
Apple & Raisin, Snack, Geobar, Traidcraft*	1 Bar/35g	127	1.7	362	3.3	76.4	4.8	2.3
Apple & Sultana, Goodness, Ryvita*	1 Bar/23g	62	0.6	268	4.3	56.4	2.8	22.0
Apricot, Dried Fruit, Sunsweet*	1 Bar/33g	96	0.0	292	3.6	72.5	0.1	0.0
Apricot & Almond, Eat Natural*	1 Serving/50g	202	8.1	403	11.2	53.3	16.1	0.0
Apricot & Almond, Yoghurt Coated, Eat Natural*	1 Bar/50g	236	12.8	471	8.3	52.0	25.5	4.3
Apricot & Peach, Multigrain, BGTY, Sainsbury's*	1 Bar/25g	71	0.6	282	6.6	58.2	2.5	23.1

B

BARS

INFO/WEIGHT	Measure	per Measure KCAL	FAT	Nutrition Values per 100g / 100ml KCAL	PROT	CARB	FAT	FIBRE
Biscuit, Chocolate, Penguin, McVitie's*	1 Bar/25g	130	6.9	520	5.2	62.4	27.7	2.4
Biscuit, Chocolate Mint, Penguin, McVitie's*	1 Bar/25g	133	6.9	531	5.4	65.0	27.7	1.5
Biscuit, Chocolate Orange, Penguin, McVitie's*	1 Bar/25g	133	6.9	531	5.4	65.0	27.7	1.5
Biscuit & Raisin, Reduced Fat, Tesco*	1 Bar/22g	90	2.8	410	4.9	69.5	12.5	1.8
Blue Riband, 99 Calories, Nestle*	1 Bar/19.3g	97	4.8	513	4.8	66.4	25.3	0.0
Blue Riband, Nestle*	1 Bar/21.1g	104	5.1	495	4.5	64.5	24.5	1.0
Blueberry, Fruit & Grain, Asda*	1 Bar/37g	124	2.6	335	4.1	64.0	7.0	3.9
Blueberry, Pistachio & Yoghurt Bar, Eat Natural*	1 Bar/45g	203	9.9	451	5.6	58.2	22.0	3.2
Blueberry & Yoghurt Nougat, Shapers, Boots*	1 Bar/23g	89	3.7	385	1.7	58.0	16.0	0.7
Boohbah, Milk & White Chocolate, M & S*	1 Bar/75g	405	24.2	540	7.9	54.7	32.3	1.2
Breakfast, Blueberry, Free From, Sainsbury's*	1 Bar/35g	163	7.8	467	3.8	62.6	22.4	0.2
Breakfast, Muesli, Country Garden Cakes*	1 Bar/25g	94	2.3	376	5.6	67.6	9.2	3.6
Breakfast, Vitality, Fruit & Fibre, Asda*	1 Bar/29g	113	2.9	390	6.0	69.0	10.0	4.1
Breakfast, with Cranberries, Asda*	1 Bar/28g	105	1.4	376	6.0	77.0	4.9	3.0
Breakfast, with Cranberries, Vitality, Asda*	1 Bar/20g	103	1.3	509	8.4	103.7	6.4	4.0
Brunch, Cranberry & Orange, Cadbury*	1 Bar/35g	154	5.6	440	5.9	67.7	15.9	0.0
Brunch, Hazelnut, Cadbury*	1 Bar/34.8g	160	7.4	460	7.0	60.5	21.4	2.2
Brunch, Snack, Raisin, Cadbury*	1 Bar/35g	151	5.4	430	5.6	66.4	15.5	1.8
Cappuccino Coll, M & S*	1 Bar/35g	185	12.3	529	6.0	50.0	35.0	1.0
Caramel, Endulge, Atkins*	1 Bar/24g	89	3.0	369	7.8	54.4	12.6	8.6
Caramel Crisp, Go Ahead, McVitie's*	1 Bar/33g	141	4.0	428	4.8	75.1	12.0	0.8
Caramel Crisp Bite, Tesco*	1 Serving/15g	72	3.5	483	4.3	64.4	23.1	1.3
Caramel Crunch, Go Ahead, McVitie's*	1 Bar/24g	106	3.3	440	4.7	76.6	13.8	0.8
Caramel Mighty, Asda*	1 Serving/40g	186	8.0	464	5.0	66.0	20.0	1.5
Caramel Nougat, Soft, Shapers, Boots*	1 Bar/25g	86	2.5	343	2.9	60.4	10.0	0.6
Cereal, Apple, Chewy, BGTY, Sainsbury's*	1 Bar/25g	85	0.5	340	4.8	76.0	2.0	2.0
Cereal, Apple & Blackberry, with Yoghurt, Alpen*	1 Bar/29g	117	3.1	404	5.4	71.8	10.6	5.0
Cereal, Apple & Cinnamon, Tesco*	1 Serving/38g	137	4.7	365	4.3	58.9	12.5	2.1
Cereal, Apple & Cinnamonr, Fruit 'n' Grain, Asda*	1 Bar/37g	131	2.6	353	4.5	68.0	7.0	2.9
Cereal, Apple & Raisin, Harvest, Quaker*	1 Bar/22g	87	2.5	396	5.0	70.0	11.5	4.0
Cereal, Apple & Raspberry, Chewy & Crisp, Tesco*	1 Bar/27g	123	5.3	456	3.3	66.7	19.6	3.0
Cereal, Apple & Raspberry, Waitrose*	1 Bar/25g	90	0.9	359	5.0	77.1	3.4	4.6
Cereal, Apple & Sultana, Go Ahead, McVitie's*	1 Bar/30g	113	2.3	375	4.1	72.9	7.5	2.8
Cereal, Apple & Sultana, Light, Alpen*	1 Bar/21g	59	0.8	281	5.7	56.2	3.8	22.4
Cereal, Apricot & Yoghurt, Shapers, Boots*	1 Bar/27g	99	1.5	366	3.7	75.0	5.7	3.3
Cereal, Balance with Fruit, Sainsbury's*	1 Bar/25g	100	2.2	401	5.8	75.2	8.6	1.9
Cereal, Cheerios & Milk Bar, Nestle*	1 Bar/24g	100	3.2	416	7.6	66.1	13.5	2.0
Cereal, Chewy, BGTY, Sainsbury's*	1 Serving/25g	85	0.5	342	4.9	75.8	2.1	1.9
Cereal, Chewy & Crisp with Choc Chips, Tesco*	1 Bar/27g	125	6.3	463	9.2	54.0	23.4	3.8
Cereal, Chewy Apple, Fruitus, Lyme Regis Foods*	1 Bar/34.9g	132	3.8	378	5.4	64.8	10.8	5.4
Cereal, Choc Chip & Nut, Chewy & Crisp, Sainsbury's*	1 Bar/27g	129	7.0	476	8.8	51.8	26.0	4.4
Cereal, Chocolate & Juicy Raisin, Shapers, Boots*	1 Bar/27g	93	2.1	345	4.2	77.0	7.8	2.7
Cereal, Chocolate & Orange, Fitnesse, Nestle*	1 Bar/23.5g	87	1.2	370	4.7	76.2	5.1	3.8
Cereal, Chocolate & Orange, Light, Alpen*	1 Bar/21g	60	1.0	286	6.1	54.9	4.6	24.6
Cereal, Chocolate & Raisin, Seeds of Change*	1 Serving/29g	107	2.3	370	5.0	69.6	7.9	3.7
Cereal, Citrus Fruits, Light, Alpen*	1 Bar/21g	59	0.9	283	5.6	55.9	4.1	22.4
Cereal, Cranberry, Eat Smart, Safeway*	1 Bar/25g	86	0.6	345	4.7	75.7	2.3	3.9
Cereal, Cranberry & Orange, BGTY, Sainsbury's*	1 Bar/26g	93	1.3	358	2.7	75.8	4.9	2.3
Cereal, Cranberry & Orange, Weight Watchers*	1 Bar/28g	102	1.1	365	4.5	77.6	4.1	2.3
Cereal, Fruit & Fibre, Asda*	1 Bar/28.5g	111	2.9	390	6.0	69.0	10.0	4.1
Cereal, Fruit & Nut, Ainsley Harriott*	1 Bar/35g	151	6.1	431	5.4	63.2	17.4	3.8
Cereal, Fruit & Nut, Alpen*	1 Bar/28g	110	2.8	394	6.6	69.6	9.9	5.0
Cereal, Fruit & Nut Break, Jordans*	1 Bar/37g	135	3.7	374	7.0	63.2	10.4	8.1

BARS

	Measure INFO/WEIGHT	per Measure KCAL	per Measure FAT	Nutrition Values per 100g / 100ml KCAL	PROT	CARB	FAT	FIBRE
Cereal, Fruit & Nut with Milk Chocolate, Alpen*	1 Bar/29g	124	4.1	427	7.1	67.8	14.1	4.0
Cereal, Frusli, Absolutely Apricot, Jordans*	1 Bar/33g	120	3.3	365	5.0	63.8	10.0	6.3
Cereal, Frusli, Blueberry Burst, Jordans*	1 Bar/33g	129	3.2	392	5.8	70.1	9.8	5.1
Cereal, Frusli, Cranberry & Apple, Jordans*	1 Bar/30g	118	3.0	393	5.7	70.0	10.0	5.3
Cereal, Frusli, Raisin & Hazelnut, Jordans*	1 Bar/30g	122	4.2	406	6.3	63.9	13.9	4.7
Cereal, Frusli, Tangy Citrus, Jordans*	1 Bar/33g	124	3.2	376	4.4	67.7	9.8	4.8
Cereal, Frusli, Wild Berries, Jordans*	1 Bar/30g	118	2.9	392	5.7	70.0	9.8	5.0
Cereal, Ginger, PB, Waitrose*	1 Bar/25.6g	90	0.5	352	4.0	79.2	2.1	3.0
Cereal, Golden Grahams, Nestle*	1 Bar/25g	106	3.4	425	6.5	68.8	13.7	0.0
Cereal, Granola, Alpen*	1 Serving/29g	119	3.1	410	5.9	72.4	10.7	0.0
Cereal, Hazelnut & Pistachio, Go Ahead, McVitie's*	1 Bar/30g	117	3.5	389	4.8	66.5	11.5	2.5
Cereal, Hazelnuts & Raisins, Organic, Tesco*	1 Bar/30g	144	8.4	481	7.2	50.3	27.9	3.8
Cereal, Maple, HL, Tesco*	1 Bar/25g	93	1.2	372	5.5	76.6	4.9	2.0
Cereal, Milk Chocolate, Weetos, Weetabix*	1 Bar/20g	88	2.9	440	5.9	70.9	14.7	1.6
Cereal, Mint Chocolate, Kellogg's*	1 Bar/21.9g	88	2.2	401	4.5	74.0	10.0	3.5
Cereal, Mixed Berry, Go Ahead, McVitie's*	1 Bar/35g	134	2.2	383	4.6	77.1	6.3	3.1
Cereal, Muesli Break, Breakfast in a Bar, Jordans*	1 Bar/46g	178	5.0	387	5.9	66.6	10.8	4.3
Cereal, Nut & Seed, Organic, Green & Black's*	1 Bar/50g	258	16.3	516	8.4	47.2	32.6	10.0
Cereal, Nutty, Free From, Sainsbury's*	1 Bar/25g	114	5.0	454	6.8	61.8	20.0	2.3
Cereal, Pomegranate, with Prebiotic, GFY, Asda*	1 Bar/22g	76	0.6	345	6.2	69.3	2.8	13.4
Cereal, Raisin & Apricot, Weight Watchers*	1 Bar/28g	100	1.3	358	6.8	72.2	4.6	3.2
Cereal, Raisin & Chocolate Chip, Fairtrade, Co-Op*	1 Bar/49g	185	4.6	378	5.3	69.2	9.4	3.7
Cereal, Strawberry, Fitness, Nestle*	1 Bar/23.5g	89	1.6	378	4.9	73.8	7.0	4.1
Cereal, Strawberry, Fruit `n` Grain, Asda*	1 Bar/37g	126	2.6	340	4.2	65.0	7.0	4.5
Cereal, Strawberry, Value, Tesco*	1 Serving/21g	80	1.1	382	5.5	77.8	5.4	3.3
Cereal, Strawberry with Yoghurt, Alpen*	1 Bar/29g	119	3.1	409	5.7	72.6	10.6	0.0
Cereal, Sultana & Honey, Jordans*	1 Bar/36g	130	3.0	361	6.0	65.9	8.2	9.2
Cereal, Summer Fruits, Light, Alpen*	1 Bar/21g	59	0.8	283	5.8	56.9	3.6	22.5
Cereal, Tropical Fruit & Nut Bar, Delicious, Boots*	1 Bar/40g	201	12.0	503	7.5	52.5	30.0	2.3
Cereal & Milk, Nesquik, Nestle*	1 Bar/25g	108	3.7	433	6.2	68.5	14.9	1.0
Cherry, Goodness, Ryvita*	1 Bar/23g	60	0.6	260	6.0	52.6	2.8	23.0
Cherry & Coconut Low Fat Fingers, Ok*	1 Bar/35g	119	0.9	339	4.1	75.0	2.5	2.0
Chocolate, Caramel, & Biscuit, Asda*	1 Bar/29.5g	152	8.4	508	8.0	56.0	28.0	2.5
Chocolate, Crisp, Weight Watchers*	1 Bar/25g	92	2.6	369	5.4	75.1	10.2	0.8
Chocolate, Crispy, Free From, Tesco*	1 Bar/30g	132	4.6	440	4.1	71.2	15.4	0.5
Chocolate, Double Cream, Nestle*	1 Bar/47g	250	14.5	531	8.5	54.8	30.9	0.0
Chocolate, Geobar, Traidcraft*	1 Bar/35g	126	1.9	360	5.2	72.6	5.4	4.8
Chocolate, Polar, Sainsbury's*	1 Bar/25g	133	7.2	533	5.5	63.0	28.6	1.2
Chocolate, Soya, Dairy Free, Free From, Sainsbury's*	1 Bar/50g	274	17.5	548	10.8	47.5	35.0	4.3
Chocolate & Orange, Crispy, Free From, Sainsbury's*	1 Bar/30g	132	4.9	440	4.8	68.2	16.2	1.2
Chocolate & Orange, Crispy, Shapers, Boots*	1 Bar/22g	94	2.6	425	3.6	77.0	12.0	0.8
Chocolate & Orange, Shapers, Boots*	1 Bar/26g	98	3.4	378	4.2	73.0	13.0	1.5
Chocolate & Peanut Butter, Atkins, Atkins*	1 Bar/60g	240	11.0	400	31.7	36.7	18.3	16.7
Chocolate & Toffee, Free From, Sainsbury's*	1 Bar/29.9g	140	5.4	465	4.8	71.0	18.0	0.8
Chocolate Brownie, Big Softies, to Go, Fox's*	1 Bar/25g	87	0.7	348	5.5	74.9	2.9	0.0
Chocolate Chip, Slim Fast*	1 Bar/26g	98	3.0	378	4.9	70.4	11.4	1.8
Chocolate Chip, Snack, Slim Fast*	1 Bar/26g	99	3.0	382	4.9	70.4	11.4	1.8
Chocolate Decadence, Atkins*	1 Bar/60g	227	12.2	378	27.1	30.7	20.4	11.6
Chocolate Hazelnut, Advantage, Atkins*	1 Bar/60g	236	12.2	393	32.3	29.0	20.3	8.3
Chocolate Heaven, Ainsley Harriott*	1 Bar/26g	141	7.8	541	7.0	60.0	30.0	2.0
Chocolate Muesli, Snack, Slim Fast*	1 Bar/26g	99	3.5	379	4.7	64.5	13.3	6.5
Chocolate Peanut, Slim Fast*	1 Bar/26g	99	3.3	382	5.4	67.8	12.6	1.1
Chocolate Truffle, M & S*	1 Bar/35g	168	11.4	480	5.9	41.7	32.5	8.3

B

BARS

	Measure INFO/WEIGHT	per Measure KCAL	FAT	Nutrition Values per 100g / 100ml KCAL	PROT	CARB	FAT	FIBRE
Club, Fruit, Jacob's*	1 Biscuit/25g	124	6.3	496	5.6	62.2	25.0	2.3
Club, Milk Chocolate, Jacob's*	1 Biscuit/24g	123	6.3	511	5.8	62.6	26.4	2.0
Club, Mint, Jacob's*	1 Biscuit/24g	124	6.5	517	5.6	62.5	27.2	1.7
Club, Orange, Jacob's*	1 Bar/22g	112	6.0	509	5.1	60.9	27.2	2.1
Coco Pops, & Milk, Kellogg's*	1 Bar/20g	85	2.6	423	7.0	70.0	13.0	1.0
Coconut Chocolate Crisp, Weight Watchers*	1 Bar/25g	89	2.6	356	3.6	71.2	10.4	3.2
Cookie, Apple Crumble, COU, M & S*	1 Bar/27g	90	0.7	335	5.8	72.6	2.6	2.3
Cookie, Maryland*	1 Bar/24.1g	120	5.4	498	7.6	60.0	22.5	0.0
Cookie, Oreo, Nabisco*	1 Bar/35g	180	10.2	514	2.0	66.0	29.0	0.0
Corn Flakes, & Chocolate Milk, Kellogg's*	1 Bar/40g	176	6.4	440	9.0	66.0	16.0	2.0
Cranberry & Honey, Soft & Chewy, Sunny Crunch*	1 Bar/30g	115	2.5	382	6.0	73.1	8.3	3.1
Cranberry & Raisin, Geobar, Traidcraft*	1 Bar/35g	131	2.8	374	3.7	72.6	8.0	2.3
Cranberry & Raisin, Goodness, Ryvita*	1 Bar/23g	60	0.6	263	5.2	54.3	2.8	22.5
Crazy Caramel, Tesco*	1 Bar/40g	192	9.2	480	3.9	64.0	23.0	1.0
Creme Brulee Chocolate, M & S*	1 Bar/36g	178	10.5	495	4.4	54.0	29.2	0.4
Crunchy Caramel, Tesco*	1 Bar/21g	98	5.3	467	4.6	56.0	25.0	1.4
Crunchy Crispy Treat, Kids, Tesco*	1 Bar/24g	109	5.0	453	3.6	62.5	20.9	1.5
Crunchy Granola, Oats 'n' Honey, Nature Valley*	1 Pack/42g	187	6.8	445	8.3	70.5	16.2	6.2
Crunchy Nut, Chocolate Peanut Crisp, Kellogg's*	1 Bar/35g	169	8.8	483	12.0	53.0	25.0	3.5
Crunchy Nut, Kellogg's*	1 Serving/30g	119	1.5	397	6.0	82.0	5.0	2.5
Crunchy Nut, Nuts About Nuts, Kellogg's*	1 Bar/40g	212	14.0	530	15.0	40.0	35.0	5.0
Date & Fig, Lyme Regis Foods*	1 Bar/42g	143	4.9	341	7.0	52.0	11.7	9.3
Date & Walnut, Eat Natural*	1 Bar/50g	221	10.1	441	8.0	57.1	20.1	3.3
Digestive, Milk Chocolate, McVitie's*	1 Bar/23g	118	5.8	511	6.6	64.6	25.1	1.9
Digestive, Milk Chocolate, Tesco*	1 Bar/19g	96	4.9	506	6.8	61.6	25.8	2.4
Digestive, Milk Chocolate, Value, Tesco*	1 Bar/19g	96	4.9	505	6.6	61.8	25.8	3.0
Double Chocolate Treat, Shapers, Boots*	1 Bar/23g	94	2.5	408	3.3	75.0	11.0	0.7
Echo, Fox's*	1 Bar/25g	128	6.7	510	7.8	59.5	26.7	1.2
Echo, Mint, Fox's*	1 Bar/25g	130	6.7	518	7.9	60.7	26.6	1.6
Echo, White Chocolate & Biscuit, Fox's*	1 Bar/26g	132	6.9	510	7.8	59.5	26.7	1.2
Fair Break, Traidcraft*	1 Bar/22g	116	6.2	528	6.0	63.0	28.0	0.0
Fig & Mango, The Food Doctor*	1 Serving/35g	113	2.7	323	9.7	53.7	7.7	13.4
Food Bar, Apple & Walnut, The Food Doctor*	1 Bar/35g	117	4.0	333	10.8	46.8	11.4	15.3
Forest Fruit & Raisin, HL, Tesco*	1 Bar/27g	95	0.7	350	4.5	76.8	2.7	3.6
Four Fruits, Organic, Trophy, The Village Bakery*	1 Bar/42.5g	152	2.5	353	3.8	71.2	5.9	4.2
Four Seeds, Organic, Trophy, The Village Bakery*	1 Bar/42.5g	166	3.7	385	8.1	68.7	8.7	2.5
Frosties, & Milk, Kellogg's*	1 Bar/25g	102	2.8	408	7.0	71.0	11.0	1.0
Frosties, Chocolate, Kellogg's*	1 Bar/25g	103	3.0	412	6.0	72.0	12.0	1.6
Fruit, Apple, Hellema*	1 Bar/33.1g	127	2.5	384	4.5	74.0	7.5	2.0
Fruit, Fig, Castus*	1 Bar/26.7g	80	1.3	300	3.0	60.0	5.0	0.0
Fruit, Nut & Seed Bars, The Village Bakery*	1 Bar/25g	93	1.6	373	5.7	73.7	6.2	0.1
Fruit, with Apricot, Castus*	1 Bar/25g	75	1.1	300	2.0	63.0	4.5	9.0
Fruit & Grain, Apple, Harvest Morn*	1 Bar/37g	129	3.0	349	4.2	65.0	8.0	4.5
Fruit & Nut, Eat Natural*	1 Bar/50g	223	11.2	446	11.6	49.8	22.3	5.3
Fruit & Nut, Multigrain, Jordans*	1 Bar/40g	164	6.5	410	7.0	59.1	16.2	5.7
Fruit & Nut, Organic, Eat Natural*	1 Bar/50g	244	15.3	488	10.2	42.9	30.6	0.0
Fruit & Nut Crisp, Go Ahead, McVitie's*	1 Bar/23.0g	99	3.2	430	5.3	71.3	13.7	1.7
Fruit 'n' Fibre, Kellogg's*	1 Bar/25g	95	2.3	380	5.0	71.0	9.0	5.0
Fruit 'n' Fibre Bakes, with Sultanas, Kellogg's*	1 Bar/40g	146	5.2	365	4.5	58.0	13.0	9.0
Fruity Cereal, Banoffee, Go, Soreen*	1 Serving/40g	143	1.9	358	6.0	72.8	4.8	0.0
Fruity Cereal, Go, Soreen*	1 Bar/40g	141	1.9	352	5.7	73.9	4.8	0.0
Fruity Cereal Bar, Free From, Sainsbury's*	1 Bar/25.1g	100	2.6	399	4.4	72.3	10.2	2.6
Ginger & Oat, Chocolate Covered, Snack, Waitrose*	1 Bar/27g	120	5.0	444	4.2	65.0	18.6	2.1

BARS

	Measure INFO/WEIGHT	per Measure KCAL	per Measure FAT	Nutrition Values per 100g / 100ml KCAL	PROT	CARB	FAT	FIBRE
Gold Bar, McVitie's*	1 Bar/23g	121	6.2	524	6.0	64.6	26.8	0.6
Goodies, Cereal & Fruit, Apricot, Organic, Organix*	1 Bar/30g	122	6.1	408	7.2	55.3	20.4	6.2
Great Greens, Juice, Crussh Juice Bars*	1 Pot/100g	65	2.1	65	5.7	5.8	2.1	2.9
Groove, Lemon, Alpen*	1 Bar/32g	124	1.9	389	5.6	78.4	5.9	1.9
Groove, Sassy Strawberry, Alpen*	1 Bar/32g	124	1.7	386	5.6	78.8	5.4	1.9
Harvest Cheweee, Apple & Raisin, Quaker*	1 Bar/22g	89	2.6	405	5.5	68.0	12.0	3.0
Harvest Cheweee, Choc Chip, Quaker*	1 Bar/22g	95	3.5	430	5.5	68.0	16.0	3.5
Harvest Cheweee, Toffee, Quaker*	1 Bar/22g	94	3.3	427	5.0	68.0	15.0	3.0
Harvest Cheweee, White Chocolate Chip, Quaker*	1 Bar/22g	94	3.4	425	6.0	67.0	15.5	3.5
Hazlenut Sandwich, Finn Crisp*	1 Bar/25g	134	8.5	535	7.0	50.0	34.0	0.0
Honey Rice Crisp, Lower Fat, Go Ahead, McVitie's*	1 Bar/21.9g	90	2.2	411	3.9	75.8	10.2	1.1
Luxury, Absolute Nut, Jordans*	1 Bar/45g	251	18.6	557	12.7	33.3	41.4	7.0
Luxury, Exotic Fruit & Nut, Jordans*	1 Bar/50g	197	2.7	393	5.0	69.1	5.4	4.8
Macadamia & Fruit, Eat Natural*	1 Bar/50g	243	15.4	485	7.3	44.6	30.8	0.0
Milk Chocolate Whirls, Asda*	1 Bar/26g	116	4.2	447	3.7	72.0	16.0	0.8
Mixed Berry, Goodness, Ryvita*	1 Bar/23g	61	0.6	264	4.8	54.8	2.8	23.2
Mixed Nut Feast, Eat Natural*	1 Bar/50g	278	20.5	555	18.8	27.9	40.9	5.5
Muesli, Cherry & Milk, Sirius*	1 Bar/25g	104	2.9	417	7.2	71.3	11.4	3.9
Multigrain, Fruit & Nut, Jordans*	1 Bar/40g	164	6.5	410	7.0	59.1	16.2	5.7
Nine Bar, Mixed Hemp Seed, Original, Wholebake*	1 Bar/50g	281	19.3	562	18.6	38.5	38.5	4.7
Nougat, Cool Mint, & Dark Chocolate, Shapers, Boots*	1 Bar/23g	83	3.2	362	2.6	70.0	14.0	1.1
Nutri-Grain, Apple, Kellogg's*	1 Bar/37g	141	3.3	380	5.0	71.0	9.0	5.0
Nutri-Grain, Blackberry & Apple, Kellogg's*	1 Bar/37g	131	3.3	355	4.0	67.0	9.0	4.0
Nutri-Grain, Blueberry, Kellogg's*	1 Bar/37g	130	3.3	351	4.0	66.0	9.0	4.0
Nutri-Grain, Cherry, Kellogg's*	1 Bar/37g	129	3.0	348	4.0	67.0	8.0	4.0
Nutri-Grain, Chocolate, Kellogg's*	1 Bar/37g	136	3.7	367	4.5	66.0	10.0	4.0
Nutri-Grain, Chocolate Chip, Chewy, Kellogg's*	1 Bar/25g	103	3.0	413	4.5	73.0	12.0	2.5
Nutri-Grain, Elevenses, Choc Chip, Kellogg's*	1 Bar/45g	179	5.9	397	4.0	66.0	13.0	2.0
Nutri-Grain, Elevenses, Ginger, Kellogg's*	1 Bar/45g	168	4.1	373	5.0	68.0	9.0	3.0
Nutri-Grain, Elevenses, Raisin, Kellogg's*	1 Bar/45g	164	4.1	364	5.0	66.0	9.0	3.5
Nutri-Grain, Honey Oat & Raisin, Chewy, Kellogg's*	1 Bar/24.9g	98	2.0	393	3.5	78.0	8.0	2.5
Nutri-Grain, Oat Bakes, Cherry, Kellogg's*	1 Bar/50g	204	7.0	408	4.5	66.0	14.0	2.5
Nutri-Grain, Oat Bakes, Totally Oaty, Kellogg's*	1 Bar/50g	206	7.5	411	5.0	64.0	15.0	3.0
Nutri-Grain, Raspberry, Kellogg's*	1 Bar/37g	131	3.3	355	4.0	67.0	9.0	4.0
Nutri-Grain, Strawberry, Kellogg's*	1 Bar/37g	131	3.3	355	4.0	67.0	9.0	3.5
Nutty Crunch Surprise, Wonka*	1 Bar/37g	202	11.9	543	4.9	58.7	32.1	0.9
Nutty Nougat Caramel, Tesco*	1 Bar/20g	99	5.4	493	8.5	54.0	27.0	2.4
Oat, Mixed Berry, Quaker*	1 Bar/38g	137	3.3	360	6.8	64.5	8.8	8.0
Oat, Original with Golden Syrup, Quaker*	1 Bar/38g	139	3.6	366	7.1	64.5	9.5	7.9
Oat, Quaker*	1 Bar/38.1g	137	3.4	360	6.8	64.5	8.8	8.0
Optivita, Berry Oat, Kellogg's*	1 Bar/28.1g	101	2.0	360	7.0	68.0	7.0	9.0
Orange Crunch, Go Ahead, McVitie's*	1 Bar/23g	99	2.9	430	4.1	78.0	12.8	0.8
Original, Crunchy, Honey & Almond, Jordans*	1 Bar/30g	139	6.8	463	8.3	56.7	22.7	6.7
Pecan Apricot & Peach, M & S*	1 Bar/50g	255	17.8	510	9.3	38.2	35.5	4.9
Penguin, Chukka, McVitie's*	1 Bar/28g	135	6.1	481	6.1	65.1	21.8	0.0
Raisin & Apricot, Geobar, Traidcraft*	1 Bar/35g	132	3.1	376	5.3	69.0	8.8	3.5
Raisin & Oatmeal, Breakfast Snack, Tesco*	1 Bar/37.5g	135	4.4	355	5.6	56.8	11.7	2.8
Rice Krispies & Milk, Kellogg's*	1 Bar/20g	83	2.4	416	7.0	71.0	12.0	0.3
Roasted Nut, Chewy & Crisp, Sainsbury's*	1 Bar/27g	120	6.6	446	10.1	46.6	24.3	3.9
Roasted Peanut, Weight Watchers*	1 Bar/25g	104	3.2	415	9.6	65.3	12.8	3.7
Sandwich, Chocolate Viennese, Fox's*	1 Biscuit/14g	76	4.4	542	6.9	57.4	31.6	1.6
Sandwich, Milk Chocolate, Value, Tesco*	1 Bar/25.8g	130	6.4	504	5.4	64.5	24.9	2.4
Sandwich, Milk Chocolate Orange, Tesco*	1 Biscuit/25.3g	136	7.4	536	6.2	62.2	29.1	1.8

	Measure INFO/WEIGHT	per Measure KCAL	FAT	Nutrition Values per 100g / 100ml KCAL	PROT	CARB	FAT	FIBRE
BARS								
School, Apple, Fruit Bowl*	1 Bar/20g	67	0.6	337	0.7	75.0	3.0	6.0
School, Apricot, Fruit Bowl*	1 Bar/20g	67	0.6	337	0.7	75.0	3.0	6.0
School, Blackcurrant, Fruit Bowl*	1 Bar/20g	67	0.6	337	0.7	75.0	3.0	2.0
School, Cherry, Fruit Bowl*	1 Bar/20g	67	0.6	337	0.7	75.0	3.0	6.0
Sesame Snaps, Anglo-Dal*	1 Pack/30g	163	9.5	542	2.8	61.8	31.5	0.0
Sesame Snaps, in Chocolate, Anglo-Dal*	1 Pack/40g	211	11.9	527	9.3	55.6	29.7	0.0
Sesame Snaps, with Coconut, Anglo-Dal*	1 Pack/30g	155	8.8	517	9.7	52.9	29.5	0.0
Slow Mango, Apple & Almond, Southern Alps*	1 Bar/45g	214	11.7	476	10.4	50.7	26.0	0.0
Smarties, Nestle*	1 Bar/45g	238	13.5	528	6.2	58.2	30.0	0.9
Special Fruit Muesli, Jordans*	1 Bar/40g	140	2.4	349	5.0	68.8	6.0	5.0
Special K, Apple & Pear, Kellogg's*	1 Bar/23g	92	1.8	400	8.0	73.0	8.0	2.0
Special K, Bliss Bar, Raspberry & Chocolate, Kellogg's*	1 Bar/22g	88	2.2	399	4.0	74.0	10.0	4.0
Special K, Chocolate Chip, Kellogg's*	1 Bar/22.4g	90	1.6	401	9.0	76.0	7.0	1.5
Special K, Fruits of the Forest, Kellogg's*	1 Bar/22g	87	1.8	397	8.0	74.0	8.0	2.5
Special K, Original, Kellogg's*	1 Bar/23g	92	1.8	402	8.0	75.0	8.0	2.0
Special K, Peach & Apricot, Kellogg's*	1 Bar/23g	92	2.1	400	8.0	73.0	9.0	2.5
Special K, Red Fruits, Kellogg's*	1 Bar/21.5g	86	1.1	390	8.0	78.0	5.0	1.5
Strawberry, Morning Shine, Atkins*	1 Bar/37g	145	8.0	392	28.9	24.9	21.6	14.1
Strawberry, Shapers, Boots*	1 Bar/22g	75	2.4	343	2.5	77.0	11.0	0.9
Strawberry Nougat, Shapers, Boots*	1 Bar/23g	84	13.0	365	11.7	317.4	56.5	2.6
Superfoods, Jordans*	1 Bar/45g	171	4.9	379	7.0	63.3	10.9	6.7
Titan*	1 Bar/40.1g	192	9.2	479	3.9	64.0	23.0	1.0
Tracker, Forest Fruits, Mars*	1 Bar/26g	123	5.8	474	4.6	64.1	22.2	0.0
Tracker, Roasted Nut, Master Foods*	1 Bar/37g	181	9.9	489	8.9	54.9	26.8	0.0
Vyomax Lite, Vyomax*	1 Bar/45g	170	6.0	378	33.3	32.4	13.3	7.6
Wafer, Chocolate Flavour Crisp, Carbolite*	1 Bar/25g	120	8.7	482	8.5	52.3	34.8	2.0
Wafer Biscuit, Milk Chocolate Coated, Value, Tesco*	1 Bar/24g	126	6.7	526	6.9	61.4	28.1	1.7
Wild & Whippy, Tesco*	1 Bar/26.7g	120	4.3	450	3.7	72.0	16.0	0.8
BASIL								
Dried, Ground	1 Tsp/1.4g	3	0.0	251	14.4	43.2	4.0	0.0
Fresh, Average	1 Tbsp/5.3g	2	0.0	40	3.1	5.1	0.8	0.0
BASKETS								
Brandy Snap, Askeys*	1 Basket/20g	98	4.3	490	1.9	72.7	21.3	0.0
BATTER MIX								
for Pancakes & Yorkshire Puddings, McDougalls*	1 Pancake/38g	83	4.0	218	6.3	24.8	10.4	1.9
for Yorkshire Puddings & Pancakes, Made Up, Morrisons*	1 Pudding/30g	43	0.8	143	6.4	23.1	2.8	4.1
for Yorkshire Puddings & Pancakes, Tesco*	1 Serving/17g	34	0.3	200	2.3	43.3	1.5	2.5
Green's*	1 Bag/125g	296	9.0	237	8.7	34.3	7.2	0.0
Made Up with Water & Egg, Safeway*	1 Serving/100g	143	2.8	143	6.4	23.1	2.8	4.1
Pancake, Buttermilk, Krusteaz*	3 Pancakes/16.2g	56	0.8	352	11.3	66.0	4.7	3.4
Pancake, Sainsbury's*	1 Pancake/63g	96	1.1	152	6.5	27.4	1.8	3.1
SmartPrice, Asda*	1 Pack/128g	268	5.8	209	8.0	34.0	4.5	2.7
Tesco*	1 Pack/130g	467	1.8	359	12.3	74.4	1.4	7.7
BAY LEAVES								
Dried, Average	1 Tsp / 0.6g	2	0.1	313	7.6	48.6	8.4	0.0
BEAN SPROUTS								
Aduki, Aconbury Sprouts*	1 Serving/100g	157	1.8	157	12.0	23.3	1.8	0.0
Mung, Canned, Drained, Average	1 Serving/90g	9	0.1	10	1.6	0.8	0.1	0.7
Mung, Raw, Average	1oz/28g	9	0.1	31	2.9	4.0	0.5	1.5
Mung, Stir-Fried in Blended Oil, Average	1 Serving/90g	65	5.5	72	1.9	2.5	6.1	0.9
BEANFEAST								
Bolognese Style, Dry, Batchelors*	1 Pack/120g	362	6.7	302	23.9	39.0	5.6	13.5
Mexican Chilli, Batchelors*	1 Serving/65g	203	3.2	312	24.3	42.7	4.9	13.6

BEANS

INFO/WEIGHT	Measure	per Measure		Nutrition Values per 100g / 100ml				
		KCAL	FAT	KCAL	PROT	CARB	FAT	FIBRE
& Meatballs, in Tomato Sauce, Sainsbury's*	½ Can/200g	216	7.2	108	5.5	13.3	3.6	2.6
Aduki, Cooked in Unsalted Water, Average	1 Tbsp/30g	37	0.1	123	9.3	22.5	0.2	5.5
Aduki, Dried, Raw	1 Tbsp/30g	82	0.2	272	19.9	50.1	0.5	11.1
Baked, & Jumbo Sausages, Asda*	1 Serving/210g	317	14.7	151	7.0	15.0	7.0	2.6
Baked, & Pork Sausages, Co-Op*	1 Sml Tin/220g	231	4.4	105	7.0	14.0	2.0	4.0
Baked, & Pork Sausages, Sainsbury's*	1 Serving/210g	248	9.2	118	5.7	13.9	4.4	3.4
Baked, & Pork Sausages, Tesco*	½ Can/210g	231	5.7	110	5.5	15.6	2.7	3.0
Baked, & Sausages, Asda*	½ Can/205g	252	8.0	123	6.0	16.0	3.9	3.0
Baked, & Sausages, Basics, Sainsbury's*	1 Serving/175g	149	2.6	85	4.8	13.1	1.5	2.6
Baked, & Sausages, GFY, Asda*	1 Serving/217g	178	5.6	82	4.7	10.0	2.6	1.8
Baked, & Sausages, Meatfree, Sainsbury's*	1 Can/420g	500	16.8	119	8.0	12.6	4.0	2.7
Baked, & Sausages, Value, Tesco*	½ Can/276.2g	290	10.2	105	5.7	11.8	3.7	3.6
Baked, Barbecue, Smokey, Heinz*	½ Can/270g	213	0.5	79	4.8	14.3	0.2	3.8
Baked, Cheezy, Heinz*	1oz/28g	53	1.4	189	11.6	24.5	4.9	6.2
Baked, Curried, Average	½ Can/210g	203	1.9	97	4.9	17.2	0.9	3.6
Baked, in Tomato Sauce, Average	1 Can/400g	346	1.8	86	4.8	16.0	0.5	3.3
Baked, in Tomato Sauce, Healthy Range, Average	½ Can/210g	143	0.5	68	3.9	12.8	0.2	2.8
Baked, in Tomato Sauce, Red Sugar & Salt, Average	½ Can/210g	159	0.7	76	4.6	13.7	0.3	3.8
Baked, Jalfrezi, Heinz*	1 Serving/195g	135	2.5	69	4.5	9.8	1.3	3.6
Baked, Mexican, Heinz*	1 Serving/195g	137	0.6	70	4.5	12.3	0.3	3.6
Baked, Sweet Chilli, Heinz*	½ Can/195g	142	0.6	73	4.5	13.0	0.3	3.6
Baked, Tikka, Heinz*	1 Serving/195g	172	5.9	88	4.8	10.6	3.0	3.5
Baked, with Chicken Nuggets, Heinz*	1 Can/200g	210	6.3	105	6.8	12.5	3.2	3.2
Baked, with Spicy Meatballs, Heinz*	1/207.5g	193	5.0	93	5.8	12.0	2.4	2.9
Black, Cooked, Average	1 Cup/172g	227	0.9	132	8.8	23.7	0.5	8.7
Blackeye, Canned, Average	1 Can/172g	206	1.3	120	8.5	19.8	0.8	3.3
Blackeye, Dried, Raw	1oz/28g	87	0.4	311	23.5	54.1	1.6	8.2
Borlotti, Canned, Average	1oz/28g	29	0.1	103	7.6	16.9	0.5	4.7
Borlotti, Dried, Raw, Average	1 Serving/100g	335	1.2	335	23.0	60.1	1.2	24.7
Broad, Canned, Average	1oz/28g	25	0.2	91	8.4	13.1	0.8	4.4
Broad, Canned, Drained, Average	1 Can /195g	134	1.5	69	6.8	8.9	0.8	6.2
Broad, Crispy, Wasabi Flavoured, Khao Shong*	1 Serving/30g	116	3.0	386	17.0	57.0	10.0	7.0
Broad, Dried, Raw, Average	1oz/28g	69	0.6	245	26.1	32.5	2.1	27.6
Broad, Frozen, Sainsbury's*	1 Serving/100g	80	0.6	80	7.9	10.7	0.6	6.5
Broad, Weighed with Pod, Raw, Average	1oz/28g	17	0.3	59	5.7	7.2	1.0	6.1
Butter, Canned, Average	1oz/28g	22	0.1	79	5.9	12.9	0.5	4.1
Butter, Dried, Boiled, Average	1oz/28g	30	0.2	106	7.2	18.7	0.6	5.2
Butter, Dried, Raw, Average	1oz/28g	81	0.5	290	19.1	52.9	1.7	16.0
Cannellini, Canned, Average	1oz/28g	26	0.1	94	7.2	15.0	0.5	5.7
Cannellini, with Chorizo & Red Peppers, Morrisons*	½ Pack/100g	155	10.0	155	6.9	9.2	10.0	2.8
Chilli, Canned, Average	1 Can/420g	381	3.1	91	5.2	15.9	0.7	4.4
Dwarf, Sainsbury's*	1oz/28g	7	0.1	25	1.9	3.1	0.5	2.2
Edamame, Sainsbury's*	1 Serving/150g	212	9.6	141	12.3	6.8	6.4	4.2
Flageolet, Canned, Average	1 Can/265g	235	1.6	89	6.8	14.1	0.6	3.5
French, Boiled, Average	1 Serving/150g	38	0.0	25	2.3	3.8	0.0	3.7
French, Canned, Average	1oz/28g	6	0.1	22	1.7	3.5	0.3	2.5
French, Raw	1oz/28g	7	0.1	24	1.9	3.2	0.5	2.2
Green, Cut, Average	1oz/28g	6	0.1	22	1.7	3.7	0.2	2.1
Green, Fine, Average	1 Serving/75g	18	0.3	25	1.8	3.4	0.4	2.6
Green, Sliced, Average	1oz/28g	6	0.1	23	1.9	3.5	0.2	2.1
Green, Sliced, Frozen, Average	1 Serving/50g	13	0.2	26	1.8	4.4	0.1	4.1
Green, Whole, Average	1oz/28g	6	0.1	22	1.6	3.0	0.4	1.7
Haricot, Canned, in Salted Water, Safeway*	1 Can/265g	257	1.3	97	6.6	16.6	0.5	4.9

	Measure INFO/WEIGHT	per Measure KCAL	per Measure FAT	Nutrition Values per 100g / 100ml KCAL	PROT	CARB	FAT	FIBRE
BEANS								
Haricot, Dried, Boiled in Unsalted Water	1oz/28g	27	0.1	95	6.6	17.2	0.5	6.1
Haricot, Dried, Raw	1oz/28g	80	0.4	286	21.4	49.7	1.6	17.0
Kidney, Red, Canned, Average	½ Can/90g	92	0.5	102	7.8	16.7	0.6	5.6
Kidney, Red, Dried, Boiled in Unsalted Water	1oz/28g	29	0.1	103	8.4	17.4	0.5	6.7
Kidney, Red, Dried, Raw	1oz/28g	74	0.4	266	22.1	44.1	1.4	15.7
Kidney, Red, in Chilli Sauce, Sainsbury's*	1 Can/420g	340	1.7	81	5.1	14.3	0.4	4.3
Kidney, White, Dry, Raw, Unico*	½ Cup Dry/80g	270	0.9	338	22.5	61.3	1.1	21.3
Macaroni, Lean Cuisine*	1 Meal/269g	310	9.0	115	7.4	14.1	3.4	1.1
Mixed, Canned, Average	1 Can/300g	300	3.5	100	6.8	15.7	1.2	4.1
Mixed, Spicy, Average	1 Serving/140g	109	0.7	78	4.9	13.4	0.5	3.9
Mixed, with Lentils, Waitrose*	1 Pack/300g	399	21.9	133	5.1	11.6	7.3	3.1
Mixed, with Passata, Tesco*	1 Can/300g	237	2.1	79	6.0	12.1	0.7	3.9
Mung, Whole, Dried, Boiled in Unsalted Water	1oz/28g	25	0.1	91	7.6	15.3	0.4	3.0
Mung, Whole, Dried, Raw	1oz/28g	78	0.3	279	23.9	46.3	1.1	10.0
Pinto, Dried, Boiled in Unsalted Water	1oz/28g	38	0.2	137	8.9	23.9	0.7	0.0
Pinto, Dried, Raw	1oz/28g	92	0.4	327	21.1	57.1	1.6	0.0
Refried, Average	1 Serving/215g	162	1.5	76	4.6	12.7	0.7	1.8
Runner, Average	1 Serving/100g	20	0.4	20	1.4	2.8	0.4	2.2
Soya, Dried, Average	1oz/28g	104	5.1	370	34.2	15.4	18.3	19.6
Soya, Dried, Boiled in Unsalted Water	1oz/28g	39	2.0	141	14.0	5.1	7.3	6.1
Soya, Frozen, Birds Eye*	1 Serving/80g	120	5.0	150	12.3	11.0	6.3	4.0
Soya, in Water, Salt Added, Sainsbury's*	1 Serving/100g	102	7.3	102	4.0	5.1	7.3	6.1
BEEF								
Aberdeen Angus, Winter Herb Butter, M & S*	1 Serving/188g	310	17.5	165	19.6	0.2	9.3	1.9
Braised, with Mashed Potato, Sainsbury's*	1 Pack/450g	473	17.6	105	7.7	10.3	3.9	0.8
Brisket, Raw, Lean	1oz/28g	39	1.7	139	21.1	0.0	6.1	0.0
Brisket, Raw, Lean & Fat	1oz/28g	61	4.5	218	18.4	0.0	16.0	0.0
Cooked, Sliced, From Supermarket, Average	1 Slice/35g	35	0.8	101	17.4	2.6	2.4	0.4
Crispy, Chilli, Tesco*	1 Pack/250g	473	17.3	189	10.8	21.0	6.9	0.5
Crispy Chilli, Cantonese, Chilled, Sainsbury's*	1 Pack/250g	683	38.8	273	11.4	22.1	15.5	1.9
Crispy Chilli, M & S*	1 Pack/250g	625	31.3	250	9.7	25.0	12.5	2.0
Escalope, Healthy Range, Average	1 Serving/170g	233	6.7	137	24.2	1.2	4.0	0.4
Flank, Pot-Roasted, Lean	1oz/28g	71	3.9	253	31.8	0.0	14.0	0.0
Flank, Pot-Roasted, Lean & Fat	1oz/28g	87	6.2	309	27.1	0.0	22.3	0.0
Flank, Raw, Lean	1oz/28g	49	2.6	175	22.7	0.0	9.3	0.0
Flank, Raw, Lean & Fat	1oz/28g	74	5.8	266	19.7	0.0	20.8	0.0
for Casserole, Diced, Lean, Sainsbury's*	1 Serving/100g	136	5.1	136	22.5	0.0	5.1	0.0
for Casserole, Lean, Diced, Average	1oz/28g	35	1.1	126	23.0	0.0	3.8	0.0
Fore Rib, Lean & Fat, Average	1oz/28g	40	1.8	144	21.7	0.1	6.3	0.2
Fore Rib, Raw, Lean	1oz/28g	41	1.8	145	21.5	0.0	6.5	0.0
Fore Rib, Roasted, Lean	1oz/28g	66	3.2	236	33.3	0.0	11.4	0.0
Fore Rib, Roasted, Lean & Fat	1oz/28g	84	5.7	300	29.1	0.0	20.4	0.0
Grill Steak, Average	1 Steak/170g	501	39.5	295	19.3	2.1	23.2	0.1
Grill Steak, Peppered, Average	1 Serving/172g	419	24.4	244	23.7	5.3	14.2	0.3
Joint, for Roasting, Average	1oz/28g	38	1.0	134	24.5	1.4	3.5	0.2
Joint, Roasting, BGTY, Sainsbury's*	1 Serving/150g	161	3.2	107	22.1	0.1	2.1	0.0
Joint, Sirloin, Roasted, Lean	1oz/28g	53	1.8	188	32.4	0.0	6.5	0.0
Joint, Sirloin, Roasted, Lean & Fat	1oz/28g	65	3.5	233	29.8	0.0	12.6	0.0
Mince, Cooked, Average	1 Serving/75g	214	15.3	286	24.0	0.0	20.3	0.0
Mince, Extra Lean, Raw, Average	1 Serving/100g	131	5.3	131	21.0	0.0	5.3	0.0
Mince, Extra Lean, Stewed	1oz/28g	50	2.4	177	24.7	0.0	8.7	0.0
Mince, Raw, Average	1oz/28g	67	5.0	239	18.7	0.3	18.0	0.1
Mince, Steak, Extra Lean, Average	1oz/28g	37	1.6	131	20.5	0.4	5.6	0.0

BEEF

INFO/WEIGHT	Measure	per Measure KCAL	FAT	Nutrition Values per 100g / 100ml KCAL	PROT	CARB	FAT	FIBRE
Mince, Steak, Raw, Average	1 Serving/125g	195	9.7	156	21.6	0.0	7.7	0.0
Mince, Stewed	1oz/28g	59	3.8	209	21.8	0.0	13.5	0.0
Peppered, Sliced, Average	1 Slice/20g	26	1.1	129	18.2	1.3	5.6	1.0
Roast, Sliced, Average	1 Slice/35g	48	1.3	136	26.1	0.4	3.6	0.2
Salt, Average	1 Serving/70g	80	1.7	114	21.7	1.0	2.5	0.1
Salted, Dried, Raw	1oz/28g	70	0.4	250	55.4	0.0	1.5	0.0
Silverside, Pot-Roasted, Lean	1oz/28g	54	1.8	193	34.0	0.0	6.3	0.0
Silverside, Pot-Roasted, Lean & Fat	1oz/28g	69	3.8	247	31.0	0.0	13.7	0.0
Silverside, Raw, Lean	1oz/28g	38	1.2	134	23.8	0.0	4.3	0.0
Silverside, Raw, Lean & Fat	1oz/28g	60	4.1	215	20.4	0.0	14.8	0.0
Silverside, Salted, Boiled, Lean	1oz/28g	52	1.9	184	30.4	0.0	6.9	0.0
Silverside, Salted, Boiled, Lean & Fat	1oz/28g	63	3.5	224	27.9	0.0	12.5	0.0
Silverside, Salted, Raw, Lean	1oz/28g	39	2.0	140	19.2	0.0	7.0	0.0
Silverside, Salted, Raw, Lean & Fat	1oz/28g	64	5.0	227	16.3	0.0	18.0	0.0
Steak, Braising, Braised, Lean	1oz/28g	63	2.7	225	34.4	0.0	9.7	0.0
Steak, Braising, Braised, Lean & Fat	1oz/28g	69	3.6	246	32.9	0.0	12.7	0.0
Steak, Braising, Lean, Raw, Average	1oz/28g	40	1.4	145	24.8	0.0	5.0	0.0
Steak, Braising, Raw, Lean & Fat	1oz/28g	45	2.4	160	20.7	0.0	8.6	0.0
Steak, Economy, Average	1oz/28g	53	2.4	190	26.9	1.2	8.7	0.4
Steak, Fillet, Cooked, Average	1oz/28g	54	2.4	191	28.6	0.0	8.5	0.0
Steak, Fillet, Lean, Average	1oz/28g	42	2.0	150	21.0	0.0	7.3	0.0
Steak, Fillet, Lean, Cooked, Average	1oz/28g	52	2.2	186	28.7	0.0	8.0	0.0
Steak, Frying, Average	1 Steak/110g	128	2.7	116	23.7	0.0	2.5	0.0
Steak, Peppered, & Mash, HL, Tesco*	1 Pack/450g	347	5.9	77	6.4	8.7	1.3	0.8
Steak, Rump, Cooked, Average	1oz/28g	69	4.0	246	29.1	0.5	14.1	0.0
Steak, Rump, Lean, Cooked, Average	1oz/28g	50	1.7	179	31.0	0.0	6.1	0.0
Steak, Rump, Marinated Strips, Asda*	1oz/28g	66	5.1	235	17.6	0.1	18.3	0.1
Steak, Rump, Raw, Lean	1oz/28g	35	1.1	125	22.0	0.0	4.1	0.0
Steak, Rump, Raw, Lean & Fat	1oz/28g	49	2.8	174	20.7	0.0	10.1	0.0
Steak, Sirloin, Fried, Rare, Lean	1oz/28g	53	2.3	189	28.8	0.0	8.2	0.0
Steak, Sirloin, Fried, Rare, Lean & Fat	1oz/28g	65	3.9	233	26.8	0.0	14.0	0.0
Steak, Sirloin, Grilled, Medium-Rare, Lean	1oz/28g	49	2.2	176	26.6	0.0	7.7	0.0
Steak, Sirloin, Grilled, Medium-Rare, Lean & Fat	1oz/28g	60	3.5	213	24.8	0.0	12.6	0.0
Steak, Sirloin, Grilled, Rare, Lean	1oz/28g	46	1.9	166	26.4	0.0	6.7	0.0
Steak, Sirloin, Grilled, Rare, Lean & Fat	1oz/28g	60	3.6	216	25.1	0.0	12.8	0.0
Steak, Sirloin, Grilled, Well-Done, Lean	1oz/28g	63	2.8	225	33.9	0.0	9.9	0.0
Steak, Sirloin, Grilled, Well-Done, Lean & Fat	1oz/28g	72	4.0	257	31.8	0.0	14.4	0.0
Steak, Sirloin, Raw, Lean	1oz/28g	38	1.3	135	23.5	0.0	4.5	0.0
Steak, Sirloin, Raw, Lean & Fat	1oz/28g	56	3.6	201	21.6	0.0	12.7	0.0
Steak, Tender, Quick Cook, Average	1oz/28g	36	1.0	127	21.2	2.3	3.7	0.3
Stewed Steak, Average	1 Serving/220g	258	10.1	117	15.8	3.3	4.6	0.0
Stewing Steak, Lean & Fat, Raw, Average	1oz/28g	41	1.8	146	22.1	0.1	6.4	0.1
Stewing Steak, Raw, Lean	1oz/28g	34	1.0	122	22.6	0.0	3.5	0.0
Stewing Steak, Stewed, Lean	1oz/28g	52	1.8	185	32.0	0.0	6.3	0.0
Stewing Steak, Stewed, Lean & Fat	1oz/28g	57	2.7	203	29.2	0.0	9.6	0.0
Stir Fry Strips, Raw, Average	1 Serving/125g	146	3.1	117	23.6	0.0	2.5	0.3
Topside, Lean & Fat, Average	1oz/28g	61	3.4	220	27.5	0.0	12.2	0.0
Topside, Raw, Lean	1oz/28g	32	0.8	116	23.0	0.0	2.7	0.0
Wafer Thin, Finest, Tesco*	1 Pack/100g	181	6.5	181	30.4	0.1	6.5	0.0
Wafer Thin Sliced, Cooked, Average	1 Slice/10g	13	0.3	129	24.5	0.5	3.2	0.2

BEEF &

INFO/WEIGHT	Measure	per Measure KCAL	FAT	Nutrition Values per 100g / 100ml KCAL	PROT	CARB	FAT	FIBRE
Beer, Princes*	½ Can/205g	215	6.2	105	14.0	5.5	3.0	0.0
Black Bean, Sizzling, Oriental Express*	1 Pack/400g	420	8.4	105	7.2	14.0	2.1	2.1

	Measure INFO/WEIGHT	per Measure KCAL	FAT	Nutrition Values per 100g / 100ml KCAL	PROT	CARB	FAT	FIBRE
BEEF &								
Chips, Steak, HE, Tesco*	1 Pack/450g	473	12.2	105	6.3	13.8	2.7	0.5
Onions, Minced, Asda*	½ Can/196g	314	19.6	160	13.0	4.6	10.0	0.1
Onions, with Gravy, Minced, Lean, Sainsbury's*	1 Sm Tin/198g	285	13.9	144	17.0	3.1	7.0	0.2
Yorkshire Pudding, Minced, Sainsbury's*	1 Pack/350g	375	11.9	107	8.4	10.7	3.4	1.1
BEEF BORDELAISE								
Sainsbury's*	1 Pack/400.8g	525	25.7	131	8.7	9.7	6.4	1.0
BEEF BOURGUIGNON								
Extra Special, Asda*	1 Serving/300g	279	11.0	93	9.3	5.7	3.7	0.7
Finest, Tesco*	½ Pack/300g	247	7.8	82	9.9	4.8	2.6	0.5
BEEF BRAISED								
& New Potatoes, GFY, Asda*	1 Pack/448.1g	242	6.3	54	8.1	2.2	1.4	3.1
& Vegetables, with Mash, Eat Smart, Morrisons*	1 Pack/400g	224	2.8	56	5.2	7.1	0.7	2.5
Steak, & Cabbage, COU, M & S*	1 Pack/380g	323	9.9	85	8.3	6.7	2.6	1.9
Steak, & Carrots, Mini Favourites, M & S*	1 Serving/200g	140	5.0	70	8.0	4.2	2.5	1.3
Steak, & Mash, GFY, Asda*	1 Pack/400g	260	3.2	65	3.4	11.0	0.8	0.7
Steak, & Mash, HL, Tesco*	1 Pack/450g	419	12.2	93	7.0	10.2	2.7	0.7
Steak, & Red Wine, Veg Mash, HL, Tesco*	1 Pack/500g	360	13.5	72	5.1	6.9	2.7	1.2
Steak, with Colcannon Mash, Tesco*	1 Pack/450g	477	15.8	106	9.5	9.0	3.5	0.9
with Parsnip Mash, Eat Smart, Safeway*	1 Pack/400g	300	4.8	75	6.8	8.2	1.2	1.1
BEEF CANTONESE								
Sainsbury's*	½ Pack/175g	200	2.3	114	5.5	20.1	1.3	0.5
BEEF CHASSEUR								
& Potato Mash, BGTY, Sainsbury's*	1 Pack/450g	387	10.8	86	7.8	8.4	2.4	1.3
Somerfield*	1 Serving/275g	287	7.4	104	14.8	5.2	2.7	2.1
BEEF DINNER								
British Cuisine, Tesco*	1 Pack/433g	390	10.0	90	6.3	10.0	2.3	2.3
Roast, Frozen, Birds Eye*	1 Pack/340g	367	8.8	108	8.8	12.3	2.6	1.4
Roast, Iceland*	1 Serving/340g	354	12.6	104	8.5	9.1	3.7	1.6
Roast, in Gravy, Yorkshire Pudding & Veg, Birds Eye*	1 Pack/340g	367	8.8	108	8.8	12.3	2.6	1.4
Tesco*	1 Pack/400g	380	11.2	95	6.1	10.1	2.8	1.7
BEEF ESCALOPE								
BGTY, Sainsbury's*	1 Serving/300g	321	6.3	107	22.1	0.1	2.1	0.1
BEEF HOT & SOUR								
Chef's Selection, M & S*	1 Pack/329g	395	17.4	120	9.2	8.4	5.3	1.3
with Garlic Rice, BGTY, Sainsbury's*	1 Pack/400g	428	6.8	107	5.9	17.0	1.7	0.6
with Vegetable Rice, COU, M & S*	1 Pack/400g	360	5.6	90	5.5	14.4	1.4	0.6
BEEF IN								
Ale Gravy, Chunky, Birds Eye*	1 Pack/340g	272	6.8	80	7.4	8.3	2.0	1.5
Ale with Mushrooms, BGTY, Sainsbury's*	1 Pack/250.6g	193	3.8	77	10.2	5.6	1.5	0.4
Black Bean, with Egg Noodles, M & S*	1 Pack/400g	460	6.0	115	8.6	16.7	1.5	1.8
Black Bean Sauce, Chinese, Tesco*	1 Pack/400g	396	12.4	99	9.1	8.7	3.1	0.5
Black Bean Sauce, M & S*	1 Pack/350g	403	22.4	115	8.9	5.7	6.4	1.1
Black Pepper Sauce & Egg Fried Rice, Tesco*	1 Pack/450.7g	622	24.8	138	7.0	15.2	5.5	1.2
Burgundy Red Wine, GFY, Asda*	1 Pack/405g	348	8.1	86	8.0	9.0	2.0	1.1
Creamy Peppercorn Sauce, Steak, Tesco*	1 Steak/150g	189	8.3	126	16.5	2.6	5.5	0.1
Gravy, Roast, Birds Eye*	1 Pack/114g	140	6.8	123	13.2	4.0	6.0	0.5
Gravy, Sliced, Sainsbury's*	1 Serving/125g	100	2.3	80	13.5	2.6	1.8	0.2
Gravy, Sliced, Tesco*	1 Serving/200g	152	4.2	76	11.3	3.1	2.1	0.2
Madeira & Mushroom Gravy, Sliced, Finest, Tesco*	1 Pack/400g	536	24.8	134	15.2	4.3	6.2	1.0
Oriental Sauce, Lean Cuisine, Findus*	1 Pack/350g	420	8.8	120	4.5	20.0	2.5	1.5
Oyster Sauce, Asda*	1 Serving/100g	82	4.0	82	7.0	4.4	4.0	1.7
Red Wine, Spinach Mash, PB, Waitrose*	1 Pack/400g	380	10.4	95	7.4	10.1	2.6	0.8
Red Wine, Spinach Mash, PB, Waitrose*	1 Pack/400g	380	10.4	95	7.4	10.1	2.6	0.8

	Measure INFO/WEIGHT	per Measure KCAL	FAT	Nutrition Values per 100g / 100ml KCAL	PROT	CARB	FAT	FIBRE
BEEF IN								
Red Wine Sauce, Milson's Kitchen, Aldi*	1 Pack/400g	256	6.0	64	5.6	9.6	1.5	2.1
Red Wine with Rice, HL, Tesco*	1 Pack/450g	405	7.7	90	4.4	14.1	1.7	0.2
Tuscan Chianti, Bighams*	½ Pack/300g	132	10.8	44	5.1	4.3	3.6	1.4
BEEF MEAL								
Roast, Mini Favourite, M & S*	1 Pack/200g	140	2.6	70	9.1	6.0	1.3	0.7
BEEF SZECHUAN								
Sizzling Hot Spicy, Oriental Express*	1 Pack/400g	380	7.6	95	6.4	13.2	1.9	2.0
BEEF TERIYAKI								
with Noodles, BGTY, Sainsbury's*	1 Pack/400g	320	4.0	80	7.7	10.1	1.0	1.0
BEEF WELLINGTON								
Extra Special, Asda*	1 Serving/218.4g	604	37.1	277	11.0	20.0	17.0	0.9
Finest, Tesco*	1/3 Pack/216g	525	33.9	243	13.0	12.3	15.7	1.5
Sainsbury's*	1 Wellington/175g	473	27.1	270	14.7	18.0	15.5	0.4
BEEF WITH								
Black Bean Sauce, Chilli, Sainsbury's*	1 Pack/300g	336	14.4	112	8.7	8.6	4.8	1.0
Diane Sauce, Rump Steak, Tesco*	1 Steak/165g	182	8.1	110	15.1	1.1	4.9	0.3
Honey & Black Pepper, Waitrose*	1 Pack/350g	326	7.4	93	9.1	9.4	2.1	1.8
Onion & Gravy, Minced, Princes*	1 Serving/200g	342	24.4	171	9.9	5.5	12.2	0.0
Onions & Gravy, Minced, Tesco*	1 Can/198g	224	10.1	113	14.0	2.8	5.1	0.8
Oyster Sauce, Ooodles of Noodles, Oriental Express*	1 Pack/425g	378	5.5	89	4.9	14.2	1.3	1.5
Oyster Sauce, Oriental Express*	1 Pack/425g	378	5.5	89	4.9	14.2	1.3	1.5
Peppercorn Sauce, Rib Eye Joint, Sainsbury's*	1 Serving/181.8g	300	12.7	165	22.2	3.4	7.0	0.1
Peppercorn Sauce, Steak, Just Cook, Sainsbury's*	½ Pack/128g	174	7.3	136	17.7	3.4	5.7	1.2
Red Wine Sauce, Rump Steak, Tesco*	1 Serving/150g	180	8.6	120	17.2	0.1	5.7	3.3
Red Wine Sauce, Steaks, Just Cook, Sainsbury's*	½ Pack/70.3g	83	2.3	118	20.0	2.0	3.3	0.2
Shiraz Wine Sauce, Pot Roast, Finest, Tesco*	1 Pack/350g	350	9.1	100	14.1	5.1	2.6	0.9
Vegetables, Tesco*	1 Pot/300g	102	3.0	34	2.9	3.3	1.0	1.1
Vegetables & Gravy, Minced, Birds Eye*	1 Pack/178g	155	6.1	87	9.1	5.1	3.4	0.6
Whisky, Collops, Sainsbury's*	1 Pack/450g	513	32.9	114	8.0	4.1	7.3	1.2
BEER								
Bitter, Canned, Average	1 Can/440ml	141	0.0	32	0.3	2.3	0.0	0.0
Bitter, Draught, Average	1 Pint/568ml	182	0.0	32	0.3	2.3	0.0	0.0
Bitter, Keg, Average	1 Pint/568ml	176	0.0	31	0.3	2.3	0.0	0.0
Bitter, Low Alcohol, Average	1 Pint/568ml	74	0.0	13	0.2	2.1	0.0	0.0
Brown Ale, Bottled, Average	1 Bottle/330ml	99	0.0	30	0.3	3.0	0.0	0.0
Conditioned Ale, Freeminer, Co-Op*	1 Bottle/500ml	155	0.1	31	0.4	0.4	0.0	0.0
Extra Light, Sleeman Breweries*	1 Bottle/341ml	90	0.0	26	0.0	0.7	0.0	0.0
Guinness*, Draught	1 Pint/568ml	210	0.3	37	0.3	3.2	0.1	0.0
Guinness*, Stout	1 Pint/568ml	170	0.0	30	0.4	3.0	0.0	0.0
Guinness* Extra Stout, Bottled	1 Bottle/500ml	215	0.0	43	4.0	0.0	0.0	0.0
Low Calorie, Low Carb, Cobra*	1 Bottle/330ml	96	0.0	29	0.1	1.3	0.0	0.0
Mackeson, Stout	1 Pint/568ml	205	0.0	36	0.4	4.6	0.0	0.0
Mild, Draught, Average	1 Pint/568ml	136	0.0	24	0.2	1.6	0.0	0.0
Non Alcoholic, Cobra*	1 Bottle/330ml	79	0.0	24	0.8	2.0	0.0	0.0
Resolution, Low Carb, Marstons*	1 Glass/250ml	78	0.3	31	0.3	0.6	0.1	0.0
Ultra, Michelob*	1 Bottle/275ml	88	0.0	32	0.0	0.9	0.0	0.0
Weissbier, Alcohol Free, Erdinger*	1 Bottle/500ml	125	0.0	25	0.4	5.3	0.0	0.0
Wheat, Tesco*	1 Bottle/500ml	155	0.0	31	0.5	0.4	0.0	0.0
BEETROOT								
& Roasted Red Onion, M & S*	1 Serving/125g	94	2.6	75	1.5	12.6	2.1	2.5
Baby, Pickled, Average	1oz/28g	10	0.0	37	1.7	7.3	0.1	1.2
Cooked, Boiled, Drained, Average	1 Serving/100g	44	0.2	44	1.7	10.0	0.2	2.0
Pickled, in Sweet Vinegar, Average	1oz/28g	16	0.0	57	1.2	12.8	0.1	1.5

B

	Measure INFO/WEIGHT	per Measure KCAL	per Measure FAT	KCAL	PROT	CARB	FAT	FIBRE
BEETROOT								
Pickled, in Vinegar, Average	1 Serving/50g	19	0.0	37	1.6	7.5	0.1	1.2
Raw, Average	1oz/28g	9	0.0	32	1.6	6.0	0.1	1.9
BHAJI								
Aubergine & Potato, Fried in Vegetable Oil, Average	1oz/28g	36	2.5	130	2.0	12.0	8.8	1.7
Bhajia Selection, Occasions, Sainsbury's*	1 Serving/15g	32	1.9	211	4.8	19.7	12.6	3.2
Cabbage & Pea, Fried in Vegetable Oil, Average	1oz/28g	50	4.1	178	3.3	9.2	14.7	3.4
Cauliflower, Fried in Vegetable Oil, Average	1oz/28g	60	5.7	214	4.0	4.0	20.5	2.0
Mushroom, Fried in Vegetable Oil, Average	1oz/28g	46	4.5	166	1.7	4.4	16.1	1.3
Mushroom, M & S*	½ Pack/112g	140	11.9	125	2.8	4.4	10.6	5.6
Okra, Bangladeshi, Fried in Butter Ghee, Average	1oz/28g	27	1.8	95	2.5	7.6	6.4	3.2
Onion, Asda*	1 Bhaji/49g	96	4.9	196	6.0	20.0	10.0	2.0
Onion, Indian, Mini, Asda*	1 Piece/17.5g	33	1.8	186	4.9	19.0	10.0	6.0
Onion, Indian Meal for One, Tesco*	1 Bhaji/100g	204	7.3	204	5.5	29.2	7.3	1.3
Onion, Indian Starter Selection, M & S*	1 Bhaji/22g	65	5.1	295	5.7	15.8	23.3	2.8
Onion, Mini, Asda*	1 Bhajis/35.2g	63	2.8	179	4.8	22.0	8.0	4.4
Onion, Mini, Snack Selection, Sainsbury's*	1 Bhaji/21.7g	49	3.4	226	4.1	17.4	15.5	3.5
Onion, Mini, Snack Selection, Sainsbury's*, Sainsbury's*	1 Bhaji/21.7g	49	3.4	226	4.1	17.4	15.5	3.5
Onion, Mini, Tesco*	1 Serving/23g	48	1.9	210	7.3	26.7	8.2	1.3
Onion, Mini Indian Selection, Tesco*	1 Bhaji/23g	40	2.2	172	6.1	15.4	9.5	4.6
Onion, Morrisons*	1 Bhaji/55g	152	8.5	277	7.0	27.3	15.5	4.7
Onion, Sainsbury's*	1 Bhaji/42.5g	109	6.5	256	7.3	22.2	15.4	4.1
Onion, Tesco*	1 Bhaji/47g	85	4.9	181	5.7	16.2	10.4	4.3
Onion, Waitrose*	1 Bhaji/45g	124	9.4	276	4.7	17.5	20.8	2.5
Onion, with Tomato & Chilli Dip, M & S*	2 Bhajis/107.5g	221	12.6	205	4.1	21.1	11.7	3.6
Potato, Onion & Mushroom, Fried in Oil, Average	1oz/28g	58	4.9	208	2.0	12.0	17.5	1.5
Potato, Onion & Mushroom, Fried in Vegetable Oil, Average	1oz/28g	58	4.9	208	2.0	12.0	17.5	1.5
Potato, Spinach & Cauliflower, Fried in Oil, Average	1oz/28g	47	4.2	169	2.2	7.1	15.1	1.4
Potato & Onion, Fried in Oil, Average	1oz/28g	45	2.8	160	2.1	16.6	10.1	1.6
Potato & Onion, Fried in Vegetable Oil, Average	1oz/28g	45	2.8	160	2.1	16.6	10.1	1.6
Spinach, Fried in Oil, Average	1oz/28g	23	1.9	83	3.3	2.6	6.8	2.4
Spinach, Fried in Vegetable Oil, Average	1oz/28g	23	1.9	83	3.3	2.6	6.8	2.4
Spinach & Potato, Fried in Oil, Average	1oz/28g	53	3.9	191	3.7	13.4	14.1	2.3
Turnip & Onion, Fried in Vegetable Oil, Average	1oz/28g	36	3.1	128	1.3	7.1	10.9	2.2
Vegetable, Fried in Oil, Average	1oz/28g	59	5.2	212	2.1	10.1	18.5	2.4
Vegetable, Fried in Vegetable Oil, Average	1oz/28g	59	5.2	212	2.1	10.1	18.5	2.4
BHUNA								
Chicken, Curry, Tesco*	1 Serving/300g	396	22.8	132	11.4	4.5	7.6	0.5
Chicken, Hyderabadi, Sainsbury's*	1 Pack/400g	472	20.8	118	12.6	5.2	5.2	1.3
Chicken, Indian Takeaway, Tesco*	1 Pack/350g	438	27.7	125	8.3	4.6	7.9	2.2
Chicken, with Naan Bread, Sharwood's*	1 Pack/375g	465	19.1	124	6.8	12.8	5.1	2.8
Chicken & Rice, Sainsbury's*	1 Pack/500.7g	696	31.6	139	7.3	13.3	6.3	1.5
Chicken Tikka, Tesco*	1 Pack/350g	438	23.5	125	11.3	5.0	6.7	0.9
Lamb, & Rice, Sainsbury's*	1 Pack/500g	619	26.5	124	7.4	11.6	5.3	2.0
Prawn, Tandoori, Indian, Sainsbury's*	½ Pack/200g	152	8.0	76	5.5	4.5	4.0	1.7
BIERWURST								
Average	1 Slice/10g	25	2.1	253	14.5	1.0	21.2	0.1
BILBERRIES								
Fresh, Raw	1oz/28g	8	0.1	30	0.6	6.9	0.2	1.8
BILTONG								
Average	1 Serving/25g	64	1.0	256	50.0	0.0	4.0	0.0
BIRYANI								
Chicken, COU, M & S*	1 Pack/400g	360	8.4	90	6.9	10.8	2.1	1.9
Chicken, Easy Steam, HL, Tesco*	1 Pack/400g	424	7.2	106	7.0	15.5	1.8	0.6

	Measure INFO/WEIGHT	per Measure KCAL	FAT	Nutrition Values per 100g / 100ml KCAL	PROT	CARB	FAT	FIBRE
BIRYANI								
Chicken, Indian, Asda*	1 Pack/450g	779	22.5	173	9.0	23.0	5.0	0.7
Chicken, Rice Bowl, Eat Smart, Safeway*	1 Pack/300g	255	4.8	85	5.5	11.3	1.6	2.4
Chicken, Tesco*	1 Pack/475g	575	16.8	121	7.2	14.8	3.5	2.0
Chicken, Weight Watchers*	1 Pack/330g	308	3.7	93	6.2	14.6	1.1	0.6
Chicken, with Rice, Tesco*	1 Pack/475g	518	16.6	109	7.2	12.1	3.5	1.0
Chicken Tikka, BGTY, Sainsbury's*	1 Pack/450g	432	4.5	96	7.1	14.6	1.0	1.5
Chicken Tikka, HL, Tesco*	1 Pack/450g	482	3.6	107	6.4	18.6	0.8	1.0
Chicken Tikka, Northern Indian, Sainsbury's*	1 Pack/450g	698	25.7	155	9.4	16.5	5.7	1.2
Chicken Tikka, with Basmati Rice, Sharwood's*	1 Pack/373g	481	16.0	129	6.3	16.2	4.3	0.9
Seafood, M & S*	1 Pack/450g	619	25.7	138	7.1	14.4	5.7	1.7
Vegetable, HL, Tesco*	1 Pack/450g	455	9.5	101	2.7	17.9	2.1	1.6
Vegetable, PB, Waitrose*	1 Serving/350g	238	0.7	68	2.6	14.0	0.2	2.7
Vegetable, PB, Waitrose*	1 Serving/350g	238	0.7	68	2.6	14.0	0.2	2.7
Vegetable, Sainsbury's*	1 Serving/225g	329	17.8	146	2.4	16.3	7.9	1.1
Vegetable, Waitrose*	1 Pack/450g	486	18.0	108	2.8	15.2	4.0	2.2
Vegetable, with Rice, Patak's*	½ Pack/125g	194	1.9	155	3.6	32.9	1.5	1.2
Vegetable & Rice, Sainsbury's*	½ Pack/125.0g	229	5.0	183	4.4	32.4	4.0	0.7
BISCOTTI								
Almond, Pan Ducale*	1 Serving/30g	130	5.0	433	10.0	60.0	16.7	3.3
BISCUITS								
Abbey Crunch, McVitie's*	1 Biscuit/9g	43	1.6	477	6.0	72.8	17.9	2.5
Abernethy, Simmers*	1 Biscuit/12.4g	61	2.7	490	5.7	69.2	21.9	0.0
After Eight, Nestle*	1 Biscuit/5g	26	1.4	525	6.5	62.6	27.7	1.5
All Butter, Tesco*	1 Biscuit/9g	44	2.1	486	6.3	63.5	23.0	1.9
Almond Butter Thins, Extra Special, Asda*	1 Biscuit/4g	15	0.5	375	5.0	60.0	12.5	2.5
Almond Fingers, Tesco*	1 Finger/46g	180	6.8	391	6.2	58.4	14.7	1.0
Almond Thins, All Butter, TTD, Sainsbury's*	1 Biscuit/3.5g	18	0.6	450	6.7	72.8	14.7	3.1
Amaretti, Doria*	1 Biscuit/4g	17	0.3	433	6.0	84.8	7.8	0.0
Amaretti, M & S*	1 Biscuit/6g	30	1.1	480	9.6	71.3	17.2	3.8
Animals, Milk Chocolate, Cadbury*	1 Biscuit/19g	94	4.0	493	6.6	69.8	20.9	0.0
Animals, Mini Packs, Cadbury*	1 Pack/25g	123	5.1	491	6.7	70.7	20.2	0.0
Animals, Minis, Cadbury*	1 Biscuit/2.1g	10	0.4	480	6.5	68.5	20.1	0.0
Apple & Cinnamon Thins, Finest, Tesco*	1 Biscuit/4.7g	22	0.8	470	5.9	71.7	17.5	1.5
Apple & Sultana, Go Ahead, McVitie's*	1 Biscuit/15g	56	1.1	386	6.0	72.7	7.9	3.3
Arrowroot, Thin, Crawfords*	1 Biscuit/7.4g	33	1.1	473	7.4	76.7	15.2	2.2
Belgian Chocolate, Selection, Finest, Tesco*	1 Biscuit/10g	52	2.7	515	6.0	62.0	27.0	3.0
Belgian Chocolate, Thins, Extra Special, Asda*	1 Biscuit/8.7g	45	2.1	503	7.0	67.0	23.0	0.2
Bisc & Bounty, Master Foods*	1 Bar/25g	132	8.3	526	4.8	52.3	33.0	0.0
Bisc & Twix, Master Foods*	1 Bar/27g	140	7.6	520	5.2	61.1	28.3	0.0
Bn, Chocolate Flavour, McVitie's*	1 Biscuit/18g	83	3.0	460	6.6	71.0	16.7	2.6
Bn, Strawberry Flavour, McVitie's*	1 Biscuit/18g	71	1.2	395	5.6	78.0	6.8	0.0
Boasters, Hazelnut & Choc Chip, McVitie's*	1 Biscuit/16g	88	5.3	549	7.0	55.5	33.3	2.4
Bourbon, Trufree*	1 Biscuit/12g	61	2.9	512	4.0	70.0	24.0	2.0
Bourbon Creams, Asda*	1 Biscuit/13.9g	67	3.1	482	5.0	66.0	22.0	3.4
Bourbon Creams, Sainsbury's*	1 Biscuit/13g	60	2.4	476	5.7	70.4	19.1	1.7
Bourbon Creams, Tesco*	1 Biscuit/14g	68	3.0	485	5.4	66.2	21.6	3.4
Bourbon Creams, Value, Multipack, Tesco*	1 Biscuit/13g	62	2.9	494	5.9	68.0	22.8	1.7
Brandy Snaps	1oz/28g	122	5.7	437	2.5	64.0	20.3	0.8
Brandy Snaps, All Butter, Fox's*	1 Pack/100g	465	14.6	465	3.0	79.2	14.6	1.0
Butter, Crinkle Crunch, Fox's*	1 Biscuit/10.9g	50	1.9	460	5.8	69.8	17.5	2.4
Cantucci, with Honey, Loyd Grossman*	1 Biscuit/7g	32	1.1	450	9.5	66.3	16.3	0.9
Cantuccini, Sainsbury's*	1 Biscotti/8g	35	1.3	440	10.4	63.1	16.2	4.4
Cantuccini, with Almonds, Average	1 Biscotti/30g	130	5.0	433	10.0	60.0	16.7	3.3

B

BISCUITS

	Measure INFO/WEIGHT	per Measure		Nutrition Values per 100g / 100ml				
		KCAL	FAT	KCAL	PROT	CARB	FAT	FIBRE
Caramelised, Lotus*	1 Biscuit/9g	44	1.8	488	5.0	72.0	20.0	0.8
Caramels, Milk Chocolate, McVitie's*	1 Serving/17g	81	3.6	478	5.6	65.8	21.4	1.8
Cheddars, Real Cheddar Cheese, Jacob's*	1 Biscuit/3.8g	20	1.1	509	11.6	53.2	27.7	2.7
Cheese Melts, Carr's*	1 Biscuit/4.6g	22	1.0	479	11.9	58.2	22.0	2.2
Cheese Sandwich, Ritz*	1 Biscuit/9.4g	50	2.8	530	9.5	55.0	30.2	2.0
Cheese Savouries, Sainsbury's*	1 Serving/50g	268	15.3	536	11.6	53.3	30.6	2.5
Choc Chip, Paterson's*	1 Biscuit/16.67g	79	3.6	474	5.6	64.0	21.6	3.1
Choco Leibniz, Milk, Bahlsen*	1 Biscuit/10g	52	2.6	515	7.9	63.4	25.5	0.0
Choco Leibniz, Orange Flavour, Bahlsen*	1 Biscuit/14g	70	3.7	504	7.9	58.5	26.4	0.0
Chocolate & Coconut, Duchy Originals*	1 Biscuit/12.5g	71	4.5	543	6.3	52.1	34.4	2.6
Chocolate Chip & Peanut, Trufree*	1 Cookie/11g	55	2.6	496	4.0	66.0	24.0	2.0
Chocolate Fingers, Caramel, Cadbury*	1 Finger/8g	39	1.9	490	5.8	63.2	23.8	0.0
Chocolate Fingers, Milk, Cadbury*	1 Biscuit/6g	31	1.6	515	6.8	60.8	27.1	1.7
Chocolate Fingers, Milk, Extra Crunchy, Cadbury*	1 Biscuit/5g	25	1.2	505	6.6	66.2	23.6	0.0
Chocolate Fingers, Plain, Cadbury*	1 Biscuit/6g	30	1.6	508	6.2	60.6	26.8	0.0
Chocolate Fingers, White, Cadbury*	1 Finger/5.6g	30	1.7	535	6.1	60.7	29.6	1.3
Chocolate Florentine, M & S*	1 Serving/39g	195	9.7	500	7.4	64.5	24.9	1.7
Chocolate Ginger, Organic, Duchy Originals*	1 Biscuit/12.4g	62	3.5	518	4.6	59.7	29.0	2.1
Chocolate Kimberley, Jacob's*	1 Biscuit/20g	86	3.4	428	3.9	64.4	17.2	1.1
Chocolate Nibbles, High Lights, Cadbury*	1 Pack/16.1g	75	2.6	465	6.2	73.4	16.1	1.7
Chocolate Orange Thins, Anna's*	1 Serving/150g	690	25.5	460	5.8	70.0	17.0	2.2
Chocolate Toffee, Crunch, Moments, McVitie's*	1 Biscuit/17g	89	4.7	520	5.6	62.3	27.6	1.7
Chocolate Viennese, Fox's*	1 Biscuit/16g	85	4.9	530	6.7	56.6	30.7	1.7
Chocolinis, Milk Chocolate, Go Ahead, McVitie's*	1 Biscuit/12g	56	1.7	466	7.7	77.2	14.0	2.0
Christmas Shapes, Assorted, Sainsbury's*	1 Biscuit/14.60g	77	4.4	525	5.2	59.0	29.8	1.7
Classic, Creams, Fox's*	1 Biscuit/14g	72	3.6	516	4.4	65.2	25.8	1.7
Classic, Fox's*	1 Biscuit/15g	71	3.7	473	4.8	58.0	24.6	2.5
Classic, Milk Chocolate, Fox's*	1 Biscuit/13g	67	3.1	517	6.1	64.9	24.0	1.6
Coconut Crinkle, Sainsbury's*	1 Biscuit/11g	54	2.8	500	6.4	59.6	26.2	3.7
Coconut Ring, Asda*	1 Biscuit/7.6g	39	1.8	486	6.0	66.0	22.0	2.6
Coconut Rings, Tesco*	1 Biscuit/9g	44	2.0	485	6.2	66.1	21.7	2.6
Cracked Black Pepper, Savoury, Weight Watchers*	1 Serving/16g	71	3.1	446	8.3	59.2	19.5	9.4
Cranberry & Pumpkin Seed, BGTY, Sainsbury's*	1 Biscuit/16.6g	68	2.8	410	7.2	56.6	17.1	13.9
Custard Creams, 25% Less Fat, Asda*	1 Biscuit/10g	47	1.8	474	6.0	72.0	18.0	1.2
Custard Creams, 25% Less Fat, Sainsbury's*	1 Biscuit/13g	59	2.2	469	5.8	72.7	17.3	1.3
Custard Creams, 25% Less Fat, Tesco*	1 Biscuit/12.5g	61	2.3	473	5.8	72.2	17.9	1.2
Custard Creams, Asda*	1 Biscuit/11.9g	59	2.7	495	5.0	67.0	23.0	2.0
Custard Creams, BGTY, Sainsbury's*	1 Biscuit/12g	57	2.1	473	5.8	72.2	17.9	1.2
Custard Creams, Crawfords*	1 Biscuit/11g	57	2.7	517	5.9	69.2	24.1	1.5
Custard Creams, Jacob's*	1 Biscuit/16g	77	3.3	481	5.3	68.0	20.9	1.6
Custard Creams, Sainsbury's*	1 Biscuit/13g	67	3.0	514	5.5	70.4	23.4	1.6
Custard Creams, SmartPrice, Asda*	1 Biscuit/12.6g	63	2.7	486	6.0	69.0	21.0	1.6
Custard Creams, Tesco*	1 Biscuit/12.7g	65	3.1	510	5.7	65.7	24.7	1.5
Custard Creams, Trufree*	1 Biscuit/12g	60	2.8	501	3.5	70.0	23.0	1.0
Custard Creams, Value, Tesco*	1 Biscuit/11.4g	51	1.6	450	7.2	72.5	14.3	3.0
Dark Chocolate & Stem Ginger, TTD, Sainsbury's*	1 Biscuit/22.2g	112	5.9	504	4.4	62.3	26.4	1.8
Dark Chocolate All Butter, M & S*	1 Biscuit/15g	72	4.1	480	6.9	52.4	27.2	11.4
Dark Chocolate Ginger, M & S*	1 Biscuit/20.8g	105	5.7	505	5.0	58.8	27.6	4.2
Dark Chocolate Gingers, Border*	1 Biscuit/16.7g	76	3.4	445	4.4	61.4	20.1	2.9
Digestive, 25% Less Fat, Asda*	1 Biscuit/16g	73	2.6	455	7.3	69.8	16.3	2.6
Digestive, 25% Less Fat, Tesco*	1 Biscuit/14g	65	2.3	462	7.3	71.0	16.5	3.8
Digestive, BGTY, Sainsbury's*	1 Biscuit/15g	70	2.6	468	7.4	71.0	17.2	3.8
Digestive, Caramels, Milk Chocolate, McVitie's*	1 Biscuit/16.9g	81	3.7	478	5.6	65.1	21.7	2.3

BISCUITS

	Measure INFO/WEIGHT	per Measure		Nutrition Values per 100g / 100ml				
		KCAL	FAT	KCAL	PROT	CARB	FAT	FIBRE
Digestive, Caramels, Plain Chocolate, McVitie's*	1 Biscuit/17g	82	3.8	481	5.7	65.5	22.1	2.1
Digestive, Chocolate	1 Biscuit/ 17g	84	4.1	493	6.8	66.5	24.1	2.2
Digestive, Chocolate, Cadbury*	1 Biscuit/17.2g	84	4.1	495	6.8	62.3	24.4	0.0
Digestive, Chocolate Chip, Asda*	1 Biscuit/13.8g	69	3.2	491	6.0	65.0	23.0	2.9
Digestive, Cracker Selection, Tesco*	1 Biscuit/12g	56	2.3	464	7.1	65.2	19.4	4.3
Digestive, Crawfords*	1 Biscuit/12g	58	2.4	484	7.1	68.8	20.0	3.4
Digestive, Creams, McVitie's*	1 Biscuit/12g	60	2.8	502	5.6	68.2	23.0	2.1
Digestive, Dark Chocolate, McVitie's*	1 Biscuit/17g	82	4.0	487	6.0	61.6	24.0	4.0
Digestive, Economy, Sainsbury's*	1 Biscuit/13g	65	3.0	498	6.8	66.3	22.8	3.3
Digestive, Fingers, Morrisons*	1 Biscuit/8g	39	1.8	482	6.8	63.6	22.2	3.2
Digestive, High Fibre, Reduced Sugar, M & S*	1 Biscuit/13g	60	2.8	460	6.5	59.3	21.7	9.4
Digestive, Hovis*	1 Biscuit/6.0g	27	1.1	447	10.2	60.0	18.5	4.4
Digestive, Jacob's*	1 Biscuit/14g	67	3.0	479	6.6	65.7	21.1	3.4
Digestive, Light, McVitie's*	1 Biscuit/15g	67	2.4	445	7.1	67.9	16.1	3.5
Digestive, McVitie's*	1 Biscuit/15g	71	3.2	470	7.2	62.7	21.5	3.6
Digestive, Milk Chocolate, 25% Less Fat, Tesco*	1 Biscuit/17g	79	3.0	466	7.4	69.0	17.8	2.6
Digestive, Milk Chocolate, GFY, Asda*	1 Biscuit/17g	78	2.9	457	7.0	69.0	17.0	3.2
Digestive, Milk Chocolate, M & S*	1 Biscuit/16.8g	85	4.4	505	6.1	62.2	26.0	2.6
Digestive, Milk Chocolate, McVitie's*	1 Biscuit/17.2g	83	4.0	487	6.7	62.6	23.3	2.9
Digestive, Milk Chocolate, Mini, McVitie's*	1 Bag/50g	248	12.4	496	6.6	61.9	24.7	2.9
Digestive, Milk Chocolate, Sainsbury's*	1 Biscuit/17g	87	6.3	511	6.9	65.9	36.8	2.5
Digestive, Milk Chocolate, Tesco*	1 Biscuit/17g	84	4.2	497	6.8	62.4	24.5	2.7
Digestive, Milk Chocolate Homewheat, McVitie's*	1 Biscuit/17g	86	4.1	505	6.8	65.8	23.9	2.3
Digestive, Organic, Sainsbury's*	1 Biscuit/12.4g	58	2.8	483	6.6	60.9	23.7	5.8
Digestive, Organic, Tesco*	1 Biscuit/13g	60	2.7	464	7.7	66.3	20.8	4.6
Digestive, Plain	1 Biscuit/14g	66	2.9	471	6.3	68.6	20.9	2.2
Digestive, Plain, M & S*	1 Biscuit/16.3g	80	3.9	490	6.5	62.7	23.8	3.3
Digestive, Plain Chocolate, Asda*	1 Biscuit/17g	84	4.0	500	7.0	64.0	24.0	3.2
Digestive, Plain Chocolate, McVitie's*	1 Biscuit/17.5g	86	4.3	480	5.7	60.6	24.0	4.0
Digestive, Plain Chocolate, Tesco*	1 Biscuit/17g	85	4.1	499	6.2	63.5	24.4	2.8
Digestive, Plain Chocolate, Value, Tesco*	1 Biscuit/14g	71	3.5	497	6.5	62.2	24.7	3.1
Digestive, Reduced Fat, M & S*	1 Biscuit/15.6g	77	2.8	480	7.2	73.3	17.5	3.4
Digestive, Reduced Fat, McVitie's*	1 Biscuit/15g	70	2.4	467	7.1	72.8	16.3	3.4
Digestive, Reduced Fat, Tesco*	1 Biscuit/15.5g	70	2.6	453	7.0	69.1	16.6	3.4
Digestive, SmartPrice, Asda*	1 Biscuit/14.4g	67	2.9	465	6.0	65.3	20.0	3.1
Digestive, Sweetmeal, Asda*	1 Biscuit/13.6g	70	3.2	499	7.0	66.0	23.0	3.5
Digestive, Sweetmeal, Sainsbury's*	1 Biscuit/14g	72	3.3	498	6.0	66.4	23.1	3.3
Digestive, Sweetmeal, Tesco*	1 Biscuit/18g	80	2.6	444	8.4	70.0	14.5	3.1
Digestive, Trufree*	1 Biscuit/10g	45	2.1	454	2.1	71.0	21.0	2.4
Digestive, Value, Tesco*	1 Biscuit/15g	74	3.4	490	6.9	64.0	22.4	3.3
Double Choc Chip, Trufree*	1 Biscuit/11g	58	3.0	523	3.0	67.0	27.0	1.8
Extremely Chocolatey Orange, M & S*	1 Biscuit/23.5g	120	6.2	510	7.5	59.9	26.5	2.7
Figfuls, Go Ahead, McVitie's*	1 Biscuit/15.2g	54	0.7	355	4.2	76.8	4.6	2.9
Fruit Shortcake, McVitie's*	1 Biscuit/8g	37	1.6	464	5.7	65.1	20.1	2.7
Fruit Shortcake, Sainsbury's*	1 Biscuit/8g	39	1.6	483	5.9	69.6	20.1	2.1
Fruit Shortcake, Tesco*	1 Biscuit/9g	43	1.7	473	5.8	70.1	18.8	1.9
Garibaldi, Asda*	1 Biscuit/10.4g	39	0.9	375	4.7	68.5	9.1	2.2
Garibaldi, Sainsbury's*	1 Biscuit/9g	35	1.0	389	5.7	67.1	10.9	3.3
Garibaldi, Tesco*	1 Biscuit/10g	40	0.9	400	4.7	74.0	9.1	2.2
Ginger, Traditional, Fox's*	1 Biscuit/8.2g	32	0.9	404	4.4	70.1	11.7	1.4
Ginger Crinkle, Sainsbury's*	1 Biscuit/11g	53	2.5	486	6.2	63.8	22.9	2.9
Ginger Crinkle Crunch, Fox's*	1 Biscuit/11.5g	48	1.4	435	4.7	75.3	12.5	1.6
Ginger Crunch, Hand Baked, Border*	1 Cookie/11.5g	52	2.2	470	4.7	71.4	20.4	0.0

B

BISCUITS

INFO/WEIGHT	Measure		per Measure		Nutrition Values per 100g / 100ml				
			KCAL	FAT	KCAL	PROT	CARB	FAT	FIBRE
Ginger Crunch Creams, Fox's*	1 Biscuit/14g		73	3.7	518	4.6	64.8	26.7	0.0
Ginger Nuts, Asda*	1 Biscuit/10g		45	1.5	447	5.0	73.0	15.0	0.0
Ginger Nuts, McVitie's*	1 Biscuit/12g		55	2.0	456	5.8	70.9	16.5	2.2
Ginger Nuts, Tesco*	1 Biscuit/8g		36	1.2	450	5.8	73.1	14.7	2.0
Ginger Snap, BGTY, Sainsbury's*	1 Biscuit/12g		51	1.2	427	6.5	78.2	9.8	1.8
Ginger Snap, Fox's*	1 Biscuit/8g		35	1.0	443	4.6	77.1	12.8	1.5
Ginger Snap, Less Than 10% Fat, Sainsbury's*	1 Biscuit/12.0g		51	1.1	424	6.5	78.9	9.1	1.9
Ginger Snap, Sainsbury's*	1 Biscuit/10.6g		47	1.6	445	5.3	73.0	14.7	2.2
Ginger Thins, Anna's*	1 Biscuit/2g		10	0.4	480	6.0	67.0	20.0	0.4
Ginger Thins, Asda*	1 Biscuit/5g		23	0.8	462	6.0	73.0	16.0	1.9
Gingernut	1 Biscuit/11g		50	1.7	456	5.6	79.1	15.2	1.4
Golden Crunch, Paterson's*	1 Biscuit/15g		69	3.3	474	5.1	62.5	22.6	4.8
Golden Crunch Creams, Fox's*	1 Biscuit/14.6g		77	3.9	515	4.7	64.8	26.3	1.2
Golden Shortie, Jacob's*	1 Biscuit/11g		54	2.6	492	6.0	64.9	23.2	0.0
Happy Faces, Jacob's*	1 Biscuit/16g		78	3.6	485	4.8	66.1	22.3	1.6
Hazelnut Meringue, Sainsbury's*	1 Biscuit/6g		24	1.4	404	5.0	43.0	23.5	1.1
Hob Nobs, Chocolate Creams, McVitie's*	1 Biscuit/12g		60	3.1	503	6.7	60.3	26.1	4.0
Hob Nobs, Light, 25% Reduced Fat, McVitie's*	1 Biscuit/14.3g		61	2.3	435	8.1	64.6	16.1	6.2
Hob Nobs, Milk Chocolate, McVitie's*	1 Biscuit/19.2g		92	4.5	479	6.8	60.7	23.3	4.5
Hob Nobs, Milk Chocolate, Mini, McVitie's*	1 Pack/20g		97	4.7	483	6.6	61.3	23.5	4.4
Hob Nobs, Plain Chocolate, McVitie's*	1 Biscuit/16.2g		80	3.9	498	6.7	63.3	24.3	4.2
Hob Nobs, Vanilla Creams, McVitie's*	1 Biscuit/12g		60	3.0	501	6.1	62.3	25.2	3.6
Honeycomb Nibbles, High Lights, Cadbury*	1 Bag/16.1g		75	2.6	465	6.2	73.4	16.2	1.8
Iced Gems, Jacob's*	1 Portion/30g		116	0.9	388	5.0	85.5	2.9	1.5
Jaffa Cakes, Asda*	1 Biscuit/11.7g		43	1.0	368	4.7	67.5	8.8	1.9
Jaffa Cakes, Blackcurrant, McVitie's*	1 Cake/12.1g		45	1.0	371	4.8	69.7	8.1	2.3
Jaffa Cakes, Dark Chocolate, M & S*	1 Biscuit/11.4g		45	1.5	395	3.7	64.9	13.2	2.8
Jaffa Cakes, Dark Chocolate, Mini, M & S*	1 Cake/4.9g		21	0.8	410	3.9	62.8	15.8	1.9
Jaffa Cakes, Lunch Box, McVitie's*	1 Cake/6.6g		28	0.6	395	4.2	74.3	9.0	1.4
Jaffa Cakes, McVitie's*	1 Biscuit/12g		45	1.0	374	4.8	70.6	8.0	2.1
Jaffa Cakes, Mini, Asda*	1 Cake/5g		21	0.8	412	3.9	63.0	16.0	1.9
Jaffa Cakes, Mini, Bags, McVitie's*	1 Cake/5.9g		24	0.8	396	4.2	65.0	13.1	3.5
Jaffa Cakes, Mini, Orange Pods, McVitie's*	1 Pod/39.5g		150	3.4	380	4.3	71.2	8.7	3.5
Jaffa Cakes, Mini, Tesco*	1 Serving/5g		19	0.6	380	4.0	64.0	12.0	2.0
Jaffa Cakes, Mini Roll, McVitie's*	1 Roll/30g		115	3.3	382	3.5	67.2	11.0	1.3
Jaffa Cakes, Mini Roll Xl, McVitie's*	1 Cake/44g		169	5.0	384	3.5	66.9	11.4	0.0
Jaffa Cakes, Plain Chocolate, Sainsbury's*	1 Cake/13g		46	1.0	384	4.4	73.3	8.1	1.3
Jaffa Cakes, Sainsbury's*	1 Serving/11g		41	1.0	373	4.3	69.3	8.8	2.0
Jaffa Cakes, SmartPrice, Asda*	1 Cake/11g		43	1.0	379	4.4	70.0	9.0	1.4
Jaffa Cakes, Tesco*	1 Cake/12g		44	1.1	370	4.7	67.5	8.9	1.9
Jaffa Cakes, Value, Tesco*	1 Cake/11.3g		42	1.0	370	4.8	67.6	8.8	1.9
Jam Creams, Jacob's*	1 Biscuit/15.4g		75	3.4	486	5.0	67.4	21.8	1.6
Jam Rings, Crawfords*	1 Biscuit/12g		56	2.1	470	5.5	73.0	17.2	1.9
Jam Sandwich Creams, M & S*	1 Biscuit/16.5g		80	3.7	485	5.7	64.5	22.6	1.8
Jam Sandwich Creams, Sainsbury's*	1 Biscuit/16g		77	3.4	486	5.0	67.0	21.8	1.6
Jammie Dodgers, Minis. Lunchbox, Burton's*	1 Pack/20g		90	2.9	452	5.5	72.7	14.7	2.5
Jammie Dodgers, Original, Burton's*	1 Biscuit/19g		83	3.0	437	5.1	69.5	15.9	1.9
Kimberley, Bolands*	1 Biscuit/16g		72	1.7	449	5.1	82.6	10.9	1.4
Lemon Puff, Jacob's*	1 Biscuit/13g		69	4.1	533	4.3	58.8	31.2	2.8
Lemon Thins, Sainsbury's*	1 Biscuit/10g		47	1.7	468	5.6	72.3	17.3	1.7
Malted Milk, Asda*	1 Biscuit/8g		39	1.8	490	7.0	66.0	22.0	2.0
Malted Milk, Chocolate, Tesco*	1 Biscuit/10g		52	2.5	500	6.7	64.4	24.0	1.9
Malted Milk, Milk Chocolate, Asda*	1 Biscuit/11g		56	2.8	509	7.0	64.0	25.0	1.7

BISCUITS

	Measure INFO/WEIGHT	per Measure KCAL	FAT	Nutrition Values per 100g / 100ml KCAL	PROT	CARB	FAT	FIBRE
Malted Milk, Sainsbury's*	1 Biscuit/8g	40	1.8	488	7.1	65.5	21.9	2.0
Malted Milk, Tesco*	1 Biscuit/8.7g	43	1.9	490	6.6	66.7	21.8	2.0
Marie, Crawfords*	1 Biscuit/7g	33	1.1	475	7.5	76.3	15.5	2.3
Melts, Carr's*	1 Biscuit/4.33g	20	0.9	468	11.0	58.3	21.2	4.9
Milk Chocolate, All Butter, M & S*	1 Biscuit/14.3g	70	3.6	490	7.9	57.4	25.5	1.4
Milk Chocolate, Assortment, Cadbury*	1 Serving/10g	51	2.6	510	6.8	61.0	26.4	0.0
Milk Chocolate, M & S*	1 Serving/50g	260	14.5	520	7.5	57.0	29.0	1.9
Milk Chocolate, Tesco*	1 Biscuit/25.3g	134	7.3	535	6.4	62.1	29.0	1.8
Mini Assortment, M & S*	4 Biscuits/10g	48	2.3	480	6.1	63.9	22.5	2.8
Mint, Plain Chocolate, Tesco*	1 Biscuit/25.3g	135	7.4	538	5.1	63.0	29.5	1.7
Mint, Viscount*	1 Biscuit/13.2g	73	3.8	552	5.1	60.6	28.8	1.3
Morning Coffee, Asda*	1 Biscuit/4.8g	23	0.8	455	8.0	72.0	15.0	2.4
Morning Coffee, Tesco*	1 Biscuit/4.8g	23	0.7	450	7.6	72.3	14.5	2.4
Nice, Asda*	1 Biscuit/8g	38	1.7	480	6.0	68.0	21.0	2.4
Nice, Cream, Tesco*	1 Serving/10g	50	2.4	503	5.3	66.2	24.1	1.9
Nice, Fox's*	1 Biscuit/8.7g	39	1.7	450	6.3	62.4	19.4	5.0
Nice, Jacob's*	1 Biscuit/7g	33	1.3	471	6.1	68.5	19.2	1.8
Nice, Sainsbury's*	1 Biscuit/8g	34	1.5	485	6.5	68.0	20.8	2.4
Nice, Value, Multipack, Tesco*	1 Biscuit/8g	39	1.7	485	6.5	68.0	20.8	2.4
Nice, Value, Tesco*	1 Biscuit/5g	24	1.1	489	6.9	64.6	22.6	2.4
Nobbles, Milk Chocolate, Trufree*	1 Biscuit/13g	71	4.2	544	6.3	58.0	32.0	3.6
Oat, Fruit & Spice, Nairn's*	1 Biscuit/10g	41	1.3	412	8.6	65.3	12.9	8.0
Oat, Mixed Berries, Nairn's*	1 Biscuit/10g	43	1.5	430	7.7	67.0	14.6	5.9
Oat, Stem Ginger, Nairn's*	1 Biscuit/10g	43	1.5	434	8.3	66.6	14.9	5.5
Oat & Wholemeal, Crawfords*	1 Biscuit/14g	67	3.0	482	7.7	64.2	21.6	4.8
Oat & Wholemeal, Dbc Foodservice*	1 Biscuit/14.4g	67	3.1	466	7.1	60.8	21.7	5.5
Oat Crunch, Weight Watchers*	2 Biscuits/23g	103	4.1	448	7.4	65.2	17.8	6.1
Oaten, Organic, Duchy Originals*	1 Biscuit/16g	71	2.7	441	9.8	62.3	16.9	5.3
Oatmeal, Asda*	1 Biscuit/11g	54	2.5	470	6.0	62.0	22.0	6.0
Oatmeal Crunch, Jacob's*	1 Biscuit/8g	37	1.5	458	6.8	65.9	18.6	3.6
Orange Chocolate, Organic, Duchy Originals*	1 Biscuit/12.6g	66	3.6	509	5.5	60.0	28.0	3.0
Orange Sultana, Go Ahead, McVitie's*	1 Biscuit/14.5g	60	1.2	400	5.1	75.7	8.1	3.0
Parmesan Cheese, Sainsbury's*	3 Biscuits/10g	53	2.9	553	14.7	56.4	29.9	1.8
Party Rings, Iced, Fox's*	1 Biscuit/6g	29	0.9	459	5.1	75.8	15.0	0.0
Peanut Butter, American Style, Sainsbury's*	1 Biscuit/12.5g	66	3.0	504	5.2	68.7	23.1	2.2
Peanut Butter Cups, Mini, Hershey*	5 Pieces/39g	220	12.0	564	10.3	56.4	30.8	2.6
Pink Wafers, Crawfords*	1 Biscuit/7g	36	1.9	521	2.5	68.6	26.5	1.1
Pink Wafers, Sainsbury's*	1 Biscuit/8g	36	1.8	486	4.6	64.2	23.4	1.7
Puffin, Chocolate, Asda*	1 Biscuit/25g	133	7.3	533	5.0	63.0	29.0	1.2
Puffin, Orange, Asda*	1 Biscuit/25g	133	7.3	529	5.0	62.0	29.0	2.2
Rich Shorties, Asda*	1 Biscuit/10.3g	49	2.2	486	6.0	66.0	22.0	2.0
Rich Shorties, Crawfords*	1 Biscuit/10g	48	2.2	481	6.1	65.3	21.7	2.6
Rich Tea, 25% Less Fat, Tesco*	1 Biscuit/10g	44	1.1	435	7.1	77.0	11.0	1.3
Rich Tea, Asda*	1 Biscuit/10g	45	1.5	447	7.0	71.0	15.0	2.3
Rich Tea, Basics, Sainsbury's*	1 Biscuit/7.8g	35	1.2	450	7.1	71.3	15.2	2.9
Rich Tea, BGTY, Sainsbury's*	1 Biscuit/10g	39	1.0	430	7.8	75.9	10.6	2.4
Rich Tea, Classic, McVitie's*	1 Biscuit/8.4g	36	1.2	453	7.1	71.2	15.5	2.9
Rich Tea, Light, McVitie's*	1 Biscuit/8.4g	36	0.9	431	7.5	75.0	11.3	3.1
Rich Tea, Low Fat, M & S*	1 Biscuit/9.2g	40	1.0	435	8.3	76.7	10.5	2.4
Rich Tea, Milk Chocolate, Sainsbury's*	1 Biscuit/13.1g	66	3.0	504	6.3	68.5	22.7	2.1
Rich Tea, Milk Chocolate Covered, Cadbury*	1 Biscuit/12.2g	59	2.6	490	6.6	67.6	21.4	0.0
Rich Tea, Sainsbury's*	1 Biscuit/7.7g	34	1.0	440	7.2	72.7	13.4	3.0
Rich Tea, Tesco*	1 Biscuit/10g	45	1.5	454	7.4	71.5	15.4	2.3

B

BISCUITS

	Measure INFO/WEIGHT	per Measure KCAL	FAT	Nutrition Values per 100g / 100ml KCAL	PROT	CARB	FAT	FIBRE
Rich Tea, Value, Tesco*	1 Biscuit/7.8g	36	1.2	453	7.2	72.4	15.0	2.3
Rich Tea Creams, Fox's*	1 Biscuit/11.4g	50	2.2	456	5.3	62.7	20.4	1.4
Rich Tea Finger, Tesco*	1 Biscuit/5g	23	0.7	451	7.4	72.9	14.4	2.3
Rich Tea Fingers, M & S*	1 Finger/4.4g	20	0.6	450	7.2	72.5	14.3	3.0
Rich Tea Fingers, Morrisons*	1 Finger/4g	18	0.6	448	7.2	72.5	14.3	3.0
Rocky, Chocolate, Fox's*	1 Biscuit/24.5g	125	6.6	510	7.3	58.7	27.0	1.7
Rocky, Chocolate & Caramel, Fox's*	1 Biscuit/30g	152	5.8	507	6.9	60.3	19.3	15.5
Rocky Rounds, Caramel, Fox's*	1 Biscuit/15g	72	3.4	480	6.2	62.3	22.9	1.1
Rolo, Nestle*	1 Biscuit/22g	110	5.6	498	5.4	62.0	25.4	0.6
Rosemary & Thyme, Savoury, Weight Watchers*	2 Biscuits/16g	67	3.0	419	8.1	55.0	18.8	13.1
Savoury, Gluten, Wheat & Dairy Free, Sainsbury's*	1 Biscuit/16.5g	75	2.8	467	11.7	65.1	17.7	2.4
Shortcake, Asda*	1 Biscuit/14g	73	3.6	518	5.0	66.0	26.0	2.0
Shortcake, Caramel, Delicious, Boots*	1 Shortcake/75g	329	12.8	439	5.0	67.0	17.0	0.8
Shortcake, Caramel, Mini, Finest, Tesco*	1 Serving/15g	74	4.2	493	4.3	56.3	27.8	1.0
Shortcake, Caramel, Mini, Thorntons*	1 Shortcake/17.5g	86	5.6	492	4.8	46.3	31.9	0.6
Shortcake, Caramel, Mr Kipling*	1 Shortcake/36g	177	10.1	506	4.2	57.6	28.8	1.3
Shortcake, Caramel, Squares, M & S*	1 Square/40g	190	9.6	475	5.5	59.7	23.9	1.0
Shortcake, Caramel, Squares, Tesco*	1 Square/54g	274	16.4	507	4.6	54.1	30.4	0.4
Shortcake, Caramel, Tesco*	1 Shortcake/45g	217	11.6	482	4.6	57.8	25.8	0.5
Shortcake, Chocolate Caramel, TTD, Sainsbury's*	1 Shortcake/41g	211	13.4	515	4.6	50.3	32.8	1.4
Shortcake, Cranberry & Caramel, TTD, Sainsbury's*	1 Serving/40g	192	10.8	480	4.0	55.4	26.9	1.3
Shortcake, Crawfords*	1 Biscuit/10.3g	52	2.4	518	6.4	68.1	24.4	2.0
Shortcake, Dairy Milk Chocolate, Cadbury*	1 Bar/49g	252	13.5	515	7.5	59.2	27.5	0.0
Shortcake, Dutch, M & S*	1 Biscuit/17g	90	5.2	530	5.7	58.2	30.6	0.9
Shortcake, Organic, Waitrose*	1 Biscuit/13g	64	3.2	495	5.8	63.0	24.4	1.8
Shortcake, Sainsbury's*	1 Biscuit/11g	53	2.3	484	7.2	66.6	21.0	2.0
Shortcake, Snack, Cadbury*	1 Biscuit/10g	52	2.7	520	7.0	62.6	26.8	0.0
Shortcake, Value, Tesco*	1 Biscuit/10g	49	2.1	486	7.1	66.5	21.2	2.1
Shortcake, with Real Milk Chocolate, Cadbury*	1 Biscuit/15g	75	3.5	500	6.3	65.8	23.5	0.0
Shortcake Ring, Creations, Fox's*	1 Biscuit/20g	105	5.6	515	7.8	59.1	27.4	1.0
Shorties, Cadbury*	1 Biscuit/15g	77	3.6	511	6.5	67.3	24.0	0.0
Shorties, Fruit, Value, Tesco*	1 Serving/10g	46	1.7	457	5.7	69.3	17.4	3.0
Shorties, Rich, Tesco*	1 Biscuit/10g	48	2.2	484	6.4	65.6	21.8	2.0
Shorties, Sainsbury's*	1 Biscuit/10g	50	2.2	500	6.4	69.8	21.8	2.0
Signature Collection, Cadbury*	1 Biscuit/15g	80	4.4	530	6.2	60.1	29.5	0.0
Sports, Fox's*	1 Biscuit/8.5g	41	1.7	483	6.7	67.0	20.0	2.0
Stem Ginger, Brakes*	2 Biscuits/25g	124	6.2	495	5.6	62.6	24.7	0.0
Strawberry Marshmallows, Go Ahead, McVitie's*	1 Biscuit/19.7g	80	2.3	401	4.7	69.7	11.5	0.9
Sultana & Cinnamon, Weight Watchers*	2 Cookies/23g	101	3.5	441	4.3	72.3	15.0	3.0
Taxi, McVitie's*	1 Biscuit/26.5g	131	6.8	504	4.2	63.3	26.0	0.7
Toffee Chip Crinkle Crunch, Fox's*	1 Biscuit/11g	51	2.0	460	4.6	69.6	18.2	0.0
Treacle Crunch Creams, Fox's*	1 Biscuit/13g	65	3.2	502	4.5	65.3	24.8	1.4
Triple Chocolate, Fox's*	1 Biscuit/20.9g	100	5.3	478	5.7	57.3	25.1	2.5
Viennese, All Butter, M & S*	1 Biscuit/8.8g	45	2.3	510	6.0	63.2	25.9	2.1
Viennese, Bronte*	2 Biscuits/50g	212	12.4	424	4.4	45.6	24.8	0.0
Viennese, Jaffa, M & S*	1 Biscuit/17.2g	79	3.7	465	5.9	61.1	21.7	0.9
Viennese, Sandwich, Chocolate, M & S*	1 Biscuit/15g	80	4.6	535	7.2	58.0	30.6	1.7
Viennese Creams, Raspberry, M & S*	1 Biscuit/17.3g	88	4.9	520	4.6	60.4	28.6	1.3
Viennese Creams, Strawberry, M & S*	1 Biscuit/16.5g	78	3.6	485	6.4	63.0	22.2	1.7
Viennese Whirl, Chocolate, Border*	1 Biscuit/18.7g	97	4.4	512	6.5	61.9	23.2	0.0
Viennese Whirl, Fox's*	1 Biscuit/25g	130	7.0	518	6.7	60.1	27.8	0.0
Wafer, Vanilla, Loacker*	1 Pack/45g	231	12.6	514	7.5	58.0	28.0	0.0
Water, Asda*	1 Biscuit/6.1g	25	0.5	412	10.0	75.0	8.0	3.3

	Measure INFO/WEIGHT	per Measure KCAL	FAT	Nutrition Values per 100g / 100ml KCAL	PROT	CARB	FAT	FIBRE
BISCUITS								
Water, Average	1oz/28g	123	3.5	440	10.8	75.8	12.5	3.1
Water, Carr's*	1 Biscuit/8g	35	0.6	434	10.3	79.1	7.6	3.2
Water, High Bake, Jacob's*	1 Biscuit/5.3g	21	0.4	414	10.5	76.4	7.4	3.0
Water, High Bake, Sainsbury's*	1 Biscuit/5g	21	0.4	412	9.8	76.3	7.5	3.2
Water, High Bake, Tesco*	1 Biscuit/5.3g	22	0.4	415	11.0	75.6	7.3	4.2
Water, Table, Carr's*	1 Biscuit/3.4g	12	0.2	406	10.1	74.2	7.6	4.2
Water, Table, Lge, Carr's*	1 Biscuit/8g	35	0.6	434	10.3	79.1	7.6	3.2
Water, Table, Sm, Carr's*	1 Biscuit/3.4g	13	0.2	438	10.4	80.0	7.7	3.3
Wholemeal Brans, Fox's*	1 Biscuit/20g	90	4.0	451	8.5	58.8	20.2	7.5
Yorkie, Nestle*	1 Biscuit/25g	128	6.7	510	6.7	60.4	26.8	1.3
Yumbles, McVitie's*	1 Biscuit/10.6g	53	2.9	498	5.5	58.4	26.9	2.8
Yumbles, Oat Nibbles, Organic, McVitie's*	1 Bisbuit/11.2g	50	2.5	449	7.9	53.2	22.7	6.6
BITES								
Cheese & Garlic, M & S*	1 Bite/11g	40	3.1	350	8.3	17.2	27.3	5.8
Ciabatta, Fried Onion, Occasions, Sainsbury's*	1 Bite/12g	44	2.3	368	10.9	37.6	19.3	1.0
Ciabatta, Garlic & Herb, Occasions, Sainsbury's*	1 Bite/12g	48	2.6	398	8.9	42.2	21.5	3.2
Cornflake, Chocolate, Mini, Tesco*	1 Bite/14g	62	2.5	446	7.1	64.1	17.9	5.9
Crispy Potato, Salt & Vinegar, BGTY, Sainsbury's*	1 Bag/19.9g	71	0.5	356	5.9	77.4	2.5	4.4
Egg & Bacon, Mini, Savoury, Tesco*	1 Bite/18g	55	3.8	305	8.8	20.2	21.0	2.7
Milk Chocolate, Mini, Luxury, Holly Lane*	1 Mini Bite/15g	72	3.9	479	5.1	55.5	26.3	2.5
BITTER LEMON								
Fever-Tree*	1 Glass/200ml	77	0.0	38	0.0	9.2	0.0	0.0
Low Calorie, Tesco*	1 Glass/200ml	6	0.0	3	0.0	0.8	0.0	0.0
Sainsbury's*	1 Glass/250ml	45	0.3	18	0.1	4.4	0.1	0.1
Schweppes*	1 Glass/250ml	85	0.0	34	0.0	8.2	0.0	0.0
BLACK GRAM								
Urad Gram, Dried, Raw	1oz/28g	77	0.4	275	24.9	40.8	1.4	0.0
BLACK PUDDING								
Average	1 Pudding/40g	101	6.0	252	10.2	19.0	14.9	0.6
BLACKBERRIES								
Fresh, Raw, Average	1oz/28g	8	0.1	30	0.8	6.0	0.3	1.6
in Fruit Juice, Average	½ Can/145g	52	0.3	36	0.6	7.9	0.2	1.3
BLACKCURRANTS								
Fresh, Raw	1oz/28g	8	0.0	28	0.9	6.6	0.0	3.6
in Fruit Juice, Average	1 Serving/30g	11	0.0	38	0.7	8.6	0.2	2.5
Stewed with Sugar	1oz/28g	16	0.0	58	0.7	15.0	0.0	2.8
Stewed without Sugar	1oz/28g	7	0.0	24	0.8	5.6	0.0	3.1
BLINIS								
Cocktail, M & S*	1 Blini/13.5g	26	0.3	190	6.3	35.9	2.3	2.0
Sausage, Cocktail, Waitrose*	1 Blini/16g	30	0.4	190	6.3	35.9	2.3	2.0
Smoked Salmon, M & S*	1oz/28g	67	3.6	240	11.9	18.9	13.0	1.8
BLUEBERRIES								
Chocolate Covered, Waitrose*	1 Serving/25g	120	5.6	481	4.0	65.6	22.4	3.0
Dried, Whitworths*	1 Pack/75g	226	0.1	301	0.9	74.2	0.1	11.4
Fresh, Raw, Sainsbury's*	½ Pack/150g	66	0.2	44	0.9	10.2	0.1	3.2
Organic, Waitrose*	1 Pack/150g	77	0.6	51	0.8	11.1	0.4	2.1
BOAR								
Wild, Raw, Average	1 Serving/200g	244	6.7	122	21.5	0.0	3.3	0.0
BOILED SWEETS								
Average	1oz/28g	92	0.0	327	0.0	87.1	0.0	0.0
Blackcurrant & Liquorice, Co-Op*	1 Sweet/8g	32	0.4	405	0.9	91.0	5.0	0.0
Cherry Drops, Bassett's*	1 Sweet/5g	18	0.0	390	0.0	98.1	0.0	0.0
Clear Fruits, Sainsbury's*	1 Sweet/7g	26	0.0	372	0.1	92.9	0.0	0.0

B

	Measure INFO/WEIGHT	per Measure KCAL	FAT	Nutrition Values per 100g / 100ml KCAL	PROT	CARB	FAT	FIBRE
BOILED SWEETS								
Fruit Drops, Co-Op*	1 Sweet/6g	24	0.0	395	0.2	98.0	0.0	0.0
Fruit Rocks, Assorted, M & S*	1oz/28g	107	0.0	381	0.0	95.2	0.0	0.0
Fruit Sherbets, Assorted, M & S*	1 Sweet/8g	34	0.6	425	0.0	89.7	7.3	0.0
Lockets, Mars*	1 Pack/43g	165	0.0	383	0.0	95.8	0.0	0.0
Pear Drops, Bassett's*	1 Sweet/4g	16	0.0	390	0.0	96.4	0.0	0.0
BOK CHOY								
Tesco*	1 Serving/100g	11	0.2	11	1.0	1.4	0.2	1.2
BOLOGNESE								
Beef, Asda*	1 Pack/392g	412	19.6	105	8.0	7.0	5.0	0.0
Extra Meaty, M & S*	1oz/28g	25	0.8	90	10.4	5.5	2.7	0.0
Fusilli, Ready Meals, M & S*	1oz/28g	38	1.7	135	7.0	13.1	6.2	1.0
Pasta Shells, 98% Fat Free, BGTY, Sainsbury's*	½ Can/200g	174	4.2	87	5.5	11.5	2.1	0.7
Pasta Shells, Canned, 98% Fat Free, BGTY, Sainsbury's*	½ Can/200g	174	4.2	87	5.5	11.5	2.1	0.7
Penne, Heinz*	1 Pack/300g	213	2.7	71	3.8	11.8	0.9	0.6
Shells, Italiana, Canned, Weight Watchers*	1 Can/395g	280	5.1	71	5.2	9.6	1.3	0.7
BOMBAY ALOO								
M & S*	1 Pack/200g	340	20.6	170	2.2	16.6	10.3	2.2
BOMBAY MIX								
Average	1oz/28g	141	9.2	503	18.8	35.1	32.9	6.2
BON BONS								
Apple, Lemon & Strawberry, Co-Op*	¼ Bag/50g	203	2.5	405	1.0	88.0	5.0	0.0
Fruit, Bassett's*	1 Serving/6.6g	27	0.0	380	0.1	94.2	0.0	0.0
Lemon, Bassett's*	4 Sweets/28.2g	119	2.7	425	0.0	83.7	9.8	0.0
BOOST								
Treat Size, Cadbury*	1 Bar/24.3g	128	7.3	535	5.3	59.6	30.5	0.0
with Glucose, Cadbury*	1 Bar/60.5g	315	17.8	521	5.6	58.0	29.4	4.0
with Glucose & Guarana, Cadbury*	1 Bar/61g	314	18.0	515	5.5	56.7	29.5	0.0
BOUILLON								
Beef, Benedicta*	1fl oz/30ml	22	0.2	73	7.5	9.5	0.5	0.0
Chicken, Benedicta*	1 fl oz/30ml	23	0.9	75	4.0	8.0	3.0	5.6
Fish, Benedicta*	1 fl oz/30ml	21	0.1	69	7.5	9.0	0.3	0.0
Powder, Miso, Marigold*	1 Tsp/5g	12	0.5	248	7.0	34.0	9.3	1.4
Powder, Swiss Vegetable, Green Tub, Marigold*	1 Tsp/5g	12	0.4	243	10.5	29.4	8.1	0.7
Vegetable, Benedicta*	1 fl oz/30ml	30	0.1	101	7.5	17.0	0.3	0.0
Vegetable, Herbamare Concentre*	1 Serving/5g	15	1.3	298	4.6	13.5	25.4	0.3
BOUNTY								
Dark, Mars*	1 Funsize/29g	137	7.8	471	3.2	54.1	26.8	0.0
Milk, Mars*	1 Funsize/29g	137	7.4	471	3.7	56.4	25.6	0.0
BOVRIL								
Beef Extract, Bovril*	1 Tsp/5g	10	0.2	197	10.8	29.3	4.1	0.0
Chicken Savoury Drink, Bovril*	1 Serving/12.5g	15	0.2	129	9.7	19.4	1.4	2.1
BOYSENBERRIES								
Canned, in Syrup	1oz/28g	25	0.0	88	1.0	20.4	0.1	1.6
BRANDY								
37.5% Volume, Average	1 Pub Shot/35ml	72	0.0	207	0.0	0.0	0.0	0.0
40% Volume, Average	1 Pub Shot/35ml	78	0.0	222	0.0	0.0	0.0	0.0
Cherry, Average	1 Pub Shot/35ml	89	0.0	255	0.0	32.6	0.0	0.0
BRAZIL NUTS								
Average	6 Whole/20g	137	13.7	687	15.5	2.9	68.3	4.9
Milk Chocolate, Tesco*	1 Nut/8g	47	3.5	585	9.9	38.0	43.7	1.9
BREAD								
50/50, Wholemeal & White, Med Sliced, Kingsmill*	1 Slice/40g	90	0.9	225	9.9	41.2	2.3	4.9
Bagel, Caramelised Onion & Poppyseed, Waitrose*	1 Bagel/86g	222	2.2	258	9.7	49.2	2.5	2.4

BREAD

	Measure INFO/WEIGHT	per Measure KCAL	FAT	Nutrition Values per 100g / 100ml KCAL	PROT	CARB	FAT	FIBRE
Bagel, Cinnamon & Raisin, New York Bagel Co*	1 Bagel/85g	215	1.7	253	7.7	51.1	2.0	4.5
Bagel, Cinnamon & Raisin, Tesco*	1 Bagel/85g	207	1.4	243	9.3	47.5	1.7	2.3
Bagel, Fruit & Spice, Sainsbury's*	1 Bagel/85.1g	234	1.8	275	9.7	54.3	2.1	3.8
Bagel, Granary, Bagel Factory*	1 Bagel/99.9g	288	2.1	288	11.9	57.4	2.1	4.5
Bagel, High Bran & Seed, The Food Doctor*	1 Bagel/85g	187	1.7	220	10.6	43.2	2.0	9.7
Bagel, Mini, Sainsbury's*	1 Bagel/25g	67	0.4	268	11.2	52.4	1.6	2.8
Bagel, Multigrain, Sainsbury's*	1 Bagel/113g	293	3.5	259	10.0	49.6	3.1	2.0
Bagel, Onion, New York Bagel Co*	1 Bagel/85g	222	1.6	261	10.6	50.4	1.9	3.1
Bagel, Onion, Tesco*	1 Bagel/85g	233	2.0	274	10.5	52.4	2.4	1.9
Bagel, Onion & Poppy Seed, Tesco*	1 Bagel/85g	217	2.6	255	10.0	46.7	3.1	3.6
Bagel, Original, Organic, New York Bagel Co*	1 Bagel/85g	220	1.2	259	9.3	52.2	1.4	4.1
Bagel, Plain, Asda*	1 Bagel/85g	226	2.0	265	15.0	46.0	2.3	2.9
Bagel, Plain, Average	1 Bagel/78g	215	1.2	276	10.7	53.6	1.5	0.0
Bagel, Plain, Bagel Factory*	1 Bagel/150g	318	1.3	212	9.4	41.6	0.9	2.1
Bagel, Plain, New York Bagel Co*	1 Bagel/84.7g	216	1.6	255	9.1	50.4	1.9	2.9
Bagel, Plain, Organic, Tesco*	1 Bagel/85g	216	2.3	254	9.0	48.4	2.7	3.6
Bagel, Plain, So Organic, Sainsbury's*	1 Bagel/85g	216	2.3	254	9.0	48.4	2.7	3.6
Bagel, Plain, Tesco*	1 Bagel/85g	220	1.8	259	9.8	50.2	2.1	1.8
Bagel, Poppy Seed, New York Bagel Co*	1 Bagel/85g	233	2.4	274	11.4	50.8	2.8	3.2
Bagel, Sesame, M & S*	1 Bagel/87.3g	239	2.8	275	10.2	51.2	3.2	2.1
Bagel, Sesame, New York Bagel Co*	1 Bagel/84g	221	2.6	264	9.8	49.4	3.1	2.8
Bagel, Sesame Seed, GFY, Asda*	1 Bagel/83.8g	228	2.1	271	11.0	51.0	2.5	2.6
Bagel, White, Asda*	1 Bagel/86g	227	2.7	264	10.0	49.0	3.1	0.0
Bagel, Wholemeal, Multiseed, M & S*	1 Bagel/84g	215	5.6	255	13.1	35.4	6.6	8.3
Bagels, Cinnamon & Raisin, Morrisons*	1 Bagel/85g	215	1.7	253	7.7	51.1	2.0	4.5
Baguette, Budgens*	1 Baguette/125g	335	1.5	268	8.5	55.7	1.2	2.3
Baguette, Cheese, & Onion, Asda*	¼ Slice/42g	154	7.4	366	12.0	39.8	17.6	1.3
Baguette, Crusty Brown, M & S*	½ Loaf/71.1g	160	1.1	225	9.8	42.7	1.6	6.3
Baguette, French, Tesco*	1 Serving/60g	144	0.7	240	7.8	49.5	1.2	3.4
Baguette, Granary, Co-Op*	1 Serving/60g	150	1.5	250	20.0	46.0	2.5	6.0
Baguette, Harvester, French Style, Somerfield*	1 Serving/110g	276	2.1	251	10.6	47.9	1.9	3.7
Baguette, Homebake, Half, Tesco*	1 Serving/60g	141	0.5	235	7.8	49.1	0.8	1.2
Baguette, Mediterranean Herb, Sainsbury's*	1 Serving/60g	203	9.4	339	8.5	40.8	15.7	2.3
Baguette, Part Baked, Half, Tesco*	½ Baguette/75g	180	0.9	240	7.8	49.5	1.2	3.4
Baguette, Ready to Bake, Sainsbury's*	½ Baguette/62g	150	0.8	242	7.8	49.7	1.3	2.8
Baguette, Soft Bake, Somerfield*	1 Serving/60g	170	0.9	284	10.3	57.3	1.5	1.9
Baguette, White, Half, Crusty, M & S*	1 Baguette/162g	420	1.8	260	8.4	53.5	1.1	2.3
Baguette, White, Homebake, Tesco*	1 Baguette/135g	331	1.8	245	7.8	49.7	1.3	2.5
Baguette, White, Ready to Bake, Asda*	1 Serving/60g	168	1.1	280	10.0	56.0	1.8	2.6
Baguette, White, Sainsbury's*	1 Serving/50g	132	0.8	263	9.3	53.1	1.5	2.7
Baguette, White, Sandwich, Somerfield*	1 Serving/60g	155	0.8	259	9.4	52.1	1.4	1.7
Baguette, Wholemeal, Part Baked, Asda*	½ Baguette/75g	176	1.0	235	8.2	47.7	1.3	3.0
Baps, Brown, Lge, Asda*	1 Bap/58g	140	0.9	242	10.0	47.0	1.6	0.0
Baps, Brown, Malted Grain, Lge, Tesco*	1 Bap/93g	228	3.1	245	9.9	42.7	3.3	5.3
Baps, Cheese Top, Sainsbury's*	1 Bap/75g	218	6.4	291	12.1	41.6	8.5	2.0
Baps, Cheese Topped, White, Tesco*	1oz/28g	86	2.0	307	12.2	48.0	7.0	0.7
Baps, Floured, M & S*	1 Bap/60g	168	3.7	280	11.5	46.8	6.2	2.0
Baps, Giant Malted, Sainsbury's*	1 Bap/108.5g	281	5.2	260	8.6	45.7	4.8	5.7
Baps, Malted, Lge, Co-Op*	1 Bap/85g	208	2.6	245	10.2	44.3	3.1	5.0
Baps, Multigrain, Tesco*	1 Serving/97.5g	239	3.1	244	8.7	45.1	3.2	1.9
Baps, White, Floured, Waitrose*	1 Bap/60g	147	1.2	244	8.0	48.6	2.0	1.1
Baps, White, Giant, Sainsbury's*	1 Bap/86g	235	3.2	273	8.3	51.7	3.7	3.4
Baps, White, Giant, Waitrose*	1 Bap/104g	261	4.0	251	8.8	45.3	3.8	2.1

BREAD

	Measure INFO/WEIGHT	per Measure KCAL	FAT	Nutrition Values per 100g / 100ml KCAL	PROT	CARB	FAT	FIBRE
Baps, White, Lge, Tesco*	1 Bap/95g	252	4.3	265	8.7	46.2	4.5	2.4
Baps, White, Med, Morrisons*	1 Bap/65.8g	160	1.4	243	9.1	46.6	2.2	2.3
Baps, White, Sliced, Lge, Asda*	1 Bap/58g	148	1.0	255	10.0	50.0	1.7	0.0
Baps, White, Soft, Floured, M & S*	1 Bap/63g	176	3.9	280	11.5	46.8	6.2	2.0
Baps, White, Warburton's*	1 Bap/57g	144	2.5	252	9.8	43.4	4.3	2.7
Baps, White Sandwich, Kingsmill*	1 Bap/80g	209	3.2	261	10.1	46.2	4.0	2.2
Baps, White Soft, Giant, Somerfield*	1 Bap/105.2g	261	4.0	249	9.1	44.7	3.8	2.3
Baps, Wholemeal, Brace's*	1 Bap/58.5g	137	2.6	234	10.5	42.5	4.4	4.3
Baps, Wholemeal, Country Oven*	1 Bap/40g	92	1.3	231	9.5	41.0	3.3	4.1
Baps, Wholemeal, Giant, Rathbones*	1 Roll/110g	230	2.1	209	9.4	39.0	1.9	8.0
Baps, Wholemeal, Giant, Sainsbury's*	1 Bap/107.8g	248	3.4	230	10.3	40.1	3.2	4.5
Baps, Wholemeal, Lge, Tesco*	1 Bap/95g	223	3.9	235	10.5	39.1	4.1	7.6
Baps, Wholemeal, Sainsbury's*	1 Bap/107.8g	248	3.4	230	10.3	40.1	3.2	4.5
Baps, Wholemeal, Tesco*	1 Bap/46g	104	2.4	227	9.6	41.4	5.3	5.6
Baps, Wholemeal, Village Green*	1 Bap/65g	151	2.3	232	10.0	40.0	3.5	3.8
Baps, Wholemeal, Waitrose*	1 Bap/66.7g	157	3.2	234	10.6	37.2	4.8	6.7
Best of Both, Farmhouse, Hovis*	1 Slice/44g	99	1.4	226	9.5	40.0	3.1	4.9
Best of Both, White, Wheatgerm, Hovis*	1 Med Slice/40g	88	0.9	220	9.1	40.9	2.2	4.6
Black Olive, Finest, Tesco*	1 Serving/72g	184	4.6	255	9.7	39.7	6.4	2.9
Bloomer, COU, M & S*	1 Slice/33g	78	0.5	235	9.5	45.5	1.5	3.6
Bloomer, Multi Seed, Organic, Sainsbury's*	1 Serving/60g	160	4.1	266	10.9	40.3	6.8	8.8
Bloomer, Multi Seed, Sliced, M & S*	1 Slice/53.6g	151	3.9	280	10.5	43.6	7.2	3.1
Bloomer, Soft Grain, M & S*	1 Slice/34g	80	0.5	235	9.5	45.5	1.5	3.6
Bloomer, Vienna, M & S*	1oz/28g	79	0.6	281	9.6	55.8	2.1	2.7
Bloomer, White, Bake Off, Somerfield*	1oz/28g	69	0.8	246	9.0	47.0	3.0	0.0
Bloomer, White, Seeded, Bake Off, Somerfield*	1oz/28g	68	0.8	243	9.0	46.0	3.0	0.0
Bloomer, Wholemeal, Organic, M & S*	1 Slice/50g	110	2.1	220	10.2	35.5	4.2	6.4
Breadcakes, Big Brown, Morrisons*	1 Breadcake/63g	154	2.1	245	9.0	44.6	3.4	4.3
Brioche, Continental Classics*	1 Roll/35g	122	3.3	349	8.2	58.3	9.3	0.0
Brioche, Finest, Tesco*	1 Bun/52g	207	11.6	398	10.8	38.3	22.4	2.0
Brioche, Loaf, Butter, Sainsbury's*	1/8 Loaf/50g	174	5.3	347	8.0	55.0	10.5	2.2
Brioche, Rolls, Butter, Tesco*	1 Serving/35g	127	4.0	363	8.6	56.0	11.4	3.7
Brioche, Rolls, Chocolate Chip, Tesco*	1 Serving/35g	131	5.6	374	8.6	49.1	16.0	6.0
Brioche, Rolls, Tesco*	1 Roll/26g	92	2.9	349	8.5	54.0	11.0	0.0
Brown	1 Med Slice/34g	74	0.7	218	8.5	44.3	2.0	3.5
Brown, Danish, Sliced, Weight Watchers*	1 Slice/20g	44	0.4	216	11.3	38.7	2.0	7.4
Brown, Danish, Warburton's*	1 Slice/20.7g	45	0.4	213	11.1	38.9	1.9	7.2
Brown, Farmhouse, Linwoods*	1 Slice/25g	56	0.4	225	7.3	44.4	1.7	5.8
Brown, Good Health, Warburton's*	1 Slice/34.8g	79	1.0	226	10.3	39.6	2.9	7.2
Brown, Granary Malted, thick Sliced, Waitrose*	1 Slice/40g	95	0.9	238	9.4	44.8	2.3	5.1
Brown, Harvest, M & S*	1oz/28g	67	0.8	240	8.8	44.5	2.7	3.7
Brown, High Fibre, Ormo*	1 Slice/24g	57	0.6	239	9.2	42.9	2.6	7.5
Brown, Honey & Oat Bran, Vogel*	1 Serving/100g	220	4.5	220	7.9	39.2	4.5	5.7
Brown, Irwin's*	1 Slice/64g	137	0.4	214	10.4	41.8	0.6	6.1
Brown, Kingsmill Gold, Seeds & Oats, Kingsmill*	1 Slice/45g	126	4.4	280	12.2	35.6	9.8	4.9
Brown, Malted, Farmhouse Gold, Morrisons*	1 Slice/38g	94	0.5	248	8.2	49.6	1.4	3.0
Brown, Med Sliced, Asda*	1 Slice/36.1g	78	0.6	216	8.0	42.0	1.8	4.1
Brown, Med Sliced, Premium, Warburton's*	1 Slice/23.7g	59	0.9	249	10.5	43.2	3.7	4.3
Brown, Med Sliced, Sainsbury's*	1 Slice/36g	81	0.7	225	8.2	43.8	1.9	3.9
Brown, Med Sliced, Tesco*	2 Slices/72g	157	1.6	218	8.0	41.6	2.2	4.5
Brown, Mixed Grain, Original, Vogel*	1 Slice/45g	102	0.6	227	9.8	47.1	1.3	6.4
Brown, Premium Gold Malted, TTD, Sainsbury's*	1 Slice/43g	93	1.0	217	8.5	40.3	2.4	2.4
Brown, Sainsbury's*	1 Slice/34g	81	0.7	239	8.4	46.8	2.1	4.2

BREAD

INFO/WEIGHT	Measure	per Measure		Nutrition Values per 100g / 100ml				
		KCAL	FAT	KCAL	PROT	CARB	FAT	FIBRE
Brown, Seeded Batch, Lge Loaf, Warburton's*	1 Slice/45.8g	132	4.1	288	12.3	39.7	8.9	6.0
Brown, Sliced, Free From, Tesco*	1 Slice/45g	121	3.7	268	5.4	43.2	8.2	3.6
Brown, Soda, M & S*	1 Slice/40g	92	1.4	229	9.2	43.6	3.6	4.9
Brown, Soy & Linseed, Vogel*	1 Slice/50g	116	2.5	232	11.2	33.3	4.9	7.0
Brown, Sunflower & Barley, Vogel*	1 Slice/50g	120	3.1	240	8.8	39.9	6.1	5.4
Brown, Thick, Warburton's*	1 Slice/37.9g	80	0.7	211	9.4	39.2	1.8	6.2
Brown, Thick Slice, Tesco*	1 Serving/50g	110	1.3	219	10.3	38.9	2.5	5.3
Brown, Thin Sliced, Sainsbury's*	1 Slice/28.9g	65	0.6	225	8.2	43.8	1.9	3.9
Brown, Toasted, Average	1 Med Slice/24g	65	0.5	272	10.4	56.5	2.1	4.5
Brown, Toastie, Thick Sliced, Kingsmill*	1 Slice/43.9g	101	1.5	230	9.5	40.5	3.3	4.7
Bun, Burger, with Sesame Seeds, Bestway*	1 Bun/75g	209	4.1	278	8.0	49.0	5.5	0.0
Buns, White, Burger, Waitrose*	1 Serving/64g	169	2.5	264	10.0	47.2	3.9	2.7
Challah, Average	1 Slice/50g	143	3.6	286	8.9	53.6	7.1	3.6
Cheese, Morrisons*	1 Serving/96g	297	13.6	311	9.9	35.9	14.2	3.0
Cheese, Onion & Garlic, Tear & Share, Waitrose*	¼ Bread/112g	326	14.6	290	9.4	33.9	13.0	2.1
Cheese, Tear & Share, Tesco*	¼ Loaf/72.5g	225	7.8	310	8.8	44.0	10.7	0.8
Cheese & Garlic, Pizza Style, Sainsbury's*	¼ Bread/62.5g	200	8.2	318	10.7	39.7	13.0	2.2
Cheese & Garlic, Slices, Morrisons*	1 Slice/32.5g	120	5.3	368	9.6	45.9	16.3	2.7
Cheese & Garlic, Stonebaked, Morrisons*	¼ Bread/68.8g	228	9.9	331	10.9	39.5	14.4	1.9
Cheese & Onion, Tear & Share, Sainsbury's*	¼ Bread/71g	202	6.6	285	9.8	40.6	9.3	1.9
Cheese & Onion, Toastie, Warburton's*	1 Slice/42g	120	5.8	286	7.5	33.1	13.7	0.0
Cheese & Tomato, Tear & Share, Sainsbury's*	¼ Bread/72g	211	9.5	293	8.0	35.7	13.2	1.5
Cholla, Average	1/10 Loaf/154g	421	14.3	274	6.9	40.9	9.3	1.0
Ciabatta, Black Olive, Part Baked, Sainsbury's*	¼ Ciabatta/67g	172	2.5	257	8.8	46.8	3.8	2.4
Ciabatta, Extra Special, Asda*	1/6 Loaf/44.5g	122	2.7	274	10.0	45.0	6.0	2.7
Ciabatta, Finest, Tesco*	1/6 Loaf/45g	124	2.7	275	10.4	44.8	5.9	2.7
Ciabatta, Garlic, Roll, Asda*	1 Roll/93g	333	16.7	358	9.0	40.0	18.0	2.3
Ciabatta, Garlic & Herb, GFY, Asda*	¼ Loaf/59.6g	137	1.4	230	8.8	43.2	2.4	1.0
Ciabatta, Green Olive, Tesco*	¼ Loaf/70g	155	3.1	222	7.4	38.2	4.4	1.9
Ciabatta, Half, Heat & Serve, TTD, Sainsbury's*	½ Ciabatta/67g	182	3.9	274	10.4	44.8	5.9	2.7
Ciabatta, Half, M & S*	1 Loaf/135g	354	5.5	262	10.3	48.1	4.1	2.1
Ciabatta, Half, Organic, Sainsbury's*	½ Roll/63g	152	0.6	241	9.1	48.7	1.0	2.3
Ciabatta, Half, Tesco*	½ Loaf/67.5g	176	2.4	260	8.9	47.7	3.5	2.2
Ciabatta, Italian Style, Safeway*	¼ Loaf/75g	194	2.6	258	8.9	47.7	3.5	2.2
Ciabatta, Italian Style, Waitrose*	1 Roll/89g	231	1.2	260	10.7	51.2	1.3	2.2
Ciabatta, Olive, Safeway*	1 Serving/25g	60	0.9	238	8.2	43.7	3.4	2.3
Ciabatta, Oregano & Feta, TTD, Sainsbury's*	½ Loaf/200g	574	22.0	287	10.4	36.5	11.0	2.4
Ciabatta, Organic, Tesco*	1/3 Loaf/100g	240	3.6	240	8.7	43.2	3.6	2.4
Ciabatta, Part Baked, Half, Sainsbury's*	½ Loaf/67g	174	2.5	260	8.9	47.7	3.7	2.2
Ciabatta, Plain, Tesco*	¼ Loaf/73g	174	2.8	240	9.8	41.5	3.9	2.4
Ciabatta, Ready to Bake, M & S*	1 Serving/150g	393	6.2	262	10.3	48.1	4.1	2.1
Ciabatta, Ready to Bake, Sainsbury's*	½ Ciabatta/66g	172	2.4	260	8.9	47.7	3.7	2.2
Ciabatta, Rolls, M & S*	1 Roll/80g	210	3.3	262	10.3	48.1	4.1	2.1
Ciabatta, Sun Dried Tomato & Basil, Tesco*	¼ Loaf/75g	193	4.3	257	8.9	42.4	5.7	2.4
Ciabatta, Sun Dried Tomato & Olive, TTD, Sainsbury's*	1 Serving/62g	161	4.2	260	10.0	39.7	6.8	2.5
Ciabatta Stick, Organic, M & S*	1 Stick/140g	315	2.0	225	8.9	48.5	1.4	4.2
Cottage Loaf, Stonebaked, Asda*	1 Serving/67g	155	0.9	232	10.0	45.0	1.3	3.2
Country Grain, Thick Sliced, COU, M & S*	1 Slice/25g	60	0.6	240	11.1	42.8	2.5	5.5
Danish, White, Med Sliced, Tesco*	1 Slice/20g	47	0.3	234	9.4	45.4	1.7	3.3
Danish, White, Thick Sliced, Tesco*	1 Slice/24g	60	0.6	250	9.7	47.4	2.3	2.9
Farmhouse, Poppy Seed, Crusty, Loaf, M & S*	1 Slice/40g	104	1.3	260	9.4	47.6	3.3	2.3
Flatbread, Garlic, BGTY, Sainsbury's*	¼ Bread/56g	177	5.7	316	9.6	46.6	10.1	2.7
Flatbread, Garlic, Tesco*	1 Serving/82.5g	251	8.6	302	6.7	45.3	10.4	3.0

BREAD

INFO/WEIGHT	Measure	per Measure KCAL	FAT	Nutrition Values per 100g / 100ml KCAL	PROT	CARB	FAT	FIBRE
Flatbread, Garlic & Herb, Tear & Share, Sainsbury's*	¼ Flatbread/68g	201	6.3	297	10.9	42.5	9.3	3.7
Flatbread, Tomato & Garlic, Sainsbury's*	1/3 Bread/73g	191	4.9	261	8.4	41.7	6.7	3.4
Focaccia, Onion & Herb, Tesco*	½ Pack/190g	547	23.8	288	8.7	35.2	12.5	3.7
Focaccia, Roast Cherry Tomato & Olive, GFY, Asda*	½ Pack/148g	350	6.0	237	9.0	41.0	4.1	2.8
Focaccia, Roasted Onion & Cheese, M & S*	1 Serving/88.9g	240	4.1	270	10.4	45.7	4.6	2.8
Focaccia, Safeway*	1/6 Slice/47g	131	2.8	279	9.5	46.9	5.9	3.4
Foccacia, Mixed Herb, TTD, Sainsbury's*	1 Serving/67g	179	5.8	269	9.7	38.0	8.7	3.8
Foccacia, Tomato & Cheese, TTD, Sainsbury's*	1 Serving/67g	167	5.0	251	10.4	35.5	7.5	3.8
French, Safeway*	1/5 Slice/41g	110	0.2	268	9.8	58.5	0.5	2.4
French, Sliced, Parisian*	2 Slices/39g	100	1.0	256	5.1	48.7	2.6	0.0
French Stick, Average	1 Serving/60g	162	1.6	270	9.6	55.4	2.7	1.5
Fruit, Raisin Swirl, Sun-Maid*	1 Slice/33.1g	95	1.9	287	8.3	50.4	5.8	2.6
Fruit & Cinnamon Loaf, Finest, Tesco*	1 Slice/37g	134	4.9	363	6.4	54.6	13.2	1.5
Fruit Loaf, Apple, M & S*	1 Slice/39.2g	99	0.6	255	8.5	51.9	1.5	3.3
Fruit Loaf, Apple & Cinnamon, Soreen*	1 Serving/10g	31	0.4	307	6.9	60.5	4.2	0.0
Fruit Loaf, Banana, Soreen*	1 Slice/25g	78	1.2	313	6.8	60.9	4.7	0.0
Fruit Loaf, Mother's Pride*	1 Slice/36g	92	1.0	256	8.2	49.3	2.9	2.6
Fruit Loaf, Sliced, Asda*	1 Serving/33.1g	89	1.2	269	8.0	51.0	3.7	2.9
Fruit Loaf, Sliced, Sainsbury's*	1 Slice/40g	104	1.4	260	8.9	47.9	3.6	2.4
Fruit Loaf, Sliced, Tesco*	1 Slice/36g	100	1.8	278	6.9	51.2	5.1	3.7
Fruit Loaf, Sultana & Cherry, Sainsbury's*	1 Slice/50g	179	6.1	357	2.7	59.0	12.2	1.7
Fruit Loaf, with Orange, Warburton's*	1 Slice/33.3g	88	1.1	268	7.7	51.5	3.4	3.0
Fruited, Malt Loaf, Weight Watchers*	1 Serving/23g	68	0.4	294	8.9	60.2	1.9	3.6
Fruited, Richly, Waitrose*	1 Serving/34g	95	1.5	279	10.4	49.3	4.5	3.1
Garlic, & Cheese, Tesco*	1 Serving/143g	490	24.0	343	9.4	38.5	16.8	2.0
Garlic, & Herb, Tear & Share, Tesco*	1 Serving/73g	218	9.2	300	6.3	40.0	12.7	1.7
Garlic, & Parsley, Tesco*	1 Loaf/230g	699	26.7	304	9.0	41.0	11.6	2.7
Garlic, & Red Onion, Somerfield*	1 Serving/60g	177	6.7	295	9.6	38.9	11.1	2.1
Garlic, & Tomato, Pizza, Italiano, Tesco*	½ Bread/140g	405	15.1	289	7.5	40.5	10.8	2.5
Garlic, 25% Less Fat, Sainsbury's*	½ Baguette/85g	268	11.9	315	7.8	39.4	14.0	3.1
Garlic, 30% Less Fat, Morrisons*	1 Serving/80g	231	7.4	289	7.9	43.8	9.2	2.7
Garlic, Asda*	1 Serving/100g	364	20.0	364	7.0	39.0	20.0	3.4
Garlic, Baguette, 25% Less Fat, Tesco*	1 Serving/100g	292	11.3	292	7.0	40.7	11.3	1.8
Garlic, Baguette, 50% Less Fat, Asda*	¼ Baguette/43g	123	3.0	287	10.0	46.0	7.0	2.5
Garlic, Baguette, Asda*	¼ Baguette/62g	209	8.6	337	7.1	46.1	13.8	2.2
Garlic, Baguette, Extra Strong, Sainsbury's*	½ Baguette/85g	278	12.6	327	8.4	40.0	14.8	3.4
Garlic, Baguette, Frozen, GFY, Asda*	¼ Baguette/48g	133	4.3	277	7.0	42.0	9.0	2.7
Garlic, Baguette, GFY, Asda*	¼ Baguette/43g	106	2.7	249	8.1	39.9	6.3	2.1
Garlic, Baguette, HL, Tesco*	1/3 Baguette/66g	172	4.4	260	8.9	41.3	6.6	2.9
Garlic, Baguette, Italian, Asda*	¼ Baguette/48g	173	9.5	364	7.0	39.0	20.0	3.4
Garlic, Baguette, Italiano, Tesco*	1 Serving/60g	213	11.3	355	6.9	39.2	18.8	2.4
Garlic, Baguette, Morrisons*	½ Baguette/95g	295	14.3	311	6.3	37.8	15.0	1.5
Garlic, Baguette, Organic, Tesco*	1 Serving/60g	192	8.1	320	8.5	41.1	13.5	2.5
Garlic, Baguette, Reduced Fat, Waitrose*	½ Baguette/85g	230	6.8	270	8.1	41.5	8.0	2.7
Garlic, Baguette, Sainsbury's*	½ Baguette/85g	342	16.3	403	8.9	48.6	19.2	2.3
Garlic, Baguette, Slices, Tesco*	1 Serving/60g	187	9.2	312	9.8	33.8	15.3	1.7
Garlic, Baguette, TTD, Sainsbury's*	½ Baguette/95g	301	11.1	317	8.3	44.5	11.7	2.8
Garlic, Baguette, Value, Tesco*	½ Baguette/85g	270	11.1	318	8.1	42.0	13.1	2.3
Garlic, Baguette, Waitrose*	½ Baguette/85g	290	15.2	341	7.1	37.8	17.9	0.0
Garlic, Baguette, White, Homebake, Tesco*	1/3 Baguette/55g	160	5.5	290	7.0	43.1	10.0	1.9
Garlic, BGTY, Sainsbury's*	½ Baguette/95g	261	7.3	275	7.6	43.3	7.7	3.0
Garlic, Caramelised, TTD, Sainsbury's*	¼ Bread/75g	218	7.1	290	9.8	41.5	9.4	3.0
Garlic, Ciabatta, & Herb Butter, Sainsbury's*	½ Loaf/105g	345	16.3	329	8.5	38.8	15.5	0.0

BREAD

INFO/WEIGHT	Measure	per Measure		Nutrition Values per 100g / 100ml				
		KCAL	FAT	KCAL	PROT	CARB	FAT	FIBRE
Garlic, Ciabatta, Finest, Tesco*	1 Serving/65g	205	8.9	316	8.1	40.1	13.7	2.4
Garlic, Ciabatta, HL, Tesco*	¼ Bread/60g	151	2.5	251	8.6	44.6	4.2	2.6
Garlic, Ciabatta, Italian, Sainsbury's*	1 Serving/145g	454	17.1	313	10.0	41.6	11.8	2.9
Garlic, Ciabatta, Italiano, Tesco*	1 Serving/65g	211	9.4	324	7.7	40.9	14.4	2.2
Garlic, Finest, Tesco*	¼ Loaf/60g	187	7.9	311	7.7	40.3	13.2	1.8
Garlic, Focaccia, & Herb, Safeway*	1/6 Focaccia /50g	154	5.6	308	9.1	42.9	11.1	2.1
Garlic, Focaccia, & Rosemary, Sainsbury's*	¼ Focaccia/75g	219	7.4	292	8.0	43.0	9.8	2.8
Garlic, Foccacia, & Herb, Italian Style, Morrisons*	1/6 Focaccia/76g	259	10.9	341	8.5	44.7	14.3	2.5
Garlic, Foccacia, & Rosemary, Tesco*	¼ Loaf/73g	193	4.9	266	9.0	42.1	6.8	3.7
Garlic, GFY, Asda*	1 Slice/20g	70	0.9	350	12.0	65.0	4.5	4.0
Garlic, Italian Style Stone Baked, Morrisons*	½ Pack/115g	420	22.0	365	7.9	40.4	19.1	1.9
Garlic, Organic, Waitrose*	1 Baguette/170g	536	23.3	315	8.7	39.1	13.7	1.8
Garlic, Pizza Bread, Co-Op*	1 Pizza/240g	756	31.2	315	8.0	41.0	13.0	2.0
Garlic, Reduced Fat, Waitrose*	1 Pack/170g	551	18.7	324	6.9	49.4	11.0	0.9
Garlic, Slices, & Parsley, Frozen, Sainsbury's*	1 Slice/26g	102	4.7	393	8.7	49.3	17.9	20.8
Garlic, Slices, BGTY, Sainsbury's*	1 Slice/27g	82	2.2	305	9.4	48.9	8.0	2.9
Garlic, Slices, Chilled, Sainsbury's*	1 Pack/368g	1369	60.0	372	9.1	47.3	16.3	3.2
Garlic, Slices, GFY, Asda*	1 Slice/31g	80	1.0	259	8.9	48.1	3.3	3.0
Garlic, Slices, HL, Tesco*	1 Slice/52g	131	2.2	251	8.6	44.6	4.2	2.6
Garlic, Slices, Italian, Chilled, Tesco*	1 Slice/27g	110	6.0	415	6.2	46.8	22.4	2.7
Garlic, Slices, Morrisons*	1 Slice/30g	82	2.7	272	7.3	40.2	9.1	2.6
Garlic, Stonebaked, M & S*	1 Loaf/85g	264	10.1	310	9.3	41.4	11.9	3.1
Garlic, Tear & Share, Chilled, Sainsbury's*	½ Bread/110g	372	15.4	338	8.0	44.9	14.0	2.2
Garlic, with Cheese, Asda*	1 Slice/34g	130	6.1	382	11.0	44.0	18.0	0.0
Granary	1 Slice/25g	59	0.7	235	9.3	46.3	2.7	4.3
Granary, Baps, Lge, Asda*	1 Bap/64g	143	1.4	224	10.0	41.0	2.2	4.3
Granary, Country, Multiseeded, Hovis*	1 Slice/44g	96	1.3	218	11.1	37.0	2.9	6.5
Granary, M & S*	1 Slice/30g	75	0.9	250	9.5	46.4	3.1	3.2
Granary, Malted, Med Brown, Asda*	1 Slice/35g	81	0.9	231	9.0	43.0	2.6	3.3
Granary, Oatmeal, Hovis*	1 Slice/44.1g	104	0.9	236	9.2	45.3	2.1	3.1
Granary, Original, Med Sliced, Hovis*	1 Slice/36g	83	0.6	231	9.2	44.8	1.7	3.8
Granary, Original, Thick Sliced, Hovis*	1 Slice/44.2g	102	0.8	231	9.2	44.8	1.7	3.8
Granary, Seeded, Sunflower, Hovis*	1 Slice/44g	119	2.5	271	10.1	44.9	5.7	2.9
Granary, Thick Slice, COU, M & S*	1 Slice/25g	60	0.6	240	10.5	44.1	2.2	6.0
Granary, Waitrose*	1 Slice/40g	88	1.0	220	9.4	39.9	2.5	4.3
Granary, White, Seeded, Med Sliced, Hovis*	1 Slice/44g	109	1.8	248	10.9	41.7	4.2	3.8
Granary, White, Seeded, Sm Loaf, Hovis*	1 Slice/33.1g	82	1.4	248	10.9	41.7	4.2	3.8
Granary, Wholemeal, Hovis*	1 Slice/44g	96	1.3	218	11.1	37.1	3.0	6.6
Granary, Wholemeal, Seeded, Med Sliced, Hovis*	1 Slice/33g	72	1.0	218	11.1	37.0	2.9	6.5
Hi Bran, M & S*	1 Slice/26.2g	55	0.8	210	12.6	32.5	3.0	6.3
Irish Barm Brack, Tesco*	1 Serving/75g	233	5.2	310	16.0	47.6	6.9	3.0
Irish Brown Soda, Tesco*	1 Serving/50g	110	1.9	219	9.2	36.2	3.8	6.4
Irish Cottage Wheaten, Tesco*	1 Serving/40g	79	0.8	198	9.1	35.4	1.9	6.1
Italian Style Pesto, TTD, Sainsbury's*	¼ Bread/99g	247	6.0	249	9.1	39.4	6.1	4.4
Malt Loaf, Family, Asda*	1 Serving/20g	54	0.3	270	8.0	56.0	1.5	5.0
Malt Loaf, Fruity, Sliced, Soreen*	1 Slice/33g	103	0.7	312	7.7	65.9	2.0	0.0
Malt Loaf, Fruity, Unsliced, Soreen*	1 Serving/42g	130	0.8	310	7.4	65.6	2.0	2.7
Malt Loaf, Organic, Tesco*	1 Slice/28g	82	0.6	292	7.2	61.2	2.0	2.3
Malt Loaf, Sticky, M & S*	3 Slices/47.5g	139	1.1	295	6.9	64.9	2.3	3.1
Malt Loaf, Tesco*	1 Slice/50g	146	1.4	291	8.6	58.0	2.7	4.8
Malt Loaf, Value, Tesco*	1 Slice/25g	72	0.4	289	8.9	60.2	1.4	3.3
Malted, & Seeded, Batch, Organic, Waitrose*	1 Slice/50g	118	2.0	236	10.9	39.5	3.9	6.2
Malted, Crusty, Sainsbury's*	1 Slice/42.1g	109	1.4	259	8.6	48.6	3.3	4.4

BREAD

	Measure INFO/WEIGHT	per Measure KCAL	FAT	Nutrition Values per 100g / 100ml KCAL	PROT	CARB	FAT	FIBRE
Malted, Farmhouse, Morrisons*	1 Serving/40g	94	0.7	235	9.1	45.6	1.8	4.7
Malted, Wheat Loaf, Crusty, Finest, Tesco*	1 Slice/50g	115	0.8	230	9.8	44.2	1.5	4.4
Malted Brown, Thick Sliced, Organic, Tesco*	1 Slice/44.4g	111	0.9	249	8.9	48.8	2.0	3.5
Malted Brown, TTD, Sainsbury's*	1 Slice/44g	103	1.3	234	8.8	42.9	3.0	3.1
Malted Danish, Weight Watchers*	1 Slice/19.1g	46	0.3	241	12.3	44.5	1.7	4.3
Malted Grain, Good As Gold, Kingsmill*	1 Slice/46.9g	114	1.2	243	9.5	45.4	2.6	4.2
Malted Wholegrain, Nimble*	1 Slice/22g	49	0.3	222	10.4	41.9	1.4	6.7
Mediterranean Olive, Waitrose*	1 Slice/30g	82	2.8	273	7.4	40.1	9.2	4.9
Mediterranean Style, M & S*	1/6 Loaf/47.6g	151	5.3	315	10.9	42.5	11.1	1.2
Milk Roll, Warburton's*	1 Slice/18g	46	0.5	253	11.0	45.1	2.7	2.7
Mixed Seed, Organic, Duchy Originals*	2 Slices/85g	229	6.9	269	10.9	39.1	8.1	5.3
Multi Seed, Somerfield*	1 Slice/44.7g	105	1.7	235	11.0	38.2	3.7	8.1
Multigrain, Batch, Finest, Tesco*	1 Slice/49.8g	117	1.4	235	10.8	40.4	2.9	5.5
Multigrain, Batch, Tesco*	2 Slices/100g	235	2.9	235	10.8	40.4	2.9	5.5
Multigrain, Brown, Farmhouse Baker's, M & S*	1 Slice/51.1g	115	2.8	225	13.0	31.2	5.4	5.1
Multigrain, Crusty, Finest, Tesco*	1 Slice/40g	98	1.4	245	9.0	44.7	3.4	5.0
Multigrain, M & S*	1 Slice/50g	120	2.9	240	11.3	35.3	5.7	8.8
Multigrain, Soft Batch, Sainsbury's*	1 Slice/44g	106	2.9	242	11.3	34.5	6.5	5.6
Multigrain, Sunblest*	1 Slice/30g	76	0.8	254	9.0	47.0	2.5	4.5
Multigrain, Tesco*	1 Slice/31g	66	1.0	214	11.1	36.8	3.2	8.9
Multigrain, Thick Sliced, Tesco*	1 Slice/50g	113	1.3	225	8.4	42.2	2.5	3.9
Multigrain, TTD, Sainsbury's*	1 Slice/44g	106	2.8	242	10.2	35.9	6.4	5.3
Multiseeded, Loaf, TTD, Sainsbury's*	1 Slice/35g	97	1.5	277	13.7	46.4	4.2	5.1
Naan, Bombay Brasserie, Sainsbury's*	1 Naan/140g	372	4.3	266	9.8	49.6	3.1	2.9
Naan, Fresh, BGTY, Sainsbury's*	1 Serving/150g	368	4.7	245	9.4	44.9	3.1	2.2
Naan, Garlic & Coriander, Asda*	1 Naan/158.7g	428	7.3	269	8.0	49.0	4.6	2.3
Naan, Garlic & Coriander, Free From, Tesco*	1 Naan/89.6g	215	6.0	240	5.1	38.7	6.7	4.9
Naan, Garlic & Coriander, Fresh, Sharwood's*	1oz/28g	71	0.9	252	7.7	47.8	3.3	2.2
Naan, Garlic & Coriander, Lge, TTD, Sainsbury's*	½ Naan/70g	188	3.7	269	7.8	46.7	5.3	3.5
Naan, Garlic & Coriander, Mini, Asda*	1 Naan/49.7g	165	7.0	330	7.0	44.0	14.0	1.2
Naan, Garlic & Coriander, Mini, Sharwood's*	1 Naan/59g	144	2.0	244	7.1	46.2	3.4	2.0
Naan, Garlic & Coriander, Sainsbury's*	1 Naan/49.8g	128	2.3	257	8.2	45.8	4.6	3.6
Naan, Garlic & Coriander, Tesco*	½ Naan/82.5g	235	6.4	285	7.6	45.6	7.7	2.6
Naan, Garlic & Coriander Mini, Tesco*	1 Naan/65g	185	5.0	285	7.6	45.6	7.7	2.6
Naan, HL, Tesco*	½ Naan/70g	179	1.5	255	7.5	50.7	2.2	2.3
Naan, Indian Meal for Two, Sainsbury's*	1 Naan//125g	357	9.3	285	8.7	45.9	7.4	1.9
Naan, Keema, Sainsbury's*	1 Naan/150g	381	10.4	254	9.7	38.2	6.9	2.2
Naan, Mini, Plain, HL, Tesco*	1 Naan/65g	150	1.8	230	8.1	42.5	2.8	2.9
Naan, Peshwari, Fresh, Sharwood's*	1oz/28g	67	1.4	240	6.8	41.9	5.0	2.5
Naan, Peshwari, Long Life, Sharwood's*	1oz/28g	71	1.8	252	6.2	42.0	6.6	2.6
Naan, Peshwari, M & S*	1 Serving/127g	394	12.8	310	9.2	45.8	10.1	1.9
Naan, Peshwari, Sainsbury's*	1 Naan/166g	511	18.3	308	7.1	45.1	11.0	4.7
Naan, Peshwari, Sharwood's*	1 Naan/130g	334	6.9	257	7.2	45.1	5.3	2.5
Naan, Peshwari, Tesco*	1 Naan/215.0g	684	26.7	318	7.5	48.9	12.4	4.8
Naan, Plain, Average	1 Naan/160g	538	20.0	336	8.9	50.1	12.5	1.9
Naan, Plain, Finest, Tesco*	½ Naan/90g	293	14.0	325	7.6	37.6	15.6	3.3
Naan, Plain, Lge, Sainsbury's*	½ Naan/70g	191	4.6	273	7.1	46.2	6.6	3.0
Naan, Plain, Mini, Asda*	1 Naan/58g	156	2.7	269	8.0	49.0	4.6	2.3
Naan, Plain, Mini, BGTY, Sainsbury's*	1 Naan/50g	113	1.1	226	8.2	43.2	2.2	3.3
Naan, Plain, Mini, Tesco*	1 Naan/50g	138	2.9	276	10.7	45.4	5.7	2.9
Naan, Plain, Patak's*	1 Naan/140g	391	8.3	279	8.9	47.6	5.9	2.9
Naan, Plain, Sharwood's*	1 Bread/120g	326	8.9	272	8.5	42.9	7.4	2.4
Naan, Plain, Tesco*	1 Naan/150g	392	6.9	261	8.4	46.4	4.6	2.3

BREAD

	Measure INFO/WEIGHT	per Measure KCAL	FAT	Nutrition Values per 100g / 100ml KCAL	PROT	CARB	FAT	FIBRE
Naan, Plain, TTD, Sainsbury's*	1 Naan/140g	352	7.2	251	8.2	43.1	5.1	2.9
Naan, Take Away, Tesco*	1 Naan/39g	97	1.3	248	8.7	45.6	3.4	1.7
Naan, Tandoori, Sharwood's*	1 Bread/130g	330	6.5	254	7.3	45.0	5.0	2.0
Naan, Tandoori Baked, Waitrose*	1 Naan/139.8g	372	4.3	266	9.8	49.6	3.1	2.9
Oatmeal, Batch, Finest, Tesco*	1 Slice/50g	128	2.2	255	10.3	43.7	4.3	4.8
Oatmeal, Farmhouse, Soft, M & S*	1 Slice/45g	110	2.0	245	11.1	39.5	4.4	5.2
Oatmeal, Sliced Loaf, Tesco*	1 Slice/50g	111	1.7	222	7.4	40.5	3.4	2.8
Olive, Waitrose*	1 Slice/28g	86	3.0	306	9.0	43.6	10.6	2.0
Pain Au Raisin, M & S*	1 Pain/74.1g	215	9.5	290	5.3	38.7	12.8	1.2
Pave, Mixed Olive, Waitrose*	1oz/28g	59	0.5	209	6.3	41.6	1.9	2.6
Pave, Sundried Tomato, Waitrose*	1oz/28g	76	0.4	271	10.8	53.4	1.6	3.3
Pave, Walnut, Sainsbury's*	1 Serving/50g	140	4.8	280	9.0	40.0	9.5	3.5
Petit Pain, Homebake, Mini, Tesco*	1 Roll/50g	120	0.6	240	7.8	48.5	1.2	3.4
Petit Pain, White, Part Baked, Asda*	1 Roll/128g	330	2.0	258	8.0	53.0	1.6	2.0
Petit Pain, White, Soft, Somerfield*	1 Roll/68g	186	1.2	274	8.5	56.1	1.7	2.1
Petits Pains, White, Ready to Bake, Sainsbury's*	1 Roll/50.4g	122	0.7	242	7.8	49.7	1.3	2.8
Pitta, Bakersfield*	1 Pitta/67g	167	0.7	250	7.0	52.0	1.0	1.5
Pitta, Brown, Organic, Waitrose*	1 Pitta/60g	137	0.8	228	6.4	47.5	1.4	6.6
Pitta, Garlic, Morrisons*	1 Pitta/60g	149	1.1	249	9.7	51.1	1.8	0.0
Pitta, Garlic, Sainsbury's*	1 Pitta/60g	153	0.6	255	9.5	52.0	1.0	2.5
Pitta, Garlic & Coriander, Asda*	1 Pitta/54.7g	116	0.5	212	7.0	44.0	0.9	1.8
Pitta, Garlic & Herb, Tesco*	1 Pitta/60g	134	1.2	223	9.6	44.6	2.0	3.0
Pitta, Mini, Morrisons*	1 Pitta/17.9g	47	0.3	262	10.1	51.2	1.9	2.6
Pitta, Organic, Tesco*	1 Pitta/60g	124	0.8	206	8.3	40.2	1.4	5.7
Pitta, Pockets, Sainsbury's*	1 Serving/75g	188	0.8	250	8.5	52.0	1.0	3.5
Pitta, Sun Dried Tomato & Feta, TTD, Sainsbury's*	1 Pitta/71g	195	3.1	274	11.3	47.4	4.4	2.9
Pitta, White, Average	1 Pitta/75g	199	0.9	265	9.2	57.9	1.2	2.2
Pitta, White, Co-Op*	1 Pitta/63.2g	151	0.6	239	9.3	48.4	0.9	3.2
Pitta, White, Free From, Tesco*	1 Pitta/75g	221	5.2	295	4.9	52.9	6.9	4.1
Pitta, White, Greek Style, Asda*	1 Pitta/50g	127	1.0	253	8.0	51.0	1.9	0.0
Pitta, White, M & S*	1 Pitta/61g	146	1.2	240	9.3	46.9	2.0	3.6
Pitta, White, Mini, Sainsbury's*	1 Pitta/30g	75	0.4	249	10.3	49.3	1.2	3.5
Pitta, White, Mini, Tesco*	1 Pitta/30g	84	0.6	280	9.8	55.1	2.1	3.4
Pitta, White, Morrisons*	1 Pitta/60.2g	145	0.7	241	9.3	51.2	1.2	2.9
Pitta, White, Organic, Sainsbury's*	1 Pitta/59g	150	0.6	254	10.3	50.7	1.1	2.5
Pitta, White, Sainsbury's*	1 Pitta/59g	147	0.7	249	10.3	49.3	1.2	3.5
Pitta, White, Somerfield*	1 Pitta/55.8g	147	1.1	262	10.1	51.2	1.9	2.6
Pitta, White, Tesco*	1 Pitta/60g	170	1.3	283	9.8	55.2	2.2	3.3
Pitta, White, Value, Tesco*	1 Pitta/50g	140	1.1	280	9.8	55.1	2.1	3.4
Pitta, White Picnic, Waitrose*	1 Pitta/30g	75	0.4	249	10.3	49.3	1.2	3.5
Pitta, Wholemeal, Asda*	1 Pitta/56g	133	0.9	238	12.0	44.0	1.6	6.0
Pitta, Wholemeal, HE, Co-Op*	1 Pitta/63g	135	1.3	215	12.0	37.0	2.0	9.0
Pitta, Wholemeal, Hollyland Bakery*	1 Pitta/20g	48	0.3	242	13.1	43.7	1.6	6.0
Pitta, Wholemeal, Lemon, TTD, Sainsbury's*	1 Pitaa/80g	199	5.0	249	10.0	38.0	6.3	6.8
Pitta, Wholemeal, M & S*	1 Pitta/60.9g	137	1.8	225	9.8	39.7	3.0	6.7
Pitta, Wholemeal, Mini, M & S*	1 Pitta/17.4g	40	0.5	230	11.1	39.2	3.1	7.0
Pitta, Wholemeal, Sainsbury's*	1 Pitta/55g	130	0.8	237	9.9	45.9	1.5	5.3
Pitta, Wholemeal, So Organic, Sainsbury's*	1 Pitta/60g	140	1.0	233	9.8	44.8	1.6	8.1
Pitta, Wholemeal, Tesco*	1 Pitta/60g	165	1.4	275	11.0	51.5	2.3	7.3
Pitta, Wholemeal, Waitrose*	1 Pitta/60g	145	0.5	242	12.4	46.0	0.9	3.1
Pitta White, Speciality Breads, Waitrose*	1 Pitta/60g	149	0.7	249	10.3	49.3	1.2	3.5
Plum Fruit Loaf, Lincolnshire, Soreen*	1 Slice/25g	65	0.9	261	8.4	49.3	3.4	2.1
Potato & Rosemary, M & S*	1 Serving/40g	108	2.7	270	9.4	42.2	6.8	2.3

B

BREAD

	Measure INFO/WEIGHT	per Measure KCAL	FAT	Nutrition Values per 100g / 100ml KCAL	PROT	CARB	FAT	FIBRE
Potato Farls, Irish, Rankin Selection, Irwin's*	1 Serving/60g	101	0.8	168	3.2	35.8	1.3	2.5
Pumpernickel, Organic, Bavarian Pumpernickel*	1 Slice/50g	90	0.5	180	6.0	38.0	1.0	10.0
Pumpernickel Rye, Kelderman*	1 Slice/50g	93	0.5	185	6.0	38.0	1.0	0.0
Raisin Loaf with Cinnamon, Warburton's*	1 Slice/35.8g	96	1.3	267	7.2	51.1	3.7	3.2
Roasted Onion, M & S*	1 Slice/50g	125	1.7	250	9.0	46.7	3.3	2.1
Rolls, 3 Seeded, Sandwich, Warburton's*	1 Bun/77g	242	6.7	314	13.3	41.2	8.7	6.0
Rolls, American Style Deli, Tesco*	1 Roll/65g	162	2.2	249	7.8	46.8	3.4	1.6
Rolls, Batched Sandwich, Warburton's*	1 Roll/60g	148	2.5	246	9.6	42.7	4.1	0.0
Rolls, Best of Both, Hovis*	1 Roll/65g	154	3.1	237	10.2	38.4	4.8	5.2
Rolls, Brioche, Plain Chocolate Chip, Sainsbury's*	1 Roll/35g	131	5.6	374	8.5	49.0	16.0	5.9
Rolls, Brioche, Sainsbury's*	1 Roll/32g	116	3.7	362	8.5	56.0	11.5	3.6
Rolls, Brown, Crusty	1 Roll/50g	128	1.4	255	10.3	50.4	2.8	3.5
Rolls, Brown, Lge, Asda*	1 Roll/57g	138	0.9	242	10.0	47.0	1.6	0.0
Rolls, Brown, M & S*	1 Roll/105g	242	6.4	230	9.2	37.3	6.1	4.4
Rolls, Brown, Malted Grain, Tesco*	1 Roll/58g	144	1.9	248	8.7	46.2	3.2	1.9
Rolls, Brown, Mini, M & S*	1 Serving/32.7g	81	2.5	245	9.8	35.5	7.6	3.8
Rolls, Brown, Morning, Farmfoods*	1 Roll/50g	135	1.9	269	12.0	47.0	3.7	4.2
Rolls, Brown, Old Fashioned, Waitrose*	1 Roll/63g	152	2.6	241	9.6	41.3	4.1	4.7
Rolls, Brown, Seeded, Organic, Sainsbury's*	1 Roll/70g	166	3.2	237	9.9	39.1	4.6	6.5
Rolls, Brown, Snack, Allinson*	1 Roll/44g	119	2.9	270	10.8	41.6	6.7	5.6
Rolls, Brown, Soft, Average	1 Roll/50g	134	1.9	268	10.0	51.8	3.8	3.5
Rolls, Brown, Soft, Organic, Sainsbury's*	1 Serving/70g	166	3.2	237	9.9	39.1	4.6	6.6
Rolls, Brown, Soft, Tesco*	1 Roll/50g	118	1.8	235	9.0	41.6	3.6	4.5
Rolls, Brown, Square, M & S*	1 Roll/105g	242	6.4	230	9.2	37.3	6.1	4.4
Rolls, Cheese & Tomato, Seeded, White, M & S*	1 Pack/160g	480	25.0	300	13.7	26.1	15.6	2.1
Rolls, Cheese Topped, Sandwich Rolls, Warburton's*	1 Roll/62g	168	4.0	270	12.1	40.7	6.5	2.6
Rolls, Cheese Topped, Village Green*	1 Roll/56g	159	4.1	284	13.1	41.2	7.4	4.8
Rolls, Ciabatta, Cheese Topped, Mini, Finest, Tesco*	1 Roll/30g	85	2.4	282	11.5	40.9	8.1	3.8
Rolls, Ciabatta, Finest, Tesco*	1 Roll/75g	206	4.4	275	16.4	44.8	5.9	2.7
Rolls, Ciabatta, Mini, Finest, Tesco*	1 Roll/30g	89	2.0	297	9.9	49.1	6.8	4.1
Rolls, Ciabatta, Mixed Olive, TTD, Sainsbury's*	1 Roll/73g	216	7.8	296	10.3	39.6	10.7	3.3
Rolls, Ciabatta, Ready to Bake, TTD, Sainsbury's*	1 Roll/72g	197	4.2	274	10.4	44.8	5.9	2.7
Rolls, Ciabatta, Tesco*	1 Serving/80g	208	2.5	260	8.6	48.2	3.1	3.3
Rolls, Country Grain, Mini, M & S*	1 Serving/30.9g	85	3.0	275	10.2	38.9	9.7	3.8
Rolls, Crisp, Original, Organic, Kallo*	1 Roll/8.7g	35	0.5	390	11.0	74.0	5.6	3.0
Rolls, Crusty, French, M & S*	1 Roll/65g	159	0.8	245	8.1	50.5	1.2	3.3
Rolls, Crusty, Part-Baked, Budgens*	1 Roll/50g	148	0.7	296	9.4	61.4	1.4	2.5
Rolls, Finger, Morrisons*	1 Roll/46g	119	0.8	259	10.7	50.0	1.8	2.3
Rolls, Finger, White, Sainsbury's*	1 Roll/40g	96	1.0	240	9.0	45.2	2.6	3.2
Rolls, Focaccia, Tesco*	1 Serving/75g	227	7.1	302	8.7	45.6	9.4	3.8
Rolls, for Hamburgers	1 Roll/50g	132	2.5	264	9.1	48.8	5.0	1.5
Rolls, Gluten Free, Antoinette Savill*	1 Serving/70g	157	1.5	224	1.9	48.8	2.2	1.5
Rolls, Granary, Bakers Premium, Tesco*	1 Roll/65g	158	0.8	243	9.9	47.8	1.3	2.3
Rolls, Granary, Mini, Tesco*	1 Roll/34g	92	2.2	271	10.0	43.5	6.5	3.8
Rolls, Granary, Waitrose*	1 Roll/59g	160	3.8	271	10.0	47.2	6.4	3.8
Rolls, Granary Malted Wheatgrain, Soft, M & S*	1 Roll/80g	208	3.1	260	9.3	47.2	3.9	2.3
Rolls, Green Olive, M & S*	1 Roll/75g	210	4.5	280	11.2	44.0	6.0	1.8
Rolls, Hot Dog, Sliced, Asda*	1 Roll/84g	197	2.8	234	7.0	44.0	3.3	0.0
Rolls, Hot Dog, Tesco*	1 Roll/85g	200	2.8	235	7.3	44.0	3.3	1.9
Rolls, Hot Dog, Value, Tesco*	1 Serving/40g	93	0.8	232	8.7	45.0	1.9	2.2
Rolls, Hot Dog, Wheat, Brownberry*	1 Roll/43g	120	2.0	279	9.3	48.8	4.7	2.3
Rolls, Malted Grain, Sainsbury's*	1 Roll/68g	190	2.9	280	8.7	51.6	4.3	4.2
Rolls, Malted Grain, Soft, Weight Watchers*	1 Roll/56.5g	142	1.0	251	11.7	47.1	1.8	4.2

BREAD

INFO/WEIGHT	Measure	per Measure		Nutrition Values per 100g / 100ml				
		KCAL	FAT	KCAL	PROT	CARB	FAT	FIBRE
Rolls, Malted Grain, Submarine, M & S*	1 Serving/109g	300	4.7	275	8.9	53.6	4.3	3.0
Rolls, Malted Wheat, Sub, Organic, Tesco*	1 Serving/108g	279	4.4	258	10.1	45.2	4.1	4.8
Rolls, Mediterranean Style, TTD, Sainsbury's*	1 Roll/75g	192	4.5	256	8.5	41.9	6.0	5.8
Rolls, Mini Submarine, M & S*	1 Roll/23g	63	1.1	275	11.4	47.7	4.9	1.1
Rolls, Morning, Tesco*	1 Roll/48g	117	1.2	243	10.4	44.8	2.5	4.7
Rolls, Multigrain, Torpedo, Sainsbury's*	1 Roll/111.9g	328	7.5	293	10.5	47.7	6.7	6.3
Rolls, Multigrain, TTD, Sainsbury's*	1 Roll/110g	327	10.3	297	11.7	41.5	9.4	6.4
Rolls, Oatmeal, Soft, M & S*	1 Roll/80g	224	5.1	280	12.3	43.4	6.4	2.7
Rolls, Pane Rustica, Waitrose*	1 Roll/114g	283	1.4	248	9.4	50.0	1.2	1.8
Rolls, Panini, M & S*	1 Roll/84.7g	250	6.3	295	10.5	46.7	7.4	2.6
Rolls, Panini, Sainsbury's*	1 Roll/90g	249	5.6	276	11.0	44.1	6.2	3.0
Rolls, Panini, White, Tesco*	1 Roll/75g	210	4.6	280	10.1	45.2	6.1	2.7
Rolls, Part Baked, Mini, Tesco*	1 Serving/50g	120	0.6	240	7.8	49.5	1.2	3.4
Rolls, Poppy Seeded Knot, Waitrose*	1 Roll/60g	169	3.2	282	10.3	48.3	5.3	2.2
Rolls, Rye, Toasting, Good & Hot*	1 Roll/65g	143	0.7	220	7.3	44.6	1.1	7.1
Rolls, Scottish Morning, Morrisons*	1 Roll/60g	157	1.3	261	11.3	51.4	2.2	2.4
Rolls, Seeded, Mixed Mini Loaf Pack, M & S*	1 Roll/76g	220	7.3	290	10.6	39.7	9.6	4.0
Rolls, Seeded, Sandwich, Warburton's*	1 Roll/77g	242	6.7	314	13.3	41.2	8.7	6.0
Rolls, Snack, Mini, Tesco*	1 Roll/35g	95	2.1	271	19.0	43.0	6.0	4.0
Rolls, Submarine, Sainsbury's*	1 Roll/117g	305	4.6	261	9.1	47.4	3.9	2.4
Rolls, Sun Dried Tomato, Homebake, Tesco*	1 Roll/50g	123	1.5	246	11.3	44.0	3.0	0.0
Rolls, Sunflower Seed, Toasting, Good & Hot*	1 Roll/65g	163	3.3	250	8.5	41.0	5.0	8.0
Rolls, White, Basics, Somerfield*	1 Roll/44g	107	0.7	243	8.9	48.2	1.6	2.1
Rolls, White, BGTY, Sainsbury's*	1 Roll/50g	114	0.5	227	9.1	45.3	1.0	3.0
Rolls, White, Cheese Topped, Asda*	1 Roll/46g	121	2.0	264	10.0	46.0	4.4	2.0
Rolls, White, Cheese Topped, Sainsbury's*	1 Roll/75g	218	6.4	291	12.1	41.6	8.5	2.0
Rolls, White, Chunky, Hovis*	1 Roll/73g	173	2.4	237	9.4	41.7	3.3	2.5
Rolls, White, Crusty, Average	1 Roll/50g	140	1.2	280	10.9	57.6	2.3	1.5
Rolls, White, Crusty, Morning, M & S*	1 Roll/75g	203	1.0	270	8.8	53.8	1.3	2.7
Rolls, White, Finger, SmartPrice, Asda*	1 Roll/50g	121	0.8	242	9.0	48.0	1.6	2.1
Rolls, White, Finger, Tesco*	1 Roll/68g	170	2.4	250	8.5	45.8	3.5	2.1
Rolls, White, Finger, Value, Tesco*	1 Roll/50g	116	1.0	232	8.7	45.0	1.9	2.2
Rolls, White, Floured, Batch, Tesco*	1 Roll/76g	193	2.5	254	8.8	47.3	3.3	2.2
Rolls, White, Floured, Warburton's*	1 Roll/50g	124	1.9	247	9.8	43.3	3.8	2.7
Rolls, White, Floury, Roberts Bakery*	1 Roll/63.0g	160	1.6	254	8.4	49.5	2.5	2.0
Rolls, White, Floury Batch, Sainsbury's*	1 Roll/68g	168	1.9	247	8.3	47.2	2.8	2.2
Rolls, White, Hot Dog, Jumbo, Sainsbury's*	1 Roll/85g	239	5.2	281	7.5	49.1	6.1	2.9
Rolls, White, Hot Dog, Tesco*	1 Roll/85g	221	3.1	260	9.6	46.1	3.7	3.2
Rolls, White, Kingsmill*	1 Roll/60g	151	2.5	252	9.3	44.5	4.1	2.4
Rolls, White, Lge, Sliced, Warburton's*	1 Serving/89g	230	4.0	258	10.1	44.4	4.5	2.7
Rolls, White, Low Price, Sainsbury's*	1 Roll/44g	107	0.7	243	8.9	48.2	1.6	2.1
Rolls, White, Milk, Warburton's*	1 Serving/18.3g	45	0.5	251	10.8	45.3	3.0	2.8
Rolls, White, Morning, Co-Op*	1 Roll/47g	134	1.4	285	12.0	53.0	3.0	2.0
Rolls, White, Old Fashioned, Waitrose*	1 Roll/57g	157	2.6	275	8.8	49.8	4.5	2.8
Rolls, White, Organic, Sainsbury's*	1 Roll/65g	170	2.0	262	8.7	49.9	3.0	1.0
Rolls, White, Part Baked, Morrisons*	1 Roll/75g	227	1.1	303	9.6	63.0	1.4	2.6
Rolls, White, Ploughman's, Sainsbury's*	1 Roll/65g	185	2.5	285	8.6	54.1	3.8	2.3
Rolls, White, Premium, Brown Hill Bakery*	1 Roll/74g	206	2.2	279	11.0	51.5	3.0	2.3
Rolls, White, Premium, Hovis*	1 Roll/62g	154	3.0	249	9.5	41.9	4.8	2.3
Rolls, White, Premium Soft, Rathbones*	1 Roll/65g	190	3.9	293	9.3	50.3	6.0	2.7
Rolls, White, Sandwich, Lge, Warburton's*	1 Roll/88.3g	224	3.5	254	10.2	44.3	4.0	2.5
Rolls, White, Sandwich, Regular, Warburton's*	1 Roll/57.5g	143	2.5	249	9.7	42.6	4.4	2.4
Rolls, White, Scottish, Morning, Safeway*	1 Roll/40g	113	0.7	283	10.4	56.4	1.8	1.6

BREAD

	Measure INFO/WEIGHT	per Measure		Nutrition Values per 100g / 100ml				
		KCAL	FAT	KCAL	PROT	CARB	FAT	FIBRE
Rolls, White, Scottish, Tesco*	1 Roll/48g	117	1.2	243	10.4	44.8	2.5	4.7
Rolls, White, Seeded, Sainsbury's*	1 Roll/80g	217	4.7	271	10.9	43.4	5.9	4.8
Rolls, White, SmartPrice, Asda*	1 Roll/35.8g	76	0.8	212	9.0	39.0	2.2	2.3
Rolls, White, Snack, Sainsbury's*	1 Roll/67g	159	0.7	237	7.9	49.2	1.0	2.3
Rolls, White, Soft, Average	1 Roll/45g	121	1.9	268	9.2	51.6	4.2	1.5
Rolls, White, Soft, COU, M & S*	1 Roll/37g	94	1.0	255	10.7	47.1	2.7	1.5
Rolls, White, Soft, Farmhouse, Warburton's*	1 Roll/59g	148	2.6	250	9.7	43.0	4.4	2.5
Rolls, White, Soft, Hovis*	1 Roll/64.8g	164	3.0	253	8.8	44.2	4.6	3.7
Rolls, White, Soft, Kingsmill*	1 Roll/58g	145	2.4	250	9.3	44.0	4.1	2.9
Rolls, White, Soft, M & S*	1 Roll/60g	150	1.9	250	10.3	45.2	3.1	2.7
Rolls, White, Soft, Morrisons*	1 Roll/42g	100	0.8	238	9.1	46.4	1.9	2.4
Rolls, White, Soft, Tesco*	1 Roll/72g	175	1.8	243	7.6	46.7	2.5	2.8
Rolls, White, Softgrain, GFY, Asda*	1 Roll/54.0g	128	1.0	237	9.0	46.0	1.9	2.9
Rolls, White, Split, Asda*	1 Roll/45g	113	1.5	251	10.0	45.0	3.4	2.8
Rolls, White, Sub, Tesco*	1 Roll/100g	258	4.0	258	11.1	44.4	4.0	2.8
Rolls, White, Submarine, M & S*	1 Serving/109g	300	5.5	275	11.0	47.0	5.0	1.0
Rolls, White, Tesco*	1 Roll/65g	180	2.5	277	8.7	52.0	3.8	2.7
Rolls, White, Value, Tesco*	1 Roll/35g	81	0.6	231	8.0	45.7	1.8	2.3
Rolls, White, Warburton's*	1 Roll/57g	141	2.4	248	9.7	42.8	4.2	0.0
Rolls, White, Weight Watchers*	1 Roll/54g	135	1.0	251	11.7	47.1	1.8	4.2
Rolls, Wholemeal	1 Roll 45g	108	1.3	241	9.0	48.3	2.9	5.9
Rolls, Wholemeal, Asda*	1 Roll/58g	131	1.6	225	11.0	39.0	2.8	6.0
Rolls, Wholemeal, COU, M & S*	1 Roll/110g	226	3.1	205	11.3	33.4	2.8	7.1
Rolls, Wholemeal, Deli, Tesco*	1 Serving/65g	156	3.1	240	9.0	40.2	4.8	5.7
Rolls, Wholemeal, Finger, Soft, M & S*	1 Roll/69g	179	4.7	260	11.9	37.4	6.8	4.4
Rolls, Wholemeal, Floury Batch, Sainsbury's*	1 Roll/68g	152	2.3	223	9.9	37.8	3.4	6.5
Rolls, Wholemeal, Golden, Hovis*	1 Roll/50g	112	2.0	223	10.5	36.5	3.9	6.8
Rolls, Wholemeal, Great Everyday, Kingsmill*	1 Roll/68.1g	158	2.6	232	10.6	38.8	3.8	6.5
Rolls, Wholemeal, HL, Tesco*	1 Roll/67.5	155	1.4	230	10.4	41.3	2.1	6.6
Rolls, Wholemeal, Kingsmill*	1 Roll/68g	167	2.7	245	10.7	41.5	4.0	5.1
Rolls, Wholemeal, Mini, Assorted, Waitrose*	1 Roll/35.6g	85	1.9	236	9.0	38.1	5.3	5.2
Rolls, Wholemeal, Mini, Tesco*	1 Roll/34g	82	1.9	240	10.9	36.4	5.6	5.8
Rolls, Wholemeal, Morrisons*	1 Roll/67.1g	155	2.7	231	10.2	38.6	4.0	6.3
Rolls, Wholemeal, Old Fashioned, Waitrose*	1 Roll/57g	135	2.7	236	11.1	37.2	4.8	6.6
Rolls, Wholemeal, Organic, Sainsbury's*	1 Roll/66g	152	1.8	230	10.7	41.0	2.7	6.6
Rolls, Wholemeal, Organic, Tesco*	1 Roll/65g	177	4.0	273	10.3	44.1	6.2	5.5
Rolls, Wholemeal, Ploughman's, Sainsbury's*	1 Roll/67g	153	2.1	229	10.7	39.3	3.2	8.6
Rolls, Wholemeal, Sainsbury's*	1 Serving/64.8g	153	2.1	236	10.7	40.8	3.3	7.4
Rolls, Wholemeal, Soft, Sainsbury's*	1 Roll/60g	133	2.0	221	9.9	37.8	3.4	6.5
Rolls, Wholemeal, Soft, Seeded, Sainsbury's*	1 Roll/75g	193	5.6	257	11.8	35.6	7.4	6.2
Rolls, Wholemeal, Submarine, Tesco*	1 Roll/100g	221	3.1	221	9.3	39.0	3.1	5.2
Rolls, Wholemeal, Submarine, Warburton's*	1 Serving/94g	231	4.1	246	10.9	40.6	4.4	6.3
Rolls, Wholemeal, Sunflower & Honey, Sainsbury's*	1 Roll/85g	225	4.3	265	9.2	45.4	5.1	4.5
Rolls, Wholemeal, Tesco*	1 Roll/58g	146	2.3	250	10.9	41.8	4.0	7.5
Rolls, Wholemeal & White, Kingsmill*	1 Roll/60g	151	2.5	251	9.5	43.7	4.2	3.5
Rolls, Wholemeal with Cracked Wheat, Allinson*	1 Roll/58g	134	2.3	231	11.0	38.0	3.9	7.0
Roti, Tesco*	1 Bread/95g	256	5.2	269	8.4	46.4	5.5	3.2
Rye, Average	1 Slice/25g	55	0.4	219	8.3	45.8	1.7	4.4
Rye, Baltic, Organic, The Village Bakery*	1oz/28g	68	0.4	243	8.0	50.3	1.4	2.9
Rye, Dark, Sliced, Trianon*	1 Slice/41g	74	0.6	180	6.5	35.0	1.5	0.0
Rye, German Style, Bolletje*	1 Slice/60g	114	1.2	190	6.0	35.0	2.0	9.5
Rye, German Style, Kelderman*	1 Slice/57g	88	0.8	155	5.6	30.2	1.4	7.7
Rye, Light, Finest, Tesco*	1 Slice/20g	47	0.4	237	10.4	44.3	2.0	3.7

BREAD

	Measure INFO/WEIGHT	per Measure KCAL	FAT	Nutrition Values per 100g / 100ml KCAL	PROT	CARB	FAT	FIBRE
Rye, Organic, Waitrose*	1 Serving/100g	207	1.2	207	6.4	42.7	1.2	5.1
Rye, Swedish Style, Kelderman*	1 Slice/50g	93	1.6	185	7.2	31.5	3.2	4.3
Rye, Wholemeal, Organic, House Of Westphalia*	1 Slice/75g	122	0.9	162	5.1	32.8	1.2	7.8
Rye, Wholemeal, Organic, Mestemacher*	1 Slice/79g	145	1.9	184	5.7	34.9	2.4	8.0
Rye, with Sunflower Seeds, Mestemacher*	1 Slice/80g	146	2.5	182	6.1	32.3	3.1	0.0
Rye with Sunflower Seeds, Organic, Sunnyvale*	1 Slice/25g	50	1.6	198	5.1	30.3	6.3	0.0
Seeded, Batch, Finest, Tesco*	1 Slice/65g	168	4.0	259	9.3	41.8	6.1	6.1
Soda	1oz/28g	72	0.7	258	7.7	54.6	2.5	2.1
Soda, Fruit, M & S*	1 Slice/40.4g	104	1.8	260	5.9	51.3	4.6	2.5
Soda, M & S*	1 Slice/40g	82	0.6	205	8.7	39.2	1.6	4.2
Soda Farls, Tesco*	1 Farl/142g	325	4.5	229	7.1	42.2	3.2	2.6
Softgrain, Mighty White*	1 Slice/36g	81	0.5	224	7.2	45.5	1.5	3.7
Soya & Linseed, Burgen*	1 Slice/36g	99	3.6	274	15.9	29.8	10.1	6.8
Soya & Linseed, Vogel*	1 Slice/45g	107	2.7	238	12.2	34.0	5.9	5.4
Stoneground, Sm Loaf, Organic, Sainsbury's*	1 Slice/24g	50	0.5	208	10.0	37.9	2.1	7.9
Sunflower, Multi-Grain, Allinson*	1 Slice/47.1g	113	2.2	240	9.8	39.6	4.7	3.9
Sunflower & Honey, M & S*	1 Serving/67g	206	9.0	308	12.9	34.0	13.4	5.6
Sunflower & Honey, Organic, Cranks*	1 Slice/30g	65	0.9	215	11.6	37.2	3.0	8.3
Sunflower & Pumpin Seed, Batch, Organic, Tesco*	1 Slice/30g	73	2.2	243	11.0	33.1	7.4	5.2
Three Grain, Organic, Schneider Brot*	1 Slice/71.5g	132	1.7	184	5.7	34.9	2.4	8.0
Tiger Loaf, Tesco*	1 Slice/40g	96	0.8	239	8.7	46.6	2.0	2.6
Toaster, White, Rathbones*	2 Slices/76g	185	1.0	243	9.1	48.6	1.3	2.3
Tomato, & Herb, Tear & Share, Tesco*	¼ Pack/73g	164	3.2	226	6.3	40.2	4.4	2.1
Tomato & Garlic, Italian Style, Morrisons*	½ Pack/155g	355	12.4	229	5.8	33.4	8.0	2.5
Walnut, Waitrose*	1 Slice/38g	129	5.8	339	10.0	40.6	15.2	5.9
Wheaten, M & S*	1 Slice/33g	74	1.2	225	9.3	42.9	3.5	3.9
Wheatgerm, Hovis, Soft, Sliced, M & S*	1 Slice/23g	50	0.7	220	10.1	38.5	3.0	4.6
Wheatgerm, Original, Med Sliced, Hovis*	1 Slice/39.7g	85	0.9	214	10.0	38.6	2.2	5.3
Wheatgerm, Original, Sm Loaf, Hovis*	1 Slice/33g	71	0.7	214	10.0	38.6	2.2	5.3
Wheatgrain, Robertson*	1 Slice/30g	90	1.2	300	9.3	57.3	4.0	4.0
White, Average	1 Med Slice/25g	59	0.5	235	8.4	49.3	1.9	1.5
White, Batch, Warburton's*	1 Slice/42g	98	0.9	233	9.8	43.6	2.1	2.7
White, Batch Loaf, Extra Special, Asda*	1 Slice/47g	109	0.9	233	9.0	45.0	1.9	2.2
White, Brace's*	1 Med Sl/31.7g	73	0.5	227	9.6	43.4	1.7	2.2
White, Classic, Med Sliced, Hovis*	1 Slice/37.9g	91	0.9	240	11.4	40.3	2.3	6.5
White, Classic, Thick Sliced, Hovis*	1 Slice/50g	120	2.3	240	9.2	40.5	4.5	3.1
White, COU M & S*	1 Slice/26g	60	0.6	231	10.6	41.9	2.3	4.6
White, Crusty, Finest, Tesco*	1oz/28g	70	0.8	250	8.9	49.0	3.0	2.0
White, Crusty, Gold, Kingsmill*	1 Slice/27g	70	0.8	258	9.4	48.5	2.9	2.7
White, Crusty, Hovis*	1 Slice/44g	103	1.0	233	8.8	44.3	2.2	2.1
White, Crusty, Sliced, Premium, Budgens*	1 Slice/50g	121	1.1	242	8.8	46.9	2.2	2.2
White, Crusty, Sliced Loaf, Tesco*	1 Slice/50g	117	1.1	233	7.4	46.0	2.1	2.0
White, Danish, Med Sliced, BFY, Morrisons*	1 Slice/17g	42	0.3	245	10.2	49.1	1.8	2.2
White, Danish, Sliced, Weight Watchers*	1 Slice/19g	45	0.3	238	10.5	45.8	1.4	2.3
White, Danish, Warburton's*	1 Slice/25.8g	61	0.4	238	10.5	45.8	1.4	2.3
White, Extra Thick Sliced, Kingsmill*	1 Slice/58g	135	1.4	232	8.8	43.8	2.4	2.8
White, Farmhouse, Hovis*	1 Slice/44g	99	0.7	226	8.2	44.6	1.6	3.2
White, Farmhouse, Seeded, Waitrose*	1 Serving/75g	192	4.1	256	10.8	40.9	5.5	5.6
White, Farmhouse, Soft, Warburton's*	1 Slice/26g	61	0.7	236	9.9	43.4	2.5	2.7
White, Farmhouse Crusty, M & S*	1 Slice/34g	82	0.7	240	8.9	46.6	2.2	3.0
White, Farmhouse Gold Premium, Morrisons*	1 Slice/38g	90	0.5	236	8.9	47.4	1.2	2.2
White, Fried in Blended Oil	1 Slice/28g	141	9.0	503	7.9	48.5	32.2	1.6
White, High Fibre, Nimble*	1 Slice/22g	48	0.4	219	10.1	40.6	1.8	7.5

B

BREAD

Measure INFO/WEIGHT	per Measure KCAL	FAT	Nutrition Values per 100g / 100ml KCAL	PROT	CARB	FAT	FIBRE

	Measure INFO/WEIGHT	per Measure KCAL	FAT	KCAL	PROT	CARB	FAT	FIBRE
White, Invisible Crust, Hovis*	1 Slice/40g	90	0.6	226	8.8	44.1	1.6	2.4
White, Loaf, Crusty, Premium, Warburton's*	1 Slice/30.5g	76	0.7	249	10.6	46.5	2.3	2.6
White, Loaf, Danish, Asda*	1 Serving/22.5g	52	0.5	236	9.0	45.0	2.2	2.0
White, Med, Stayfresh, Tesco*	1 Slice/45g	108	0.7	240	8.2	47.8	1.5	3.0
White, Med Sliced	1 Med Slice/39g	93	0.6	238	7.5	48.5	1.6	1.8
White, Med Sliced, Asda*	1 Slice/36.7g	80	0.6	218	8.0	43.0	1.5	3.3
White, Med Sliced, Basics, Sainsbury's*	1 Slice/35.9g	83	0.5	231	8.0	46.4	1.5	2.1
White, Med Sliced, Budgens*	1 Slice/35.8g	82	0.6	229	8.0	45.6	1.6	3.0
White, Med Sliced, Co-Op*	1 Slice/36g	80	0.6	222	8.3	44.4	1.7	2.8
White, Med Sliced, Great Everyday, Kingsmill*	1 Slice/40g	93	0.8	232	9.0	44.6	2.0	2.7
White, Med Sliced, Long Life, Asda*	1 Slice/36g	82	0.6	228	8.0	45.0	1.8	2.7
White, Med Sliced, Makes Sense, Somerfield*	1 Slice/36.3g	81	0.4	226	7.5	46.4	1.2	2.4
White, Med Sliced, Mother's Pride*	1 Slice/36g	82	0.6	229	8.0	45.6	1.6	3.0
White, Med Sliced, Sainsbury's*	1 Slice/36.1g	78	0.7	216	8.7	41.1	1.9	7.1
White, Med Sliced, Sm Loaf, Warburton's*	1 Slice/23g	55	0.4	239	10.3	45.1	1.9	2.7
White, Med Sliced, SmartPrice, Asda*	1 Slice/36g	81	0.5	226	7.0	46.0	1.5	2.8
White, Med Sliced, Soft, Danish, Somerfield*	1 Slice/21g	48	0.3	229	8.6	44.8	1.4	2.4
White, Med Sliced, Stay Fresh, Tesco*	2 Slices/69g	170	1.4	246	8.9	48.1	2.0	0.8
White, Med Sliced, Superlife, Morrisons*	1 Slice/30g	79	1.2	263	9.6	47.4	3.9	2.5
White, Med Sliced, Tesco*	1 Slice/36g	86	0.5	240	8.2	47.8	1.5	3.0
White, Med Sliced, Value, Tesco*	1 Slice/36g	81	0.4	225	7.9	46.1	1.0	2.1
White, Med Sliced, Warburton's*	1 Slice/40.3g	94	0.8	234	9.9	43.8	2.0	2.6
White, Med Sliced, Weight Watchers*	1 Slice/12g	30	0.2	247	12.5	45.2	1.9	3.2
White, Oatmeal, Allinson*	1 Slice/47g	111	1.4	237	9.0	43.5	3.0	2.7
White, Organic, Hovis*	1 Slice/43.9g	108	1.4	246	8.6	45.8	3.2	2.3
White, Organic, M & S*	1 Slice/35g	95	1.7	270	12.1	45.2	4.8	2.2
White, Organic, Sainsbury's*	1 Slice/35.9g	84	0.6	234	8.9	45.5	1.8	2.3
White, Plain, Scottish, Sunblest*	1 Slice/57g	133	1.5	233	10.1	42.3	2.6	2.8
White, Premium Farmhouse, Lidl*	1 Slice/44g	99	0.7	225	7.4	45.4	1.5	2.5
White, Premium Gold, TTD, Sainsbury's*	1 Slice/44g	103	0.8	233	8.4	45.6	1.9	2.2
White, Sandwich, Bakery, Sainsbury's*	1 Slice/50g	121	0.3	242	10.3	49.0	0.6	2.9
White, Sandwich, Kingsmill*	1 Slice/42g	97	1.0	232	8.8	43.8	2.4	2.8
White, Scottish Plain, Mother's Pride*	1 Med Slice/50g	114	0.8	227	8.7	44.6	1.5	3.0
White, Sliced, Gluten & Wheat Free, Sainsbury's*	1 Slice/33g	75	2.8	227	1.9	35.5	8.6	1.0
White, Sliced, Roberts Bakery*	1 Slice/34.9g	87	0.7	249	10.0	48.0	2.1	2.5
White, Sm Loaf, Classic, Hovis*	1 Slice/32.9g	75	0.8	228	11.4	40.3	2.3	6.5
White, Soft, Batch Loaf, Sliced, Tesco*	1 Slice/50g	117	1.1	233	7.5	46.1	2.1	2.1
White, Soft, Farmhouse, M & S*	1 Slice/25g	60	0.8	239	9.8	42.6	3.3	2.5
White, Soft, Gold, Kingsmill*	1 Slice/46.9g	112	1.5	239	8.2	44.5	3.1	2.7
White, Soft, Great Everyday, Thick Sliced, Kingsmill*	1 Slice/47.0g	109	0.9	232	9.0	44.6	2.0	2.7
White, Soft, M & S*	1 Slice/46.7g	105	0.8	225	7.3	46.1	1.7	2.4
White, Soft, Milk Roll, Warburton's*	1 Slice/18g	46	0.5	251	10.8	45.3	3.0	2.8
White, Soft Batch, Sliced, Sainsbury's*	1 Slice/44.0g	102	0.8	232	8.2	45.4	1.9	2.3
White, Soft Crusty, M & S*	1 Slice/25g	64	0.6	256	9.3	49.0	2.5	2.4
White, Softgrain, Sliced, Tesco*	1 Med Slice/36g	81	0.5	224	7.2	45.5	1.5	3.7
White, Square, Extra Thick Sliced, Hovis*	1 Slice/67.1g	155	1.3	231	8.5	44.7	2.0	2.6
White, Square, Med Sliced, Hovis*	1 Slice/40g	92	0.8	231	8.5	44.7	2.0	2.6
White, Square, Thick Sliced, Hovis*	1 Slice/50.2g	116	1.0	231	8.5	44.7	2.0	2.6
White, Square Cut, Kingsmill*	1 Slice/41.8g	97	1.0	232	8.8	43.8	2.4	2.8
White, Stay Fresh, Tesco*	1 Slice/40g	100	1.0	249	8.6	48.3	2.4	1.5
White, Sunblest*	1 Med Slice/33g	77	0.6	232	7.4	46.4	1.9	2.1
White, Super Toastie, Warburton's*	1 Serving/57g	134	1.0	235	10.1	44.6	1.8	2.7
White, Thick, So Organic, Sainsbury's*	1 Slice/44.2g	102	1.0	231	8.2	44.6	2.2	3.1

B

BREAD

INFO/WEIGHT	Measure	per Measure		Nutrition Values per 100g / 100ml				
		KCAL	FAT	KCAL	PROT	CARB	FAT	FIBRE
White, Thick Sliced, Asda*	1 Slice/44g	96	0.7	218	8.0	43.0	1.5	3.3
White, Thick Sliced, Bakers Gold, Asda*	1 Slice/44g	101	0.8	229	8.0	45.0	1.9	2.3
White, Thick Sliced, Brace's*	1 Slice/38.3g	90	0.5	235	9.5	46.6	1.2	2.6
White, Thick Sliced, Budgens*	1 Slice/40g	89	0.5	223	7.4	45.3	1.3	2.5
White, Thick Sliced, Healthy, Warburton's*	1 Slice/38g	84	0.7	222	10.3	41.2	1.8	4.1
White, Thick Sliced, Long Life, Somerfield*	1 Slice/44g	100	0.8	227	7.5	44.9	1.9	2.4
White, Thick Sliced, M & S*	1 Slice/42g	96	0.5	228	7.3	46.7	1.3	2.8
White, Thick Sliced, Organic, Tesco*	1 Slice/44g	108	0.9	245	8.5	46.8	2.1	3.1
White, Thick Sliced, Premium, Tesco*	1 Slice/44.4g	98	0.3	222	8.7	45.2	0.7	1.5
White, Thick Sliced, Sainsbury's*	1 Slice/44g	95	0.8	216	8.7	41.1	1.9	7.1
White, Thick Sliced, Square Cut, Asda*	1 Slice/43.9g	101	0.7	230	8.0	46.0	1.5	2.1
White, Thick Sliced, Staysoft, Rathbones*	2 Slices/76g	173	1.0	228	8.5	45.5	1.3	2.7
White, Thick Sliced, Sunblest*	1 Slice/40g	91	0.6	228	8.0	45.7	1.5	2.8
White, Thick Sliced, Super Toastie, Morrisons*	1 Slice/50g	129	1.5	257	8.7	48.9	3.0	2.1
White, Thick Sliced, Tesco*	1 Slice/44g	106	0.7	240	8.2	47.8	1.5	3.0
White, Thick Sliced, Value, Tesco*	1 Slice/44g	106	0.7	240	8.2	47.8	1.5	3.0
White, Thick Sliced, Warburton's*	1 Slice/28g	65	0.6	233	9.8	43.6	2.1	2.7
White, Thin Sliced, Sainsbury's*	1 Slice/29g	66	0.4	228	7.1	46.4	1.5	2.8
White, Thin Sliced, Tesco*	2 Slices/59g	135	0.8	228	9.5	44.5	1.3	3.4
White, Toasted, Average	1 Med Slice/33g	87	0.5	265	9.3	57.1	1.6	1.8
White, Toastie, 800g Loaf, Warburton's*	1 Slice/47.4g	111	0.9	234	9.9	43.9	1.9	2.5
White, Toastie, Thick, Love to Toast, Kingsmill*	1 Slice/50g	116	1.0	232	9.0	44.6	2.0	2.7
White, Toastie, Thick Cut, Hovis*	1 Slice/50g	115	1.0	230	8.5	44.8	2.0	2.5
White, Weight Watchers*	1 Serving/5g	12	0.1	246	12.3	45.1	1.6	3.3
White, Whole, Kingsmill*	1 Slice/38g	87	1.0	230	9.0	42.9	2.5	3.4
White, Wholesome, Loaf, Sainsbury's*	1 Serving/36g	81	0.7	224	9.4	42.5	1.8	4.4
White, Wholesome, Med Sliced, Asda*	1 Slice/35.0g	78	0.9	223	7.0	43.0	2.6	5.0
White, Wholesome, Med Sliced, Premium, Tesco*	1 Slice/36.6g	86	0.9	232	8.9	43.9	2.3	4.2
White, Wholesome, Thick Sliced, Tesco*	1 Serving/80g	177	1.5	221	10.5	40.5	1.9	4.8
Whole & White, Med Sliced, Sainsbury's*	1 Slice/36g	80	0.9	222	8.9	41.3	2.4	6.2
Whole Grain, Batch, Finest, Tesco*	1oz/28g	71	0.8	254	9.8	47.7	2.7	4.2
Whole Grain, Brennans*	1 Slice/39g	79	0.6	203	9.0	40.0	1.5	4.9
Whole Wheat, Nature's Own*	1 Slice/28g	66	1.0	236	14.3	39.3	3.6	10.7
Wholegrain, & White, Kingsmill*	1 Slice/46.9g	107	1.2	228	9.0	42.3	2.5	4.0
Wholegrain, Med Sliced, Irish Pride*	1 Slice/38g	90	0.8	237	9.2	46.6	2.1	7.6
Wholemeal, & Oat Flakes, Gold, Kingsmill*	1 Slice/46.8g	103	1.6	220	10.0	37.3	3.4	7.0
Wholemeal, Allinson*	1 Slice/47.2g	102	1.4	216	12.5	34.8	3.0	7.4
Wholemeal, Average	1 Slice/25g	54	0.6	215	9.2	41.6	2.5	5.8
Wholemeal, Batch, Organic, Waitrose*	1 Slice/40g	88	1.0	219	10.0	38.8	2.6	7.2
Wholemeal, BGTY, Sainsbury's*	1 Slice/20g	41	0.2	207	12.6	36.8	1.0	7.3
Wholemeal, Brennans*	1 Slice/40g	76	0.8	190	8.6	36.2	1.9	8.0
Wholemeal, COU, M & S*	1 Slice/21g	45	0.5	213	13.6	33.7	2.6	7.0
Wholemeal, Crusty, Finest, Tesco*	1 Slice/50g	103	0.9	206	10.8	37.0	1.7	6.9
Wholemeal, Crusty, Kingsmill*	1 Slice/42g	104	1.8	247	11.2	41.1	4.2	7.0
Wholemeal, Danish, BFY, Morrisons*	1 Slice/17g	39	0.3	228	11.2	47.9	1.8	6.2
Wholemeal, Danish, Warburton's*	1 Slice/25g	57	0.6	229	13.3	38.5	2.4	7.2
Wholemeal, Economy, Sainsbury's*	1 Slice/28g	61	0.7	217	10.3	38.4	2.5	6.5
Wholemeal, Farmhouse, Hovis*	1 Slice/44g	91	1.0	207	11.0	36.0	2.2	7.1
Wholemeal, Farmhouse Gold, Organic, Morrisons*	1 Slice/35g	67	0.9	191	8.0	34.0	2.6	5.1
Wholemeal, Farmhouse Soft Golden, M & S*	1 Slice/30g	65	0.9	215	11.0	35.1	3.1	7.4
Wholemeal, Fresher for Longer, Sainsbury's*	1 Slice/44.1g	98	1.6	222	10.9	36.2	3.7	6.5
Wholemeal, Gold, Kingsmill*	1 Slice/44g	95	1.3	217	10.9	36.8	2.9	7.0
Wholemeal, Golden, M & S*	1 Slice/30.2g	65	0.9	215	11.0	35.1	3.1	7.4

BREAD

INFO/WEIGHT	Measure	per Measure		Nutrition Values per 100g / 100ml				
		KCAL	FAT	KCAL	PROT	CARB	FAT	FIBRE
Wholemeal, Golden Wheat, Kingsmill*	1 Slice/44g	97	1.3	221	10.9	37.8	2.9	6.0
Wholemeal, Greggs*	1 Slice/36g	77	0.9	215	9.2	41.6	2.5	5.8
Wholemeal, Loaf, Crusty, Farmhouse, M & S*	1 Serving/32.6g	76	0.9	230	10.1	40.7	2.7	6.3
Wholemeal, Longer Life, Sainsbury's*	1 Med Slice/36g	85	1.2	237	10.7	41.0	3.4	6.2
Wholemeal, Makes Sense, Somerfield*	1 Slice/36g	78	0.8	217	10.7	38.6	2.2	6.6
Wholemeal, Med, 400g Loaf, Warburton's*	1 Slice/23.8g	55	0.6	231	10.4	40.7	2.5	6.5
Wholemeal, Med, 800g Loaf, Warburton's*	1 Slice/40.3g	93	1.0	231	10.2	39.6	2.5	6.5
Wholemeal, Med Slice, Co-Op*	1 Slice/36g	75	0.7	208	8.3	38.9	1.9	5.6
Wholemeal, Med Sliced, Asda*	1 Slice/36g	80	1.2	223	9.0	39.0	3.4	6.0
Wholemeal, Med Sliced, Great Everyday, Kingsmill*	1 Slice/40g	91	1.5	227	10.5	37.7	3.8	6.2
Wholemeal, Med Sliced, Hovis*	1 Slice/40g	91	0.9	228	11.4	40.3	2.3	6.5
Wholemeal, Med Sliced, M & S*	1 Slice/40g	80	1.2	200	10.5	32.7	3.1	6.7
Wholemeal, Med Sliced, Morrisons*	1 Slice/32g	68	0.8	214	9.9	38.0	2.5	5.8
Wholemeal, Med Sliced, Organic, Asda*	1 Slice/43.3g	93	1.0	217	9.0	40.0	2.3	6.0
Wholemeal, Med Sliced, Organic, Tesco*	2 Slices/53g	111	1.5	209	9.2	37.2	2.8	6.0
Wholemeal, Med Sliced, Premium, Tesco*	2 Slices/72g	141	0.4	196	9.8	37.8	0.6	7.2
Wholemeal, Med Sliced, Sainsbury's*	1 Slice/36g	77	0.9	214	10.3	37.8	2.4	7.4
Wholemeal, Med Sliced, Tesco*	1 Slice/36g	81	0.8	225	11.0	39.1	2.2	6.6
Wholemeal, Med Sliced, The Village Bakery*	1 Slice/33g	69	0.7	209	9.8	38.0	2.0	6.0
Wholemeal, Med Sliced, Waitrose*	1 Slice/35.7g	77	0.9	213	10.1	37.6	2.4	7.0
Wholemeal, Multigrain, Sliced, Finest, Tesco*	1 Serving/50g	123	2.1	246	10.1	42.1	4.1	6.5
Wholemeal, Multigrain, Soft Batch, Sainsbury's*	1 Slice/44g	106	2.9	242	11.3	34.5	6.5	5.6
Wholemeal, Multiseed, Orgainic, Sainsbury's*	1 Slice/26g	75	2.5	289	13.8	36.6	9.7	6.0
Wholemeal, Nimble*	1 Slice/20g	44	0.5	219	12.2	37.0	2.5	6.8
Wholemeal, Organic, 400g Loaf, Warburton's*	1 Slice/28.2g	63	0.9	223	10.3	37.9	3.2	6.7
Wholemeal, Organic, Hovis*	1 Slice/44g	92	1.3	209	10.2	35.6	2.9	7.6
Wholemeal, Organic, M & S*	1 Slice/34.1g	75	1.5	220	10.4	34.1	4.3	7.6
Wholemeal, Premium, Thick Slice, M & S*	1 Slice/50g	95	1.5	190	9.8	30.8	3.0	6.4
Wholemeal, Rustic, Tin, Tesco*	1 Slice/37g	92	1.3	249	12.2	44.0	3.5	3.1
Wholemeal, Sliced, Gluten Free, Glutano*	1 Slice/56g	107	1.7	191	7.0	34.0	3.0	0.0
Wholemeal, Sm Loaf, Hovis*	1 Slice/32.9g	75	0.8	228	11.4	40.3	2.3	6.5
Wholemeal, Soft, Med Sliced, Morrisons*	1 Slices/30.6g	72	0.7	235	10.2	42.0	2.4	6.8
Wholemeal, Stayfresh, Tesco*	2 Slices/68.9g	155	1.5	225	11.0	39.1	2.2	6.0
Wholemeal, Stoneground, 800g Loaf, Warburton's*	1 Slice/45.3g	95	1.2	210	10.4	35.8	2.7	6.8
Wholemeal, Stoneground, Organic, Sainsbury's*	1 Slice/29g	61	0.6	210	10.2	37.9	1.9	7.8
Wholemeal, Stoneground, Organic, Waitrose*	1 Sm Slice/25g	57	0.9	228	10.8	38.2	3.6	7.1
Wholemeal, Stoneground, Thick Sliced, Sainsbury's*	1 Slice/43.8g	92	0.8	210	10.2	37.9	1.9	7.8
Wholemeal, Thick Sliced, 800g Loaf, Tesco*	1 Slice/44g	99	1.0	225	11.0	39.1	2.2	6.6
Wholemeal, Thick Sliced, Asda*	1 Slice/43.8g	91	1.0	208	10.0	37.0	2.2	6.0
Wholemeal, Thick Sliced, Bakers Gold, Asda*	1 Slice/44g	99	1.4	225	12.0	37.0	3.2	6.0
Wholemeal, Thick Sliced, COU, M & S*	1 Slice/26g	56	0.7	215	13.6	33.7	2.6	7.0
Wholemeal, Thick Sliced, Great Everyday, Kingsmill*	1 Slice/44.1g	100	1.7	227	10.5	37.7	3.8	6.2
Wholemeal, Thick Sliced, HL, Co-Op*	1 Slice/44g	95	0.9	215	11.0	38.0	2.0	7.0
Wholemeal, Thick Sliced, Hovis*	1 Slice/50g	114	1.2	228	11.4	40.3	2.3	6.5
Wholemeal, Thick Sliced, Organic, Tesco*	1 Slice/44g	98	1.2	220	8.8	38.8	2.8	5.9
Wholemeal, Thick Sliced, Premium, Tesco*	1 Serving/44g	95	0.7	214	10.0	40.1	1.5	5.7
Wholemeal, Thick Sliced, Sainsbury's*	1 Slice/44g	94	1.1	214	10.3	37.8	2.4	7.4
Wholemeal, Thick Sliced, Waitrose*	1 Slice/44g	94	1.1	213	10.1	37.6	2.4	7.0
Wholemeal, Toasted, Average	1 Med Slice/26g	58	0.6	224	8.6	42.3	2.2	5.8
Wholemeal, Toastie, 800g Loaf, Warburton's*	1 Slice/45.1g	101	1.1	224	9.7	39.3	2.4	6.6
Wholemeal, Unsliced, Organic, Dove's Farm*	1 Med Slice/35g	73	0.9	208	8.5	40.5	2.5	6.4
Wholemeal, Value, Tesco*	1 Slice/36g	78	0.9	217	10.3	38.4	2.5	6.5

B

	Measure INFO/WEIGHT	per Measure KCAL	FAT	Nutrition Values per 100g / 100ml KCAL	PROT	CARB	FAT	FIBRE
BREAD & BUTTER PUDDING								
5% Fat, M & S*	1 Pudding/237g	367	10.0	155	4.4	24.8	4.2	0.4
Average	1 Portion/190g	304	14.8	160	6.2	17.5	7.8	0.3
BGTY, Sainsbury's*	1 Serving/120g	121	2.8	101	6.3	13.4	2.3	5.4
Finest, Tesco*	1 Serving/153g	379	22.0	248	4.9	24.6	14.4	0.9
Individual, M & S*	1 Pudding/130g	280	16.4	215	4.4	21.4	12.6	0.5
Sainsbury's*	½ Pudding/115g	223	11.2	194	4.8	21.9	9.7	0.4
Sticky Toffee, M & S*	1oz/28g	83	3.0	295	4.1	46.3	10.6	2.2
Tesco*	½ Pack	494	31.8	250	5.0	20.8	16.1	0.4
BREAD MIX								
Brown, Sunflower, Sainsbury's*	1 Serving/60g	151	3.7	251	10.0	38.9	6.1	4.0
Cheese & Onion, Dry Mix, Sainsbury's*	1 Serving/100g	311	2.8	311	11.9	59.5	2.8	2.6
Crusty White, Made Up, Tesco*	1 Slice/126g	316	2.3	251	9.4	49.3	1.8	2.5
Focaccia, Garlic & Herb, Asda*	1 Serving/125g	385	10.0	308	11.0	48.0	8.0	3.3
Italian Ciabatta, Sainsbury's*	1 Slice/45g	96	0.9	213	8.7	40.0	2.0	2.4
Mixed Grain, Sainsbury's*	1 Serving/45g	103	0.7	228	7.7	46.0	1.5	4.4
Sun Dried Tomato & Parmesan, Sainsbury's*	1 Serving/100g	247	1.7	247	8.1	50.1	1.7	2.5
White Loaf, Asda*	1 Slice/60g	150	0.9	250	10.0	49.0	1.5	3.1
Wholemeal, Crusty, Tesco*	1 Serving/45g	95	1.0	210	8.8	38.2	2.2	7.8
BREADCRUMBS								
Average	1oz/28g	98	0.5	350	10.8	74.8	1.9	2.6
BREADFRUIT								
Canned, Drained	1oz/28g	18	0.1	66	0.6	16.4	0.2	1.7
Raw	1oz/28g	27	0.1	95	1.3	23.1	0.3	0.0
BREADSTICKS								
Asda*	1 Serving/5g	21	0.4	412	12.0	73.0	8.0	2.9
Chive & Onion Twists, Tesco*	3 Twists/24g	115	5.3	480	11.6	57.6	22.1	2.2
GFY, Asda*	1 Breadstick/5g	19	0.1	378	13.7	77.3	1.6	3.8
Grissini, Italian, Sainsbury's*	1 Breadstick/5g	20	0.4	408	11.6	72.9	7.8	2.9
Grissini, Thin, with Olive Oil, Forno Bianco*	1 Stick/5g	21	0.4	420	11.0	77.0	7.5	0.0
Mini, Sainsbury's*	1 Breadstick/2g	8	0.1	404	15.6	68.7	7.4	4.8
Original, Italian, Tesco*	1 Stick/5.5g	23	0.4	410	11.6	72.9	7.8	2.9
Original, Organic, Kallo*	1 Breadstick/6g	24	0.5	393	11.8	69.5	7.6	4.7
PB, Waitrose*	1 Breadstick/5g	20	0.1	378	13.7	77.3	1.6	3.8
Plain, Asda*	1 Stick/5g	21	0.4	412	12.0	73.0	8.0	2.9
Sesame Seed Grissini, Sainsbury's*	1 Breadstick/5g	21	0.6	419	12.7	65.5	11.8	3.2
BREAK POT								
Pasta Break, Tomato & Herb Flavour, Asda*	1 Pot/209.3g	180	1.0	86	2.3	18.0	0.5	1.3
Rice Break, Balti, Asda*	1 Serving/60g	209	1.0	348	13.3	70.0	1.7	0.0
BREAKFAST								
All Day, Kershaws*	1 Pack/280g	392	22.4	140	7.3	9.6	8.0	1.6
All Day, with Baked Beans, Heinz*	1 Pack/403g	463	17.3	115	5.8	13.3	4.3	2.4
Farmhouse, Ready Meals, Waitrose*	½ Pack/250g	385	25.0	154	2.9	11.0	10.0	1.2
Pack, Lorne, Sausage, Asda*	1 Serving/54g	96	7.6	178	6.0	7.0	14.0	0.0
BREAKFAST CEREAL								
3 in One, Raisin & Apple, Jordans*	1 Serving/50g	170	2.2	340	7.6	67.4	4.4	9.8
3 in One, Strawberry, Jordans*	1 Serving/50g	181	2.9	362	9.4	68.0	5.8	11.9
Advantage, Weetabix*	1 Serving/30g	105	0.7	350	10.2	72.0	2.4	9.0
All Bran, Asda*	1 Serving/40g	110	1.4	276	15.0	46.0	3.5	27.0
All Bran, Bran Flakes, & Fruit, Kellogg's*	1 Serving/40g	143	2.4	358	8.0	68.0	6.0	9.0
All Bran, Bran Flakes, Chocolate, Kellogg's*	1 Serving/30g	106	1.8	354	10.0	65.0	6.0	13.0
All Bran, Bran Flakes, Kellogg's*	1 Serving/30g	98	0.6	326	10.7	67.0	2.0	15.0
All Bran, Bran Flakes, Yoghurty, Kellogg's*	1 Serving/40g	141	2.0	353	10.0	67.0	5.0	12.0
All Bran, Fibre Plus, Kellogg's*	1 Serving/40g	112	1.4	280	14.0	48.0	3.5	27.0

B

BREAKFAST CEREAL

	Measure INFO/WEIGHT	per Measure KCAL	FAT	Nutrition Values per 100g / 100ml				
				KCAL	PROT	CARB	FAT	FIBRE
All Bran, Fruitful, Kellogg's*	1 Serving/40g	136	3.0	340	12.5	57.5	7.5	0.0
All Bran, High Fibre, Morrisons*	1 Serving/40g	109	1.4	273	14.8	45.5	3.5	27.0
All Bran, Original, High Fibre, Kellogg's*	1 Serving/40g	112	1.4	280	14.0	48.0	3.5	27.0
Apple & Cinnamon Flakes, M & S*	1 Serving/30g	111	0.6	370	6.0	82.7	1.9	3.4
Apricot Wheats, Whole Grain, Tesco*	1 Serving/40g	130	0.6	326	7.6	70.6	1.4	8.0
Balance, Sainsbury's*	1 Serving/30g	111	0.5	370	11.4	77.7	1.5	3.2
Balance with Red Fruit, Sainsbury's*	1 Serving/40g	148	0.8	369	9.9	78.1	1.9	3.1
Banana & Toffee Crisp, Mornflake*	1 Serving/30g	133	4.8	443	5.7	68.8	16.1	5.4
Benefit Flakes, Harvest Morn*	1 Serving/40g	148	0.6	370	11.4	77.7	1.5	3.2
Berries, Cherries & Flakes, COU, M & S*	1 Serving/40g	152	0.8	380	8.5	82.2	1.9	3.2
Blackberry & Apple, Alpen*	1 Serving/40g	140	1.5	349	9.2	69.4	3.8	8.3
Bran Flakes, Asda*	1 Serving/47g	157	1.5	333	11.0	65.0	3.2	14.0
Bran Flakes, Crunchy Nut, Sainsbury's*	1 Serving/40g	203	3.8	508	19.8	85.8	9.5	11.0
Bran Flakes, HL, Tesco*	1 Serving/30g	101	0.7	335	10.2	67.0	2.4	14.1
Bran Flakes, Honey Nut, Tesco*	1 Serving/40g	143	1.8	358	9.6	70.0	4.4	11.0
Bran Flakes, Morrisons*	1 Serving/25g	83	0.8	331	11.1	64.6	3.2	14.5
Bran Flakes, Organic, Asda*	1 Serving/30g	99	0.7	330	10.0	67.0	2.4	14.0
Bran Flakes, Organic, Sainsbury's*	1 Serving/30g	100	0.7	332	10.2	67.4	2.4	14.1
Bran Flakes, Organic, Tesco*	1 Serving/30g	101	0.7	335	10.2	67.4	2.4	13.8
Bran Flakes, Sultana, Dry, Sainsbury's*	1 Serving/30g	98	0.6	325	8.3	68.6	1.9	12.1
Bran Flakes, Sultana Bran, Kellogg's*	1 Serving/30g	95	0.6	318	8.0	67.0	2.0	13.0
Bran Flakes, Tesco*	1 Serving/30g	99	0.7	331	10.2	67.1	2.4	14.1
Bran Flakes, Value, Tesco*	1 Serving/50g	160	1.2	320	11.4	63.2	2.4	17.1
Bran Flakes, Whole Grain, Sainsbury's*	1 Serving/30g	99	0.7	331	10.2	67.1	2.4	14.1
Breakfast Biscuits, Aldi*	4 Biscuits/60g	213	1.5	355	13.7	69.5	2.5	7.5
Caribbean Crunch, Alpen*	1 Serving/40g	155	3.6	388	8.8	67.9	9.0	4.6
Cheerios, Honey Nut, Nestle*	1 Serving/40g	150	1.5	374	7.0	78.3	3.7	5.2
Cheerios, Nestle*	1 Serving/40g	148	1.6	369	8.1	75.2	3.9	6.6
Choco Crackles, Morrisons*	1 Serving/30g	115	0.7	383	5.5	84.8	2.4	1.9
Choco Flakes, Asda*	1 Serving/50g	187	0.4	374	6.0	86.0	0.7	2.6
Choco Flakes, Kellogg's*	1 Serving/30g	114	0.9	380	5.0	84.0	3.0	2.5
Choco Hoops, Aldi*	1 Serving/30g	116	1.4	385	7.0	79.1	4.5	0.0
Choco Hoops, Asda*	1 Serving/40g	154	1.8	385	7.0	79.0	4.5	4.0
Choco Snaps, Asda*	1 Serving/30g	115	0.7	382	5.0	85.0	2.4	1.9
Choco Snaps, Tesco*	1 Serving/30g	115	0.7	383	5.5	84.8	2.4	1.9
Choco Squares, Asda*	1 Serving/30g	130	4.2	434	10.0	67.0	14.0	4.0
Chocolate Crisp, Minis, Weetabix*	1 Serving/36g	134	1.9	371	9.0	71.7	5.3	8.5
Chocolate Wheats, Kellogg's*	1 Serving/40g	148	3.6	369	10.0	62.0	9.0	12.0
Cinnamon Grahams, Nestle*	1 Serving/40g	164	3.9	411	4.7	76.1	9.8	4.2
Clusters, Nestle*	1 Serving/40g	149	2.3	372	9.4	70.6	5.8	8.4
Coco Pops, Crunchers, Kellogg's*	1 Serving/30g	114	1.1	380	7.0	81.0	3.5	3.0
Coco Pops, Kellogg's*	1 Serving/30g	116	0.9	387	5.0	85.0	3.0	2.0
Coco Pops, Mega Munchers, Kellogg's*	1 Serving/30g	113	0.8	375	8.0	80.0	2.5	4.5
Coco Pops, Straws, Kellogg's*	1 Tube/12.6g	58	1.9	459	9.0	72.0	15.0	2.0
Coco Snaps, Value, Tesco*	1 Serving/30g	117	0.7	390	7.0	84.1	2.4	2.4
Corn Flakes, Asda*	1 Serving/30g	111	0.2	370	7.0	84.0	0.7	3.0
Corn Flakes, Co-Op*	1 Serving/30g	113	0.3	375	8.0	84.0	1.0	1.0
Corn Flakes, Crispy Nut, Asda*	1 Serving/30g	117	1.3	390	7.0	81.0	4.2	2.5
Corn Flakes, Hint of Honey, Kellogg's*	1 Serving/30g	113	0.2	377	6.0	87.0	0.6	2.5
Corn Flakes, Honey Nut, Morrisons*	1 Serving/30g	116	1.3	387	7.1	80.0	4.3	3.0
Corn Flakes, Honey Nut, Sainsbury's*	1 Serving/30g	119	1.4	397	7.4	81.7	4.5	2.5
Corn Flakes, Honey Nut, Tesco*	1 Serving/30g	118	1.3	392	7.4	81.2	4.2	2.5
Corn Flakes, Kellogg's*	1 Serving/30g	112	0.3	372	7.0	84.0	0.9	3.0

B

BREAKFAST CEREAL

INFO/WEIGHT	Measure	per Measure		Nutrition Values per 100g / 100ml				
		KCAL	FAT	KCAL	PROT	CARB	FAT	FIBRE
Corn Flakes, Morrisons*	1 Serving/30g	111	0.2	371	7.3	83.8	0.7	3.0
Corn Flakes, Organic, Whole Earth*	1 Serving/40g	154	0.4	386	8.6	84.2	1.0	3.0
Corn Flakes, Sainsbury's*	1 Serving/25g	93	0.2	371	7.3	83.8	0.7	3.0
Corn Flakes, Tesco*	1 Serving/25g	93	0.2	371	7.3	83.8	0.7	3.0
Country Crisp, Four Nut Combo, Jordans*	1 Serving/50g	240	12.4	480	8.9	55.4	24.7	6.9
Country Crisp, Raspberries, Jordans*	1 Serving/50g	215	7.9	429	7.5	64.1	15.8	7.1
Country Crisp, Strawberries, Jordans*	1 Serving/40g	171	6.3	428	7.5	64.1	15.7	7.1
Country Crisp, Wild Berries, Jordans*	1 Serving/50g	222	7.9	443	7.5	68.0	15.7	5.7
Cranberry Wheats, Tesco*	1 Serving/40g	130	0.6	325	7.3	70.9	1.4	7.7
Crispy Rice & Wheat Flakes, Asda*	1 Serving/50g	185	0.8	370	11.0	78.0	1.5	3.2
Crunchy Bran, Weetabix*	1 Serving/40g	122	1.4	306	11.9	56.6	3.6	20.0
Crunchy Nut, Clusters, Kellogg's*	1 Serving/40g	174	6.3	435	8.0	67.0	15.7	5.0
Crunchy Nut, Corn Flakes, Kellogg's*	1 Serving/30g	118	1.2	392	6.0	83.0	4.0	2.5
Crunchy Oat with Tropical Fruits, Tesco*	1 Serving/35g	146	4.8	417	7.8	65.3	13.8	6.1
Crunchy Oats, Tropical Fruits, Jordans*	1 Serving/75g	319	11.0	425	8.1	65.4	14.6	6.7
Crunchy Rice & Wheat Flakes, Co-Op*	1 Serving/30g	111	0.6	370	11.0	78.0	2.0	3.0
Eat Natural*	1 Serving/40g	180	10.0	450	12.0	45.0	25.0	6.0
Fitnesse & Fruits, Nestle*	1 Serving/40g	148	0.4	370	6.6	83.4	1.1	3.4
Frosted Flakes, Sainsbury's*	1 Serving/30g	112	0.1	374	4.9	87.8	0.4	2.4
Frosted Flakes, Tesco*	1 Serving/30g	112	0.1	374	4.9	87.8	0.4	2.4
Frosted Wheats, Kellogg's*	1 Serving/30g	104	0.6	346	10.0	72.0	2.0	9.0
Frosties, Kellogg's*	1 Serving/30g	111	0.2	371	4.5	87.0	0.6	2.0
Frosties, Reduced Sugar, Kellogg's*	1 Serving/30g	111	0.2	369	6.0	85.0	0.6	2.5
Fruit & Fibre, Asda*	1 Serving/35g	129	2.3	368	8.0	69.1	6.6	7.7
Fruit & Fibre, Flakes, Waitrose*	1 Serving/40g	143	2.5	357	8.2	67.2	6.2	9.9
Fruit & Fibre, Harvest Morn*	1 Serving/30g	109	1.7	363	8.7	69.0	5.7	8.0
Fruit & Fibre, Lidl*	1 Serving/25g	91	1.2	363	8.8	70.9	4.9	8.0
Fruit & Fibre, Morrisons*	1 Serving/30g	110	2.2	366	8.8	66.5	7.2	8.5
Fruit & Fibre, Somerfield*	1 Serving/40g	144	2.4	361	8.1	68.7	6.0	8.9
Fruit & Fibre, Tesco*	1 Serving/30g	111	2.0	370	8.0	69.1	6.6	7.7
Fruit & Fibre, Value, Tesco*	1 Serving/40g	144	2.2	359	11.4	65.7	5.6	8.0
Fruit & Fibre, Whole Grain, Sainsbury's*	1 Serving/30g	108	1.8	361	8.1	68.7	6.0	8.9
Fruit & Nut Crisp, Minis, Weetabix*	1 Serving/36g	129	1.7	359	9.3	70.0	4.6	8.9
Fruit 'n' Fibre, Kellogg's*	1 Serving/40g	143	2.4	358	8.0	68.0	6.0	9.0
Fruit Nuts & Flakes, M & S*	1 Serving/30g	117	2.6	391	9.1	69.6	8.5	3.5
Golden Honey Puffs, Tesco*	1 Serving/30g	115	0.4	382	6.6	86.3	1.2	3.0
Golden Nuggets, Nestle*	1 Serving/40g	152	0.3	381	6.2	87.4	0.7	1.5
Granola, Low Fat, Home Farm*	1 Serving/55g	180	3.0	328	7.3	69.0	5.4	9.0
Granola, Quaker*	1 Serving/48g	210	7.0	438	10.4	72.9	14.6	6.3
Granola, Superfoods, Jordans*	1 Serving/50g	208	6.7	415	9.0	64.7	13.4	8.6
Grape Nuts, Kraft*	1 Serving/45g	155	0.9	345	11.5	70.0	2.0	11.0
Hawaiian Crunch, Asda*	1 Serving/50g	221	8.5	441	8.0	64.0	17.0	6.0
Hawaiian Crunch, Mornflake*	1 Serving/60g	247	7.4	411	8.1	66.8	12.4	6.8
Hi-Fibre Bran, Tesco*	1 Serving/40g	110	1.4	275	14.7	45.5	3.5	27.0
High Fibre Bran, Co-Op*	1 Serving/40g	110	1.6	275	15.0	46.0	4.0	27.0
High Fibre Bran, Sainsbury's*	1 Serving/40g	109	1.4	272	14.7	45.5	3.5	27.0
High Fibre Bran, Tesco*	1 Serving/40g	28	0.4	275	14.7	45.5	3.5	27.0
Honey & Nut Crisp, Mini, Weetabix*	1 Serving/36g	132	1.8	368	9.9	70.6	5.1	9.0
Honey Loops, Kellogg's*	1 Serving/30g	110	0.9	367	8.0	77.0	3.0	6.0
Hoops, Multigrain, Asda*	1 Serving/30g	113	1.2	376	6.5	78.4	4.0	4.6
Hoops, Multigrain, Tesco*	1 Serving/30g	113	1.1	375	6.5	78.6	3.8	4.6
Hot Oat, Harvest Morn*	1 Serving/40g	142	3.3	356	11.6	58.8	8.3	8.9
Hot Oats, Instant, Tesco*	1 Serving/30g	108	2.6	360	11.8	58.4	8.7	7.9

BREAKFAST CEREAL

	Measure INFO/WEIGHT	per Measure KCAL	FAT	Nutrition Values per 100g / 100ml KCAL	PROT	CARB	FAT	FIBRE
Just Right, Kellogg's*	1 Serving/40g	145	1.0	363	7.0	78.0	2.5	4.5
Malt Crunchies, Co-Op*	1 Serving/50g	168	1.0	335	10.0	69.0	2.0	10.0
Malted Wheaties, Asda*	1 Serving/50g	171	1.5	342	10.0	69.0	2.9	10.0
Malted Wheats, Waitrose*	1 Serving/32g	110	0.6	343	9.7	71.7	1.9	9.9
Malties, Sainsbury's*	1 Serving/40g	137	1.2	343	10.0	69.2	2.9	10.0
Malty Flakes, with Red Berries, Tesco*	1 Serving/30g	111	0.6	369	9.9	78.1	1.9	3.1
Malty Flakes with Rasberries, M & S*	1 Serving/40g	148	1.4	370	7.4	77.5	3.5	3.2
Maple & Pecan, Crisp, Asda*	1 Serving/30g	135	5.7	451	8.0	62.0	19.0	6.0
Maple & Pecan, Sainsbury's*	1 Serving/60g	318	13.2	530	13.3	69.7	22.0	5.3
Maple & Pecan Crisp, Sainsbury's*	1 Serving/50g	226	9.8	452	7.9	61.3	19.5	5.4
Maple & Pecan Crisp, Tesco*	1 Serving/50g	215	7.6	430	10.5	62.5	15.2	10.2
Maple Frosted Flakes, Whole Earth*	1 Serving/30g	113	0.3	375	6.2	85.6	1.0	1.6
Mini Wheats, Sainsbury's*	1 Serving/45g	157	1.0	348	11.8	69.9	2.3	11.8
Minibix, Weetabix*	1 Serving/40g	134	1.5	335	8.8	71.2	3.8	8.1
Muddles, Kellogg's*	1 Serving/30g	110	1.1	368	8.0	76.0	3.5	8.0
Muesli, Base, Nature's Harvest*	1 Serving/50g	179	2.6	358	11.0	71.2	5.1	7.4
Muesli, COU, M & S*	1 Serving/60g	201	1.5	335	7.6	70.2	2.5	8.1
Muesli, Crunchy, Organic, Sainsbury's*	1 Serving/40g	168	5.8	420	10.6	62.0	14.4	9.2
Muesli, Crunchy Bran, Nature's Harvest*	1 Serving/50g	176	5.0	352	8.8	62.9	9.9	6.4
Muesli, Fruit, 55%, Asda*	1 Serving/35g	111	1.0	318	6.0	67.0	2.9	7.0
Muesli, Fruit, GFY, Asda*	1 Serving/50g	152	0.9	304	8.0	64.0	1.8	10.0
Muesli, Fruit, Luxury, Weight Watchers*	1 Serving/40g	127	0.8	318	7.2	67.7	2.0	8.1
Muesli, Fruit, Sainsbury's*	1 Serving/40g	132	1.8	330	8.1	64.3	4.5	9.6
Muesli, Fruit, Tesco*	1 Serving/50g	173	2.4	345	7.4	67.2	4.8	5.0
Muesli, Fruit, Waitrose*	1 Serving/30g	101	1.4	338	7.2	66.8	4.7	6.8
Muesli, Fruit & Bran, Unsweetened, M & S*	1 Serving/50g	160	1.6	320	8.2	64.8	3.1	8.3
Muesli, Fruit & Nut, 55%, Asda*	1 Serving/40g	151	5.6	378	9.0	54.0	14.0	7.0
Muesli, Fruit & Nut, COU, M & S*	1 Serving/40g	128	1.1	320	7.4	74.5	2.8	7.4
Muesli, Fruit & Nut, Jordans*	1 Serving/50g	189	5.9	378	7.3	60.6	11.8	6.7
Muesli, Fruit & Nut, Luxury, Co-Op*	1 Serving/40g	150	4.0	375	8.0	64.0	10.0	6.0
Muesli, Fruit & Nut, Luxury, Lidl*	1 Serving/57g	205	5.6	360	8.0	60.0	9.8	7.5
Muesli, Fruit & Nut, Luxury, M & S*	1 Serving/40g	140	3.1	350	7.7	62.2	7.7	7.3
Muesli, Fruit & Nut, Luxury, Waitrose*	1 Serving/40g	145	3.8	363	9.0	60.3	9.5	6.5
Muesli, Fruit & Nut, M & S*	1 Serving/40g	128	1.1	320	7.4	74.5	2.8	7.4
Muesli, Fruit & Nut, Organic, M & S*	1 Serving/50g	167	3.0	333	8.2	61.6	6.0	7.6
Muesli, Fruit & Nut, Sainsbury's*	1 Serving/30g	121	5.2	402	10.4	51.3	17.2	9.2
Muesli, Fruit & Nut, Tesco*	1 Serving/50g	190	5.7	380	8.4	60.3	11.3	5.3
Muesli, Fruit & Nut, Traidcraft*	1 Serving/28g	100	2.2	358	10.0	63.0	8.0	6.0
Muesli, HL, Tesco*	1 Serving/40g	133	0.9	333	6.9	71.1	2.3	5.3
Muesli, Less Than 3% Fat, BGTY, Sainsbury's*	1 Serving/50g	164	1.0	328	6.7	71.0	1.9	5.4
Muesli, Luxury, Jordans*	1 Serving/40g	154	5.0	384	9.6	58.4	12.5	8.2
Muesli, Luxury Fruit, Harvest Morn*	1 Serving/50g	158	1.7	315	6.8	64.5	3.3	6.9
Muesli, Luxury Fruit, Sainsbury's*	1 Serving/50g	162	1.7	324	7.1	66.4	3.3	7.0
Muesli, No Added Sugar, Waitrose*	1 Serving/40g	146	2.5	364	12.0	64.9	6.3	6.7
Muesli, Organic, Waitrose*	1 Serving/50g	188	0.8	375	10.3	59.6	1.6	8.3
Muesli, Original, Sainsbury's*	1 Serving/60g	226	5.0	376	9.3	65.7	8.4	7.1
Muesli, Really Nutty, Dorset Cereals*	1 Serving/70g	253	6.1	362	9.8	61.1	8.7	6.3
Muesli, Simply Delicious, Dorset Cereals*	1 Serving/70g	256	6.7	366	10.8	59.2	9.5	7.4
Muesli, Special, Fruit, Jordans*	1 Serving/50g	162	1.4	323	6.6	68.0	2.7	8.4
Muesli, Special, Jordans*	1 Serving/40g	146	4.3	366	7.9	59.5	10.7	8.5
Muesli, Super High Fibre, Dorset Cereals*	1 Serving/60g	214	5.6	357	8.0	60.1	9.4	8.4
Muesli, Superfoods, Jordans*	1 Serving/50g	173	3.7	346	9.2	60.9	7.3	10.2
Muesli, Swiss, Bettabuy, Morrisons*	1 Serving/50g	170	2.5	340	11.0	62.8	5.0	9.4

BREAKFAST CEREAL

	Measure INFO/WEIGHT	per Measure KCAL	FAT	Nutrition Values per 100g / 100ml KCAL	PROT	CARB	FAT	FIBRE
Muesli, Swiss, Harvest Morn*	1 Serving/50g	180	3.3	359	9.8	65.3	6.5	8.3
Muesli, Swiss, Organic, Whole Earth*	1 Serving/50g	170	3.3	340	10.5	59.5	6.6	9.6
Muesli, Swiss, Sainsbury's*	1 Serving/50g	181	2.9	361	9.2	68.1	5.8	7.1
Muesli, Swiss, SmartPrice, Asda*	1 Serving/60g	222	3.6	370	9.0	70.0	6.0	10.0
Muesli, Swiss, Waitrose*	1 Serving/40g	144	2.3	361	9.2	68.1	5.8	7.1
Muesli, Swiss, with Fruit, Tesco*	1 Serving/40g	144	2.1	360	10.4	67.4	5.3	7.4
Muesli, Tropical, Tesco*	1 Serving/50g	173	2.4	346	7.8	68.2	4.7	9.1
Muesli, Unsweetened, M & S*	1 Serving/40g	129	1.1	322	8.1	68.0	2.7	9.4
Muesli, Value, Tesco*	1 Serving/50g	163	2.6	325	10.7	58.3	5.1	14.9
Muesli, Whole Wheat, Sainsbury's*	1 Serving/40g	144	3.2	359	11.5	60.5	7.9	8.5
Muesli, Wild-Berry, Amaranth, Allos*	1 Serving/40g	160	4.2	401	12.5	63.3	10.6	4.3
Multi Fruit & Flake, COU, M & S*	1 Serving/39g	142	0.4	365	6.5	81.8	1.1	4.0
Multigrain, Balanced Lifestyle, Aldi*	1 Serving/30g	108	0.7	360	7.5	77.1	2.4	4.5
Multigrain, Fitnesse, Nestle*	1 Serving/30g	109	0.4	363	8.0	79.8	1.3	5.1
Nesquik, Chocolatey Corn & Rice, Nestle*	1 Serving/30g	114	1.2	380	7.2	79.1	3.9	5.1
No Added Sugar, Alpen*	1 Serving/40g	142	2.4	354	10.5	64.6	6.0	7.7
Nutty Crunch, Alpen*	1 Serving/40g	159	4.5	398	10.7	63.6	11.2	6.5
Nutty Crunch, Deliciously, M & S*	1 Serving/50g	238	11.3	476	8.8	59.6	22.5	4.4
Oat, Crunchy, Sainsbury's*	1 Serving/50g	227	10.2	453	8.2	59.3	20.3	6.6
Oat Crisp, Quaker*	1 Serving/30g	109	2.0	364	10.6	60.8	6.8	12.7
Oat Granola, Quaker*	1 Bowl/50g	206	4.4	411	8.6	73.0	8.8	5.2
Oat Krunchies, Quaker*	1 Serving/30g	118	2.1	393	9.5	72.0	7.0	5.5
Oatibix, Bitesize, Original, Weetabix*	1 Serving/36g	133	2.4	370	10.6	66.5	6.8	10.1
Oatibix, Weetabix*	2 Biscuits/48g	181	3.8	377	12.5	63.7	8.0	7.3
Oats, Golden Syrup, Made Up, Tesco*	1 Serving/199g	226	4.6	114	4.0	19.1	2.3	1.2
Oats, Jumbo, Organic, Waitrose*	1 Serving/50g	181	4.1	361	11.0	61.1	8.1	7.8
Oats, Original, Instant, Hot, Waitrose*	1 Sachet/27g	97	2.2	359	11.0	60.4	8.1	8.5
Oats, Ready, Asda*	1 Serving/30g	108	2.7	361	12.0	58.0	9.0	8.0
Oats, Superfast, Mornflake*	1 Serving/40g	144	3.2	359	11.0	60.4	8.1	8.5
Oats, Tesco*	1 Serving/40g	142	3.2	356	11.0	60.0	8.0	8.0
Oatso Simple, Fruit Muesli, Quaker*	1 Sachet/39g	136	2.3	348	8.0	66.1	5.8	6.8
Oatso Simple, Golden Syrup, Quaker*	1 Sachet/36g	132	2.2	366	8.4	68.7	6.2	6.8
Oatso Simple, Original, Quaker*	1 Sachet/27g	98	2.3	363	11.1	60.0	8.5	9.3
Optimum Power, Nature's Path*	1 Serving/30g	109	2.0	363	15.3	60.0	6.7	12.6
Organic, Weetabix*	2 Biscuits/35g	116	0.8	331	10.9	66.8	2.2	11.0
Original, Ready Brek*	1 Serving/40g	144	3.5	359	11.8	58.5	8.7	7.9
Perfect Balance, Weight Watchers*	1 Serving/30g	90	0.5	300	7.8	63.3	1.7	15.6
Porridge, Chocolate, Oatibix, Weetabix*	1 Pack/40.1g	149	3.9	372	9.9	61.3	9.7	6.2
Porridge, Free From, Sainsbury's*	1 Serving/50g	174	1.5	348	8.6	72.0	3.0	3.4
Porridge, Instant, Quaker*	1 Serving/34g	124	2.9	364	11.0	60.0	8.5	9.0
Porridge, Multigrain, Jordans*	1 Serving/40g	134	2.2	335	10.4	60.9	5.5	10.0
Porridge, Original, Oatibix, Weetabix*	1 Sachet/30g	104	2.5	347	12.5	55.6	8.3	10.1
Porridge, Original, Simply Porridge, Asda*	1 Sachet/27g	96	2.2	356	11.0	60.0	8.0	8.0
Porridge, Ready Made, COU, M & S*	1 Pot/200g	180	4.4	90	3.9	13.3	2.2	0.9
Porridge, Superfoods, Jordans*	1 Serving/40g	145	3.6	362	10.4	59.8	9.0	8.3
Porridge, Take Heart, Quaker*	1 Serving/32g	194	5.7	606	30.9	80.3	17.8	7.8
Porridge Flakes, Organic, Barkat*	1 Serving/30g	109	0.9	362	8.5	74.1	3.0	0.0
Porridge Oats, Co-Op*	1 Serving/40g	144	3.2	360	12.0	61.0	8.0	9.0
Porridge Oats, Dry Weight, Value, Tesco*	1 Serving/50g	180	4.1	359	11.0	60.4	8.1	8.5
Porridge Oats, Mornflake*	1 Serving/50g	180	4.1	359	11.0	60.4	8.1	8.5
Porridge Oats, Organic, Jordans*	1 Serving/45g	164	4.2	364	11.7	58.4	9.3	9.0
Porridge Oats, Organic, Tesco*	1 Serving/28g	100	2.3	358	11.0	60.4	8.1	8.5
Porridge Oats, Original, Scotts*	1 Serving/45g	160	3.6	356	11.0	60.0	8.0	9.0

BREAKFAST CEREAL

	Measure INFO/WEIGHT	per Measure		Nutrition Values per 100g / 100ml				
		KCAL	FAT	KCAL	PROT	CARB	FAT	FIBRE
Porridge Oats, Quaker*	1 Serving/40g	142	3.2	356	11.0	60.0	8.0	4.0
Porridge Oats, Quick, M & S*	1 Serving/40g	148	3.5	370	14.2	58.4	8.7	8.2
Porridge Oats, Quick & Easy, Morrisons*	1 Serving/40g	144	3.2	359	11.0	60.4	8.1	8.5
Porridge Oats, Rolled, Tesco*	1 Serving/50g	180	4.1	359	11.0	60.4	8.1	8.5
Porridge Oats, Scottish, Tesco*	1 Serving/50g	180	4.1	359	11.0	60.4	8.1	8.5
Porridge Oats, SmartPrice, Asda*	1 Serving/50g	178	4.0	356	11.0	60.0	8.0	8.0
Porridge Oats, So Easy, Scotts*	1 Serving/30g	109	2.6	364	11.0	60.0	8.5	9.0
Porridge Oats, Somerfield*	1 Serving/40g	154	2.8	385	12.0	68.0	7.0	0.0
Porridge Oats, Whole Oats, Jordans*	1 Serving/40g	146	3.7	364	11.7	58.4	9.3	9.0
Porridge Oats, with Wheat Bran, Tesco*	1 Serving/50g	167	3.6	334	12.3	55.0	7.2	13.0
Porridge Oats & Bran, Co-Op*	1 Serving/40g	141	2.8	353	12.5	60.0	7.0	12.0
Puffed Wheat, Quaker*	1 Serving/15g	49	0.2	328	15.3	62.4	1.3	5.6
Puffed Wheat, Tesco*	1 Serving/28g	104	0.9	373	13.9	72.2	3.2	5.7
Quaker Oats Crunch, Quaker*	1 Serving/40g	146	2.0	366	9.1	71.1	5.0	7.4
Raisin, Bran Flakes, Asda*	1 Serving/50g	166	1.5	331	7.0	69.0	3.0	10.0
Raisin, Honey & Almond Crunch, Asda*	1 Serving/60g	220	6.8	366	9.2	56.6	11.4	15.5
Raisin & Almond, Crunchy, Jordans*	1 Serving/56g	230	7.0	411	8.4	66.0	12.5	5.0
Raisin & Coconut, Crunchy, Jordans*	1 Serving/40g	165	5.4	412	8.4	64.2	13.5	7.1
Raisin Wheats, Kellogg's*	1 Serving/30g	99	0.6	330	9.0	70.0	2.0	8.0
Raisin Wheats, Sainsbury's*	1 Serving/50g	166	0.8	332	8.2	71.5	1.5	8.0
Ready Brek, Original, Weetabix*	1 Serving/40g	158	3.5	395	11.8	58.4	8.7	7.9
Rice Krispies, Honey, Kellogg's*	1 Serving/30g	114	0.2	380	4.0	89.0	0.7	1.0
Rice Krispies, Kellogg's*	1 Serving/30g	114	0.3	381	6.0	87.0	1.0	1.0
Rice Krispies, Multigrain Shapes, Kellogg's*	1 Serving/30g	111	0.8	370	8.0	77.0	2.5	8.0
Rice Pops, Sainsbury's*	1 Serving/30g	114	0.4	381	7.4	84.8	1.3	1.5
Rice Snaps, Asda*	1 Serving/28g	105	0.4	376	7.0	84.0	1.3	1.5
Rice Snaps, Tesco*	1 Serving/35g	135	0.5	385	7.4	84.8	1.3	1.5
Ricicles, Kellogg's*	1 Serving/30g	114	0.2	381	4.5	89.0	0.8	0.8
Right Balance, Morrisons*	1 Serving/50g	181	1.1	362	6.9	78.6	2.2	5.3
Shredded Wheat, Bitesize, Nestle*	1 Serving/45g	158	1.2	350	11.8	69.9	2.6	11.9
Shredded Wheat, Fruitful, Nestle*	1 Serving/40g	140	2.1	351	8.8	67.2	5.2	3.7
Shredded Wheat, Honey Nut, Nestle*	1 Serving/40g	151	2.6	378	11.2	68.8	6.5	9.4
Shredded Wheat, Nestle*	2 Biscuits/45g	153	1.1	340	11.6	67.8	2.5	11.8
Shredded Wheat, Triple Berry, Nestle*	1 Serving/40g	138	0.8	344	10.6	70.6	2.1	11.1
Shreddies, Coco, Nestle*	1 Serving/45g	161	0.9	358	8.4	76.5	2.0	8.6
Shreddies, Frosted, Kellogg's*	1 Serving/50g	162	0.9	323	0.7	78.5	1.8	4.7
Shreddies, Frosted, Nestle*	1 Serving/45g	164	0.7	365	7.4	80.7	1.5	6.4
Shreddies, Malt Wheats, Tesco*	1 Serving/45g	151	0.9	335	8.3	70.7	2.1	9.7
Shreddies, Nestle*	1 Bowl/50g	176	1.0	351	9.9	73.7	1.9	9.8
Special Crunchy Luxury, Jordans*	1 Serving/50g	206	7.0	411	7.6	63.8	13.9	6.5
Special Flakes, Tesco*	1 Serving/20g	74	0.3	371	11.0	78.4	1.5	4.3
Special K, Choco, Kellogg's*	1 Serving/40g	160	2.8	400	14.0	70.0	7.0	3.5
Special K, Kellogg's*	1 Serving/30g	112	0.3	373	16.0	75.0	1.0	2.5
Special K, Peach & Apricot, Kellogg's*	1 Serving/30g	112	0.3	373	14.0	77.0	1.0	2.5
Special K, Purple Berries, Kellogg's*	1 Serving/30g	112	0.3	374	13.0	77.0	1.0	3.5
Special K, Red Berries, Kellogg's*	1 Serving/30g	112	0.3	373	14.0	77.0	1.0	3.0
Special K, Yoghurty, Kellogg's*	1 Serving/30g	115	0.9	383	14.0	75.0	3.0	2.5
Start, Kellogg's*	1 Serving/30g	113	0.8	375	8.0	80.0	2.5	5.0
Strawberry & Almond Crunch, M & S*	1 Serving/40g	186	7.4	465	8.0	66.0	18.6	4.9
Strawberry Crisp, Asda*	1 Serving/30g	129	4.7	431	8.1	64.7	15.5	5.9
Strawberry Crisp, Tesco*	1 Serving/50g	200	5.3	400	10.2	66.2	10.5	10.2
Sugar Puffs, Quaker*	1 Serving/30g	116	0.3	387	6.5	86.5	1.0	3.0
Sultana Bran, Asda*	1 Serving/30g	98	0.9	327	9.0	66.0	3.0	11.0

	Measure INFO/WEIGHT	per Measure KCAL	FAT	Nutrition Values per 100g / 100ml KCAL	PROT	CARB	FAT	FIBRE
BREAKFAST CEREAL								
Sultana Bran, Co-Op*	1 Serving/40g	130	1.2	325	9.0	66.0	3.0	11.0
Sultana Bran, HL, Tesco*	1 Serving/30g	98	0.6	325	8.2	68.0	1.9	12.0
Sultana Bran, Morrisons*	1 Serving/30g	98	0.9	325	8.8	65.8	3.0	11.4
Sultana Bran, Sainsbury's*	1 Serving/30g	97	0.6	324	8.2	68.6	1.9	11.6
Sultana Bran, Somerfield*	1 Serving/30g	97	0.6	324	8.2	68.6	1.9	11.6
Sultana Bran, Waitrose*	1 Serving/30g	97	0.6	324	8.2	68.6	1.9	11.6
Superfoods, Breakfast Flakes, Jordans*	1 Bowl/75g	256	3.1	341	8.7	67.2	4.1	11.3
Triple Chocolate Crisp, Sainsbury's*	1 Serving/40g	180	7.3	451	7.7	63.8	18.3	6.0
Triple Chocolate Crunch, M & S*	1 Serving/50g	228	10.1	455	8.6	60.0	20.1	6.2
Vitality, Asda*	1 Serving/30g	111	0.5	370	11.0	78.0	1.5	3.2
Vitality, with Red Fruit, Asda*	1 Serving/30g	110	0.5	366	11.0	77.0	1.6	3.8
Weetaflakes, Weetabix*	1 Serving/30g	102	0.4	340	8.9	72.9	1.4	11.0
Weetos, Chocolate, Weetabix*	1 Serving/30g	113	1.5	378	8.4	75.1	4.9	5.8
Wheat Biscuits, HE, Tesco*	2 Biscuits/37.5g	127	0.8	338	11.5	68.4	2.0	10.0
Wheat Biscuits, Morrisons*	2 Biscuits/38g	129	1.0	340	11.2	67.6	2.7	10.5
Wheat Biscuits, Sainsbury's*	1 Biscuit/15g	51	0.3	342	11.5	68.4	2.0	10.0
Wheat Biscuits, Somerfield*	2 Biscuits/38g	129	1.0	339	11.2	67.6	2.7	10.5
Wheat Flakes, Alpen*	1 Serving/40g	140	1.0	350	10.2	72.0	2.4	9.0
Whole Wheat Biscuits, Waitrose*	2 Biscuits/37g	124	0.7	336	11.8	68.0	1.9	10.1
Whole Wheat Bisks, Asda*	2 Biscuits/37.5g	127	0.8	338	11.5	68.4	2.0	10.0
Yoghurt & Raspberry, Crisp, Sainsbury's*	1 Serving/45g	199	7.4	442	7.5	66.0	16.4	5.4
BRESAOLA								
Della Valtellina, Sainsbury's*	1 Slice/14g	23	0.4	163	34.7	0.1	2.6	0.1
Finest, Tesco*	1 Serving/35g	64	1.4	182	36.0	0.5	4.0	0.0
M & S*	1oz/28g	56	1.9	200	34.6	0.0	6.8	0.0
BRIE								
French, Mild, Waitrose*	1 Serving/30g	90	7.2	300	21.0	0.0	24.0	0.0
BROCCOLI								
& Cauliflower, Floret Mix, Fresh, Tesco*	1 Portion/75g	26	0.7	34	3.9	2.5	0.9	2.7
& Cauliflower, Floret Mix, Iceland*	1 Serving/100g	26	0.7	26	2.6	2.2	0.7	2.4
& Cheese, Morrisons*	1 Pack/350g	406	24.9	116	6.2	6.6	7.1	0.8
Cauliflower & Carrots, Frozen, Great Value, Asda*	1 Serving/100g	25	0.6	25	2.2	2.6	0.6	5.0
Green, Boiled, Average	1 Serving/90g	22	0.7	24	3.1	1.1	0.8	2.3
Green, Raw, Average	1 Serving/17g	5	0.1	31	3.7	2.1	0.8	2.4
Purple Sprouting, Boiled, Average	1 Serving/90g	17	0.5	19	2.1	1.3	0.6	2.3
Purple Sprouting, Raw	1oz/28g	10	0.3	35	3.9	2.6	1.1	3.5
Tenderstem, Finest, Tesco*	½ Pack/100g	31	0.2	31	4.2	3.2	0.2	3.1
BROWN SAUCE								
Asda*	1 Serving/10g	10	0.0	97	0.7	23.0	0.2	0.4
Bottled	1 Tsp/6g	6	0.0	99	1.1	25.2	0.0	0.7
Iceland*	1 Serving/20g	16	0.0	82	0.7	19.3	0.2	1.1
Tesco*	1 Tsp/10g	10	0.0	104	0.7	25.1	0.1	0.6
BROWNIES								
Chocolate, Belgian, Starbucks*	1 Slice/75g	318	16.2	424	4.8	53.2	21.6	1.3
Chocolate, Cadbury*	1 Brownie/36g	145	5.7	403	6.1	59.7	15.8	0.0
Chocolate, Chewy, M & S*	1 Brownie/28.6g	132	6.1	455	6.5	59.8	21.1	2.0
Chocolate, Chunky, Belgian, M & S*	1 Brownie/55g	242	11.2	440	6.2	57.7	20.3	2.5
Chocolate, Fudgy, M & S*	1 Brownie/87g	400	21.9	460	4.8	56.9	25.2	3.0
Chocolate, Gu*	1 Brownie/45g	200	12.0	444	6.7	44.4	26.6	5.0
Chocolate, Mini Bites, Asda*	1 Brownie/15g	62	3.0	420	5.0	55.0	20.0	1.4
Chocolate, Sainsbury's*	1 Brownie/60g	265	13.6	442	4.6	55.0	22.6	1.6
Chocolate, Slices, M & S*	1 Brownie/36g	158	8.7	440	5.3	51.1	24.1	1.3
Chocolate, Tesco*	1 Brownie/46g	201	9.8	438	6.6	55.1	21.2	1.5

B

	Measure INFO/WEIGHT	per Measure KCAL	FAT	Nutrition Values per 100g / 100ml KCAL	PROT	CARB	FAT	FIBRE
BROWNIES								
Chocolate, Topped with M & M's, McVitie's*	1 Brownie/79.4g	355	17.5	447	4.6	57.7	22.0	0.0
Chocolate, Waitrose*	1 Brownie/45g	192	8.9	426	6.3	55.6	19.8	2.7
Chocolate, Weight Watchers*	1 Brownie/47g	143	1.8	304	4.8	62.5	3.8	3.2
Chocolate Orange, Organic, The Village Bakery*	1 Brownie/30g	126	6.7	421	5.0	50.5	22.2	0.9
Double Chocolate, Mini Bites, Sainsbury's*	1 Bite/15g	49	2.5	326	5.8	38.9	16.4	1.6
Praline, Mini, Finest, Tesco*	1 Brownie/12g	59	3.1	492	4.2	60.0	25.8	0.8
BRUSCHETTA								
Cheese & Cranberry, Brunchetta, Golden Vale*	1 Pack/95g	200	8.6	211	8.2	24.8	9.0	1.3
Pane Italia*	1 Serving/75g	367	18.8	489	12.4	53.6	25.1	1.4
Ploughman's Relish, Brunchetta, Golden Vale*	1 Pack/90g	261	15.5	290	14.2	20.2	17.2	1.6
Red Pepper & Onion, Brunchetta, Golden Vale*	1 Pack/90g	266	17.1	296	14.6	17.0	19.0	1.3
Safeway*	¼ Pack/115g	420	6.7	365	11.8	65.5	5.8	2.8
Toasted, Olive Oil & Sea Salt, Tesco*	1 Serving/30g	126	4.7	420	11.5	58.7	15.5	4.5
BRUSSELS SPROUTS								
& Sweet Chestnuts, Asda*	1 Serving/100g	73	1.7	73	3.1	11.0	1.7	4.2
Boiled, Average	1 Serving/90g	32	1.2	35	3.1	3.2	1.3	3.5
Button, Raw, Average	1oz/28g	10	0.4	37	3.5	2.9	1.3	3.2
Canned, Drained	1oz/28g	8	0.3	28	2.6	2.4	1.0	2.6
Raw, Average	1oz/28g	10	0.3	37	3.5	3.3	1.1	3.0
BUBBLE & SQUEAK								
Aunt Bessie's*	1 Serving/100g	145	7.1	145	2.7	17.5	7.1	1.3
Fried in Vegetable Oil	1oz/28g	35	2.5	124	1.4	9.8	9.1	1.5
Morrisons*	1 Serving/110g	168	9.6	153	2.2	16.3	8.7	0.7
Safeway*	1 Serving/200g	160	6.6	80	1.8	10.7	3.3	1.4
Tesco*	½ Pack/325g	293	12.7	90	1.6	11.3	3.9	0.9
Waitrose*	½ Pack/225g	167	5.2	74	1.4	11.9	2.3	2.2
BUCKWHEAT								
Average	1oz/28g	102	0.4	364	8.1	84.9	1.5	2.1
BULGAR WHEAT								
Dry Weight, Average	1oz/28g	99	0.5	353	9.7	76.3	1.7	8.0
BUNS								
American, Safeway*	1 Bun/60.1g	152	2.6	253	8.9	44.5	4.4	3.7
Bath, M & S*	1 Bun/71g	217	5.7	305	8.3	49.8	8.0	1.9
Belgian, Asda*	1 Bun/133g	464	19.9	350	4.8	49.0	15.0	2.2
Belgian, Co-Op*	1 Bun/118g	413	15.3	350	5.0	54.0	13.0	2.0
Belgian, Dairy Cream, Somerfield*	1 Serving/120.8g	401	13.4	331	5.2	52.6	11.1	2.0
Belgian, Sainsbury's*	1 Bun/110g	398	11.3	362	6.1	61.3	10.3	1.9
Belgian, Tesco*	1 Bun/123g	438	15.7	356	5.2	54.9	12.8	2.2
Burger, American Style, Sainsbury's*	1 Bun/50g	131	2.1	261	10.5	45.6	4.1	3.6
Burger, Cheese & Onion Topped, Finest, Tesco*	1 Serving/105g	309	10.0	294	10.2	41.9	9.5	2.8
Burger, Giant, Sainsbury's*	1 Bun/95g	249	4.9	262	8.7	45.2	5.2	2.9
Burger, Sainsbury's*	1 Bun/56g	154	2.9	275	9.2	47.8	5.2	4.1
Burger, Sesame, American Style, Sainsbury's*	1 Serving/60g	162	3.8	270	7.3	46.2	6.3	2.2
Burger, Sesame, Sliced, Tesco*	1 Bun/60g	168	4.0	280	7.9	47.3	6.6	2.1
Burger, with Sesame Seeds, Co-Op*	1 Bun/55g	143	2.8	260	9.0	44.0	5.0	2.0
Chelsea	1 Bun/78g	285	10.8	366	7.8	56.1	13.8	1.7
Chelsea, Sainsbury's*	1 Bun/85g	239	4.4	281	6.9	51.6	5.2	2.9
Chelsea, Tesco*	1 Bun/85g	269	6.5	316	7.9	53.9	7.6	2.3
Choux, Caramel, Asda*	1 Bun/189g	745	51.0	394	4.3	33.5	27.0	1.3
Choux, Custard, M & S*	1 Bun/85g	234	18.7	275	4.2	15.0	22.0	0.3
Choux, Fresh Cream, Tesco*	1 Bun/95g	340	23.7	358	4.9	28.5	24.9	0.9
Choux, M & S*	1oz/28g	89	6.2	317	5.4	25.6	22.2	0.3
Currant	1 Bun/60g	178	4.5	296	7.6	52.7	7.5	0.0

	Measure INFO/WEIGHT	per Measure KCAL	per Measure FAT	Nutrition Values per 100g / 100ml KCAL	PROT	CARB	FAT	FIBRE
BUNS								
Currant, Sainsbury's*	1 Bun/72g	197	3.7	274	7.0	50.0	5.1	2.8
Dairy Cream, Somerfield*	1 Bun/98g	304	10.7	310	6.0	46.9	10.9	0.0
Fruit, Waitrose*	1 Bun/54g	155	2.3	287	8.1	54.0	4.3	1.6
Hevva, Somerfield*	1 Bun/75g	298	12.0	397	5.4	57.8	16.0	1.5
Hot Cross	1 Bun/50g	155	3.4	310	7.4	58.5	6.8	1.7
Hot Cross, 25% Reduced Fat, Asda*	1 Bun/60.5g	152	1.4	253	9.0	49.0	2.3	3.0
Hot Cross, Apple & Cinnamon, M & S*	1 Bun/71g	170	1.2	240	7.6	48.7	1.7	3.1
Hot Cross, Asda*	1 Bun/60g	190	3.8	317	10.0	55.0	6.3	3.3
Hot Cross, BGTY, Sainsbury's*	1 Bun/70g	160	1.6	229	7.6	44.4	2.3	2.7
Hot Cross, Classics, M & S*	1 Bun/65g	159	1.2	245	8.5	49.1	1.8	2.2
Hot Cross, Co-Op*	1 Bun/60g	165	3.6	275	8.0	47.0	6.0	3.0
Hot Cross, Finest, Tesco*	1 Bun/75g	210	4.1	280	7.8	49.5	5.4	2.8
Hot Cross, Fruity, TTD, Sainsbury's*	1 Bun/72g	201	4.8	279	6.9	47.9	6.7	3.8
Hot Cross, HE, Tesco*	1 Bun/60g	155	1.5	258	8.6	50.3	2.5	2.6
Hot Cross, HL, Tesco*	1 Serving/70g	176	1.9	251	6.7	50.3	2.7	2.6
Hot Cross, Less Than 3% Fat, M & S*	1 Bun/70g	175	1.3	250	8.1	49.8	1.8	2.2
Hot Cross, Luxury, M & S*	1 Bun/79g	201	3.2	255	8.6	46.2	4.0	2.1
Hot Cross, Mini, M & S*	1 Bun/37.3g	91	0.7	245	8.5	49.1	1.8	2.2
Hot Cross, Mini, Tesco*	1 Bun/36g	99	2.0	274	7.9	48.1	5.5	2.7
Hot Cross, Morrisons*	1 Bun/62g	164	2.6	265	7.1	50.0	4.2	2.6
Hot Cross, Reduced Fat, GFY, Asda*	1 Bun/61g	136	1.3	223	8.0	43.0	2.1	2.4
Hot Cross, Sainsbury's*	1 Bun/67.8g	158	1.3	233	7.1	47.0	1.9	3.9
Hot Cross, Somerfield*	1 Bun/60g	151	3.2	252	8.0	43.0	5.3	2.4
Hot Cross, Tesco*	1 Bun/70g	186	1.9	265	7.4	51.8	2.7	3.6
Hot Cross, Wholemeal, Organic, Tesco*	1 Bun/55g	140	2.7	254	7.6	44.8	4.9	4.5
Hot Cross, Wholemeal, Tesco*	1 Bun/69.4g	170	1.7	245	9.0	46.1	2.4	5.6
Iced, Filled with Raspberry Jam, M & S*	1 Bun/48.4g	154	3.2	320	6.4	58.9	6.6	1.9
Iced, Sainsbury's*	1 Bun/39.8g	127	3.1	319	4.4	57.9	7.7	2.3
Iced, Spiced Fruit, M & S*	1 Bun/90g	270	3.3	300	7.0	60.3	3.7	1.5
Iced, Tesco*	1 Bun/35g	117	3.4	334	7.0	54.8	9.6	2.5
Iced & Spiced Soft, M & S*	1 Bun/90g	270	3.3	300	7.0	60.3	3.7	1.5
Iced Finger, Tesco*	1 Bun/95g	314	8.1	330	55.5	56.8	8.5	1.7
Vanilla Iced, Soft, M & S*	1 Bun/41g	131	3.3	320	7.6	54.9	8.0	2.9
White, Stay Fresh, Tesco*	1 Bun/56g	152	3.7	271	7.5	45.5	6.6	0.0
BURGERS								
Aberdeen Angus, Virgin Trains*	1 Burger/240g	695	37.6	290	13.5	23.8	15.7	0.0
Aberdeen Angus Beef, Mega, Birds Eye*	1 Burger/101g	279	22.6	276	16.3	2.4	22.4	0.1
American Style, Asda*	1 Burger/41.7g	157	10.9	374	25.0	10.0	26.0	1.1
American Style, Tesco*	1 Burger/125g	250	9.1	200	13.0	20.4	7.3	3.9
Beef, 100%, Birds Eye*	1 Burger/41g	120	10.2	292	17.3	0.0	24.8	0.0
Beef, 100%, Grilled, Tesco*	1 Burger/88g	250	18.4	284	16.3	6.8	20.9	0.6
Beef, 100%, Half Pounders, Sainsbury's*	1 Burger/147.6g	463	33.2	313	26.0	1.7	22.4	0.2
Beef, 100%, Mega, Birds Eye*	1 Burger/95.6g	281	23.9	293	17.3	0.0	24.9	0.0
Beef, 100%, Quarter Pounders, Aldi*	1 Burger/114g	320	23.3	282	24.3	0.1	20.5	1.3
Beef, 100%, Quarter Pounders, Prime, Asda*	1 Burger/113g	316	19.0	280	31.5	0.6	16.8	0.8
Beef, 100%, Quarter Pounders, Ross*	1 Burger/73.8g	223	18.9	301	16.8	1.1	25.5	0.0
Beef, 100%, Sainsbury's*	1 Burger/44g	133	10.4	302	21.4	0.9	23.6	0.9
Beef, 100%, Somerfield*	1 Burger/113.5g	329	27.4	289	17.0	1.0	24.0	0.0
Beef, 100%, with Seasoning, No Onion, Birds Eye*	1 Burger/41g	134	11.9	326	16.1	0.2	29.0	0.0
Beef, 100%, without Onion, Sainsbury's*	1 Burger/43g	133	10.4	308	21.9	0.8	24.1	0.8
Beef, 100% Pure, Ross*	1 Burger/56g	128	9.6	229	17.1	1.4	17.1	0.0
Beef, Aberdeen Angus, Asda*	1 Burger/112g	249	13.3	222	22.2	6.7	11.9	0.9
Beef, Aberdeen Angus, Finest, Tesco*	1 Burger/130g	280	17.3	215	17.6	5.4	13.3	0.8

BURGERS

	Measure INFO/WEIGHT	per Measure KCAL	FAT	Nutrition Values per 100g / 100ml KCAL	PROT	CARB	FAT	FIBRE
Beef, Aberdeen Angus, Fresh, Waitrose*	1 Burger/113g	269	21.0	238	16.4	1.2	18.6	0.0
Beef, Aberdeen Angus, M & S*	1 Burger/142g	298	18.9	210	18.3	4.1	13.3	0.1
Beef, Asda*	1 Burger/114g	304	18.6	267	26.8	3.2	16.3	0.7
Beef, Barbecue, New York Style, Tesco*	1oz/28g	64	6.2	227	12.5	7.1	22.1	0.2
Beef, Barbecue, Tesco*	1 Burger/113.5g	259	19.8	227	16.4	1.3	17.4	1.2
Beef, BGTY, Sainsbury's*	1 Burger/110g	177	6.1	161	20.8	7.1	5.5	1.1
Beef, Chargrill, Tesco*	1 Burger/113.5g	247	18.5	217	17.0	0.8	16.2	2.5
Beef, Chargrilled, Quarter Pounder, Morrisons*	1 Burger/227g	590	45.2	260	15.0	5.3	19.9	0.2
Beef, Farmfoods*	1 Burger/50g	128	9.8	255	14.4	5.4	19.6	0.1
Beef, Flame Grilled, Dalepak*	1 Burger/44g	131	11.2	304	15.3	2.1	26.0	0.4
Beef, Frozen, Safeway*	1 Burger/44g	123	8.9	279	21.3	1.3	20.2	0.0
Beef, Giant Chargrilled, Farmfoods*	1 Burger/170g	352	21.8	207	17.3	5.6	12.8	1.2
Beef, in a Bun, HE, Tesco*	1 Pack/189g	282	2.5	149	13.6	20.7	1.3	2.1
Beef, Mega, Birds Eye*	1 Burger/109g	300	25.1	275	14.3	2.7	23.0	0.3
Beef, Morrisons*	1 Burger/56.7g	170	14.4	298	12.3	5.5	25.2	0.6
Beef, Organic, M & S*	1 Burger/110g	239	17.6	217	18.2	0.0	16.0	0.2
Beef, Organic, Tesco*	1 Burger/84g	134	6.8	160	17.9	3.7	8.1	0.5
Beef, Original & Best, Birds Eye*	1 Burger/45.6g	115	8.9	252	14.1	5.1	19.5	0.4
Beef, Quarter Pound, Somerfield*	1 Burger/113.9g	295	20.6	259	20.9	3.0	18.1	0.0
Beef, Quarter Pounder, HL, Tesco*	1 Burger/88g	123	6.0	140	17.4	2.0	6.8	0.7
Beef, Quarter Pounder, Somerfield*	1 Burger/113.9g	295	20.6	259	20.9	3.0	18.1	0.0
Beef, Quarter Pounders, BGTY, Sainsbury's*	1 Burger/83g	171	7.8	205	26.6	3.8	9.3	0.9
Beef, Quarter Pounders, Birds Eye*	1 Burger/113.5g	287	22.2	252	14.1	5.1	19.5	0.4
Beef, Quarter Pounders, Chilled, Morrisons*	1 Burger/115g	228	13.9	198	17.2	4.4	12.1	0.2
Beef, Quarter Pounders, Farmfoods*	1 Burger/113g	289	22.1	256	14.4	5.4	19.6	0.1
Beef, Quarter Pounders, Flame Grilled, Rustlers*	1 Burger/190g	557	28.7	293	14.9	24.3	15.1	0.0
Beef, Quarter Pounders, Flame Grilled, Tesco*	1 Burger/88g	246	20.4	280	13.1	4.8	23.2	0.8
Beef, Quarter Pounders, Good Intentions, Somerfield*	1 Burger/96.3g	183	11.5	191	18.9	1.9	12.0	0.8
Beef, Quarter Pounders, HL, Tesco*	1 Burger/88g	123	6.0	140	17.4	2.0	6.8	0.7
Beef, Quarter Pounders, Morrisons*	1 Burger/113.5g	340	28.7	298	12.3	5.5	25.2	0.6
Beef, Quarter Pounders, Reduced Fat, Tesco*	1 Burger/95g	171	12.4	180	14.0	1.8	13.0	0.8
Beef, Quarter Pounders, Safeway*	1 Burger/100g	227	12.8	227	22.2	5.7	12.8	0.6
Beef, Quarter Pounders, Somerfield*	1 Burger/113.9g	295	20.6	259	20.9	3.0	18.1	0.0
Beef, Quarter Pounders, Steak Country*	1 Burger/68g	188	15.1	276	16.3	2.4	22.2	0.1
Beef, Quarter Pounders, Tesco*	1 Burger/113g	292	23.1	258	17.8	0.7	20.4	1.3
Beef, Quarter Pounders, with Onion, BGTY, Sainsbury's*	1 Burger/83g	171	7.8	205	26.6	3.8	9.3	0.9
Beef, Quarter Pounders, with Onion, Birds Eye*	1 Burger/113.5g	287	22.2	252	14.1	5.1	19.5	0.4
Beef, Quarter Pounders, with Onion, Sainsbury's*	1 Burger/113g	306	22.4	271	18.0	5.1	19.8	1.5
Beef, Sainsbury's*	1 Burger/57g	150	8.9	267	29.6	1.3	15.9	1.5
Beef, Scotch, 5oz, TTD, Sainsbury's*	1 Burger/142g	317	17.0	223	23.7	4.9	12.0	1.4
Beef, Tesco*	1 Burger/47g	120	7.9	255	23.2	0.4	16.8	0.9
Beef, with Herbs, Finest, Tesco*	1 Burger/105.3g	200	11.8	190	17.3	4.5	11.2	0.7
Beef, with Herbs, Grilled, Finest, Tesco*	1 Burger/85g	157	9.4	185	17.1	4.2	11.1	0.5
Beef, with Jalapeno Chilli, Finest, Tesco*	1 Burger/113.5g	205	12.4	181	17.0	3.4	10.9	0.4
Beef, with Onion, Cooked, Ross*	1 Burger/41.2g	116	9.8	284	14.7	2.8	23.8	0.4
Beef, with Peppermix, Danish Crown*	1 Burger/100g	250	19.0	250	19.0	0.0	19.0	0.0
Beef, with Red Onion & Mustard, Finest, Tesco*	1 Burger/130g	308	24.2	237	17.2	0.2	18.6	2.6
Beef & Onion, Grilled, Asda*	1 Burger/81g	201	11.5	248	23.1	6.9	14.2	0.5
Beef with Onion, Sainsbury's*	1 Burger/42g	102	6.2	243	20.7	6.9	14.8	1.0
Cheeseburger, American, Tesco*	1 Burger/275g	660	26.3	240	13.6	24.9	9.6	1.6
Cheeseburger, Bacon, with Bun, Chargrilled, Tesco*	1 Burger/265g	726	42.1	274	13.0	19.6	15.9	1.0
Cheeseburger, Micro Snack, Tesco*	1 Burger/115g	309	14.5	269	12.6	26.4	12.6	0.0
Cheeseburger, SmartPrice, Asda*	1 Burger/150g	374	14.0	249	13.3	28.0	9.3	1.4

BURGERS

	Measure INFO/WEIGHT	per Measure KCAL	FAT	Nutrition Values per 100g / 100ml KCAL	PROT	CARB	FAT	FIBRE
Cheeseburger, with Sesame Seed Bun, Tesco*	1 Burger/275g	644	32.2	234	12.2	20.1	11.7	2.0
Cheeseburger, Wth Relish, American Style, Tesco*	1 Burger/61.4g	131	6.0	215	14.2	17.5	9.8	4.2
Chicken, Breaded, Asda*	1 Burger/55.3g	109	5.0	197	15.0	14.0	9.0	1.6
Chicken, Breaded, Iceland*	1 Burger/58g	142	7.1	245	14.4	19.1	12.3	1.1
Chicken, Crispy Crumb, Farmfoods*	1 Burger/242g	707	45.5	292	10.5	20.2	18.8	1.1
Chicken, Crunch Crumb, Tesco*	1 Burger/57g	161	10.8	282	12.3	15.6	18.9	0.0
Chicken, Fillet, Cajun, Cooked, Birds Eye*	1 Burger/91.5g	129	4.3	140	20.1	4.8	4.7	0.2
Chicken, Fillet, Cajun, Weighed After Cooking, Birds Eye*	1 Burger/91.5g	129	4.3	140	20.1	4.8	4.7	0.2
Chicken, Fresh, Non Coated, Waitrose*	1 Burger/100g	141	4.0	141	16.0	10.4	4.0	0.9
Chicken, in Breadcrumbs, Frozen, Birds Eye*	1 Burger/56g	130	6.9	232	13.8	16.4	12.4	0.3
Chicken, in Bun, Morrisons*	1 Burger/110g	250	4.7	228	12.7	38.1	4.3	3.8
Chicken, in Golden Breadcrumbs, Birds Eye*	1 Burger/56g	130	6.9	232	13.8	16.4	12.4	0.3
Chicken, Quarter Pounders, Birds Eye*	1 Burger/117g	280	16.1	239	13.5	15.2	13.8	0.6
Chicken, Sainsbury's*	1 Burger/46g	115	7.0	247	15.6	12.2	15.1	1.3
Chicken, Southern Fried, Sainsbury's*	1 Burger/52g	154	10.3	297	12.6	17.2	19.8	1.3
Chicken, Spar*	1 Burger/67g	163	7.5	244	16.1	20.8	11.2	1.5
Chicken, with Sesame Seed Bun, Breaded, Tesco*	1 Burger/205g	588	32.2	287	10.2	26.2	15.7	2.9
Chicken Cajun, Fillet, Birds Eye*	1 Pack/180g	275	8.8	153	21.5	5.8	4.9	0.3
Chicken Crunch & Fries, M & S*	1 Pack/425g	915	47.6	215	8.8	20.8	11.2	2.1
Chicken Fillet, Weight After Cooking, Birds Eye*	1 Burger/90g	126	4.1	140	20.0	5.1	4.6	0.2
Chilli, Quarter Pounders, Asda*	1 Burger/87.7g	222	14.1	252	25.0	2.0	16.0	0.0
Chilli, Quarter Pounders, Farmfoods*	1 Burger/115g	285	23.3	248	13.5	2.9	20.3	0.9
Chilli, Quarter Pounders, Iceland*	1 Burger/84g	265	20.1	316	18.6	6.5	23.9	0.4
Classic, Eddie Rockets*	1 Burger/295g	620	35.0	210	10.9	14.9	11.9	0.0
Economy, SmartPrice, Asda*	1 Burger/48.5g	141	10.1	293	14.0	12.0	21.0	1.1
Gemüse, Alnatura*	1 Burger/30g	44	0.8	148	5.1	25.7	2.8	0.0
Hamburger, Tinned, Westlers*	1 Burger/109g	119	6.2	109	5.7	8.8	5.7	0.7
Lamb, Minted, Asda*	1 Burger/100g	234	14.0	234	22.0	4.9	14.0	0.3
Lamb, Minted, Tesco*	1 Burger/113.5g	221	15.2	195	15.2	2.5	13.4	1.2
Lamb, Quarter Pounders, Birds Eye*	1 Burger/112g	232	16.9	207	13.9	3.8	15.1	0.3
Lamb, Quarter Pounders, Farmfoods*	1oz/28g	76	6.1	272	12.3	6.6	21.8	1.0
Lamb, Waitrose*	1 Burger/66.9g	99	4.7	148	15.7	5.4	7.0	0.9
Less Than 7% Fat, Sainsbury's*	1 Burger/102g	164	5.6	161	20.8	7.1	5.5	1.1
Low Fat, Iceland*	1 Burger/85g	148	4.1	174	27.8	5.0	4.8	1.1
Meat Free, Sainsbury's*	1 Burger/57g	86	2.9	151	22.0	4.4	5.0	3.4
Nacho, Chicken & Sweetcorn, Asda*	½ Pack/143.9g	249	13.0	173	14.0	9.0	9.0	2.3
Pork, Quarter Pounders, Birds Eye*	1 Burger/122g	292	23.2	239	13.9	3.2	19.0	0.2
Quarter Pounder, with Onion, Tesco*	1 Burger/87g	213	16.2	245	16.0	3.0	18.6	0.5
Quarter Pounder with Cheese & Buns, Sainsbury's*	1 Burger/198g	471	22.8	238	15.6	19.1	11.5	1.4
Quarter Pounders, 95% Fat Free, Good Choice, Iceland*	1 Burger/86g	150	4.1	174	27.8	5.0	4.8	1.1
Quarter Pounders, Beef, BGTY, Sainsbury's*	1 Burger/113.5g	266	13.1	166	16.9	6.1	8.2	1.0
Quarter Pounders, Big Country*	1 Burger/90g	271	20.8	301	22.1	1.8	23.1	0.0
Quarter Pounders, Chargrilled, BGTY, Sainsbury's*	1 Burger/114g	184	6.3	161	20.8	7.1	5.5	1.1
Quarter Pounders, Highlander*	1 Burger/113.5g	335	26.3	295	21.7	4.2	23.2	0.0
Quarter Pounders, Iceland*	1 Burger/83g	253	18.8	305	20.4	5.1	22.6	0.6
Quarter Pounders, Scotch Beef, Sainsbury's*	1 Burger/113.5g	257	15.5	225	22.2	3.5	13.6	0.5
Quarter Pounders, with Cheese & Bun, Sainsbury's*	1 Burger/198g	471	22.8	238	15.6	19.1	11.5	1.4
Salmon, Quarter Pounders, Morrisons*	1 Burger/109.8g	235	13.0	214	21.4	5.5	11.8	1.7
Salmon, Quarter Pounders, Tesco*	1 Burger/114g	145	2.7	128	15.9	10.6	2.4	1.2
Spicy Bean, Ainsley Harriott*	1 Burger/200g	302	7.5	151	7.3	23.5	3.8	5.2
Spicy Bean, Sainsbury's*	1 Burger/110g	262	13.5	240	5.0	27.1	12.4	2.0
Spreadable, Slightly Salted, Lurpak*	1 Thin Spread/7g	51	5.6	728	1.0	1.0	80.0	0.0
Spreadable, Unsalted, Lurpak*	1 Thin Spread/7g	51	5.6	726	1.0	0.5	80.0	0.0

	Measure INFO/WEIGHT	per Measure KCAL	FAT	Nutrition Values per 100g / 100ml KCAL	PROT	CARB	FAT	FIBRE
BURGERS								
Super Sized Beef, Big Bite, Birds Eye*	1 Burger/122.1g	320	25.2	262	13.1	6.0	20.6	1.0
Tuna, Quarter Pounder, Asda*	1 Burger/113g	212	11.3	188	21.0	3.4	10.0	0.0
Tuna, Quarter Pounders, Sainsbury's*	1 Serving/100g	179	4.8	179	24.0	10.0	4.8	0.4
Tuna, Quarter Pounders, Tesco*	1 Burger/114g	132	1.8	116	18.8	6.7	1.6	0.9
Tuna, Sainsbury's*	1 Serving/105g	194	10.3	185	20.8	3.4	9.8	1.2
Turkey, Crispy Crumb, Bernard Matthews*	1 Burger/71g	222	14.1	313	11.3	19.3	19.8	0.9
Turkey Cheese, Somerfield*	1oz/28g	79	5.0	281	14.0	16.0	18.0	0.0
Turkey Cheeseburgers, Tesco*	1 Burger/105g	252	14.8	240	15.4	12.8	14.1	1.3
Unsalted, Lurpak*	1 Serving/10g	75	8.2	749	1.0	0.8	82.4	0.0
Unsalted, Organic, Yeo Valley*	1 Serving/6g	45	4.9	745	0.6	0.6	82.2	0.0
Value, Farmfoods*	1 Burger/49g	138	10.8	282	11.4	9.6	22.1	0.9
Venison, Finnebrougue Estate*	1 Burger/142g	170	7.0	120	19.9	4.2	4.9	0.5
with Crushed Garlic, Lurpak*	1 Serving/10g	70	7.5	700	1.0	4.0	75.0	0.0
BURGERS MEAT FREE								
Vegetable & Cheese, Tesco*	1 Burger/75g	143	5.3	190	7.7	23.6	7.1	1.4
BURGERS VEGETARIAN								
Bean Burgers, Mexican Style, Quarter Pounders, Tesco*	1 Burger/113.5g	250	12.0	220	5.0	25.0	10.6	2.4
Black Bean, Organic, Cauldron*	1 Burger/88g	170	10.1	193	9.2	13.1	11.5	8.5
Cheese & Spring Onion, Tesco*	1 Burger/87.3g	178	10.3	204	4.4	20.0	11.8	3.2
Flame Grilled, Linda McCartney*	1 Burger/60g	104	3.1	174	17.9	13.8	5.2	3.3
Meat Free, Asda*	1 Burger/60g	138	6.0	230	24.0	11.0	10.0	0.3
Meat Free, Sainsbury's*	1 Burger/57g	92	4.2	161	19.6	3.9	7.4	4.8
Meat Free, Spicy, Bean & Nacho, Asda*	1 Burger/113.4g	288	17.7	254	5.0	23.3	15.6	3.9
Mexican Style, Bean, Meat Free, Tesco*	1 Burger/93.6g	206	8.7	220	4.9	28.2	9.3	3.9
Mushroom, Cauldron*	1 Burger/87.5g	126	5.5	143	5.5	16.1	6.3	2.6
Mushroom, Meat Free, Tesco*	1 Burger/87g	151	9.5	173	3.6	15.3	10.8	3.7
Mushroom, Organic, Cauldron*	1 Burger/87.5g	137	7.3	156	7.1	18.2	8.3	2.3
Quarter Pounders, Chargrilled, Tesco*	1 Burger/113.5g	187	9.1	164	16.0	7.0	8.0	2.5
Quarter Pounders, HL, Tesco*	1 Burger/102g	117	1.7	114	4.0	20.7	1.7	2.0
Savoury, Cauldron*	1 Burger/75g	125	6.9	166	108.0	7.9	9.2	2.4
Spicy Bean, BGTY, Sainsbury's*	1 Burger/85g	123	2.3	145	6.9	23.3	2.7	3.1
Spicy Bean, Cauldron*	1 Burger/87.5g	203	9.8	232	5.4	27.4	11.2	6.2
Spicy Bean, Linda McCartney*	1 Burger/85g	190	9.5	223	4.3	26.2	11.2	2.9
Spicy Bean, Quarter Pounder, Dalepak*	1 Burger/115g	237	12.5	206	4.6	22.3	10.9	2.6
Spicy Vegetable & Bean, ¼lb, Asda*	1 Burger/108.6g	228	11.7	210	5.0	23.3	10.8	5.2
Tesco*	1 Burger/56g	92	4.5	164	16.0	7.0	8.0	2.5
Vegetable, Captains, Birds Eye*	1 Burger/48g	96	4.2	200	4.7	25.5	8.8	2.0
Vegetable, Organic, Goodlife*	1 Burger/67.1g	114	3.9	170	3.2	26.3	5.8	2.6
Vegetable, Organic, Tesco*	1 Burger/90g	108	3.9	120	2.6	17.6	4.3	2.1
Vegetable, Quarter Pounders, Tesco*	1 Burger/108g	227	13.1	211	4.4	20.8	12.2	2.7
Vegetable, Spicy, Asda*	1 Burger/56g	108	6.2	193	3.4	20.0	11.0	0.0
with Tofu, Organic, Evernat*	1oz/28g	52	2.3	186	7.9	16.9	8.3	0.0
BUTTER								
Basics, Sainsbury's*	1 Serving/10g	74	8.2	737	0.5	0.1	81.7	0.0
Brandy, Tesco*	1oz/28g	152	10.8	543	0.3	48.3	38.7	0.5
Brandy, with Cognac, Sainsbury's*	1/8 Pot/25g	137	9.4	549	0.2	44.1	37.6	0.0
Cornish, Finest, Tesco*	1 Serving/15g	111	12.3	737	0.5	0.0	81.7	0.0
Creamery, Average	1 Serving/10g	74	8.1	736	0.5	0.4	81.4	0.0
Fresh, Average	1 Thin Spread/7g	51	5.7	735	0.6	0.4	81.3	0.0
Garlic, Somerfield*	1oz/28g	192	21.0	686	1.0	2.0	75.0	0.0
Pure Irish, Salted, Kerrygold*	1 Serving/10g	72	8.0	720	0.4	0.0	80.0	0.0
Reduced Fat, Fresh, Average	1 Thin Spread/7g	26	2.8	368	2.3	1.2	39.4	0.2
Salted, Average	1 Thin Spread/7g	51	5.7	729	0.4	0.3	81.1	0.0

	Measure INFO/WEIGHT	per Measure KCAL	FAT	Nutrition Values per 100g / 100ml KCAL	PROT	CARB	FAT	FIBRE
BUTTER								
Slightly Salted, Lurpak*	1 Serving/10g	74	8.2	742	1.0	1.0	81.5	0.0
Spreadable, Fresh, Average	1 Thin Spread/7g	51	5.7	730	0.4	0.3	80.8	0.0
Spreadable, Reduced Fat, Average	1 Thin Spread/7g	38	4.2	540	0.5	0.5	60.0	0.0
BUTTERMILK								
Average	1 Mug/400ml	177	1.3	44	4.2	5.9	0.3	0.0
BUTTERNUT SQUASH								
with Spinach & Goats' Cheese Cannelloni, Tesco*	Pack/350g	490	29.4	140	5.1	10.7	8.4	1.9
BUTTONS								
Dairy Milk, Milk Chocolate, Cadbury*	1 Pack/32.4	170	9.7	525	7.7	56.7	29.9	0.7
Milk Chocolate, Asda*	1 Bag/70g	368	21.0	526	7.0	57.0	30.0	1.5
Milk Chocolate, Giant, Cadbury*	1 Button/2.9g	16	0.9	525	7.6	56.2	29.9	0.0
Milk Chocolate, Tesco*	1 Bag/70g	359	19.3	513	7.1	59.1	27.6	2.1
White Chocolate, Cadbury*	1 Pack/32.4g	180	11.0	555	4.5	58.4	33.8	0.0
White Chocolate, Co-Op*	½ Pack/35g	186	9.8	530	7.0	64.0	28.0	0.0
White Chocolate, Tesco*	1 Bag/70g	388	23.5	554	5.1	58.0	33.5	0.0

B

	Measure INFO/WEIGHT	per Measure KCAL	per Measure FAT	Nutrition Values per 100g / 100ml KCAL	PROT	CARB	FAT	FIBRE
CABBAGE								
& Leek, Crunchy Mix, Ready to Cook, Sainsbury's*	1 Serving/125g	34	0.6	27	1.9	3.7	0.5	2.6
Boiled, Average	1 Serving/90g	14	0.3	15	1.0	2.2	0.3	1.7
Greens, Trimmed, Average	1oz/28g	8	0.1	29	2.9	3.0	0.5	3.4
Raw, Average	1 Serving/100g	21	0.5	21	1.3	3.2	0.5	1.9
Red, Average	1 Serving/90g	19	0.2	21	1.0	3.7	0.3	2.2
Red, Braised with Red Wine, M & S*	½ Pack/150g	180	7.2	120	1.4	17.1	4.8	1.0
Red, with Apple, Braised, Sainsbury's*	½ Pack/117g	91	4.1	78	0.8	10.8	3.5	1.7
Red, with Apple, Finest, Tesco*	½ Pack/150g	177	8.9	118	1.6	14.7	5.9	4.6
Red, with Apple, Frozen, Sainsbury's*	1 Serving/75g	38	0.0	50	1.8	10.8	0.0	2.2
Red, with Apple & Cranberry, TTD, Sainsbury's*	½ Pack/200g	166	5.8	83	1.3	12.8	2.9	1.4
Savoy, Boiled in Salted Water, Average	1 Serving/90g	15	0.5	17	1.1	2.2	0.5	2.0
Savoy, Raw, Average	1 Serving/90g	24	0.5	27	2.1	3.9	0.5	3.1
Sweetheart, Tesco*	1 Serving/100g	20	0.7	20	1.9	1.6	0.7	2.6
White, Raw, Average	1oz/28g	8	0.1	27	1.4	5.0	0.2	2.1
CAKE								
Alabama Chocolate Fudge, Farmfoods*	1/6 Cake/61g	201	5.9	329	4.7	55.7	9.7	2.7
Alabama Chocolate Fudge, Morrisons*	1/6 Cake/58g	195	6.4	337	4.5	55.1	11.0	2.3
Almond Flavoured Rounds, Country Garden Cakes*	1 Cake/45.4g	181	6.6	403	4.3	62.4	14.7	2.3
Almond Slices, GFY, Asda*	1 Slice/25g	67	0.8	268	4.0	56.0	3.1	0.7
Almond Slices, Lyons*	1 Slice/26.8g	115	7.0	426	7.1	41.3	25.8	1.6
Almond Slices, Mr Kipling*	1 Slice/35g	141	4.9	403	6.3	63.4	14.0	2.0
Almond Slices, Sainsbury's*	1 Serving/27g	120	7.1	444	5.9	45.9	26.3	1.5
Angel, Sainsbury's*	1/8 Cake/41g	171	8.1	417	4.1	55.7	19.8	0.8
Angel Layer, Tesco*	1 Serving/25g	101	4.3	403	4.5	57.4	17.3	0.9
Angel Slices, Mr Kipling*	1 Slice/38g	153	7.0	403	2.9	58.8	18.3	0.6
Apple, Bramley, & Blackberry Crumble, M & S*	1/8 Cake/56g	221	10.0	395	4.4	54.1	17.9	1.5
Apple, Home Style, M & S*	1 Cake/54g	189	7.9	350	5.3	49.4	14.7	1.5
Apple Bakes, Go Ahead, McVitie's*	1 Cake/34.9g	126	2.7	361	2.6	70.0	7.8	2.0
Apple Slice, Delightful, Mr Kipling*	1 Slice/25.5g	81	1.0	317	4.4	66.2	3.9	1.3
Apple Sponge Sandwich, M & S*	1/6 Cake/67.3g	165	8.5	245	3.2	29.1	12.6	0.6
Apricot & Almond, Bakers Delight*	1oz/28g	106	4.5	379	5.5	53.2	16.0	1.8
Bakewell, The Handmade Flapjack Company*	1 Cake/75g	311	17.1	415	4.5	47.4	22.8	0.0
Bakewell Slices, Mr Kipling*	1 Slice/36g	163	7.3	454	4.2	63.4	20.4	1.2
Banana, The Handmade Flapjack Company*	1 Cake/75g	290	10.8	387	5.3	59.2	14.4	0.0
Banana & Walnut, Handmade, Delicious, Boots*	1 Pack/60g	209	10.8	348	5.6	41.0	18.0	1.9
Banana Loaf, Organic, Respect Organics*	1 Serving/100g	391	21.0	391	3.9	48.6	21.0	1.5
Banana Loaf, Waitrose*	1 Slice/70g	236	7.5	337	5.0	55.2	10.7	1.7
Battenberg, Lyons*	1/6 Cake/38.3g	166	4.4	433	6.3	73.7	11.4	1.3
Battenberg, Mini, Mr Kipling*	1 Cake/35g	144	3.9	410	4.6	76.2	11.0	1.3
Battenberg, Mr Kipling*	1 Serving/38.2g	160	4.6	421	5.0	73.3	12.0	1.6
Birthday, M & S*	1 Serving/60g	240	7.1	400	2.3	70.9	11.9	0.8
Birthday Present, Tesco*	1 Serving/79g	347	13.9	439	3.5	66.6	17.6	0.4
Bites, Caramel, Mr Kipling*	1 Bite/13.8g	68	3.8	492	5.9	55.3	27.4	0.8
Bites, Jaffa Cake Roll, Mini, McVitie's*	1 Cake/15.9g	62	1.9	389	3.7	66.7	12.0	1.4
Butterfly, Mr Kipling*	1 Cake/29g	114	6.4	392	4.4	43.4	22.2	0.6
Buttons, Happy Birthday, Cadbury*	1 Cake/25g	118	6.8	470	4.1	52.8	27.1	0.0
Caramel, Milk Chocolate, Holly Lane*	1 Cake/25g	110	5.1	441	6.9	57.6	20.3	1.1
Caramel Slice, M & S*	1 Slice/64g	304	16.1	475	4.9	60.4	25.2	2.6
Carrot, Amo*	1 Slice/45g	153	6.8	340	4.0	47.0	15.0	0.0
Carrot, Entenmann's*	1 Serving/40g	156	8.2	391	4.1	47.4	20.5	1.5
Carrot, Farmfoods*	1/8 Cake/59g	187	10.5	317	3.7	35.4	17.8	1.6
Carrot, Handmade, Delicious, Boots*	1 Slice/75g	292	13.5	389	4.1	53.0	18.0	1.4
Carrot, Iced, Tesco*	1 Serving/61g	246	12.0	404	3.1	53.7	19.6	1.6

CAKE

	Measure INFO/WEIGHT	per Measure KCAL	FAT	Nutrition Values per 100g / 100ml KCAL	PROT	CARB	FAT	FIBRE
Carrot, M & S*	Slice/83g	274	16.3	330	5.5	33.0	19.6	2.7
Carrot, Organic, Respect Organics*	1 Slice/45g	179	10.1	398	3.1	47.4	22.4	1.5
Carrot, Slices, Eat Smart, Morrisons*	1 Cake/27g	84	0.6	312	3.0	70.0	2.2	2.3
Carrot, The Handmade Flapjack Company*	1 Cake/75g	295	13.0	393	6.4	53.0	17.3	0.0
Carrot, Traditional, Farringford Foods*	1oz/28g	115	7.1	412	4.4	44.8	25.2	0.0
Carrot, Ultimate, Entenmann's*	1/8 Cake/63.8g	235	10.1	367	4.7	51.4	15.8	0.3
Carrot & Apple, Safeway*	1 Serving/50g	158	5.6	315	3.2	50.4	11.2	0.8
Carrot & Orange, Extra Special, Asda*	1/6 Cake/65g	240	11.7	369	4.7	47.0	18.0	0.9
Carrot & Orange, Finest, Tesco*	1/8 Cake/50g	205	10.3	410	4.6	51.2	20.5	2.1
Carrot & Orange, Waitrose*	1/6 Cake/47g	165	7.4	350	5.3	46.8	15.7	1.8
Carrot & Orange Slices, GFY, Asda*	1 Serving/23.1g	77	0.6	334	3.4	74.0	2.7	1.0
Carrot & Orange Slices, HL, Tesco*	1 Slice/29g	90	0.8	310	6.6	64.8	2.8	2.8
Carrot & Pecan, M & S*	1 Slice/90.4g	329	14.6	365	6.4	48.7	16.2	2.3
Carrot & Walnut, Layered, Asda*	1 Serving/42g	172	8.0	409	4.6	55.0	19.0	1.0
Carrot & Walnut, Mini Classics, Mr Kipling*	1 Cake/39g	172	9.8	440	4.5	48.6	25.2	1.0
Carrot & Walnut, TTD, Sainsbury's*	1 Slice/58.1g	208	10.0	358	3.6	47.3	17.2	0.9
Carrot Slices, Weight Watchers*	1 Slice/27g	71	0.7	263	3.0	56.7	2.7	1.9
Carrot Wedge, Tesco*	1 Pack/175g	532	27.7	304	3.9	36.6	15.8	1.5
Celebration, Sainsbury's*	1/12 Cake/100g	265	9.2	265	2.1	43.6	9.2	0.3
Cherry, Asda*	1 Slice/37.3g	130	4.4	351	4.7	56.0	12.0	0.6
Cherry, Co-Op*	1/8 Cake/47g	190	8.5	405	4.0	57.0	18.0	0.8
Cherry, M & S*	1 Serving/75g	285	9.5	380	5.0	60.6	12.7	0.8
Cherry Bakewell, M & S*	1 Cake/44g	185	7.8	420	4.5	61.7	17.7	1.0
Cherry Bakewell, Safeway*	1 Bakewell/47g	203	9.5	432	3.5	58.7	20.3	3.9
Cherry Bakewell, Sainsbury's*	1 Cake/46g	200	8.1	436	3.1	66.3	17.6	1.4
Cherry Bakewell, Somerfield*	1 Cake/50g	216	10.2	431	3.5	58.7	20.3	3.9
Cherry Bakewell, Tesco*	1 Cake/39g	171	7.5	439	3.2	63.3	19.2	1.1
Cherry Bakewell, Weight Watchers*	1 Cake/43g	157	4.3	365	3.6	65.4	9.9	3.6
Cherry Bakewell Slices, GFY, Asda*	1 Slice/29.1g	96	0.7	331	3.3	74.0	2.4	0.7
Cherry Bakewells, Delightful, Mr Kipling*	1 Cake/45.1g	176	5.8	390	3.9	66.4	12.9	1.2
Cherry Bakewells, Mr Kipling*	1 Cake/45g	193	8.3	428	3.9	61.3	18.5	1.4
Cherry Genoa, M & S*	1oz/28g	99	3.1	355	4.5	59.3	10.9	1.6
Chocolate	1oz/28g	128	7.4	456	7.4	50.4	26.4	0.0
Chocolate, Big, Tesco*	1 Slice/79g	311	13.1	396	7.4	54.1	16.7	1.8
Chocolate, Birthday, Tesco*	1 Serving/54g	229	13.2	425	5.9	45.5	24.4	2.1
Chocolate, Caterpillar, Tesco*	1 Serving/53g	248	13.2	468	5.7	55.3	24.9	1.1
Chocolate, Fudge, The Cake Shop*	1 Cake/37.1g	178	10.8	480	3.7	50.5	29.2	1.3
Chocolate, Happy Birthday, Tesco*	1 Serving/58g	241	13.2	415	4.7	46.9	22.7	2.9
Chocolate, Iced, Tesco*	1 Serving/40g	158	6.3	395	4.7	58.5	15.8	1.8
Chocolate, Individual, with Mini Eggs, Cadbury*	1 Cake/26.2g	118	6.0	455	4.6	57.5	23.1	1.3
Chocolate, Lge, Happy Birthday, Tesco*	1/18 Cake/63g	249	12.2	396	6.2	49.3	19.3	1.8
Chocolate, Loaf, Moist, McVitie's*	1 Sm Slice/30g	119	6.1	398	4.8	49.0	20.3	1.9
Chocolate, Morrisons*	1 Serving/31.5g	157	10.0	505	5.3	48.0	32.4	1.2
Chocolate, Part of Tea Time Selection, Iceland*	1 Cake/31g	144	7.9	464	4.5	54.1	25.5	2.0
Chocolate, Party, Tesco*	1 Slice/62g	244	13.1	394	4.6	46.3	21.2	0.9
Chocolate, Sainsbury's*	1 Serving/30g	119	5.6	395	4.1	52.6	18.5	1.3
Chocolate, Sara Lee*	1/4 Cake/88g	339	14.8	385	4.1	54.3	16.8	0.0
Chocolate, Smarties, Celebration, Lge, Nestle*	1/16 Cake/71.3g	308	17.4	432	5.4	48.9	24.4	1.2
Chocolate, Thorntons*	1 Serving/87g	408	25.1	469	5.2	47.1	28.8	0.6
Chocolate, TTD, Sainsbury's*	1 Serving/207g	749	32.1	362	4.4	50.9	15.5	1.3
Chocolate, Ultimate, TTD, Sainsbury's*	1 Serving/70g	263	11.5	375	5.4	51.5	16.4	1.9
Chocolate & Orange Rolls, M & S*	1 Roll/60g	228	17.0	380	3.6	27.0	28.4	1.3
Chocolate & Sweetest, Beetroot, Battle Bakehouse*	1/6 Cake/48.8g	185	8.7	379	5.2	48.6	17.9	4.0

C

CAKE

	Measure INFO/WEIGHT	per Measure KCAL	FAT	Nutrition Values per 100g / 100ml KCAL	PROT	CARB	FAT	FIBRE
Chocolate Birthday, Asda*	Slice/61.9g	283	16.9	457	4.5	48.2	27.3	1.1
Chocolate Birthday, M & S*	10th Cake/57.6g	245	9.6	425	2.8	67.2	16.6	1.8
Chocolate Box, Asda*	1 Serving/60g	263	13.8	439	5.0	53.0	23.0	0.7
Chocolate Brownie, Fudge, Entenmann's*	1/8 Cake/55g	168	2.4	306	4.0	62.7	4.4	1.5
Chocolate Button, Cakes For The Connoisseur*	1 Cake/30g	145	9.8	485	5.2	42.1	32.8	2.3
Chocolate Chip, Co-Op*	1/6 Cake/62.5g	273	16.7	440	5.0	44.0	27.0	0.5
Chocolate Chip, The Cake Shop*	1 Cake/35g	178	11.0	508	4.7	50.2	31.5	1.1
Chocolate Fudge, & Vanilla Cream, M & S*	1/6 Cake/69g	306	17.7	450	5.2	49.8	26.0	1.3
Chocolate Fudge, Classics, M & S*	1 Serving/70.9g	195	7.5	275	2.8	42.8	10.6	1.1
Chocolate Fudge, Entenmann's*	1 Serving/48g	173	7.2	361	4.4	51.8	15.1	0.9
Chocolate Fudge, M & S*	1oz/28g	109	5.2	390	5.3	50.2	18.4	1.1
Chocolate Fudge, Morrisons*	1 Portion/40g	169	8.1	423	2.7	57.2	20.3	1.4
Chocolate Fudge, Pizza Express*	1 Cake/100g	395	17.0	395	4.0	57.2	17.0	0.0
Chocolate Fudge, Sainsbury's*	1/8 Cake/98g	402	21.9	410	5.5	47.3	22.3	1.9
Chocolate Fudge, Tea Time Treats, Asda*	1 Cake/37.0g	157	8.1	424	3.6	53.0	22.0	1.7
Chocolate Fudge Slice, Waitrose*	1 Slice/60g	230	9.7	383	4.7	54.6	16.2	1.5
Chocolate Heaven, Extra Special, Asda*	1/6 Cake/65.7g	256	13.2	388	4.0	48.0	20.0	1.0
Chocolate Indulgence, Finest, Tesco*	1 Slice/52g	221	11.2	425	5.3	51.9	21.5	1.8
Chocolate Loaf, Somerfield*	1oz/28g	111	6.2	396	6.0	44.0	22.0	0.0
Chocolate Log, Fresh Cream, Finest, Tesco*	1 Slice/85g	301	15.4	354	4.5	43.2	18.1	1.4
Chocolate Orange, Sponge, Asda*	1 Serving/70g	298	18.2	425	4.9	42.9	26.0	3.0
Chocolate Party, M & S*	1 Serving/60.8g	241	12.7	395	4.6	46.9	20.8	1.1
Chocolate Rice Crispy, Knightsbridge*	1 Cake/24g	88	4.2	368	3.9	48.7	17.5	0.1
Chocolate Roll, Sainsbury's*	1 Slice/50g	210	10.2	420	5.0	54.0	20.4	3.3
Chocolate Sensation, Sainsbury's*	1 Serving/92.0g	320	17.7	348	3.7	40.0	19.2	2.3
Chocolate Slices, Mr Kipling*	1 Slice/32.5g	132	6.7	406	5.6	50.4	20.6	2.7
Chocolate Sponge, Budgens*	1/6 Cake/76g	297	13.6	392	3.8	55.9	18.0	2.1
Chocolate Sponge, Morrisons*	1 Serving/59g	179	7.6	303	4.4	42.5	12.8	0.7
Chocolate Sponge, Tesco*	1 Serving/35g	129	5.1	373	5.3	54.4	14.9	1.5
Chocolate Sponge Sandwich, Co-Op*	1 Slice/39g	140	5.0	360	4.6	57.6	12.7	2.3
Chocolate Truffle, Extra Special, Asda*	1 Serving/103g	402	26.8	390	5.0	34.0	26.0	1.8
Chocolate Truffle, Mini, Finest, Tesco*	1 Cake/28g	125	6.6	448	5.9	52.9	23.7	0.3
Chocolate Truffle, So Good, Somerfield*	1 Slice/80g	328	18.6	410	6.4	44.0	23.2	1.0
Chocolate Victoria Sponge, Co-Op*	1 Slice/61g	201	9.8	330	5.0	42.0	16.0	1.0
Chocolate with Butter Icing, Average	1oz/28g	135	8.3	481	5.7	50.9	29.7	0.0
Chorley, Asda*	1 Cake/60g	269	12.6	449	6.0	59.0	21.0	2.2
Christmas, M & S*	1 Serving/60g	207	4.1	345	3.4	67.4	6.8	3.8
Christmas, Rich Fruit, All Iced, Sainsbury's*	1/16 Cake/85g	307	7.6	361	4.0	66.4	8.9	1.5
Christmas, Rich Fruit, Free From, Tesco*	1 Serving/100g	301	7.3	301	2.9	56.0	7.3	0.9
Christmas, Rich Fruit, Organic, Tesco*	1 Serving/75.5g	284	7.6	374	3.9	67.1	10.0	2.0
Christmas, Rich Fruit, Tesco*	1 Serving/75g	257	5.6	342	3.9	64.3	7.4	3.1
Christmas Slices, Mr Kipling*	1 Slice/52g	190	4.6	366	3.0	68.0	8.9	0.9
Classic Lemon Drizzle, M & S*	1/6 Cake/67.5g	255	10.4	375	4.7	55.0	15.3	0.6
Coconut	1 Slice/70g	304	16.7	434	6.7	51.2	23.8	2.5
Coconut & Raspberry, M & S*	1 Serving/52g	231	13.9	445	5.0	45.5	26.8	2.3
Coconut Delight, Burton's*	1 Cake/21g	89	3.5	424	4.0	63.0	16.9	2.0
Coconut Snowball, Bobby's*	1 Cake/18.3g	78	4.0	436	2.2	57.3	22.1	0.0
Coconut Sponge, Mini Classics, Mr Kipling*	1 Cake/38g	155	8.7	409	3.7	47.0	22.9	0.9
Coffee, Entenmann's*	1 Portion/41g	159	7.1	388	4.0	54.7	17.3	0.6
Coffee, Iced, M & S*	1 Slice/33g	135	6.5	410	4.4	54.5	19.6	1.6
Coffee & Walnut, Classics, M & S*	1 Serving/70.8g	309	17.3	435	4.3	50.3	24.3	1.6
Coffee & Walnut, Mrs Beeton's*	1 Slice/54g	219	13.5	405	3.7	41.4	25.0	0.3
Coffee & Walnut, Somerfield*	1oz/28g	123	7.3	440	5.0	46.0	26.0	0.0

CAKE

	Measure INFO/WEIGHT	per Measure KCAL	FAT	Nutrition Values per 100g / 100ml KCAL	PROT	CARB	FAT	FIBRE
Coffee & Walnut Slices, HE, Tesco*	1 Slice/23g	69	0.5	301	4.4	65.7	2.3	2.8
Colin the Caterpillar, M & S*	1 Slice/60g	234	12.8	390	5.3	57.2	21.3	1.3
Cornflake, Bobby's*	1/6 Cake/45g	207	9.2	461	3.9	65.5	20.4	0.0
Cornflake, Chocolate Clusters, Asda*	1 Cluster/13.9g	64	2.6	460	8.2	65.2	18.5	2.7
Country Farmhouse, Waitrose*	1 Serving/80g	308	12.1	385	4.7	57.5	15.1	1.4
Country Slices, Mr Kipling*	1 Slice/31.8	121	4.8	380	4.4	56.7	15.0	1.2
Cream Slices, M & S*	1 Slice/80g	310	18.3	387	2.3	45.7	22.9	0.6
Date & Walnut Loaf, Sainsbury's*	1/10 Slice/40g	148	8.2	371	6.7	40.1	20.4	1.0
Double Chocolate Ganache, M & S*	1/12 Cake/61g	281	16.8	460	5.9	46.1	27.6	2.5
Double Chocolate Wedge, Tesco*	1 Piece/100g	416	20.3	416	5.0	53.4	20.3	0.9
Dundee, Co-Op*	1/8 Cake/71g	238	7.8	335	5.0	53.0	11.0	2.0
Eccles	1 Cake/45g	214	11.9	475	3.9	59.3	26.4	1.6
Fairy, Co-Op*	1oz/28g	105	5.9	375	4.0	43.0	21.0	0.8
Fairy, Holly Lane*	1 Cake/25.7g	120	6.8	460	3.7	52.5	26.1	3.5
Fairy, Iced, Somerfield*	1 Cake/15.1g	59	2.0	392	4.9	62.9	13.4	1.4
Fairy, Lemon Iced, Tesco*	1 Cake/24g	94	3.3	393	4.4	63.2	13.6	1.1
Fairy, Mini, Kids, Tesco*	1 Cake/12g	54	2.8	435	5.3	53.3	22.3	1.1
Fairy, Mini, Tesco*	1 Cake/13g	53	2.5	424	6.1	54.6	20.1	1.3
Fairy, Plain, Sainsbury's*	1 Cake/19.9g	84	4.3	422	4.9	46.4	21.5	1.2
Fairy, Plain, Somerfield*	1 Serving/16g	70	3.5	436	6.1	53.7	21.9	1.0
Fairy, Plain, Value, Tesco*	1 Cake/15g	52	1.3	348	5.3	62.4	8.6	0.9
Fairy, SmartPrice, Asda*	1 Cake/15g	66	3.3	438	6.0	54.0	22.0	1.0
Fairy, Strawberry Iced, Tesco*	1 Cake/24g	94	3.2	392	4.9	62.9	13.4	1.4
Fairy, Value, Tesco*	1 Cake/16g	70	3.5	436	6.1	53.7	21.9	1.0
Fairy, Vanilla Iced, Tesco*	1 Cake/24g	93	2.9	388	4.4	65.1	12.2	1.2
Farmhouse Fruit, Bakers Delight*	1oz/28g	107	4.3	381	5.2	55.5	15.3	2.1
Flake, Cadbury*	1 Cake/20.2g	90	4.5	445	6.3	54.5	22.3	0.0
Fondant Fancies, Lemon, Waitrose*	1 Cake/40g	176	7.1	441	2.5	67.9	17.7	0.6
Fondant Fancies, M & S*	1 Cake/34.5g	148	4.6	435	2.4	76.5	13.4	0.5
Fondant Fancies, Sainsbury's*	1 Cake/27g	95	2.4	353	2.4	65.7	9.0	0.4
French Fancies, Mr Kipling*	1 Cake/28g	103	2.6	369	2.8	68.3	9.4	0.6
Fruit, Fully Iced, Luxury Rich, Co-Op*	1oz/28g	99	2.5	355	3.0	64.0	9.0	4.0
Fruit, Healthy Selection, Somerfield*	1oz/28g	73	0.6	260	5.0	55.0	2.0	0.0
Fruit, Plain, Average	1 Slice/90g	319	11.6	354	5.1	57.9	12.9	0.0
Fruit, Rich, Average	1 Slice/70g	225	8.8	322	4.9	50.7	12.5	1.7
Fruit, Rich, Iced	1 Slice/70g	249	8.0	356	4.1	62.7	11.4	1.7
Fruit, Rich, M & S*	1 Serving/50g	158	3.3	315	3.1	60.9	6.5	4.3
Fruit, Slices, Value, Tesco*	1 Slice/22.6g	85	4.1	372	4.0	48.7	17.7	1.3
Fruit & Nut Cluster, Finest, Tesco*	1 Slice/77g	262	10.3	338	4.5	50.1	13.3	2.7
Fruit Cake with Marzipan & Icing, Asda*	1/12 Slice/76g	280	6.8	369	3.9	68.0	9.0	0.0
Fudge Brownie, The Handmade Flapjack Company*	1 Cake/75g	286	9.2	381	4.9	62.8	12.3	0.0
Genoa, Tesco*	1 Slice/0.7g	2	0.1	325	3.6	60.9	7.4	4.0
Ginger, M & S*	1/6 Of Cake/38g	143	4.3	375	5.3	63.1	11.3	0.2
Ginger Drizzle, Iced, Co-Op*	1/6 Cake/64.5g	226	7.7	350	3.0	58.0	12.0	1.0
Ginger Orange, The Handmade Flapjack Company*	1 Cake/75g	289	15.2	385	4.3	46.3	20.3	0.0
Happy Birthday, Sainsbury's*	1 Slice/50g	207	8.1	414	2.8	64.5	16.1	0.6
Holly Hedgehog, Tesco*	1 Serving/55g	227	7.9	413	2.0	69.0	14.3	0.8
Iced Madeira, Sainsbury's*	1/8 Cake/47g	182	6.6	388	3.6	61.6	14.1	0.7
Jamaica Ginger, McVitie's*	1 Cake/291g	1048	31.4	360	3.5	62.2	10.8	1.4
Jammy Strawberry Rolls, Mini, Cadbury*	1 Roll/29g	119	4.8	411	4.9	59.8	16.5	0.5
Lemon, Home Bake, McVitie's*	1oz/28g	108	5.1	384	4.6	53.9	18.2	1.0
Lemon & Orange, Finest, Tesco*	1 Serving/53g	216	10.7	410	4.5	52.4	20.3	1.1
Lemon Bakewell, Mr Kipling*	1 Cake/48g	195	7.3	407	2.6	65.0	15.2	0.7

CAKE

	Measure INFO/WEIGHT	per Measure KCAL	FAT	Nutrition Values per 100g / 100ml KCAL	PROT	CARB	FAT	FIBRE
Lemon Buttercream & Lemon Curd, The Cake Shop*	1 Cake/28g	124	7.8	444	3.5	43.4	27.8	0.6
Lemon Drizzle, M & S*	1/6 Cake/63g	230	8.8	365	4.2	55.8	13.9	1.4
Lemon Drizzle, Slices, HL, Tesco*	1 Slice/24.2g	75	0.6	310	4.2	67.4	2.5	1.9
Lemon Drizzle Cake, Asda*	1 Serving/50g	150	6.0	299	2.8	45.0	12.0	0.4
Lemon Iced Madeira, Co-Op*	1 Cake/290g	1131	52.2	390	4.0	53.0	18.0	0.6
Lemon Madeira, Half Moon, Dan Cake*	1 Slice/50g	215	10.0	430	3.5	59.0	20.0	0.0
Lemon Slices, Eat Smart, Morrisons*	1 Slice/26g	81	0.7	312	3.9	68.1	2.7	1.9
Lemon Slices, Low Fat, Weight Watchers*	1 Slice/26.1g	79	0.5	303	3.1	68.1	2.0	2.2
Lemon Slices, Mr Kipling*	1 Slice/29.1g	120	4.8	413	4.2	61.9	16.6	0.7
Madeira	1 Slice/40g	157	6.8	393	5.4	58.4	16.9	0.9
Madeira, All Butter, Sainsbury's*	1 Serving/30g	116	5.9	388	5.2	47.4	19.7	0.8
Madeira, Cherry, Tesco*	¼ Cake/100g	342	11.2	342	4.3	55.9	11.2	2.6
Madeira, Iced, Tesco*	1/16 Cake/56g	218	6.8	389	2.6	67.2	12.2	0.4
Madeira, Lemon Iced, Tesco*	1 Slice/30g	122	5.3	407	4.5	57.8	17.5	0.9
Madeira, Tesco*	1 Serving/50g	197	7.8	394	5.5	57.9	15.6	1.2
Manor House, Mr Kipling*	1 Serving/69.2g	276	13.8	400	5.3	49.7	20.0	1.4
Marble, Tesco*	1/8 Cake/45g	185	8.4	410	4.4	55.9	18.7	1.5
Mini Rolls, Cadbury*	1 Roll/27g	120	6.1	445	4.4	56.4	22.5	1.3
Mini Rolls, Chocolate, Tesco*	1 Roll/31g	144	7.2	465	5.5	58.1	23.1	1.3
Mini Rolls, Chocolate, Weight Watchers*	1 Roll/26g	87	3.4	334	4.6	58.1	13.2	3.7
Mini Rolls, Easter Selection, Cadbury*	1oz/28g	122	5.8	434	5.5	55.6	20.6	0.0
Mini Rolls, Milk Chocolate, Cadbury*	1 Roll/27g	120	6.0	445	4.4	56.5	22.2	0.0
Mini Rolls, Rolo, Nestle*	1 Cake/29g	111	5.4	388	4.8	49.5	19.0	1.0
Party, Asda*	1 Serving/56.5g	240	9.1	421	2.3	67.0	16.0	0.4
Party Bake, M & S*	1/15 Cake/59.7g	231	12.1	385	4.0	46.6	20.2	0.9
Piece of Cake, Birthday, M & S*	1 Serving/85g	395	24.4	465	4.3	39.7	28.7	0.9
Raisin, Sainsbury's*	1 Cake/40g	161	7.6	403	4.7	53.5	18.9	3.0
Raisin, Tesco*	1 Cake/38g	158	7.6	417	5.6	53.8	19.9	1.4
Rich Choc Roll, Cadbury*	1/6 Portion/39g	149	6.1	381	4.8	50.2	15.6	1.0
Rich Fruit, Sainsbury's*	1 Serving/100g	321	8.5	321	3.9	57.3	8.5	2.1
Rich Fruit Slices, Free From, Sainsbury's*	1 Slice/40g	144	5.0	361	4.5	57.4	12.6	3.7
Rock	1 Sm Cake/40g	158	6.6	396	5.4	60.5	16.4	1.5
Rock, Tesco*	1 Serving/87g	311	8.4	357	7.4	60.1	9.7	1.6
Seriously Chocolatey Celebration, Sainsbury's*	1/8 Cake/77g	336	19.8	437	6.3	45.0	25.7	0.3
Snowballs, Tesco*	1 Snowball/18g	79	4.0	432	2.5	55.8	22.1	5.4
Sponge	1 Slice/53g	243	13.9	459	6.4	52.4	26.3	0.9
Sponge, Fatless	1 Slice/53g	156	3.2	294	10.1	53.0	6.1	0.9
Sponge, Fresh Cream & Strawberry, Asda*	1 12th/60g	170	6.0	284	4.6	44.0	10.0	1.1
Sponge, Iced, M & S*	1 Serving/100g	400	17.0	400	3.4	58.4	17.0	1.3
Sponge, Jam Filled	1 Slice/65g	196	3.2	302	4.2	64.2	4.9	1.8
Sponge Roll, Chocolate, M & S*	¼ Cake/66g	251	12.1	380	3.9	50.5	18.4	1.8
Sponge Roll, Coffee, M & S*	1 Serving/40g	150	6.9	375	3.5	51.1	17.3	0.6
Sponge with Butter Icing	1 Slice/65g	319	19.9	490	4.5	52.4	30.6	0.6
Strawberry Sponge Roll, M & S*	1/6 Cake/48.5g	158	4.6	330	2.8	58.0	9.5	0.8
Sultana, Apple & Cranberry, 99% Fat Free, Trimlyne*	1/6 Cake/66.6g	130	0.6	195	4.6	45.5	0.9	3.3
Sultana, Fair Trade, Co-Op*	1/8 Cake/45g	155	4.1	345	5.0	60.0	9.0	1.0
Sultana & Cherry, Tesco*	1 Cake/37g	124	4.0	334	4.7	54.4	10.8	2.5
Sultana & Cherry Slice, Co-Op*	1oz/28g	87	3.4	310	3.0	48.0	12.0	2.0
Swiss Roll, Average	1oz/28g	77	1.2	276	7.2	55.5	4.4	0.8
Swiss Roll, Chocolate, Lyons*	1 Serving/50g	190	9.7	379	4.3	47.0	19.3	0.9
Swiss Roll, Chocolate, M & S*	1 Serving/46g	168	11.1	365	4.6	32.6	24.2	1.2
Swiss Roll, Chocolate, Mini, Tesco*	1 Roll/22g	87	3.3	396	4.6	61.0	14.8	0.0
Swiss Roll, Chocolate, Morrisons*	1/6 Roll/26g	103	4.9	401	4.4	56.4	18.9	3.1

CAKE

INFO/WEIGHT	per Measure KCAL	FAT	Nutrition Values per 100g / 100ml KCAL	PROT	CARB	FAT	FIBRE
Swiss Roll, Chocolate, Value, Tesco*	1 Serving/20g	81	3.7	404	5.0	54.1	18.7	2.1
Swiss Roll, Chocolate Flavour, Value, Tesco*	1 Slice/20g	79	3.9	394	5.5	49.2	19.5	1.4
Swiss Roll, Raspberry, Asda*	1/6 Roll/34.9g	104	0.7	298	3.0	66.9	2.0	0.4
Swiss Roll, Raspberry, Lyons*	1 Roll/175g	485	2.5	277	5.2	60.6	1.4	0.0
Swiss Roll, Raspberry, Sainsbury's*	1 Serving/35g	105	0.7	301	3.5	67.0	2.1	1.1
Swiss Roll, Raspberry & Vanilla, Morrisons*	1 Serving/28g	98	2.7	350	4.2	61.8	9.5	0.0
Swiss Roll, Raspberry Jam, Mr Kipling*	1/6 Cake/51.8g	184	5.3	355	2.8	63.0	10.2	1.0
Tangy Lemon Trickle, M & S*	1 Slice/75g	281	14.1	375	4.7	47.4	18.8	1.1
Tiffin, Chocolate, Sainsbury's*	1 Cake/61g	184	11.6	301	2.7	29.8	19.0	1.3
Toffee, Iced, Tesco*	1 Serving/35g	132	5.2	376	3.3	57.2	14.9	1.6
Toffee, Slices, HL, Tesco*	1 Cake/24g	76	0.6	315	4.5	65.0	2.6	1.6
Toffee, Thorntons*	1/6 Cake/70.1g	302	16.8	431	4.6	49.2	24.0	0.8
Toffee & Pecan Slices, M & S*	1 Slice/36g	160	8.5	445	4.7	54.0	23.7	1.3
Toffee Flavour Slices, Low Fat, Weight Watchers*	1 Slice/27g	80	0.7	297	4.2	63.9	2.6	3.2
Tray Bake, Crunchy Granola, Waitrose*	1/6 Tray/42g	187	10.1	445	5.8	51.2	24.1	4.5
Vanilla Sponge, Fresh Cream, Sainsbury's*	1 Slice/50g	152	5.1	304	7.5	45.6	10.2	0.4
Victoria Sandwich, Classic, Lge, M & S*	1/10 Cake/65.8g	261	12.9	395	5.1	49.5	19.6	2.3
Victoria Sandwich, Co-Op*	1oz/28g	101	4.8	360	4.0	48.0	17.0	1.0
Victoria Slices, Mr Kipling*	1 Slice/28.2g	122	4.4	432	3.9	68.8	15.7	0.4
Victoria Sponge, Fresh Cream, Tesco*	¼ Of Cake/69.6g	240	12.1	345	3.9	42.5	17.4	0.6
Victoria Sponge, Fresh Cream, Value, Tesco*	1 Serving/50g	169	8.7	337	4.4	40.7	17.4	0.6
Victoria Sponge, Lemon, Co-Op*	1 Slice/42g	151	8.0	360	4.0	44.0	19.0	0.7
Victoria Sponge, Mini, Mr Kipling*	1 Cake/36.2g	152	6.9	420	3.9	58.5	19.0	0.8
Victoria Sponge, TTD, Sainsbury's*	1 Serving/69g	255	11.3	370	4.3	51.4	16.4	1.1
Victoria Sponge Sandwich, Somerfield*	1oz/28g	112	5.3	400	4.0	53.0	19.0	0.0
Viennese Whirl, Lemon, Mr Kipling*	1 Cake/28g	115	4.5	409	4.2	62.2	15.9	0.7
Viennese Whirl, Mr Kipling*	1 Whirl/28g	142	8.5	507	4.1	53.9	30.5	1.3
Walnut, Sandwich, Sainsbury's*	1/8 Cake/48g	182	8.3	379	5.4	53.8	17.3	1.3
Walnut & Coffee, Co-Op*	¼ Cake/65g	254	13.0	390	5.0	47.0	20.0	0.7
Walnut & Coffee, TTD, Sainsbury's*	1 Slice/68g	269	14.7	396	4.4	45.9	21.6	0.7
Walnut Layer, Somerfield*	¼ Cake/77.5g	295	15.5	381	6.0	45.0	20.0	0.0
Welsh, Average	1oz/28g	121	5.5	431	5.6	61.8	19.6	1.5
Yorkshire Parkin, Bakers Delight*	1oz/28g	111	4.1	395	5.1	60.3	14.8	1.5

CAKE BAR

INFO/WEIGHT	per Measure KCAL	FAT	KCAL	PROT	CARB	FAT	FIBRE
Bounty, McVitie's*	1 Cake/36g	166	8.8	461	5.1	55.2	24.5	0.0
Caramel, Cadbury*	1 Bar/26g	107	4.4	411	6.4	57.0	16.8	0.0
Caramel, Weight Watchers*	1 Bar/22.8g	86	3.1	377	5.6	58.2	13.5	3.9
Carrot, Tesco*	1 Bar/68g	239	12.6	351	4.7	41.4	18.5	2.4
Chocolate, High Lights, Cadbury*	1 Bar/25g	95	3.5	380	5.5	58.8	14.0	1.1
Chocolate, Snack Cakes, Penguin, McVitie's*	1 Bar/24g	122	7.2	510	4.8	54.6	30.2	1.6
Chocolate, Tesco*	1 Serving/26g	113	6.0	435	5.2	51.9	23.0	5.4
Chocolate Chip, Mr Kipling*	1 Bar/33g	156	8.7	472	5.3	53.5	26.3	1.2
Chocolate Chip, Sainsbury's*	1 Cake Bar/25g	108	5.6	430	6.1	51.2	22.3	0.6
Chocolate Chip, Tesco*	1 Cake/30g	124	5.9	415	7.0	51.4	19.7	2.3
Crunchie, Cadbury*	1 Cake Bar/32g	147	7.2	460	5.9	58.3	22.6	0.0
Double Chocolate, Free From, Sainsbury's*	1 Cake/50.1g	196	7.9	391	4.2	58.2	15.7	1.0
Flake, Cadbury*	1 Cake/22g	97	5.1	442	6.5	51.8	23.3	0.5
Fudge, Cadbury*	1 Pack/52.4g	218	9.2	420	5.7	60.3	17.6	0.0
Galaxy, McVitie's*	1oz/28g	138	7.6	494	5.1	57.5	27.0	0.3
Galaxy Caramel, McVitie's*	1 Cake/31g	137	6.5	441	5.5	57.4	21.1	0.0
Jaffa Cake, McVitie's*	1 Cake Bar/31g	126	5.4	408	3.9	59.1	17.4	29.0
Jamaica Ginger, McVitie's*	1 Mini Cake/33g	128	4.9	388	3.5	60.2	14.7	1.2
Milk Chocolate, Cadbury*	1 Bar/34.9g	150	7.6	430	5.6	53.3	21.7	1.2

	Measure INFO/WEIGHT	per Measure KCAL	FAT	Nutrition Values per 100g / 100ml KCAL	PROT	CARB	FAT	FIBRE
CAKE BAR								
Milk Chocolate Orange, Sandwich Bar, Lyons*	1 Bar/27.5g	144	8.1	516	5.0	62.0	29.0	0.0
Milky Way, McVitie's*	1 Cake/28.2g	144	8.7	511	5.0	53.9	30.7	0.0
CAKE MIX								
Carrot Cake, Betty Crocker*	¼ Pack/125g	504	8.4	403	5.8	78.9	6.7	1.5
Cheesecake, Original, Made Up, Asda*	1/6 Cake/85g	228	10.2	268	4.1	36.0	12.0	1.4
Cheesecake, Strawberry, Real, Green's*	1 Serving/100g	254	12.8	253	3.9	30.6	12.8	0.6
Cheesecake, Tesco*	1 Serving/76g	199	7.9	262	4.1	38.0	10.4	1.6
Christmas, Mini, Jane Asher*	1oz/28g	104	3.4	372	5.2	65.8	12.0	1.3
Dennis, Green's*	1 Cake/17.3g	54	1.3	319	4.6	57.8	7.7	0.0
Free From, Sainsbury's*	1 Serving/50g	173	0.2	346	1.3	84.4	0.3	2.2
Yellow, Super Moist, Betty Crocker*	1 Cake/128.0g	517	9.5	404	3.3	81.6	7.4	1.1
CALZONE								
Bolognese, Weight Watchers*	1 Calzone/88.1g	178	3.0	202	11.7	31.2	3.4	4.3
Cheese & Tomato, Weight Watchers*	1 Calzone/88g	191	3.8	217	11.3	33.4	4.3	3.4
Ham & Gruyere, Asda*	1 Serving/280g	661	22.4	236	10.0	31.0	8.0	2.7
CANAPES								
Caponata, Puff Pastry, Occasions, Sainsbury's*	1 Square/12g	30	1.9	249	4.1	22.9	15.7	2.1
Smoked Salmon, Youngs*	1 Canape/10g	21	1.5	210	15.9	2.0	15.2	0.7
CANNELLONI								
Beef, BGTY, Sainsbury's*	1 Pack/300g	249	6.9	83	5.5	10.1	2.3	1.7
Beef, Finest, Tesco*	½ Pack/300g	399	22.2	133	7.1	9.4	7.4	1.9
Beef, Great Value, Asda*	1 Pack/400g	384	10.8	96	6.0	12.0	2.7	1.6
Beef, HL, Tesco*	1 Pack/340g	323	8.2	95	6.4	11.9	2.4	1.5
Beef, Italian, Sainsbury's*	1 Pack/400g	498	26.2	125	5.9	10.5	6.6	1.6
Beef, Italian, Tesco*	1 Pack/400g	520	26.8	130	5.3	11.6	6.7	0.9
Beef, Sainsbury's*	1 Pack/400g	372	17.6	93	4.4	8.8	4.4	1.6
Beef & Red Wine, Waitrose*	½ Pack/170g	355	16.0	209	17.5	13.8	9.4	1.0
Chicken & Pesto, Italian, Sainsbury's*	1 Pack/450g	675	33.8	150	6.1	14.4	7.5	1.1
Iceland*	1 Pack/400g	584	28.8	146	7.2	13.0	7.2	0.6
M & S*	1 Pack/400g	540	32.4	135	7.4	7.8	8.1	2.1
Mediterranean Vegetable, Waitrose*	1 Serving/170g	330	15.3	194	9.7	18.7	9.0	1.9
Mushroom, Italian, Sainsbury's*	1 Pack/449.6g	599	31.1	133	5.2	12.5	6.9	0.5
Parmesan & Basil, M & S*	1 Pack/360g	504	28.4	140	5.9	11.4	7.9	0.8
Plain, Dry, Barilla*	1 Pack/250g	875	3.8	350	11.5	72.7	1.5	0.0
Pork, M & S*	1 Pack/400g	460	24.8	115	6.2	8.7	6.2	1.1
Ricotta & Spinach, Co-Op*	1 Pack/400g	420	20.0	105	4.0	12.0	5.0	2.0
Ricotta & Spinach, COU, M & S*	1 Pack/400g	320	8.0	80	5.3	9.7	2.0	2.8
Ricotta & Spinach, Eat Smart, Morrisons*	1 Pack/400g	328	8.0	82	5.2	10.9	2.0	1.6
Ricotta & Spinach, Fresh, Waitrose*	½ Pack/170g	207	12.4	122	5.1	8.8	7.3	1.2
Ricotta & Spinach, PB, Waitrose*	1 Pack/400g	272	9.2	68	3.8	7.7	2.3	1.4
Ricotta & Spinach, PB, Waitrose*	1 Pack/400g	272	9.2	68	3.8	7.7	2.3	1.4
Smoked Salmon & Spinach, Sainsbury's*	1 Pack/450g	599	27.9	133	5.7	13.5	6.2	0.4
Spinach & Cheese, Finest, Tesco*	1 Pack/350g	532	31.9	152	5.4	12.1	9.1	1.5
Spinach & Ricotta, BGTY, Sainsbury's*	1 Pack/300g	246	6.9	82	4.7	10.7	2.3	3.8
Spinach & Ricotta, Finest, Tesco*	1 Portion/120g	247	15.7	206	8.1	13.9	13.1	2.6
Spinach & Ricotta, Frozen, Sainsbury's*	1 Pack/350g	513	25.8	147	6.1	13.9	7.4	1.1
Spinach & Ricotta, Good Intentions, Somerfield*	1 Serving/400g	366	9.6	92	5.3	12.2	2.4	2.1
Spinach & Ricotta, HL, Tesco*	1 Pack/400g	320	11.2	80	4.0	10.0	2.8	1.1
Spinach & Ricotta, Italian Style, Co-Op*	1 Pack/450g	540	27.0	120	5.0	12.0	6.0	2.0
Spinach & Ricotta, Ross*	1 Pack/299g	296	8.1	99	3.3	15.2	2.7	1.6
Spinach & Ricotta, Somerfield*	1 Pack/300g	393	21.0	131	5.0	13.0	7.0	0.0
Spinach & Wild Mushroom, Linda McCartney*	1 Pack/340g	381	13.6	112	4.9	14.1	4.0	1.7
Tubes, Dry, Sainsbury's*	2 Tubes/16g	55	0.3	357	12.3	73.1	1.7	2.5

	Measure INFO/WEIGHT	per Measure KCAL	FAT	Nutrition Values per 100g / 100ml KCAL	PROT	CARB	FAT	FIBRE
CANNELLONI								
Value, Tesco*	1 Serving/250g	320	17.0	128	6.6	10.0	6.8	1.4
CAPERS								
Caperberries, Spanish, Waitrose*	1 Serving/55g	9	0.3	17	1.1	2.1	0.5	2.5
Capucines, Sainsbury's*	1 Tsp/6g	1	0.0	14	1.4	1.3	0.3	2.2
CAPPELLETTI								
Goats Cheese & Red Pesto, Waitrose*	½ Pack/125g	374	10.9	299	11.6	43.5	8.7	2.2
Meat, Italian, Somerfield*	½ Pack/125g	331	7.9	265	13.6	38.5	6.3	2.4
Parma Ham, Fresh, Waitrose*	½ Pack/125g	368	11.5	294	14.1	38.6	9.2	2.2
Prosciutto, Fresh, Waitrose*	½ Pack/125g	369	11.5	295	14.1	38.6	9.2	2.2
CAPRI SUN								
Orange	1 Pouch/200ml	90	0.0	45	0.0	11.0	0.0	0.0
CARAMAC								
Nestle*	1 Bar/30g	163	10.4	563	5.8	54.4	35.8	0.0
CARAMBOLA								
Average	1oz/28g	9	0.1	32	0.5	7.3	0.3	1.3
CARAMEL								
Egg, Cadbury*	1 Egg/39g	191	10.2	490	4.3	58.9	26.1	0.0
CARBONARA								
Frozen, Tesco*, Carbonara, Iceland*	1 Pack/400g	404	14.4	101	5.9	11.4	3.6	0.8
Frozen, Tesco*, Carbonara, Italiano, Tesco*	1 Serving/325g	757	37.4	233	8.6	23.8	11.5	1.2
Frozen, Tesco*, Carbonara, Low Fat, Bertorelli*	1 Pack/350g	301	7.7	86	5.3	12.0	2.2	0.9
Frozen, Tesco*, Carbonara, Naturally Less 5% Fat, Asda*	1 Pack/400g	440	9.6	110	4.2	18.0	2.4	0.8
Frozen, Tesco*, Carbonara, PB, Waitrose*	1 Pack/350g	357	12.6	102	5.3	12.1	3.6	0.7
Frozen, Tesco*, Carbonara, PB, Waitrose*	1 Pack/350g	357	12.6	102	5.3	12.1	3.6	0.7
Frozen, Tesco*, Carbonara, Safeway*	1 Serving/298g	277	8.3	93	3.7	13.2	2.8	0.6
Frozen, Tesco*, Chicken, Italia, M & S*	1 Pack/360g	342	6.5	95	8.1	12.1	1.8	1.2
Frozen, Tesco*, Chicken, Italian, Sainsbury's*	1 Pack/450g	567	15.8	126	6.5	17.0	3.5	2.6
Frozen, Tesco*, Chicken & Mushroom, GFY, Asda*	1 Pack/400g	359	7.0	90	7.3	11.3	1.8	0.7
Frozen, Tesco*, Chicken & Tomato, Eat Smart, Safeway*	1 Pack/400g	360	5.6	90	7.5	10.8	1.4	1.1
Frozen, Tesco*, Chicken & Tomato, Italiano, Tesco*	1 Pack/400g	416	8.4	104	6.6	14.8	2.1	0.8
Frozen, Tesco*, Dry, Average	1 Serving/100g	357	1.8	357	12.6	72.4	1.8	1.1
Frozen, Tesco*, Egg, Dry, Average	1 Serving/75g	272	2.5	362	14.3	68.8	3.3	2.3
Frozen, Tesco*, Egg, Fresh, Dry, Average	1 Serving/125g	345	3.5	276	10.6	53.0	2.8	2.1
Frozen, Tesco*, Egg & Spinach, M & S*	1 Serving/100g	365	2.7	365	15.5	69.6	2.7	3.0
Frozen, Tesco*, Egg & Spinach, Safeway*	1 Serving/83g	289	2.4	348	13.2	67.3	2.9	2.9
Frozen, Tesco*, Fresh, Dry, Average	1 Serving/75g	211	2.0	281	11.4	53.3	2.6	2.6
Frozen, Tesco*, Garlic & Herb, Cooked, Sainsbury's*	1oz/28g	41	0.5	147	6.5	26.3	1.8	1.9
Frozen, Tesco*, Garlic & Herb, Fresh, Asda*	½ Pack/150.7g	202	6.0	134	3.5	21.0	4.0	2.1
Frozen, Tesco*, Garlic & Herb, Fresh, Sainsbury's*	1 Serving/125g	184	2.3	147	6.5	26.2	1.8	1.9
Frozen, Tesco*, Garlic & Herb, Fresh, Tesco*	1 Serving/125g	361	4.6	289	12.0	51.8	3.7	1.5
Frozen, Tesco*, Garlic & Herb, Fresh, Waitrose*	1 Serving/125g	328	3.1	262	11.8	48.1	2.5	2.1
Frozen, Tesco*, Garlic & Herb, Italiano, Tesco*	1 Serving/85g	236	2.3	278	11.4	52.0	2.7	2.4
Frozen, Tesco*, Garlic & Herb, Safeway*	1 Serving/125g	175	2.3	140	5.7	25.5	1.8	1.9
Frozen, Tesco*, Garlic & Herbs, Cooked, Pasta Reale*	1 Pack/250g	390	2.8	156	6.2	30.4	1.1	1.0
Frozen, Tesco*, Garlic Mushroom, BGTY, Sainsbury's*	1 Pack/400g	416	9.2	104	4.7	16.2	2.3	2.0
Frozen, Tesco*, Garlic Mushroom, Italiano, Tesco*	1 Pack/450g	738	41.0	164	5.2	15.2	9.1	0.6
Frozen, Tesco*, Ham & Mushroom, Asda*	1 Pack/340g	469	12.9	138	6.0	20.0	3.8	0.2
Frozen, Tesco*, Ham & Mushroom, BFY, Morrisons*	1 Pack/350g	326	13.3	93	5.3	9.4	3.8	0.8
Frozen, Tesco*, Ham & Mushroom, BGTY, Sainsbury's*	1 Pack/450g	486	14.4	108	5.3	14.5	3.2	0.8
Frozen, Tesco*, Ham & Mushroom, Co-Op*	1 Pack/300g	270	9.0	90	6.0	10.0	3.0	2.0
Frozen, Tesco*, Ham & Mushroom, COU, M & S*	1 Pack/400g	720	17.6	180	9.2	25.9	4.4	1.5
Frozen, Tesco*, Ham & Mushroom, Eat Smart, Safeway*	1 Pack/400g	380	10.0	95	5.0	13.0	2.5	1.2
Frozen, Tesco*, Ham & Mushroom, GFY, Asda*	1 Pack/398.8g	323	9.2	81	5.4	9.6	2.3	0.7

	Measure INFO/WEIGHT	per Measure KCAL	FAT	Nutrition Values per 100g / 100ml KCAL	PROT	CARB	FAT	FIBRE
CARBONARA								
Frozen, Tesco*, Ham & Mushroom, HL, Tesco*	1 Pack/400g	460	10.4	115	7.2	15.4	2.6	1.1
Frozen, Tesco*, Ham & Mushroom, Italian, Tesco*	1 Pack/430g	516	18.5	120	5.6	14.7	4.3	0.7
Frozen, Tesco*, Ham & Mushroom, Morrisons*	1 Meal/450.4g	635	26.1	141	6.4	15.7	5.8	1.5
CARIBBEAN TWIST								
Halewood International*	1 Serving/500ml	430	0.0	86	0.0	13.7	0.0	0.0
CAROB POWDER								
Average	1 Tsp/2g	3	0.0	159	4.9	37.0	0.1	0.0
CARROT & SWEDE								
Diced, for Mashing, Average	½ Pack/250g	58	0.7	23	0.6	4.7	0.3	1.9
Mash, From Supermarket, Average	1 Serving/150g	138	7.5	92	1.3	10.4	5.0	1.3
Mash, Healthy Range, Average	1 Serving/150g	98	4.2	66	1.3	8.6	2.8	2.1
CARROTS								
& Peas, Sainsbury's*	1 Serving/200g	100	1.0	50	3.3	8.3	0.5	3.8
Baby, Canned, Average	1 Can/195g	40	0.5	21	0.5	4.2	0.3	2.1
Baby, Fresh, Average	1 Serving/60g	17	0.2	29	0.7	5.8	0.3	1.7
Baby, with Fine Beans, Tesco*	1 Pack/200g	58	1.0	29	1.3	4.7	0.5	2.3
Baby Corn, & Mange Tout, Safeway*	1 Pack/200g	48	0.6	24	2.1	3.2	0.3	0.0
Batons, Fresh, Average	½ Pack/150g	41	0.5	28	0.6	5.7	0.3	2.6
Boiled, Average	1oz/28g	6	0.1	22	0.6	4.4	0.4	2.3
Canned, Average	1oz/28g	6	0.1	22	0.6	4.4	0.3	2.1
Chantenay, Tesco*	1oz/28g	7	0.1	24	0.6	4.4	0.4	2.3
Sliced, Canned, Average	1 Serving/180g	36	0.2	20	0.7	4.1	0.1	1.5
Sliced, Fresh, Average	1 Serving/60g	17	0.2	28	0.7	5.7	0.3	2.0
Whole, Raw, Peeled, Average	1 Carrot/75g	21	0.2	29	0.6	6.4	0.3	2.2
with Parsley & English Butter, M & S*	½ Pack/100g	65	3.9	65	0.6	7.1	3.9	2.4
CASHEW NUTS								
Plain, Average	¼ Pack/25g	146	12.2	585	15.7	18.8	48.9	3.4
Roasted & Salted, Average	1 Serving/50g	306	25.6	612	18.8	19.6	51.1	3.1
CASHEWS & PEANUTS								
Honey Roasted, Average	1 Serving/50g	290	21.5	579	21.6	26.6	42.9	4.2
CASSAVA								
Baked, Average	1oz/28g	43	0.1	155	0.7	40.1	0.2	1.7
Boiled in Unsalted Water, Average	1oz/28g	36	0.1	130	0.5	33.5	0.2	1.4
Gari, Average	1oz/28g	100	0.1	358	1.3	92.9	0.5	0.0
Raw, Average	1oz/28g	40	0.1	142	0.6	36.8	0.2	1.6
Steamed, Average	1oz/28g	40	0.1	142	0.6	36.8	0.2	1.6
CASSEROLE								
Bean, & Lentil, Morrisons*	1 Can/410g	287	1.6	70	4.1	12.5	0.4	0.0
Bean, Spicy, BGTY, Sainsbury's*	1 Pack/300g	171	2.7	57	3.0	9.1	0.9	4.2
Beef, & Ale, Finest, Tesco*	½ Pack/300g	234	4.2	78	11.5	5.0	1.4	1.1
Beef, & Ale, with Dumplings, Sainsbury's*	1 Pack/450g	711	32.9	158	7.7	15.4	7.3	0.6
Beef, & Ale, with Mashed Potato, HL, Tesco*	1 Pack/450g	365	11.3	81	5.1	10.9	2.5	0.6
Beef, & Dumplings, Safeway*	1 Pack/390g	215	7.6	55	1.6	7.5	1.9	1.2
Beef, & Onion, Minced, British Classics, Tesco*	1 Pack/340g	367	19.0	108	5.0	9.3	5.6	0.8
Beef, & Red Wine, BGTY, Sainsbury's*	1 Pack/300g	192	1.8	64	8.0	6.7	0.6	0.9
Beef, & Vegetable, Ready Meals, Waitrose*	1oz/28g	32	1.5	114	4.1	12.8	5.2	0.9
Beef, Canned, Waitrose*	1 Tin/400g	372	10.0	93	10.5	7.0	2.5	1.8
Beef, M & S*	1 Pack/454g	522	22.7	115	9.6	7.5	5.0	0.9
Beef, Meal for One, Tesco*	1 Pack/450g	425	18.9	94	3.6	10.6	4.2	1.7
Beef, Mini Favourites, M & S*	1 Pack/200g	210	8.4	105	7.1	9.3	4.2	1.4
Beef, Traditional British, TTD, Sainsbury's*	1 Serving/100g	136	5.1	136	22.5	0.1	5.1	0.1
Beef, with Dumplings, Eat Smart, Safeway*	1 Pack/390.9g	215	7.4	55	1.6	7.3	1.9	1.2
Beef, with Dumplings, GFY, Asda*	1 Pack/400g	416	8.8	104	11.0	10.0	2.2	0.9

CASSEROLE

INFO/WEIGHT	Measure	per Measure KCAL	FAT	Nutrition Values per 100g / 100ml KCAL	PROT	CARB	FAT	FIBRE
Beef, with Herb Dumplings, COU, M & S*	1 Pack/400g	400	10.0	100	9.6	11.0	2.5	1.2
Beef, with Herb Potatoes, Tesco*	1 Serving/475g	504	17.1	106	6.8	11.5	3.6	1.6
Chicken, & Asparagus, HL, Tesco*	1 Serving/450g	342	10.4	76	6.3	8.3	2.3	0.5
Chicken, & Asparagus, in White Wine, Finest, Tesco*	1 Pack/350.3g	683	42.4	195	10.0	11.6	12.1	0.3
Chicken, & Asparagus in White Wine, Tesco*	½ Pack/300g	444	23.7	148	11.5	7.7	7.9	0.8
Chicken, & Dumplings, HL, Tesco*	1 Pack/450g	441	12.2	98	7.4	11.1	2.7	0.6
Chicken, & Dumplings, Morrisons*	1 Pack/300g	291	12.6	97	3.4	11.4	4.2	1.3
Chicken, & Dumplings, Sainsbury's*	1 Serving/450g	612	32.4	136	6.8	11.0	7.2	0.6
Chicken, & Herb Dumplings, BGTY, Sainsbury's*	1 Pack/450g	446	18.5	99	6.1	9.5	4.1	0.6
Chicken, & Red Wine, Duchy Originals*	½ Pack/175g	187	7.5	107	14.0	5.1	4.3	1.6
Chicken, & Tomato, Asda*	¼ Pack/273g	569	41.0	208	16.0	2.2	15.0	0.5
Chicken, & Vegetable, Apetito*	1 Pack/330g	286	9.9	87	6.3	9.4	3.0	1.6
Chicken, & Vegetable, Long Life, Sainsbury's*	1 Pack/300g	186	4.5	62	4.6	7.4	1.5	0.8
Chicken, & White Wine, BGTY, Sainsbury's*	1 Serving/300g	216	6.6	72	7.2	5.9	2.2	1.3
Chicken, Catalan, TTD, Sainsbury's*	½ Pack/300g	324	15.6	108	10.8	4.4	5.2	0.6
Chicken, Fillets, Safeway*	½ Pack/172.2g	155	2.2	90	15.6	2.9	1.3	0.6
Chicken, GFY, Asda*	1 Pack/400g	356	9.6	89	8.2	8.7	2.4	1.9
Chicken, Green Isle*	1 Pack/400g	300	6.8	75	5.7	9.2	1.7	1.0
Chicken, Leek & Mushroom, Tesco*	1 Pack/350g	382	22.1	109	4.5	8.6	6.3	1.0
Chicken, Mediterranean, Tesco*	1 Pack/400g	260	9.2	65	6.7	4.5	2.3	0.9
Chicken, Mini, M & S*	1 Pack/200g	210	9.6	105	6.7	9.1	4.8	2.3
Chicken, PB, Waitrose*	1 Pack/400g	392	14.4	98	6.6	9.8	3.6	1.2
Chicken, PB, Waitrose*	1 Pack/400g	392	14.4	98	6.6	9.8	3.6	1.2
Chicken, with Dumplings, M & S*	½ Pack/227g	261	10.0	115	9.7	9.0	4.4	0.9
Chicken, with Herb Dumpling, BGTY, Sainsbury's*	1 Pack/400g	252	5.2	63	5.3	7.4	1.3	2.9
Chicken, with Sage & Onion Dumplings, COU, M & S*	1 Pack/400g	380	8.8	95	9.2	10.2	2.2	1.0
Cowboy, Iceland*	1 Pack/400g	500	26.0	125	5.8	10.9	6.5	1.7
Lamb, & Rosemary, Eat Well, M & S*	1 Pack/380g	325	11.0	86	7.6	7.0	2.9	2.2
Lamb, BGTY, Sainsbury's*	1 Serving/200g	242	8.6	121	20.7	0.1	4.3	0.1
Lamb, Braised, British Classics, Tesco*	1 Pack/350g	333	18.2	95	7.5	4.6	5.2	1.2
Lamb, M & S*	1 Pack/200g	230	9.4	115	8.5	9.5	4.7	1.8
Lamb, with Mint Dumplings, Minced, Sainsbury's*	1 Pack/450g	558	30.6	124	5.4	10.4	6.8	1.1
Minced Beef, with Dumplings, M & S*	1 Pack/193g	299	16.6	155	10.7	9.2	8.6	0.9
Mushroom, & Onion, Iceland*	1 Pack/400g	272	12.4	68	1.3	8.8	3.1	1.9
Pork, & Apple, with Boiled Potatos & Vegetables, Apetito*	1 Pack/350g	251	3.9	72	5.1	8.5	1.1	1.1
Pork, Normandy Style, Finest, Tesco*	1 Pack/450g	405	21.6	90	7.6	4.1	4.8	2.3
Pork, with Apple & Cider, Safeway*	1 Pack/450g	729	37.8	162	8.3	13.4	8.4	1.1
Rabbit, Average	1oz/28g	29	1.4	102	11.6	2.6	5.1	0.4
Sausage, & Potato, M & S*	1 Serving/200g	190	11.8	95	3.3	7.5	5.9	0.9
Steak, & Ale, British Classics, Tesco*	1 Serving/100g	93	3.4	93	11.2	4.5	3.4	1.1
Steak, & Ale, Sainsbury's*	1 Pack/300g	288	10.5	96	10.6	5.6	3.5	0.4
Steak, & Mushroom, Asda*	½ Pack/304.4g	410	30.4	135	7.0	4.2	10.0	0.3
Steak, & Mushroom with Mustard Mash, Finest, Tesco*	1 Pack/550g	523	21.5	95	5.9	9.0	3.9	1.1
Steak, Prime, Sainsbury's*	1oz/28g	34	1.0	122	22.6	0.1	3.5	0.1
Steak & Kidney, Mini, Favourites, M & S*	1 Pack/200g	240	10.8	120	7.9	9.5	5.4	1.5
Vegetable, Chunky, M & S*	1 Bag/450g	90	1.4	20	0.7	3.4	0.3	1.4
Vegetable, Country, Sainsbury's*	1 Can/400g	300	10.0	75	2.2	11.0	2.5	1.1
Vegetable, Mixed, Farmfoods*	1oz/28g	8	0.1	29	0.8	5.8	0.3	2.1
Vegetable, Mixed, Safeway*	1 Serving/100g	17	0.3	17	0.7	3.0	0.3	2.1
Vegetable, Tesco*	1 Serving/220g	66	0.7	30	0.8	6.1	0.3	1.5
Vegetable, with Herb Dumplings, COU, M & S*	1 Pack/450g	270	5.4	60	1.6	10.1	1.2	1.0
Vegetable, with Potato Crush, Safeway*	1 Pack/450g	293	14.0	65	1.3	7.7	3.1	2.0
Venison, Scottish Wild, & Beaujolais, Tesco*	1 Pack/425g	366	8.9	86	11.9	4.9	2.1	0.6

C

	Measure INFO/WEIGHT	per Measure		Nutrition Values per 100g / 100ml				
		KCAL	FAT	KCAL	PROT	CARB	FAT	FIBRE
CASEROLE MIX								
Beef, Authentic, Schwartz*	1 Pack/43g	111	0.4	257	7.4	54.5	1.0	0.4
Beef, Colman's*	1/3 Pack/13.3g	40	0.2	308	7.5	66.0	1.5	2.5
Beef & Ale, Colman's*	1 Pack/45g	144	0.9	320	9.2	66.3	2.0	2.3
Chicken, Authentic, Schwartz*	1 Pack/36g	131	1.5	363	10.4	70.7	4.3	2.0
Chicken, Traditional, Colman's*	1/3 Pack/13g	40	0.2	311	5.7	69.4	1.3	1.5
Chicken Chasseur, Asda*	1 Pack/80g	273	0.8	341	9.0	74.0	1.0	1.4
Chicken Chasseur, Morrisons*	1 Pack/40g	115	0.5	288	9.2	59.8	1.2	0.0
Farmhouse Sausage, Schwartz*	1 Pack/39g	124	1.1	317	8.1	64.6	2.9	0.5
Honey Chicken, Colman's*	1 Pack/50g	129	0.6	257	3.4	58.3	1.1	1.8
Lamb, Authentic, Schwartz*	1 Pack/35g	116	1.2	332	7.7	68.0	3.3	1.3
Liver & Bacon, Colman's*	1 Pack/40g	121	0.7	303	10.3	61.6	1.7	4.7
Moroccan Lamb, Schwartz*	½ Pack/17.5g	62	1.0	354	6.2	74.1	5.7	4.5
Peppered Beef, Schwartz*	1 Serving/80g	258	3.9	323	7.0	62.9	4.9	7.3
Pork, Colman's*	1/3 Pack/13.4g	44	0.2	328	6.7	72.0	1.4	2.8
Pork, Morrisons*	1 Pack/36g	118	0.5	327	8.1	70.6	1.4	0.0
Sausage, Asda*	¼ Pack/25g	80	1.0	321	6.0	65.0	4.1	3.0
Sausage, Classic, Schwartz*	1 Pack/39g	107	1.1	275	12.4	50.1	2.7	14.9
Sausage, Colman's*	1 Pack/40g	144	0.6	361	8.9	77.7	1.6	1.6
Sausage & Onion, Colman's*	1 Pack/45g	143	1.2	318	9.6	64.2	2.6	2.6
Somerset Pork, Colman's*	1 Serving/23g	74	0.3	321	7.1	70.2	1.3	2.2
Somerset Pork, Schwartz*	1 Pack/36g	115	1.4	320	9.4	61.9	3.8	7.7
Spicy Chicken, Colman's*	1 Pack/45g	151	0.8	336	6.5	73.4	1.8	1.5
Turkey, Colman's*	1 Pack/50g	157	1.0	313	5.9	68.0	1.9	3.5
CATFISH								
Cooked, Average	1 Fillet/87g	199	11.6	229	18.1	8.1	13.3	0.7
Raw, Average	1oz/28g	27	0.8	96	17.6	0.0	2.8	0.0
CAULIFLOWER								
& Broccoli Florets, Tesco*	1 Bag/350g	119	3.2	34	3.9	2.5	0.9	2.7
Boiled, Average	1 Serving/80g	22	0.7	28	2.9	2.1	0.9	1.6
Florets, Peas & Carrots, Frozen, Asda*	1 Serving/100g	37	0.6	37	3.0	5.0	0.6	2.8
Peas & Carrots, Birds Eye*	1oz/28g	9	0.1	32	2.2	4.8	0.4	2.6
Raw, Average	1 Serving/100g	31	0.8	31	3.3	2.7	0.8	1.6
CAULIFLOWER CHEESE								
& Bacon, Gastropub, M & S*	1 Pack/300g	318	21.0	106	6.3	4.5	7.0	1.0
& Broccoli, Morrisons*	1 Serving/500g	355	16.5	71	3.7	6.6	3.3	0.9
& Broccoli, Sainsbury's*	1 Serving/130g	83	2.1	64	4.8	7.6	1.6	2.7
Asda*	1 Pack/450g	486	36.0	108	4.6	4.3	8.0	1.5
BFY, Morrisons*	1 Pack/300g	231	12.3	77	4.5	5.4	4.1	1.2
BGTY, Sainsbury's*	½ Pack/225.5g	115	5.6	51	3.6	3.5	2.5	2.4
Birds Eye*	1 Pack/329g	354	21.0	108	4.8	7.7	6.4	0.8
Budgens*	1 Pack/450g	284	18.9	63	5.3	4.0	4.2	1.0
Eat Smart, Morrisons*	1 Pack/300g	192	6.0	64	4.9	6.7	2.0	1.5
Eat Smart, Safeway*	1 Pack/300g	165	6.3	55	4.5	4.0	2.1	1.0
Finest, Tesco*	1 Serving/250g	318	21.3	127	6.5	6.1	8.5	0.4
Frozen, Tesco*	1 Pack/450g	428	30.2	95	4.2	4.3	6.7	1.3
Great Value, Asda*	1 Pack/396g	352	23.8	89	3.9	4.9	6.0	0.8
Grills, Dalepak*	1 Grill/94.1g	240	15.4	255	5.0	22.0	16.4	2.6
Grills, Meat Free, Tesco*	1 Grill/91.4g	160	7.4	175	5.3	20.0	8.1	2.9
Iceland*	1 Pack/500g	350	14.0	70	3.4	7.9	2.8	1.1
M & S*	1 Serving/150g	150	9.2	100	5.5	5.9	6.1	1.1
Made with Half Fat Cheese, HL, Tesco*	1 Pack/400g	228	10.4	57	6.5	2.0	2.6	2.2
Made with Semi-Skimmed Milk	1oz/28g	28	1.8	100	6.0	5.2	6.4	1.3
Made with Skimmed Milk	1oz/28g	27	1.7	97	6.0	5.2	6.0	1.3

	Measure INFO/WEIGHT	per Measure KCAL	FAT	Nutrition Values per 100g / 100ml KCAL	PROT	CARB	FAT	FIBRE
CAULIFLOWER CHEESE								
Made with Whole Milk	1oz/28g	29	1.9	105	6.0	5.2	6.9	1.3
Morrisons*	1 Pack/350g	399	29.8	114	5.5	3.8	8.5	1.4
Ross*	1 Pack/300g	300	19.8	100	4.9	5.5	6.6	0.1
Safeway*	½ Pack/185g	205	15.0	111	5.7	3.7	8.1	1.5
Sainsbury's*	1 Pack/300g	357	20.7	119	6.4	7.8	6.9	0.9
Somerfield*	1 Serving/402.5g	322	22.2	80	4.6	3.1	5.5	1.8
TTD, Sainsbury's*	½ Pack/150g	252	18.0	168	6.9	8.0	12.0	0.9
Waitrose*	1 Pack/450g	329	21.6	73	4.1	3.3	4.8	1.6
with Crispy Bacon, Finest, Tesco*	1/3 Pack/166g	211	14.1	127	6.5	6.1	8.5	0.4
with Roasted Potatoes, M & S*	1 Serving/200g	260	13.0	130	5.3	12.0	6.5	1.8
CAVATELLI								
Egg, Asda*	1 Serving/100g	203	3.4	203	9.0	34.0	3.4	3.0
King Prawn & Scallop, M & S*	1 Pack/400g	600	22.4	150	6.4	18.0	5.6	1.3
CAVIAR								
Average	1oz/28g	26	1.3	92	12.0	0.5	4.7	0.0
CELERIAC								
Boiled in Salted Water, Average	1oz/28g	4	0.1	15	0.9	1.9	0.5	3.2
Raw, Average	1 Serving/100g	42	0.3	42	1.5	9.2	0.3	1.8
CELERY								
Boiled in Salted Water	1 Med Serving/50g	4	0.2	8	0.5	0.8	0.3	1.2
Raw, Average	1 Med Stalk/40g	3	0.1	8	0.7	1.0	0.2	1.7
CELLANTANI								
Dry Weight, Buitoni*	1 Serving/195g	706	3.3	362	12.2	74.4	1.7	0.0
CHAMPAGNE								
Average	1 Glass/120ml	89	0.0	76	0.3	1.4	0.0	0.0
CHANNA MASALA								
Indian, Sainsbury's*	1 Serving/149g	165	7.3	111	4.2	12.4	4.9	3.3
M & S*	1 Pack/225g	360	23.7	160	5.6	11.2	10.5	8.2
Safeway*	1 Pack/400g	540	21.6	135	5.3	16.2	5.4	2.5
CHAPATIS								
Brown Wheat Flour, Waitrose*	1 Chapatis/42g	128	3.4	305	8.6	49.4	8.0	4.6
Elephant Atta*	1 Chapati/44.9g	129	2.9	287	7.5	53.1	6.4	3.2
Indian Style, Asda*	1 Chapatis/43g	95	0.4	221	8.0	45.0	1.0	2.9
Made with Fat	1 Chapatis/60g	197	7.7	328	8.1	48.3	12.8	0.0
Made without Fat	1 Chapatis/55g	111	0.6	202	7.3	43.7	1.0	0.0
Morrisons*	1 Chapatis/40g	105	2.7	269	8.6	49.8	6.9	0.0
Plain, Wraps, Original, Patak's*	1 Chapatis/42g	115	3.2	273	9.4	48.8	7.5	0.0
Wholemeal, Patak's*	1 Chapatis/42g	130	4.0	310	11.2	44.9	9.5	9.0
CHEDDARS								
Baked, Mini, Cheddar Cheese, McVitie's*	1 Bag/30g	155	9.1	518	10.2	51.4	30.2	2.5
Baked, Mini, Cheese & Ham Flavour, McVitie's*	1 Bag/30g	160	8.9	534	11.0	55.5	29.8	2.0
Baked, Mini, Cheese & Onion Flavour, McVitie's*	1 Pack/25g	130	7.5	518	9.2	53.2	29.9	2.8
Baked, Mini, Peperami, McVitie's*	1 Bag/30g	160	9.1	532	9.7	55.2	30.2	2.0
Baked, Mini, Tangy Salsa, McVitie's*	1 Bag/50g	266	15.0	532	11.0	54.7	29.9	2.1
Smokey BBQ, McVitie's*	1 Sm Pack/30g	155	8.9	516	9.3	52.8	29.8	2.6
CHEESE								
Ail & Fines Herbes, Boursin*	1oz/28g	116	11.8	414	7.0	2.0	42.0	0.0
Appenzellar, Sainsbury's*	1 Serving/25g	97	7.9	386	25.4	0.0	31.6	0.0
Applewood, Somerfield*	1oz/28g	119	9.8	426	28.0	0.0	35.0	0.0
Asiago, M & S*	1oz/28g	105	7.6	375	33.0	0.1	27.0	0.0
Babybel, Emmental, Fromageries Bel*	1 Serving/20g	63	4.9	316	23.0	1.0	24.5	0.0
Babybel, Light, Mini, Fromageries Bel*	1 Cheese/20g	42	2.4	208	25.0	0.2	12.0	0.0
Babybel, Original, Mini, Fromageries Bel*	1 Cheese/20g	63	5.0	315	22.5	0.2	25.0	0.0

CHEESE

INFO/WEIGHT	Measure	per Measure		Nutrition Values per 100g / 100ml				
		KCAL	FAT	KCAL	PROT	CARB	FAT	FIBRE
Babybel, with Cheddar, Mini, Fromageries Bel*	1 Cheese/19g	69	5.7	362	23.0	0.2	30.0	0.0
Bavarian, Smoked, Slices, Asda*	1 Slice/18g	50	4.1	277	17.0	0.4	23.0	0.0
Bavarian, Smoked, with Ham, Sainsbury's*	1 Serving/30g	89	7.2	298	19.4	0.8	24.1	0.0
Bavarian Smoked, Processed, Somerfield*	1oz/28g	85	5.9	302	29.0	0.0	21.0	0.0
Biscuits & Chutney, Delicious, Boots*	1 Pack/133.6g	290	14.7	217	9.0	19.0	11.0	2.3
Bleu D' Auvergne, Sainsbury's*	1 Serving/25g	84	6.6	335	22.0	2.0	26.5	0.0
Blue, Castello, Soft, Castello*	¼ Pack/37.5g	162	15.6	432	14.0	0.5	41.5	0.0
Bresse Bleu, M & S*	1oz/28g	99	8.7	355	19.0	0.3	31.0	0.0
Brie, Average	1 Serving/25g	74	6.0	296	19.7	0.3	24.0	0.0
Brie, Reduced Fat, Average	1 Serving/50g	99	5.7	198	23.0	0.8	11.4	0.0
Caerphilly, Average	1 Serving/50g	187	15.7	374	23.0	0.1	31.3	0.0
Cambazola, Tesco*	1 Serving/30g	128	12.3	425	13.5	0.5	41.0	0.0
Camembert, Average	1 Serving/50g	141	11.1	283	20.5	0.1	22.2	0.0
Camembert, Breaded, Average	1 Serving/90g	307	20.9	342	16.7	14.3	23.3	0.5
Camembert, French, Morrisons*	1 Pack/250g	665	50.0	266	21.0	0.5	20.0	0.0
Cantal, French, Sainsbury's*	1 Serving/30g	106	8.7	353	23.0	0.1	29.0	0.0
Cantenaar, M & S*	1 Serving/28g	84	5.4	300	32.2	0.1	19.2	0.0
Chaumes, M & S*	1oz/28g	85	7.3	305	20.2	1.0	26.0	0.0
Cheddar, Canadian, Average	1 Serving/30g	123	10.3	409	25.0	0.1	34.3	0.0
Cheddar, Davidstow, Mature, Average	1 Serving/28g	115	9.6	410	25.0	0.1	34.4	0.0
Cheddar, Extra Mature, Average	1 Serving/30g	123	10.3	410	25.1	0.1	34.4	0.0
Cheddar, Extra Mature, Pilgrims Choice*	1 Serving/30g	123	10.3	410	25.0	0.1	34.4	0.0
Cheddar, Fingers, Great Stuff, Asda*	1 Finger/20g	75	6.2	375	23.0	0.1	31.0	0.0
Cheddar, Grated, Average	1 Serving/50g	206	17.2	413	24.4	1.5	34.3	0.0
Cheddar, Mature, Average	1 Serving/30g	123	10.3	410	25.0	0.1	34.4	0.0
Cheddar, Mature, Grated, Average	1 Serving/28g	113	9.3	404	24.7	1.6	33.2	0.0
Cheddar, Mature, Lighter, Cathedral City*	1 Serving/30g	93	6.5	311	28.6	0.1	21.8	0.0
Cheddar, Mature, Reduced Fat, Average	1 Serving/25g	68	4.2	271	30.0	0.1	16.7	0.0
Cheddar, Mature Yet Mellow, Cathedral City*	1 Slice/10g	42	3.5	416	25.4	0.1	34.9	0.0
Cheddar, Medium, Average	1 Serving/30g	123	10.4	411	24.9	0.2	34.5	0.0
Cheddar, Mild, Average	1 Serving/30g	123	10.3	409	25.0	0.1	34.3	0.0
Cheddar, Mild, Slices, Morrisons*	1 Slice/20g	82	6.9	410	25.0	0.1	34.4	0.0
Cheddar, Reduced Fat, Average	1 Serving/30g	76	4.2	255	32.2	0.1	14.0	0.0
Cheddar, Smoked, Average	1 Serving/30g	123	10.3	411	25.3	0.1	34.4	0.0
Cheddar, West Country Farmhouse, Average	1 Serving/28g	115	9.6	410	25.0	0.1	34.4	0.0
Cheddar, Wexford, Average	1 Serving/20g	82	6.9	410	25.0	0.1	34.4	0.0
Cheddar, with Caramelised Onion, Sainsbury's*	1 Serving/28g	109	8.7	391	22.8	5.1	31.0	0.0
Cheddar, with Caramelised Onion, Tesco*	1 Serving/50g	183	14.0	366	21.4	7.1	28.0	0.4
Cheddar, with Onion & Chives, Davidson*	1 Serving/25g	100	8.3	400	24.3	0.6	33.3	0.0
Cheddar, with Winter Berries, Christmas, Tesco*	1oz/28g	106	8.5	378	22.9	3.4	30.3	0.2
Cheddar & Mozzarella, Spicy, Grated, Tesco*	1 Serving/40g	140	10.5	350	26.0	2.5	26.2	0.0
Cheestrings, Cheddar, Original, Golden Vale*	1 Stick/21g	69	5.0	328	28.0	0.0	24.0	0.0
Cheestrings, Double Cheese, Golden Vale*	1 Stick/21g	69	5.0	328	28.0	0.0	24.0	0.0
Cheshire	1oz/28g	106	8.8	379	24.0	0.1	31.4	0.0
Chevre Pave D'affinois, Finest, Tesco*	1 Pack/150g	404	32.6	269	18.5	0.0	21.7	0.0
Cotswold, Full Fat with Herbs, Somerfield*	1oz/28g	113	9.5	405	25.0	0.0	34.0	0.0
Cottage, & Chargrilled Vegetables, BGTY, Sainsbury's*	1oz/28g	25	0.3	88	12.1	7.8	0.9	0.6
Cottage, Arla*	1 Serving/25g	23	1.0	90	12.0	2.0	4.0	0.0
Cottage, Bettabuy, Morrisons*	1 Tub/200g	210	10.0	105	11.0	5.0	5.0	0.0
Cottage, BFY, Morrisons*	1 Pot/125g	110	1.1	88	13.0	6.9	0.9	0.0
Cottage, Crunchy Vegetable, GFY, Asda*	1 Serving/50g	37	0.7	74	11.0	4.5	1.3	0.6
Cottage, Danone*	1 Serving/100g	89	3.9	89	11.2	2.3	3.9	0.0
Cottage, Garlic & Herb, Diet, Yoplait*	1 Pot/225g	180	4.3	80	12.0	3.9	1.9	0.0

C

CHEESE

	Measure INFO/WEIGHT	per Measure KCAL	FAT	Nutrition Values per 100g / 100ml KCAL	PROT	CARB	FAT	FIBRE
Cottage, Healthy Choice, Asda*	1oz/28g	25	0.6	88	13.0	4.0	2.0	0.0
Cottage, Healthy Choice, Nisa Heritage*	1 Pot/227g	175	4.1	77	11.8	3.4	1.8	0.3
Cottage, Iceland*	1 Serving/100g	77	1.8	77	11.8	3.4	1.8	0.3
Cottage, Jocca, Kraft*	1 Serving/50g	55	2.8	109	9.3	5.0	5.5	0.0
Cottage, Less Than 5% Fat, Sainsbury's*	½ Pot/125g	131	5.3	105	12.3	4.4	4.2	0.0
Cottage, Lidl*	1 Tub/200g	210	9.0	105	12.5	3.0	4.5	0.0
Cottage, Light Choices, Tesco*	1 Serving/60g	48	0.9	80	12.2	4.5	1.5	0.0
Cottage, Low Fat, Balanced Lifestyle, Aldi*	1 Serving/100g	85	1.3	85	14.6	3.6	1.3	0.1
Cottage, Low Fat, Longley Farm*	1oz/28g	32	1.7	114	11.5	3.4	6.0	0.0
Cottage, Low Fat, with Onion & Chive, Safeway*	1 Pot/250g	210	4.8	84	12.0	4.2	1.9	0.1
Cottage, Natural, 95% Fat Free, M & S*	1oz/28g	28	1.1	99	11.6	3.5	4.0	0.0
Cottage, Natural, Asda*	¼ Pot/113g	118	4.7	104	12.0	4.0	4.2	0.0
Cottage, Natural, BGTY, Sainsbury's*	1 Serving/125g	105	1.1	84	12.0	6.9	0.9	0.0
Cottage, Natural, COU, M & S*	½ Pot/125g	100	2.3	80	11.9	3.3	1.8	0.3
Cottage, Natural, Deliciously Creamy, M & S*	½ Pot/125g	138	6.6	110	11.7	4.0	5.3	0.0
Cottage, Natural, GFY, Asda*	1 Serving/113g	95	2.0	84	13.0	3.9	1.8	0.3
Cottage, Natural, HE, Tesco*	1 Pot/125g	98	2.3	78	11.9	3.6	1.8	0.0
Cottage, Natural, Healthy Choice, Safeway*	1oz/28g	24	0.6	87	12.7	4.0	2.0	0.0
Cottage, Natural, Healthy Choice, Somerfield*	½ Tub/125.6g	98	1.9	78	11.0	5.2	1.5	0.0
Cottage, Natural, HL, Co-Op*	1 Pot/250g	188	5.0	75	10.0	4.0	2.0	0.0
Cottage, Natural, HL, Tesco*	1 Serving/150g	128	2.3	85	14.3	3.4	1.5	0.3
Cottage, Natural, Kwik Save*	1 Serving/25g	22	0.2	89	13.0	6.9	0.9	0.0
Cottage, Natural, Less Than 5% Fat, Sainsbury's*	½ Pot/125g	124	6.0	99	11.0	3.0	4.8	0.0
Cottage, Natural, Loseley*	½ Tub/100g	115	7.1	115	9.4	2.9	7.1	0.0
Cottage, Natural, Morrisons*	1 Serving/100g	88	0.9	88	13.0	6.9	0.9	0.0
Cottage, Natural, Organic, Sainsbury's*	1 Pot/201g	185	3.6	92	12.8	6.3	1.8	0.0
Cottage, Natural, Organic, Tesco*	1 Serving/60g	48	1.1	80	12.3	3.3	1.8	0.0
Cottage, Natural, Simply, Kwik Save*	1 Pot/200g	158	2.2	79	11.7	5.5	1.1	0.0
Cottage, Natural, SmartPrice, Asda*	½ Pot/100g	86	2.0	86	12.0	4.3	2.0	0.0
Cottage, Natural, Somerfield*	1 Serving/100g	105	4.2	105	12.3	4.4	4.2	0.0
Cottage, Natural, Tesco*	1 Serving/50g	49	1.8	98	12.4	3.2	3.5	0.4
Cottage, Natural, Waitrose*	½ Pot/125g	120	4.4	96	12.4	3.6	3.5	0.4
Cottage, Onion & Chive, Waitrose*	1 Serving/20g	18	0.6	91	10.8	4.9	3.1	0.3
Cottage, Onion & Chives, Light Choices, Tesco*	1 Serving/60g	51	0.9	85	11.4	4.8	1.5	0.1
Cottage, Pineapple, Light Choices, Tesco*	1 Serving/60g	54	0.8	90	9.8	8.5	1.3	0.4
Cottage, Pineapple, PB, Waitrose*	½ Pot/125g	107	1.8	85	8.4	9.7	1.4	0.5
Cottage, Plain	1oz/28g	27	1.1	98	13.8	2.1	3.9	0.0
Cottage, Plain, Reduced Fat	1oz/28g	22	0.4	78	13.3	3.3	1.4	0.0
Cottage, Red Onion & Garlic, Sainsbury's*	½ Tub/125g	91	1.1	73	10.4	5.8	0.9	0.6
Cottage, Slimline*	1 Serving/70g	43	0.1	62	12.0	3.0	0.2	0.0
Cottage, Stilton & Celery, BGTY, Sainsbury's*	½ Pot/125g	99	2.8	79	10.8	4.0	2.2	1.5
Cottage, Tropical, Westacre*	1 Serving/100g	89	1.2	89	13.1	6.4	1.2	1.4
Cottage, Tuna & Sweetcorn, GFY, Asda*	½ Pot/113g	104	2.7	92	12.4	5.3	2.4	0.3
Cottage, Tuna & Sweetcorn, Morrisons*	¼ Tub/63g	59	0.8	94	12.8	8.2	1.2	0.0
Cottage, Very Low Fat, Nisa Heritage*	1 Tub/227g	193	3.2	85	13.8	4.4	1.4	0.0
Cottage, Virtually Fat Free, Eden Vale*	1oz/28g	22	0.1	80	12.9	6.5	0.3	0.0
Cottage, Virtually Fat Free, Longley Farm*	½ Pot/125g	84	0.1	67	13.4	3.0	0.1	0.0
Cottage, Virtually Fat Free, Sainsbury's*	1oz/28g	22	0.1	80	12.9	6.5	0.3	0.0
Cottage, West Country, Low Fat 1.5%, Waitrose*	1 Serving/100g	77	1.5	77	11.8	4.4	1.5	0.0
Cottage, West Country, Waitrose*	1 Serving/100g	113	6.1	113	6.1	3.3	6.1	0.0
Cottage, with Black Pepper, HE, Tesco*	1 Pot/125g	101	2.3	81	12.1	4.0	1.8	0.0
Cottage, with Chives, Good Intentions, Somerfield*	1 Pot/125g	101	3.5	81	10.8	3.2	2.8	0.0
Cottage, with Chives, Low Fat, Westacre*	1 Pot/100g	81	1.4	81	13.7	3.5	1.4	1.2

CHEESE

	Measure INFO/WEIGHT	per Measure KCAL	FAT	Nutrition Values per 100g / 100ml KCAL	PROT	CARB	FAT	FIBRE
Cottage, with Chives, M & S*	1oz/28g	28	1.1	100	11.9	3.5	3.9	0.0
Cottage, with Chives, Somerfield*	1oz/28g	29	1.1	105	12.0	5.0	4.0	0.0
Cottage, with Coronation Chicken, BGTY, Sainsbury's*	1oz/28g	25	0.3	91	11.3	8.7	1.2	0.1
Cottage, with Cucumber & Mint, BGTY, Sainsbury's*	½ Pot/125g	103	1.1	82	12.0	6.6	0.9	0.0
Cottage, with Cucumber & Mint, COU, M & S*	1 Pot/113g	85	1.7	75	11.6	3.1	1.5	0.2
Cottage, with Cucumber & Mint, GFY, Asda*	1 Serving/75g	54	1.0	72	11.0	4.1	1.3	0.5
Cottage, with Cucumber & Mint, HE, Tesco*	½ Pot/125g	91	2.1	73	10.7	3.8	1.7	0.1
Cottage, with Lime & Coriander, Low Fat, Safeway*	½ Pot/126g	113	2.5	90	12.2	5.2	2.0	0.0
Cottage, with Mango, COU, M & S*	1 Serving/100g	100	1.1	100	10.3	11.0	1.1	0.5
Cottage, with Mango & Peach, HE, Tesco*	1 Pot/250g	188	4.0	75	10.4	4.8	1.6	0.1
Cottage, with Mango & Pineapple, BGTY, Sainsbury's*	½ Pot/125g	113	0.9	90	10.7	10.4	0.7	0.2
Cottage, with Mango & Pineapple, Morrisons*	1 Pot/125g	113	0.9	90	10.7	10.4	0.7	0.0
Cottage, with Onion & Chive, BFY, Morrisons*	1oz/28g	23	0.3	83	12.4	6.4	0.9	0.0
Cottage, with Onion & Chive, BGTY, Sainsbury's*	1 Serving/50g	42	0.5	83	12.4	6.4	0.9	0.1
Cottage, with Onion & Chive, GFY, Asda*	1 Serving/50g	43	1.0	85	12.0	4.4	1.9	0.1
Cottage, with Onion & Chive, Good Choice, Iceland*	1 Serving/100g	74	1.6	74	11.1	3.8	1.6	0.3
Cottage, with Onion & Chive, Healthy Choice, Asda*	1oz/28g	23	0.6	82	12.0	4.0	2.0	0.1
Cottage, with Onion & Chive, HL, Tesco*	1 Serving/65g	55	1.0	85	13.9	3.6	1.5	0.3
Cottage, with Onion & Chive, Iceland*	½ Pot/100g	81	1.3	81	8.5	8.9	1.3	0.3
Cottage, with Onion & Chive, Low Fat, Sainsbury's*	1oz/28g	28	1.1	99	11.6	4.4	4.0	0.1
Cottage, with Onion & Chive, M & S*	¼ Pot/65g	88	5.5	135	10.4	4.0	8.5	0.1
Cottage, with Onion & Chive, Nisa Heritage*	1 Pot/227g	168	3.6	74	11.1	3.8	1.6	0.3
Cottage, with Peach & Mango, COU, M & S*	1 Pot/113g	96	1.1	85	9.1	9.7	1.0	0.4
Cottage, with Pineapple, Asda*	1oz/28g	31	1.1	109	10.0	8.0	3.9	0.0
Cottage, with Pineapple, BGTY, Sainsbury's*	1 Serving/125g	105	0.9	84	10.5	8.9	0.7	0.1
Cottage, with Pineapple, GFY, Asda*	1 Pot/227g	193	2.3	85	9.0	10.0	1.0	0.5
Cottage, with Pineapple, HE, Tesco*	1oz/28g	25	0.4	90	12.5	6.8	1.3	0.4
Cottage, with Pineapple, Healthy Choice, Safeway*	1oz/28g	25	0.5	89	10.8	6.9	1.8	0.0
Cottage, with Pineapple, HL, Tesco*	½ Pot/125g	113	1.6	90	12.5	6.8	1.3	0.4
Cottage, with Pineapple, Iceland*	½ Pot/100g	81	1.3	81	8.5	8.9	1.3	0.3
Cottage, with Pineapple, Low Fat, Waitrose*	1 Serving/40g	34	0.7	84	10.4	6.7	1.7	0.2
Cottage, with Pineapple, Morrisons*	1 Pot/300g	291	10.2	97	10.0	6.8	3.4	0.0
Cottage, with Pineapple, Shape, Danone*	1oz/28g	20	0.1	73	9.8	8.0	0.2	0.1
Cottage, with Pineapple, Somerfield*	1oz/28g	27	0.8	97	10.0	7.0	3.0	0.0
Cottage, with Pineapple, Tesco*	1 Serving/150g	158	5.0	105	9.1	9.8	3.3	0.1
Cottage, with Poached Salmon & Dill, GFY, Asda*	1/3 Pot/75g	65	2.0	86	12.0	2.3	2.7	0.6
Cottage, with Prawn, GFY, Asda*	1oz/28g	22	0.5	79	10.0	6.0	1.7	0.3
Cottage, with Prawn & Cucumber, Safeway*	1 Serving/200g	184	5.0	92	12.0	4.7	2.5	0.1
Cottage, with Prawn Cocktail, BGTY, Sainsbury's*	1oz/28g	25	0.3	91	12.3	8.3	0.9	0.1
Cottage, with Prawns, M & S*	½ Pot/125g	175	10.5	140	12.7	3.8	8.4	0.0
Cottage, with Salmon & Dill, HE, Tesco*	1oz/28g	25	0.7	89	12.0	4.7	2.5	0.5
Cottage, with Smoked Cheese & Onion, GFY, Asda*	1 Serving/50g	39	0.8	78	12.0	3.9	1.6	0.4
Cottage, with Sweet Chilli Chicken, M & S*	1 Serving/200g	190	4.2	95	13.8	4.7	2.1	0.5
Cottage, with Tuna & Cucumber, Safeway*	1 Serving/40g	35	1.0	87	12.0	3.7	2.5	0.1
Cottage, with Tuna & Pesto, Asda*	1 Serving/170g	184	10.2	108	10.0	3.5	6.0	0.7
Cottage, with Tuna & Sweetcorn, HL, Tesco*	1 Serving/150g	137	3.2	91	12.8	4.8	2.1	0.4
Cream, Average	1 Portion/30g	132	14.2	439	3.1	0.0	47.4	0.0
Cream, Garlic & Herbs, Light, Boursin*	1 Portion/20g	28	1.8	140	12.0	2.5	9.0	0.0
Cream, Reduced Fat, Average	1 Seving/20g	23	1.1	117	13.0	4.0	5.3	0.1
Cream, with Onion & Chives, Morrisons*	1 Serving/20g	38	3.0	190	11.0	3.0	15.0	0.0
Cream, with Pineapple, Asda*	1 Serving/40g	77	5.2	193	8.0	11.0	13.0	0.0
Cream, with Red Peppers & Onion, GFY, Asda*	1 Serving/32.3g	42	1.9	130	13.0	6.0	6.0	0.0
Creamy Chaumes, M & S*	1oz/28g	80	6.6	287	17.6	1.0	23.6	0.0

CHEESE

INFO/WEIGHT	Measure	per Measure		Nutrition Values per 100g / 100ml				
		KCAL	FAT	KCAL	PROT	CARB	FAT	FIBRE
Creme De Saint Agur, Saint Agur*	1 Sm Piece/10g	36	3.4	363	16.0	0.2	33.5	0.0
Dairylea, Light, Slices, Kraft*	1 Slice/22.5g	46	2.4	205	17.0	8.6	10.5	0.0
Dairylea, Rippers, Straight, Kraft*	1 Ripper/21g	60	3.9	285	28.0	1.0	18.5	0.0
Dairylea, Slices, Kraft*	1 Slice/25g	69	5.1	275	13.0	8.6	20.5	0.0
Danish Blue, Average	1 Serving/30g	106	8.7	352	20.8	0.0	29.1	0.0
Demi Pont L'eveque, Finest, Tesco*	1 Serving/46g	138	10.6	301	21.1	0.4	23.0	0.0
Dolcelatte, Average	1 Serving/30g	110	9.7	366	17.8	0.4	32.3	0.4
Double Gloucester, Average	1 Serving/30g	121	10.2	405	24.5	0.1	34.0	0.0
Doux De Montagne, Average	1 Serving/25g	88	7.1	352	22.9	1.5	28.3	0.0
Edam, Average	1 Serving/10g	33	2.5	326	25.3	0.0	24.9	0.0
Edam, Dutch, Garlic & Herb Wedge, Asda*	1 Serving/60g	197	15.0	329	26.0	0.0	25.0	0.0
Edam, Reduced Fat, Average	1 Serving/30g	69	3.3	230	32.4	0.1	11.1	0.0
Edam, Slices, Average	1 Slice/30g	96	7.2	320	25.0	0.4	24.1	0.0
Emmental, Average	1 Serving/10g	37	2.8	369	28.4	0.0	28.4	0.0
Emmental, Light, Slices, President*	1 Slice/20g	60	3.6	298	34.0	0.0	18.0	0.0
Farmhouse, Reduced Fat, Healthy Range, Average	1 Serving/30g	78	4.6	261	30.4	0.1	15.4	0.0
Feta, Average	1 Serving/30g	79	6.4	262	16.3	1.0	21.5	0.0
Feta, with Green Olives, for Salad, Discover*	1oz/28g	75	5.9	267	19.0	1.0	21.0	0.0
Feta, with Herbs & Spices, for Salad, Discover*	1oz/28g	75	5.9	267	19.0	1.0	21.0	0.0
Feta, with Kalamata Olives, for Salad, Discover*	1oz/28g	75	5.9	267	19.0	1.0	21.0	0.0
Feta, with Red Pepper, for Salad, Discover*	1oz/28g	75	5.9	267	19.0	1.0	21.0	0.0
Fontina, Average	1 Serving/28g	109	9.0	389	25.0	0.0	32.1	0.0
for Pizza, Grated, Average	1 Serving/50g	163	12.2	326	25.0	1.6	24.4	0.0
Goats, Average	1 Tsp/10g	26	2.1	262	13.8	3.8	21.2	0.0
Goats, Breaded, Bites, Sainsbury's*	1 Bite/24.9g	84	6.3	337	13.0	15.1	25.0	0.8
Goats, French, Mild, Average	1 Serving/30g	49	3.5	163	11.3	3.0	11.8	0.0
Goats, Premium, Average	1 Serving/30g	98	7.8	327	20.5	0.6	26.1	0.0
Goats, Soft, Asda*	1 Pack/125g	376	31.3	301	15.5	3.5	25.0	0.0
Goats, Welsh, with Garlic & Chives, Tesco*	1 Serving/32g	93	7.7	290	15.1	3.3	24.1	0.1
Goats, Welsh, with Herbs, Sainsbury's*	1 Serving/30g	90	7.4	299	15.3	3.6	24.8	0.1
Goats, with Roasted Vegetables, Somerfield*	1oz/28g	55	2.0	196	8.0	26.0	7.0	0.0
Gorgonzola, Average	1 Serving/30g	100	8.1	334	20.0	0.1	27.0	0.0
Gouda, Average	1 Serving/30g	113	9.5	376	24.0	0.0	31.5	0.0
Grana Padano, Italian Cheese, Waitrose*	1 Serving/14g	54	4.0	388	33.0	0.0	28.4	0.0
Greek Style, 50% Less Fat, BGTY, Sainsbury's*	½ Pack/50g	84	4.0	168	24.0	0.1	8.0	0.1
Gruyere	1oz/28g	115	9.3	409	27.2	0.0	33.3	0.0
Halloumi, Average	1 Serving/80g	253	19.7	316	20.8	1.6	24.7	0.0
Halloumi, Light, Pittas*	1 Pack/225g	590	36.0	262	27.0	2.5	16.0	0.0
Havarti, Danish, Sainsbury's*	1 Serving/100g	426	38.0	426	20.0	1.0	38.0	0.0
Italian, Grated, Average	1 Serving/30g	144	10.0	481	44.0	1.1	33.4	0.0
Jarlsberg, Slices, Average	1 Slice/15g	54	4.1	360	27.0	0.0	27.0	0.0
Lancashire	1oz/28g	104	8.7	373	23.3	0.1	31.0	0.0
Light Salad, Discover*	1oz/28g	61	3.6	216	24.0	1.0	13.0	0.0
Manchego	1 Serving/70g	340	30.8	485	22.2	0.1	44.0	0.0
Mascarpone, 25% Less Fat, Sainsbury's*	1 Portion/30g	95	9.0	316	6.7	4.8	30.0	0.0
Mascarpone, Average	1 Serving/30g	131	13.1	437	5.6	4.1	43.6	0.0
Mild, Reduced Fat, Grated, Average	1 Serving/30g	70	3.3	235	31.5	2.2	11.1	0.0
Monterey Jack, Shredded, Kraft*	¼ Cup/28g	101	8.1	360	22.0	3.6	28.8	0.0
Morbier, Sainsbury's*	1 Serving/10g	33	2.4	330	28.0	0.1	24.2	0.0
Mozzarella, Average	1 Serving/50g	137	10.3	275	21.2	1.2	20.6	0.0
Mozzarella, Reduced Fat, Average	1 Serving/50g	92	5.1	184	21.2	1.0	10.3	0.0
Mozzarella & Cheddar, Grated, Tesco*	1 Serving/40g	131	9.6	327	25.0	2.5	24.1	0.0
Norvegia, Light, Sliced, Tine*	1 Slice/10g	27	1.6	272	32.0	0.0	16.0	0.0

C

CHEESE

	Measure INFO/WEIGHT	per Measure KCAL	FAT	Nutrition Values per 100g / 100ml KCAL	PROT	CARB	FAT	FIBRE
Parmesan, Average	1 Tbsp/10g	40	2.9	401	35.2	0.0	29.4	0.0
Pecorino, Italian, Tesco*	1 Serving/30g	119	9.9	397	22.0	0.0	33.0	0.0
Philadelphia, for Salad, Kraft*	1 Pot/50g	158	15.3	315	6.6	2.6	30.5	0.5
Poivre, Boursin*	1oz/28g	116	11.8	414	7.0	2.0	42.0	0.0
Port Salut, M & S*	1oz/28g	90	7.3	322	21.0	1.0	26.0	0.0
Provolone Piccante, Sainsbury's*	1 Serving/30g	119	9.9	398	25.0	0.2	33.0	0.0
Quark, Average	1 Serving/20g	13	0.0	66	11.9	4.0	0.2	0.0
Red Leicester, Average	1 Serving/30g	120	10.1	400	23.8	0.1	33.7	0.0
Red Leicester, Reduced Fat, Average	1 Serving/30g	78	4.6	261	30.2	0.1	15.4	0.0
Ricotta, Average	1 Serving/50g	67	4.8	134	9.3	2.9	9.5	0.0
Roquefort, Average	1oz/28g	105	9.2	375	19.7	0.0	32.9	0.0
Roule, French, Sainsbury's*	1 Serving/30g	96	9.2	321	8.5	3.0	30.5	0.0
Roule, Garlic, with Herbs, Somerfield*	1oz/28g	92	8.7	329	10.0	3.0	31.0	0.0
Roule, Garlic & Parsley, Light, BGTY, Sainsbury's*	1 Serving/30g	51	3.2	171	16.4	2.6	10.6	0.0
Sage Derby	1oz/28g	113	9.5	402	24.2	0.1	33.9	0.0
Saint Agur, M & S*	1 Serving/25g	91	8.4	363	16.0	0.2	33.5	0.0
Savoury, Light, President*	1 Slice/21g	40	2.3	192	22.0	1.0	11.0	0.0
Selles Sur Cher, TTD, Sainsbury's*	1 Serving/30g	89	7.2	296	20.0	0.1	24.0	0.0
Shropshire, Blue, Average	1 Serving/50g	196	17.1	391	21.1	0.1	34.3	0.0
Slices, 17% Fat, Lightlife, Leerdammer*	1 Slice/25g	70	4.3	280	31.0	0.1	17.0	0.0
Slices, Bettabuy, Morrisons*	1 Slice/17g	47	3.8	274	14.0	4.0	22.5	0.0
Slices, BFY, Morrisons*	1 Slice/20g	39	2.0	196	21.0	5.4	10.0	0.0
Slices, Farmfoods*	1 Slice/17g	49	3.7	286	18.0	4.0	22.0	0.0
Slices, Fol Epi*	1 Slice/22g	75	5.9	339	25.0	0.5	27.0	0.0
Slices, Good Intentions, Somerfield*	1 Slice/20g	39	2.0	195	19.2	7.1	10.0	0.0
Slices, Half Fat, Asda*	1 Slice/20g	39	2.0	194	20.6	5.4	10.0	0.0
Slices, Kraft*	1 Slice/20g	56	4.3	280	13.5	6.6	21.5	0.0
Slices, Light, Aldi*	1 Slice/19.9g	41	2.1	206	20.1	8.1	10.4	0.9
Slices, Light, The Laughing Cow, Fromageries Bel*	1 Slice/20g	41	2.1	203	21.0	6.0	10.5	0.0
Slices, Low Fat, HL, Tesco*	1 Slice/27g	52	0.7	193	36.1	6.0	2.7	0.0
Slices, Mature, GFY, Asda*	1 Slice/20.4g	53	3.3	260	29.0	0.1	16.0	0.0
Slices, Mature, HE, Tesco*	1 Slice/30g	78	4.5	260	30.9	0.1	15.0	0.0
Slices, Reduced Fat, GFY, Asda*	1 Slice/19.9g	38	2.0	191	21.0	4.2	10.0	0.0
Slices, SmartPrice, Asda*	1 Slice/16.6g	48	3.9	283	14.0	5.0	23.0	0.0
Slices, Smoked, with Ham, Aldi*	1 Slice/21g	66	5.3	313	21.0	1.0	25.0	0.1
Slices, Tesco*	1 Slice/20g	55	4.2	275	14.2	7.2	21.0	0.0
Slimline, Avonmore*	1oz/28g	47	2.2	169	30.0	0.1	8.0	0.0
Soft, & Creamy with Onions & Garlic, GFY, Asda*	1 Serving/25g	32	1.5	126	13.0	5.0	6.0	0.0
Soft, & Creamy with Pineapple, Asda*	1 Serving/32g	62	4.2	193	8.0	11.0	13.0	0.0
Soft, Blue, Philadelphia, Kraft*	1 Serving/28g	76	7.1	270	6.8	3.4	25.5	0.2
Soft, Cracked Pepper, Less Than 5% Fat, M & S*	1 Serving/30g	30	1.4	100	11.0	4.2	4.5	0.3
Soft, Double Gloucester, & Chives, M & S*	1oz/28g	100	7.5	358	20.0	9.2	26.8	0.0
Soft, Extra Light, Average	1 Serving/20g	25	1.2	125	14.3	3.6	5.9	0.1
Soft, Fruit & Rum Halo, Discover*	1 Serving/25g	104	8.5	414	8.6	11.7	34.1	0.0
Soft, Full Fat, Average	1 Serving/50g	156	15.2	312	8.2	1.7	30.3	0.0
Soft, Garlic & Herb, Extra Light, HE, Tesco*	1 Serving/30g	39	1.9	130	12.3	5.1	6.3	0.3
Soft, Garlic & Herb, Lite, Somerfield*	½ Pot/100g	191	15.0	191	9.0	4.9	15.0	0.0
Soft, Garlic & Herb, M & S*	1oz/28g	58	5.0	206	8.5	2.7	18.0	0.0
Soft, Garlic & Herb, Medium Fat, Safeway*	1 Serving/10g	20	1.5	195	9.3	4.9	15.0	0.0
Soft, Goats Milk	1oz/28g	55	4.4	198	13.1	1.0	15.8	0.0
Soft, Herbs & Garlic, Creamery, Light, Sainsbury's*	1 Serving/30g	54	4.7	180	7.2	3.4	15.5	0.3
Soft, Light, Average	1 Serving/30g	54	3.9	179	12.1	3.2	13.1	0.0
Soft, Medium Fat, Average	1 Serving/30g	62	5.4	207	8.4	3.0	17.9	0.0

CHEESE

	Measure INFO/WEIGHT	per Measure		Nutrition Values per 100g / 100ml				
		KCAL	FAT	KCAL	PROT	CARB	FAT	FIBRE
Soft, Onion & Chive, Low Fat, BGTY, Sainsbury's*	1 Serving/30g	35	1.5	115	13.5	4.0	5.0	1.0
Soft, Onion & Chives, Less Than 5% Fat, M & S*	¼ Pack/37.5g	38	1.8	100	10.7	4.4	4.7	1.2
Soft, Philadelphia, Extra Light, Kraft*	1 Serving/30g	33	1.5	110	11.0	4.5	5.1	0.5
Soft, Philadelphia, Garlic & Herb, Light, Kraft*	1 Serving/30g	47	3.5	156	8.2	3.9	11.5	0.4
Soft, Philadelphia, Kraft*	1 Serving/30g	77	7.2	255	5.9	3.2	24.0	0.2
Soft, Philadelphia, Mini Tubs, Extra Light, Kraft*	1 Tub/35g	39	1.8	111	11.0	4.8	5.2	0.4
Soft, Philadelphia, Mini Tubs, Light, Kraft*	1 Tub/35g	57	4.9	163	7.1	2.9	14.0	0.0
Soft, Philadelphia, Tomato & Basil, Light, Kraft*	1 Tbsp/20g	38	3.2	190	7.6	4.3	16.0	0.5
Soft, Philadelphia, with Chive & Onion, Kraft*	1 Serving/25g	73	7.3	290	6.5	6.5	29.0	0.0
Soft, Philadelphia, with Chives, Light, Kraft*	1 Serving/30g	48	3.6	160	8.4	4.2	12.0	0.5
Soft, Philadelphia, with Ham, Light, Kraft*	1oz/28g	52	4.2	184	7.9	4.3	15.0	0.2
Soft, Philadelphia Light, Kraft*	1 Serving/30g	47	3.5	157	8.7	4.0	11.7	0.3
Soft, Pineapple, Light, Safeway*	1 Serving/25g	48	3.1	190	7.6	10.8	12.5	0.0
Soft, Pineapple Halo, Discover*	1 Serving/25g	101	8.2	404	7.2	16.6	32.6	1.2
Soft, with Black Pepper, Light, Sainsbury's*	½ Pack/100g	205	16.5	205	11.0	3.0	16.5	0.0
Soft, with Garlic & Herbs, Full Fat, Deli, Boursin*	1 Serving/28g	84	8.3	299	3.5	5.0	29.5	0.0
Soft, with Garlic & Herbs, Medium Fat, Westacre*	1 Serving/30g	56	4.8	188	8.0	3.0	16.0	0.1
Soft, with Garlic & Herbs, Sainsbury's*	1 Serving/33g	89	8.6	269	6.1	2.7	26.0	0.0
Soft, with Onion & Chives, BGTY, Sainsbury's*	1 Serving/20g	23	1.0	115	13.5	4.0	5.0	1.0
Soft, with Shallots & Chives, BGTY, Sainsbury's*	1 Serving/20g	47	4.5	235	5.8	2.2	22.5	0.0
Soft & Smooth, Extra Light, HL, Tesco*	1 Serving/30g	39	1.8	130	14.2	3.7	6.0	0.0
Soya	1oz/28g	89	7.6	319	18.3	0.0	27.3	0.0
Stilton, Average	1 Serving/30g	123	10.7	410	22.4	0.1	35.5	0.0
Stilton, Blue, Average	1 Serving/30g	124	10.7	412	22.8	0.1	35.7	0.0
Stilton, White, & Apricot, M & S*	1oz/28g	94	6.5	337	13.8	18.5	23.1	0.0
Stilton, White, & Cranberry, M & S*	1oz/28g	101	7.1	362	18.2	15.5	25.3	0.0
Stilton, White, Average	1oz/28g	101	8.8	362	19.9	0.1	31.3	0.0
Stilton, White, with Apricot, Somerfield*	1oz/28g	103	8.4	369	16.0	8.0	30.0	0.0
Stilton, White, with Cranberries, Tesco*	1 Serving/50g	184	14.9	368	15.8	9.5	29.7	0.7
Stilton, White, with Mango & Ginger, Tesco*	1/3 Pack/65g	228	14.0	350	13.1	25.8	21.6	0.6
Substitute, Mozzarella Style, Grated, Value, Tesco*	1 Serving/40g	120	8.4	300	25.0	2.5	21.1	0.0
Supreme Des Ducs, Ligne Et Plaisir*	1 Serving/50g	100	6.0	200	21.0	2.0	12.0	0.0
Wedge, Leerdammer*	1 Serving/30g	112	8.6	373	28.3	0.0	28.6	0.0
Wensleydale, Average	1 Serving/25g	92	7.8	369	22.5	0.1	31.0	0.1
Wensleydale with Cranberries, Sainsbury's*	1 Serving/50g	180	13.9	359	20.7	6.4	27.8	0.0
White, Slices, 85% Fat Free, Kerry*	1 Slice/20g	54	3.0	270	33.0	0.1	15.0	0.0
White, Slices, 85% Fat Free, Kerry*	1 Slice/20g	54	3.0	270	33.0	0.1	15.0	0.0

CHEESE ALTERNATIVE

Cheezly, Nacho Style, Redwood*	1 Serving/25g	42	2.0	169	3.3	21.1	7.9	0.0

CHEESE ON TOAST

Average	1oz/28g	106	7.4	380	13.8	23.8	26.3	0.7

CHEESE PUFFS

Cheeky, Tesco*	1 Bag/20g	108	7.0	542	6.7	50.2	34.9	0.0
Farmfoods*	1 Bag/18g	96	5.7	532	7.0	54.3	31.9	1.0
Morrisons*	1 Bag/25g	136	8.7	542	6.7	50.2	34.9	1.1
Sainsbury's*	1 Pack/100g	530	32.0	530	9.1	51.4	32.0	1.9
Shapers, Boots*	1 Bag/16g	80	3.8	500	7.1	64.0	24.0	0.9
SmartPrice, Asda*	1 Bag/16g	84	4.9	527	6.7	56.3	30.6	0.8
Value, Tesco*	1 Pack/16g	84	4.6	525	6.3	60.0	28.8	0.6

CHEESE SINGLES

50% Less Fat, Asda*	1 Single/20g	38	2.0	190	19.0	6.0	10.0	0.0
50% Less Fat, BGTY, Sainsbury's*	1 Single/20g	39	2.0	195	19.2	7.1	10.0	0.0
American, 2% Milk, Kraft*	1 Single/19g	45	3.0	237	21.0	5.3	15.8	0.0

	Measure INFO/WEIGHT	per Measure		Nutrition Values per 100g / 100ml				
		KCAL	FAT	KCAL	PROT	CARB	FAT	FIBRE
CHEESE SINGLES								
Half Fat, Co-Op*	1 Single/20g	47	2.4	235	25.0	7.0	12.0	0.0
HL, Tesco*	1 Single/20g	39	2.0	195	19.2	7.1	10.0	0.0
Kraft*	1 Single/20g	52	3.7	260	13.5	7.6	18.5	0.0
Light, Kraft*	1 Single/20g	43	2.3	215	19.0	6.9	11.5	0.0
CHEESE SPREAD								
60% Less Fat, Asda*	1 Serving/30g	52	2.7	174	16.0	7.3	9.0	0.0
Asda*	1 Serving/33g	92	7.9	280	9.0	7.0	24.0	0.0
BFY, Morrisons*	1 Serving/25g	43	2.1	172	13.5	6.5	8.5	0.0
BGTY, Sainsbury's*	1 Serving/25g	28	1.4	111	11.0	4.3	5.5	0.4
Cheese & Garlic, Primula*	1 Serving/20g	49	3.7	247	15.7	4.3	18.6	0.0
Cream, Light, Sainsbury's*	1 Serving/50g	94	7.8	187	7.8	4.1	15.5	0.3
Creamery, Light, Sainsbury's*	1 Serving/25g	46	3.8	185	9.0	3.5	15.0	0.0
Dairylea, Light, Tub, Kraft*	1 Serving/33g	49	2.3	147	14.5	6.1	7.0	0.0
Dairylea, Tub, Kraft*	1 Serving/25g	60	4.9	240	11.0	5.3	19.5	0.0
Garlic & Herb, Soft, Free From, Sainsbury's*	1 Serving/30g	91	9.0	302	2.5	5.5	30.0	0.1
Garlic & Herbs, Light, Benecol*	1 Serving/20g	35	2.8	174	7.8	4.2	14.0	0.7
Light, Primula*	1oz/28g	39	1.5	141	18.8	4.1	5.5	0.5
Low Fat, Weight Watchers*	1 Serving/50g	56	1.5	112	18.1	3.4	2.9	1.2
Morrisons*	1 Serving/3g	7	0.5	225	10.0	7.0	17.5	0.0
Plain, Original, Primula*	1 Serving/30g	68	5.6	227	12.9	2.1	18.7	0.6
Soft, Low Fat, M & S*	1 Pack/100g	111	4.5	111	13.0	4.2	4.5	0.3
Squeeze, Light, The Laughing Cow*	1 Portion/30g	42	2.1	139	12.0	7.0	7.0	5.0
Squeeze, Original, The Laughing Cow*	1 Portion/30g	71	6.0	236	9.0	5.0	20.0	0.0
Triangles, Extra Light, The Laughing Cow*	1 Triangle/18g	21	0.5	116	15.0	6.5	3.0	0.0
Triangles, Light, The Laughing Cow*	1 Triangle/18g	25	1.3	141	13.0	6.5	7.0	0.0
Triangles, Original, The Laughing Cow*	1 Triangle/17.5g	42	3.3	239	11.0	6.0	19.0	0.0
with Chives, Primula*	1 Serving/30g	76	6.3	253	15.0	1.0	21.0	0.0
with Ham, Primula*	1 Serving/30g	70	5.6	232	13.5	2.1	18.8	0.3
with Shrimp, Primula*	1 Tbsp/15g	38	3.2	253	15.0	1.0	21.0	0.0
CHEESE STRAWS								
Cheddar, M & S*	1 Straw/11g	59	3.8	535	14.9	40.1	34.9	2.4
Cheese Twists, Tesco*	1 Serving/20g	99	5.6	494	14.0	46.4	28.0	4.2
Finest, Tesco*	1 Straw/7g	39	2.6	558	13.3	41.5	37.6	1.5
Fudges*	1 Serving/10g	53	3.5	534	14.9	40.1	34.9	0.0
Homemade Or Bakery, Average	1 Straw/41g	173	12.6	422	12.0	24.2	30.7	0.7
Selection, Sainsbury's*	1 Straw/7g	41	2.9	558	16.6	34.5	39.3	2.8
CHEESE TRIANGLES								
Average	1 Triangle/14g	35	2.8	247	10.6	6.6	19.9	0.0
HL, Tesco*	1 Triangle/17.5g	30	1.2	170	17.5	8.5	7.0	0.0
Reduced Fat, Average	1 Triangle/18g	30	1.6	170	14.8	7.4	9.0	0.0
Tri-Bites, Dairylea, Kraft*	1 Triangle/20g	60	4.6	300	20.0	3.2	23.0	0.0
CHEESE TWISTS								
All Butter, M & S*	1 Pack/125g	625	33.4	500	14.2	50.2	26.7	3.2
Asda*	1 Stick/8g	42	2.4	500	14.0	48.0	28.0	5.0
CHEESECAKE								
American Red White & Blueberry, Sainsbury's*	1/6th/83g	264	15.4	318	3.8	35.1	18.5	0.4
Apricot, Co-Op*	1 Cake/100g	230	11.0	230	4.0	29.0	11.0	0.9
Average	1 Slice/115g	490	40.8	426	3.7	24.6	35.5	0.4
Belgian Chocolate, M & S*	1 Slice/100g	385	23.9	385	5.3	39.2	23.9	2.5
Belgian Chocolate Truffle, TTD, Sainsbury's*	1/6 Cake/91.6g	365	24.6	399	4.2	35.6	26.9	3.5
Blackcurrant, M & S*	1oz/28g	82	5.0	293	3.3	29.4	17.9	0.9
Blackcurrant, PB, Waitrose*	1 Slice/106g	227	3.8	214	4.0	39.6	3.6	2.4
Blackcurrant, Sainsbury's*	1oz/28g	75	4.2	267	3.2	29.5	15.1	1.1

CHEESECAKE

	Measure INFO/WEIGHT	per Measure KCAL	FAT	Nutrition Values per 100g / 100ml KCAL	PROT	CARB	FAT	FIBRE
Blackcurrant, Value, Tesco*	1 Serving/70g	174	8.6	248	2.8	31.4	12.3	1.0
Blackcurrant Devonshire, McVitie's*	1/6 Cake/67g	190	11.3	288	3.8	29.7	17.1	1.7
Cherry, BGTY, Sainsbury's*	1 Serving/91g	181	3.9	199	4.6	35.5	4.3	0.5
Cherry, Low Fat, Tesco*	1 Serving/91g	185	3.7	203	3.4	38.0	4.1	0.9
Chocolate, & Irish Cream Liqueur, Tesco*	1 Serving/93g	385	28.0	414	5.0	30.7	30.1	0.8
Chocolate, Baked, Ultimate, Entenmann's*	1 Serving/100g	331	19.0	331	5.7	34.2	19.0	2.8
Chocolate, M & S*	1oz/28g	106	6.0	380	6.5	40.3	21.5	0.4
Chocolate, Tesco*	1 Serving/91g	317	17.4	348	6.2	37.8	19.1	1.5
Chocolate Chip, M & S*	1oz/28g	109	6.6	391	5.1	39.7	23.6	0.2
Devonshire Strawberry, McVitie's*	1/6 Portion/66g	192	10.7	291	4.4	31.8	16.2	3.6
Double Chocolate Wedge, Sainsbury's*	1 Portion/75g	327	24.8	436	5.7	29.0	33.0	1.7
Homestyle Chocolate, M & S*	1oz/28g	105	6.2	376	6.0	38.0	22.2	0.7
Lemon, BGTY, Sainsbury's*	1/6 Cake/71g	142	2.7	200	4.4	37.0	3.8	0.5
Lemon, Creamy & Light, M & S*	1/6 Cake/67.5g	238	13.9	350	3.5	32.3	20.4	0.4
Lemon, Sainsbury's*	1 Serving/180g	650	37.1	361	4.0	39.9	20.6	1.3
Lemon, Tesco*	1 Slice/93g	315	21.0	339	5.2	28.6	22.6	0.3
Lemon, Value, Tesco*	1 Serving/78.6g	222	11.9	281	4.3	32.2	15.0	4.2
Mandarin, Co-Op*	1 Slice/99g	297	16.8	300	4.0	32.0	17.0	0.3
Mandarin, GFY, Asda*	1 Sixth/92g	178	4.0	194	3.6	35.0	4.4	1.2
Mandarin, Low Fat, Tesco*	1 Serving/70g	145	3.3	207	3.3	37.0	4.7	1.4
Mandarin, Morrisons*	1 Serving/135g	335	16.9	248	3.8	32.2	12.5	0.8
Pizza Express*	1 Slice/100g	347	24.8	347	5.9	24.8	24.8	0.0
Raspberry, BGTY, Sainsbury's*	1 Pot/94.5g	154	2.5	163	6.6	28.2	2.6	2.8
Raspberry, M & S*	1 Slice/105g	331	21.5	315	5.0	32.2	20.5	1.0
Raspberry & Mascarpone, Best, Morrisons*	1 Serving/84g	257	14.0	306	3.9	34.8	16.7	1.0
Raspberry & Strawberry, M & S*	1 Slice/104.6g	340	21.1	325	3.9	33.4	20.2	1.2
Raspberry Brulee, M & S*	1 Serving/100g	255	12.9	255	5.7	29.7	12.9	2.1
Raspberry Rapture, Slices, Tesco*	1 Slice/110g	341	20.4	310	4.2	30.8	18.5	1.8
Raspberry Ripple, M & S*	1oz/28g	84	4.4	300	5.9	32.8	15.6	0.3
Raspberry Swirl, Heinz*	1 Serving/100g	266	14.5	266	3.9	30.1	14.5	2.8
Rhubarb Crumble, Sainsbury's*	1 Serving/114g	268	10.6	235	3.1	34.8	9.3	2.4
Sticky Toffee, Iceland*	1/6th/78g	230	10.9	295	5.3	36.9	14.0	0.5
Sticky Toffee, Tesco*	1 Slice/66g	248	16.0	375	4.0	35.3	24.2	0.5
Strawberries & Cream, Finest, Tesco*	1 Serving/104.2g	324	22.4	312	4.3	25.3	21.5	0.5
Strawberry, Finest, Tesco*	1 Slice/113g	383	25.1	339	4.8	30.1	22.2	0.9
Strawberry, Fresh, M & S*	¼ Cake/125g	300	19.3	240	2.8	23.1	15.4	1.1
Strawberry, Frozen, Sainsbury's*	1/6 Cake/93.4g	310	15.9	332	4.3	40.4	17.0	2.3
Strawberry, Heinz*	1 Pack/245g	588	31.1	240	3.4	28.1	12.7	2.4
Strawberry, Tesco*	1 Serving/100g	254	12.0	254	3.9	32.5	12.0	0.0
Strawberry Shortcake, Sara Lee*	1/6 Slice/68.2g	229	15.6	337	4.9	27.6	23.0	0.5
Summerfruit, GFY, Asda*	1 Sixth/92g	175	3.8	191	3.7	34.5	4.2	1.4
The Ultimate New York Baked, Entenmann's*	1 Cake/100g	347	21.3	347	4.2	35.7	21.3	0.9
Toffee, American Style, Asda*	1 Serving/75g	269	15.8	359	4.5	38.0	21.0	3.8
Toffee, Asda*	1 Cake/87g	295	19.1	339	4.3	31.0	22.0	3.5
Toffee, M & S*	1 Serving/105g	357	22.6	340	5.2	37.2	21.5	0.9
Toffee, Morrisons*	1 Serving/100g	341	17.4	341	5.5	40.4	17.4	0.0
Toffee, Tesco*	1 Serving/100g	265	12.9	265	4.3	33.1	12.9	0.8
Toffee & Banana, M & S*	1oz/28g	88	4.7	315	5.0	35.7	16.7	0.2
Toffee & Pecan, Wedge, Sainsbury's*	1 Serving/75g	296	21.8	395	5.4	28.1	29.0	3.1
Vanilla, Tesco*	1 Serving/115g	417	28.4	363	5.7	29.4	24.7	0.6
Zesty Lemon, M & S*	1/6 Cake/97g	325	18.9	335	4.0	38.7	19.5	2.6

CHEETOS

	Measure INFO/WEIGHT	per Measure KCAL	FAT	Nutrition Values per 100g / 100ml KCAL	PROT	CARB	FAT	FIBRE
Cheese, Walkers*	1 Bag/24g	120	6.2	500	6.5	61.0	26.0	1.3

	Measure INFO/WEIGHT	per Measure		Nutrition Values per 100g / 100ml				
		KCAL	FAT	KCAL	PROT	CARB	FAT	FIBRE
CHERRIES								
Black, Fresh, Average	1 Serving/80g	41	0.1	51	0.9	11.5	0.1	1.6
Black, in Syrup, Average	1 Serving/242g	160	0.0	66	0.6	16.0	0.0	0.7
Dried, Sainsbury's*	2 Tbsp/28g	89	0.4	319	3.8	72.4	1.5	6.2
Glace, Average	1oz/28g	79	0.0	281	0.4	71.2	0.2	1.1
Raw, Average	1oz/28g	14	0.0	49	0.9	11.3	0.1	1.5
Stewed, with Sugar, Average	1oz/28g	23	0.0	82	0.7	21.0	0.1	0.7
Stewed, without Sugar, Average	1oz/28g	12	0.0	42	0.8	10.1	0.1	0.8
CHESTNUTS								
Average	1 Nut/10g	17	0.3	170	2.0	36.6	2.7	4.1
CHEWING GUM								
Airwaves, Sugar Free, Wrigleys*	1 Pack/15g	23	0.0	155	0.0	62.0	0.0	0.0
Extra, Peppermint, Sugar Free, Wrigleys*	2 Pieces/4g	6	0.0	155	0.0	39.0	0.0	0.0
Splash, Rapberry & Peach, Trident*	1 Gum/2g	4	0.0	180	1.6	68.5	0.5	0.0
CHICK PEAS								
Dried, Average	1 Serving/100g	319	5.4	319	21.7	47.4	5.4	8.0
Dried, Boiled, Average	1 Serving/75g	85	1.7	114	7.3	16.4	2.2	2.6
in Salted Water, Canned, Average	1 Can/179g	204	5.2	114	7.2	14.9	2.9	4.1
in Water, Canned, Average	1 Can/250g	283	6.6	113	7.2	15.3	2.6	4.8
CHICKEN								
& Veg, Deli Style Pieces, Redwood*	1 Serving/40g	116	6.9	290	24.4	4.6	17.2	0.3
Balls, Crispy, M & S*	1 Ball/16g	35	1.3	220	13.3	23.7	8.1	0.5
Balls, Lemon, Asda*	1 Ball/15g	42	2.6	279	14.0	19.0	17.0	1.6
Bites, Battered, Tesco*	1 Pack/200g	440	28.6	220	15.2	7.6	14.3	2.0
Bites, in Light Batter, Captain Birds Eye, Birds Eye*	5 Bites/80g	168	10.0	210	18.6	5.8	12.5	0.2
Bites, Mexican, Somerfield*	1 Pack/227g	508	15.9	224	26.0	15.0	7.0	0.0
Bites, Southern Fried, Tesco*	1 Pack/300g	720	33.3	240	18.1	16.9	11.1	2.1
Bites, Tikka, Average	1 Serving/50g	96	5.3	193	20.7	3.8	10.5	1.9
Breast, Chargrilled, Lime & Coriander, Asda*	1 Breast/159.5g	260	11.2	163	25.0	0.1	7.0	1.5
Breast, Chargrilled, Premium, Average	1 Piece/10g	20	1.1	197	21.6	1.5	11.2	0.3
Breast, Chargrilled, Sliced, Average	1 Slice/19g	24	0.5	124	24.4	0.5	2.7	0.4
Breast, Chunks, Chilli, Safeway*	1 Serving/100g	142	3.2	142	22.2	6.3	3.2	0.0
Breast, Chunks, Hot, Rogan Josh, Sainsbury's*	½ Pack/114g	143	2.0	126	23.6	3.9	1.8	1.0
Breast, Chunks, Korma, Sainsbury's*	1 Serving/227g	354	9.3	156	28.0	1.7	4.1	0.8
Breast, Crispy, 100%, Birds Eye*	1 Portion/95g	220	13.0	228	14.6	12.0	13.5	0.1
Breast, Diced, Average	1 Serving/188g	215	3.8	114	25.0	0.1	2.0	0.1
Breast, Eastern Spices, Birds Eye*	1 Portion/175g	308	20.8	176	13.5	3.8	11.9	1.5
Breast, Escalope, Pesto Chargrilled, M & S*	1 Serving/100g	135	6.2	135	19.6	0.7	6.2	0.6
Breast, Escalope, Plain, Average	1 Serving/100g	110	2.2	110	22.3	0.7	2.2	0.5
Breast, Fillets, Breaded, Average	1 Fillet/112g	246	11.6	220	17.6	14.0	10.4	1.3
Breast, Fillets, Breaded, Lemon & Pepper, Average	1 Fillet/89g	133	2.0	150	22.0	10.1	2.3	1.3
Breast, Fillets, Cajun, Average	1 Fillet/93g	124	2.6	134	23.6	3.5	2.8	0.3
Breast, Fillets, Chargrilled, Average	1 Serving/100g	120	1.1	120	27.3	0.3	1.1	0.3
Breast, Fillets, Cheesy Salsa, Safeway*	½ Pack/163.6g	180	4.9	110	17.9	2.2	3.0	1.1
Breast, Fillets, Chinese Style, Sliced, GFY, Asda*	1 Pack/140g	178	1.8	127	23.2	5.7	1.3	0.1
Breast, Fillets, Garlic & Herb, Mini, Morrisons*	1 Pack/300g	336	3.0	112	20.2	4.9	1.0	0.5
Breast, Fillets, Garlic & Herb, Tesco*	1 Fillet/135g	290	12.2	215	18.9	14.4	9.0	1.3
Breast, Fillets, Korma Style, Average	1 Serving/100g	132	2.8	132	27.4	0.8	2.8	0.6
Breast, Fillets, Lemon Parsley, M & S*	½ Pack/145g	232	3.5	160	14.3	20.7	2.4	4.3
Breast, Fillets, Lime & Coriander, Just Add, M & S*	1 Pack/140g	182	2.4	130	26.1	2.7	1.7	0.1
Breast, Fillets, Mini, Raw, Average	1oz/28g	34	0.4	121	26.9	0.2	1.5	0.1
Breast, Fillets, Organic, Average	1 Serving/150g	153	1.1	102	24.0	0.0	0.8	0.0
Breast, Fillets, Skinless & Boneless, Raw, Average	1 Serving/100g	126	2.3	126	25.1	1.2	2.3	0.2
Breast, Fillets, Smokey Maple, Roast, Waitrose*	1 Fillet/96g	140	1.9	146	27.9	4.2	2.0	0.1

CHICKEN

Measure INFO/WEIGHT		per Measure		Nutrition Values per 100g / 100ml				
		KCAL	FAT	KCAL	PROT	CARB	FAT	FIBRE
Breast, Fillets, Smoky Chilli, Tesco*	1 Fillet/91.7g	111	1.2	121	21.2	6.0	1.3	0.1
Breast, Fillets, Sundried Tomato & Basil, M & S*	½ Pack/110g	165	4.5	150	22.5	4.7	4.1	1.1
Breast, Fillets, Tikka, Mini, Ready to Eat, Tesco*	1 Pack/200g	230	2.0	115	23.4	2.2	1.0	0.2
Breast, Garlic & Herb, Bernard Matthews*	1 Serving/50g	51	1.3	101	17.9	1.6	2.5	1.8
Breast, Garlic & Herb Flavour, Co-Op*	1 Serving/170g	281	15.3	165	19.0	2.0	9.0	0.3
Breast, Joint, Free Range, M & S*	1oz/28g	36	1.1	130	22.0	3.9	4.1	0.6
Breast, Joint, Just Cook, Sainsbury's*	1/3 Pack/126g	194	9.1	154	22.4	0.1	7.2	0.1
Breast, Joint, Lemon & Tarragon, Finest, Tesco*	1 Serving/175g	247	11.0	141	18.8	2.3	6.3	0.2
Breast, Latino Style, Asda*	1 Breast/65g	99	2.0	152	27.0	4.1	3.1	0.5
Breast, Lemon Pepper, Cooked, Birds Eye*	1 Piece/100.5g	261	14.1	260	15.0	19.0	14.0	0.9
Breast, Lime & Coriander, Summer Eating, Asda*	½ Pack/112g	164	4.5	146	26.0	1.6	4.0	0.5
Breast, Meat & Skin, Weighed with Bone, Raw, Av	1oz/28g	46	2.1	165	24.2	0.0	7.6	0.0
Breast, Mediterranean Style Coating, Tesco*	1 Breast/195g	283	13.1	145	20.4	0.7	6.7	0.0
Breast, Pieces, Tikka, Average	1 Serving/100g	154	3.4	154	28.2	2.8	3.4	0.4
Breast, Roast, Sage & Onion Stuffing, M & S*	1 Slice/16.5g	27	1.1	165	24.1	3.0	6.5	0.0
Breast, Roast, Sliced, From Supermarket, Average	1 Slice/13g	17	0.4	139	25.0	1.8	3.5	0.2
Breast, Roast, with Pork Stuffing, M & S*	1 Serving/100g	165	6.5	165	24.1	3.0	6.5	0.0
Breast, Roast, without Skin, Average	1oz/28g	42	1.3	149	25.4	1.1	4.7	0.2
Breast, Roll, Average	1 Slice/10g	17	1.0	167	16.1	3.2	10.0	0.2
Breast, Sage & Onion, Slices, Sainsbury's*	1 Pack/140g	158	2.5	113	23.1	1.0	1.8	0.5
Breast, Sage & Onion, Wafer, Bernard Matthews*	1 Serving/25g	30	0.8	120	19.8	3.5	3.0	0.1
Breast, Sliced, Mexican Style, Asda*	½ Pack/117g	153	1.6	131	27.0	2.6	1.4	0.5
Breast, Sliced, Mexican Style, Cooked, Asda*	1 Pack/234g	307	5.1	131	25.5	4.3	2.2	0.1
Breast, Sliced, Tex, Mex, Sainsbury's*	1 Serving/140g	185	1.5	132	26.7	3.8	1.1	0.0
Breast, Smoked, Sliced, Average	1 Slice/20g	22	0.5	110	20.7	0.9	2.6	0.1
Breast, Southern Fried, Bernard Matthews*	1 Serving/60g	70	1.7	117	19.6	3.1	2.9	0.6
Breast, Strips, Raw, Average	1 Serving/280g	358	5.7	128	27.1	0.4	2.1	0.3
Breast, Tandoori Style, Average	1 Serving/180g	237	6.8	132	22.3	2.3	3.8	1.0
Breast, Tikka, Sliced, Average	1oz/28g	34	0.5	120	24.9	2.0	1.7	0.6
Breast, with Skin, Raw, Average	1oz/28g	51	2.0	181	24.3	4.9	7.2	0.6
Breasts, Chilli & Ginger, COU, M & S*	1 Breast/120g	156	2.4	130	19.5	8.6	2.0	1.7
Breasts, Cracked Pepper, Birds Eye*	1 Portion/95g	192	10.7	203	20.1	5.1	11.3	0.2
Breasts, Garlic Lemon & Thyme, M & S*	½ Pack/197.5g	356	18.2	180	22.2	1.9	9.2	0.1
Breasts, Grilled, Sun Valley*	1 Serving/100g	148	2.2	148	32.0	0.0	2.2	0.0
Chargrilled, & Quinoa Salad, Shapers, Boots*	1 Pack/185g	139	1.9	75	6.2	10.0	1.0	1.8
Chargrills, Garlic, Raw, Birds Eye*	1 Piece/76g	152	8.6	200	20.3	4.2	11.3	0.1
Chargrills, Original, Raw, Birds Eye*	1 Chargrill/90g	148	8.1	164	17.5	3.2	9.0	0.1
Chicksticks, Captain Birds Eye, Birds Eye*	1 Chickstick/25g	64	4.0	257	13.3	15.0	16.0	0.8
Coated, Baked, Tesco*	1 Serving/101g	148	8.5	146	13.8	4.6	8.4	0.0
Cooked, Sliced, Average	1 Slice/15g	18	0.4	118	22.4	1.6	2.4	0.1
Cracked Pepper Seasoned, Birds Eye*	1 Portion/97g	165	8.6	166	17.4	4.4	8.7	0.2
Dippers, Crispy, Average	5 Dippers/93g	231	14.3	249	13.2	14.4	15.4	0.6
Drumsticks, & Thighs, Garlic & Herb, Sainsbury's*	1 Serving/120g	184	10.7	153	16.6	1.5	8.9	0.1
Drumsticks, BBQ Flavour, Average	1 Serving/200g	348	16.0	174	22.6	3.1	8.0	0.4
Drumsticks, Breaded, Fried, Average	1oz/28g	70	4.1	248	19.7	9.9	14.6	0.6
Drumsticks, Chinese Style, Average	1 Drumstick/100g	178	8.1	178	22.6	3.6	8.1	0.7
Drumsticks, Hoi Sin, Co-Op*	1 Pack/750g	1013	42.0	135	19.8	1.3	5.6	1.3
Drumsticks, Roast, without Skin, Average	1 Serving/100g	163	7.8	163	22.6	0.5	7.8	0.2
Drumsticks, Southern Fried, Sainsbury's*	1 Serving/87g	190	8.6	218	20.8	11.2	9.9	0.7
Drumsticks, with Skin, Average	1 Drumstick/125g	269	16.6	215	22.1	1.8	13.3	0.3
Escalope, Breaded, Average	1 Escalope/128g	361	21.6	282	13.4	19.1	16.9	0.7
Escalope, Cheese Topped, Asda*	1 Serving/173.4g	410	22.5	237	12.0	18.0	13.0	1.9
Escalope, Lemon & Pepper, Sainsbury's*	1 Serving/143g	428	27.6	299	12.8	18.7	19.3	1.9

CHICKEN

Measure INFO/WEIGHT		per Measure		Nutrition Values per 100g / 100ml				
		KCAL	FAT	KCAL	PROT	CARB	FAT	FIBRE
Escalope, Tomato & Basil, Safeway*	1 Escalope/150g	242	11.3	161	21.2	2.2	7.5	1.2
Fillet Strips, Barbeque, Birds Eye*	4 Strips/100g	180	8.7	179	18.9	6.5	8.6	0.2
Fillet Strips, Dijon Mustard, Birds Eye*	1 Serving/4 Strips	155	5.9	137	18.9	3.7	5.2	0.1
Fillet Strips, Red Pesto, Birds Eye*	4 Strips/100g	135	5.1	135	19.1	3.2	5.1	0.2
Fillet Strips, Tomato & Basil, Birds Eye*	1 Portion/4 Strips	150	5.4	149	19.4	5.6	5.4	0.3
Fillets, Battered, Average	1 Fillet/90g	199	10.4	221	16.1	13.3	11.5	0.5
Fillets, Breaded, Average	1 Piece/98g	214	10.5	219	14.2	15.9	10.7	1.9
Fillets, Chinese Style, Average	1oz/28g	37	0.5	132	24.4	4.6	1.8	0.5
Fillets, Coronation, BGTY, Sainsbury's*	1 Fillet/100g	136	2.6	136	27.1	2.4	2.6	1.0
Fillets, Hickory Barbecue & Chilli, BGTY, Sainsbury's*	1 Fillet/100g	133	1.2	133	26.9	3.6	1.2	0.9
Fillets, Honey & Maple, Roast, Mini, Waitrose*	½ Pack/100g	131	0.5	131	23.0	8.6	0.5	1.5
Fillets, Honey & Mustard, Average	1 Serving/100g	138	3.7	138	18.4	7.5	3.7	0.8
Fillets, Honey & Mustard, Mini, M & S*	1 Serving/105g	142	2.1	135	24.9	3.9	2.0	1.3
Fillets, Honey & Mustard, Somerfield*	1 Serving/100g	117	1.0	117	22.2	4.9	1.0	1.8
Fillets, Hot & Spicy, Average	1oz/28g	58	3.1	206	16.4	10.5	11.0	1.1
Fillets, in Provencal Sauce, M & S*	½ Pack/186.4g	205	7.8	110	13.8	4.0	4.2	1.1
Fillets, Lime & Coriander, Mini, Average	1 Fillet/42g	49	0.5	118	24.3	2.6	1.3	0.6
Fillets, Mango Salsa, Mini, Sainsbury's*	½ Pack/100g	132	1.2	132	24.7	5.6	1.2	0.0
Fillets, Red Pepper, Mini, BGTY, Sainsbury's*	1 Serving/100g	126	0.6	126	26.5	3.7	0.6	0.7
Fillets, Red Thai, Mini, Average	1oz/28g	36	0.6	128	21.7	5.5	2.1	0.6
Fillets, Roast, Sweet Chilli, Mini, Waitrose*	1 Pack/200g	216	0.4	108	23.0	3.8	0.2	0.9
Fillets, Salsa, Mini, BGTY, Sainsbury's*	1 Pack/200g	240	3.6	120	23.5	2.2	1.8	0.3
Fillets, Southern Fried, Average	1 Piece/100g	222	12.0	222	16.4	12.2	12.0	1.1
Fillets, Sweet Chilli, Mini, Sainsbury's*	½ Pack/100g	119	1.1	119	21.8	5.4	1.1	0.9
Fillets, Sweet Chilli & Lime, Mini, M & S*	1 Serving/50g	78	1.1	155	28.3	5.1	2.2	0.0
Fillets, Tandoori Style, Mini, Average	1 Serving/100g	128	2.1	128	24.7	2.6	2.1	0.4
Fillets, Thai, COU, M & S*	1 Fillet/120g	160	1.9	133	19.5	10.4	1.6	1.3
Fillets, Tikka, Average	1 Serving/100g	141	5.0	141	22.4	1.7	5.0	1.1
Fillets, Tikka, Mini, Average	1oz/28g	35	0.6	124	25.1	1.3	2.2	1.2
Fillets, Tomato & Basil, Mini, Average	1oz/28g	34	0.6	123	23.5	2.5	2.1	0.4
Fillets, with Peppers, M & S*	½ Pack/209.5g	220	8.0	105	12.2	6.0	3.8	2.3
Fingers, Average	1 Serving/75g	188	9.9	250	13.7	18.8	13.3	1.2
Garlic, Frozen, Tesco*	1 Serving/94.9g	182	8.3	192	15.6	12.9	8.7	1.0
Garlic Basted, Morrisons*	1 Serving/100g	231	13.1	231	23.3	0.7	13.1	0.4
Goujons, Breaded, Average	1 Serving/114g	293	17.1	258	15.8	15.2	15.0	1.0
Goujons, Breast, Fresh, Average	1oz/28g	36	0.5	127	28.0	0.0	1.7	0.0
Goujons, Cracked Black Pepper, American, Asda*	1 Serving/150g	333	21.0	222	16.0	8.0	14.0	2.5
Goujons, Garlic & Herb, Breaded, American, Asda*	½ Pack/150g	377	22.5	251	17.0	12.0	15.0	2.1
Goujons, Hot & Spicy, Sainsbury's*	½ Pack/125g	253	9.6	202	20.0	13.1	7.7	1.2
Griddlers, BBQ, Captain Birds Eye, Birds Eye*	1 Griddlers/77g	161	9.6	209	18.3	5.7	12.5	0.5
Honey & Mustard Seasoned Portions, Birds Eye*	1 Portion/97.5g	155	7.5	159	17.4	5.0	7.7	0.1
Honey Roast, Sliced, Average	1 Slice/13g	15	0.3	117	21.6	2.2	2.5	0.1
Leg, Meat Only, Raw, Average	1oz/28g	34	1.1	120	20.1	0.0	3.8	0.0
Leg, Meat Only, Raw, Weighed with Skin & Bone	1oz/28g	38	1.2	134	22.5	0.0	4.3	0.0
Leg, Roast, Skin, Weighed without Bone, Average	1 Quarter/120g	244	15.3	203	21.6	0.3	12.7	0.2
Leg, with Skin, Raw, Average	1oz/28g	48	2.9	172	19.1	0.0	10.4	0.0
Leg, with Skin, Roasted, Average	1oz/28g	66	4.6	234	21.5	0.1	16.4	0.0
Leg Or Thigh, Hot & Spicy, Average	1oz/28g	50	3.0	179	19.4	1.0	10.8	0.4
Lemon, Crispy, M & S*	½ Pack/175g	341	15.1	195	10.6	18.7	8.6	2.0
Light Meat, Raw	1oz/28g	30	0.3	106	24.0	0.0	1.1	0.0
Light Meat, Roasted	1oz/28g	43	1.0	153	30.2	0.0	3.6	0.0
Meat, Roasted, Average	1oz/28g	50	2.1	177	27.3	0.0	7.5	0.0
Meat & Skin, Raw, Average	1oz/28g	64	5.0	230	17.6	0.0	17.7	0.0

CHICKEN	Measure INFO/WEIGHT	per Measure KCAL	per Measure FAT	Nutrition Values per 100g / 100ml KCAL	PROT	CARB	FAT	FIBRE
Meat & Skin, Roasted, Average	1oz/28g	60	3.9	216	22.6	0.0	14.0	0.0
Meat & Skin Portions, Deep Fried, Average	1oz/28g	73	4.7	259	26.9	0.0	16.8	0.0
Mince, Average	1oz/28g	39	1.7	140	20.9	0.1	6.1	0.2
Nuggets, Battered, Average	1 Nugget/20g	50	2.9	251	13.5	16.9	14.4	0.9
Nuggets, Breaded, Average	1 Nugget/14g	37	2.0	263	14.8	19.8	13.8	1.9
Nuggets, Free From Gluten & Wheat, Sainsbury's*	4 Nuggets/75g	187	9.8	251	13.4	19.7	13.2	0.8
O'S, Captain Birds Eye, Birds Eye*	10 Pieces/48g	119	6.9	248	13.2	16.4	14.4	0.8
Pieces, Garlic, Crunchy, Birds Eye*	1 Piece/99g	259	15.0	262	14.4	16.9	15.2	0.9
Pieces, Spicy, Mexican, Birds Eye*	1 Piece/103g	254	14.0	247	14.6	16.5	13.6	0.6
Roasted, in a Sugar Marinade, M & S*	1 Serving/100g	130	1.0	130	29.8	0.6	1.0	0.5
Seasoned & Basted, M & S*	1oz/28g	38	1.3	137	17.3	6.7	4.5	0.5
Skewers, BBQ, George Foreman's Lean Mean Grillers*	1 Skewer/59.6g	68	0.8	114	20.0	5.5	1.4	0.4
Skewers, with Chorizo, Bighams*	1 Skewer/94.9g	129	6.5	136	17.1	1.5	6.9	0.5
Soy Brasied, M & S*	1 Serving/100g	130	7.0	130	13.1	3.4	7.0	0.7
Spatchcock, Poussin, Sainsbury's*	1 Serving/122g	168	6.6	138	21.1	0.1	5.4	0.2
Spatchcock, Salt & Cracked Pepper, Sainsbury's*	1 Serving/122g	168	6.6	138	21.1	0.1	5.4	0.2
Spicy, Fried, Sainsbury's*	1 Serving/150g	414	24.9	276	28.8	2.9	16.6	2.1
Steaks, Average	1 Serving/100g	205	9.4	205	21.1	9.0	9.4	0.7
Steaks, Garlic & Herb, Tesco*	1 Serving/138g	354	23.2	257	14.1	12.2	16.9	1.7
Strips, Mexican, Sliced, M & S*	½ Pack/70g	77	0.4	110	24.3	2.3	0.6	0.5
Strips Or Tenders, Chinese Style, Average	1oz/28g	41	1.1	145	19.7	8.0	4.1	1.1
Tenders, Tex Mex, Jumbo, M & S*	1 Serving/200g	250	6.8	125	22.8	0.7	3.4	0.6
Thigh, Meat & Skin, Average	1 Serving/100g	218	14.7	218	21.4	0.0	14.7	0.0
Thigh, Meat & Skin, Casseroled, Average	1oz/28g	65	4.6	233	21.5	0.0	16.3	0.0
Thigh, Meat Only, Diced, Casseroled	1oz/28g	50	2.4	180	25.6	0.0	8.6	0.0
Thigh, Meat Only, Raw, Average	1 Thigh/90g	113	4.9	126	19.5	0.0	5.5	0.0
Thigh, Roast, Average	1 Serving/100g	238	15.7	238	23.9	0.4	15.7	0.0
Wafer Thin, Average	1 Slice/10g	12	0.4	120	19.0	2.8	3.6	0.2
Wafer Thin, Coronation, Sainsbury's*	½ Pack/50g	68	2.3	135	19.1	4.5	4.5	0.1
Whole, Roast, Average	1oz/28g	59	3.7	211	21.2	1.5	13.4	0.2
Whole, Roasted, Brown Sugar Marinade, Tesco*	1 Serving/100g	195	11.3	195	22.1	0.1	11.3	0.1
Whole, Rotisserie, M & S*	1oz/28g	62	3.9	220	23.7	0.4	14.0	0.4
Wing, Breaded, Fried, Average	1oz/28g	82	5.2	294	18.4	14.0	18.5	0.4
Wing, Meat & Skin, Cooked, Average	1oz/28g	67	4.4	241	23.3	1.9	15.6	0.3
Wing Quarter, Meat Only, Casseroled	1oz/28g	46	1.8	164	26.9	0.0	6.3	0.0
Wings, BBQ Flavour, Average	1oz/28g	61	3.5	220	20.3	6.6	12.5	0.6
Wings, Chinese Style, Average	1oz/28g	72	4.3	256	24.2	5.1	15.5	0.6
Wings, Hickory Smoke Flavour, Sainsbury's*	1 Wing/100g	245	15.3	245	23.5	3.5	15.3	0.5
Wings, Hot & Spicy, Average	1oz/28g	65	3.8	231	21.9	5.2	13.7	0.9
Wings, Meat & Skin, Raw, Average	1oz/28g	52	3.3	184	19.0	0.5	11.8	0.2
Zingy, with Peri Peri Hot Sauce, Rustlers*	1 Burger/131g	282	8.4	215	15.2	24.2	6.4	2.7
CHICKEN &								
& Veg, Deli Style Pieces, Redwood*	1 Serving/40g	116	6.9	290	24.4	4.6	17.2	0.3
Apricot Rice, COU, M & S*	1 Pack/400g	360	3.6	90	9.4	10.6	0.9	0.7
Asparagus, Baby Potatoes, Creamy, Sainsbury's*	1 Pack/450g	473	19.8	105	8.0	8.3	4.4	0.9
Asparagus, BGTY, Sainsbury's*	1 Pack/400g	428	5.6	107	9.1	14.5	1.4	0.9
Asparagus, in a Champagne Sauce, Finest, Tesco*	1 Pack/500g	615	33.5	123	8.8	7.0	6.7	0.9
Asparagus, Long Grain & Wild Rice, BGTY, Sainsbury's*	1 Pack/451g	555	9.0	123	9.2	17.1	2.0	0.8
Bacon, Al Forno, Safeway*	½ Pack/400g	420	11.6	105	6.1	13.3	2.9	1.1
Bacon, Easy Steam, Tesco*	1 Pack/400g	728	36.4	182	11.7	13.6	9.1	0.8
Bacon Parcels, Finest, Tesco*	1 Pack/232.5g	380	21.7	163	16.1	3.7	9.3	0.5
Bacon Parcels, Sainsbury's*	½ Pack/170g	406	28.6	239	21.9	0.1	16.8	0.0
Balsamic Roasted Pepper Pasta, M & S*	1 Pack/310g	419	11.5	135	7.8	17.2	3.7	1.7

CHICKEN &

	Measure INFO/WEIGHT	per Measure KCAL	FAT	Nutrition Values per 100g / 100ml KCAL	PROT	CARB	FAT	FIBRE
Black Bean, Chinese, Tesco*	1 Pack/350g	382	17.2	109	8.9	7.4	4.9	0.7
Black Bean, Chinese Takeaway, Tesco*	1 Serving/200g	190	6.6	95	8.3	8.0	3.3	0.5
Black Bean, Safeway*	1 Pack/350g	263	5.6	75	10.3	4.4	1.6	2.5
Black Bean, Special Fried Rice, HL, Tesco*	1 Pack/450g	360	6.3	80	6.8	9.5	1.4	0.9
Black Bean, with Chinese Rice, COU, M & S*	1 Pack/400g	320	9.6	80	7.4	7.6	2.4	1.1
Black Bean, with Noodles, Tesco*	1 Pack/475g	470	7.6	99	7.6	13.6	1.6	0.2
Black Bean, with Rice, Chinese, Tesco*	1 Serving/450g	459	9.5	102	5.3	15.4	2.1	0.5
Black Bean, with Rice, HL, Tesco*	1 Pack/450g	464	7.2	103	6.9	19.6	1.6	0.6
Black Bean Noodles, Sainsbury's*	1 Serving/130g	155	0.9	119	4.3	23.9	0.7	0.8
Black Bean Sauce, & Egg Fried Rice, BGTY, Sainsbury's*	1 Pack/450g	527	14.9	117	7.2	14.7	3.3	0.5
Broccoli, with Herb Potatoes, Tesco*	1 Pack/475g	499	10.9	105	7.8	12.5	2.3	1.5
Cashew Nuts, Asda*	1 Pack/400g	528	36.4	132	8.2	4.2	9.1	0.8
Cashew Nuts, Chinese, Cantonese, Sainsbury's*	½ Pack/175g	172	8.8	98	8.4	4.9	5.0	1.3
Cashew Nuts, Chinese, Tesco*	1 Pack/350g	378	19.6	108	9.5	4.9	5.6	0.6
Cashew Nuts, COU, M & S*	1 Pack/400g	380	8.8	95	8.2	11.2	2.2	1.9
Cashew Nuts, Easy Steam, Tesco*	1 Serving/400g	460	19.2	115	8.7	9.2	4.8	1.0
Cashew Nuts, Oriental, HL, Tesco*	1 Pack/450g	437	4.5	97	7.0	15.1	1.0	0.7
Cashew Nuts, PB, Waitrose*	1 Pack/400g	400	8.8	100	6.9	13.2	2.2	1.7
Cashew Nuts, with Egg Fried Rice, HL, Tesco*	1 Pack/450g	441	5.9	98	8.9	12.7	1.3	1.3
Cashew Nuts, with Egg Fried Rice, Somerfield*	1 Pack/340g	435	17.0	128	7.0	13.0	5.0	0.0
Cashew Nuts, with Egg Rice, GFY, Asda*	1 Pack/396g	396	8.7	100	7.0	13.0	2.2	1.3
Cashew Nuts, with Rice, Eat Smart, Safeway*	1 Serving/400g	400	9.2	100	6.6	12.6	2.3	2.0
Chargrilled Vegetable Roll, HL, Tesco*	1 Pack/221.1g	336	6.0	152	10.1	21.8	2.7	2.3
Chips, BBQ, BGTY, Sainsbury's*	1 Pack/381g	423	6.9	111	7.9	15.9	1.8	2.5
Chorizo Paella, Go Cook, Asda*	½ Pack/475g	591	10.5	124	12.2	15.9	2.2	2.6
Cous Cous, HE, Tesco*	1 Pack/351g	263	1.8	75	10.3	7.3	0.5	1.4
Cranberry, PB, Waitrose*	1 Pack/240g	161	1.0	67	11.8	4.1	0.4	1.1
Fries, Southern Fried, Sainsbury's*	½ Pack/250g	563	21.8	225	10.5	26.2	8.7	0.8
Fries, Southern Fried Style, Tesco*	1 Pack/500g	930	40.0	186	11.5	16.0	8.0	1.4
Gravy, COU, M & S*	1 Pack/300g	216	3.9	72	7.2	7.8	1.3	1.6
Herb Pasta with Lemon, HL, Tesco*	1 Pack/400g	520	8.0	130	8.2	18.8	2.0	1.6
King Prawn Special Fried Rice, Finest, Tesco*	1 Pack/450g	734	32.0	163	7.7	17.0	7.1	0.7
Mushroom, Chinese, Iceland*	1 Pack/400g	276	9.2	69	8.2	3.8	2.3	0.4
Mushroom, Chinese, Sainsbury's*	½ Pack/175g	116	3.5	66	7.6	4.4	2.0	0.9
Mushroom, Chinese, Tesco*	1 Pack/460g	474	12.9	103	5.7	13.8	2.8	1.0
Mushroom, in White Wine Sauce, GFY, Asda*	1 Pack/400g	272	7.2	68	6.0	7.0	1.8	1.2
Mushroom, with Egg Fried Rice, Iceland*	1 Pack/500g	410	6.0	82	4.9	13.0	1.2	0.7
Mushroom, with Vegetable Rice, BGTY, Sainsbury's*	1 Pack/400g	376	7.2	94	6.4	13.0	1.8	0.9
Noodles, Chinese Style, HE, Tesco*	1 Pack/370g	422	6.3	114	8.5	15.9	1.7	1.5
Peppers, in a Black Bean Sauce, M & S*	1 Pack/320g	256	4.8	80	9.4	7.3	1.5	1.2
Peppers, M & S*	1 Serving/240g	264	10.8	110	14.7	2.3	4.5	0.6
Pineapple, Chilled, Tesco*	1 Pack/350g	364	8.4	104	9.6	11.1	2.4	5.5
Pineapple, with Egg Fried Rice, HL, Tesco*	1 Pack/450g	414	3.2	92	6.0	15.4	0.7	0.6
Pineapple, with Egg Fried Rice, Tesco*	1 Pack/450g	450	10.8	100	7.6	12.1	2.4	1.2
Pineapple, with Rice, HL, Tesco*	1 Pack/450g	401	7.2	89	6.6	12.0	1.6	1.0
Pineapple, with Vegetable Rice, M & S*	1 Pack/400g	400	7.6	100	7.2	13.0	1.9	1.6
Red Pepper Dressing, Simple Solutions, Tesco*	1 Serving/140g	228	13.3	163	19.2	0.1	9.5	0.5
Tomato & Basil, COU, M & S*	½ Pack/200g	180	4.6	90	14.3	3.4	2.3	0.8
Tomato Saag, with Pilau Rice, BGTY, Sainsbury's*	1 Pack/400g	404	4.0	101	7.3	15.6	1.0	1.0
Vegetable Medley, Chargrilled, HE, Tesco*	1 Pack/450g	270	5.4	60	6.5	5.8	1.2	0.9
Vegetable Savoury Rice, Safeway*	½ Pack/185g	231	2.0	125	2.9	25.9	1.1	0.8
White Wine, with Rice, HE, Tesco*	1 Pack/450g	450	6.3	100	7.1	14.8	1.4	1.0

	Measure INFO/WEIGHT	per Measure		Nutrition Values per 100g / 100ml				
		KCAL	FAT	KCAL	PROT	CARB	FAT	FIBRE
CHICKEN A L' ORANGE								
Lean Cuisine, Findus*	1 Pack/334g	384	7.0	115	5.6	18.0	2.1	0.4
CHICKEN ALFREDO								
Al Forno, Sainsbury's*	1 Pack/900g	1026	22.5	114	6.5	16.4	2.5	1.4
BGTY, Sainsbury's*	1 Serving/200g	208	5.4	104	18.0	1.9	2.7	0.5
HL, Tesco*	1 Serving/377g	388	9.8	103	9.4	10.6	2.6	0.9
CHICKEN ARRABBIATA								
Bistro, Waitrose*	½ Pack/175g	156	5.3	89	12.9	2.5	3.0	0.5
Easy Steam, HL, Tesco*	1 Pack/400g	284	3.2	71	8.4	7.6	0.8	1.2
GFY, Asda*	1 Pack/447.7g	394	3.1	88	5.2	15.1	0.7	1.1
M & S*	1 Pack/500g	350	10.7	70	5.4	7.4	2.1	0.7
PB, Waitrose*	1 Serving/240g	211	5.8	88	12.4	4.0	2.4	0.6
PB, Waitrose*	1 Serving/240g	211	5.8	88	12.4	4.0	2.4	0.6
CHICKEN BANG BANG								
Oriental Express*	½ Pack/200g	170	3.4	85	6.4	11.0	1.7	3.2
Waitrose*	1 Pack/350g	368	17.2	105	9.4	5.9	4.9	1.2
CHICKEN BARBECUE								
with Potato Wedges, Eat Smart, Morrisons*	1 Pack/350g	368	4.9	105	8.5	14.5	1.4	1.5
CHICKEN BBQ								
& Chips, Sainsbury's*	1 Serving/380g	422	6.8	111	7.9	15.9	1.8	2.5
CHICKEN BUTTER								
Curry, Fresh, Tesco*	1 Pack/350g	487	24.5	139	11.8	7.1	7.0	1.8
Rich & Aromatic, Sainsbury's*	1 Pack/400g	592	36.4	148	12.1	4.4	9.1	1.2
Safeway*	1 Pack/350g	473	25.6	135	12.0	4.1	7.3	2.5
Tesco*	1 Pack/350g	515	33.0	147	11.7	3.7	9.4	0.7
CHICKEN CAJUN								
& Pasta, Safeway*	1 Pack/455g	501	15.5	110	8.6	10.5	3.4	2.1
& Potato Hash, HL, Tesco*	1 Pack/450g	428	6.3	95	6.5	14.1	1.4	1.5
Breast, Chargrilled, Iceland*	1 Serving/80g	114	1.5	143	27.4	3.9	1.9	0.0
HE, Tesco*	1 Pack/365g	412	4.7	113	7.9	17.3	1.3	0.7
CHICKEN CALYPSO								
with Turmeric Rice, BGTY, Sainsbury's*	1 Pack/450g	495	9.5	110	6.7	16.3	2.1	1.0
CHICKEN CANTONESE								
& Rice, Sizzler, Tesco*	1 Serving/450g	639	25.7	142	7.7	14.9	5.7	0.9
Breast, Fillets, Sainsbury's*	1 Serving/154.1g	168	2.3	109	20.3	3.6	1.5	0.6
Chinese, Tesco*	½ Pack/175g	196	6.5	112	10.3	9.4	3.7	0.4
Honey, Sesame, Sainsbury's*	1/3 Pack/135g	116	3.6	86	9.8	5.5	2.7	0.8
Honey Pepper, Sainsbury's*	½ Pack/175g	124	3.9	71	6.6	6.1	2.2	0.9
CHICKEN CARIBBEAN								
Fruity, with Rice & Peas, New, BGTY, Sainsbury's*	1 Pack/400g	352	3.6	88	6.9	13.1	0.9	2.2
Somerfield*	1 Pack/400g	554	16.8	139	8.7	16.5	4.2	1.7
Style, Breasts, COU, M & S*	1 Serving/205g	205	3.1	100	14.6	7.3	1.5	1.3
with Potato & Toasted Coconut Rosti, TTD, Sainsbury's*	½ Pack/200g	320	14.6	160	13.8	9.7	7.3	0.6
with Rice & Peas, BGTY, Sainsbury's*	1 Pack/400g	352	3.6	88	6.9	13.1	0.9	2.2
CHICKEN CHASSEUR								
BGTY, Sainsbury's*	1 Pack/320g	243	3.5	76	6.8	9.5	1.1	1.0
Breast Fillets, Morrisons*	1 Pack/380g	384	11.4	101	15.7	2.9	3.0	0.8
Finest, Tesco*	½ Pack/200g	200	6.4	100	14.3	2.4	3.2	1.1
CHICKEN CHAUSSEUR								
Mix, Colman's*	1 Pack/38g	120	0.4	316	8.6	68.2	1.0	3.7
CHICKEN CHILLI								
& Lemongrass, with Egg Noodles, BGTY, Sainsbury's*	1 Pack/450g	500	15.3	111	10.0	10.2	3.4	1.2
Sweet, & Egg Fried Rice, HL, Tesco*	1 Serving/450g	446	8.1	99	5.7	15.0	1.8	0.4
Sweet, Findus*	1 Pack/350g	420	12.3	120	6.0	15.0	3.5	1.5

	Measure INFO/WEIGHT	per Measure KCAL	FAT	Nutrition Values per 100g / 100ml KCAL	PROT	CARB	FAT	FIBRE
CHICKEN CHILLI								
Sweet, Just Cook, Sainsbury's*	½ Pack/190.5g	200	1.3	105	15.2	9.4	0.7	0.5
Sweet, with Noodles, Frozen, HL, Tesco*	1 Pack/450g	473	6.3	105	4.9	17.3	1.4	1.4
with Lime, Breast, Simple Solutions, Tesco*	1 Pack/400g	564	21.2	141	22.5	0.8	5.3	1.4
CHICKEN CHINESE								
& Prawns, Sizzler, House Special, Tesco*	1 Serving/450g	684	23.4	152	7.5	18.8	5.2	1.2
Battered, with Plum Sauce, Tesco*	1 Pack/350g	648	20.3	185	6.7	26.5	5.8	0.8
Crispy Aromatic, Half, Tesco*	1 Serving/233g	524	24.2	225	16.3	16.7	10.4	1.2
Fillets, with Sweet Chilli Sauce, Tesco*	1 Serving/350g	592	22.1	169	8.8	19.2	6.3	0.7
Stir Fry, Morrisons*	1 Serving/319g	341	5.4	107	5.7	17.0	1.7	1.5
Style, & Noodles, HE, Tesco*	1 Pack/370g	278	4.1	75	6.9	9.4	1.1	0.7
Style Sauce, Breast Fillets, Morrisons*	½ Pack/200g	162	2.0	81	13.5	4.6	1.0	1.2
with Ginger & Spring Onion, Tesco*	1 Serving/350g	299	10.1	85	7.6	7.3	2.9	0.6
CHICKEN CIDER								
COU, M & S*	1 Pack/400g	300	9.2	75	7.2	6.7	2.3	0.8
with Colcannon, PB, Waitrose*	1 Pack/401.1g	353	12.4	88	6.2	8.9	3.1	1.1
CHICKEN CORDON BLEU								
Breast, Fillets, Sainsbury's*	1 Serving/150g	304	14.3	203	17.5	11.5	9.5	1.6
TTD, Sainsbury's*	1 Fillet/140g	339	15.7	242	21.3	14.1	11.2	1.1
Waitrose*	1 Serving/160g	325	15.4	203	20.1	9.1	9.6	2.4
CHICKEN CORONATION								
M & S*	1 Serving/200g	420	26.4	210	12.6	10.6	13.2	1.3
CHICKEN CURRIED								
with Vegetables, Plumrose*	1 Serving/196g	253	16.1	129	5.8	8.0	8.2	0.0
CHICKEN DINNER								
Breast, with Pork, Sage & Onion Stuffing, Tesco*	1 Serving/180g	277	14.8	154	19.4	0.7	8.2	0.5
Kershaws*	1 Pack/350g	210	3.5	60	4.3	8.4	1.0	1.2
Tesco*	1 Serving/400g	388	7.2	97	9.2	10.9	1.8	1.2
with Gravy, The Crafty Cook*	1 Serving/320g	330	6.7	103	5.6	15.3	2.1	1.9
CHICKEN EN CROUTE								
Asda*	½ Pack/174g	393	17.4	226	14.0	20.0	10.0	1.5
Breast, Tesco*	1 Serving/215g	555	33.1	258	9.4	20.4	15.4	0.6
Just Cook, Sainsbury's*	1 Serving/180g	481	27.2	267	16.8	15.9	15.1	0.4
CHICKEN ESCALOPE								
Creamy Peppercorn, Sainsbury's*	1 Serving/150g	367	24.5	245	13.3	11.2	16.3	1.1
Ham & Cheese, Bernard Matthews*	1 Escalope/132g	351	19.5	266	12.2	21.0	14.8	0.7
Lemon, & Herb, Waitrose*	1 Serving/200g	202	4.4	101	19.2	1.0	2.2	1.4
Sour Cream & Chive, Tesco*	1 Escalope/143g	390	24.8	274	13.3	16.1	17.4	2.0
Southern Fried, Bernard Matthews*	1 Escalope/130g	234	11.2	180	17.9	7.8	8.6	2.7
Southern Fried, Crispy, Bernard Matthews*	1 Escalope/130g	234	11.2	180	17.9	7.8	8.6	2.7
Spinach & Ricotta, Sainsbury's*	1 Escalope/150g	354	22.9	236	13.1	11.5	15.3	0.9
Topped with Cheese, Ham & Mushrooms, Asda*	½ Pack/149.4g	216	8.9	145	22.0	0.8	6.0	0.4
CHICKEN FLORENTINE								
Asda*	1 Serving/200g	322	18.0	161	18.0	2.1	9.0	0.9
Finest, Tesco*	½ Pack/225g	358	19.1	159	11.0	9.7	8.5	1.3
HL, Tesco*	1 Pack/400g	340	10.8	85	12.1	3.0	2.7	0.9
CHICKEN FORRESTIERE								
COU, M & S*	1 Serving/220g	187	3.7	85	14.5	2.2	1.7	0.6
GFY, Asda*	½ Pack/225g	205	5.2	91	15.0	2.5	2.3	0.3
CHICKEN FU YUNG								
Chinese Takeaway, Tesco*	1 Pack/350g	315	3.5	90	5.6	14.5	1.0	0.8
CHICKEN GINGER								
& Lemon, with Apricot Rice, BGTY, Sainsbury's*	1 Pack/401.8g	438	5.6	109	9.7	14.5	1.4	0.3
& Lemon, with Rice, East Smart, Safeway*	1 Pack/395g	395	6.7	100	7.3	13.4	1.7	1.4

	Measure INFO/WEIGHT	per Measure		Nutrition Values per 100g / 100ml				
		KCAL	FAT	KCAL	PROT	CARB	FAT	FIBRE
CHICKEN GINGER								
& Plum, with Rice, PB, Waitrose*	1 Pack/400g	492	2.0	123	6.3	23.5	0.5	1.0
& Spring Onion, with Rice, Sharwood's*	1 Pack/375g	347	6.4	93	5.1	14.2	1.7	1.7
CHICKEN GLAZED								
Balsamic, HL, Tesco*	1 Pack/400g	288	3.6	72	5.1	10.8	0.9	0.9
CHICKEN HARISSA								
BGTY, Sainsbury's*	1 Serving/250g	211	3.0	84	10.4	8.0	1.2	1.5
with Cous Cous, PB, Waitrose*	1 Pack/400g	348	8.0	87	7.6	9.5	2.0	1.7
CHICKEN HAWAIIAN								
with Rice, Birds Eye*	1 Pack/350g	406	5.3	116	5.5	20.2	1.5	0.6
CHICKEN HERB								
Steam Cuisine, M & S*	1 Pack/400g	280	6.4	70	8.2	6.0	1.6	0.9
CHICKEN HONEY & MUSTARD								
HL, Tesco*	1 Serving/375g	424	8.6	113	5.8	17.3	2.3	1.4
Shapers, Boots*	1 Pack/241g	304	5.8	126	7.0	19.0	2.4	1.7
with Baby Potatoes, BGTY, Sainsbury's*	1 Pack/450g	392	3.2	87	8.5	11.7	0.7	0.8
with Spring Vegetable Rice, Slim Fast*	1 Pack/375g	375	5.3	100	5.8	15.5	1.4	0.8
with Vegetable Medley, BGTY, Sainsbury's*	Pack/400g	252	2.0	63	9.0	5.5	0.5	0.8
CHICKEN IN								
a Curry Sauce, Fillets, Safeway*	1 Serving/124g	180	7.9	145	17.2	3.9	6.4	0.6
Bacon, Mushroom & Red Wine Sauce, Asda*	1 Serving/151g	145	3.9	96	16.0	2.2	2.6	0.5
Barbeque Sauce, HE, Tesco*	1 Breast/170g	177	2.4	104	18.3	4.5	1.4	0.9
Basil Sauce, with Pasta, Easy Steam, BGTY, Sainsbury's*	1 Pack/380g	429	6.8	113	9.7	14.4	1.8	1.3
BBQ Sauce, Breast, Sainsbury's*	1 Serving/170g	199	1.2	117	14.5	13.1	0.7	1.3
BBQ Sauce, Chargrilled, Breast, GFY, Asda*	1 Serving/166g	214	6.1	129	19.0	5.0	3.7	1.0
BBQ Sauce, GFY, Asda*	1 Pack/380g	494	2.7	130	18.0	13.0	0.7	0.2
BBQ Sauce, Weight Watchers*	1 Pack/339g	332	11.9	98	5.8	10.8	3.5	0.9
Black Bean, with Egg Fried Rice, HL, Tesco*	1 Pack/450g	468	4.1	104	6.8	17.1	0.9	0.5
Black Bean, with Egg Fried Rice, Tesco*	1 Pack/450g	653	26.1	145	7.0	16.1	5.8	1.2
Black Bean Sauce, Budgens*	1 Pack/350g	333	14.0	95	9.9	4.9	4.0	0.9
Black Bean Sauce, Canned, BGTY, Sainsbury's*	1 Can/400g	308	3.6	77	9.3	7.9	0.9	0.7
Black Bean Sauce, Chinese Takeaway, Iceland*	1 Pack/400g	348	12.8	87	9.3	5.3	3.2	0.7
Black Bean Sauce, Frozen, BGTY, Sainsbury's*	1 Pack/400g	380	4.4	95	4.5	16.6	1.1	0.5
Black Bean Sauce, M & S*	1 Pack/350g	298	7.0	85	8.7	8.0	2.0	1.1
Black Bean Sauce, Safeway*	1 Pack/350g	284	4.6	81	9.4	7.9	1.3	1.0
Black Bean Sauce, Sainsbury's*	1 Pack/465g	484	7.9	104	5.0	17.3	1.7	0.3
Black Bean Sauce, Somerfield*	½ Pack/175g	133	1.8	76	10.7	6.1	1.0	1.9
Black Bean Sauce, Tinned, Tesco*	1 Serving/200g	164	2.6	82	10.0	7.7	1.3	1.1
Black Bean Sauce, Waitrose*	1 Pack/300g	243	3.6	81	10.9	6.6	1.2	0.8
Black Bean Sauce, with Egg Fried Rice, GFY, Asda*	1 Serving/416g	320	4.2	77	5.0	12.0	1.0	0.9
Black Bean Sauce, with Egg Fried Rice, Somerfield*	1 Pack/340g	384	13.6	113	7.0	13.0	4.0	0.0
Black Bean Sauce, with Noodles, Pro Cuisine*	1 Pack/600g	366	3.6	61	5.6	8.5	0.6	0.0
Black Bean Sauce, with Rice, Asda*	1 Pack/400g	500	7.6	125	7.0	20.0	1.9	0.6
Black Bean Sauce, with Rice, Iceland*	1 Pack/400g	388	6.0	97	5.1	15.8	1.5	0.8
Broccoli & Mushroom, Good Choice, Iceland*	1 Pack/500g	590	11.0	118	6.4	18.1	2.2	0.6
Broccoli & Mushroom, with Rice, HE, Tesco*	1 Pack/400g	440	4.8	110	7.5	17.1	1.2	0.7
Cheese & Bacon, Wrapped, Breast, Tesco*	1 Serving/300g	474	23.4	158	20.7	1.2	7.8	0.5
Cheesy Salsa, Fillets, Safeway*	½ Pack/175g	193	5.3	110	17.9	2.2	3.0	1.1
Chilli & Lemon Grass with Rice, Sainsbury's*	1 Pack/450g	527	11.3	117	6.2	17.4	2.5	0.7
Coconut, Sizzler, HL, Tesco*	1 Pack/350g	280	7.7	80	9.8	4.5	2.2	2.1
Coriander & Lime Marinade, Chargrilled, Asda*	½ Pack/163.4g	285	14.7	175	23.0	0.5	9.0	0.0
Creamy Madeira Sauce, HL, Tesco*	1 Pack/400g	320	6.8	80	12.8	2.3	1.7	1.0
Creamy Mushroom Sauce, HL, Tesco*	1 Pack/400g	296	6.0	74	13.2	1.8	1.5	0.5
Creamy Mustard Sauce, GFY, Asda*	1 Pack/400g	468	9.2	117	6.0	18.0	2.3	0.4

C

	Measure INFO/WEIGHT	per Measure KCAL	per Measure FAT	Nutrition Values per 100g / 100ml KCAL	PROT	CARB	FAT	FIBRE
CHICKEN IN								
Creamy Thai Sauce, Somerfield*	1 Pack/440g	748	35.2	170	22.0	2.0	8.0	0.0
Creamy Tikka Style Sauce, Tesco*	1 Breast/190g	215	10.5	113	15.1	0.7	5.5	0.8
Creamy Tomato & Mascarpone Sauce, Waitrose*	1 Serving/400g	492	23.2	123	7.9	9.9	5.8	0.8
Creamy White Wine Sauce, Sainsbury's*	1 Pack/324g	285	12.0	88	8.9	4.7	3.7	1.0
Garlic & Cream Sauce, Breast Fillet, Morrisons*	1 Serving/179.5g	261	15.8	146	14.9	1.8	8.8	0.6
Garlic & Herbs, Breast, Sainsbury's*	1 Serving/200g	316	5.2	158	28.3	5.4	2.6	0.1
Ginger & Chilli with Veg Noodles, COU, M & S*	1 Pack/400g	300	2.4	75	6.4	10.7	0.6	1.1
Gravy, Breast, Sainsbury's*	1 Box/200g	124	1.0	62	11.8	2.9	0.5	0.2
Gravy, Chunky, M & S*	1 Can/489g	465	19.1	95	13.6	1.4	3.9	0.8
Hot Ginger Sauce, & Thai Sticky Rice, Sainsbury's*	1 Pack/450g	603	20.7	134	6.8	16.3	4.6	0.5
Hot Ginger Sauce, with Jasmine Rice, BGTY, Sainsbury's*	1 Pack/400g	400	5.6	100	6.6	15.4	1.4	0.5
Hot Ginger Sauce, with Thai Sticky Rice, Sainsbury's*	1 Pack/450g	603	20.7	134	6.8	16.3	4.6	0.5
Leek & Bacon Sauce, Chilled, Co-Op*	1 Pack/400g	460	20.0	115	15.0	2.0	5.0	0.2
Leek & Bacon Sauce, with Mash, HL, Tesco*	1 Pack/450g	338	8.1	75	6.7	8.0	1.8	1.6
Lemon Flavour Sauce, Breast Fillets, Safeway*	1 Fillet/92g	200	8.6	217	17.0	16.0	9.4	1.4
Lemon Sauce, Breast, HE, Tesco*	1 Pack/385g	385	7.3	100	15.9	4.7	1.9	0.5
Lemon Sauce with Rice, Sainsbury's*	1 Pack/450g	513	6.8	114	8.1	17.0	1.5	0.7
Mango Ginger Marinade, Breast, Chargrilled, GFY, Asda*	½ Pack/190g	234	2.3	123	17.0	11.0	1.2	0.5
Mediterranean Sauce, Iceland*	1 Pack/500g	640	6.0	128	7.4	21.8	1.2	0.5
Mediterranean Style Sauce, Breasts, BGTY, Sainsbury's*	½Pack/170g	148	3.4	87	14.5	2.7	2.0	0.9
Mexican Salsa, Tesco*	1 Pack/320g	368	8.6	115	19.5	3.1	2.7	0.6
Mexican Style Sauce, Tesco*	1 Serving/180g	128	1.4	71	13.3	2.6	0.8	0.7
Mushroom & Ham Sauce with Rice, BGTY, Sainsbury's*	1 Pack/450g	581	7.2	129	9.7	18.9	1.6	0.3
Mushroom & Red Wine Sauce, Breast Fillets, Morrisons*	1 Serving/176.9g	184	4.4	104	15.7	4.6	2.5	0.7
Mushroom & White Wine Sauce, Fillets, Morrisons*	1 Serving/190g	243	10.5	128	18.8	0.9	5.5	0.5
Mushroom Sauce with Mash, HL, Tesco*	1 Pack/400g	384	10.8	96	9.9	8.0	2.7	0.6
Oyster Sauce, & Mushrooms, Tesco*	1 Pack/350g	252	5.6	72	8.0	6.3	1.6	0.7
Oyster Sauce, with Mushrooms, Tesco*	1 Pack/350g	189	3.2	54	8.0	3.5	0.9	0.8
Peppercorn Sauce, GFY, Asda*	1 Serving/399.1g	431	7.2	108	6.0	17.0	1.8	0.5
Peppercorn Sauce, Safeway*	1 Pack/395.2g	415	8.7	105	8.8	12.2	2.2	1.6
Peppers, Fillets, Sainsbury's*	1 Pack/360g	378	13.3	105	13.7	4.2	3.7	1.1
Pesto Style Dressing, Asda*	1 Serving/150g	210	10.0	140	18.7	1.3	6.7	0.0
Red Pepper Dressing, Tesco*	1 Serving/140g	228	13.3	163	19.2	0.1	9.5	0.5
Red Thai Marinade, Breasts, Mini, HE, Tesco*	1 Serving/200g	276	5.0	138	26.8	2.0	2.5	0.5
Red Thai Sauce, Breasts, HE, Tesco*	1 Pack/350g	368	9.5	105	17.0	3.1	2.7	0.2
Red Wine, with Mash, Eat Smart, Morrisons*	1 Serving/400g	288	5.2	72	9.1	6.1	1.3	1.4
Red Wine & Bacon Sauce, Breast, Somerfield*	1 Breast/150g	131	3.0	87	14.0	3.0	2.0	0.0
Red Wine Sauce, Fillets, Safeway*	1 Serving/175g	210	6.8	120	17.7	2.9	3.9	0.7
Red Wine with Mash, Eat Smart, Safeway*	1 Pack/400g	300	5.2	75	9.1	6.1	1.3	1.4
Satay Sauce, Safeway*	1 Serving/250g	363	20.0	145	10.5	7.1	8.0	1.4
Shiraz Wine Sauce, Finest, Tesco*	1 Pack/600g	420	9.6	70	10.9	2.9	1.6	1.3
Smoky Barbeque Sauce, Tesco*	1 Serving/185g	229	3.9	124	16.3	9.9	2.1	1.0
Spicy Chilli Sauce, Topped with Cheese, Breast, Asda*	½ Pack/190g	241	7.0	127	20.0	3.4	3.7	0.0
Sun Dried Tomato & Basil Sauce, Breast, Iceland*	1 Serving/155.8g	134	2.5	86	14.6	3.3	1.6	1.0
Tarragon Sauce, Lean Cuisine*	1 Pack/337.5g	270	6.8	80	4.0	11.0	2.0	1.5
Tomato & Basil, & Roast Potatoes, BGTY, Sainsbury's*	1 Pack/450g	419	4.1	93	8.1	13.1	0.9	2.3
Tomato & Basil, with Roasted Potatoes, BGTY, Sainsbury's*	1 Pack/450g	419	4.1	93	8.1	13.1	0.9	2.3
Tomato & Basil Sauce, Asda*	1 Breast/189.3g	231	6.0	122	22.0	1.2	3.2	2.0
Tomato & Basil Sauce, BGTY, Sainsbury's*	1 Fillet/175g	177	2.6	101	20.6	1.2	1.5	0.6
Tomato & Basil Sauce, Breast, Fillets, BGTY, Sainsbury's*	1 Fillet/175g	177	2.6	101	20.6	1.2	1.5	0.6
Tomato & Basil Sauce, Breast, GFY, Asda*	1 Pack/392g	447	13.3	114	12.0	9.0	3.4	1.5
Tomato & Basil Sauce, Breast Fillets, Morrisons*	½ Pack/171g	231	7.5	135	21.3	2.5	4.4	1.4
Tomato & Basil Sauce, Chargrilled, M & S*	1 Serving/235g	223	8.9	95	12.9	2.1	3.8	1.3

	Measure INFO/WEIGHT	per Measure KCAL	FAT	Nutrition Values per 100g / 100ml KCAL	PROT	CARB	FAT	FIBRE
CHICKEN IN								
Tomato & Basil Sauce, Eat Smart, Safeway*	1 Serving/235.7g	165	3.8	70	10.3	2.4	1.6	1.3
Tomato & Basil Sauce, GFY, Asda*	½ Pack/189.3g	231	6.1	122	22.0	1.2	3.2	2.0
Tomato & Basil Sauce, Good Choice, Iceland*	½ Pack/170g	153	4.4	90	13.3	3.3	2.6	0.6
Tomato & Basil Sauce, HL, Tesco*	1 Breast/200g	154	2.4	77	12.4	4.2	1.2	0.6
Tomato & Basil Sauce, Safeway*	1 Serving/175g	201	6.3	115	16.7	3.8	3.6	1.1
Tomato & Herb Sauce, Breasts, Tesco*	½ Pack/172.5g	155	2.4	90	15.0	3.6	1.4	0.5
Tomato & Wine Sauce, Potatoes, SteamFresh, Birds Eye*	1 Pack/400g	280	5.6	70	7.7	6.7	1.4	1.6
White Sauce, BGTY, Sainsbury's*	1 Can/200g	162	4.2	81	1.2	2.4	2.1	1.1
White Sauce, Canned, Asda*	½ Can/400g	644	44.0	161	12.0	3.5	11.0	0.0
White Sauce, Canned, HL, Tesco*	½ Can/200g	180	5.8	90	14.3	1.3	2.9	5.4
White Sauce, Low Fat, Breast, Safeway*	1 Serving/200g	190	9.0	95	11.5	2.1	4.5	0.2
White Wine, with Pasta, PB, Waitrose*	1 Pack/400g	400	10.0	100	8.2	12.1	2.5	2.5
White Wine, with Rice, Eat Smart, Safeway*	1 Serving/400g	400	4.0	100	8.9	13.6	1.0	1.1
White Wine, with Rice, HE, Tesco*	1 Serving/450g	513	12.2	114	7.1	15.3	2.7	0.7
White Wine & Asparagus Panzerotti, Asda*	½ Pack/150g	239	2.6	159	8.0	28.0	1.7	0.0
White Wine & Mushroom Sauce, Breasts, Asda*	1 Breast/167.9g	217	8.4	129	20.0	1.0	5.0	0.4
White Wine & Mushroom Sauce, M & S*	1 Serving/200g	260	13.6	130	15.6	1.6	6.8	1.0
White Wine & Tarragon Sauce, Breasts, Finest, Tesco*	½Pack/200g	326	20.2	163	16.8	1.3	10.1	0.0
White Wine & Tarragon Sauce, Somerfield*	½ Pack/136g	163	6.8	120	18.1	0.6	5.0	0.6
White Wine & Tarragon Sauce, Waitrose*	½ Pack/225g	281	17.3	125	10.7	3.1	7.7	0.3
White Wine Sauce, Breasts, Tesco*	1 Serving/370g	389	14.1	105	16.9	0.8	3.8	0.6
White Wine Sauce, Simple Solutions, Tesco*	½ Pack/200g	198	4.0	99	19.3	0.9	2.0	0.5
White Wine Sauce, Wild Rice, Birds Eye*	1 Pack/450g	335	5.9	74	7.1	8.4	1.3	2.1
White Wine Sauce, with Rice, HL, Tesco*	1 Pack/450g	500	7.1	111	7.1	17.0	1.6	0.8
Wild Mushroom Sauce, Breasts, HL, Tesco*	1 Serving/212g	191	5.1	90	15.1	2.1	2.4	1.5
Wild Mushroom Sauce, Extra Special, Asda*	1 Serving/225g	319	19.0	142	14.2	2.2	8.4	0.3
Zesty Orange Sauce, Asda*	1 Serving/200g	340	12.0	170	16.0	13.0	6.0	0.4
Zesty Orange Sauce, Breast, Asda*	1 Serving/200g	326	14.0	163	16.0	9.0	7.0	0.0
CHICKEN INDIAN								
Style, Fillets, Sainsbury's*	1 Pack/200g	233	9.2	112	13.7	4.4	4.4	1.2
CHICKEN ITALIAN								
Good Choice, Iceland*	1 Pack/400g	388	2.0	97	4.7	18.3	0.5	0.6
Iceland*	1 Pack/250g	208	2.5	83	13.6	4.8	1.0	0.5
Style, BGTY, Sainsbury's*	1 Pack/400g	364	4.4	91	6.0	14.5	1.1	0.9
Style, Dinner, Asda*	1 Pack/400g	244	4.0	61	6.0	7.0	1.0	1.1
Style, Meal, Asda*	1 Pack/408g	241	3.3	59	6.0	7.0	0.8	0.8
Style, Sainsbury's*	½ Pack/190g	222	7.6	117	16.3	3.9	4.0	0.1
with a Spicy Tomato, Chilli & Herb Sauce, Slim Fast*	1 Pack/371.4g	390	4.1	105	7.1	16.6	1.1	0.4
CHICKEN JEERA								
Sainsbury's*	½ Pack/200.8g	247	14.1	123	10.5	4.6	7.0	1.8
CHICKEN KUNG PO								
Chinese, Tesco*	1 Pack/350g	406	20.0	116	7.2	9.0	5.7	0.7
Sainsbury's*	½ Pack/175g	131	4.4	75	9.2	4.0	2.5	1.0
Waitrose*	1 Pack/350g	319	3.9	91	8.2	12.1	1.1	1.2
with Egg Fried Rice, Asda*	1 Pack/450g	689	22.5	153	6.0	21.0	5.0	1.0
CHICKEN LEMON								
Battered, Cantonese, Sainsbury's*	1 Pack/350g	560	19.6	160	10.7	16.6	5.6	0.9
Battered, Chinese Meal for Two, Tesco*	½ Portion/175g	294	13.0	168	6.6	18.8	7.4	2.0
Battered, HE, Tesco*	1 Pack/350g	399	9.1	114	8.8	13.9	2.6	0.4
Breast, Fillets, BGTY, Sainsbury's*	1 Fillet/112.5g	195	2.4	173	18.4	19.9	2.1	1.9
Cantonese, Sainsbury's*	½ Pack/140g	217	8.8	156	11.0	13.9	6.3	0.6
Cantonese Style, with Egg Fried Rice, Farmfoods*	1 Pack/324g	486	15.6	150	4.9	21.8	4.8	0.1
Chinese, Tesco*	1 Serving/350g	564	11.2	161	7.0	26.0	3.2	0.3

	Measure INFO/WEIGHT	per Measure KCAL	per Measure FAT	Nutrition Values per 100g / 100ml KCAL	PROT	CARB	FAT	FIBRE
CHICKEN LEMON								
COU, M & S*	1 Pack/150g	150	1.4	100	17.9	5.6	0.9	0.8
Steam Cuisine, COU, M & S*	1 Pack/400g	420	8.8	105	9.8	11.8	2.2	2.0
Tesco*	½ Pack/175g	214	7.4	122	11.0	10.1	4.2	0.6
Waitrose*	1 Serving/400g	596	23.2	149	12.7	11.7	5.8	0.9
with Rice, HL, Tesco*	1 Pack/450g	477	12.2	106	5.9	14.4	2.7	0.9
with Vegetable Rice, BGTY, Sainsbury's*	1 Pack/400g	428	6.4	107	6.5	16.8	1.6	0.8
CHICKEN LUNCH								
French Style, Light, John West*	1 Pack/240g	194	6.5	81	7.2	6.9	2.7	2.1
Italian Style, Light, John West*	1 Pack/240g	209	6.2	87	6.9	9.0	2.6	0.7
CHICKEN MANGO								
Tesco*	1 Pack/455g	687	30.9	151	7.3	15.3	6.8	1.2
CHICKEN MEAL								
American, Fillets, Asda*	1 Pack/345g	838	38.0	243	9.0	27.0	11.0	2.3
Roast, M & S*	1 Pack/250g	375	19.3	150	14.6	5.3	7.7	0.1
CHICKEN MEDITERRANEAN								
Style, Somerfield*	1 Pot/215g	455	28.2	212	7.4	16.0	13.1	1.0
with Trotolle Pasta, Easy Steam, BGTY, Sainsbury's*	1 Pack/400g	284	4.4	71	7.8	7.5	1.1	2.9
CHICKEN MEXICAN								
Style, BGTY, Sainsbury's*	1 Serving/260g	255	6.5	98	6.9	12.1	2.5	2.2
Style, Combo, Asda*	1 Pack/380g	562	16.7	148	21.0	6.0	4.4	2.0
Style, GFY, Asda*	½ Pack/200g	256	10.0	128	17.0	3.7	5.0	0.3
Style, with Rice, BFY, Morrisons*	1 Pack/400g	360	5.2	90	5.1	14.1	1.3	0.8
CHICKEN MOROCCAN								
Apricots & Pine Nuts, TTD, Sainsbury's*	1 Pack/400g	444	19.6	111	12.3	4.3	4.9	2.3
Style, Sainsbury's*	½ Pack/269g	334	7.0	124	14.7	10.4	2.6	3.1
Style, with Spicy Cous Cous, BGTY, Sainsbury's*	1 Serving/225g	304	3.8	135	9.2	20.6	1.7	0.0
with Apricots & Pine Nuts, TTD, Sainsbury's*	1 Pack/400g	444	19.6	111	12.3	4.3	4.9	2.3
with Cous Cous, BGTY, Sainsbury's*	1 Pack/400g	440	8.0	110	10.0	13.1	2.0	2.6
with Cous Cous, GFY, Asda*	1 Serving/450g	414	5.9	92	8.0	12.0	1.3	0.8
with Cous Cous & Fruity Sauce, BGTY, Sainsbury's*	1 Pack/400g	440	8.0	110	10.0	13.1	2.0	2.6
CHICKEN MUSTARD								
with Creme Fraiche Mash, PB, Waitrose*	1 Pack/400g	408	16.0	102	7.2	9.4	4.0	0.8
with Gratin Potatoes, HL, Tesco*	1 Pack/450g	464	12.2	103	9.0	10.7	2.7	2.5
CHICKEN ORIENTAL								
& Pineapple, HL, Tesco*	1 Serving/450g	414	3.2	92	6.0	15.4	0.7	0.6
Slim Fast*	1 Pack/385g	385	2.3	100	5.7	18.6	0.6	0.6
with Noodles, SteamFresh, Birds Eye*	1 Pack/399g	335	8.8	84	7.1	9.0	2.2	0.3
CHICKEN PAPRIKA								
& Savoury Rice, BGTY, Sainsbury's*	1 Pack/400g	384	2.0	96	7.2	15.6	0.5	1.1
COU, M & S*	1 Pack/400g	380	6.4	95	9.0	11.7	1.6	2.0
with Savoury Vegetables & Rice, BGTY, Sainsbury's*	1 Pack/451g	555	11.7	123	7.2	17.8	2.6	0.8
CHICKEN PARMESAN								
& Sun Dried Tomato, Fillets, Mini, Sainsbury's*	1 Pack/200g	278	5.8	139	22.1	6.0	2.9	0.5
Sun Dried Tomato, Fillets, BGTY, Sainsbury's*	½ Pack/100g	138	2.9	138	22.1	6.0	2.9	0.5
CHICKEN PENANG								
Waitrose*	1 Pack/400g	364	10.8	91	10.1	6.6	2.7	0.8
CHICKEN PEPPER								
Fry, Sainsbury's*	1 Pack/400g	508	24.8	127	15.0	2.9	6.2	1.6
Hot, & Hash, HL, Tesco*	1 Pack/450g	396	8.6	88	7.0	10.7	1.9	1.0
Hot, with Minted Mash, BGTY, Sainsbury's*	1 Serving/450g	333	5.4	74	7.3	8.4	1.2	1.3
CHICKEN PEPPERCORN								
BGTY, Sainsbury's*	1 Pack/251.8g	214	6.6	85	11.0	4.5	2.6	0.9

C

	Measure INFO/WEIGHT	per Measure		Nutrition Values per 100g / 100ml				
		KCAL	FAT	KCAL	PROT	CARB	FAT	FIBRE
CHICKEN PICCATA								
HE, Tesco*	1 Pack/405g	518	15.4	128	15.7	7.7	3.8	0.5
CHICKEN PIRI PIRI								
Breast, Fillets, Mini, Tesco*	1 Pack/200g	250	2.2	125	22.7	4.9	1.1	0.8
GFY, Asda*	1 Pack/400g	360	1.6	90	4.7	17.0	0.4	0.5
M & S*	1 Pack/300g	420	23.1	140	10.0	7.3	7.7	1.3
Morrisons*	1 Pack/350g	357	15.4	102	12.7	2.9	4.4	2.8
Safeway*	1 Serving/350g	455	24.5	130	11.6	4.7	7.0	2.4
Sainsbury's*	½ Pack/200g	248	10.8	124	14.0	4.8	5.4	0.5
with Rice, BGTY, Sainsbury's*	1 Serving/399g	395	4.4	99	10.3	11.9	1.1	1.6
CHICKEN RENDANG								
Sainsbury's*	1 Pack/350g	690	53.6	197	9.6	5.1	15.3	1.7
CHICKEN ROAST								
in a Pot, Sainsbury's*	1 Pack/450g	477	13.1	106	9.6	10.3	2.9	0.7
Meal, Blue Parrot Cafe, Sainsbury's*	1 Pack/285g	259	9.7	91	6.9	8.1	3.4	1.5
CHICKEN ROLL								
Broccoli & Mushroom, Sainsbury's*	1 Roll/355g	895	47.2	252	8.7	24.3	13.3	1.2
Value, Tesco*	1 Slice/13g	30	2.2	223	15.4	3.9	16.2	0.1
with Pork, Sage & Onion Stuffing, Value, Tesco*	1 Roll/125g	166	8.9	133	9.4	7.8	7.1	0.5
CHICKEN SAFFRON								
& Rice, M & S*	1 Pack/400g	360	4.8	90	7.6	11.6	1.2	1.1
CHICKEN SALSA								
Breast, Chunks, Roast, Waitrose*	1oz/28g	36	0.3	127	25.9	3.6	1.0	1.1
CHICKEN SICILIAN								
Somerfield*	1 Serving/400g	384	15.6	96	7.5	7.8	3.9	1.0
CHICKEN SIZZLER								
GFY, Asda*	1 Pack/350g	289	5.0	83	12.9	4.6	1.4	1.4
HL, Tesco*	1 Serving/350g	273	7.0	78	11.1	3.8	2.0	4.3
CHICKEN SPANISH								
Style, Asda*	½ Pack/275.2g	322	13.5	117	14.0	4.1	4.9	0.7
CHICKEN STUFFED								
Asparagus & Ricotta, with Herb Rice, BGTY, Sainsbury's*	1 Pack/400g	444	10.4	111	8.1	13.8	2.6	0.3
Breast, with Mushrooms, HE, Tesco*	1 Serving/175g	152	3.2	87	16.3	1.5	1.8	0.2
with Moroccan Style Cous Cous, GFY, Asda*	½ Pack/180g	259	4.9	144	20.0	10.0	2.7	0.0
with Mushrooms, Finest, Tesco*	1 Serving/150g	177	7.7	118	15.9	2.0	5.1	0.6
CHICKEN SUPREME								
BGTY, Sainsbury's*	1 Pack/350g	417	4.9	119	9.4	17.2	1.4	0.5
Breast, Sainsbury's*	1 Serving/187g	421	29.5	225	20.6	0.3	15.8	0.6
with Rice, Asda*	1 Pack/450g	617	31.5	137	15.0	3.4	7.0	1.1
with Rice, Birds Eye*	1 Pack/376g	470	9.8	125	6.6	18.8	2.6	0.5
with Rice, HE, Tesco*	1 Pack/400g	384	6.4	96	4.9	15.6	1.6	1.5
with Rice, Weight Watchers*	1 Pack/300g	255	4.8	85	5.6	11.9	1.6	0.5
CHICKEN SZECHUAN								
Chilli & Peppercorn, Sainsbury's*	1 Pack/400g	352	16.0	88	9.9	3.2	4.0	0.5
Tesco*	1 Pack/350g	385	10.5	110	7.2	13.6	3.0	0.3
with Noodles, Sainsbury's*	1 Pack/450g	423	14.0	94	6.0	10.4	3.1	0.9
CHICKEN TAGINE								
with Cous Cous, BGTY, Sainsbury's*	1 Pack/450g	626	17.6	139	10.1	15.9	3.9	1.5
CHICKEN TANDOORI								
GFY, Asda*	1 Pack/420g	420	15.1	100	9.0	8.0	3.6	1.4
Masala, & Rice, HL, Tesco*	1 Serving/450g	410	7.7	91	6.6	12.9	1.7	0.6
Masala, Asda*	1 Pack/400g	580	20.0	145	7.0	18.0	5.0	1.3
Masala, Indian, Tesco*	1 Serving/350g	431	25.9	123	10.2	4.0	7.4	1.8
Masala, Sainsbury's*	1 Pack/400g	536	27.2	134	13.2	5.0	6.8	0.5

	Measure INFO/WEIGHT	per Measure KCAL FAT		Nutrition Values per 100g / 100ml KCAL PROT CARB FAT FIBRE				

CHICKEN TANDOORI

	Measure INFO/WEIGHT	per Measure KCAL	FAT	KCAL	PROT	CARB	FAT	FIBRE
CHICKEN TANDOORI								
Safeway*	1 Pack/350g	595	36.1	170	13.7	5.7	10.3	1.3
Sizzler, HL, Tesco*	1 Pack/350g	275	7.0	79	11.1	3.8	2.0	4.3
Sizzler, Sainsbury's*	1 Pack/400g	536	29.2	134	12.8	4.3	7.3	1.7
Sizzler, Tesco*	1 Serving/175g	243	11.6	139	10.0	10.0	6.6	1.0
Tesco*	1 Serving/175g	198	8.6	113	10.6	6.7	4.9	1.0
with Rice, Easy Steam, Tesco*	1 Pack/400g	484	12.0	121	8.7	14.7	3.0	0.7
with Spicy Potatoes & Dip, HE, Tesco*	1 Pack/370g	322	3.0	87	9.7	10.3	0.8	1.3
with Spicy Vegatable Rice, Eat Smart, Safeway*	1 Serving/350g	368	7.7	105	9.7	11.1	2.2	7.0
CHICKEN TERIYAKI								
& Noodles, Asda*	½ Pack/340g	445	8.8	131	9.0	18.0	2.6	0.9
Asda*	1 Pack/360g	299	5.0	83	9.1	8.6	1.4	0.8
Japanese, with Ramen Noodles, Sainsbury's*	1 Pack/450g	482	9.5	107	6.5	15.5	2.1	0.8
with Ramen Noodles, Sainsbury's*	1 Pack/450g	482	9.5	107	6.5	15.5	2.1	0.8
CHICKEN THAI								
& Siu Mai Dumplings, M & S*	1 Dumpling/20.6g	36	1.6	170	16.0	9.4	7.6	0.8
Chiang Mai, & Noodles, BGTY, Sainsbury's*	1 Pack/448g	484	17.9	108	6.9	11.0	4.0	1.7
Green, Fillets, Mini, Sainsbury's*	½ Pack/100g	130	1.6	130	27.9	0.9	1.6	0.8
Marinated in Lemongrass, Lime Leaves & Chilli, Waitrose*	1 Serving/390g	323	9.4	83	8.0	7.2	2.4	9.5
Style, with Noodles, Tesco*	1 Pack/400g	332	6.8	83	7.5	9.5	1.7	1.0
Style Marinade, Breast, Chargrilled, GFY, Asda*	½ Pack/178g	178	5.3	100	17.0	1.3	3.0	0.5
with Rice, SteamFresh, Birds Eye*	1 Serving/400g	380	7.6	95	6.8	12.8	1.9	0.9
CHICKEN TIKKA								
& Coriander Rice, Weight Watchers*	1 Pack/457.1g	400	2.7	88	6.2	14.3	0.6	1.6
& Cous Cous, Boots*	1 Pack/160g	307	17.6	192	6.2	17.0	11.0	1.3
& Lemon Rice, Deli Meal, M & S*	1 Pack/360g	342	7.2	95	9.8	10.2	2.0	0.7
BGTY, Sainsbury's*	1 Serving/188g	265	3.0	141	10.5	21.2	1.6	0.0
Creamy, Breast, Tesco*	1 Breast/190g	215	10.5	113	15.1	0.7	5.5	0.8
Pinwheels, BGTY, Sainsbury's*	1 Serving/213.9g	261	4.7	122	9.6	16.0	2.2	0.0
Strips, Iceland*	1 Serving/100g	113	1.5	113	22.9	1.9	1.5	0.5
with Basmati Rice, GFY, Asda*	1 Pack/400g	592	7.2	148	9.0	24.0	1.8	1.6
CHICKEN TOPPED								
with Cheese, Ham & Mushroom, Breast Fillet, Morrisons*	1 Serving/175g	222	10.2	127	17.8	0.8	5.8	0.2
CHICKEN TUSCAN								
Style, Somerfield*	½ Pack/175g	222	10.3	127	15.7	2.5	5.9	0.2
CHICKEN VINDALOO								
Asda*	1 Pack/411g	649	24.7	158	7.0	19.0	6.0	0.0
Indian Takeaway, Tesco*	1 Pack/350g	438	20.0	125	8.3	9.0	5.7	3.0
Sainsbury's*	1 Pack/400g	460	16.8	115	14.6	4.8	4.2	0.6
Waitrose*	1 Pack/340g	398	18.4	117	10.6	6.4	5.4	1.6
CHICKEN WITH								
a Sea Salt & Black Pepper Crust, Breasts, Asda*	1 Serving/153.7g	186	4.3	121	19.0	5.0	2.8	0.0
a Sticky Honey & Chilli Sauce, Breast, Asda*	1 Serving/175g	247	5.6	141	20.0	8.0	3.2	0.0
Apricots & Almonds, HE, Tesco*	1 Pack/500g	465	9.5	93	11.8	7.3	1.9	0.5
Asparagus & Rice, BGTY, Sainsbury's*	1 Pack/400g	428	5.6	107	9.1	14.5	1.4	0.9
Bacon & Leeks, & Mash Potato, BGTY, Sainsbury's*	1 Pack/450g	435	11.3	97	8.4	10.1	2.5	0.7
Bacon & Leeks, GFY, Asda*	1 Pack/400g	328	8.0	82	13.0	3.0	2.0	0.6
Bacon & Leeks, with Mashed Potato, BGTY, Sainsbury's*	1 Pack/450g	435	11.3	97	8.4	10.1	2.5	0.7
Black Bean Sauce, Green Peppers, & Rice, Farmfoods*	1 Meal/324g	408	12.6	126	5.5	17.1	3.9	0.4
Black Bean Sauce & Noodles, Eat Smart, Safeway*	1 Pack/369g	295	2.6	80	7.2	10.5	0.7	1.2
Broccoli & Pesto Pasta, BGTY, Sainsbury's*	1 Pack/300.9g	328	5.1	109	10.3	13.2	1.7	2.5
Cheddar & Bacon Filling, Breast, Just Cook, Sainsbury's*	1 Serving/180g	346	14.6	192	23.2	6.5	8.1	0.1
Cheese, Ham & Mushrooms, Sainsbury's*	1 Serving/175g	206	9.1	118	17.2	0.6	5.2	0.6
Cheese, Leek & Bacon, Breasts, Stuffed, Safeway*	1 Serving/159.0g	310	15.7	195	24.3	1.0	9.9	0.6

CHICKEN WITH

	Measure INFO/WEIGHT	per Measure KCAL	FAT	Nutrition Values per 100g / 100ml KCAL	PROT	CARB	FAT	FIBRE
Cheese & Bacon, Tesco*	1 Pack/450g	540	23.9	120	10.9	6.8	5.3	0.5
Cheese & Chive Sauce, Carb Control, Tesco*	1 Serving/400g	400	25.6	100	8.4	2.0	6.4	1.6
Cheese Croutons & Onion, Asda*	1 Serving/200g	200	6.4	100	16.0	2.0	3.2	0.9
Cheesy Salsa, Safeway*	1 Serving/100g	180	4.9	180	29.2	3.6	4.9	1.8
Chorizo, & Patatas Bravas, COU, M & S*	1 Pack/400g	380	9.2	95	7.8	10.8	2.3	1.7
Chorizo & Tomato Sauce, Catalan, Bighams*	1 Pack/479g	407	15.8	85	10.9	2.8	3.3	0.7
Con Carne, Fluffy White Rice, COU, M & S*	1 Pack/400g	360	7.6	90	5.7	12.3	1.9	1.5
Con Carne, Frozen, Co-Op*	1 Pack/340g	306	3.4	90	6.0	15.0	1.0	1.0
Con Carne, Good Choice, Iceland*	1 Pack/400g	476	4.0	119	5.5	21.9	1.0	1.0
Con Carne, Homepride*	1 Can/390g	234	2.3	60	2.5	11.2	0.6	0.0
Con Carne, M & S*	1 Pack/285g	285	10.5	100	8.7	7.4	3.7	2.0
Con Carne, Recipe Mix, Colman's*	1 Pack/50g	158	1.3	316	10.4	62.9	2.5	6.8
Con Carne, Restaurant, Sainsbury's*	1 Serving/100g	80	2.7	80	6.9	7.0	2.7	1.5
Con Carne, Sainsbury's*	1 Pack/376.2g	459	6.0	122	7.4	19.6	1.6	1.0
Con Carne, Silverado Beef, Stagg*	1 Tin/410g	406	11.1	99	7.8	10.9	2.7	1.5
Con Carne, Slim Fast*	1 Pack/375g	394	7.1	105	5.5	16.2	1.9	1.5
Con Carne, Tesco*	1 Pack/100g	110	5.7	110	7.8	6.4	5.7	4.7
Con Carne, Tinned, Morrisons*	1 Tin/392g	368	11.8	94	8.8	8.0	3.0	2.4
Con Carne, with Rice, Birds Eye*	1 Pack/285g	291	7.1	102	3.3	16.6	2.5	0.8
Con Carne, with Rice, Eat Smart, Morrisons*	1 Pack/400g	328	5.2	82	5.3	12.2	1.3	1.4
Con Carne, with Rice, Tesco*	1 Pack/480g	562	14.4	117	6.9	15.6	3.0	2.0
Coriander & Lime, Asda*	1 Serving/105g	122	0.9	116	24.0	2.9	0.9	0.2
Cranberry & Orange Stuffing, Sainsbury's*	1 Serving/100g	201	10.3	201	23.0	4.1	10.3	0.8
Cranberry Stuffing, Breast, Finest, Tesco*	½ Pack/200g	252	4.8	126	16.2	9.9	2.4	0.9
Creamy Mushroom Sauce, Eat Smart, Safeway*	1 Serving/250g	213	6.0	85	12.8	2.7	2.4	0.9
Creamy Mushroom Sauce & Mash, HL, Tesco*	1 Pack/400g	384	10.8	96	10.0	8.0	2.7	0.6
Creamy Spinach & Parmesan, M & S*	1 Pack/390g	468	17.2	120	10.8	12.3	4.4	2.5
Fusilli & Courgette, Sainsbury's*	1 Pack/450g	675	28.8	150	8.6	14.6	6.4	0.5
Garlic & Herb, Breasts, COOK!, M & S*	½ Pack/130g	143	2.5	110	22.7	0.4	1.9	0.0
Garlic & Herbs, Asda*	1 Slice/25g	29	0.4	114	23.9	1.1	1.5	0.0
Garlic & Mushrooms, Somerfield*	½ Pack/100g	145	5.5	145	23.9	0.0	5.5	1.6
Garlic Mushrooms, Asda*	1 Serving/320g	342	16.0	107	13.8	1.8	5.0	2.3
Garlic Mushrooms, Breasts, Simply Cook, Tesco*	1 Serving/155g	245	14.4	158	17.9	0.8	9.3	0.5
Garlic Mushrooms, Simply Cook, Tesco*	½ Pack/155g	245	14.4	158	17.9	0.8	9.3	0.5
Grapes & Asparagus, Sainsbury's*	½ Pack/200g	240	13.2	120	13.3	1.8	6.6	1.0
Gravy & Stuffing, Breasts, Tesco*	½ Pack/173g	257	11.1	149	14.4	8.3	6.4	2.2
Gravy & Stuffing, Mini Classics, Tesco*	1 Pack/300g	255	8.1	85	6.1	8.7	2.7	1.2
Gruyere & Smoked Garlic, Breast, TTD, Sainsbury's*	½ Pack/200g	444	30.2	222	17.3	4.2	15.1	0.1
Gruyere & Smoked Garlic, TTD, Sainsbury's*	½ Pack/200g	444	30.2	222	17.3	4.2	15.1	0.1
Ham & Vegetables, Creamy, Eat Smart, Safeway*	1 Pack/370g	241	6.7	65	6.5	5.5	1.8	1.4
Hoi Sin Sauce, Ooodles of Noodles, Oriental Express*	1 Pack/425g	400	9.4	94	5.3	13.2	2.2	1.7
Leek, Cheese & Bacon, Breasts, Simple Solutions, Tesco*	1 Serving/200g	296	16.8	148	17.6	0.5	8.4	0.3
Lemon Grass, Thai Greens & Baby Corn, Sainsbury's*	1 Serving/200g	196	6.8	98	10.0	6.9	3.4	1.4
Lime & Coriander, Chargrilled, Asda*	1 Serving/190g	352	17.1	185	24.0	2.0	9.0	1.1
Lime & Coriander, Easy, Waitrose*	½ Pack/168g	203	7.9	121	18.9	0.7	4.7	0.5
Lime & Coriander Marinade, Chargrilled, Asda*	1 Portion/163.4g	285	14.7	175	23.0	0.5	9.0	0.0
Lime & Tequila, Asda*	1 Serving/150g	194	2.7	129	24.0	4.3	1.8	0.5
Lyonnaise Potatoes, M & S*	½ Pack/260g	286	8.1	110	12.6	8.0	3.1	0.9
Mango Salsa & Potato Wedges, BGTY, Sainsbury's*	1 Pack/400g	336	6.4	84	7.0	10.4	1.6	1.5
Mascarpone, Bacon & Roasted Onions, Finest, Tesco*	1 Serving/200g	312	17.6	156	14.5	4.7	8.8	0.5
Medium, Uncle Ben's*	1 Jar/500g	305	4.0	61	1.8	11.1	0.8	0.0
Mexican, with Potato Wedges, Weight Watchers*	1 Pack/300g	249	8.7	83	4.6	9.6	2.9	1.3
Mexican Chilli with Potato Wedges, Weight Watchers*	1 Pack/300g	249	8.7	83	4.6	9.6	2.9	1.3

C

CHICKEN WITH

INFO/WEIGHT	Measure	per Measure		Nutrition Values per 100g / 100ml				
		KCAL	FAT	KCAL	PROT	CARB	FAT	FIBRE
Mexican Style, Aldi*	½ Can/196g	231	10.2	118	8.7	9.2	5.2	2.1
Minced, Master Foods*	1 Teaspoon/7g	7	0.1	103	1.6	20.8	1.4	0.0
Mixed Vegetable, Tesco*	1 Pack/400g	352	11.6	88	3.9	11.0	2.9	3.2
Mushroom & Bacon, Fillets, M & S*	½ Pack/187.5g	226	11.3	120	15.5	0.5	6.0	1.7
Mushroom & Garlic, Breast Fillets, Just Cook, Sainsbury's*	½ Pack/165.8g	330	17.1	199	20.0	4.6	10.3	0.1
Mushroom & Garlic Butter, Breasts, Sainsbury's*	½ Pack/180g	388	20.1	199	20.0	4.6	10.3	0.1
Mushroom & Madeira Ragout, TTD, Sainsbury's*	½ Pack/225g	218	7.0	97	13.6	3.7	3.1	0.1
Mushroom & Tomato Sauce, GFY, Asda*	1 Serving/175g	180	3.7	103	19.0	2.0	2.1	2.7
Mushroom Pilaff, BGTY, Sainsbury's*	1 Serving/400g	320	2.0	80	8.1	10.5	0.5	1.4
Mushroom Risotto, M & S*	1 Pack/365g	493	27.0	135	6.9	10.4	7.4	1.3
Mushroom Sauce & Herby Rice, Fillets, M & S*	1 Pack/380g	475	19.4	125	7.7	12.0	5.1	1.3
Mushrooms, & Madeira Sauce, Finest, Tesco*	½ Pack/200g	320	15.6	160	15.0	7.2	7.8	1.0
Mushrooms, in Madeira Sauce, HE, Tesco*	½ Pack/200g	182	2.0	91	15.0	5.4	1.0	0.4
Non Carne, Linda McCartney*	1 Pack/340g	275	7.8	81	5.8	9.2	2.3	1.7
Pancakes & Plum Sauce, COU, M & S*	1 Pack/245g	257	5.6	105	7.9	12.7	2.3	0.3
Pancetta & Mozzarella, Finest, Tesco*	½ Pack/225g	349	16.9	155	14.8	5.8	7.5	0.8
Pasta, Chianti & Balsamic, BGTY, Sainsbury's*	1 Pack/400g	372	7.6	93	9.4	9.5	1.9	1.9
Pesto & Linguine Pasta, Birds Eye*	1 Pack/400g	440	16.0	110	8.5	10.0	4.0	1.3
Pesto & Linguine Pasta, Steamfresh Meal, Birds Eye*	1 Pack/400g	440	16.0	110	8.5	10.0	4.0	1.3
Plum Sauce, Battered, Tesco*	1 Serving/175g	324	10.2	185	6.7	26.5	5.8	0.8
Plum Tomatoes & Basil, Breast, Birds Eye*	1 Portion/172.4g	200	8.1	116	13.3	5.0	4.7	0.6
Pork, Parsnip Herb Stuffing, Sainsbury's*	1 Serving/100g	181	9.0	181	22.9	2.1	9.0	0.7
Pork, Sage & Onion Stuffing, Breast, TTD, Sainsbury's*	1 Pack/150g	222	8.7	148	22.7	1.3	5.8	0.9
Pork, Sage & Onion Stuffing, Mini Roasts, Tesco*	1 Serving/240g	353	20.6	147	14.7	2.6	8.6	0.2
Pork, Sage & Onion Stuffing, TTD, Sainsbury's*	1 Pack/150g	222	8.7	148	22.7	1.3	5.8	0.9
Pork Stuffing & Chipolatas, Breast Joint, Tesco*	½ Pack/340g	524	27.9	154	16.7	3.4	8.2	0.5
Potato & Smoked Bacon Topping, M & S*	1 Serving/175g	228	8.4	130	17.8	3.2	4.8	1.2
Prosciutio, Dolcelatte & 3 Cheese Sauce, Asda*	½ Pack/195g	355	11.7	182	30.0	1.9	6.0	1.2
Red Wine & Mushroooms, Breasts, Tesco*	1 Breast/195g	154	3.7	79	12.0	3.5	1.9	0.8
Rice, Breast, Chargrilled, Spicy, Asda*	1 Pack/400g	372	2.4	93	6.0	16.0	0.6	1.0
Rice, Fiesta, Weight Watchers*	1 Pack/330g	307	6.6	93	6.1	12.8	2.0	0.4
Rice 'n' Peas, Sainsbury's*	1 Pack/300g	489	18.3	163	12.5	14.4	6.1	2.1
Roast Potatoes, Eat Smart, Safeway*	1 Serving/363.2g	345	6.5	95	8.5	10.1	1.8	1.5
Sage & Onion Stuffing & Chipolatas, Breast Joint, Tesco*	½ Pack/280g	507	32.8	181	16.2	2.8	11.7	1.9
Salsa & Potato Wedges, GFY, Asda*	1 Serving/400g	327	7.0	82	6.0	10.5	1.8	1.8
Spicy Bean & Vegetable, Safeway*	1 Pack/311g	196	4.0	63	3.3	9.6	1.3	2.5
Spinach, Honey Mustard, American Style, Asda*	1 Serving/240g	394	24.0	164	14.0	4.4	10.0	0.3
Spinach & Pasta, M & S*	1oz/28g	64	4.2	228	9.4	14.0	15.0	1.3
Spring Vegetables, Chargrilled, COU, M & S*	1 Pack/414g	290	3.7	70	8.8	7.3	0.9	1.8
Stilton & Port Sauce, Breasts, Finest, Tesco*	1 Serving/400g	668	34.4	167	18.5	3.9	8.6	0.7
Stuffing, Butter Basted, Co-Op*	1 Slice/23.1g	30	0.9	130	21.0	2.0	4.0	1.0
Sun Dried Tomato & Basil Butter, Sainsbury's*	1 Breast/185g	363	17.6	196	25.0	2.5	9.5	0.2
Sun Dried Tomato & Basil Sauce, Bistro, Waitrose*	½ Pack/175g	254	14.2	145	14.2	3.7	8.1	0.3
Sweet Chilli & Garlic, Chinese, Asda*	1 Serving/400g	436	2.4	109	8.0	18.0	0.6	2.1
Sweet Chilli Noodles, Eat Smart, Morrisons*	1 Pack/380g	236	4.2	62	5.9	7.1	1.1	1.3
Sweet Potato Mash, Jerk, Sainsbury's*	1 Pack/400g	284	4.4	71	6.1	9.2	1.1	2.2
Sweet Potato Mash, Jerk, Super Naturals, Sainsbury's*	1 Pack/400g	284	4.4	71	6.1	9.2	1.1	2.2
Tagine, Cous Cous, PB, Waitrose*	1 Pack/400g	516	14.0	129	8.2	16.2	3.5	1.0
Tagine, Cous Cous, PB, Waitrose*	1 Pack/400g	516	14.0	129	8.2	16.2	3.5	1.0
Tangy Lemon Sauce, Breasts, Just Cook, Sainsbury's*	1 Serving/164g	244	3.0	149	16.2	16.9	1.8	0.1
Tomato & Basil, GFY, Sainsbury's*	1 Pack/400g	300	3.2	75	13.6	3.4	0.8	1.4
Tomato & Basil, HE, Tesco*	1 Serving/225g	189	3.8	84	11.2	6.1	1.7	1.2
Tomato & Basil, Steam Cuisine, M & S*	1 Pack/400g	460	13.6	115	9.6	11.6	3.4	2.0

	Measure INFO/WEIGHT	per Measure KCAL	FAT	Nutrition Values per 100g / 100ml KCAL	PROT	CARB	FAT	FIBRE
CHICKEN WITH								
Tomato & Basil Pasta, M & S*	1 Pack/205g	420	24.2	205	8.7	16.0	11.8	1.0
Tomato & Basil Sauce, Breasts, HL, Tesco*	1 Serving/200g	146	2.2	73	12.0	3.9	1.1	0.6
Tomato & Basil Sauce, Carb Control, Tesco*	1 Serving/400g	316	18.8	79	7.4	1.7	4.7	1.6
Tomato Sauce & Basil Mash, COU, M & S*	1 Pack/400g	360	10.4	90	7.6	8.5	2.6	1.1
Uncle Ben's*	1oz/28g	17	0.2	59	1.8	11.1	0.8	0.0
Vegetable	1oz/28g	16	0.2	57	3.0	10.8	0.6	2.6
Vegetable, Canned, Sainsbury's*	1 Can/400g	368	2.0	92	5.1	16.7	0.5	4.9
Vegetable, Chesswood*	½ Can/200g	138	0.6	69	3.3	13.3	0.3	2.1
Vegetable, Retail	1oz/28g	20	0.6	70	4.0	9.4	2.1	0.0
Vegetable, Tinned, GFY, Asda*	½ Can/200g	140	1.8	70	3.5	12.0	0.9	3.5
Vegetable & Rice, BGTY, Sainsbury's*	1 Pack/450g	410	5.0	91	3.5	16.7	1.1	3.5
Vegetable & Rice, Good Intentions, Somerfield*	1 Serving/400g	336	4.4	84	2.7	15.8	1.1	2.1
Vegetable & Rice, HE, Tesco*	1 Pack/450g	392	5.4	87	2.8	16.1	1.2	1.5
Vegetable & Rice, Safeway*	1 Pack/500g	530	4.0	106	3.4	21.2	0.8	1.7
Vegetable Garden, Stagg*	1 Can/410g	254	2.1	62	3.6	10.8	0.5	2.3
Vegetarian, & Rice, Meat Free, Tesco*	1 Pack/450g	455	8.1	101	4.2	17.0	1.8	1.7
Vegetarian, with Rice, Tesco*	1 Pack/500g	575	13.0	115	4.0	19.0	2.6	1.8
with Caramelised Peppers, Chargrilled, M & S*	½ Pack/237g	225	9.0	95	12.9	2.1	3.8	1.3
with Cous Cous, Lemon & Herb, Finest, Tesco*	1 Pack/370g	492	18.5	133	10.5	11.5	5.0	0.9
CHICORY								
Fresh, Raw, Average	1 Av Head/150g	30	0.9	20	0.6	2.8	0.6	0.9
CHILLI								
& Lemongrass Prawns with Noodles, BGTY, Sainsbury's*	1 Pack/400g	328	2.8	82	5.0	13.8	0.7	1.3
& Potato Wedges, Good Choice, Iceland*	1 Pack/400g	368	13.6	92	5.5	9.8	3.4	1.2
& Potato Wedges, Sainsbury's*	1 Pack/370g	393	15.2	106	7.2	10.1	4.1	2.2
& Rice, Birds Eye*	1 Serving/285g	305	7.7	107	3.4	17.2	2.7	1.0
& Rice, Frozen, Sainsbury's*	1 Pack/400g	436	7.6	109	4.8	18.4	1.9	0.6
& Rice, GFY, Asda*	1 Pack/400g	352	1.6	88	5.0	16.0	0.4	1.8
& Rice, Morrisons*	1 Serving/500g	630	15.5	126	5.7	18.9	3.1	1.1
& Spicy Wedges, Good Intentions, Somerfield*	1 Serving/400g	340	9.2	85	5.6	10.5	2.3	1.1
& Wedges, BBQ, HL, Tesco*	1 Pack/420g	391	10.9	93	5.4	12.2	2.6	1.9
Beef, & Potato Crush, Weight Watchers*	1 Pack/400g	232	6.0	58	5.0	5.9	1.5	3.4
Beef, Asda*	½ Pack/200g	190	7.8	95	7.0	8.0	3.9	1.2
Beef, with Potato Wedges, Naturally Good Food, Tesco*	1 Pack/440g	352	12.3	80	7.2	6.2	2.8	1.8
Beef, with Potato Wedges, Tesco*	1 Pack/440g	352	12.3	80	7.2	6.2	2.8	1.8
Beef, with Rice, GFY, Asda*	1 Serving/402.3g	354	6.0	88	4.7	14.0	1.5	0.9
Beef, with Rice, Sainsbury's*	1 Serving/300g	360	5.1	120	5.6	20.6	1.7	1.1
Beef & Chilli Sauce, Chinese Takeaway, Farmfoods*	1oz/28g	66	3.6	234	6.7	20.0	13.0	0.3
Bowl, American Style, Sainsbury's*	½ Pack/300g	255	10.5	85	8.8	4.6	3.5	2.0
Bowl, Safeway*	1 Pack/300g	327	13.5	109	8.8	8.3	4.5	2.7
Chicken Grande, Stagg*	1 Serving/204.9g	168	1.2	82	9.7	9.4	0.6	1.6
Con Carne, Asda*	1 Can/392g	376	13.7	96	7.0	9.0	3.5	0.0
Con Carne, BGTY, Sainsbury's*	1 Serving/377g	430	6.4	114	6.9	17.8	1.7	0.8
Con Carne, Canned, Co-Op*	1 Can/392g	392	15.7	100	8.0	8.0	4.0	3.0
Con Carne, Canned, la Caldera*	¼ Can/200g	240	12.8	120	6.9	8.6	6.4	0.0
Con Carne, Classic, Stagg*	½ Can/205g	226	10.3	110	7.2	9.1	5.0	2.2
Con Carne, Dynamite Hot, Stagg*	1 Serving/250g	310	15.5	124	7.6	9.6	6.2	2.5
Con Carne & Potato Wedges, Morrisons*	1 Pack/400g	324	10.0	81	4.5	9.9	2.5	2.6
Con Carne & Rice, HL, Co-Op*	1 Pack/400g	400	6.8	100	7.8	13.9	1.7	2.1
Con Carne & Rice, Somerfield*	1 Pack/500g	490	5.0	98	5.0	18.0	1.0	0.0
Con Carne with Potato Wedges, BGTY, Sainsbury's*	1 Pack/366.3g	359	12.1	98	4.6	12.6	3.3	3.0
Con Carne with Rice, BGTY, Sainsbury's*	1 Pack/400g	448	6.0	112	6.0	18.8	1.5	1.8
Con Carne with Rice, Eat Smart, Safeway*	1 Pack/400g	340	5.2	85	5.3	12.2	1.3	1.4

C

	Measure INFO/WEIGHT	per Measure KCAL	FAT	Nutrition Values per 100g / 100ml KCAL	PROT	CARB	FAT	FIBRE
CHILLI								
Con Carne with Rice, GFY, Asda*	1 Serving/400g	456	6.4	114	6.0	19.0	1.6	0.9
Con Carne with Rice, Healthy Choice, Asda*	1 Pack/400g	412	8.4	103	6.0	15.0	2.1	0.9
Con Carne with Rice, Organic, Sainsbury's*	1 Pack/400g	472	10.8	118	5.0	18.5	2.7	1.8
Con Carne with Rice, PB, Waitrose*	1 Pack/401g	405	7.2	101	5.8	15.3	1.8	1.7
CHILLIES								
Crushed, Schwartz*	1 Tsp/0.5g	2	0.1	425	15.9	56.4	15.1	0.3
CHINESE LEAF								
Fresh, Raw, Asda*	4 Leafs/125g	14	0.3	11	1.0	1.4	0.2	1.2
Fresh, Raw, Tesco*	1 Serving/200g	36	0.6	18	3.5	0.3	0.3	2.6
CHINESE MEAL								
Cantonese Take Away, to Share, M & S*	1/3 Pack/433g	671	24.2	155	5.9	21.8	5.6	1.3
for One, GFY, Asda*	1 Pack/570g	946	16.5	166	7.0	28.0	2.9	0.0
for One, Morrisons*	1 Pack/550g	495	5.5	90	6.5	13.7	1.0	1.1
for Two, Tesco*	1 Pack/500g	480	8.0	96	4.4	16.0	1.6	1.1
House Special, HL, Tesco*	1 Pack/450g	369	7.2	82	6.5	10.5	1.6	1.1
House Special, with Egg Fried Rice, Tesco*	1 Pack/450g	563	8.6	125	7.2	19.7	1.9	0.8
My Very Own, Asda*	1 Pack/297g	416	5.3	140	7.0	24.0	1.8	0.6
CHIPLETS								
Salt & Vinegar, Potato & Maize Snack, M & S*	1 Pack/50g	219	9.5	438	5.7	61.3	18.9	4.7
CHIPS								
& Curry Sauce, Tesco*	1 Serving/400g	440	20.0	110	2.1	14.1	5.0	1.0
11mm Fresh, Deep Fried, McCain*	1oz/28g	66	3.0	235	3.2	31.8	10.6	0.0
14mm Fresh, Deep Fried, McCain*	1oz/28g	59	1.9	209	2.7	34.2	6.8	0.0
14mm Friers Choice, Deep Fried, McCain*	1oz/28g	56	2.2	199	3.5	29.3	8.0	0.0
3 Way Cook, Somerfield*	1 Serving/96g	145	4.8	151	2.5	24.0	5.0	1.6
9/16" Straight Cut Caterpack, Deep Fried, McCain*	1oz/28g	63	2.6	225	3.1	32.1	9.4	0.0
American Style, Oven, Co-Op*	1 Serving/150g	255	9.0	170	2.0	26.0	6.0	3.0
American Style, Oven, Safeway*	1 Serving/125g	288	8.5	230	4.1	38.2	6.8	3.0
American Style, Oven, Sainsbury's*	1 Serving/165g	314	13.7	190	5.4	23.6	8.3	1.3
American Style, Thin, Oven, Tesco*	1 Serving/125g	210	8.1	168	2.7	24.6	6.5	2.1
Basics, Sainsbury's*	1 Serving/165g	277	7.6	168	1.8	29.7	4.6	0.3
Beefeater, Deep Fried, McCain*	1oz/28g	71	2.8	253	3.3	37.7	9.9	0.0
Beefeater, Oven Baked, McCain*	1oz/28g	55	1.6	195	4.0	32.2	5.6	0.0
British Classics, HL, Tesco*	½ Pack/200g	250	1.6	125	2.6	26.9	0.8	1.3
Chippy, Microwave, McCain*	1oz/28g	49	2.0	176	2.6	25.2	7.2	1.7
Chunky, Baked, Organic, M & S*	1 Serving/100g	150	3.7	150	1.7	27.1	3.7	2.2
Chunky, COU, M & S*	1 Serving/150g	158	2.4	105	2.1	20.5	1.6	2.3
Chunky, Eat Smart, Safeway*	1 Serving/158g	150	2.5	95	1.6	18.3	1.6	1.4
Chunky, Fresh, Chilled, Finest, Tesco*	½ Pack/200g	270	8.0	135	2.1	22.3	4.0	2.7
Chunky, Ready to Bake, M & S*	1 Serving/200g	310	8.4	155	2.2	26.8	4.2	2.0
Chunky, Waitrose*	1 Portion/155g	200	8.8	129	1.9	17.6	5.7	2.8
Chunky Oven, Harry Ramsden's*	1 Serving/150g	185	5.4	123	2.8	19.9	3.6	1.6
Crinkle Cut, Frozen, Fried in Corn Oil	1oz/28g	81	4.7	290	3.6	33.4	16.7	2.2
Crinkle Cut, M & S*	1 Serving/150g	270	8.1	180	3.3	29.5	5.4	2.4
Crinkle Cut, Oven, Asda*	1 Serving/100g	134	3.8	134	2.0	23.0	3.8	8.0
Crinkle Cut, Oven Baked, Aunt Bessie's*	1 Serving/100g	206	9.2	206	2.9	28.0	9.2	3.2
Family Fries Oven, Tesco*	1 Serving/125g	164	4.6	131	2.0	22.4	3.7	1.8
Fat, with Fluffy Centres, M & S*	1 Serving/200g	210	9.0	105	1.6	14.2	4.5	1.8
Fine Cut, Frozen, Fried in Blended Oil	1oz/28g	102	6.0	364	4.5	41.2	21.3	2.4
Fine Cut, Frozen, Fried in Corn Oil	1oz/28g	102	6.0	364	4.5	41.2	21.3	2.7
Fried, Average	1 Serving/130g	296	12.4	228	4.4	33.3	9.5	1.7
Fried, Chip Shop, Average	1 Serving/400g	956	49.6	239	3.2	30.5	12.4	2.2
Frying, Crinkle Cut, Tesco*	1 Serving/125g	161	4.1	129	2.6	22.2	3.3	1.9

CHIPS

INFO/WEIGHT	per Measure KCAL	FAT	KCAL	PROT	CARB	FAT	FIBRE
CHIPS							
Frying, Value, Tesco*	1 Serving/125g	376	19.9	301	4.3	35.4	15.9	2.5
Homefries, Chunky, Weighed Baked, McCain*	1 Serving/165g	252	5.1	153	3.2	28.0	3.1	2.3
Homefries, Chunky, Weighed Frozen, McCain*	1 Serving/100g	123	2.5	123	2.5	22.6	2.5	1.6
Homefries, Crinkle Cut, Weighed Baked, McCain*	1 Serving/225g	443	14.6	197	3.0	31.7	6.5	2.5
Homefries, Crinkle Cut, Weighed Frozen, McCain*	1 Serving/100g	197	6.5	197	3.0	31.7	6.5	2.5
Homefries, Extra Chunky, Weighed Baked, McCain*	1 Serving/100g	195	4.6	195	3.7	34.7	4.6	2.3
Homefries, Jacket Oven, McCain*	1 Serving/100g	220	7.4	220	3.9	37.9	7.4	0.0
Homefries, Straight Cut, Weighed Baked, McCain*	1 Serving/60g	109	3.7	181	3.1	28.1	6.2	2.4
Homefries, Straight Cut, Weighed Frozen, McCain*	1 Serving/200g	268	9.2	134	2.2	21.0	4.6	1.7
Homefries, Thin & Crispy, Weighed Frozen, McCain*	1 Serving/100g	143	4.1	143	2.6	24.0	4.1	1.5
Homemade, Fried in Blended Oil, Average	1oz/28g	53	1.9	189	3.9	30.1	6.7	2.2
Homemade, Fried in Corn Oil, Average	1oz/28g	53	1.9	189	3.9	30.1	6.7	2.2
Homemade, Fried in Dripping, Average	1oz/28g	53	1.9	189	3.9	30.1	6.7	2.2
Homestyle, Frozen, Aunt Bessie's*	1 Serving/200g	260	11.2	130	2.2	17.6	5.6	2.7
Homestyle, Oven Cooked, Aunt Bessie's*	1 Serving/100g	191	7.8	191	3.1	27.0	7.8	2.9
Homestyle Oven, Sainsbury's*	1 Serving/125g	206	5.4	165	2.4	29.2	4.3	2.1
Just Bake, Low Fat, M & S*	1oz/28g	37	1.0	133	2.0	24.7	3.7	1.7
Micro, Asda*	1 Serving/112g	221	7.8	197	3.5	30.0	7.0	4.0
Micro Chips, Crinkle Cut, Cooked, McCain*	1 Pack/100g	166	4.2	166	2.9	28.9	4.2	2.4
Micro Chips, Straight Cut, Cooked, McCain*	1 Pack/100g	163	4.8	163	2.3	27.7	4.8	2.0
Microwave, Cooked	1oz/28g	62	2.7	221	3.6	32.1	9.6	2.9
Oven, American Style, Champion*	1 Serving/200g	372	14.4	186	2.2	28.2	7.2	2.0
Oven, Best in the World, Iceland*	1 Serving/175g	333	11.7	190	3.4	28.9	6.7	3.5
Oven, Champion*	1 Pack/133g	210	6.0	158	2.5	27.0	4.5	0.0
Oven, Chunky, Ross*	1 Serving/100g	177	6.5	177	3.1	26.6	6.5	3.9
Oven, Cooked, Value, Tesco*	1 Serving/125g	308	9.8	246	4.5	39.5	7.8	2.9
Oven, Crinkle Cut, 5% Fat, Weighed Baked, McCain*	1 Serving/100g	163	4.3	163	3.1	27.9	4.3	3.0
Oven, Crinkle Cut, 5% Fat, Weighed Frozen, McCain*	1 Serving/100g	134	3.6	134	2.4	23.2	3.6	2.4
Oven, Crinkle Cut, Co-Op*	1oz/28g	38	1.1	135	2.0	22.0	4.0	3.0
Oven, Crinkle Cut, Oven Baked, Tesco*	1oz/28g	50	1.5	180	3.3	29.5	5.4	2.4
Oven, Crinkle Cut, Safeway*	1 Serving/130g	234	7.0	180	3.3	29.5	5.4	2.4
Oven, Crinkle Cut, Sainsbury's*	1 Serving/165g	297	9.1	180	3.3	29.5	5.5	2.4
Oven, Curly, Safeway*	1 Serving/125g	376	20.8	301	3.8	34.0	16.6	4.1
Oven, Frozen, Baked	1oz/28g	45	1.2	162	3.2	29.8	4.2	2.0
Oven, Frozen, BGTY, Sainsbury's*	1 Serving/165g	226	4.6	137	2.9	25.0	2.8	2.7
Oven, Frozen, Value, Tesco*	1 Serving/125g	189	5.8	151	2.8	24.7	4.6	1.9
Oven, Good Choice, Iceland*	1 Serving/150g	266	3.2	177	3.6	35.8	2.1	4.5
Oven, Healthy Choice, Safeway*	1 Serving/150g	227	5.3	151	2.8	27.1	3.5	2.1
Oven, Morrisons*	1 Serving/100g	134	3.9	134	2.4	22.2	3.9	0.0
Oven, Organic, Waitrose*	1 Serving/165g	233	6.3	141	1.5	25.1	3.8	1.6
Oven, Original, McCain*	1 Serving/100g	158	3.8	158	2.5	28.5	3.8	2.3
Oven, Original, Straight Cut, 5% Fat, Cooked, McCain*	1 Serving/84g	144	4.1	172	3.4	32.4	4.9	2.3
Oven, Original, Straight Cut, 5% Fat, Frozen, McCain*	1 Serving/250g	345	10.0	138	2.5	26.2	4.0	1.9
Oven, Reduced Fat, Waitrose*	1oz/28g	37	0.8	133	2.3	24.3	3.0	1.6
Oven, Safeway*	1oz/28g	42	1.0	151	2.8	27.1	3.5	2.1
Oven, Steak Cut, Asda*	1 Serving/100g	153	4.1	153	2.0	27.0	4.1	2.5
Oven, Steak Cut, Frozen, Champion*	1 Serving/100g	130	3.5	130	1.9	22.6	3.5	3.3
Oven, Steak Cut, Sainsbury's*	1 Serving/165g	266	7.8	161	2.6	27.1	4.7	2.8
Oven, Steak Cut, Somerfield*	1 Serving/180g	265	9.0	147	2.4	23.0	5.0	1.5
Oven, Steak Cut, Waitrose*	1 Serving/165g	218	5.6	132	2.7	22.7	3.4	1.7
Oven, Steakhouse, Frozen, Tesco*	1 Serving/125g	165	4.3	132	2.7	22.7	3.4	1.7
Oven, Straight, Waitrose*	1 Serving/165g	219	6.1	133	2.0	23.0	3.7	1.7
Oven, Straight Cut, 4% Fat, HE, Tesco*	1oz/28g	35	0.9	124	2.3	21.8	3.1	1.9

C

CHIPS

	Measure INFO/WEIGHT	per Measure KCAL	FAT	Nutrition Values per 100g / 100ml KCAL	PROT	CARB	FAT	FIBRE
Oven, Straight Cut, 5% Fat, Sainsbury's*	1 Serving/165g	281	8.1	170	3.4	28.0	4.9	2.5
Oven, Straight Cut, Asda*	1 Serving/100g	199	5.0	199	3.5	35.0	5.0	3.0
Oven, Straight Cut, Budgens*	1 Portion/180g	205	3.4	114	2.3	21.9	1.9	2.7
Oven, Straight Cut, Frozen Weight, HL, Tesco*	1 Serving/125g	133	2.4	106	2.1	20.0	1.9	2.3
Oven, Straight Cut, GFY, Asda*	1oz/28g	42	1.0	150	2.6	27.0	3.5	2.4
Oven, Straight Cut, HE, Tesco*	1oz/28g	30	0.5	106	2.1	20.0	1.9	2.3
Oven, Straight Cut, Iceland*	1 Serving/100g	197	6.2	197	3.6	31.6	6.2	2.3
Oven, Straight Cut, Low Fat, HL, Tesco*	1 Serving/100g	132	2.8	132	2.7	23.9	2.8	2.8
Oven, Straight Cut, Reduced Fat, Tesco*	1 Serving/100g	127	3.0	127	2.3	22.7	3.0	2.1
Oven, Straight Cut, Safeway*	1 Serving/125g	226	6.5	181	3.6	30.0	5.2	2.5
Oven, Straight Cut, Tesco*	1oz/28g	46	1.4	166	2.6	27.8	4.9	1.7
Oven, Stringfellows, McCain*	1oz/28g	72	2.9	256	4.1	37.0	10.2	0.0
Oven, Thick Cut, Frozen, Baked	1oz/28g	44	1.2	157	3.2	27.9	4.4	1.8
Oven, Thin Cut, American Style, Asda*	1 Serving/100g	240	10.0	240	3.4	34.0	10.0	3.0
Oven, Thin Fries, Morrisons*	1 Serving/100g	161	6.1	161	2.9	23.6	6.1	1.2
Oven, Weight Watchers*	1 Serving/100g	150	3.0	150	2.8	33.7	3.0	5.9
Potato, Lights, Reduced Fat, Lay's*	1 Serving/25g	118	5.5	470	7.5	60.0	22.0	5.0
Southern Fried, Amercan Style, Iceland*	1 Serving/150g	369	18.6	246	3.5	30.3	12.4	2.8
Steak, Cut Frying, Safeway*	1 Serving/125g	289	15.1	231	3.3	27.1	12.1	2.2
Steak Cut, Frying, Asda*	1 Serving/96.8g	181	6.8	187	2.9	28.0	7.0	2.8
Steak Cut, Oven, Tesco*	1 Serving/165.2g	233	6.4	141	2.0	24.4	3.9	2.0
Steakhouse, Fry, Tesco*	1 Serving/125g	278	15.1	222	3.1	25.2	12.1	2.0
Straight Cut, Frozen, Fried in Blended Oil	1oz/28g	76	3.8	273	4.1	36.0	13.5	2.4
Straight Cut, Frozen, Fried in Corn Oil	1oz/28g	76	3.8	273	4.1	36.0	13.5	2.4
Straight Cut, Low Fat, Tesco*	1 Serving/125g	159	3.8	127	2.3	22.7	3.0	2.1
Straight Cut, Microwave Baked, McCain*	1oz/28g	70	3.0	251	3.5	35.0	10.7	0.0
The Big Chip, Frozen, Tesco*	1 Serving/200g	220	4.8	110	1.8	20.3	2.4	2.1
Thick Cut, Caterpack, Deep Fried, McCain*	1oz/28g	60	2.7	215	3.1	28.8	9.7	0.0
Thick Cut, Frozen, Fried in Corn Oil, Average	1oz/28g	66	2.9	234	3.6	34.0	10.2	2.4
Three Way Cook, Skinny, Co-Op*	1 Serving/100g	175	7.0	175	2.0	26.0	7.0	3.0
Vending 3/8" Straight Cut, Deep Fried, McCain*	1oz/28g	62	2.7	220	3.3	29.6	9.8	0.0
Waffle, Birds Eye*	1 Serving/75g	156	8.4	208	2.5	24.3	11.2	2.6

CHIPSTICKS

Ready Salted, Smiths, Walkers*	1 Bag/25g	120	5.8	480	6.5	62.0	23.0	3.0
Salt 'n' Vinegar, Walkers*	1 Pack/22.5g	107	5.2	475	6.0	61.0	23.0	3.0

CHIVES

Fresh, Average	1 Tsp/2g	0	0.0	23	2.8	1.7	0.6	1.9

CHOC ICES

Average	1 Ice/50g	139	8.8	277	3.5	28.1	17.5	0.0
Belgian Milk, Sainsbury's*	1 Serving/80ml	170	10.7	212	1.9	21.1	13.4	0.5
Chunky, Wall's*	1 Ice/81g	162	10.6	200	2.6	18.9	13.1	0.0
Dark, Sainsbury's*	1 Ice/43.2g	135	9.5	315	3.8	25.5	22.0	0.4
Dark, Somerfield*	1 Ice/62ml	186	13.0	300	3.0	25.0	21.0	0.0
Dark, Tesco*	1 Ice/43.4g	140	9.0	325	2.8	30.2	21.0	0.1
Light, Safeway*	1 Ice/43.5g	136	9.5	310	2.8	25.9	21.6	0.9
Light, Sainsbury's*	1 Ice/43g	135	9.2	313	3.2	27.0	21.4	0.3
Light, Waitrose*	1 Serving/70ml	141	10.0	201	1.7	17.0	14.3	0.3
Mini Mix, Eis Stern*	1 Ice/38.6g	130	9.0	334	4.2	29.0	23.0	0.0
Morrisons*	1 Ice/31g	86	6.0	279	3.0	24.7	19.3	0.4
Neapolitan, Safeway*	1 Ice/41.4g	119	8.0	290	2.6	25.4	19.5	0.3
Neapolitan Chocolate, Co-Op*	1 Ice/62g	120	8.2	194	2.0	16.9	13.2	0.4
Real Plain, Sainsbury's*	1 Ice/48.4g	149	9.6	310	2.9	29.5	20.0	2.2
SmartPrice, Asda*	1 Ice/31g	81	5.9	262	2.8	20.0	19.0	0.0

	Measure INFO/WEIGHT	per Measure KCAL	FAT	Nutrition Values per 100g / 100ml KCAL	PROT	CARB	FAT	FIBRE
CHOC ICES								
Vanilla, Co-Op*	1 Ice/70g	130	12.0	186	3.6	3.6	17.1	0.0
CHOCOLATE								
Advent Calendar, Dairy Milk, Cadbury*	1 Window/4.2g	22	1.3	525	7.5	56.6	30.1	0.7
Advent Calendar, Maltesers, Mars*	1 Piece/4g	21	1.2	537	6.8	57.9	30.9	0.0
Almond & Honey, Dairy Milk, Cadbury*	1 Sm Bar/54g	281	15.6	520	8.0	57.1	28.9	1.0
Animal Bar, Nestle*	1 Bar/19g	97	5.0	513	5.8	63.6	26.1	0.0
Baking, Belgian, Milk, Luxury, Sainsbury's*	1 Chunk/8g	44	2.7	556	7.6	56.5	33.3	1.5
Baking, Continental, Luxury, Tesco*	1 Pack/150g	822	67.7	548	2.7	27.7	45.1	0.9
Baking, Milk, Luxury, Tesco*	1 Pack/150g	839	54.3	559	7.0	51.4	36.2	1.7
Bar, Cappuccino, Thorntons*	1 Bar/38g	201	13.2	529	5.2	49.7	34.7	0.5
Bar, Dark, Thorntons*	1 Sm Bar/48g	250	17.7	521	7.3	39.9	36.9	10.9
Bar, Dark, with Ginger, Thorntons*	1 Bar/100g	509	35.1	509	5.8	44.3	35.1	8.8
Bar, Lemon Mousse, Continental, Thorntons*	1 Bar/40g	200	11.6	500	3.8	55.4	29.1	0.7
Bar, Lemon Mousse, Thorntons*	1oz/28g	141	8.2	503	4.1	55.3	29.3	0.0
Bar, Milk, Thorntons*	1 Sm Bar/50g	269	16.0	538	7.5	54.8	32.0	1.0
Bar, Viennese, Continental, Thorntons*	1 Bar/38g	206	13.0	542	4.2	54.0	34.2	0.8
Bar, White, Thorntons*	1 Bar/50g	274	15.7	547	6.5	59.5	31.3	0.0
Bars, Alpini, Continental, Thorntons*	1 Bar/35.6g	194	11.5	538	6.9	55.3	32.0	2.7
Bars, Chocolate, Cherry, Lindt*	1 Bar/100g	470	22.8	470	4.5	61.7	22.8	0.0
Bars, Chocolate, Strawberry, Lindt*	1 Bar/100g	470	22.8	470	4.5	61.6	22.8	0.0
Bars, Milk Chocolate, Gold, Lindt*	1 Bar/300g	1605	92.9	535	6.6	58.7	31.0	0.0
Bars, Milk Chocolate, Hazelnut, Gold, Lindt*	1 Bar/300g	1665	108.2	555	7.9	50.7	36.1	0.0
Bars, Milk Chocolate, Hazelnut, Lindt*	1 Bar/100g	570	38.8	570	8.5	47.0	38.8	0.0
Bars, Milk Chocolate, Lindt*	1 Bar/100g	535	31.0	535	6.6	57.7	31.0	0.0
Bars, Milk Chocolate, Raisin & Hazelnut, Lindt*	1 Bar/ 100g	530	31.6	530	3.1	54.7	31.6	0.0
Beans, Coffee, Dark, Solid, M & S*	1 Serving/10g	53	3.8	532	4.7	42.4	37.6	11.6
Belgian, Kschocolat*	4 Pieces/40g	212	12.2	530	6.0	57.5	30.5	2.3
Black Magic, Nestle*	1oz/28g	128	5.8	456	4.4	62.6	20.8	1.6
Breakaway, Nestle*	1 Bar/21.4g	107	5.5	500	6.2	61.1	25.6	2.4
Bubbly, Dairy Milk, Cadbury*	1 Bar/35.2g	184	10.4	525	7.7	56.9	29.7	0.7
Bunny, Lindt*	1 Bunny/84g	480	29.1	572	7.5	57.5	34.6	0.0
Caramel, Chunk, Dairy Milk, Cadbury*	1 Chunk/33g	158	7.6	480	5.0	63.0	23.0	0.0
Caramel, Dairy Milk, Cadbury*	1 Bar/50g	240	11.8	480	4.9	62.1	23.5	0.4
Choco Swing, Milka*	1 Square/16g	89	5.5	555	5.7	54.0	34.5	0.0
Chocolat Noir, Lindt*	1/6 Bar/17g	87	5.4	510	6.0	50.0	32.0	0.0
Chomp, Cadbury*	1 Bar/24g	112	4.8	465	3.3	67.9	20.0	0.2
Christmas Tree Decoration, Cadbury*	1 Decoration/12g	60	3.4	525	7.6	56.2	29.9	0.0
Chunk Bar, Dairy Milk, Cadbury*	1 Chunk/6.7g	35	2.0	525	7.5	57.0	29.8	0.1
Chunky Hazelnut Bar, M & S*	1 Bar/52g	293	19.4	563	8.8	48.1	37.3	1.7
Coins, Milk, Sainsbury's*	1 Coin/5g	26	1.4	502	5.5	58.8	27.1	2.5
Cream, Fry's*	1 Bar/50g	208	7.0	415	2.8	69.9	13.9	0.0
Crispies, Dairy Milk, Cadbury*	1 Bar/49g	250	13.4	510	7.6	58.6	27.4	0.0
Crispy, Sainsbury's*	4 Squares/19g	99	5.4	521	9.1	56.9	28.5	2.1
Dairy Milk, Cadbury*	1 Bar/49g	257	14.6	525	7.7	56.9	29.7	0.7
Dark, 70% Cocoa Solida, Extra Fine, Lindt*	1 Square/10g	54	4.1	537	8.0	33.0	41.0	0.0
Dark, 85% Cocoa, Excellence, Lindt*	1 Serving/40g	208	18.4	521	11.0	19.0	46.0	0.0
Dark, 85% Cocoa, TTD, Sainsbury's*	1 Piece/10g	56	5.1	562	9.5	16.4	50.9	13.0
Dark, Belgian, Extra Special, Asda*	2 Squares/20g	102	8.0	508	11.0	26.0	40.0	16.0
Dark, Belgian, Luxury Continental, Sainsbury's*	1 Bar/100g	490	38.7	490	11.1	24.2	38.7	7.4
Dark, Classic, Bournville, Cadbury*	1 Bar/17.5g	87	4.6	495	4.0	61.1	26.3	6.0
Dark, Espresso, with Real Coffee, Green & Black's*	1 Bar/150g	824	62.4	549	9.8	33.8	41.6	11.7
Dark, Extra Fine, Swiss, M & S*	1 Square/13g	72	5.9	555	7.8	30.4	45.3	12.0
Dark, Fair Trade, Co-Op*	1 Bar/45g	214	13.1	475	4.0	49.0	29.0	6.0

C

CHOCOLATE

	Measure INFO/WEIGHT	per Measure KCAL	FAT	Nutrition Values per 100g / 100ml KCAL	PROT	CARB	FAT	FIBRE
Dark, Hazelnuts & Currant, Green & Black's*	1 Bar/100g	513	33.5	513	7.6	45.4	33.5	9.2
Dark, Luxury Continental, Sainsbury's*	½ Bar/50g	252	20.0	504	10.7	25.5	40.0	16.1
Dark, Plain, Average	1oz/28g	143	7.8	510	5.0	63.5	28.0	2.5
Dark, Plain, Rich, Co-Op*	1 Bar/200g	1010	58.0	505	4.0	57.0	29.0	6.0
Dark, Plain, Rich, Sainsbury's*	1oz/28g	144	8.3	514	3.7	65.0	29.5	0.9
Dark, Raspberry, Ruffles, Jameson's*	1oz/28g	123	5.3	441	1.9	65.9	18.9	4.4
Dark, Rich, Tesco*	1 Serving/20g	98	6.1	491	5.8	60.0	30.4	11.5
Dark, Soft Mint Centre, Green & Black's*	1 Bar/100g	478	27.3	478	7.4	50.5	27.3	8.6
Dark, TTD, Sainsbury's*	1 Square/10g	57	4.6	569	7.2	31.2	46.3	10.9
Dark, Whole Nut, Tesco*	1 Serving/13g	67	4.5	539	6.1	48.3	35.7	6.5
Divine, Milk, Co-Op*	1 Bar/45g	243	14.4	540	7.0	57.0	32.0	2.0
Drops, Plain, Sainsbury's*	1 Serving/125g	638	34.5	510	5.3	60.1	27.6	4.0
Eggs, Party, Mini, Safeway*	1 Egg/20.3g	64	4.4	320	11.2	18.4	21.9	0.7
Extra Dark, Bournville, 76%, Cadbury*	1 Sm Bar/17.5g	95	7.8	545	7.9	27.8	44.8	11.1
Ferrero Rocher, Ferrero*	1 Chocolate/12.5g	74	5.1	593	7.0	49.0	41.0	0.0
Freddo, Caramel, Dairy Milk, Cadbury*	1 Bar/19.6g	95	4.8	485	5.5	60.2	24.6	0.0
Freddo, Dairy Milk, Cadbury*	1 Freddo/20g	105	6.0	525	7.5	57.0	29.8	0.7
Fruit & Nut, Cadbury*	1 Bar/49g	240	12.9	490	8.0	55.7	26.3	0.0
Fruit & Nut, Dark, Tesco*	4 Squares/25g	124	7.0	494	5.8	54.8	27.9	6.5
Fruit & Nut Assortment, M & S*	1oz/28g	148	9.6	527	7.6	49.8	34.3	1.3
Fudge, Keto Bar*	1 Serving/65g	250	7.0	385	36.9	36.9	10.8	32.3
Golf Balls, Milk Chocolate, Lindt*	1 Packet/110g	619	39.5	563	6.5	53.6	35.9	0.0
Kinder, Bueno Bar, Ferrero*	1 Bar/21.5g	121	8.1	563	9.8	46.6	37.5	0.0
Kinder, Riegel, Ferrero*	1 Bar/21g	117	7.1	558	10.0	53.0	34.0	0.0
Kinder Maxi, Ferrero*	1 Bar/21g	116	7.1	550	10.0	51.0	34.0	0.0
Kinder Surprise, Ferrero*	1 Egg/20g	110	6.8	550	10.0	51.0	34.0	0.4
King Size, Dairy Milk, Cadbury*	1 Serving/85g	446	25.2	525	7.6	56.4	29.7	0.0
Lait Intense, Experiences, Cote D'or*	3 Squares/100g	575	40.0	575	7.2	44.5	40.0	5.0
Light & Whippy, Bite Sized, Sainsbury's*	1 Bar/15.0g	66	2.4	439	3.3	69.7	16.3	0.1
Milk, & Hazelnut, Bar, Swiss, M & S*	1oz/28g	156	10.1	556	6.4	51.9	36.0	3.3
Milk, Average	1oz/28g	146	8.6	520	7.7	56.9	30.7	0.8
Milk, Bars, M & S*	1 Bar/40g	214	12.8	535	7.8	54.0	32.0	1.9
Milk, Belgian, TTD, Sainsbury's*	2 Squares/20g	110	7.0	549	9.6	48.8	35.0	1.8
Milk, Bubbly, Swiss, M & S*	1 Serving/40g	218	13.7	545	8.0	52.0	34.3	2.5
Milk, Excellence, Lindt*	1 Sm Bar/35g	196	13.0	560	6.0	51.0	37.0	0.0
Milk, Exra Fine, Swiss, M & S*	1 Bar/124g	700	45.5	565	7.2	50.9	36.7	2.3
Milk, Extra Au Lait, Milch Extra, Lindt*	½ Bar/50g	268	15.5	535	6.5	57.0	31.0	0.0
Milk, Extra Creamy, Excellence, Lindt*	1 Bar/100g	560	37.1	560	6.0	51.1	37.1	0.0
Milk, Fair Trade, Co-Op*	1 Bar/45g	248	16.7	550	8.0	47.0	37.0	2.0
Milk, Fimbles Bar, Kinnerton*	1 Bar/12.1g	65	3.8	539	5.8	57.0	31.8	1.9
Milk, Lindor, Lindt*	1 Square/11g	68	5.2	615	4.7	43.0	47.0	0.0
Milk, Organic, Tesco*	1 Serving/25g	140	9.1	558	6.3	51.4	36.3	2.3
Milk, Sainsbury's*	4 Squares/25g	133	7.7	533	9.2	54.6	30.8	2.2
Milk, Santas, Tesco*	1 Bag/90g	433	21.8	481	4.5	61.4	24.2	1.4
Milk, SmartPrice, Asda*	1 Square/6g	32	1.9	536	8.0	54.0	32.0	1.8
Milk, Swiss, M & S*	4 Squares/33.3g	186	12.2	560	7.4	50.7	36.7	2.3
Milk, Swiss Made, Organic, Traidcraft*	4 Squares/16.6g	94	5.8	550	7.0	50.0	34.0	0.0
Milk, Tesco*	1 Serving/25g	133	7.7	533	9.5	54.7	30.7	2.2
Milk, Value, Tesco*	1/6 Bar/16g	83	4.5	520	6.8	60.0	28.0	2.3
Milk, Whole Nut, Tesco*	1 Serving/25g	129	8.5	517	8.7	53.4	33.8	9.0
Milk, with Crisped Rice, Dubble*	1 Bar/40g	211	11.8	528	6.4	59.6	29.4	0.0
Mini, Toblerone*	1 Serving/6g	32	1.8	525	5.6	57.5	30.0	3.5
Mini Bites, Chunky, Moments, Fox's*	1 Roll/20g	90	4.9	450	5.7	52.4	24.6	2.2

CHOCOLATE

	Measure INFO/WEIGHT	per Measure KCAL	FAT	KCAL	PROT	CARB	FAT	FIBRE
				Nutrition Values per 100g / 100ml				
Mini Eggs, Cadbury*	1 Egg/3.3g	15	0.7	455	4.6	64.7	20.0	0.5
Mint Creme, Sainsbury's*	1 Serving/20g	93	4.9	467	2.8	62.7	24.5	2.1
Mint Crisp, Cadbury*	1oz/28g	141	6.2	505	6.4	70.3	22.2	0.0
Mint Truffle, Bar, M & S*	1 Bar/35g	189	11.3	540	6.8	55.6	32.4	2.0
Mints, Twilight, Terry's*	1 Chocolate/8g	38	2.1	475	2.5	56.3	26.3	3.8
Mountain Bar, Swiss, M & S*	1 Bar/100g	555	35.3	555	6.5	55.2	35.3	0.2
Nutty Nougat, Bite Sized, Sainsbury's*	1 Bar/23.1g	111	5.5	481	7.6	59.0	23.8	0.6
Orange, Sainsbury's*	4 Squares/19g	100	5.8	531	9.2	54.3	30.7	2.2
Orange Cream, Fry's*	1 Bar/50g	210	6.9	420	2.8	72.3	13.7	0.0
Peanut Butter Cup, Big Cup, Reese's, Hershey*	1 Cup/39g	210	12.0	538	10.3	53.9	30.8	2.6
Peanut Butter Cup, Miniature, Reese's, Hershey*	1 Cup/7g	36	2.1	514	10.0	55.7	30.0	4.3
Peanut Butter Cup, Reese's, Hershey*	1 Cup/17g	90	5.0	529	11.8	58.8	29.4	5.9
Peppermint, Ritter Sport*	1 Bar/100g	483	26.0	483	3.0	60.0	26.0	0.0
Peppermint Cream, Fry's*	1 Bar/51g	217	7.9	425	2.6	68.8	15.4	0.0
Peppermint Patty, Hershey*	3 Patties/41g	160	3.0	390	2.4	80.5	7.3	0.0
Plain, 50% Cocoa Solids Minimum, Tesco*	4 Squares/22g	115	6.2	523	7.4	60.0	28.1	1.8
Plain, 72% Cocoa Solids, Finest, Tesco*	1 Square/10g	60	4.4	603	7.7	44.0	44.0	3.7
Plain, Continental, Waitrose*	1 Square/4.1g	22	1.8	558	7.7	32.9	44.0	5.9
Plain, Dark, Fruit & Nut, Rich, Sainsbury's*	4 Squares/25g	117	6.7	489	5.2	53.9	27.9	5.7
Plain, Organic, Tesco*	2 Squares/20g	114	7.5	570	10.5	48.0	37.5	11.5
Plain, Whole Nut, Belgian, Waitrose*	4 Squares/25g	135	9.5	540	6.3	45.4	38.0	7.8
Plain, with Ginger, Belgian, TTD, Sainsbury's*	2 Squares/20g	114	9.3	571	7.2	31.2	46.4	10.9
Plain, with Hazelnuts, Tesco*	4 Squares/25g	135	8.9	539	6.1	48.3	35.7	6.5
Planets, Mars*	1 Pack/37g	178	8.3	481	4.9	65.4	22.4	0.0
Praline, M & S*	1 Bar/34g	185	12.0	545	7.3	49.6	35.2	3.1
Rafaello, Roche, Ferrero*	1 Sweet/10g	60	4.7	600	9.7	35.4	46.6	0.0
Shots, Cadbury*	1 Pack/160g	752	37.1	470	5.9	59.7	23.2	0.0
Snack Size, Dairy Milk, Cadbury*	1 Bar/30g	159	9.0	530	7.8	57.1	29.9	0.0
Snaps, Milk, Cadbury*	1 Snap/3g	15	0.8	505	6.3	60.5	27.0	1.0
Snaps, Orange, Cadbury*	1 Snap/3g	15	0.8	505	6.3	60.4	27.0	1.0
Tasters, Dairy Milk, Cadbury*	1 Bag/45g	239	13.7	530	7.6	56.4	30.5	0.0
Treatsize, Dairy Milk, Cadbury*	1 Bar/14g	74	4.2	525	7.5	57.0	29.8	0.7
Triple Delight, Weight Watchers*	1 Dessert/110.2g	183	2.9	166	4.9	30.8	2.6	2.6
Truffle, Dark Chocolate, Balls, Lindor, Lindt*	1 Ball/12g	76	6.2	630	3.4	38.5	51.4	0.0
Turkish Delight, Large Bar, Dairy Milk, Cadbury*	4 Chunks/33g	155	7.1	470	5.6	63.2	21.4	0.5
White, Average	1oz/28g	148	8.7	529	8.0	58.3	30.9	0.0
White, Belgian, Sugar Less, Sweet' N Low*	25g	128	9.6	512	5.8	63.1	38.3	0.0
White, Creamy, Safeway*	4 Squares/21g	113	6.2	537	6.9	59.9	29.5	0.0
White, Creamy, Tesco*	1 Serving/25g	139	8.7	557	5.1	55.7	34.9	3.3
White, Creamy Vanilla, Green & Black's*	1 Serving/20g	115	7.3	573	7.4	53.5	36.6	0.1
White, Crispy, Fair Trade, Co-Op*	½ Bar/50g	278	17.5	555	9.0	51.0	35.0	0.1
White, Nestle*	4 Pieces/40g	220	13.0	550	7.5	55.0	32.5	0.0
White, Value, Tesco*	1 Serving/10g	55	3.1	548	4.7	62.0	31.2	0.0
Whole Nut, Dairy Milk, Cadbury*	1 Bar/49.1g	270	17.4	550	8.9	49.5	35.4	1.7
Wildlife Bar, Cadbury*	1 Bar/21g	109	6.2	520	7.8	56.8	29.3	0.0
with Crunchie Bits, Dairy Milk, Cadbury*	1 Bar/200g	1000	48.8	500	6.2	63.3	24.4	0.0
with Shortcake Biscuit, Dairy Milk, Cadbury*	1 Square/6g	31	1.7	520	7.5	59.0	28.0	0.0

CHOCOLATE DROPS

Plain, Asda*	1 Serving/100g	489	29.0	489	7.0	50.0	29.0	10.0
White, for Cooking, Sainsbury's*	1oz/28g	152	8.6	544	6.5	60.3	30.8	0.0

CHOCOLATE NUTS

Peanuts, Belgian Coated, M & S*	1 Serving/20g	109	7.6	545	14.7	35.6	38.0	5.8
Peanuts, Milk, Tesco*	1 Bag/227g	1221	86.0	538	17.5	31.8	37.9	4.4

	Measure INFO/WEIGHT	per Measure KCAL	FAT	Nutrition Values per 100g / 100ml KCAL	PROT	CARB	FAT	FIBRE
CHOCOLATE ORANGE								
Bar, Montana*	1 Serving/25g	131	6.9	523	7.0	62.2	27.4	0.0
Crunchball, Terry's*	1 Segment/8.7g	47	2.5	520	6.9	59.8	28.1	2.0
Dark, Terry's*	1 Segment/9g	45	2.6	511	4.3	57.0	29.3	6.2
Milk, Mini Segments, Terry's*	1 Segment/8g	42	2.4	527	7.7	57.9	29.4	2.1
Milk, Terry's*	1 Orange/175g	931	51.6	532	7.4	57.8	29.5	2.1
Milk Bar, Terry's*	1 Segment/6.6g	37	2.1	530	7.3	58.0	29.5	2.1
Plain, Terry's*	1 Orange/175g	889	51.5	508	3.8	56.8	29.4	6.2
Segsations, Terry's*	1 Segsation/8.2g	42	2.3	520	6.9	58.5	28.5	2.8
CHOCOLATE RAISINS								
Assorted, Thorntons*	1 Bag/140g	601	27.6	429	4.2	58.8	19.7	2.9
Bonds Sweetstars*	1 Serving/28g	109	4.5	391	4.7	57.0	16.0	0.0
Californian, Tesco*	¼ Bag/56.8g	268	11.7	472	5.2	66.2	20.7	1.3
Coated, Californian, M & S*	1 Bag/130g	520	19.1	400	4.3	63.2	14.7	1.9
Co-Op*	¼ Pack/50g	205	7.5	410	4.0	64.0	15.0	1.0
Jameson's*	1 Serving/23g	96	3.8	418	4.7	62.7	16.5	1.4
Milk, Asda*	1 Serving/28g	127	5.6	452	6.0	62.0	20.0	1.2
Milk, Co-Op*	½ Bag/100g	420	17.0	420	5.0	63.0	17.0	6.0
Milk, Tesco*	1 Lge Bag/227g	933	35.0	411	4.8	63.3	15.4	0.9
CHOCOLATE SPREAD								
Average	1 Tsp/12g	68	4.5	569	4.1	57.1	37.6	0.0
with Nuts	1 Tsp/12g	66	4.0	549	6.2	60.5	33.0	0.8
CHOCOLATES								
All Gold, Dark, Terry's*	1 Serving/30g	152	8.7	505	4.0	57.5	29.0	4.3
All Gold, Milk, Terry's*	1 Serving/30g	158	9.2	525	4.8	58.0	30.5	1.5
Almond Marzipan, Milk Chocolate, Thorntons*	1 Chocolate/13g	60	2.9	464	6.6	59.4	22.6	5.6
Almond Mocca Mousse, Thorntons*	1 Chocolate/14g	76	5.3	543	8.5	40.7	37.9	2.9
Alpini, Thorntons*	1 Chocolate/13g	70	4.2	538	7.0	54.6	32.3	2.3
Bittermint, Bendicks*	1 Mint/18.2g	79	2.9	440	4.3	68.9	16.3	2.4
Brandy Liqueurs, Asda*	1 Chocolate/8.3g	33	1.4	409	4.0	60.0	17.0	0.8
Caramels, Sainsbury's*	1 Sweet/11.6g	57	2.6	490	3.5	69.0	22.2	0.2
Celebrations, Mars*	1 Sweet/8g	41	2.2	512	5.7	61.5	27.0	1.7
Cherry Liqueur, M & S*	1 Chocolate/10g	40	1.8	395	2.9	52.8	17.8	4.3
Chocolate Mousse, Thorntons*	1 Chocolate/13g	67	4.7	515	7.5	40.0	36.2	3.1
Classic Collection, Thorntons*	1 Chocolate/12.3g	58	2.8	472	4.3	62.7	22.8	2.4
Coffee Creme, Milk, Thorntons*	1 Chocolate/13g	52	1.3	400	2.8	74.6	10.0	0.8
Continental, Belgian, Thorntons*	1 Chocolate/13g	67	3.9	514	5.8	53.5	30.3	2.9
Continental, Thorntons*	1 Chocolate/15g	76	4.4	506	5.6	54.5	29.3	2.7
Country Caramel, Milk, Thorntons*	1 Chocolate/9g	45	2.4	500	4.6	62.2	26.7	0.0
Dairy Box, Milk, Nestle*	1 Serving/10g	46	1.9	456	4.4	65.9	19.4	0.7
Dark, Swiss Thins, Lindt*	1 Pack/125g	681	46.2	545	4.8	49.2	37.0	0.0
Italian Collection, Amaretto, M & S*	1 Chocolate/12.5g	62	3.3	480	4.4	59.7	25.1	2.3
Italian Collection, Favourites, M & S*	1 Chocolate/14g	74	4.7	530	5.7	50.4	33.7	1.6
Italian Collection, Panna Cotta, M & S*	1 Chocolate/12.8g	71	4.7	545	5.3	49.4	36.4	0.1
Liquers, Cognac Truffle, Thorntons*	1 Chocolate/14g	65	3.8	464	7.3	40.0	27.1	2.9
Liqueur, Elizabeth Shaw*	1 Sweet/8.2g	36	1.6	441	2.5	57.3	19.9	3.8
Milk, Discs, Swiss, M & S*	1 Disc/5g	28	1.8	553	8.9	50.4	35.3	2.4
Milk Tray, Cadbury*	1 Chocolate/9.4g	47	2.4	495	4.7	61.5	25.8	0.7
Mingles, Bendicks*	1 Chocolate/5g	27	1.6	540	6.5	58.6	31.3	0.1
Mint Crisp, Bendicks*	1 Mint/7.7g	40	2.4	494	5.2	55.0	29.9	0.0
Mint Crisp, Dark, Elizabeth Shaw*	1 Chocolate/6g	27	1.2	458	1.9	68.0	20.7	0.0
Mint Crisp, Milk, Elizabeth Shaw*	1 Chocolate/6g	30	1.3	493	4.0	70.9	21.4	0.0
Mint Crisp, Thorntons*	1 Chocolate/7g	34	2.2	486	7.7	40.0	31.4	4.3
Misshapes, Assorted, Cadbury*	1 Chocolate/8g	41	2.3	515	5.2	57.5	29.1	0.0

	Measure INFO/WEIGHT	per Measure		Nutrition Values per 100g / 100ml				
		KCAL	FAT	KCAL	PROT	CARB	FAT	FIBRE
CHOCOLATES								
Orange Crisp, Elizabeth Shaw*	1 Chocolate/6g	29	1.3	478	2.9	68.2	21.5	0.0
Praline, Coffee, Thorntons*	1 Chocolate/7g	37	2.4	529	7.0	47.1	34.3	2.9
Praline, Hazelnut, Thorntons*	1 Chocolate/5g	27	1.8	540	7.0	48.0	36.0	4.0
Praline, Marzipan, Thorntons*	1 Chocolate/14g	63	3.0	450	5.9	58.6	21.4	2.1
Praline, Roast Hazelnut, Thorntons*	1 Chocolate/13g	70	4.4	538	6.0	51.5	33.8	3.1
Quality Street, Nestle*	1 Sweet/8.5g	39	1.7	464	4.0	66.3	20.3	0.8
Rocher, Continental, Thorntons*	1 Chocolate/15g	76	5.0	507	6.8	45.3	33.3	2.0
Roses, Cadbury*	1 Chocolate/14g	69	3.5	495	4.8	62.6	25.3	0.7
Sea Shells, Belgian, Guylian*	1 Shell/11.3g	65	4.4	574	8.0	49.0	39.0	0.0
Seashells, Belgian, Woolworths*	1 Box/63g	347	19.6	550	5.5	52.9	31.1	0.0
Strawberrys & Cream, Thorntons*	1 Chocolate/12g	64	3.9	533	5.1	54.2	32.5	0.8
Swiss Tradition, Mixed, Lindt*	1 Pack/392g	2215	149.4	565	6.1	49.8	38.1	0.0
Truffle, Amaretto, Thorntons*	1 Chocolate/14g	66	3.6	471	5.5	55.0	25.7	2.9
Truffle, Brandy, Thorntons*	1 Chocolate/14g	68	3.8	486	6.1	52.1	27.1	0.7
Truffle, Caramel, Thorntons*	1 Chocolate/14g	67	3.6	479	4.2	57.9	25.7	2.1
Truffle, Cherry, Thorntons*	1 Chocolate/14g	58	3.0	414	4.2	50.7	21.4	1.4
Truffle, Continental Champagne, Thorntons*	1 Chocolate/16g	78	4.5	488	6.1	51.3	28.0	0.6
Truffle, Grand Marnier, Thorntons*	1 Chocolate/15g	77	5.1	513	7.2	40.7	34.0	4.0
Truffle, Hazelnut, Balls, Lindor, Lindt*	1 Ball/12g	76	6.1	632	5.0	39.1	50.6	0.0
Truffle, Lemon, White, Thorntons*	1 Chocolate/14g	63	3.5	450	4.6	64.3	25.0	0.7
Truffle, Milk Chocolate, Balls, Lindor, Lindt*	1 Ball/12g	74	5.7	617	4.9	43.1	47.2	0.0
Truffle, Rum, Average	1 Truffle/11g	57	3.7	521	6.1	49.7	33.7	1.9
Truffle, Rum, Thorntons*	1 Chocolate/13g	63	3.2	485	4.8	58.5	24.6	4.8
Truffle, Selection, Tesco*	1 Chocolate/14g	75	4.2	539	5.1	62.0	29.8	0.5
Truffle, Seville, Thorntons*	1 Chocolate/14g	76	4.7	543	7.1	53.6	33.6	1.4
Truffle, Thorntons*	1 Chocolate/7g	33	1.9	471	6.0	48.6	27.1	1.4
Truffle, Vanilla, Thorntons*	1 Chocolate/13g	64	3.5	492	4.8	57.7	26.9	1.5
Truffle, Viennese, Dark, Thorntons*	1 Chocolate/10g	53	3.6	530	5.9	47.0	36.0	3.0
Truffle, Viennese, Milk, Thorntons*	1 Chocolate/10g	56	3.6	560	4.9	54.0	36.0	0.0
Truffle, White Chocolate, Balls, Lindor, Lindt*	1 Ball/12g	78	6.2	649	5.2	40.2	51.9	0.0
Truffles, Belgian, Flaked, Tesco*	1 Truffle/14g	81	5.4	575	4.4	52.7	38.5	2.3
Truffles, Belgian, TTD, Sainsbury's*	1 Truffle/12.5g	75	5.1	579	4.3	51.9	39.3	0.0
Truffles, Belgian Milk, Waitrose*	1 Truffle/14g	74	4.8	525	5.8	52.9	34.1	1.2
Valentine, Thorntons*	1 Chocolate/11g	60	3.8	542	5.7	52.0	34.5	2.1
Winter Selection, Thorntons*	1 Chocolate/10g	51	3.1	506	6.2	51.3	30.6	3.8
CHOP SUEY								
Chicken, with Noodles, Sainsbury's*	1 Pack/300g	300	7.5	100	5.7	13.6	2.5	1.2
Chinese, Vegetable, Stir Fry, Sharwood's*	1 Pack/310g	223	3.4	72	1.5	13.9	1.1	0.6
CHOW MEIN								
Beef, Sainsbury's*	1 Pack/450g	500	11.3	111	6.6	15.5	2.5	0.8
Cantonese Vegetable Stir Fry, Sainsbury's*	¼ Pack/100g	85	3.8	85	2.2	10.6	3.8	1.2
Char Sui, Cantonese, Sainsbury's*	½ Pack/225g	205	7.0	91	5.7	10.0	3.1	1.1
Chicken, Ainsley Harriott*	1 Serving/250g	447	11.8	179	14.0	21.2	4.7	2.0
Chicken, Asda*	1 Pack/401.1g	373	10.0	93	5.0	12.7	2.5	1.2
Chicken, BGTY, Sainsbury's*	1 Pack/450g	360	10.8	80	6.1	8.5	2.4	1.8
Chicken, Cantonese, Sainsbury's*	½ Pack/225g	198	4.5	88	5.7	11.7	2.0	1.2
Chicken, Chinese Takeaway, Sainsbury's*	1 Pack/316g	338	8.5	107	9.1	11.6	2.7	0.7
Chicken, Chinese Takeaway, Tesco*	1 Serving/350g	294	8.4	84	8.1	7.5	2.4	1.1
Chicken, COOK!, M & S*	1 Pack/375g	356	7.9	95	7.9	10.5	2.1	1.7
Chicken, Co-Op*	1 Pack/300g	270	9.0	90	8.0	9.0	3.0	0.9
Chicken, COU, M & S*	1 Pack/200g	180	4.6	90	9.3	8.1	2.3	1.1
Chicken, Frozen, Sainsbury's*	1 Pack/403.8g	424	12.1	105	6.1	13.4	3.0	0.9
Chicken, Great Value, Asda*	1 Pack/400g	408	11.6	102	5.0	14.0	2.9	0.8

	Measure INFO/WEIGHT	per Measure		Nutrition Values per 100g / 100ml				
		KCAL	FAT	KCAL	PROT	CARB	FAT	FIBRE
CHOW MEIN								
Chicken, HL, Tesco*	1 Pack/450g	338	3.2	75	7.3	9.2	0.7	1.0
Chicken, Morrisons*	1 Pack/400g	368	9.2	92	5.8	13.0	2.3	1.1
Chicken, New, BGTY, Sainsbury's*	1 Pack/450g	374	6.3	83	6.0	11.4	1.4	1.1
Chicken, New Improved Recipe, Sainsbury's*	1 Pack/449g	395	9.0	88	5.7	11.7	2.0	1.2
Chicken, Sainsbury's*	1 Serving/400g	364	8.4	91	5.2	12.9	2.1	1.0
Chicken, Sizzling Stir Fry, Oriental Express*	1 Bag/312g	293	6.2	94	6.5	12.3	2.0	2.4
Chicken, Tesco*	1 Pack/450g	383	5.4	85	7.7	10.3	1.2	1.2
Chicken, Waitrose*	1 Serving/400g	384	11.6	96	6.0	11.4	2.9	1.3
Chicken with Vegetable Spring Roll, Oriental Express*	1 Pack/300g	213	1.8	71	5.5	12.4	0.6	1.9
Chinese Style, Safeway*	1 Serving/150g	167	6.6	111	4.0	13.0	4.4	1.1
Pork, PB, Waitrose*	½ Pack/310g	332	2.8	107	7.6	17.2	0.9	1.6
Special, COU, M & S*	1 Pack/400g	320	4.0	80	7.4	9.9	1.0	1.0
Special, GFY, Asda*	1 Pack/398.9g	367	2.4	92	7.0	14.6	0.6	1.3
Special, HL, Tesco*	1 Pack/450g	351	5.4	78	6.3	10.6	1.2	0.6
Special, M & S*	1 Pack/400g	400	13.6	100	6.5	11.3	3.4	2.2
Special, PB, Waitrose*	1 Pack/400g	316	4.4	79	7.4	10.0	1.1	0.9
Special, Somerfield*	1 Pot/300g	357	10.2	119	6.5	16.2	3.4	0.6
Special Chinese, Farmfoods*	1 Pack/400g	276	11.2	69	4.3	6.7	2.8	0.8
Stir Fry, Asda*	1 Pack/350g	270	17.5	77	2.1	6.0	5.0	0.0
Stir Fry, Somerfield*	1 Pack/300g	474	3.0	158	6.0	32.0	1.0	0.0
Stir Fry, Tesco*	½ Pack/240g	180	3.4	75	2.8	12.0	1.4	1.6
Stir Fry with Veg & Noodles, Somerfield*	1 Serving/200g	234	12.0	117	2.8	12.9	6.0	1.3
Vegetable, Asda*	1 Pack/400g	520	15.2	130	2.4	21.5	3.8	3.0
Vegetable, HE, Tesco*	1 Pack/350g	221	1.8	63	6.8	7.9	0.5	1.3
Vegetable, Take Away, Meal for One, Tesco*	1 Serving/345g	262	7.6	76	6.7	7.3	2.2	1.3
Vegetable & Cashew Nut, Eat Smart, Safeway*	1 Pack/380g	323	4.6	85	7.0	11.4	1.2	1.1
Vegetables & Noodles in Sauce, Safeway*	1 Serving/200g	110	0.4	55	3.7	9.5	0.2	1.3
CHRISTMAS PUDDING								
Average	1oz/28g	81	2.7	291	4.6	49.5	9.7	1.3
CHUNKY								
Finest, Tesco*, Youngs*	1oz/28g	42	1.5	150	5.0	20.3	5.4	1.7
CHUTNEY								
Albert's Victorian, Baxters*	1 Serving/25g	38	0.0	150	35.0	6.0	0.1	0.0
Apple, Spiced, TTD, Sainsbury's*	1 Serving/10g	15	0.0	153	0.4	36.9	0.4	1.6
Apple, Tomato & Sultana, Tesco*	1 Serving/50g	88	0.1	176	1.1	42.4	0.2	1.3
Apricot, Sharwood's*	1 Tsp/16g	21	0.0	131	0.6	32.0	0.1	2.3
Bengal Spice Mango, Sharwood's*	1 Tsp/5g	12	0.0	236	0.5	58.0	0.2	1.2
Caramalised Onion, Sainsbury's*	1 Serving/25g	28	0.4	111	1.1	23.5	1.4	1.1
Caramelised Red Onion, Loyd Grossman*	1 Serving/10g	11	0.0	111	0.5	27.2	0.0	0.5
Caramelised Red Onion, M & S*	1 Serving/40g	94	0.4	235	1.4	55.1	1.1	1.0
Cranberry & Caramelised Red Onion, Baxters*	1 Serving/20g	31	0.0	154	0.3	38.0	0.1	0.3
Fruit, Spiced, Baxters*	1 Tsp/16g	23	0.0	143	6.0	34.8	0.1	0.0
Fruit, Traditional, M & S*	1oz/28g	43	0.1	155	0.9	37.2	0.3	1.7
Indian Appetisers, Pot, Waitrose*	1 Pot/158g	330	2.2	209	1.8	47.3	1.4	1.8
Lime & Chilli, Geeta's*	1 Serving/25g	69	0.4	277	2.0	64.0	1.4	1.9
Mango, Green Label, Sharwood's*	1 Tsp/10g	23	0.0	234	0.3	57.8	0.2	0.9
Mango, Hot, Patak's*	1 Jar/340g	877	0.7	258	0.4	67.1	0.2	0.7
Mango, Hot, TTD, Sainsbury's*	1 Tbsp/15g	36	0.3	240	0.7	54.7	2.0	2.0
Mango, Major Grey, Patak's*	1 Tbsp/15g	38	0.0	255	0.4	66.0	0.2	0.7
Mango, Premium, Geeta's*	1 Serving/50g	131	0.2	262	0.8	63.0	0.3	0.9
Mango, Sensations, Walkers*	¼ Jar/57g	122	0.1	214	0.3	53.0	0.1	0.6
Mango, Spiced, M & S*	1 Serving/15g	26	0.1	175	1.2	42.3	0.4	3.2
Mango, Spicy, Sainsbury's*	1 Tbsp/15g	24	0.1	160	0.7	37.0	0.7	1.3

	Measure INFO/WEIGHT	per Measure KCAL	per Measure FAT	Nutrition Values per 100g / 100ml KCAL	PROT	CARB	FAT	FIBRE
CHUTNEY								
Mango, Sweet	1 Tbsp/16g	30	0.0	189	0.7	48.3	0.1	0.0
Mango, Tesco*	1 Serving/20g	45	0.0	224	0.4	55.5	0.1	1.3
Mango & Apple, Sharwood's*	1oz/28g	65	0.0	233	0.4	57.6	0.1	1.1
Mango & Ginger, Baxters*	1 Jar/320g	598	0.6	187	5.0	45.7	0.2	0.9
Mango & Lime, Sharwood's*	1oz/28g	58	0.1	206	0.4	50.5	0.3	0.8
Mixed Fruit	1 Serving/16g	25	0.0	155	0.6	39.7	0.0	0.0
Onion, TTD, Sainsbury's*	1 Serving/20g	55	0.1	277	0.9	67.2	0.5	1.4
Peach, Spicy, Waitrose*	1 Serving/20g	43	0.3	215	1.0	49.0	1.5	1.5
Ploughman's Plum, EPC*	1 Tsp/10g	16	0.0	160	1.3	38.1	0.2	1.6
Spicy Fruit, Baxters*	1 Serving/15g	22	0.0	146	0.6	35.4	0.2	0.0
Spicy Fruit, Safeway*	1 Tsp/16g	16	0.0	109	0.5	25.5	0.1	0.1
Sweet Mango, Patak's*	1 Tbsp/15g	39	0.0	259	0.3	67.4	0.1	0.7
Sweet Tomato & Chilli, EPC*	1 Tsp/10g	19	0.0	189	0.9	46.0	0.2	1.7
Tomato	1 Serving/16g	20	0.0	128	1.2	31.0	0.2	1.3
Tomato, TTD, Sainsbury's*	1 Tbsp/15g	29	0.2	193	2.0	44.7	1.3	2.7
Tomato & Red Pepper, Baxters*	1 Jar/312g	512	1.2	164	2.0	38.0	0.4	1.5
CIABATTA								
Cheese, & Ham, Asda*	¼ Bread/74g	231	9.0	312	11.6	38.9	12.2	1.2
Chicken, & Herb, Shapers, Boots*	1 Pack/168g	290	4.7	173	11.9	25.0	2.8	1.7
Chicken Tomato & Basil, Boots*	1 Pack/207g	499	26.9	241	11.0	20.0	13.0	3.0
Tuna, Crunch, Eat Smart, Safeway*	1 Serving/200g	280	2.2	140	10.7	21.7	1.1	1.5
CIDER								
Diamond White*	1 fl oz/30ml	11	0.0	36	0.0	2.6	0.0	0.0
Dry, Average	1 Pint/568ml	205	0.0	36	0.0	2.6	0.0	0.0
Dry, French, So Good, Somerfield*	1 Bottle/500ml	150	0.0	30	0.0	0.3	0.0	0.0
Dry, Strongbow*	1 Bottle/375ml	161	0.0	43	0.0	3.4	0.0	0.0
Low Alcohol	1 Pint/568ml	97	0.0	17	0.0	3.6	0.0	0.0
Low Carb, Stowford*	1 Bottle/500ml	140	0.0	28	0.0	0.2	0.0	0.0
Magner's*	½ Pint/284ml	105	0.0	37	0.0	2.0	0.0	0.0
Medium Sweet, Somerfield*	1 Pint/568ml	233	0.0	41	0.0	5.0	0.0	0.0
Sweet, Average	1 Pint/568ml	239	0.0	42	0.0	4.3	0.0	0.0
Vintage	1 Pint/568ml	574	0.0	101	0.0	7.3	0.0	0.0
CINNAMON								
Ground, Average	1 Tsp/3g	8	0.1	261	3.9	55.5	3.2	0.0
CLAMS								
in Brine, Average	1oz/28g	22	0.2	79	16.0	2.5	0.6	0.0
Raw, Average	20 Sm/180g	133	1.7	74	12.8	2.6	1.0	0.0
CLEMENTINES								
Raw, Weighed with Peel, Average	1 Med/60g	27	0.1	44	0.8	11.3	0.1	1.6
Raw, Weighed without Peel, Average	1 Med/46g	22	0.1	47	0.9	12.0	0.2	1.7
COCKLES								
Boiled	1 Cockle/4g	2	0.0	53	12.0	0.0	0.6	0.0
Bottled in Vinegar, Drained	1oz/28g	17	0.2	60	13.3	0.0	0.7	0.0
COCKTAIL								
Alcoholic, Juice Based, Average	1 Glass/200ml	464	29.2	232	6.4	18.7	14.6	1.4
Bucks Fizz, Premixed, M & S*	1 Glass/250ml	152	0.0	61	0.0	9.0	0.0	0.0
Grenadine, Oange Juice, Pineapple Juice	1 Serving/200ml	158	0.3	79	0.5	19.2	0.1	0.2
Mai Tai, Average	1 Serving/200ml	209	0.1	105	0.2	13.9	0.1	0.1
Pina Colada	1 Glass/250ml	593	20.0	237	1.0	28.0	8.0	0.0
COCOA BUTTER								
Average	1oz/28g	251	27.9	896	0.0	0.0	99.5	0.0
COCOA POWDER								
Cadbury*	1 Tbsp/16g	52	3.3	322	23.1	10.5	20.8	0.0

C

	Measure INFO/WEIGHT	per Measure		Nutrition Values per 100g / 100ml				
		KCAL	FAT	KCAL	PROT	CARB	FAT	FIBRE
COCOA POWDER								
Organic, Green & Black's*	1 Tbsp/15g	53	3.3	350	23.6	13.6	22.3	0.0
Valrhona*	1 Tsp/5g	23	1.0	450	25.0	45.0	20.0	30.0
COCONUT								
Creamed, Average	1oz/28g	186	19.2	666	6.0	6.7	68.4	7.0
Desiccated, Average	1oz/28g	169	17.4	604	5.6	6.4	62.0	13.7
Fresh, Flesh Only, Average	1oz/28g	98	10.1	351	3.2	3.7	36.0	7.3
Ice, Average	1oz/28g	104	3.6	371	1.7	66.7	12.7	2.6
Milk, BGTY, Sainsbury's*	¼ Can/100ml	96	8.6	96	1.0	3.6	8.6	0.0
Milk, Blue Dragon*	1 Can/400g	716	68.0	179	2.2	4.0	17.0	0.2
Milk, Light, Reduced Fat, Blue Dragon*	1 Can/400ml	408	39.2	102	0.9	2.4	9.8	0.0
Milk, Low Fat, Tiger Tiger*	½ Tin/200ml	200	20.0	100	1.0	0.7	10.0	0.2
Milk, Reduced Fat, Amoy*	1 Serving/100g	115	11.0	115	1.2	2.9	11.0	0.0
Milk, Reduced Fat, Barts*	1 Serving/100ml	94	8.6	94	0.7	3.6	8.6	0.0
Milk, Rich Creamy, Amoy*	1 Can/400ml	684	68.0	171	2.0	2.5	17.0	0.0
COD								
Baked, Average	1oz/28g	27	0.3	96	21.4	0.0	1.2	0.0
Dried, Salted, Average	10g	29	0.2	290	62.8	0.0	2.4	0.0
Dried, Salted, Boiled, Average	1oz/28g	39	0.3	138	32.5	0.0	0.9	0.0
Fillets, Battered, Average	1 Serving/90g	158	7.3	176	12.6	13.0	8.2	1.1
Fillets, BGTY, Sainsbury's*	1 Slice/125g	190	3.1	152	15.3	17.0	2.5	1.4
Fillets, Breaded, Average	1 Portion/97g	200	9.4	206	13.0	16.7	9.8	1.0
Fillets, Breaded, Chunky, Average	1 Piece/135g	204	8.0	151	13.7	10.9	5.9	1.4
Fillets, Breaded, Light, Healthy Range, Average	1 Fillet/135g	209	6.9	154	13.6	13.3	5.1	1.2
Fillets, Chunky, Average	1 Fillet/198g	267	7.3	135	17.1	8.2	3.7	0.8
Fillets, Chunky, Breaded, Northern Catch, Aldi*	1 Fillet/125.3g	228	9.3	182	13.5	15.3	7.4	2.3
Fillets, Skinless & Boneless, Raw, Average	1 Portion/92g	90	1.6	98	17.8	2.7	1.8	0.4
Fillets, Smoked, Average	1 Serving/150g	152	2.4	101	21.6	0.0	1.6	0.0
Fillets, Smoked, Raw, Line Caught, Icelandic, Waitrose*	1 Fillet/130g	82	0.7	63	14.6	0.0	0.5	0.0
Fillets, with Fish Pesto, COOK!, M & S*	½ Pack/165g	210	5.1	127	16.4	8.4	3.1	4.2
Loins, Average	1 Serving/145g	116	1.2	80	17.9	0.1	0.8	0.2
Mediterranean, PB, Waitrose*	1 Serving/370g	255	3.7	69	13.1	1.9	1.0	1.2
Poached, Average	1oz/28g	26	0.3	94	20.9	0.0	1.1	0.0
Provencale, Cote Table*	1 Serving/281g	185	5.6	66	8.6	3.4	2.0	0.0
Smoked, Raw, Average	1oz/28g	22	0.2	79	18.3	0.0	0.6	0.0
Steaks, Battered, Chip Shop Style, Average	1 Serving/150g	321	18.0	214	12.5	14.3	12.0	1.1
Steamed, Average	1oz/28g	23	0.3	83	18.6	0.0	0.9	0.0
COD &								
Cauliflower Bake, Asda*	1 Pack/400g	492	28.0	123	9.5	5.5	7.0	1.0
Cauliflower Cheese, Fillets, Iceland*	½ Pack/176g	234	13.5	133	12.7	3.3	7.7	1.7
Chips, Oven Baked, Safeway*	1 Pack/250g	523	21.0	209	8.4	25.0	8.4	3.5
Parsley Sauce, Frozen, M & S*	1 Pack/184g	156	7.2	85	11.1	1.9	3.9	1.0
Salmon, Steam Cuisine, COU, M & S*	1 Pack/400g	340	7.2	85	6.8	8.9	1.8	1.2
COD IN								
a Sweet Red Pepper Sauce, Fillets, GFY, Asda*	½ Pack/170g	143	2.7	84	15.0	2.3	1.6	0.1
Butter Sauce, Filet, Portions, Asda*	1 Portion/150.6g	125	5.0	83	9.8	3.5	3.3	0.4
Butter Sauce, Portions, Ocean Trader*	1 Pack/150g	137	6.2	91	10.3	3.3	4.1	0.1
Butter Sauce, Ross*	1 Serving/150g	126	5.9	84	9.1	3.2	3.9	0.1
Butter Sauce, Steaks, Birds Eye*	1 Pack/170g	185	9.4	109	9.8	5.0	5.5	0.1
Butter Sauce, Steaks, Frozen, Asda*	1 Pouch/152.3g	163	4.0	107	16.0	5.0	2.6	0.8
Butter Sauce, Steaks, Morrisons*	1 Steak/170g	153	5.6	90	10.9	4.1	3.3	0.4
Butter Sauce, Steaks, Sainsbury's*	1 Serving/170g	184	10.0	108	10.5	3.1	5.9	0.3
Butter Sauce, Tesco*	1 Pack/150g	123	5.4	82	9.4	2.9	3.6	0.5
Cheese & Parsley Sauce with Vegetables, HL, Tesco*	1 Pack/450g	270	5.9	60	5.8	6.2	1.3	1.5

INFO/WEIGHT	Measure	per Measure		Nutrition Values per 100g / 100ml				
	INFO/WEIGHT	KCAL	FAT	KCAL	PROT	CARB	FAT	FIBRE

COD IN

Cheese Sauce, BGTY, Sainsbury's*	1 Serving/170g	145	4.1	85	12.8	3.1	2.4	0.0
Cheese Sauce, Steaks, Birds Eye*	1 Pack/182g	175	6.4	96	10.9	5.2	3.5	0.1
Mushroom Sauce, BGTY, Sainsbury's*	1 Serving/170g	112	2.9	66	9.9	2.8	1.7	0.1
Parsley Sauce, BGTY, Sainsbury's*	1 Pack/170g	143	5.4	84	11.4	2.4	3.2	0.3
Parsley Sauce, COU, M & S*	1 Pack/185g	130	4.6	70	10.6	1.4	2.5	0.6
Parsley Sauce, Eat Smart, Safeway*	1 Serving/200g	150	3.8	75	11.5	2.4	1.9	0.9
Parsley Sauce, Fillets, BGTY, Sainsbury's*	1 Pack/351g	316	15.1	90	11.6	1.3	4.3	0.7
Parsley Sauce, Frozen, Morrisons*	1 Serving/170g	131	4.6	77	9.6	3.2	2.7	0.5
Parsley Sauce, GFY, Asda*	½ Pack/149g	124	5.2	83	12.0	1.5	3.5	0.6
Parsley Sauce, M & S*	½ Pack/180g	162	6.8	90	12.5	1.4	3.8	0.7
Parsley Sauce, Portions, Asda*	1 Serving/150g	116	3.0	77	11.0	3.8	2.0	0.1
Parsley Sauce, Portions, Ocean Trader*	1 Serving/120g	112	4.7	93	9.4	4.0	3.9	0.1
Parsley Sauce, Portions, Sainsbury's*	1 Pack/170g	143	5.4	84	11.4	2.4	3.2	0.3
Parsley Sauce, Steaks, Birds Eye*	1 Steak/172g	155	4.8	90	10.5	5.6	2.8	0.1
Parsley Sauce, Steaks, Iceland*	1 Serving/151.2g	130	6.9	86	9.1	2.1	4.6	0.7
Parsley Sauce, Steaks, Sainsbury's*	1 Serving/150g	126	4.8	84	11.4	2.4	3.2	0.3
Parsley Sauce, Tesco*	1 Serving/150g	122	4.7	81	10.0	3.3	3.1	0.3
Red Pepper Sauce, SteamFresh, Birds Eye*	1 Serving/125g	115	2.4	92	14.4	4.7	1.9	0.3

COD MEDITERRANEAN

Style, Fillets, GFY, Asda*	1 Pack/400g	274	9.9	69	9.0	2.5	2.5	0.9
Style, Fillets, Herb, Tesco*	1 Serving/115g	163	11.0	142	13.8	0.1	9.6	0.1

COD WITH

a Mediterranean Pepper Sauce, Fillets, Waitrose*	1 Pack/370g	241	4.8	65	12.2	1.1	1.3	0.9
a Thai Crust, PB, Waitrose*	1 Pack/280g	249	7.0	89	15.1	1.6	2.5	0.6
Chunky Chips, M & S*	1 Serving/340g	510	20.4	150	6.5	17.5	6.0	1.5
Mediterranean Butter, Sainsbury's*	1 Pack/170.4g	196	8.8	115	17.0	0.1	5.2	0.1
Parma Ham & Sardinian Chick Peas, M & S*	½ Pack/255g	268	12.5	105	9.8	5.3	4.9	0.5
Parsley Sauce, Somerfield*	1 Serving/200g	196	9.4	98	12.2	1.7	4.7	0.5
Roasted Vegetables, M & S*	1 Serving/280g	238	10.6	85	8.0	4.9	3.8	1.7
Salsa & Rosemary Potatoes, BGTY, Sainsbury's*	1 Pack/450g	356	4.1	79	4.7	13.1	0.9	1.6
Sunblush Tomato Sauce, GFY, Asda*	½ Pack/177.3g	117	2.7	66	13.0	0.1	1.5	1.0
Sweet Chilli, COU, M & S*	1 Pack/400g	360	2.0	90	7.7	13.1	0.5	1.6
Tomato Sauce, Fillets, Asda*	1 Serving/181g	210	10.9	116	13.0	2.6	6.0	2.3
Vegetables, Haches, Steaks, Peche Ocean*	1 Serving/200g	184	7.8	92	12.0	2.1	3.9	0.0

COD ZESTY

COU, M & S*	1 Serving/400g	260	6.8	65	7.2	5.2	1.7	1.2

COFFEE

Black	1 Mug/270ml	5	0.0	2	0.2	0.3	0.0	0.0
Cafe Caramel, Cafe Range, Nescafe*	1 Sachet/17g	72	2.4	423	9.2	64.6	14.1	1.3
Cafe Hazelnut, Nescafe*	1 Sachet/17g	73	2.4	428	9.3	66.0	14.1	0.0
Cafe Irish Cream, Cafe Range, Nescafe*	1 Sachet/23g	98	3.2	425	8.2	65.2	14.1	1.2
Cafe Latte, Dry, Douwe Egberts*	1 Serving/12g	58	2.6	480	10.0	60.0	22.0	0.0
Cafe Latte, Instant, Maxwell House*	1 Serving/16g	67	3.0	420	17.0	45.5	18.9	0.1
Cafe Mocha, Cafe Range, Nescafe*	1 Sachet/22g	92	2.9	418	8.5	66.6	13.1	0.0
Cafe Vanilla, Cafe Range, Nescafe*	1 Mug/18.4g	79	2.7	429	9.3	64.6	14.9	1.2
Cappuccino, Cafe Mocha, Dry, Maxwell House*	1 Serving/23g	100	2.5	434	4.3	78.2	10.8	0.0
Cappuccino, Cafe Specials, Dry, M & S*	1 Serving/14g	55	1.6	395	14.0	59.0	11.5	0.7
Cappuccino, Cappio, Iced, Kenco*	1 Can/200ml	138	6.0	69	3.0	7.0	3.0	0.0
Cappuccino, Cappio, Kenco*	1 Sachet/18g	79	1.9	439	11.7	73.9	10.6	0.6
Cappuccino, Co-Op*	1 Serving/12.5g	55	2.0	440	16.0	64.0	16.0	8.0
Cappuccino, Decaff, Instant, Made Up, Nescafe*	1 Mug/200ml	68	2.3	34	1.0	5.0	1.2	0.0
Cappuccino, Decaff, Nescafe*	1 Sachet/16g	68	2.3	428	11.6	62.6	14.6	0.0
Cappuccino, Decaff, Unsweetened, Nescafe*	1 Sachet/16g	76	3.9	472	15.1	47.4	24.6	0.0

C

COFFEE

INFO/WEIGHT	Measure	per Measure KCAL	FAT	Nutrition Values per 100g / 100ml KCAL	PROT	CARB	FAT	FIBRE
Cappuccino, Dry, Maxwell House*	1 Mug/15g	53	1.4	350	12.0	64.0	9.6	0.4
Cappuccino, Dry, Waitrose*	1 Sachet/13.2g	57	2.2	439	15.1	56.0	17.2	4.4
Cappuccino, for Filter Systems, Kenco*	1 Sachet/6g	23	0.8	375	19.0	44.0	13.5	0.0
Cappuccino, Instant, Alcafe*	1 Sachet/12.5g	49	1.7	393	12.5	55.1	13.6	0.0
Cappuccino, Instant, Asda*	1 Sachet/15g	60	2.3	399	13.0	53.0	15.2	0.9
Cappuccino, Instant, Douwe Egberts*	1 Serving/12g	48	1.9	400	11.0	53.0	16.0	0.0
Cappuccino, Instant, Kenco*	1 Sachet/20g	80	2.8	401	13.5	55.7	13.8	0.0
Cappuccino, Instant, Made Up, Maxwell House*	1 Serving/280g	123	5.3	44	0.6	5.8	1.9	0.0
Cappuccino, Low Sugar, Tesco*	1 Serving/13g	55	2.6	425	18.4	43.3	19.8	0.4
Cappuccino, M & S*	1 Serving/164g	66	2.6	40	1.5	4.4	1.6	0.1
Cappuccino, Organic Chocolate, Traidcraft*	1 Serving/25g	139	9.5	555	7.0	43.0	38.0	0.0
Cappuccino, Original, Sachets, Nescafe*	1 Sachet/18g	80	3.1	444	11.7	60.3	17.4	0.0
Cappuccino, Original Mugsticks, Maxwell House*	1 Serving/18g	73	2.8	406	14.4	52.8	15.6	0.0
Cappuccino, Reduced Sugar, Sainsbury's*	1 Serving/12g	48	2.3	418	18.0	41.0	20.0	0.0
Cappuccino, Sainsbury's*	1 Serving/12g	49	1.9	411	14.9	52.9	15.5	0.4
Cappuccino, Semi Skimmed Milk, Average	1 Serving/200ml	48	2.1	24	1.6	2.6	1.1	0.0
Cappuccino, Skinny, Nescafe*	1 Sachet/16g	58	0.8	365	23.6	56.8	4.8	0.0
Cappuccino, Swiss Chocolate, Nescafe*	1 Sachet/20g	81	2.3	404	10.5	65.3	11.5	2.9
Cappuccino, to Go, Original, Nescafe*	1 Serving/19g	84	3.3	444	11.7	60.3	17.4	0.0
Cappuccino, to Go, Unsweetened, Nescafe*	1 Serving/17g	79	4.0	464	15.0	47.3	23.8	0.0
Cappuccino, Unsweetened, Cappio, Kenco*	1 Serving/18g	73	1.8	406	12.2	66.7	10.0	0.6
Cappuccino, Unsweetened, Nescafe*	1 Serving/15.9	74	3.8	464	15.0	47.3	23.8	0.0
Cappuccino, Unsweetened Taste, Maxwell House*	1 Serving/15g	65	2.9	434	17.4	47.6	19.3	0.3
Columbian, Nescafe*	1 Serving/1.8g	2	0.0	111	16.7	11.1	0.0	5.6
Compliment*	1 Serving/14ml	20	1.8	143	1.4	6.4	12.9	0.0
Dandelion, Symingtons*	1 Serving/10g	32	0.0	320	2.8	79.3	0.0	0.0
Decaffeinated, Gold Blend, Nescafe*	1 Tsp/5g	5	0.0	101	14.9	10.0	0.2	8.4
Double Choca Mocha, Cafe Range, Nescafe*	1 Sachet/23g	94	2.5	408	9.2	68.0	11.0	2.8
Frappe Iced, Nestle*	1 Serving/25g	96	1.0	384	15.0	72.0	4.0	0.5
Ice Mocha Drink, Nescafe, Nestle*	1 Bottle/280ml	160	3.4	57	1.1	10.5	1.2	0.0
Infusion, Average with Semi-Skimmed Milk	1 Cup/220ml	14	0.4	7	0.6	0.7	0.2	0.0
Infusion, Average with Single Cream	1 Cup/220ml	31	2.6	14	0.4	0.3	1.2	0.0
Infusion, Average with Whole Milk	1 Cup/220ml	15	0.9	7	0.5	0.5	0.4	0.0
Instant, Alta Rica, Nescafe*	1 Serving/100g	98	0.3	98	13.8	10.0	0.3	21.0
Instant, Decaffeinated, Nescafe*	1 Tsp/5g	5	0.0	101	14.9	10.0	0.2	8.4
Instant, Made with Skimmed Milk	1 Serving/270ml	15	0.0	6	0.6	0.8	0.0	0.0
Instant, Made with Water & Semi-Skimmed Milk	1 Serving/350ml	25	1.4	7	0.4	0.5	0.4	0.0
Instant, Original, Nescafe*	1 Tsp/1.9g	2	0.0	103	15.4	10.0	0.2	13.4
Latte, Cafe, M & S*	1 Serving/190g	143	5.3	75	4.3	8.3	2.8	0.0
Latte, Instant, Skinny, Douwe Egberts*	1 Serving/12g	35	1.3	290	11.0	38.0	11.0	29.0
Latte, Nescafe*	1 Sachet/21g	105	6.0	498	14.5	45.7	28.5	0.0
Latte, Skinny, Nescafe*	1 Sachet/21.9g	86	1.5	393	26.9	56.3	6.7	1.0
Mocha, Instant, Skinny, Douwe Egberts*	1 Serving/12g	37	1.3	308	10.8	40.8	10.8	25.0

COFFEE MATE

INFO/WEIGHT	Measure	per Measure KCAL	FAT	Nutrition Values per 100g / 100ml KCAL	PROT	CARB	FAT	FIBRE
Original, Nestle*	1 Tsp/3.5g	19	1.2	547	2.4	56.7	34.4	0.0
Virtually Fat Free, Nestle*	2 Tsp/10g	20	0.3	200	1.0	42.0	3.0	0.0

COFFEE SUBSTITUTE

INFO/WEIGHT	Measure	per Measure KCAL	FAT	Nutrition Values per 100g / 100ml KCAL	PROT	CARB	FAT	FIBRE
Bambu, Vogel*	1 Tsp/3g	10	0.0	320	3.5	75.3	0.5	0.0

COFFEE WHITENER

INFO/WEIGHT	Measure	per Measure KCAL	FAT	Nutrition Values per 100g / 100ml KCAL	PROT	CARB	FAT	FIBRE
Half Fat, Co-Op*	1 Tsp/5g	22	0.7	430	0.9	78.0	13.0	0.0
Light, Asda*	1 Serving/3g	13	0.4	433	0.9	78.0	13.0	0.0
Light, HE, Tesco*	1 Tsp/6g	27	1.0	449	3.5	71.0	16.8	0.0
Light, Tesco*	1 Tsp/3g	13	0.4	429	0.9	77.7	12.7	0.0

	Measure INFO/WEIGHT	per Measure		Nutrition Values per 100g / 100ml				
		KCAL	FAT	KCAL	PROT	CARB	FAT	FIBRE
COFFEE WHITENER								
Morrisons*	1 Serving/10g	54	3.3	535	2.6	57.5	32.8	0.0
Tesco*	1 Tsp/3g	16	0.9	533	1.2	61.3	31.4	0.0
COGNAC								
40% Volume	1 Pub Shot/35ml	78	0.0	222	0.0	0.0	0.0	0.0
COINTREAU								
Liqueur Specialite De France	1 Serving/37g	80	0.0	215	0.0	0.0	0.0	0.0
COLA								
Average	1 Can/330ml	135	0.0	41	0.0	10.9	0.0	0.0
Coke, Cherry, Coca-Cola*	1 Bottle/500ml	225	0.0	45	0.0	11.2	0.0	0.0
Coke, Coca-Cola*	1 Can/330ml	142	0.0	43	0.0	10.7	0.0	0.0
Coke, Diet, Caffeine Free, Coca-Cola*	1 Can/330ml	1	0.0	0	0.0	0.1	0.0	0.0
Coke, Diet, Coca-Cola*	1 Can/330ml	1	0.0	0	0.0	0.0	0.0	0.0
Coke, Diet, with Cherry, Coca-Cola*	1 Bottle/500ml	5	0.0	1	0.0	0.0	0.0	0.0
Coke, with Lemon, Diet, Coca-Cola*	1 Can/330ml	5	0.0	1	0.0	0.0	0.0	0.0
Coke, with Vanilla, Diet, Coca-Cola*	1 Glass/200ml	1	0.0	0	0.0	0.1	0.0	0.0
Diet, Classic, Sainsbury's*	1 Can/330ml	1	0.0	0	0.0	0.0	0.0	0.0
Diet, Just, Asda*	1 Bottle/250ml	1	0.0	0	0.0	0.0	0.0	0.0
Diet, M & S*	1 Can/330ml	3	0.0	1	0.0	0.3	0.0	0.0
Diet, Pepsi*	1 Can/330ml	1	0.0	0	0.0	0.0	0.0	0.0
Diet, Tesco*	1 Glass/200ml	2	0.2	1	0.1	0.1	0.1	0.0
Diet, Virgin*	1 Glass/250ml	1	0.3	0	0.1	0.1	0.1	0.0
Max, Pepsi*	1 fl oz/30ml	0	0.0	1	0.1	0.1	0.0	0.0
Pepsi*	1 Can/330ml	145	0.0	44	0.0	11.1	0.0	0.0
Tesco*	1 Can/330ml	145	0.0	44	0.0	10.8	0.0	0.0
Twist, Light, Pepsi*	1 Bottle/500ml	5	0.0	1	0.0	0.1	0.0	0.0
Zero, Coca-Cola*	1 Can/330ml	2	0.0	1	0.0	0.0	0.0	0.0
COLESLAW								
20% Less Fat, Asda*	1 Serving/100g	88	6.0	88	1.5	7.0	6.0	1.7
30% Reduced Fat, Somerfield*	1 Serving/100g	90	7.5	90	0.8	4.7	7.5	2.5
50% Less Fat, Asda*	1oz/28g	17	0.8	61	2.1	6.8	2.8	0.9
99% Fat Free, Kraft*	1 Serving/40ml	50	0.4	126	1.0	28.9	1.0	0.0
Aldi*	1 Serving/100g	206	18.7	206	0.8	8.6	18.7	0.0
Apple, M & S*	1oz/28g	53	4.6	190	1.4	9.2	16.6	1.4
Asda*	1 Serving/100g	190	18.0	190	1.0	6.0	18.0	1.4
Basics, Sainsbury's*	1 Serving/25g	25	2.0	98	1.0	5.2	8.1	1.6
Bettabuy, Morrisons*	1 Serving/100g	120	10.2	120	0.7	6.4	10.2	1.1
BFY, Morrisons*	1oz/28g	17	1.0	62	1.5	6.7	3.5	0.0
BGTY, Sainsbury's*	1 Serving/60g	51	3.7	85	1.5	6.0	6.1	1.7
Bryn Wharf Food Co*	1 Serving/90g	109	9.4	121	1.4	5.7	10.4	1.8
Budgens*	1 Serving/50g	103	9.1	206	1.2	9.5	18.1	2.0
Cheese, Co-Op*	1 Serving/125g	344	31.3	275	6.0	6.0	25.0	1.0
Cheese, M & S*	1 Serving/57g	185	19.1	325	4.2	2.0	33.5	1.7
Cheese, Sainsbury's*	1 Serving/75g	174	16.4	232	3.4	5.6	21.8	0.6
Cheese, Somerfield*	¼ Pot/62.5g	141	11.9	225	4.5	8.0	19.1	1.2
Cheese, Supreme, Waitrose*	¼ Pack/87.6g	197	18.2	225	4.5	5.0	20.8	1.2
Chunky, Asda*	1oz/28g	54	5.0	194	1.0	7.1	18.0	1.6
Co-Op*	1 Serving/125g	119	8.6	95	0.9	7.7	6.9	1.8
COU, M & S*	½ Pack/125g	75	3.4	60	1.3	7.4	2.7	1.7
Creamy, 30% Less Fat, Sainsbury's*	1 Tub/300g	378	33.0	126	1.0	5.5	11.0	1.4
Creamy, Asda*	1 Serving/25g	62	6.0	248	0.9	7.0	24.0	1.8
Creamy, HL, Tesco*	1 Serving/100g	70	4.2	70	1.8	6.4	4.2	1.6
Creamy, Kwik Save*	1 Serving/10g	27	2.8	274	1.1	5.1	27.7	1.3
Creamy, Morrisons*	1 Serving/40g	111	11.1	277	1.1	5.5	27.7	1.3

C

COLESLAW

INFO/WEIGHT	Measure	per Measure KCAL	FAT	Nutrition Values per 100g / 100ml KCAL	PROT	CARB	FAT	FIBRE
Creamy, Reduced Fat, HL, Tesco*	1 Serving/100g	90	6.0	90	1.7	7.0	6.0	1.6
Crunchy, Premium, Millcroft*	1 Pack/400g	756	69.6	189	0.9	7.3	17.4	1.5
Deli Style, M & S*	1 Serving/320g	336	31.0	105	3.5	1.5	9.7	1.4
Eat Smart, Safeway*	¼ Pack/50g	30	1.3	60	1.8	7.2	2.6	1.9
Finest, Tesco*	1 Serving/25g	38	3.7	151	1.0	3.8	14.6	2.7
Fruity, Asda*	½ Pot/125g	101	6.1	81	1.3	8.0	4.9	1.7
Fruity, M & S*	1 Serving/63g	151	14.3	240	1.1	8.3	22.7	3.1
Garlic & Herb, Asda*	1 Tbsp/15g	22	2.0	147	0.9	5.8	13.3	1.7
GFY, Asda*	1 Serving/50g	28	1.5	55	1.3	6.0	2.9	2.3
Half Fat, Safeway*	1 Serving/70g	60	4.0	86	1.5	7.4	5.7	1.6
Half Fat, Waitrose*	1 Serving/100g	64	4.5	64	1.0	4.8	4.5	2.0
Healthy Choice, Safeway*	1 Pot/250g	215	14.3	86	1.5	7.4	5.7	1.6
Heinz*	1oz/28g	38	2.9	135	1.6	9.4	10.2	1.2
Iceland*	1 Serving/110g	112	8.3	102	0.7	7.8	7.5	1.6
Kwik Save*	1 Serving/50g	51	3.8	101	0.8	7.7	7.5	2.1
Light, Morrisons*	1 Tub/300g	309	21.9	103	1.3	6.4	7.3	1.8
Light, Reduced Fat, Morrisons*	1 Serving/30g	38	3.1	125	0.8	7.4	10.2	0.0
Low Fat Mayonnaise, Tesco*	1oz/28g	18	1.2	64	1.4	4.7	4.4	1.4
Luxury, Asda*	1 Serving/50g	109	10.5	217	0.9	6.0	21.0	0.0
Luxury, Lidl*	1 Serving/50g	102	9.7	203	0.9	5.9	19.4	0.0
Luxury, M & S*	1oz/28g	43	3.9	152	1.0	6.0	13.8	1.0
Luxury, Morrisons*	1 Serving/50g	137	13.5	273	1.2	6.4	27.0	0.0
M & S*	1oz/28g	50	4.6	180	1.7	6.1	16.5	1.1
Prawn, Asda*	1oz/28g	54	4.8	192	2.4	6.6	17.3	1.4
Prawn, Safeway*	1 Serving/113g	156	11.3	139	3.1	6.3	10.0	1.0
Premium, Co-Op*	1 Serving/50g	160	17.0	320	1.0	3.0	34.0	2.0
Premium, Safeway*	1 Serving/125g	334	34.0	267	1.9	3.8	27.2	2.3
Reduced Calorie, Budgens*	½ Pot/125g	124	8.6	99	1.0	8.3	6.9	2.3
Reduced Calorie, Iceland*	1 Serving/50g	51	3.8	102	0.7	7.8	7.5	1.6
Reduced Fat, Asda*	1 Pot/250g	218	15.8	87	1.5	6.0	6.3	1.6
Reduced Fat, Co-Op*	1 Serving/50g	45	3.5	90	0.9	6.0	7.0	2.0
Reduced Fat, HL, Co-Op*	1 Serving/50g	48	3.5	95	0.8	8.0	7.0	2.0
Reduced Fat, M & S*	½ Tub/112.2g	230	22.4	205	1.1	5.4	20.0	2.8
Safeway*	1 Serving/75g	128	11.7	170	0.7	6.7	15.6	0.0
Sainsbury's*	1 Serving/75g	104	9.0	138	1.4	6.1	12.0	1.7
Savers, Safeway*	1 Serving/114g	122	9.7	107	1.1	6.6	8.5	0.0
SmartPrice, Asda*	1oz/28g	30	2.2	107	0.8	8.0	8.0	2.0
So Good, Somerfield*	1 Serving/50g	105	10.0	210	1.4	6.6	20.0	1.2
Somerfield*	1/5 Tub/50g	72	6.0	144	1.2	7.8	12.0	1.6
Supreme, Waitrose*	1oz/28g	53	5.1	190	1.8	4.9	18.1	1.7
Tesco*	1 Serving/50g	79	7.2	158	2.2	5.2	14.3	1.6
The Best, Safeway*	1 Serving/10g	30	2.9	296	1.0	7.2	29.2	0.8
Three Cheese, Asda*	1 Serving/78g	203	18.7	260	5.0	6.0	24.0	1.7
Three Cheese, Safeway*	½ Pot/113g	189	16.0	168	4.5	6.2	14.2	1.1
Three Cheese, Tesco*	½ Pot/125g	230	20.6	184	4.0	4.8	16.5	1.2
Traditional, Side Salad, M & S*	¼ Tub/100g	330	33.4	330	1.2	5.8	33.4	1.7
TTD, Sainsbury's*	¼ Tub/75g	181	18.1	241	1.1	5.0	24.1	2.8
Value, Tesco*	1oz/28g	32	2.6	115	1.2	6.8	9.2	1.6
with 60% Less Fat, GFY, Asda*	1 Serving/41g	36	2.5	88	1.5	7.0	6.0	1.7
with Mayonnaise, Retail	1oz/28g	72	7.4	258	1.2	4.2	26.4	1.4
with Reduced Calorie Dressing, Retail	1oz/28g	19	1.3	67	0.9	6.1	4.5	1.4

COLESLAW MIX

INFO/WEIGHT	Measure	per Measure KCAL	FAT	Nutrition Values per 100g / 100ml KCAL	PROT	CARB	FAT	FIBRE
Shredded, Waitrose*	1 Serving/100g	29	0.2	29	1.1	5.6	0.2	2.2

	Measure INFO/WEIGHT	per Measure KCAL	FAT	Nutrition Values per 100g / 100ml KCAL	PROT	CARB	FAT	FIBRE
COLESLAW MIX								
Tesco*	1 Pack/400g	124	0.8	31	1.1	6.2	0.2	2.1
COLEY								
Portions, Raw, Average	1 Portion/92g	75	0.7	82	18.4	0.0	0.7	0.0
Steamed, Average	1oz/28g	29	0.4	105	23.3	0.0	1.3	0.0
CONCHIGLIE								
Cooked, Average	1 Serving/185g	247	1.6	134	4.9	26.7	0.9	0.6
Dry Weight, Average	1 Serving/100g	352	1.7	352	12.5	71.6	1.7	2.6
Shells, Dry, Average	1 Serving/100g	346	1.5	346	12.3	70.4	1.5	3.0
Whole Wheat, Dry Weight, Average	1 Serving/75g	237	1.5	316	12.6	62.0	2.0	10.7
CONCHIGLIONI								
Dry, Waitrose*	1 Serving/75g	256	1.0	341	12.5	69.8	1.3	3.7
CONSERVE								
Apricot, Average	1 Tbsp/15g	37	0.0	244	0.5	59.3	0.2	1.5
Apricot, Reduced Sugar, Streamline*	1 Tbsp/20g	37	0.0	184	0.5	45.0	0.2	0.0
Black Cherry, with Amaretto, Finest, Tesco*	1 Serving/10g	26	0.0	261	0.5	64.4	0.1	0.8
Blackcurrant, Average	1 Tbsp/15g	37	0.0	245	0.6	60.1	0.1	1.9
Blueberry, M & S*	1 Tsp/7.5g	16	0.0	206	0.3	51.1	0.1	1.3
Morello Cherry, Waitrose*	1 Tbsp/15g	39	0.0	258	0.4	64.2	0.0	1.4
Raspberry, Average	1 Tbsp/15g	37	0.1	249	0.6	61.0	0.3	1.3
Red Cherry, Finest, Tesco*	1 Tbsp/15g	42	0.0	277	0.6	67.6	0.1	0.8
Rhubarb & Ginger, M & S*	1 Tbsp/15g	29	0.0	194	0.3	47.9	0.1	1.0
Strawberry, 60% Fruit, Reduced Sugar, M & S*	1 Tsp/7g	9	0.0	135	0.4	30.1	0.2	1.9
Strawberry, Average	1 Tbsp/15g	37	0.0	250	0.4	61.6	0.1	0.5
Yellow Plum & Greengage, TTD, Sainsbury's*	1 Tbsp/15g	36	0.0	243	0.4	60.0	0.1	0.7
CONSOMME								
Average	1oz/28g	3	0.0	12	2.9	0.1	0.0	0.0
Beef, Canned, Sainsbury's*	1 Can/415g	46	0.0	11	2.0	0.7	0.0	0.0
Beef, Luxury, Baxters*	1 Can/415g	54	0.0	13	2.6	0.7	0.0	0.0
COOKIES								
All Butter, Almond, Italian Style, M & S*	1 Biscuit/23g	120	6.4	515	6.7	59.4	27.6	3.6
All Butter, Fruity Flapjack, M & S*	1 Cookie/23.1g	105	4.9	455	5.1	60.5	21.4	3.5
All Butter, Melting Moment, M & S*	1 Cookie/23.4g	108	6.3	470	4.5	51.5	27.5	3.4
Apple Pie, The Biscuit Collection*	1 Biscuit/19g	90	4.2	474	3.9	65.0	22.1	0.0
Big Milk Chocolate Chunk, Cookie Coach*	1 Cookie/35g	174	8.8	497	6.2	61.4	25.1	0.0
Bites, Weight Watchers*	1 Pack/21g	97	4.0	464	5.8	67.0	19.2	4.3
Brazil Nut, Organic, Traidcraft*	1 Cookie/16.6g	93	5.5	547	5.8	57.7	32.6	2.1
Butter & Sultana, Sainsbury's*	1 Cookie/13g	61	2.6	473	4.5	68.4	20.1	1.6
Choc Chip, Asda*	1 Biscuit/12g	60	3.0	500	5.2	62.8	25.3	2.6
Choc Chip, Bronte*	1 Biscuit/16.7g	79	3.6	474	5.8	64.0	21.6	0.0
Choc Chip, Cadbury*	1 Biscuit/10.9g	55	2.8	503	5.9	62.2	25.6	0.0
Choc Chip, Giant, Paterson's*	1 Cookie/60g	296	15.2	493	0.1	61.3	25.3	3.2
Choc Chip, Lyons*	1 Cookie/11.4g	57	2.7	499	5.2	68.3	23.4	1.7
Choc Chip, Maryland*	1 Cookie/11g	56	2.6	511	6.2	68.0	23.9	1.3
Choc Chip, McVitie's*	1 Cookie/10g	50	2.6	496	5.8	60.2	25.8	3.0
Choc Chip, Parkside*	1 Biscut/11.3g	56	2.7	495	5.3	64.5	23.7	0.0
Choc Chip, Reduced Fat, Maryland*	1 Cookie/10.7g	51	1.9	478	5.9	73.0	18.0	0.0
Choc Chip, Sainsbury's*	1 Biscuit/10.8g	55	2.6	508	6.2	67.0	23.9	1.3
Choc Chip & Coconut, Maryland*	1oz/28g	143	6.6	512	5.1	62.9	23.7	0.0
Choc Chip & Hazelnut, Maryland*	1 Biscuit/10g	55	2.7	513	6.3	65.3	25.0	0.0
Choc Chip 'n' Chunk, McVitie's*	1 Cookie/11g	55	2.9	498	5.8	59.2	26.4	3.5
Choc Chunk, Finest, Tesco*	1 Serving/79.8g	355	14.1	445	5.7	65.3	17.7	1.8
Choc Chunk & Hazelnut, Co-Op*	1 Cookie/17g	89	5.3	525	6.0	56.0	31.0	3.0
Choc Chunk & Hazelnut, Luxury, Cadbury*	1oz/28g	146	8.0	521	6.3	60.0	28.7	0.0

COOKIES

	Measure INFO/WEIGHT	per Measure KCAL	FAT	Nutrition Values per 100g / 100ml KCAL	PROT	CARB	FAT	FIBRE
Chocolate, Belgian, Extra Special, Asda*	1 Cookie/25.8g	139	8.1	535	6.0	58.0	31.0	2.0
Chocolate, Half Coated Triple, Finest, Tesco*	1 Biscuit/25g	131	7.3	525	5.7	58.7	29.3	2.3
Chocolate, Milk, Free From, Tesco*	1 Biscuit/20g	100	6.1	500	5.6	50.4	30.7	4.1
Chocolate, Milk, Tesco*	1 Biscuit/20g	100	6.1	500	5.6	50.4	30.7	4.1
Chocolate, Quadruple, Sainsbury's*	1 Serving/20g	117	6.6	585	6.0	66.5	33.0	1.5
Chocolate, Soft, American Style, Budgens*	1 Cookie/50g	216	9.3	431	5.1	60.8	18.6	2.2
Chocolate, Triple, Half Coated, Finest, Tesco*	1 Serving/25g	129	7.2	517	5.8	58.8	28.7	2.2
Chocolate & Orange, COU, M & S*	1 Cookie/25.7g	91	0.7	350	5.7	77.2	2.6	3.2
Chocolate Chip, Asda*	1 Biscuit/12g	57	2.9	497	5.0	63.0	25.0	2.6
Chocolate Chip, BGTY, Sainsbury's*	1 Cookie/16.8g	73	2.0	428	4.5	75.6	11.9	2.5
Chocolate Chip, Chips Ahoy*	1 Cookie/11g	55	2.8	500	6.0	65.0	25.0	3.0
Chocolate Chip, Co-Op*	1 Cookie/11g	55	2.6	500	5.0	65.0	24.0	1.0
Chocolate Chip, Handbaked, Border*	1 Cookie/15g	72	3.4	480	5.9	67.4	22.6	0.0
Chocolate Chip, Low Price, Sainsbury's*	1 Cookie/10.8g	55	2.3	500	7.0	70.1	21.3	2.5
Chocolate Chip, M & S*	1 Cookie/12g	59	3.0	495	5.7	62.1	24.8	2.7
Chocolate Chip, McVitie's*	1 Cookie/11g	54	2.8	496	5.8	60.2	25.8	3.0
Chocolate Chip, Mini, McVitie's*	1 Pack/40g	196	9.2	491	5.5	65.1	23.1	2.8
Chocolate Chip, Mini, Tesco*	1 Bag/30g	148	7.1	493	5.4	64.6	23.7	1.7
Chocolate Chip, Morrisons*	1 Cookie/10g	52	2.5	502	5.0	66.2	24.1	1.3
Chocolate Chip, Organic, Sainsbury's*	1 Cookie/16.8g	90	5.0	530	5.0	61.8	29.2	0.3
Chocolate Chip, SmartPrice, Asda*	1 Biscuit/10.4g	52	2.4	499	5.2	68.3	23.4	1.7
Chocolate Chip, Tesco*	1 Serving/11g	55	2.6	500	4.7	66.7	23.4	0.6
Chocolate Chip, Value, Tesco*	1 Cookie/11g	56	2.9	512	4.8	64.8	26.0	1.6
Chocolate Chip, Weight Watchers*	2 Biscuits/22g	97	3.8	443	7.6	65.4	17.2	4.6
Chocolate Chunk, All Butter, COU, M & S*	1 Cookie/23.9g	110	4.3	460	5.7	69.1	17.9	2.3
Chocolate Chunk, Cadbury*	1 Cookie/22g	119	6.9	540	6.5	58.0	31.2	0.0
Chocolate Chunk, Quadruple, TTD, Sainsbury's*	1 Cookie/23g	117	6.6	509	5.2	57.4	28.7	1.7
Chocolate Chunk & Hazelnut, Tesco*	1 Cookie/22g	118	6.7	538	6.2	60.2	30.3	1.9
Chocolate Fruit & Nut, Extra Special, Asda*	1 Cookie/24.6g	127	7.3	509	6.0	56.0	29.0	2.0
Coconut & Raspberry, Gluten Free, Sainsbury's*	1 Cookie/20g	102	5.9	511	5.9	56.0	29.3	6.7
Cranberry & Orange, Weight Watchers*	1 Pack/21.9g	100	3.7	456	3.8	72.2	16.9	3.5
Double Choc, Cadbury*	1 Biscuit/11g	55	2.5	485	7.3	64.3	22.2	0.0
Double Choc, Maryland*	1 Cookie/10g	46	2.3	510	5.2	64.4	25.7	0.0
Double Choc Chip, Giant, Paterson's*	1 Cookie/60g	293	15.2	489	0.3	61.3	25.3	3.7
Double Choc Chip, Mini, M & S*	1 Cookie/22g	108	5.2	490	5.3	63.6	23.7	1.8
Double Choc Chip, Tesco*	1 Cookie/11g	55	2.7	500	4.2	65.3	24.7	3.0
Double Choc Chip, Weight Watchers*	2 Biscuits/22g	97	3.8	443	7.6	65.4	17.2	4.6
Double Choc Chunk, Luxury, Cadbury*	1oz/28g	146	8.1	521	5.7	59.0	29.0	0.0
Double Chocolate, Premium, Co-Op*	1 Cookie/17g	86	4.6	505	5.0	62.0	27.0	2.0
Double Chocolate & Walnut, Soft, Tesco*	1 Serving/25g	116	6.4	463	5.8	52.1	25.7	4.7
Double Chocolate Chip, Co-Op*	1 Cookie/17g	87	4.6	510	5.0	63.0	27.0	2.0
Double Chocolate Chip, Organic, Waitrose*	1 Cookie/18g	96	5.6	535	5.1	58.6	31.0	1.9
Double Chocolate Chip, Somerfield*	1 Cookie/11g	56	2.8	513	5.2	64.9	25.8	1.3
Double Chocolate Chip, Treat Yourself, Spar*	1 Biscuit/20g	94	5.0	470	5.5	56.0	25.0	2.5
Ginger, Low Fat, M & S*	1 Cookie/23g	82	1.0	358	5.1	74.9	4.3	2.4
Ginger & Choc Chip, BGTY, Sainsbury's*	1 Biscuit/16.7g	69	3.2	415	5.8	55.3	19.0	12.1
Ginger & Lemon, Weight Watchers*	2 Cookies/23g	104	3.5	451	4.2	73.9	15.4	2.2
Hazelnut & Choc Chip 'n' Chunk, McVitie's*	1 Biscuit/10.9g	55	3.0	505	6.1	57.8	27.7	3.5
Lemon Zest, Organic, Dove's Farm*	1 Cookie/16.7g	82	3.8	489	3.6	66.8	23.0	1.4
Milk Chocolate, Classic, Millie's Cookies*	1 Cookie/45g	190	10.2	422	5.1	49.3	22.7	1.3
Oat, Giant Jumbo, Paterson's*	1 Cookie/60g	299	16.2	499	0.4	58.4	27.0	3.2
Oat & Cranberry, BGTY, Sainsbury's*	1 Cookie/28g	126	5.0	449	6.8	65.0	18.0	5.1
Oat & Raisin, Health Matters*	1 Cookie/8g	33	0.7	414	7.0	76.6	8.8	3.3

	Measure INFO/WEIGHT	per Measure KCAL	FAT	Nutrition Values per 100g / 100ml KCAL	PROT	CARB	FAT	FIBRE
COOKIES								
Oat & Raisin, Safeway*	1 Cookie/12g	50	1.1	414	7.5	77.5	8.8	0.0
Oatflake & Raisin, Waitrose*	1 Cookie/17g	80	3.8	469	5.8	61.7	22.1	4.7
Oreo, Nabisco*	3 Cookies/34g	160	7.0	471	5.9	70.6	20.6	2.9
Peanut, Hellema*	1 Cookie/14.7g	78	4.2	532	12.5	57.0	28.5	2.0
Pecan & Maple, Mini, Bronte*	1 Pack/100g	509	27.3	509	5.4	60.3	27.3	1.6
Stem Ginger, & Oatflake, TTD, Sainsbury's*	1 Cookie/17g	84	4.2	496	4.5	63.4	24.9	1.7
Stem Ginger, Free From, Sainsbury's*	1 Biscuit/17.1g	84	4.8	489	6.5	58.0	28.0	6.8
Stem Ginger, Half Coated, Finest, Tesco*	1 Cookie/25g	127	6.7	508	4.4	62.4	26.8	3.6
Stem Ginger, Reduced Fat, Waitrose*	1 Cookie/16.7g	75	2.7	448	4.5	71.0	16.2	1.6
Stem Ginger, Tesco*	1 Cookie/20g	98	4.8	489	4.2	64.0	24.0	2.0
Sultana, All Butter, M & S*	1 Cookie/16.7g	75	2.9	450	5.7	67.3	17.6	2.5
Sultana, All Butter, Reduced Fat, M & S*	1 Cookie/16.7g	71	2.4	420	4.9	68.6	14.2	2.5
Sultana, Soft & Chewy, Sainsbury's*	1 Cookie/25g	104	3.5	414	4.4	67.8	13.9	2.5
Tennessee American Style, Stiftung & Co*	1 Cookie/19g	96	4.6	504	6.0	66.0	24.0	0.0
Toffee, Weight Watchers*	2 Cookies/23g	105	3.9	456	5.2	71.1	16.8	2.9
White Chocolate, Asda*	1 Cookie/54g	256	11.9	474	5.0	64.0	22.0	2.1
White Chocolate, Maryland*	1 Biscuit/10g	51	2.5	512	5.7	64.0	25.0	0.0
White Chocolate & Raspberry, McVitie's*	1 Cookie/17g	87	4.4	512	4.7	64.1	25.9	1.8
White Chocolate & Raspberry, TTD, Sainsbury's*	I Biscuit/16.7g	81	4.1	485	5.7	60.3	24.5	2.6
COQ AU VIN								
Finest, Tesco*	1 Serving/273g	251	9.8	92	14.3	0.7	3.6	1.8
HL, Tesco*	½ Pack/200g	172	3.8	86	15.2	2.1	1.9	0.4
M & S*	1 Serving/295g	398	22.7	135	14.2	1.5	7.7	1.0
PB, Waitrose*	1 Pack/500g	445	15.5	89	12.6	2.7	3.1	0.6
PB, Waitrose*	1 Pack/500g	445	15.5	89	12.6	2.7	3.1	0.6
Sainsbury's*	1 Pack/400g	484	17.6	121	16.8	3.5	4.4	0.2
CORDIAL								
Blackcurrant & Elderberry, Diluted, TTD, Sainsbury's*	1 Glass/250ml	48	0.0	19	0.0	4.7	0.0	0.0
Elderflower, Made Up, Bottle Green*	1 Glass/200ml	46	0.0	23	0.0	5.6	0.0	0.0
Elderflower, Undiluted, Waitrose*	1 Cordial/20ml	22	0.0	110	0.0	27.5	0.0	0.0
Lime, Sainsbury's*	1 Serving/50ml	14	0.0	27	0.0	6.2	0.0	0.0
Lime Juice, Concentrated	1 Serving/20ml	22	0.0	112	0.1	29.8	0.0	0.0
Lime Juice, Diluted	1 Glass/250ml	55	0.0	22	0.0	6.0	0.0	0.0
Lime Juice, Waitrose*	1 Serving/20ml	21	0.0	104	10.0	23.7	0.0	0.0
CORIANDER								
Leaves, Dried, Average	1oz/28g	78	1.3	279	21.8	41.7	4.8	0.0
Leaves, Fresh, Average	1 Serving/5g	1	0.0	20	2.4	1.8	0.6	0.0
Seeds, Ground, Schwartz*	1 Tsp/5g	22	0.9	446	14.2	54.9	18.8	0.0
CORN								
Baby, & Asparagus Tips, Tesco*	1 Pack/150g	38	0.8	25	2.6	2.5	0.5	1.9
Baby, & Mange Tout, Tesco*	1 Serving/100g	27	0.2	27	2.9	3.3	0.2	2.1
Baby, & Sugar Snap Peas, Safeway*	½ Pack/100g	27	0.2	27	2.9	3.3	0.2	0.0
Baby, Average	1oz/28g	7	0.1	26	2.5	3.1	0.4	1.7
Cobs, Boiled, Weighed with Cob, Average	1 Ear/200g	132	2.8	66	2.5	11.6	1.4	1.3
Creamed, Green Giant*	1 Can/418g	238	2.1	57	1.2	11.9	0.5	3.0
in Brine, for Stir Fry, Braxted Hall*	1 Can/133g	25	0.0	19	1.5	3.0	0.0	1.5
CORN CAKES								
Organic, Kallo*	1 Cake/5g	16	0.2	340	12.7	74.3	4.1	11.2
Ryvita*	1 Pack/13.1g	48	0.4	366	10.0	74.3	3.2	7.2
Thick Slices, Orgran*	1 Cake/11g	42	0.4	385	13.2	79.0	3.7	14.2
CORN MEAL								
Yellow, Enriched & Degerminated, Quaker*	1 Tbsp/9g	30	0.2	333	7.4	77.8	1.9	7.4

	Measure INFO/WEIGHT	per Measure KCAL	FAT	Nutrition Values per 100g / 100ml KCAL	PROT	CARB	FAT	FIBRE
CORN NUTS								
Roasted, Kraft*	1 Serving/28g	120	4.5	429	10.7	71.4	16.1	7.1
CORN SNACKS								
Crispy, Bugles*	1 Bag/20g	102	5.6	508	4.8	60.7	28.0	1.4
Scampi, Smiths, Walkers*	1 Bag/27g	134	7.0	496	13.0	52.5	26.0	0.0
Toasted, Holland & Barrett*	1 Serving/100g	412	12.1	412	8.1	69.7	12.1	4.0
CORNED BEEF								
Average	1 Slice/35g	75	4.3	215	25.9	0.7	12.2	0.0
Lean, Healthy Range, Average	1 Slice/30g	57	2.6	191	27.0	1.0	8.7	0.0
CORNFLAKE NEST								
Crunchy Chocolate, M & S*	1 Nest/14.7g	71	3.0	475	6.3	67.2	20.2	2.2
CORNFLOUR								
Average	1oz/28g	99	0.3	355	0.7	86.9	1.2	0.1
Original, Patent, Brown & Polson*	1 Tbsp/15g	51	0.1	343	0.6	83.6	0.7	0.1
COTTAGE PIE								
Disney, Tesco*	1 Pack/280.9g	250	7.0	89	4.9	11.8	2.5	1.9
COURGETTE								
Boiled in Unsalted Water, Average	1oz/28g	5	0.1	19	2.0	2.0	0.4	1.2
Fried, Average	1oz/28g	18	1.3	63	2.6	2.6	4.8	1.2
Raw, Average	1oz/28g	5	0.1	18	1.8	1.8	0.4	0.9
COUS COUS								
& Chargrilled Vegetables, M & S*	1 Serving/200g	200	3.0	100	3.9	17.3	1.5	1.6
& Roasted Vegetables, M & S*	1 Pack/200g	320	17.2	160	3.7	17.1	8.6	2.8
& Wok Oriental, Findus*	½ Pack/300g	510	25.5	170	4.5	19.0	8.5	0.0
Balsamic Roasted Vegetable, TTD, Sainsbury's*	1 Serving/240g	281	13.0	117	2.8	14.3	5.4	1.1
Chargrilled Red & Yellow Pepper, Tesco*	1 Pack/200g	212	3.6	106	4.6	17.8	1.8	0.5
Chargrilled Vegetable, Morrisons*	1 Serving/225g	227	5.4	101	3.3	16.5	2.4	1.3
Chargrilled Vegetables, Tomato, Pepper& Chili Sainsbury's*	1 Pot/250g	295	2.8	118	4.3	22.7	1.1	2.1
Citrus Kick, Cooked, Ainsley Harriott*	1 Serving/130g	182	1.6	140	4.3	27.9	1.2	2.4
Citrus Kick, Dry, Ainsley Harriott*	½ Pack/134.3g	493	3.2	368	11.6	77.0	2.4	9.2
Cooked, Average	1 Cup/157g	249	2.9	159	4.3	31.4	1.9	1.3
Coriander & Lemon, Asda*	1 Pack/110g	150	1.3	136	4.2	27.0	1.2	1.8
Coriander & Lemon, Morrisons*	1 Serving/100g	159	3.4	159	4.4	27.7	3.4	1.4
Coriander & Lemon, Savoury, Sainsbury's*	½ Pack/137.3g	206	5.9	150	4.3	23.4	4.3	2.7
Dry, Average	1 Serving/50g	178	0.7	356	13.7	72.8	1.5	2.6
Garlic & Coriander, Dry, Waitrose*	1 Serving/70g	235	2.5	336	11.7	64.2	3.6	6.2
Harissa Style Savoury, Sainsbury's*	1 Serving/260g	434	12.0	167	4.7	26.8	4.6	1.3
Indian Style, Sainsbury's*	½ Pack/143g	204	3.9	143	4.5	25.1	2.7	1.0
Lemon & Coriander, Cooked, Tesco*	1 Serving/137g	207	3.3	151	4.0	28.3	2.4	2.0
Lemon & Coriander, Dry, Tesco*	1 Pack/110g	375	3.0	341	11.0	68.2	2.7	6.1
Mediterranean Style, Cooked, Tesco*	1 Serving/146g	215	3.8	147	4.4	26.5	2.6	1.3
Mediterranean Style, Dry, Tesco*	1 Pack/110g	369	3.3	335	11.9	65.1	3.0	5.6
Mediterranean Style, Tomato, Morrisons*	1 Serving/100g	147	2.6	147	4.4	26.4	2.6	1.3
Mediterranean Tomato, GFY, Asda*	½ Pack/141g	192	1.3	136	5.0	27.0	0.9	1.7
Mint & Coriander Flavour, Dry, Amazing Grains*	1 Sachet/99g	349	2.7	353	12.2	70.0	2.7	3.2
Moroccan Style, Finest, Tesco*	1 Tub/225g	338	10.6	150	3.7	23.6	4.7	3.9
Moroccan Style, Fruity, M & S*	1 Serving/200g	370	5.4	185	3.4	36.7	2.7	3.4
Moroccan Style, Sainsbury's*	½ Pack/150g	195	4.1	130	5.0	21.5	2.7	1.0
Moroccan Style, Savoury, Sainsbury's*	½ Pack/150.8g	196	4.1	130	5.0	21.5	2.7	1.0
Moroccan Sultana & Pine Nuts, Dry, Sammy's*	1 Serving/50g	172	1.5	343	12.0	72.0	3.0	6.0
Morrisons*	1 Serving/100g	126	1.2	126	5.5	23.2	1.2	3.5
Morrocan, Roast Chicken, Delicious, Shapers, Boots*	1 Pack/250g	248	3.8	99	9.2	12.0	1.5	2.6
Mushroom & Garlic, Cooked, Morrisons*	1 Serving/100g	164	3.0	164	5.7	28.7	3.0	1.7
Mushrooms, Onion, Garlic & Herbs, Dry, Tesco*	½ Pack/50g	167	1.3	333	11.3	66.2	2.6	4.9

COUS COUS	Measure INFO/WEIGHT	per Measure KCAL	per Measure FAT	Nutrition Values per 100g / 100ml KCAL	PROT	CARB	FAT	FIBRE
Plain, Dry Weight, Tesco*	1 Serving/100g	365	1.1	365	15.1	73.1	1.1	0.8
Red Pepper & Chilli, Waitrose*	1 Pack/200g	344	13.8	172	4.5	23.0	6.9	1.3
Roast Garlic & Olive Oil, Dry Weight, Sammy's*	1 Serving/49.9g	170	1.5	339	12.0	71.5	3.0	0.0
Roasted Vegetable, Cooked, Ainsley Harriott*	½ Pack/139.9g	193	2.1	138	5.6	25.5	1.5	2.6
Roasted Vegetable, Dry, Ainsley Harriott*	½ Sachet/140g	386	4.2	276	11.2	51.0	3.0	5.2
Roasted Vegetables, Waitrose*	1 Serving/200g	328	13.2	164	3.9	22.0	6.6	0.9
Spice Sensation, Cooked, Ainsley Harriott*	1 Serving/135g	166	1.2	123	4.3	24.5	0.9	3.4
Spice Sensation, Dry, Ainsley Harriott*	½ Sachet/50g	166	1.2	332	11.6	66.2	2.4	9.2
Spicey Vegetable, Morrisons*	½ Pack/55g	69	0.7	126	5.5	23.2	1.2	3.5
Spicy Moroccan Chicken & Veg, COU, M & S*	1 Pack/400g	380	6.8	95	9.1	10.3	1.7	1.9
Spicy Vegetable, GFY, Asda*	½ Pack/55g	71	0.6	129	4.7	25.0	1.1	2.0
Spicy Vegetable, Morrisons*	1 Pack/110g	187	5.5	170	5.1	26.2	5.0	2.9
Sun Dried Tomato, Somerfield*	1 Jar/110g	176	5.5	160	3.0	25.0	5.0	4.0
Tangy Tomato, Cooked, Ainsley Harriott*	1 Serving/132.8g	166	0.8	125	4.6	25.3	0.6	3.3
Tangy Tomato, Dry, Ainsley Harriott*	½ Sachet/50g	166	0.8	332	12.2	67.2	1.6	8.8
Tomato & Basil, Made Up, Tesco*	1 Serving/200g	348	16.6	174	3.9	21.0	8.3	3.4
Tomato & Onion, Dry Weight, Waitrose*	1 Pack/110g	376	4.0	342	12.6	64.9	3.6	5.1
Wild Mushroom & Garlic, Sainsbury's*	½ Pack/141.2g	240	5.5	170	5.0	28.7	3.9	2.0
with Chargrilled Vegetables, Sainsbury's*	1 Pack/200g	236	4.4	118	4.7	19.7	2.2	2.8
with Chickpea & Feta, Toasted, TTD, Sainsbury's*	1 Serving/150g	273	18.5	182	5.2	12.6	12.3	0.0
with Lemon & Garlic, Dry, Waitrose*	½ Pack/55g	188	1.8	341	11.8	65.9	3.3	4.5
Zesty Lemon & Coriander, Dry, Sammy's*	1 Serving/50g	171	1.4	342	13.0	74.0	2.8	6.0
CRAB								
Boiled, Meat Only, Average	1 Tbsp/40g	51	2.2	128	19.5	0.0	5.5	0.0
Claws, Asda*	1oz/28g	25	0.3	89	11.0	9.0	1.0	0.2
Cocktail, Waitrose*	1 Serving/100g	217	17.6	217	10.8	3.8	17.6	0.4
Dressed, Average	1 Can/43g	66	3.4	154	16.8	4.1	7.9	0.2
Meat, in Brine, Average	½ Can/60g	46	0.3	76	17.2	0.9	0.4	0.1
Meat, Raw, Average	1oz/28g	28	0.2	100	20.8	2.8	0.6	0.0
CRAB CAKES								
Goan, M & S*	1 Pack/190g	228	7.6	120	8.0	12.9	4.0	1.8
Iceland*	1 Serving/18g	52	3.2	288	7.2	25.6	18.0	1.3
M & S*	1 Cake/85g	174	8.1	205	9.7	20.3	9.5	1.2
Tesco*	1 Serving/130g	281	16.0	216	11.0	15.4	12.3	1.1
CRAB STICKS								
Average	1 Stick/15g	14	0.0	94	9.1	13.9	0.3	0.0
CRACKERBREAD								
High Fibre, Crackerbread, Ryvita*	1 Slice/5.2g	17	0.1	325	12.5	62.4	2.8	15.0
Rice, Ryvita*	1 Slice/5.1g	19	0.1	374	9.1	79.4	2.2	1.9
Sainsbury's*	1 Slice/5g	19	0.2	380	10.0	80.0	4.0	2.0
Wheat, Original, Ryvita*	1 Slice/5g	19	0.2	380	10.3	76.9	3.5	3.5
Wholemeal, Crackerbread, Ryvita*	1 Slice/5.6g	22	0.2	373	11.0	73.2	4.0	6.5
CRACKERS								
99% Fat Free, Rakusen's*	1 Cracker/10g	18	0.0	180	4.8	42.0	0.5	1.9
Bath Oliver, Jacob's*	1 Cracker/12g	52	1.6	432	9.6	67.6	13.7	2.6
Biscuits for Cheese, TTD, Sainsbury's*	1 Cracker/8g	39	1.9	493	8.6	61.0	23.8	3.1
Black Olive, M & S*	1 Cracker/4.1g	19	0.9	485	8.3	59.4	23.5	4.3
Bombay, Extra Spicy, Patak's*	1 Serving/30g	146	7.3	487	1.3	66.0	24.3	0.0
Bran, Jacob's*	1 Cracker/7g	32	1.3	454	9.7	62.8	18.2	3.2
Butter Puff, Sainsbury's*	1 Cracker/10g	54	2.7	523	10.4	60.7	26.5	2.5
Cheddars, McVitie's*	1 Cracker/4g	22	1.3	543	10.0	55.1	31.3	2.6
Cheese, Cheese Heads, Walkers*	1 Pack/27g	128	6.0	475	10.8	58.0	22.3	2.8
Cheese, Ritz*	1 Cracker/3.5g	19	1.0	486	10.1	55.9	24.7	2.2

C

CRACKERS

	Measure INFO/WEIGHT	per Measure KCAL	FAT	Nutrition Values per 100g / 100ml KCAL	PROT	CARB	FAT	FIBRE
Cheese, Trufree*	1 Cracker/8g	42	2.6	524	9.0	50.0	32.0	0.5
Cheese Biscuit Thins, Safeway*	1 Cracker/4g	22	1.3	545	11.9	52.6	31.9	2.5
Cheese Thins, Asda*	1 Cracker/4g	21	1.3	532	12.0	49.0	32.0	0.0
Cheese Thins, Cheddar, The Planet Snack Co*	1 Serving/30g	153	8.8	509	11.5	50.1	29.2	2.1
Cheese Thins, Co-Op*	1 Cracker/4g	21	1.3	530	12.0	49.0	32.0	3.0
Cheese Thins, Mini, Snack Rite*	1 Bag/30g	144	6.8	480	12.9	55.9	22.7	2.5
Cheese Thins, Waitrose*	1 Biscuit/4g	21	1.2	545	11.9	52.6	31.9	2.5
Chinese, Pop Pan*	2 Crackers/15g	80	5.0	533	13.3	53.3	33.3	0.0
Chives, Jacob's*	1 Cracker/6.1g	27	1.0	457	9.5	67.5	16.5	2.7
Choice Grain, Jacob's*	1 Cracker/7.5g	32	1.1	427	9.0	65.5	14.3	5.4
Corn Thins, 97% Fat Free, Real Foods*	1 Cracker/6g	19	0.2	378	10.2	81.7	3.0	8.6
Cornish Wafer, Jacob's*	1 Cracker/8.5g	45	2.7	527	8.3	53.2	31.2	3.0
Cream, Aldi*	1 Cracker/8g	36	1.2	456	9.1	71.7	14.7	3.0
Cream, Asda*	1 Cracker/8g	35	1.2	443	10.0	67.0	15.0	0.0
Cream, Average	1 Cracker/7g	31	1.1	440	9.5	68.3	16.3	2.2
Cream, BGTY, Sainsbury's*	1 Cracker/8g	32	0.6	400	10.9	71.7	7.7	3.1
Cream, Choice Grain, Jacob's*	1 Cracker/7g	30	0.9	400	9.0	64.5	11.8	7.0
Cream, Jacob's*	1 Cracker/7.9g	34	1.1	431	10.0	67.5	13.5	3.8
Cream, Light, Jacob's*	1 Biscuit/8g	31	0.5	388	10.6	72.2	6.3	4.1
Cream, Lower Fat, Tesco*	1 Cracker/5g	20	0.3	393	11.0	72.4	6.6	3.1
Cream, Morrisons*	1 Cracker/8g	36	1.2	446	9.6	68.5	14.8	2.7
Cream, Reduced Fat, Tesco*	1 Cracker/8g	31	0.5	406	10.9	74.4	7.2	2.8
Cream, Sainsbury's*	1 Cracker/8.3g	34	1.2	422	9.5	66.7	15.2	2.8
Cream, Sun Dried Tomato Flavour, Jacob's*	1 Cracker/8g	35	1.1	434	10.2	66.7	14.0	3.0
Cream, Tesco*	1 Cracker/7.7g	34	1.2	447	9.0	69.0	15.0	3.0
Cream with Flaked Salt, TTD, Sainsbury's*	1 Cracker/7.4g	35	1.6	500	8.5	64.8	22.9	2.7
Crispy Cheese, M & S*	1 Biscuit/4.3g	20	1.0	470	9.4	58.1	22.1	3.0
Extra Wheatgerm, Hovis*	1 Serving/6g	27	1.1	447	10.2	60.0	18.5	4.4
Harvest Grain, Sainsbury's*	1 Cracker/6g	27	1.1	458	8.5	64.5	18.4	4.1
Herb & Onion, 99% Fat Free, Rakusen's*	1 Cracker/5g	18	0.1	360	9.1	82.6	1.0	3.9
Herb & Onion, Trufree*	1 Cracker/6g	25	0.7	418	2.5	75.0	12.0	10.0
High Fibre, Trufree*	1 Cracker/6g	24	0.7	400	3.3	66.7	11.7	10.0
Italian, Doriano, Doria*	1 Pack/29.9g	137	4.9	458	9.3	68.2	16.4	3.3
Japanese Beef Teriyaki, Sensations, Walkers*	1 Serving/24g	118	6.3	490	1.4	62.0	26.0	3.5
Krackawheat, McVitie's*	1 Cracker/7.4g	33	1.4	446	9.7	60.0	18.6	5.8
Lightly Salted, Crispy, Sainsbury's*	1 Cracker/4.7g	27	1.4	533	7.8	62.6	27.9	2.1
Lightly Salted, Italian, Jacob's*	1 Cracker/6g	26	0.8	429	10.3	67.6	13.0	2.9
Mediterranean, Jacob's*	1 Cracker/6g	27	1.0	450	9.7	66.5	16.1	2.7
Mixed Seed, Multi Grain, Asda*	4 Crackers/25.2g	112	4.3	445	11.0	62.0	17.0	4.4
Multigrain, Tesco*	1 Cracker/6g	27	1.1	458	8.5	64.5	18.4	4.1
Olive Oil & Oregano, Mediterreaneo, Jacob's*	1 Cracker/6g	25	0.7	412	12.4	65.5	11.2	6.0
Oriental Style, Safeway*	1 Serving/25g	88	0.3	350	1.5	82.2	1.2	6.2
Peking Spare Rib & 5 Spice, Sensations, Walkers*	1 Bag/24g	116	6.2	485	1.3	62.0	26.0	3.5
Poppy & Sesame Seed, Sainsbury's*	1 Cracker/4g	21	1.1	530	9.6	58.9	28.4	3.4
Poppy & Sesame Thins, Morrisons*	1 Thin/3.1g	15	0.7	481	9.9	57.6	23.5	4.4
Ritz, Original, Jacob's*	1 Cracker/3.3g	17	1.0	509	6.9	55.6	28.8	2.0
Rye, Organic, Dove's Farm*	1 Cracker/7.1g	28	1.0	393	7.0	58.4	14.6	8.7
Salt & Black Pepper, Jacob's*	1 Cracker/6g	27	1.0	457	9.5	67.5	16.5	2.7
Salted, Ritz, Nabisco*	1 Cracker/3.4g	17	0.9	493	7.0	57.5	26.1	2.9
Selection, Finest, Tesco*	1 Serving/30g	136	4.3	452	9.6	71.0	14.4	0.0
Sesame & Poppy Thins, Tesco*	4 Crackers/16.5g	80	3.9	485	9.9	57.6	23.5	4.4
Spicy Indonesian Vegetable, Waitrose*	1 Pack/60g	295	16.3	492	1.2	60.6	27.2	2.2
Thai Spicy Vegetable, Sainsbury's*	1 Pack/50g	231	10.4	462	7.2	61.5	20.8	2.6

C

	INFO/WEIGHT	KCAL	FAT	KCAL	PROT	CARB	FAT	FIBRE
CRACKERS								
Tuc, Cheese Sandwich, Jacob's*	1 Cracker/13.6g	72	4.3	531	8.4	53.8	31.4	0.0
Tuc, Jacob's*	1 Cracker/5g	24	1.3	522	7.0	60.5	28.0	2.9
Tuc, Mini, with Sesame Seeds, Jacob's*	5 Crackers/10g	52	2.6	523	9.7	63.1	25.8	3.9
Waterthins, Wafers, Philemon*	6 Crackers/10g	39	0.4	392	10.6	77.9	3.6	5.0
Wheaten, M & S*	1 Cracker/4.4g	18	0.8	450	10.2	57.0	20.2	5.0
Wholemeal, Tesco*	1 Cracker/7g	29	1.0	414	9.4	60.6	14.9	10.4
Wholewheat, Saiwa*	1 Pack/31g	128	3.9	414	12.5	62.9	12.5	7.9
CRANBERRIES								
& Blueberries, Delicious, Boots*	1 Pack/75g	220	1.0	293	0.7	70.0	1.3	9.1
& Raisins, Dried, Sweetened, Ocean Spray*	1 Serving/50g	163	0.3	326	0.1	80.3	0.5	4.6
Dried, Sweetened, Average	1 Serving/10g	34	0.1	335	0.3	81.1	0.8	4.4
Fresh, Raw	1oz/28g	4	0.0	15	0.4	3.4	0.1	3.0
Raw	1oz/28g	19	0.2	67	14.9	0.0	0.8	0.0
CRAYFISH								
Tails, Chilli & Garlic, Asda*	1 Serving/140g	133	4.3	95	16.0	1.1	3.1	0.8
Tails, in Brine, Luxury, The Big Prawn Co*	½ Tub/90g	46	0.6	51	10.1	1.0	0.7	0.0
CREAM								
Aerosol, Average	1oz/28g	87	8.7	309	1.8	6.2	30.9	0.0
Aerosol, Real Dairy, Whipped, Sainsbury's*	1 Serving/55ml	43	4.4	79	0.4	1.4	8.0	0.0
Aerosol, Reduced Fat, Average	1 Serving/55ml	33	3.0	60	0.6	2.0	5.5	0.0
Brandy, Pourable, with Remy Martin*, Finest, Tesco*	½ Pot/125ml	460	35.5	368	2.7	19.8	28.4	0.0
Brandy, Really Thick, Finest, Tesco*	½ Pot/125ml	579	49.5	463	1.3	19.7	39.6	0.0
Clotted, Fresh, Average	1 Serving/28g	162	17.5	579	1.6	2.3	62.7	0.0
Double, Average	1 Serving/25ml	110	11.7	438	1.8	2.6	46.7	0.0
Double, Reduced Fat, Average	1 Serving/30g	73	7.0	243	2.7	5.7	23.3	0.1
Irish, Country, Tesco*	½ Pot 350mls	704	43.1	201	2.8	22.7	12.3	0.0
Oat Alternative, Dairy Free, Oatly*	1 Carton/250ml	375	32.5	150	1.0	6.0	13.0	0.8
Single, Average	1 Serving/50ml	62	5.3	123	2.7	4.4	10.5	0.1
Single, Extra Thick, Average	1 Serving/37.5ml	73	7.0	192	2.7	4.1	18.4	0.0
Single, Pouring, M & S*	1 Serving/50ml	94	9.0	188	2.6	3.9	18.0	0.0
Soured, Fresh, Average	1 Tbsp/15ml	29	2.8	191	2.7	3.9	18.4	0.0
Strawberry, Light, Real Dairy, Uht, Anchor*	1 Serving/12.5g	25	2.1	198	2.6	8.7	17.0	0.0
Thick, Sterilised, Average	1 Tbsp/15ml	35	3.5	233	2.6	3.6	23.1	0.0
Uht, Double, Average	1 Tbsp/15g	41	3.9	275	2.2	7.4	26.3	0.0
Uht, Reduced Fat, Average	1 Serving/25ml	16	1.4	62	0.6	2.3	5.7	0.0
Uht, Single, Average	1 Tbsp/15ml	29	2.8	194	2.6	4.0	18.8	0.0
Whipping, Average	1 Tbsp/15ml	52	5.5	348	2.1	3.2	36.4	0.1
CREAM HORN								
Fresh, Tesco*	1 Horn/57g	244	15.8	428	4.1	40.3	27.8	0.3
CREAM SODA								
American, with Vanilla, Tesco*	1 Glass/313ml	75	0.0	24	0.0	5.9	0.0	0.0
Diet, Sainsbury's*	1 Serving/250ml	3	0.0	1	0.0	0.0	0.0	0.0
No Added Sugar, Sainsbury's*	1 Can/330ml	2	0.3	1	0.1	0.1	0.1	0.1
Traditional Style, Tesco*	1 Can/330ml	139	0.0	42	0.0	10.4	0.0	0.0
CREME BRULEE								
Gastropub, M & S*	1 Brulee/83.8g	285	24.6	340	3.1	15.7	29.3	0.7
M & S*	1 Pot/100g	360	32.6	360	3.3	13.0	32.6	0.0
Somerfield*	1 Pot/100g	316	27.0	316	4.0	15.0	27.0	0.0
CREME CARAMEL								
Asda*	1 Pot/100g	113	2.6	113	2.4	20.0	2.6	0.0
Average	1 Portion/128g	140	2.8	109	3.0	20.6	2.2	0.0
Carmelle, Green's*	1 Pack/70g	82	2.8	117	3.0	17.0	4.0	0.0
La Laitiere*	1 Pot/100g	135	4.0	135	5.0	20.0	4.0	0.0

C

	Measure INFO/WEIGHT	per Measure KCAL	FAT	Nutrition Values per 100g / 100ml KCAL	PROT	CARB	FAT	FIBRE
CREME CARAMEL								
M & S*	1oz/28g	48	2.4	172	4.5	18.9	8.7	0.0
Morrisons*	1 Pot/100g	120	2.8	120	2.4	21.4	2.8	0.0
Sainsbury's*	1 Pot/100g	102	0.9	102	2.5	21.1	0.9	0.0
SmartPrice, Asda*	1 Pot/100g	87	0.5	87	2.5	18.0	0.5	0.0
Tesco*	1 Pot/100g	120	1.6	120	2.6	22.8	1.6	0.0
CREME EGG								
Cadbury*	1 Egg/39g	174	6.2	445	3.0	71.0	16.0	0.0
Minis, Cadbury*	1 Egg/11.2g	50	1.8	445	4.1	67.5	16.4	0.4
CREME FRAICHE								
Average	1 Pot/295g	1067	112.2	362	2.2	2.6	38.0	0.0
Cucumber & Mint, Triangles, Sainsbury's*	1 Serving/25g	105	2.4	421	11.0	72.3	9.7	2.5
Extra Light, President*	1 Tub/200g	182	10.0	91	2.7	8.7	5.0	0.0
Half Fat, Average	1 Tbsp/30g	54	4.9	181	3.1	5.5	16.3	0.0
Lemon & Rocket, Sainsbury's*	1 Serving/150g	188	17.3	125	2.2	3.0	11.5	0.5
CREPES								
Chocolate Filled, Tesco*	1 Crepe/32g	140	5.8	438	5.9	62.5	18.1	1.6
Lobster, Finest, Tesco*	1 Serving/160g	250	10.2	156	10.7	14.0	6.4	1.2
Mushroom, M & S*	1 Pack/186g	195	4.5	105	5.7	17.1	2.4	2.5
CRISPBAKES								
Bubble & Squeak, M & S*	1 Bake/46.5g	78	4.0	170	2.7	19.6	8.8	1.5
Cheese, Spring Onion & Chive, Sainsbury's*	1 Bake/113.5g	287	16.8	253	7.1	24.5	14.8	1.7
Cheese & Onion, Dalepak*	1 Bake/98.4g	239	12.6	243	7.2	24.1	12.8	1.7
Cheese & Onion, M & S*	1 Bake/114g	285	18.5	250	6.4	19.4	16.2	1.7
Cheese & Onion, Tesco*	1 Bake/109g	275	17.2	252	7.9	19.6	15.8	2.1
Chicken & Broccoli, M & S*	1 Bake/113.9g	205	10.4	180	7.4	17.1	9.1	1.7
Dutch, Asda*	1 Bake/7.8g	30	0.3	385	15.0	75.0	3.3	4.2
Dutch, HL, Tesco*	1 Bake/7.7g	30	0.2	385	14.7	74.9	2.7	4.2
Dutch, Sainsbury's*	1 Bake/9g	35	0.5	392	14.5	72.3	5.0	5.8
Minced Beef, M & S*	1 Bake/113g	226	12.3	200	10.0	15.6	10.9	1.5
Morrisons*	1 Bake/10.5g	44	0.8	420	13.7	73.5	8.0	2.2
Mushroom & Garlic, Ovenbaked, Iceland*	1 Bake/140g	241	9.4	172	4.3	23.7	6.7	2.9
Organic, Trimlyne*	1 Bake/10g	38	0.2	380	16.0	73.0	2.0	6.0
Roast Vegetable & Basil, Cauldron*	1 Bake/115g	242	11.0	210	3.5	26.0	9.6	2.9
Spinach, Cheese & Sweetcorn, Cauldron*	1 Bake/115g	233	12.2	203	5.6	21.3	10.6	2.1
Spinach, Feta & Soft Cheese, Mini, Safeway*	1 Bake/191.5g	449	25.6	235	6.6	20.8	13.4	2.5
Tuna & Sweetcorn, Lakeland*	1 Bake/170g	391	19.7	230	11.3	20.1	11.6	0.0
Vegetable, M & S*	1 Bake/114.3g	160	8.8	140	2.8	14.9	7.7	1.8
Vegetable, Sainsbury's*	1 Bake/114g	246	13.0	216	2.0	26.2	11.4	2.0
CRISPBREAD								
3 Seed, Classic, Gourmet, Dr Karg*	1 Bread/25g	108	4.9	430	16.5	46.6	19.7	10.9
Bran, Scandinavian, Gg*	2 Breads/16g	36	0.8	223	14.9	29.0	5.3	42.1
Corn, Orgran*	1 Bread/5g	18	0.1	360	7.5	83.0	1.8	3.0
Crisp 'n' Light, Wasa*	1 Crispbread/7g	24	0.1	360	12.0	73.0	2.2	5.3
Currant Crunch, Ryvita*	1oz/28g	94	0.7	334	8.7	69.9	2.5	12.8
Dark Rye, Morrisons*	1 Slice/13g	39	0.4	300	11.5	61.5	3.1	16.9
Dark Rye, Ryvita*	1 Slice/10g	31	0.2	311	8.5	65.5	1.7	18.0
Gluten Free, Dietary Specials*	1 Serving/8g	25	0.1	331	6.4	72.9	1.5	0.0
Light, M & S*	1 Bread/4.1g	15	0.2	370	10.7	71.8	4.6	5.0
Light, Ryvita*	1 Slice/5g	19	0.2	383	9.8	79.3	3.0	2.6
Minis, Apple, Ryvita*	1 Pack/30g	101	0.8	336	6.1	71.9	2.7	12.0
Minis, Cheese & Chives, Ryvita*	1 Pack/30g	103	0.9	342	8.0	71.0	2.9	11.5
Minis, Garlic & Herb, Ryvita*	1 Bag/30g	103	0.8	343	7.9	71.5	2.8	11.5
Minis, Mature Cheddar & Onion, Ryvita*	1 Bag/30g	101	0.9	337	9.3	68.2	3.0	11.5

C

CRISPBREAD

INFO/WEIGHT	Measure	per Measure KCAL	per Measure FAT	Nutrition Values per 100g / 100ml KCAL	PROT	CARB	FAT	FIBRE
Minis, Salt & Vinegar, Ryvita*	1 Pack/29.8g	93	0.8	312	6.8	64.8	2.8	12.1
Minis, Sweet Chilli, Ryvita*	1 Pack/30g	101	0.8	335	7.0	71.0	2.6	11.9
Minis, Worcester Sauce, Ryvita*	1 Pack/30g	102	0.8	339	6.9	71.9	2.6	12.0
Muesli Crunch, Ryvita*	1 Slice/15.6g	57	1.0	366	10.9	65.8	6.6	11.1
Multigrain, Ryvita*	1 Bread/11g	36	0.6	331	10.0	61.1	5.2	16.7
Original Rye, Wasa*	1 Bread/11g	35	0.2	315	9.0	67.0	1.4	14.0
Poppyseed, Wasa*	1 Bread/13g	46	1.0	350	13.0	56.0	8.0	14.0
Provita*	1 Biscuit/6g	26	0.6	416	12.5	68.4	9.9	0.0
Pumpkin Seeds & Oats, Ryvita*	1 Bread/12g	43	1.2	362	12.5	55.6	9.9	14.5
Roasted Onion, Organic, Dr Karg*	1 Bread/25g	98	3.7	390	15.8	48.5	14.8	12.9
Rounds, Multigrain, Finn Crisp*	1 Bread/8g	26	0.5	330	13.0	56.0	6.0	18.0
Rounds, Original, Rye, Finn Crisp*	1 Bread/14g	45	0.4	320	11.0	60.0	2.7	16.0
Rounds, Wholegrain Wheat, Finn Crisp*	1 Serving/50g	180	3.0	360	11.0	66.0	5.9	10.0
Rye, Original, Ryvita*	1 Bread/9g	29	0.2	317	8.5	66.6	1.7	16.5
Seeded, Spelt, Organic, Dr Karg*	1 Bread/25g	102	4.5	408	17.2	44.4	18.0	10.4
Sesame Rye, Ryvita*	1 Bread/10.5g	35	0.7	336	10.5	58.8	6.5	17.5
Snacks, Caribbean Chicken, Seasons, Quaker*	1 Pack/24g	101	2.1	421	7.9	77.1	8.9	2.1
Spelt, Sesame, Sunflower, Amisa*	1 Bread/28.5g	85	4.3	297	11.7	28.5	15.1	5.0
Sport, Wasa*	1 Slice/15g	47	0.2	310	9.0	64.0	1.5	16.0
Sunflower Seeds & Oats, Ryvita*	1 Slice/12g	42	1.1	348	10.1	57.2	8.8	16.7
Thin Crisps, Original Taste, Finn Crisp*	1 Slice/6.3g	20	0.2	320	11.0	63.0	2.4	19.0
Whole Grain, Crispy, Thin, Kavli*	3 Slices/15g	50	0.3	333	10.0	70.0	1.7	12.7
Wholemeal, Organic, Allinson*	1 Crispbread/5g	17	0.1	336	14.2	66.0	1.7	12.2
Wholemeal, Rye Sesame, Grafschafter*	1 Slice/10g	34	0.6	340	12.0	58.0	6.0	16.0
Wholemeal, Rye with Milk, Grafschafter*	1 Crispbread/9.3g	29	0.1	316	11.4	64.0	1.6	15.0
Wholemeal Rye, Organic, Kallo*	1 Slice/10g	31	0.2	314	9.7	65.0	1.7	15.4

CRISPS

INFO/WEIGHT	Measure	per Measure KCAL	per Measure FAT	Nutrition Values per 100g / 100ml KCAL	PROT	CARB	FAT	FIBRE
Apple, Thyme & Sage, M & S*	1 Bag/55g	253	13.4	460	5.5	55.3	24.3	6.1
Bacon, Shapers, Boots*	1 Bag/23g	99	3.5	431	8.0	66.0	15.0	3.0
Bacon Bites, Eat Smart, Safeway*	1 Bag/12g	41	0.2	340	10.8	70.3	1.6	3.5
Bacon Crispies, Sainsbury's*	1 Bag/25g	117	5.7	468	19.9	45.8	22.8	4.8
Bacon Flavour Rashers, BGTY, Sainsbury's*	1 Pack/10g	34	0.2	340	10.8	70.3	1.6	3.5
Bacon Flavour Rashers, Morrisons*	1 Pack/25.1g	122	6.6	487	16.3	46.4	26.3	3.8
Bacon Pillows, Light, Shapers, Boots*	1 Pack/12g	44	0.3	367	3.7	83.0	2.3	4.0
Bacon Rashers, M & S*	1 Pack/50g	238	11.6	475	8.8	57.5	23.2	2.8
Bacon Rashers, Tesco*	1 Serving/25g	125	6.4	500	7.1	59.8	25.5	4.0
Baked, Cheese & Onion, Walkers*	1 Pack/25g	99	2.1	395	6.5	73.0	8.5	5.5
Baked, Ready Salted, Walkers*	1 Pack/25g	98	2.0	390	6.0	74.0	8.0	5.5
Baked, Salt & Vinegar, Walkers*	1 Pack/25g	98	2.0	390	6.0	73.0	8.0	5.0
Baked Bean Flavour, Walkers*	1 Bag/35g	184	11.6	525	6.5	50.0	33.0	4.0
Banging BBQ, Shots, Walkers*	1 Pack/17.9g	87	4.5	485	5.5	60.0	25.0	1.3
Barbecue, Handcooked, Tesco*	1 Bag/40g	187	10.0	468	6.6	53.8	25.1	5.2
Barbecue, Snack Rite*	1 Bag/25g	131	8.3	524	5.1	51.3	33.2	0.0
Barbecue, Sunseed Oil, Walkers*	1 Pack/25g	131	8.3	525	6.5	50.0	33.0	4.0
Barbecue Beef, Select, Tesco*	1 Pack/25g	134	8.7	536	6.4	49.2	34.8	4.4
BBQ Chilli & Mesquite, Pan-Fried, TTD, Sainsbury's*	1 Pack/50g	239	13.4	478	8.0	51.3	26.7	5.4
BBQ Rib, Sunseed, Walkers*	1 Bag/25g	131	8.3	525	6.5	50.0	33.0	4.0
Beef, Squares, Walkers*	1 Bag/25g	105	4.5	420	6.0	59.0	18.0	4.6
Beef & Onion, Asda*	1 Bag/25g	129	7.8	516	5.7	53.3	31.1	3.9
Beef & Onion, Potato, M & S*	1 Bag/24.5g	133	8.6	530	6.6	48.2	34.5	5.0
Beef & Onion, Tayto*	1 Bag/35g	184	11.9	526	7.6	47.3	34.0	4.5
Beef & Onion, Walkers*	1 Bag/35g	184	11.6	525	6.5	50.0	33.0	4.0
Beefy, Smiths, Walkers*	1 Bag/25g	133	9.3	531	4.3	45.2	37.0	0.0

CRISPS

INFO/WEIGHT	Measure	per Measure		Nutrition Values per 100g / 100ml				
		KCAL	FAT	KCAL	PROT	CARB	FAT	FIBRE
Buffalo Mozzarella Tomato & Basil, Kettle Chips*	1 Pack/150g	714	38.6	476	6.7	54.4	25.7	4.9
Chargrilled Steak, Max, Walkers*	1 Bag/55g	289	18.2	525	6.5	50.0	33.0	4.0
Cheddar & Onion, McCoys*	1 Bag/50g	258	15.3	516	7.0	53.2	30.6	3.9
Cheddar & Red Onion Chutney, Sensations, Walkers*	1 Bag/40g	198	11.2	495	6.5	54.0	28.0	4.5
Cheddar & Spring Onion, 35% Less Fat, Sainsbury's*	1 Pack/20g	93	4.2	463	6.3	62.4	20.9	0.9
Cheddar & Spring Onion, TTD, Sainsbury's*	1 Serving/30g	140	8.2	465	6.7	48.3	27.2	7.8
Cheddar Cheese, Sunseed Oil, Walkers*	1 Bag/34.5g	181	11.4	525	6.5	50.0	33.0	4.0
Cheese & Branston Pickle, Walkers*	1 Bag/34.5g	181	11.4	525	6.5	50.0	33.0	4.0
Cheese & Chive Flavour, GFY, Asda*	1 Bag/25g	119	6.0	476	6.0	59.0	24.0	6.0
Cheese & Chives, Walkers*	1 Bag/35g	186	11.6	530	6.5	50.0	33.0	4.1
Cheese & Onion, 30% Less Fat, Sainsbury's*	1 Pack/25g	115	5.5	459	7.5	58.1	21.8	5.4
Cheese & Onion, Asda*	1 Bag/25g	129	7.8	517	5.7	53.6	31.1	4.0
Cheese & Onion, BGTY, Sainsbury's*	1 Bag/25g	120	6.2	479	7.0	57.0	24.8	5.7
Cheese & Onion, GFY, Asda*	1 Pack/26g	122	5.7	470	7.0	61.0	22.0	4.2
Cheese & Onion, Golden Wonder*	1 Bag/25g	131	8.4	524	6.1	49.2	33.6	2.0
Cheese & Onion, KP Snacks*	1 Bag/25g	134	8.7	534	6.6	48.7	34.8	4.8
Cheese & Onion, Lights, Walkers*	1 Bag/28g	132	5.9	470	7.5	62.0	21.0	5.0
Cheese & Onion, Limbos, Ryvita*	1 Pack/18g	63	0.5	352	12.1	69.1	3.0	9.3
Cheese & Onion, M & S*	1 Bag/25g	134	8.9	535	5.5	48.8	35.5	5.0
Cheese & Onion, Max, Walkers*	1 Pack/50g	263	16.0	525	6.8	52.0	32.0	5.2
Cheese & Onion, McCoys*	1 Bag/35g	181	10.7	517	7.1	53.1	30.6	4.0
Cheese & Onion, Morrisons*	1 Pack/25g	132	8.3	529	6.1	51.8	33.0	4.4
Cheese & Onion, Organic, Tesco*	1 Bag/25g	129	8.2	514	5.2	49.9	32.6	7.0
Cheese & Onion, Oven Baked, Tesco*	1 Bag/25g	103	1.7	410	5.3	74.7	6.6	7.7
Cheese & Onion, Potato Heads, Walkers*	1 Pack/23g	108	5.3	470	6.0	60.0	23.0	5.5
Cheese & Onion, Safeway*	1 Bag/25g	143	9.4	570	5.8	52.5	37.5	0.0
Cheese & Onion, Sainsbury's*	1 Bag/25g	132	8.7	527	4.6	48.8	34.8	3.9
Cheese & Onion, Squares, Walkers*	1 Bag/25g	108	4.5	430	6.5	61.0	18.0	5.5
Cheese & Onion, Sunseed Oil, Walkers*	1 Bag/55g	289	18.2	525	7.0	50.0	33.0	4.0
Cheese & Onion, Tayto*	1 Bag/25g	132	8.5	526	7.6	47.3	34.0	4.5
Cheese & Onion, Tesco*	1 Pack/25g	133	8.3	530	5.8	51.6	33.2	4.4
Cheese & Onion, Value, Tesco*	1 Bag/20g	108	7.2	541	6.0	48.3	36.0	4.8
Cheese & Onion Rings, Crunchy, Shapers, Boots*	1 Bag/15g	56	0.4	374	5.9	81.0	2.9	2.0
Cheese Curls, Asda*	1 Bag/14g	74	4.5	528	5.0	55.0	32.0	2.1
Cheese Curls, Morrisons*	1 Bag/14g	71	4.5	510	4.5	55.0	32.0	2.6
Cheese Curls, Shapers, Boots*	1 Pack/13.9g	68	3.8	489	4.5	57.0	27.0	2.7
Cheese Curls, Sprinters*	1 Bag/14g	68	3.8	483	4.1	56.4	26.8	0.0
Cheese Curls, Tesco*	1 Bag/14.4g	75	4.5	520	4.5	54.4	31.1	1.9
Cheese Tasters, M & S*	1 Bag/20g	103	5.9	515	8.1	55.0	29.3	1.7
Cheese XI, Golden Wonder*	1 Bag/30g	155	9.6	516	6.2	50.6	32.1	4.2
Cheesy Curls, Bobby's*	1 Bag/40g	225	14.8	563	7.6	50.1	36.9	0.0
Cheesy Puffs, Co-Op*	1 Bag/60g	321	20.4	535	3.0	54.0	34.0	2.0
Chicken, Firecracker, McCoys*	1 Bag/35g	177	10.3	506	6.2	54.0	29.5	4.0
Chicken Flavour, HE, Tesco*	1 Bag/12g	43	0.2	357	5.1	81.0	1.4	3.4
Chilli & Lemon, Walkers*	1 Pack/25g	131	8.3	525	6.3	51.0	33.0	3.8
Chilli Salsa & Lime, Handcooked, M & S*	1 Serving/40g	184	10.2	460	6.5	51.0	25.5	8.1
Chinese Sizzling Beef, McCoys*	1 Bag/35g	178	10.6	506	6.9	51.8	30.2	4.0
Chinese Spare Rib, Walkers*	1 Bag/25g	131	8.3	525	6.5	50.0	33.0	4.0
Chinese Szechaun Chicken, Hand Cooked, Asda*	1 Serving/50g	254	15.5	507	6.0	51.0	31.0	3.4
Corn Chips, Fritos*	1 Pack/42.5g	240	15.0	565	4.7	56.5	35.3	0.0
Cracked Black Pepper Seasoned, TTD, Sainsbury's*	1 Bag/30g	145	7.9	484	7.0	54.6	26.4	4.0
Cream Cheese & Chive, Waffles, Spar*	1 Pack/27g	132	6.8	488	4.2	60.7	25.3	1.3
Crispy Bacon Bites, Shapers, Boots*	1 Packet/21g	99	4.6	471	8.6	61.9	21.9	1.9

CRISPS

	Measure INFO/WEIGHT	per Measure KCAL	per Measure FAT	Nutrition Values per 100g / 100ml KCAL	PROT	CARB	FAT	FIBRE
Crunchy Twirls, Salt & Vinegar, Red Mill*	1 Pack/38g	170	7.4	447	4.7	62.4	19.5	3.4
Double Gloucester & Red Onion, Kettle Chips*	1 Serving/40g	188	9.9	471	6.6	55.5	24.7	4.8
Flame Grilled Steak, McCoys*	1 Bag/50g	258	15.4	516	7.0	53.0	30.7	4.0
Four Cheese & Red Onion, Sensations, Walkers*	1 Bag/40g	194	10.8	485	6.5	54.0	27.0	4.5
Garlic & Herbs Creme Fraiche, Kettle Chips*	1 Bag/50g	249	14.2	497	6.0	54.7	28.3	4.2
Handcooked, M & S*	1 Portion/40g	184	10.3	460	6.3	50.5	25.8	7.8
Heinz Tomato Ketchup, Sunseed, Walkers*	1 Bag/35g	182	11.2	520	6.5	51.0	32.0	4.0
Honey Roast Ham, Crinkle, Reduced Fat, M & S*	1 Pack/40g	178	8.1	445	6.3	58.7	20.3	5.6
Honey Roast Wiltshire Ham, Full on Flavour, M & S*	1 Serving/30g	153	8.8	510	6.6	53.6	29.2	6.0
Honey Roasted Ham, Sensations, Walkers*	1 Bag/40g	196	10.8	490	6.5	55.0	27.0	4.0
Lamb & Mint, Slow Roasted, Sensations, Walkers*	1 Bag/35g	170	9.5	485	6.5	54.0	27.0	4.5
Lamb & Mint, Sunseed Oil, Walkers*	1 Pack/34.5g	181	11.4	525	6.5	50.0	33.0	4.0
Lant Chips, Ikea*	1 Serving/25g	126	6.9	505	8.3	55.9	27.6	4.5
Lighly Salted, Organic, Kettle Chips*	1 Serving/40g	198	11.4	495	5.5	54.1	28.5	4.4
Lightly Salted, Baked, COU, M & S*	1 Bag/26g	91	0.6	350	8.5	76.4	2.3	5.7
Lightly Salted, Handcooked, Finest, Tesco*	½ Pack/150g	708	39.2	472	6.4	52.9	26.1	5.1
Lightly Salted, Kettle Chips*	1 Serving/50g	243	13.3	485	3.2	55.1	26.6	5.2
Lightly Salted, Low Fat, Waitrose*	1 Bag/25g	125	6.3	500	7.5	61.3	25.0	4.8
Lightly Sea Salted, Jonathan Crisp*	1 Bag/35g	176	10.2	503	6.5	52.0	29.0	5.4
Lightly Sea Salted, Potato Chips, Hand Fried, Burts*	¼ Bag/50g	252	13.9	504	6.4	57.4	27.7	0.0
Lime & Thai Spices, Sensations, Walkers*	1 Pack/40g	200	11.6	500	6.5	54.0	29.0	4.0
Mango Chilli, Kettle Chips*	1 Packet/50g	238	12.0	475	6.3	53.9	24.0	6.1
Marmite, Sunseed, Walkers*	1 Bag/34.5g	179	11.4	520	6.5	49.0	33.0	4.0
Mature Cheddar & Chive, Kettle Chips*	1 Serving/50g	239	12.7	478	8.1	54.4	25.4	5.0
Mediterranean Baked Potato, COU, M & S*	1 Pack/25g	90	0.6	360	7.6	74.0	2.4	6.8
Mexican Chilli, McCoys*	1 Bag/35g	177	10.5	511	7.1	52.8	30.2	4.1
Mexican Lime with a Hint of Chilli, Kettle Chips*	1 Serving/50g	242	13.8	484	5.0	54.1	27.5	5.4
New York Cheddar, Kettle Chips*	1 Bag/50g	242	13.4	483	6.7	53.9	26.7	4.5
Onion Rings, Asda*	1 Serving/30g	153	8.3	510	7.0	58.6	27.5	1.8
Onion Rings, Crunchy, Shapers, Boots*	1 Bag/12g	61	3.4	507	2.5	62.0	28.0	2.6
Onion Rings, M & S*	1 Pack/40g	186	8.6	465	5.2	62.1	21.5	4.3
Onion Rings, Maize Snacks, Sainsbury's*	¼ Bag/25g	122	6.6	488	5.6	56.9	26.4	1.7
Onion Rings, Maize Snacks, Value, Tesco*	1 Pack/14g	75	4.4	536	5.7	57.1	31.4	0.7
Onion Rings, Tayto*	1 Pack/16.9g	82	4.1	484	3.0	63.4	24.0	2.4
Onion Rings, Tesco*	1 Serving/16g	79	4.1	495	8.4	57.8	25.5	2.5
Paprika, Handcooked, Shapers, Boots*	1 Bag/20g	99	4.8	493	7.2	62.0	24.0	5.0
Paprika, Max, Walkers*	1 Bag/55g	286	17.5	520	6.5	52.0	31.9	5.1
Paprika, Mini Hoops, Shapers, Boots*	1 Bag/13.0g	64	3.5	494	8.7	54.0	27.0	2.2
Parsnip, Passions, Snack Rite*	1 Serving/25g	124	9.4	494	4.5	34.5	37.6	18.8
Parsnip & Black Pepper, Sainsbury's*	1 Serving/35g	166	11.1	473	3.2	43.6	31.8	15.2
Pickled Onion, Beastie Bites, Asda*	1 Bag/20g	100	5.2	498	6.0	60.0	26.0	0.0
Pickled Onion, Golden Wonder*	1 Bag/25g	131	8.5	524	5.6	49.0	34.0	2.0
Pickled Onion, M & S*	1 Bag/20.3g	69	0.3	345	5.0	81.7	1.5	3.7
Pickled Onion, Monster Bites, Sainsbury's*	1 Bag/20g	107	6.7	535	5.2	53.5	33.3	1.0
Pickled Onion, Stompers, Morrisons*	1 Pack/25g	129	7.9	518	6.1	52.2	31.6	1.3
Pickled Onion, Sunseed, Walkers*	1 Bag/35g	184	11.6	525	6.5	50.0	33.0	4.0
Pickled Onion, Tesco*	1 Bag/20g	104	7.0	520	6.5	50.0	35.0	1.0
Pickled Onion Rings, BGTY, Sainsbury's*	1 Bag/10g	35	0.2	345	5.0	81.7	1.5	3.7
Potato, Baked, COU, M & S*	1 Bag/25g	88	0.6	350	8.5	76.4	2.3	5.7
Potato, Cheddar & Onion, Hand Cooked, Aldi*	1 Pack/150g	753	41.9	502	7.7	54.9	27.9	4.0
Potato, Tyrells*	1 Pack/261g	1362	72.8	522	6.1	56.5	27.9	0.0
Potato Squares, Ready Salted, Sainsbury's*	1 Bag/50g	192	8.0	384	6.5	53.8	15.9	7.8
Potato Sticks, Ready Salted, M & S*	1 Pack/75g	398	24.8	530	6.5	52.0	33.0	4.0

CRISPS

	Measure INFO/WEIGHT	per Measure		Nutrition Values per 100g / 100ml				
		KCAL	FAT	KCAL	PROT	CARB	FAT	FIBRE
Potato Triangles, Ready Salted, Sainsbury's*	½ Pack/50g	243	11.7	486	9.4	59.7	23.4	3.4
Potato Tubes, Lightly Salted, Shapers, Boots*	1 Bag/14.9g	65	3.0	435	5.8	59.0	20.0	6.4
Prawn Cocktail, Asda*	1 Bag/25g	134	8.8	535	6.0	49.0	35.0	4.3
Prawn Cocktail, Golden Wonder*	1 Bag/25g	130	8.4	521	5.8	49.0	33.5	2.0
Prawn Cocktail, KP Snacks*	1 Bag/25g	133	8.7	531	5.9	48.4	34.9	4.7
Prawn Cocktail, Lites, Advantage, Tayto*	1 Pack/21g	96	4.1	455	5.3	65.1	19.3	3.8
Prawn Cocktail, Lites, Shapers, Boots*	1 Bag/21g	92	3.8	438	5.1	64.0	18.0	4.1
Prawn Cocktail, M & S*	1 Bag/30.1g	155	8.6	515	6.2	58.0	28.6	2.2
Prawn Cocktail, Sainsbury's*	1 Bag/25g	130	8.7	521	4.3	47.5	34.9	3.9
Prawn Cocktail, Seabrook*	1 Bag/32g	150	7.1	472	5.4	66.7	22.3	3.8
Prawn Cocktail, Snack Rite*	1 Bag/25g	129	8.3	516	5.0	49.2	33.2	0.0
Prawn Cocktail, Sunseed Oil, Walkers*	1 Bag/34.5g	181	11.4	525	6.5	50.0	33.0	4.0
Prawn Cocktail, Tayto*	1 Bag/35g	185	12.3	526	7.5	46.6	35.0	4.5
Prawn Cocktail, Tesco*	1 Pack/25g	135	8.2	540	5.2	52.0	32.8	4.0
Prawn Cocktail Flavour, Morrisons*	1 Bag/25g	131	8.3	525	5.1	51.9	33.0	4.1
Prawn Crackers, Tesco*	1 Bag/60g	316	17.5	527	3.2	62.8	29.2	0.8
Ready Salted, 30% Less Fat, Sainsbury's*	1 Serving/25g	122	5.6	486	7.3	63.7	22.4	8.2
Ready Salted, Bettabuy, Morrisons*	1 Bag/22g	119	7.8	539	4.7	50.0	35.6	4.2
Ready Salted, BGTY, Sainsbury's*	1 Bag/25g	122	6.6	486	6.8	55.7	26.2	6.6
Ready Salted, Co-Op*	1 Bag/25g	131	8.5	525	6.0	51.0	34.0	3.0
Ready Salted, GFY, Asda*	1 Bag/23g	109	5.3	475	7.0	60.0	23.0	4.3
Ready Salted, Golden Wonder*	1 Bag/25g	135	8.8	539	5.5	49.9	35.3	2.0
Ready Salted, KP Snacks*	1 Bag/24g	131	8.8	545	5.6	47.9	36.8	4.9
Ready Salted, Lidl*	1 Bag/25g	139	9.3	554	4.9	50.3	37.0	0.0
Ready Salted, M & S*	1 Bag/25g	136	9.2	545	5.6	47.8	36.6	4.9
Ready Salted, McCoys*	1 Bag/49g	253	15.4	517	6.0	52.3	31.5	4.9
Ready Salted, Morrisons*	1 Bag/25g	134	8.7	536	4.9	50.9	34.8	4.3
Ready Salted, Organic, Tesco*	1 Bag/25g	130	8.5	520	4.3	49.0	34.1	7.3
Ready Salted, Potato Chips, Tesco*	1 Bag/25g	132	8.3	526	5.6	51.7	33.0	3.8
Ready Salted, Reduced Fat, Tesco*	1 Pack/25g	114	6.2	456	6.3	52.0	24.7	5.9
Ready Salted, Safeway*	1 Serving/50g	264	16.5	528	5.6	52.2	33.0	3.8
Ready Salted, Sainsbury's*	1 Bag/25g	135	9.2	538	4.3	47.4	36.8	4.1
Ready Salted, Select, Tesco*	1 Bag/25g	136	9.2	544	6.2	47.9	36.6	4.5
Ready Salted, SmartPrice, Asda*	1 Bag/20g	111	7.4	553	5.0	50.0	37.0	3.0
Ready Salted, Snack Rite*	1 Bag/25g	136	9.0	545	4.9	50.3	36.0	0.0
Ready Salted, Squares, M & S*	1 Bag/35g	151	6.3	430	6.8	63.5	18.1	3.9
Ready Salted, Squares, Walkers*	1 Pack/25g	109	4.8	435	6.5	60.0	19.0	6.0
Ready Salted, Sunseed Oil, Walkers*	1 Bag/35g	186	11.9	530	6.5	49.0	34.0	4.0
Ready Salted, Value, Tesco*	1 Bag/21g	115	7.6	548	6.0	50.0	36.0	0.0
Red Leicester & Spring Onion, Handcooked, M & S*	1 Pack/40g	194	10.6	485	6.8	55.0	26.4	5.1
Roast Beef & Mustard, Thick Cut, Brannigans*	1 Bag/40g	203	12.0	507	7.6	51.7	30.0	3.7
Roast Chicken, Golden Wonder*	1 Bag/25g	131	8.4	522	6.2	48.6	33.6	2.0
Roast Chicken, Highlander*	1 Bag/25g	139	9.7	554	5.3	46.0	38.9	5.1
Roast Chicken, Morrisons*	1 Pack/25g	131	8.2	525	5.5	51.7	32.9	4.2
Roast Chicken, Select, Tesco*	1 Bag/25g	134	8.8	536	6.6	48.6	35.0	4.4
Roast Chicken, Snack Rite*	1 Bag/25g	132	8.3	526	5.3	51.3	33.3	0.0
Roast Chicken, Sunseed Oil, Walkers*	1 Bag/35g	184	11.6	525	6.5	50.0	33.0	4.0
Roast Chicken Flavour, Budgens*	1 Bag/25g	129	8.3	516	7.3	47.6	33.0	3.6
Roasted Lamb, Moroccan, Sensations, Walkers*	1 Bag/40g	198	11.6	495	6.0	53.0	29.0	4.5
Root Vegetable, TTD, Sainsbury's*	¼ Pack/25g	115	8.2	460	5.7	35.9	32.6	16.4
Salsa with Mesquite, Kettle Chips*	1 Serving/50g	231	12.1	462	5.8	55.2	24.2	5.7
Salt & Black Pepper, Handcooked, M & S*	1 Bag/40g	180	9.2	450	5.7	55.0	22.9	5.2
Salt & Malt Vinegar, Hunky Dorys*	1 Serving/30.1g	141	8.6	469	6.3	49.3	28.7	0.0

CRISPS

	Measure INFO/WEIGHT	per Measure KCAL	FAT	Nutrition Values per 100g / 100ml KCAL	PROT	CARB	FAT	FIBRE
Salt & Malt Vinegar, McCoys*	1 Bag/50g	256	15.2	512	6.8	52.8	30.4	3.9
Salt & Malt Vinegar Flavour, Sainsbury's*	1 Bag/25g	135	8.8	538	4.9	50.3	35.2	2.3
Salt & Shake, Walkers*	1 Bag/25g	135	8.8	540	6.5	50.0	35.0	4.0
Salt & Vinegar, 30% Less Fat, Sainsbury's*	1 Bag/25g	115	5.5	458	7.2	58.3	21.8	5.1
Salt & Vinegar, BGTY, Sainsbury's*	1 Bag/25g	121	6.3	482	6.5	57.3	25.2	5.2
Salt & Vinegar, Crinkle, M & S*	1 Pack/24.7g	121	6.0	485	6.5	61.0	24.0	3.5
Salt & Vinegar, Crinkle, Reduced Fat, M & S*	1 Pack/40g	175	8.1	438	4.8	60.0	20.3	5.5
Salt & Vinegar, Crinkle Cut, Seabrook*	1 Bag/31.8g	182	11.7	569	5.4	54.4	36.7	3.9
Salt & Vinegar, Everyday, Co-Op*	1 Bag/17g	77	3.4	455	6.0	62.0	20.0	2.0
Salt & Vinegar, GFY, Asda*	1 Bag/26g	120	5.7	466	6.0	61.0	22.0	4.1
Salt & Vinegar, Golden Lights, Golden Wonder*	1 Bag/21g	94	3.9	446	4.2	65.7	18.5	3.7
Salt & Vinegar, Golden Wonder*	1 Bag/25g	131	8.5	522	5.4	48.5	34.0	2.0
Salt & Vinegar, HE, Tesco*	1 Bag/17g	61	0.3	357	3.2	82.4	1.6	3.0
Salt & Vinegar, in Sunflower Oil, Sainsbury's*	1 Serving/25g	131	8.5	524	5.2	49.7	33.8	3.7
Salt & Vinegar, KP Snacks*	1 Bag/25g	133	8.8	532	5.5	48.7	35.0	4.7
Salt & Vinegar, Lights, Walkers*	1 Bag/28g	133	6.2	475	7.0	62.0	22.0	4.5
Salt & Vinegar, Limbos, Ryvita*	1 Pack/18g	62	0.3	344	9.8	72.0	1.9	7.8
Salt & Vinegar, Lower Fat, Asda*	1 Bag/25g	120	6.3	481	5.0	58.0	25.0	4.8
Salt & Vinegar, M & S*	1 Bag/25g	131	8.6	525	5.4	48.8	34.5	4.6
Salt & Vinegar, Max, Walkers*	1 Bag/55g	289	18.2	525	6.5	50.0	33.0	4.0
Salt & Vinegar, Morrisons*	1 Bag/25g	129	7.8	515	4.9	53.9	31.1	3.6
Salt & Vinegar, Red Mill*	1 Bag/40g	174	7.0	436	3.9	65.8	17.5	2.4
Salt & Vinegar, Sainsbury's*	1 Bag/25g	131	8.8	522	4.1	46.9	35.3	3.9
Salt & Vinegar, Select, Tesco*	1 Bag/25g	132	8.7	529	5.9	47.8	34.9	4.3
Salt & Vinegar, Snack Rite*	1 Bag/25g	127	8.3	508	4.7	48.1	33.0	0.0
Salt & Vinegar, Squares, Walkers*	1 Bag/25g	108	4.5	430	6.5	61.0	18.0	5.5
Salt & Vinegar, Sunseed Oil, Walkers*	1 Bag/35g	184	11.6	525	6.5	50.0	33.0	4.0
Salt & Vinegar, Tayto*	1 Bag/35g	184	11.9	526	7.6	47.3	34.0	4.5
Salt & Vinegar, Value, Tesco*	1 Bag/20g	109	7.4	547	5.7	47.7	37.0	4.8
Salt & Vinegar, Waitrose*	1 Pack/25g	132	8.5	529	6.3	50.5	33.8	4.4
Salt & Vinegar Flavour, Asda*	1 Bag/25g	131	8.5	522	6.0	48.0	34.0	4.2
Salt & Vinegar Flavour, Half Fat, M & S*	1 Bag/40g	168	6.8	420	5.8	61.0	17.0	7.7
Salt & Vinegar Flavour, Sprinters*	1 Bag/25g	133	8.8	532	4.8	49.1	35.2	0.0
Salt & Vinegar Fries, COU, M & S*	1 Bag/25g	85	0.4	340	5.0	80.0	1.6	4.0
Salt & Vinegar Spirals, Shapers, Boots*	1 Pack/15g	71	3.4	475	3.1	64.0	23.0	1.7
Salted Tubes, Shapers, Boots*	1 Bag/15g	67	3.0	448	5.1	62.0	20.0	3.6
Sausage & Tomato Flavour, Golden Wonder*	1 Bag/34.5g	177	10.7	505	6.1	51.3	30.6	4.5
Sea Salt, Golden Lights, Golden Wonder*	1 Bag/21g	94	3.9	448	3.9	66.4	18.5	4.4
Sea Salt, Handcooked, Extra Special, Asda*	1 Pack/31g	149	7.8	477	7.0	56.0	25.0	4.1
Sea Salt, Original, Crinkle Cut, Seabrook*	1 Bag/31.8g	182	11.7	569	5.4	54.4	36.7	3.9
Sea Salt, TTD, Sainsbury's*	1 Serving/50g	236	12.9	472	6.2	53.6	25.8	5.2
Sea Salt & Balsamic Vinegar, Kettle Chips*	1 Bag/50g	245	13.8	489	6.8	53.5	27.5	4.9
Sea Salt & Balsamic Vineger, Low Fat, Peak*	1 Serving/25g	87	0.4	348	7.4	76.6	1.4	6.7
Sea Salt & Black Pepper, Highlander*	1 Serving/25g	141	9.6	564	5.6	44.0	38.4	4.8
Sea Salt & Black Pepper, Sensations, Walkers*	1 Bag/40g	196	10.8	490	6.5	55.0	27.0	4.0
Sea Salt & Malt Vinegar, Sensations, Walkers*	1 Bag/40g	194	10.8	485	6.5	54.0	27.0	4.5
Simply Salted, Lights, Walkers*	1 Bag/24g	113	5.3	470	7.0	61.0	22.0	5.0
Sizzling Beef, Spice, McCoys*	1 Bag/35g	175	10.4	501	6.4	51.7	29.8	4.0
Smoked Ham & Pickle, Thick Cut, Brannigans*	1 Bag/40g	203	11.9	507	7.0	52.8	29.8	3.8
Smokey Bacon, Budgens*	1 Bag/25g	130	8.3	519	6.2	49.3	33.0	4.8
Smokey Bacon, Crinkle, Shapers, Boots*	1 Pack/20g	96	4.8	482	6.6	60.0	24.0	4.0
Smokey Bacon, Limbos, Ryvita*	1 Pack/18g	63	0.3	350	0.0	7.8	1.7	7.8
Smokey Bacon, Seabrook*	1 Bag/32g	181	11.7	569	5.4	54.4	36.7	3.9

	Measure INFO/WEIGHT	per Measure		Nutrition Values per 100g / 100ml				
		KCAL	FAT	KCAL	PROT	CARB	FAT	FIBRE
CRISPS								
Smokey Bacon, Select, Tesco*	1 Bag/25g	134	8.7	536	6.4	49.0	34.9	4.3
Smoky Bacon, Asda*	1 Bag/25g	133	8.5	530	6.0	50.0	34.0	4.5
Smoky Bacon, Golden Wonder*	1 Bag/25g	131	8.4	523	5.9	49.1	33.7	2.0
Smoky Bacon, Sainsbury's*	1 Bag/25g	132	8.6	529	5.7	49.5	34.2	4.4
Smoky Bacon, Snack Rite*	1 Bag/25g	131	8.3	525	5.5	51.2	33.1	0.0
Smoky Bacon, Sunseed Oil, Walkers*	1 Bag/34g	180	11.2	530	6.5	51.0	33.0	4.0
Smoky Bacon, Tayto*	1 Bag/35g	184	11.9	526	7.6	47.3	34.0	4.5
Snaps, Spicy Tomato Flavour, Walkers*	1 Bag/17.9g	91	4.8	508	1.5	65.5	26.8	0.0
Snax, Tayto*	1 Pack/17g	82	3.7	483	2.4	70.0	21.5	1.6
Sour Cream & Chive, Crinkle, Reduced Fat, M & S*	1 Bag/40g	178	8.2	445	5.6	58.8	20.6	5.6
Sour Cream & Chive, Lights, Walkers*	1 Bag/24g	114	5.3	475	7.5	62.0	22.0	5.0
Sour Cream & Chive Crinkles, Shapers, Boots*	1 Bag/20g	96	4.8	482	6.6	60.0	24.0	4.0
Sour Cream & Chive Crispy Discs, Shapers, Boots*	1 Bag/21g	94	4.0	448	5.7	61.9	19.0	4.3
Sour Cream & Chives, Jordans*	1 Bag/30g	125	3.6	417	7.3	69.9	12.0	2.7
Space Raiders, Beef, KP Snacks*	1 Bag/12.9g	62	2.9	479	7.0	61.5	22.8	3.6
Space Raiders, Cheese, KP Snacks*	1 Bag/16g	76	3.5	473	7.1	61.6	22.0	3.1
Space Raiders, Pickled Onion, KP Snacks*	1 Bag/16g	77	3.7	480	6.7	61.3	23.3	4.0
Space Raiders, Salt & Vinegar, KP Snacks*	1 Bag/16.9g	81	3.8	478	6.9	61.7	22.6	2.2
Spare Rib Flavour, Chinese, Walkers*	1 Bag/34.5g	184	11.6	525	6.5	50.0	33.0	4.0
Spiced Chilli, McCoys*	1 Bag/35g	175	10.1	500	6.1	54.2	28.8	4.2
Spicy Chilli, Sunseed, Walkers*	1 Pack/34.5g	183	11.4	530	6.5	51.0	33.0	4.0
Spring Onion, Seabrook*	1 Bag/32g	182	11.7	569	5.4	54.4	36.7	3.9
Steak & Onion, Walkers*	1 Pack/34.5g	179	11.4	520	6.5	49.0	33.0	4.0
Sweet Chilli, Hand Cooked, Asda*	1 Pack/25g	120	7.1	479	5.7	54.5	28.3	4.5
Sweet Chilli & Red Peppers, Fusion, Tayto*	1 Pack/28g	140	8.3	500	4.9	52.2	29.8	4.6
T- Bone Steak Flavour, Roysters*	1 Pack/28g	147	8.7	525	5.4	55.8	31.1	3.1
Tangy Malaysian Chutney, Sensations, Walkers*	1 Bag/24g	116	6.2	485	0.9	62.0	26.0	4.0
Tangy Toms, Red Mill*	1 Bag/15g	76	4.1	507	6.0	60.0	27.3	0.7
Thai Curry & Coriander, Tyrrell's*	1 Pack/50g	261	14.0	522	6.1	56.5	27.9	5.4
Thai Green Curry, TTD, Sainsbury's*	1 Bag/50g	235	12.4	470	6.1	55.6	24.8	5.2
Thai Sweet Chicken, McCoys*	1 Bag/35g	179	10.6	512	7.4	52.3	30.4	4.0
Thai Sweet Chilli, Sensations, Walkers*	1 Bag/40g	202	11.6	505	6.5	54.0	29.0	4.5
Tomato & Red Pepper Salsa, Sensations, Walkers*	1 Bag/35g	168	9.5	480	6.5	53.0	27.0	4.5
Tomato Sauce, Golden Wonder*	1 Bag/25g	130	8.4	521	5.7	49.2	33.5	2.0
Traditional, Hand Cooked, Finest, Tesco*	1 Bag/150g	708	39.2	472	6.4	52.9	26.1	5.1
Vegetable, Crunchy, Asda*	½ Bag/50g	251	12.0	502	1.4	70.0	24.0	6.0
Vegetable, Finest, Tesco*	1 Serving/50g	203	12.8	406	5.0	39.0	25.5	14.6
Vegetable, Waitrose*	1 Pack/100g	512	39.0	512	5.1	35.1	39.0	12.5
Waffles, Bacon Flavour, BGTY, Sainsbury's*	1 Serving/12g	41	0.2	345	6.4	79.7	1.4	2.9
Wild Chilli, McCoys*	1 Bag/50g	255	15.2	510	6.0	53.2	30.3	4.0
Worcester Sauce, Sunseed Oil, Walkers*	1 Bag/34.5g	183	11.4	530	6.5	52.0	33.0	4.0
Yoghurt & Green Onion, Kettle Chips*	1 Serving/50g	237	13.1	473	6.6	54.1	26.1	5.4
CRISPY BAKES								
Mild Cheese & Sweet Onion, Kettle Chips*	1 Bag/24g	91	1.9	379	10.6	66.7	7.8	4.3
CRISPY PANCAKE								
Beef Bolognese, Findus*	1 Pancake/65g	104	2.6	160	6.5	25.0	4.0	1.0
Chicken, Bacon & Sweetcorn, Findus*	1 Pancake/63g	101	2.5	160	5.5	26.0	4.0	1.1
Minced Beef, Findus*	1 Serving/100g	160	4.0	160	6.5	25.0	4.0	1.0
Three Cheeses, Findus*	1 Pancake/62g	118	4.0	190	7.0	25.0	6.5	0.9
CROISSANT								
All Butter, BGTY, Sainsbury's*	1 Croissant/44g	151	6.5	343	9.3	42.7	14.8	1.8
All Butter, Budgens*	1 Croissant/45g	185	11.1	412	7.9	39.7	24.6	3.3
All Butter, Finest, Tesco*	1 Croissant/77g	328	18.2	426	8.6	44.9	23.6	1.9

	Measure INFO/WEIGHT	per Measure KCAL	per Measure FAT	Nutrition Values per 100g / 100ml KCAL	PROT	CARB	FAT	FIBRE

CROISSANT

	Measure INFO/WEIGHT	KCAL	FAT	KCAL	PROT	CARB	FAT	FIBRE
All Butter, M & S*	1 Croissant/54g	224	12.9	415	7.4	45.2	23.8	1.6
All Butter, Mini, Sainsbury's*	1 Croissant/35g	150	8.6	428	9.2	42.6	24.5	1.2
All Butter, Mini, Tesco*	1 Croissant/35g	151	8.2	430	9.3	45.2	23.5	2.0
All Butter, Reduced Fat, M & S*	1 Croissant/49g	181	8.3	370	9.6	44.8	16.9	2.3
All Butter, Sainsbury's*	1 Croissant/44g	188	10.8	428	9.2	42.6	24.5	1.2
All Butter, Tesco*	1 Croissant/48g	192	10.4	400	8.5	41.7	21.6	2.6
All Butter, TTD, Sainsbury's*	1 Croissant/75g	362	24.1	483	8.3	40.2	32.1	2.9
Asda*	1 Croissant/47g	186	9.7	405	9.0	45.0	21.0	0.0
Average	1 Croissant/50g	180	10.2	360	8.3	38.3	20.3	1.6
Butter, GFY, Asda*	1 Croissant/44g	151	6.9	352	6.0	46.0	16.0	2.0
Butter, Morrisons*	1 Serving/44g	196	12.5	446	9.3	38.2	28.4	2.0
Butter, Part Baked, De Graaf*	1 Croissant/45g	170	8.4	378	7.3	45.2	18.7	0.0
Cheese & Ham, Delice de France*	1 Serving/91g	225	12.3	247	7.0	24.4	13.5	2.5
Flaky Pastry, Plain Chocolate Filling, Tesco*	1 Croissant/78g	318	19.0	408	6.5	41.0	24.3	2.0
French, Butter, Mini, Waitrose*	1 Croissant/26g	110	5.5	425	10.4	47.4	21.3	3.7
Low Fat, M & S*	1 Croissant/45g	180	9.1	400	8.2	46.0	20.2	1.8
Mini, Lidl*	1 Croissant/30g	112	5.0	373	7.8	48.0	16.6	0.0
Organic, Tesco*	1 Croissant/45g	195	11.6	433	8.2	42.0	25.8	2.2

CROQUETTES

	Measure INFO/WEIGHT	KCAL	FAT	KCAL	PROT	CARB	FAT	FIBRE
Morrisons*	1 Serving/150g	231	8.1	154	3.3	23.1	5.4	1.1
Potato, Asda*	3 Croquettes/81.4g	144	5.7	177	2.0	26.5	7.0	2.2
Potato, Bacon & Gruyere, Finest, Tesco*	1/3 Pack/75g	165	8.8	220	7.1	21.7	11.7	2.1
Potato, Birds Eye*	1 Croquette/29g	44	1.7	152	2.6	22.6	5.7	1.2
Potato, Chunky, Aunt Bessie's*	1 Serving/41g	62	2.5	152	2.3	23.9	6.1	1.8
Potato, Crispy, Chilled, Sainsbury's*	3 Croquettes/125g	245	11.5	196	2.5	25.7	9.2	1.9
Potato, Fresh, Tesco*	1 Croquette/36.6g	66	3.6	180	2.9	20.4	9.7	3.6
Potato, Fried in Blended Oil, Average	1 Croquette/80g	171	10.5	214	3.7	21.6	13.1	1.3
Potato, Frozen, Tesco*	2 Croquettes/96g	170	6.4	177	3.4	25.8	6.7	3.1
Potato, M & S*	1 Croquette/41.2g	68	3.6	165	2.4	19.3	8.8	2.2
Potato, Sainsbury's*	1 Croquette/28g	50	2.4	180	2.8	22.6	8.6	2.5
Potato, Waitrose*	1 Croquette/29.9g	47	2.4	157	3.0	17.9	8.1	1.5
Potato & Parsnip, Finest, Tesco*	½ Pack/110g	237	11.2	215	5.7	24.1	10.2	1.7
Vegetable, Sainsbury's*	1 Serving/175g	392	20.8	224	5.8	23.3	11.9	2.2

CROUTONS

	Measure INFO/WEIGHT	KCAL	FAT	KCAL	PROT	CARB	FAT	FIBRE
Cracked Black Pepper & Sea Salt, Safeway*	1 Serving/20g	77	2.0	385	11.8	61.6	10.2	4.4
Fresh, M & S*	1 Serving/10g	53	3.3	530	11.4	50.0	32.8	3.2
Garlic, Waitrose*	1 Serving/40g	209	12.0	522	10.8	52.1	30.0	2.7
Herb, Sainsbury's*	1 Serving/15g	64	1.7	429	13.4	68.2	11.4	2.8
Herb & Garlic, La Rochelle*	¼ Pack/18g	106	7.2	587	6.9	49.8	40.0	2.1
Italian Salad, Sainsbury's*	1 Pack/40g	204	10.0	510	8.5	62.7	25.0	2.5

CRUDITE

	Measure INFO/WEIGHT	KCAL	FAT	KCAL	PROT	CARB	FAT	FIBRE
Platter, Sainsbury's*	1 Pack/275g	96	0.8	35	1.4	6.6	0.3	1.6
Selection, Prepared, M & S*	1 Serving/250g	75	1.0	30	1.4	5.8	0.4	2.0

CRUMBLE

	Measure INFO/WEIGHT	KCAL	FAT	KCAL	PROT	CARB	FAT	FIBRE
Apple, Co-Op*	¼ Crumble/110g	270	7.7	245	2.0	43.0	7.0	2.0
Apple, Eat Smart, Safeway*	1 Serving/28g	85	0.7	305	5.2	64.5	2.4	1.2
Apple, Farmfoods*	½ Pack/185g	411	10.9	222	2.9	39.3	5.9	2.3
Apple, Fresh, Chilled, Tesco*	¼ Pack/150g	368	13.4	245	2.8	38.0	8.9	1.4
Apple, Frozen, Tesco*	½ Pack/300g	690	32.6	230	2.1	30.7	10.9	3.9
Apple, Sara Lee*	1 Serving/200g	606	18.0	303	2.3	53.3	9.0	1.2
Apple, Somerfield*	1 Serving/195g	454	16.4	233	2.5	36.8	8.4	1.1
Apple, Waitrose*	1 Serving/125g	310	2.9	248	2.2	54.5	2.3	1.2
Apple, with Sultanas, Weight Watchers*	1 Dessert/110g	196	4.3	178	1.4	34.2	3.9	1.3

	Measure INFO/WEIGHT	per Measure		Nutrition Values per 100g / 100ml				
		KCAL	FAT	KCAL	PROT	CARB	FAT	FIBRE
CRUMBLE								
Apple & Blackberry, Asda*	1 Serving/175g	427	15.8	244	2.7	38.0	9.0	1.2
Apple & Blackberry, M & S*	1 Serving/135g	398	15.1	295	3.5	44.9	11.2	1.6
Apple & Blackberry, Sainsbury's*	1 Serving/110g	232	6.2	211	3.0	37.1	5.6	2.1
Apple & Blackberry, Tesco*	1 Crumble/335g	737	32.2	220	2.8	30.7	9.6	2.0
Apple & Blackberry, with Custard, Somerfield*	1 Serving/120g	324	15.0	270	2.3	36.3	12.5	1.1
Apple & Custard, Asda*	1 Serving/125g	250	8.8	200	2.3	32.0	7.0	0.0
Apple & Toffee, Weight Watchers*	1 Pot/98g	190	4.5	194	1.6	36.6	4.6	0.0
Apple with Custard, Green's*	1 Serving/79g	171	5.3	216	1.9	37.0	6.7	1.2
Apple with Custard, Individual, Sainsbury's*	1 Pudding/120g	286	13.9	238	2.0	31.4	11.6	2.4
Bramley Apple, Favourites, M & S*	1 Serving/140g	390	13.8	279	4.6	43.2	9.9	1.2
Bramley Apple, M & S*	1 Serving/149g	387	13.7	260	4.3	40.3	9.2	1.1
Bramley Apple, Sainsbury's*	1 Serving/100g	248	10.9	248	2.0	35.4	10.9	2.3
Bramley Apple, Tesco*	1/3 Pack/155g	378	14.9	244	2.8	36.7	9.6	1.8
Cauliflower & Camembert, Sainsbury's*	1 Pack/400g	588	43.2	147	5.5	6.9	10.8	0.7
Fish & Prawn, Youngs*	1 Pie/375g	476	27.0	127	5.8	9.7	7.2	1.3
Fruit	1oz/28g	55	1.9	198	2.0	34.0	6.9	1.7
Gooseberry, M & S*	1 Serving/133g	379	14.2	285	3.5	43.3	10.7	1.7
Ocean, Good Choice, Iceland*	1 Pack/340g	377	9.2	111	7.2	14.4	2.7	1.1
Ocean, Low Fat, Ross*	1 Crumble/300g	219	2.4	73	5.1	11.4	0.8	0.4
Rhubarb, Asda*	½ Crumble/200g	460	24.0	230	2.4	28.0	12.0	5.0
Rhubarb, M & S*	1 Serving/133g	366	13.2	275	3.4	42.6	9.9	1.4
Rhubarb, Sainsbury's*	1 Serving/50g	112	2.8	224	3.1	40.4	5.6	1.8
Rhubarb, Tesco*	1/6 Crumble/117g	228	9.7	195	2.8	27.3	8.3	1.7
Rhubarb, with Custard, Sainsbury's*	1 Serving/120g	288	13.9	240	2.4	31.4	11.6	2.3
CRUMBLE MIX								
Luxury, Tesco*	¼ Pack/55g	243	9.0	441	5.7	67.9	16.3	3.2
CRUMBLE TOPPING								
Morrisons*	1 Serving/40g	179	6.6	448	5.4	69.5	16.5	2.8
CRUMPETS								
Asda*	1 Crumpet/45g	85	0.4	188	6.0	39.0	0.9	2.1
Co-Op*	1 Crumpet/40g	70	0.3	175	7.0	35.0	0.7	2.0
Golden Sun*	1 Crumpet/43g	83	0.7	193	7.8	37.1	1.6	1.6
Iceland*	1 Crumpet/46g	92	0.4	200	6.2	41.9	0.8	2.7
Kingsmill*	1 Crumpet/55g	99	0.4	180	5.8	37.5	0.8	1.7
Morning Fresh*	1 Crumpet/20g	36	0.3	180	7.3	34.8	1.3	5.2
Morrisons*	1 Crumpet/41g	71	0.3	174	6.6	35.3	0.7	1.8
Mother's Pride*	1 Crumpet/48g	90	0.5	187	5.6	38.9	1.0	1.7
PB, Waitrose*	1 Crumpet/55g	94	0.2	171	6.1	36.1	0.3	4.4
Premium, Sainsbury's*	1 Crumpet/50g	96	0.7	191	6.1	38.6	1.4	1.7
Premium, TTD, Sainsbury's*	1 Crumpet/56g	101	0.7	180	7.3	34.8	1.3	5.2
Sainsbury's*	1 Crumpet/46g	86	0.3	186	5.8	39.1	0.7	2.5
SmartPrice, Asda*	1 Crumpet/36g	67	0.3	188	6.0	39.0	0.9	2.1
Somerfield*	1 Crumpet/41g	79	0.4	192	5.9	39.9	1.0	2.5
Square, Spongebob Squarepants*	1 Crumpet/50g	93	0.5	186	7.0	37.2	1.0	1.0
Square, Tesco*	1 Crumpet/60g	101	0.5	168	6.3	33.8	0.8	2.7
Tesco*	1 Crumpet/47g	90	0.3	190	5.8	39.1	0.7	2.5
Toasted, Average	1 Crumpet/40g	80	0.4	199	6.7	43.4	1.0	2.0
Value, Tesco*	1 Crumpet/35g	59	0.3	168	6.4	33.9	0.8	1.8
Waitrose*	1 Crumpet/55g	99	0.7	180	7.3	34.8	1.3	5.2
Warburton's*	1 Crumpet/58g	100	0.4	172	5.5	36.0	0.7	2.2
CRUNCHIE								
Blast, Cadbury*	1 Serving/41.5g	202	8.4	480	4.7	69.6	20.1	0.7
Cadbury*	1 Bar/40g	186	7.6	465	4.0	69.5	18.9	0.5

	Measure INFO/WEIGHT	per Measure KCAL	FAT	Nutrition Values per 100g / 100ml KCAL	PROT	CARB	FAT	FIBRE
CRUNCHIE								
Nuggets, Cadbury*	1 Bag/125g	569	20.5	455	3.8	73.1	16.4	0.0
Treat Size, Cadbury*	1 Bar/17g	80	3.1	470	4.0	71.5	18.4	0.0
CRUNCHY STICKS								
Orange, Cool, Diet, Sainsbury's*	1 Can/330ml	10	0.2	3	0.1	0.6	0.1	0.1
Pineapple & Grapefruit, No Added Sugar, Morrisons*	1 Glass/250ml	10	0.0	4	0.2	1.2	0.0	0.0
Ready Salted, Tesco*	1 Serving/25g	119	5.9	475	5.6	60.3	23.5	3.0
Salt & Vinegar, Sainsbury's*	1 Bag/25g	119	6.1	474	5.9	58.0	24.3	2.4
Salt & Vinegar, Shapers, Boots*	1 Pack/21g	96	3.8	457	5.7	66.7	18.1	2.4
Salt & Vinegar, Tesco*	1 Serving/25g	118	6.1	470	6.9	55.7	24.4	2.7
Salt & Vinegar, Value, Tesco*	1 Bag/22g	109	5.8	497	6.3	58.7	26.3	2.4
CUCUMBER								
Average	1 Serving/80g	8	0.1	10	0.7	1.5	0.1	0.6
CUMIN								
Seeds, Ground, Schwartz*	1 Tsp/5g	22	1.2	446	19.0	40.3	23.2	0.0
CUPCAKES								
Assorted, Sainsbury's*	1 Cake/38g	130	2.3	341	2.2	69.3	6.1	0.4
Chocolate, Fabulous Bakin' Boys*	1 Cupcake/34g	152	8.2	448	4.0	54.0	24.0	1.0
Chocolate, Lyons*	1 Cake/39g	125	1.8	321	2.4	67.5	4.6	0.8
Pink, M & S*	1 Cupcake/39g	160	3.3	410	2.5	81.3	8.5	0.6
CURACAO								
Average	1 Pub Shot/35ml	109	0.0	311	0.0	28.3	0.0	0.0
CURLY WURLY								
Cadbury*	1 Bar/26g	117	4.6	450	3.5	69.1	17.8	0.0
Squirlies, Cadbury*	1 Squirl/3g	14	0.5	450	3.9	69.0	17.8	0.0
CURRANTS								
Average	1oz/28g	75	0.1	267	2.3	67.8	0.4	1.9
CURRY								
& Chips, Curry Sauce, Chipped Potatoes, Kershaws*	1 Sering/330g	391	8.3	119	10.0	14.0	2.5	2.0
Aubergine	1oz/28g	33	2.8	118	1.4	6.2	10.1	1.5
Beef, Hot, Canned, M & S*	1 Can/425g	446	21.7	105	12.2	2.8	5.1	1.0
Beef, Sainsbury's*	1 Serving/400g	552	32.8	138	10.7	5.4	8.2	0.9
Beef, SmartPrice, Asda*	1 Serving/392g	223	2.0	57	4.0	9.0	0.5	1.0
Beef, Thai, Finest, Tesco*	1 Serving/500g	770	29.0	154	9.0	16.5	5.8	1.2
Beef, with Rice, Asda*	1 Pack/406g	547	15.8	135	6.0	19.0	3.9	1.2
Beef, with Rice, Birds Eye*	1 Pack/388g	524	10.9	135	6.9	20.8	2.8	0.8
Beef, with Rice, Healthy Choice, Asda*	1 Pack/400g	476	10.4	119	6.0	18.0	2.6	0.9
Beef, with Rice, Iceland*	1 Pack/400g	404	6.8	101	6.7	14.7	1.7	1.0
Beef, with Rice, Morrisons*	1 Serving/400g	480	20.0	120	6.0	12.6	5.0	0.6
Beef, with Rice, Tesco*	1 Pack/400g	456	13.2	114	4.5	16.7	3.3	0.6
Beef, with Rice, Weight Watchers*	1 Pack/328g	249	3.3	76	4.2	12.5	1.0	0.3
Blackeye Bean, Gujerati	1oz/28g	36	1.2	127	7.2	16.1	4.4	2.8
Cabbage	1oz/28g	23	1.4	82	1.9	8.1	5.0	2.1
Cauliflower & Potato	1oz/28g	17	0.7	59	3.4	6.6	2.4	1.8
Chana Dall, Curry Special*	1 Pack/350g	434	22.8	124	6.0	10.5	6.5	5.9
Chick Pea, Whole	1oz/28g	50	2.1	179	9.6	21.3	7.5	4.5
Chick Pea, Whole, Basic	1oz/28g	30	1.0	108	6.0	14.2	3.6	3.3
Chick Pea, Whole & Tomato, Punjabi with Vegetable	1oz/28g	31	1.4	112	5.6	12.4	4.9	2.9
Chicken, & Rice, International Cuisine*	1 Serving/400g	420	11.6	105	3.3	16.4	2.9	0.8
Chicken, & Rice, Value, Tesco*	1 Pack/300g	399	14.1	133	6.5	16.2	4.7	1.0
Chicken, Asda*	1 Can/200g	210	10.0	105	10.0	5.0	5.0	0.0
Chicken, Canned, Sainsbury's*	1 Serving/100g	136	6.1	136	11.1	9.1	6.1	1.0
Chicken, Chinese with Egg Fried Rice, Morrisons*	1 Pack/500g	600	15.5	120	5.7	17.4	3.1	0.9
Chicken, COU, M & S*	1 Pack/200g	290	13.8	145	6.9	13.3	6.9	1.4

C

CURRENT

	Measure INFO/WEIGHT	per Measure KCAL	FAT	Nutrition Values per 100g / 100ml KCAL	PROT	CARB	FAT	FIBRE
CURRY								
Chicken, Extra Strong, M & S*	1oz/28g	28	1.1	100	13.8	2.5	3.9	1.4
Chicken, Frozen, Sainsbury's*	1 Serving/400g	528	16.4	132	5.8	18.0	4.1	0.7
Chicken, Green Thai, BGTY, Sainsbury's*	1 Pack/400g	316	10.4	79	10.6	3.4	2.6	1.9
Chicken, Green Thai, Birds Eye*	1 Pack/450g	536	19.8	119	4.7	15.2	4.4	0.3
Chicken, Green Thai, Breasts, Finest, Tesco*	1 Serving/200g	292	16.0	146	16.5	2.0	8.0	0.7
Chicken, Green Thai, Jasmine Rice, COU, M & S*	1 Pack/400g	380	6.0	95	7.8	12.5	1.5	0.8
Chicken, Green Thai, Jasmine Rice, Weight Watchers*	1 Pack/400g	364	4.0	91	6.1	14.3	1.0	0.5
Chicken, Green Thai, Safeway*	1 Pack/350g	490	28.0	140	12.5	3.5	8.0	1.4
Chicken, Green Thai, Sainsbury's*	½ Pack/200g	264	13.6	132	13.0	4.8	6.8	0.9
Chicken, Green Thai Style, & Sticky Rice, Asda*	1 Pack/450g	585	10.8	130	7.0	20.0	2.4	0.1
Chicken, Hot, Can, Tesco*	1 Can/418g	514	26.3	123	9.7	6.9	6.3	0.9
Chicken, Hot, Canned, Asda*	1 Can/398g	501	23.9	126	11.0	7.0	6.0	0.5
Chicken, Hot, Canned, Sainsbury's*	1 Can/400g	448	17.2	112	14.1	4.2	4.3	2.0
Chicken, Hot, Iceland*	1 Can/392g	492	20.4	126	10.0	9.9	5.2	0.7
Chicken, Kashmiri, Waitrose*	1 Serving/400g	640	36.4	160	14.5	5.0	9.1	0.6
Chicken, Medium Hot, M & S*	1 Serving/200g	310	14.2	155	7.8	14.3	7.1	0.8
Chicken, Mild, Asda*	½ Can/189.7g	239	11.4	126	11.0	7.0	6.0	0.5
Chicken, Mild, BGTY, Sainsbury's*	1 Serving/200g	184	5.2	92	10.0	7.2	2.6	0.5
Chicken, Mild, Canned, Bilash*	½ Can/200g	180	7.6	90	9.5	4.5	3.8	0.7
Chicken, Mild, Iceland*	½ Can/200g	234	9.0	117	10.6	8.5	4.5	0.7
Chicken, Mild, M & S*	1oz/28g	28	1.1	100	13.8	2.5	3.9	1.4
Chicken, Mild, Sainsbury's*	1 Can/400g	472	27.6	118	10.5	3.5	6.9	1.3
Chicken, Mild, Tinned, Sainsbury's*	1 Serving/200g	214	7.0	107	12.7	6.1	3.5	1.1
Chicken, Mild & Fruity, Breasts, HE, Tesco*	2 Breasts/345g	321	5.2	93	15.8	4.1	1.5	0.5
Chicken, Newgate*	1 Serving/196g	220	11.8	112	8.0	6.6	6.0	0.0
Chicken, Red Thai, 97% Fat Free, Birds Eye*	1 Pack/366g	425	7.0	116	5.7	19.0	1.9	0.5
Chicken, Red Thai, Asda*	1 Pack/360g	461	27.7	128	9.1	5.5	7.7	1.0
Chicken, Red Thai, COU, M & S*	1 Pack/400g	420	9.2	105	7.1	13.4	2.3	1.4
Chicken, Red Thai, HL, Tesco*	½ Box/175g	158	4.9	90	10.7	5.4	2.8	0.7
Chicken, Red Thai, Sainsbury's*	½ Pack/200g	270	14.8	135	13.1	4.0	7.4	0.9
Chicken, Red Thai, Tesco*	1 Serving/175g	215	11.6	123	10.5	5.5	6.6	1.4
Chicken, Red Thai, Waitrose*	1 Pack/400g	480	20.4	120	12.2	5.8	5.1	1.5
Chicken, Red Thai, with Fragrant Rice, Somerfield*	1 Pack/340g	503	17.0	148	8.0	18.0	5.0	0.0
Chicken, Red Thai, with Rice, Tesco*	1 Serving/475g	746	32.3	157	7.2	16.8	6.8	1.1
Chicken, Red Thai Style, HE, Tesco*	1 Pack/420g	423	7.1	101	7.0	14.4	1.7	0.7
Chicken, Reduced Fat, Asda*	1 Pack/400g	476	10.4	119	6.0	18.0	2.6	0.9
Chicken, SmartPrice, Asda*	1 Can/392g	282	5.1	72	4.0	11.0	1.3	1.0
Chicken, Thai, Red, GFY, Asda*	1 Serving/400g	364	8.4	91	6.0	12.0	2.1	1.6
Chicken, Thai, Tom Yum, Sainsbury's*	1 Pot/400g	416	20.4	104	11.1	3.5	5.1	1.9
Chicken, Thai, with Rice, Oriental Express*	1 Pack/340g	303	4.4	89	4.1	15.3	1.3	1.2
Chicken, Thai Green, Nutritionally Balanced, M & S*	1 Pack/400g	400	5.2	100	9.2	12.4	1.3	1.4
Chicken, Thai Mango, Sainsbury's*	½ Pack/200g	288	17.8	144	11.2	4.8	8.9	1.9
Chicken, Thai Peanut, Sainsbury's*	½ Pack/200g	314	19.2	157	12.8	4.9	9.6	1.2
Chicken, Value, Tesco*	1 Pack/300g	399	15.6	133	5.5	15.9	5.2	1.7
Chicken, with Naan Bread, Iceland*	1 Portion/260g	484	16.4	186	10.1	22.3	6.3	1.4
Chicken, with Potato Wedges, HE, Tesco*	1 Pack/450g	428	12.2	95	7.6	10.3	2.7	1.1
Chicken, with Rice, Asda*	1 Pack/400g	492	12.0	123	6.0	18.0	3.0	1.0
Chicken, with Rice, Big Value, Safeway*	1 Serving/500g	645	16.5	129	4.2	20.7	3.3	0.5
Chicken, with Rice, Birds Eye*	1 Pack/380g	388	7.6	102	6.5	14.6	2.0	7.6
Chicken, with Rice, Dunnes Stores*	1 Pack/375g	400	6.3	107	4.2	20.2	1.7	0.8
Chicken, with Rice, Fresh, Co-Op*	1 Pack/300g	270	9.0	90	3.0	13.0	3.0	1.0
Chicken, with Rice, Frozen, Tesco*	1 Pack/400g	488	15.6	122	4.6	17.2	3.9	0.7
Chicken, with Rice, Fruity, HL, Tesco*	1 Pack/450g	495	5.4	110	6.5	18.2	1.2	1.2

CURRENT

	Measure INFO/WEIGHT	per Measure KCAL	per Measure FAT	KCAL	PROT	CARB	FAT	FIBRE
				Nutrition Values per 100g / 100ml				

CURRY

	Measure INFO/WEIGHT	KCAL	FAT	KCAL	PROT	CARB	FAT	FIBRE
Chicken, with Rice, Hot, Asda*	1 Pack/400g	476	12.0	119	5.0	18.0	3.0	1.0
Chicken, with Rice, Iceland*	1 Pack/500g	566	14.8	113	5.2	16.4	3.0	1.2
Chicken, with Rice, Malaysian, Bernard Matthews*	1 Pack/400g	512	15.6	128	6.1	17.0	3.9	0.0
Chicken, with Rice, Morrisons*	1 Pack/300g	345	6.0	115	5.5	18.7	2.0	0.4
Chicken, with Rice, Quick Bite, Asda*	1 Serving/300g	294	9.9	98	5.0	12.0	3.3	0.5
Chicken, with Rice, Ross*	1 Serving/320g	272	4.2	85	3.4	14.7	1.3	0.5
Chicken, with Rice, Sainsbury's*	1 Pack/400g	500	14.8	125	5.4	17.5	3.7	0.8
Chicken, with Rice, Spar*	1 Pack/300g	372	8.1	124	4.9	19.9	2.7	1.2
Chicken, with Rice, Tesco*	1 Pack/300g	390	12.6	130	4.4	17.5	4.2	1.2
Chicken, with Vegetables, Canned, Value, Tesco*	1 Can/392g	294	10.2	75	4.2	7.9	2.6	1.4
Chicken, with Vegetables, Morrisons*	1 Can/392g	392	15.7	100	9.0	7.0	4.0	1.0
Chicken, Yellow Thai Style, HL, Tesco*	1 Pack/450g	504	12.2	112	9.3	12.6	2.7	0.5
Chicken Biryani, Recipe Mix, Schwartz*	1 Pack/30g	75	2.4	249	14.6	58.1	8.1	28.6
Chinese Chicken, Morrisons*	1 Pack/340g	347	15.6	102	10.3	5.0	4.6	0.8
Chinese Chicken, Oriental Express*	1 Pack/340g	286	2.0	84	4.8	16.2	0.6	0.8
Chinese Chicken, with Vegetable Rice, M & S*	1 Pack/400g	320	8.0	80	7.1	8.4	2.0	1.3
Cod, Red Thai, with Rice, PB, Waitrose*	1 Pack/400g	360	7.2	90	7.5	11.0	1.8	1.0
Courgette & Potato	1oz/28g	24	1.5	86	1.9	8.7	5.2	1.2
Dudhi, Kofta	1oz/28g	32	2.1	113	2.6	9.4	7.4	2.8
Fish, & Vegetable, Bangladeshi	1oz/28g	33	2.4	117	9.1	1.4	8.4	0.5
Fish, Bangladeshi	1oz/28g	35	2.2	124	12.2	1.5	7.9	0.3
Fish, Red Thai, Waitrose*	1 Pack/500g	275	11.0	55	5.2	3.7	2.2	1.0
Gobi Aloo Sag, Retail	1oz/28g	27	1.9	95	2.2	7.1	6.9	1.4
Green, Thai, with Rice, Microwaveable Meals, M & S*	1 Pot/330g	545	23.4	165	8.1	16.9	7.1	2.0
Green, Thai, with Sticky Rice, HL, Tesco*	1 Pack/450g	518	12.2	115	7.7	14.9	2.7	0.6
Green Thai, & Rice, GFY, Asda*	1 Pack/400g	356	7.6	89	7.0	11.0	1.9	1.6
King Prawn, Coconut & Lime, Sainsbury's*	½ Pack/351g	207	8.8	59	3.7	5.4	2.5	1.0
King Prawn, Goan, Eat Smart, Safeway*	1 Pack/400g	340	6.8	85	3.7	12.7	1.7	2.1
King Prawn, Malay with Rice, Sainsbury's*	1 Pack/400g	608	20.4	152	5.0	21.5	5.1	1.4
King Prawn Malay, Waitrose*	1 Pack/350g	364	19.3	104	6.6	7.1	5.5	0.9
Lamb, Extra Strong, M & S*	1oz/28g	35	1.9	125	11.5	4.6	6.9	0.9
Lamb, Hot, M & S*	½ Can/213.3g	320	19.6	150	14.9	6.0	9.2	2.3
Lamb, Kefthedes, Waitrose*	½ Pack/200g	294	17.6	147	9.0	8.0	8.8	2.1
Lamb, with Rice, Birds Eye*	1 Pack/382g	520	13.0	136	5.6	20.8	3.4	0.9
Matar Paneer, Peas & Cheese, Ashoka*	½ Pack/150g	183	10.1	122	5.3	10.0	6.7	2.0
Potato & Pea	1oz/28g	26	1.1	92	2.9	13.0	3.8	2.4
Prawn, & Mushroom	1oz/28g	47	4.0	168	7.3	2.5	14.4	1.0
Prawn, Frozen, Sainsbury's*	1 Pack/400g	500	15.6	125	3.5	19.0	3.9	0.8
Prawn, King, Goan, M & S*	1 Pack/400g	680	44.4	170	5.1	11.6	11.1	1.5
Prawn, Red Thai, Sainsbury's*	1 Pack/300g	546	39.6	182	6.3	9.4	13.2	1.7
Prawn, Red Thai Sauce, Youngs*	1 Pack/255g	197	8.7	77	4.8	6.5	3.4	0.8
Prawn, Thai, with Jasmine Rice, BGTY, Sainsbury's*	1 Serving/401g	353	6.0	88	4.2	14.5	1.5	2.0
Prawn, with Rice, Asda*	1 Pack/400g	420	10.4	105	3.5	17.0	2.6	1.1
Prawn, with Rice, Birds Eye*	1 Pack/375g	443	0.0	118	3.5	20.6	0.0	0.0
Prawn, with Rice, Iceland*	1 Pack/400g	360	9.6	90	3.2	13.8	2.4	0.9
Prawn, with Rice, Morrisons*	1 Serving/400g	484	9.2	121	3.2	21.9	2.3	0.9
Red Kidney Bean, Punjabi	1oz/28g	30	1.6	106	4.7	10.1	5.6	3.8
Red Thai, Safeway*	1 Pack/324g	369	19.8	114	10.0	4.8	6.1	1.6
Red Thai, Vegetarian, Tesco*	1 Pack/429ml	588	21.9	137	5.4	17.3	5.1	1.6
Red Thai, with Rice, Finest, Tesco*	1 Pack/500g	660	15.5	132	8.0	17.8	3.1	0.6
Salmon, Green, Waitrose*	1 Pack/400.7g	581	40.5	145	9.1	4.5	10.1	2.7
Vegetable, & Rice, Microwaveable, M & S*	1 Pot/325g	390	7.2	120	2.3	22.3	2.2	2.2
Vegetable, Asda*	1 Pack/350g	329	21.0	94	1.9	8.0	6.0	1.9

	Measure INFO/WEIGHT	per Measure KCAL	FAT	Nutrition Values per 100g / 100ml KCAL	PROT	CARB	FAT	FIBRE
CURRY								
Vegetable, Budgens*	1 Pack/350g	249	14.0	71	1.8	6.9	4.0	2.2
Vegetable, Canned, Sainsbury's*	½ Can/200g	200	12.2	100	1.4	9.8	6.1	1.8
Vegetable, Frozen, Mixed Vegetables	1oz/28g	25	1.7	88	2.5	6.9	6.1	0.0
Vegetable, in a Mild & Creamy Curry Sauce, Waitrose*	1 Pack/400g	388	26.4	97	2.6	6.9	6.6	1.5
Vegetable, in a Mild & Creamy Sauce, Waitrose*	1 Pack/400g	388	26.4	97	2.6	6.9	6.6	1.5
Vegetable, in Sweet Sauce	1 Serving/330g	162	6.9	49	1.4	6.7	2.1	1.3
Vegetable, Indian, Canned, Tesco*	½ Pack/150g	120	6.8	80	2.0	6.7	4.5	1.1
Vegetable, Indian, Tesco*	1 Serving/225g	257	17.8	114	2.1	8.6	7.9	1.6
Vegetable, Indian Meal for One, Tesco*	1 Serving/200g	218	14.4	109	2.0	9.0	7.2	1.2
Vegetable, Medium, Tesco*	1 Pack/350g	326	21.7	93	2.3	7.1	6.2	1.9
Vegetable, Mild, Tesco*	1 Can/425g	315	10.6	74	2.1	10.7	2.5	1.7
Vegetable, Mixed, Organic, Pure & Pronto*	1 Pack/400g	368	11.6	92	4.2	12.4	2.9	4.8
Vegetable, Pakistani	1oz/28g	17	0.7	60	2.2	8.7	2.6	2.2
Vegetable, Sabzi Tarkari, Patak's*	1 Pack/400g	500	31.2	125	2.5	11.1	7.8	2.2
Vegetable, Safeway*	1 Pack/275g	239	14.9	87	2.4	7.3	5.4	2.8
Vegetable, SmartPrice, Asda*	½ Can/203g	132	1.0	65	2.0	13.0	0.5	1.7
Vegetable, Takeaway	1oz/28g	29	2.1	105	2.5	7.6	7.4	0.0
Vegetable, Tesco*	½ Can/200g	278	18.6	139	3.4	10.5	9.3	3.2
Vegetable, Tinned, Asda*	½ Can/200g	206	12.0	103	2.2	10.0	6.0	2.5
Vegetable, Way to Five, Sainsbury's*	½ Pack/344g	227	3.8	66	2.5	11.6	1.1	1.4
Vegetable, with Pilau Rice, BGTY, Sainsbury's*	1 Pack/450g	329	2.7	73	1.9	14.9	0.6	1.3
Vegetable, with Pilau Rice, Linda McCartney*	1 Pack/339g	224	2.0	66	1.6	13.5	0.6	0.5
Vegetable, with Rice, Asda*	1 Pack/392.7g	432	12.2	110	2.6	18.0	3.1	1.4
Vegetable, with Rice, Birds Eye*	1 Pack/413.6g	455	9.5	110	2.3	19.6	2.3	1.1
Vegetable, with Rice, Co-Op*	1 Pack/340g	289	3.4	85	2.0	17.0	1.0	0.7
Vegetable, with Rice, HL, Tesco*	1 Pack/450g	486	12.2	108	2.7	18.2	2.7	1.1
Vegetable, with Rice, Retail	1oz/28g	29	0.8	102	3.3	16.4	3.0	0.0
Vegetable, with Rice, Tesco*	1 Pack/400g	440	12.0	110	2.1	18.7	3.0	1.0
Vegetable, with Yoghurt	1oz/28g	17	1.1	62	2.6	4.6	4.1	1.4
Vegetable, Yellow, Tesco*	1 Pack/355.6g	324	17.4	91	1.9	9.9	4.9	1.4
Vegetable, Yellow Thai, Sainsbury's*	1 Pack/400g	624	48.8	156	2.2	9.4	12.2	1.1
CURRY PASTE								
Balti, Sharwood's*	¼ Pack/72.5g	328	28.7	453	5.0	19.2	39.6	3.1
Balti, Tomato & Coriander, Original, Patak's*	1 Tbsp/15g	58	5.1	388	4.0	14.6	34.0	3.7
Bhuna, Tomato & Tamarind, Patak's*	1 Serving/10g	40	5.6	397	4.3	17.5	56.2	6.3
Garam Masala, Cinnamon & Ginger, Hot, Patak's*	1 Tbsp/25g	101	8.9	403	3.2	17.9	35.4	0.6
Green Thai, Mild, Sainsbury's*	1 Tbsp/15g	23	1.5	156	2.2	14.5	9.9	2.7
Hot, Sharwood's*	1oz/28g	123	10.7	439	5.1	18.6	38.3	2.6
Jalfrezi, Patak's*	1 Serving/35g	192	18.1	549	4.1	16.8	51.6	3.5
Korma, Coconut & Coriander, Original, Patak's*	1 Serving/30g	125	11.7	415	3.5	11.6	39.0	5.2
Madras, Cumin & Chilli, Hot, Patak's*	½ Jar/50g	293	26.8	586	4.3	21.6	53.6	5.2
Medium, Barts Spices*	1 Serving/30g	89	6.5	295	4.5	19.2	21.5	5.5
Medium, Sharwood's*	1oz/28g	122	10.9	434	4.5	16.8	38.8	2.7
Mild, Coriander & Cumin, Original, Patak's*	1 Serving/30g	169	15.8	562	4.8	16.8	52.5	2.8
Mild, Sharwood's*	1oz/28g	78	6.0	279	3.6	17.7	21.5	3.4
Red Thai, Sainsbury's*	1 Jar/250g	385	31.0	154	2.2	8.5	12.4	3.5
Rogan Josh, Tomato & Paprika, Patak's*	1 Serving/30g	119	11.0	397	4.1	12.7	36.7	5.9
Tandoori, Sharwood's*	1oz/28g	64	4.4	228	5.9	15.5	15.8	1.9
Tandoori, Tamarind & Ginger, Patak's*	1 Serving/30g	33	0.5	110	3.1	20.4	1.8	2.6
Tikka Masala, Sharwood's*	1oz/28g	53	4.3	191	3.2	9.9	15.4	2.6
CURRY POWDER								
Average	1 Tsp/2g	7	0.3	325	12.7	41.8	13.8	0.0
Mixed Flavours	1 Tsp/2g	6	0.3	316	13.0	34.7	13.9	0.0

	Measure	per Measure		Nutrition Values per 100g / 100ml				
	INFO/WEIGHT	KCAL	FAT	KCAL	PROT	CARB	FAT	FIBRE

CURRY SAUCE

Asda*	1 Tbsp/15g	62	2.1	414	13.0	59.0	14.0	1.3
Balti, Asda*	¼ Jar/125g	155	12.5	124	1.6	7.0	10.0	1.7
Balti, Loyd Grossman*	½ Jar/212.5g	346	28.5	163	1.7	8.8	13.4	1.4
Bhuna, Cooking, Shere Khan*	1 Jar/425g	344	26.8	81	1.1	5.7	6.3	1.2
Chinese Style, Cooking, Asda*	1 Jar/560g	465	24.1	83	1.5	9.6	4.3	1.7
Green Curry, Thai, Stir Fry, Blue Dragon*	1 Sachet/120g	74	4.8	62	0.9	5.7	4.0	0.5
Green Thai, Asda*	1 Jar/340g	309	27.2	91	0.5	4.3	8.0	0.2
Jalfrezi, Hot, M & S*	1 Serving/165g	107	3.8	65	1.9	8.8	2.3	1.2
Jalfrezi, Loyd Grossman*	½ Jar/212.5g	270	20.2	127	2.1	8.2	9.5	1.2
Jalfrezi, Mild, Sharwood's*	1 Serving/140g	106	4.6	76	1.3	10.2	3.3	3.3
Jalfrezi, Spicy, Cooking Sauce, Sharwood's*	1/3 Jar/140g	122	6.7	87	1.8	9.2	4.8	3.6
Jalfrezi, Tesco*	1 Jar/500g	450	32.5	90	1.3	6.6	6.5	2.4
Korma, Loyd Grossman*	½ Jar/222g	542	37.7	244	3.6	19.1	17.0	0.6
Korma, Uncle Ben's*	1 Jar/500g	630	42.0	126	1.4	11.1	8.4	0.0
Madras, Aldi*	1 Serving/113g	68	2.3	60	1.5	9.0	2.0	0.0
Madras, Chilli & Cumin, Canned, Patak's*	1 Can/283g	640	52.6	226	2.7	11.9	18.6	1.6
Madras, Cooking, Asda*	¼ Jar/141.6g	109	6.2	77	1.3	8.0	4.4	1.0
Madras, Cooking, Sharwood's*	1 Tsp/2g	2	0.1	86	1.5	6.9	5.8	1.3
Madras, Indian, Sharwood's*	1 Jar/420g	433	26.5	103	1.8	9.7	6.3	1.9
Madras, Sharwood's*	1 Jar/420g	521	38.2	124	1.7	8.9	9.1	1.4
Madras, Tesco*	½ Jar/200g	168	13.0	84	1.1	5.2	6.5	1.3
Malaysian Rendang, Loyd Grossman*	1 Serving/100g	168	12.5	168	3.1	10.7	12.5	2.2
Medium, Uncle Ben's*	1 Jar/500g	330	10.0	66	0.9	10.9	2.0	0.0
Red Thai, Cooking Sauce, Asda*	1 Jar/315g	438	36.5	139	1.6	7.1	11.6	1.3
Rogan Josh, Loyd Grossman*	1 Serving/106g	206	16.7	194	2.4	10.5	15.8	1.5
Rogan Josh, Worldwide Sauces*	1 Jar/500g	255	1.5	51	1.1	11.0	0.3	0.0
SmartPrice, Asda*	¼ Jar/110g	73	2.0	66	1.4	11.0	1.8	0.6
Tikka, Cooking, Tesco*	1 Jar/500g	617	42.2	123	1.7	10.1	8.4	2.1
Tikka Masala, Cooking, HL, Tesco*	¼ Jar/125g	94	3.8	75	2.6	8.2	3.0	1.2
Tikka Masala, COU, M & S*	½ Pack/100g	80	2.6	80	4.5	9.9	2.6	1.7
Tikka Masala, Loyd Grossman*	½ Jar/212.5g	438	34.4	206	2.6	12.5	16.2	1.0
Vindaloo, Hot, Patak's*	1 Serving/90g	107	7.7	119	1.7	8.5	8.6	2.1

CUSTARD

Banana Flavour, Ambrosia*	1 Pack/135g	136	3.9	101	2.6	16.2	2.9	0.1
Chocolate Flavour, Ambrosia*	1 Pot/150g	177	4.4	118	3.0	20.0	2.9	0.7
Dairy Free, Sainsbury's*	1 Serving/250g	210	4.3	84	3.0	14.2	1.7	0.2
Instant, Dry, Bird's*	1oz/28g	119	3.2	425	4.3	76.3	11.4	0.4
Instant, Light, Powder Dry Weight, Bird's*	1 Serving/25g	102	2.1	407	4.3	79.0	8.2	0.4
Instant, No Added Sugar, Dry, Tesco*	1 Serving/18g	73	1.5	406	5.3	77.0	8.5	0.0
Instant, No Sugar, Dry Weight, BFY, Morrisons*	1 Pack/70g	285	7.0	407	6.0	73.2	10.0	2.6
Low Fat, Average	1/3 Pot/141g	116	1.6	82	2.9	15.0	1.2	0.0
Mix, Instant, Co-Op*	1 Pack/76g	340	13.1	448	4.5	68.5	17.3	0.0
Powder	1oz/28g	99	0.2	354	0.6	92.0	0.7	0.1
Powder, Instant, Value, Tesco*	1 Serving/70g	49	0.6	70	0.8	13.5	0.9	0.0
Powder, Original, Made Up, Bird's*	1 Serving/167g	106	2.9	63	0.7	11.4	1.7	0.1
Ready to Serve, Average	1 Serving/50g	59.1	2.3	118.3	3.3	16.1	4.6	0.2
Ready to Serve, Bird's*	½ Carton/212½g	184.4	3.0	87	2.8	15.5	1.4	0.0
Strawberry Flavoured, Ambrosia*	1 Serving/135g	139	3.8	103	2.8	16.7	2.8	0.0
Vanilla, Fresh, Waitrose*	1 Serving/100g	214	15.3	214	3.2	15.8	15.3	1.1
with Strawberry Sauce, Ambrosia*	1 Pot/160g	171	3.8	107	2.4	19.0	2.4	0.1

CUTLETS

Nut, Goodlife*	1 Cutlet/88g	283	19.4	322	9.1	21.8	22.0	3.4
Nut, Vegetarian, Tesco*	1 Cutlet/87.5g	250	16.5	286	7.5	21.3	18.9	4.1

	Measure INFO/WEIGHT	per Measure KCAL	per Measure FAT	Nutrition Values per 100g / 100ml KCAL	PROT	CARB	FAT	FIBRE
CUTLETS								
Vegetable & Nut, Asda*	1 Cutlet/88.4g	295	20.2	335	10.0	22.0	23.0	4.6
CUTTLEFISH								
Raw	1oz/28g	20	0.2	71	16.1	0.0	0.7	0.0

C

	Measure INFO/WEIGHT	per Measure		Nutrition Values per 100g / 100ml				
		KCAL	FAT	KCAL	PROT	CARB	FAT	FIBRE
DAB								
Fillets, Lightly Dusted, M & S*	1 Fillet/112g	190	9.7	170	12.8	9.7	8.7	0.5
Raw	1oz/28g	21	0.3	74	15.7	0.0	1.2	0.0
DAIRYLEA DUNKERS								
Baked Crisps, Dairylea, Kraft*	1 Pack/44.9g	101	4.0	225	9.2	26.0	9.0	1.1
Jumbo Munch, Dairylea, Kraft*	1 Serving/50g	150	9.3	300	7.2	26.5	18.5	1.2
Salt & Vinegar, Dairylea, Kraft*	1 Tub/42g	116	8.2	275	6.7	17.5	19.5	0.3
DAIRYLEA LUNCHABLES								
Cheese & Pizza Crackers, Dairylea, Kraft*	1oz/28g	105	7.6	375	10.5	24.5	27.0	1.4
Cheese & Pizza Crackers, Dairylea*	1oz/28g	105	7.6	375	10.5	24.5	27.0	1.4
Double Cheese, Dairylea, Kraft*	1 Pack/110g	413	28.6	375	18.0	17.0	26.0	0.3
Double Cheese, Dairylea*	1 Pack/110g	413	28.6	375	18.0	17.0	26.0	0.3
Ham & Cheese Pizza, Dairylea, Kraft*	1 Pack/97g	247	10.7	255	11.5	26.0	11.0	1.6
Ham & Cheese Pizza, Dairylea*	1 Pack/97g	247	10.7	255	11.5	26.0	11.0	1.6
Harvest Ham, Dairylea, Kraft*	1 Pack/110g	314	18.7	285	16.5	16.5	17.0	0.3
Tasty Chicken, Dairylea, Kraft*	1 Pack/110g	314	18.2	285	17.0	17.5	16.5	0.3
DAMSONS								
Raw, Weighed with Stones, Average	1oz/28g	10	0.0	34	0.5	8.6	0.0	1.6
Raw, Weighed without Stones, Average	1oz/28g	11	0.0	38	0.5	9.6	0.0	1.8
DANDELION & BURDOCK								
Original, Ben Shaws*	1 Can/440ml	128	0.0	29	0.0	7.0	0.0	0.0
Sparkling, Diet, Morrisons*	1 Glass/200ml	2	0.0	1	0.0	0.3	0.0	0.0
DANISH PASTRY								
Apple, Bar, Sara Lee*	1/6 Bar/70g	160	4.0	229	4.3	42.1	5.7	1.7
Apple, Fresh Cream, Sainsbury's*	1 Pastry/67g	248	14.6	368	3.1	40.2	21.6	0.4
Apple, Iceland*	¼ Pastry/94.9g	223	5.0	235	5.3	41.5	5.3	2.3
Apple & Sultana, Tesco*	1 Pastry/72g	293	16.4	407	5.4	45.0	22.8	1.4
Average	1 Pastry/110g	411	19.4	374	5.8	51.3	17.6	1.6
Cherry, Bar, Sainsbury's*	¼ Bar/88g	221	10.0	252	4.2	33.2	11.4	1.7
Pecan, M & S*	1 Serving/67g	287	17.4	428	6.2	45.0	26.0	1.3
Toasted Pecan, Danish Twist, Entenmann's*	1 Slice/48g	171	7.6	351	7.0	47.2	15.6	1.4
DATES								
Dried, Average	1 Date/5g	14	0.0	272	2.8	65.4	0.4	4.2
Fresh, Raw, Yellow, Average	1 Date/30g	35	0.0	116	1.4	29.1	0.1	1.7
Medjool, Stuffed with Walnuts, Tesco*	2 Dates/40g	98	2.3	245	4.4	44.0	5.7	3.4
DELI FILLER								
Chicken, Caesar Style, Sainsbury's*	1 Pack/80g	212	18.2	265	14.0	1.0	22.7	2.6
Coronation Chicken, M & S*	1 Serving/85g	251	20.1	295	12.3	7.7	23.7	0.5
King Prawn & Avocado, M & S*	1 Pack/170g	425	38.8	250	9.5	1.4	22.8	0.5
Prawn & Mayonnaise, M & S*	1 Serving/60g	150	13.8	250	11.3	1.0	23.0	0.5
Smoked Salmon & Soft Cheese, M & S*	1 Serving/85g	208	17.3	245	11.7	3.3	20.4	0.5
DELIGHT								
Butterscotch Flavour, No Added Sugar, Tesco*	½ Pack/25g	115	5.1	460	4.8	63.3	20.5	0.0
Ravishing Raspberry, Made Up, Asda*	1/3 Pack/100g	112	3.9	112	3.2	16.0	3.9	0.0
Strawberry, Shapers, Boots*	1 Pot/121g	96	1.2	79	4.5	13.0	1.0	0.1
Strawberry Flavour, No Added Sugar, Dry, Tesco*	½ Pack/25g	111	4.5	445	4.9	65.4	17.9	0.0
DESSERT								
Baked Lemon, COU, M & S*	1 Serving/100g	140	2.5	140	6.8	22.0	2.5	0.8
Banoffee, Weight Watchers*	1 Pot/80g	152	3.0	190	4.9	34.3	3.7	1.4
Banoffee Layered, Sainsbury's*	1 Pot/115g	270	14.7	235	2.2	27.8	12.8	1.0
Blueberry Muffin, Tesco*	1 Pot/91g	265	18.7	291	2.0	24.5	20.6	3.0
Buttons, Milk Chocolate, Cadbury*	1 Pot/100g	280	14.9	280	6.2	30.8	14.9	0.0
Cappuccino, Italian, Co-Op*	1 Pack/90g	257	10.8	285	5.0	39.0	12.0	0.1
Chocolate, M & S*	1 Serving/120g	168	2.5	140	5.6	26.4	2.1	1.1

D

	Measure INFO/WEIGHT	per Measure KCAL	FAT	Nutrition Values per 100g / 100ml KCAL	PROT	CARB	FAT	FIBRE
DESSERT								
Chocolate, Weight Watchers*	1 Serving/82g	145	2.5	177	5.2	32.3	3.0	2.9
Chocolate Brownie, M & S*	¼ Pack/143.5g	612	39.6	425	4.7	39.6	27.5	1.0
Chocolate Creme, Somerfield*	1 Pot/125g	180	5.0	144	4.0	22.0	4.0	0.0
Chocolate Desire, Magnum, Wall's*	1 Dessert/85g	374	24.0	440	5.3	40.0	28.2	0.0
Chocolate Fudge Brownie, Tesco*	1 Pot/125g	374	16.6	299	4.6	40.2	13.3	1.3
Chocolate Marshmallow, Weight Watchers*	1 Serving/50g	97	2.4	194	3.2	34.5	4.7	1.3
Chocolate Muffin, Tesco*	1 Serving/104g	354	21.2	340	3.5	35.5	20.4	2.1
Chocolate Toffee, Weight Watchers*	1 Dessert/89.8g	177	4.0	197	4.3	34.9	4.5	2.2
Crazy Chocolate Overload, M & S*	1 Pot/120g	402	27.0	335	3.1	30.0	22.5	0.5
Creme Caramel, Sainsbury's*	1 Pot/100g	102	0.9	102	2.5	21.1	0.9	0.0
Crunchie, Dairy Milk, Cadbury*	1 Pot/100g	260	12.2	260	4.4	33.4	12.2	0.0
Custard, with Caramel, Layers, Ambrosia*	1 Pot/160.5g	183	4.7	114	2.5	19.6	2.9	0.0
Double Chocolate Brownies, Weight Watchers*	1 Serving/82.5g	145	2.5	177	5.2	32.3	3.0	2.9
Flake, Milk Chocolate, Cadbury*	1 Pot/100g	275	14.6	275	6.2	29.8	14.6	0.0
Gulabjam Indian, Waitrose*	1 Pot/180g	476	15.4	266	4.8	42.9	8.6	0.6
Hot Cookie Dough, Pizza Hut*	½ Bowl/172.6g	604	26.9	350	4.9	47.2	15.6	0.0
Paris Brest, Fresh Cream, TTD, Sainsbury's*	1 Cake/90g	315	22.1	350	5.9	26.2	24.6	1.0
Peach & Raspberry, COU, M & S*	1 Pot/90g	135	1.4	150	2.6	30.5	1.6	1.0
Pineapple & Passionfruit, M & S*	1 Pot/100g	130	3.8	130	0.8	21.7	3.8	0.3
Rocky Road, Sainsbury's*	1 Pot/110g	328	21.6	298	3.6	26.8	19.6	2.1
Rolo, Nestle*	1 Pot/77g	187	9.5	243	3.1	30.0	12.3	0.5
Strawberry, Value, Tesco*	1 Pot/115g	113	2.6	98	2.4	16.9	2.3	0.0
Strawberry Mousse Cake, Weight Watchers*	1 Serving/90g	124	2.4	138	3.0	25.5	2.7	0.5
Toffee, with Biscuit Pieces, Weight Watchers*	1 Pot/57.1g	93	2.7	163	2.7	26.2	4.8	0.2
Toffee & Vanilla, Weight Watchers*	1 Pot/67g	107	0.5	159	3.1	34.8	0.8	3.9
Toffee Banana Crunch, Farmfoods*	1/6 Dessert/82g	219	9.3	267	2.6	38.5	11.4	0.7
Toffee Flavour Fudge Swirl, Weight Watchers*	1 Pot/57g	82	2.5	143	2.5	22.6	4.4	0.4
Toffee Muffin, COU, M & S*	1 Serving/100g	180	2.2	180	3.7	35.8	2.2	0.3
Triple Chocolate, Delice, Sainsbury's*	1 Serving/105g	399	27.4	380	3.8	32.4	26.1	0.7
Triple Chocolate Layered, BGTY, Sainsbury's*	1 Pot/105g	147	2.9	140	4.2	24.4	2.8	0.5
Vanilla & Caramel, Petits Filous, Yoplait*	1 Pot/60g	90	3.2	150	4.7	21.0	5.3	0.2
Vanilla & Raspberry Swirl, Weight Watchers*	1 Serving/100ml	81	2.2	81	1.5	13.3	2.2	0.2
Vanilla & Strawberry Compote, Weight Watchers*	1 Pot/57g	81	2.2	142	2.5	23.4	3.9	0.2
Vanilla & Toffee, Heavenly Swirls, Tesco*	1 Pot/73g	106	1.8	145	2.5	28.1	2.5	0.5
Vanilla with Strawberries Swirl, Weight Watchers*	1 Pot/57g	46	1.3	81	1.5	13.3	2.2	0.2
DESSERT SAUCE								
Chocolate, M & S*	1 Dtsp/10.6g	35	1.0	330	2.1	59.3	9.4	1.9
Raspberry, M & S*	1 Serving/20g	24	0.1	120	0.5	28.7	0.3	2.6
Toffee, Old English, Asda*	1 Serving/28g	99	1.7	355	2.3	73.0	6.0	0.0
DHAL								
Black Gram, Average	1oz/28g	21	1.0	74	4.2	7.0	3.4	1.7
Blackeye Bean, Patak's*	1oz/28g	29	1.3	102	3.6	12.4	4.6	1.8
Chick Pea	1oz/28g	42	1.7	149	7.4	17.7	6.1	3.8
Chick Pea, Asda*	1 Serving/400g	404	12.0	101	4.5	14.0	3.0	3.0
Chick Pea, Canned, Asda*	½ Can/194g	198	6.2	102	4.3	14.0	3.2	2.9
Chick Pea, Sainsbury's*	½ Can/200g	432	18.2	216	10.8	22.7	9.1	7.1
Chickpea, Tinned, Sainsbury's*	½ Tin/432g	933	39.3	216	10.8	22.7	9.1	7.1
Lentil, Patak's*	1 Can/283g	156	2.8	55	2.8	9.3	1.0	1.0
Lentil, Red, Way to Five, Sainsbury's*	½ Pack/273.1g	254	4.1	93	5.5	14.4	1.5	1.4
Lentil, Red Masoor, Punjabi, Average	1oz/28g	39	1.3	139	7.2	19.2	4.6	2.0
Lentil, Red Masoor & Tomato with Butter, Average	1oz/28g	26	1.4	94	4.0	9.7	4.9	0.9
Lentil, Red Masoor & Vegetable, Average	1oz/28g	31	1.1	110	5.8	14.7	3.8	1.8
Lentil, Red Masoor with Vegetable Oil, Average	1oz/28g	48	2.2	172	7.6	19.2	7.9	1.8

D

	Measure INFO/WEIGHT	per Measure KCAL	FAT	Nutrition Values per 100g / 100ml KCAL	PROT	CARB	FAT	FIBRE
DHAL								
Lentil, Red Masoorl & Mung Bean, Average	1oz/28g	32	1.9	114	4.8	9.9	6.7	1.6
Lentil, Safeway*	1 Serving/200g	182	8.8	91	2.4	10.5	4.4	0.9
Lentil, Tesco*	1 Serving/200g	248	13.2	124	5.1	10.6	6.6	2.5
Mung Bean, Bengali	1oz/28g	20	0.9	73	4.2	7.4	3.3	1.7
Mung Beans, Dried, Boiled in Unsalted Water	1oz/28g	26	0.1	92	7.8	15.3	0.4	0.0
Mung Beans, Dried, Raw	1oz/28g	81	0.3	291	26.8	46.3	1.1	0.0
Regular, Eastern Essence*	1 Serving/113g	105	4.0	93	7.1	19.5	3.5	2.7
Split Peas, Yellow, Chana, Asda*	1 Serving/275g	300	19.3	109	2.6	9.0	7.0	1.8
Tarka, Asda*	½ Pack/150g	216	12.0	144	6.0	12.0	8.0	6.0
DHANSAK								
Chicken, Ready Meals, M & S*	1oz/28g	50	3.2	180	12.4	6.6	11.5	1.6
Chicken with Bagara Rice, Waitrose*	1 Pack/450g	549	8.1	122	8.2	18.2	1.8	1.2
Vegetable, Sainsbury's*	1 Serving/200g	148	5.6	74	3.1	8.9	2.8	2.8
DIJONNAISE								
Pork, Fillet, Finest, Tesco*	1 Pack/380g	536	28.6	141	16.5	1.8	7.5	0.5
DILL								
Dried	1 Tsp/1g	3	0.0	253	19.9	42.2	4.4	13.6
Fresh, Chopped, Average	1 Tbsp/3g	1	0.0	25	3.7	0.9	0.8	2.5
DIM SUM								
From Restaurant, Average	1 Piece/12g	50	2.4	433	28.9	31.3	20.4	0.0
DIME								
Terry's*	1oz/28g	154	9.5	550	4.6	68.5	33.8	0.6
DIP								
Aubergine, Fresh, Delphi*	½ Tub/85g	320	34.0	376	1.7	5.2	40.0	4.9
Aubergine, Fresh, Waitrose*	1 Serving/85g	159	12.8	187	2.5	10.5	15.0	1.7
Blue Cheese, Fresh, Sainsbury's*	1/5 Pot/34g	115	11.7	337	3.6	3.1	34.5	0.1
Caramelised Onion & Garlic, Waitrose*	¼ Pack/50g	232	24.5	464	1.5	4.4	48.9	0.5
Cheese & Chive, 50% Less Fat, Asda*	1 Pot/125g	261	21.5	209	4.5	9.0	17.2	0.0
Cheese & Chive, Asda*	1 Serving/42.5g	192	19.8	447	4.9	3.4	46.0	0.0
Cheese & Chive, Fresh, Safeway*	1 Pot/170g	877	92.1	516	4.1	3.0	54.2	0.0
Cheese & Chive, HL, Tesco*	1 Serving/50g	105	8.6	210	4.9	8.1	17.2	0.1
Cheese & Chive, Tesco*	¼ Pack/50g	268	27.6	535	4.3	4.3	55.1	0.1
Chilli, M & S*	1 Pot/35g	103	0.1	295	0.4	73.2	0.2	0.4
Chilli Cheese, Asda*	1 Serving/50g	131	11.0	262	8.0	8.0	22.0	1.1
Cucumber & Mint, Fresh, Sainsbury's*	1oz/28g	34	2.8	123	4.5	3.7	10.0	0.0
Feta Cheese, Fresh, Tesco*	1oz/28g	81	7.1	288	6.8	7.9	25.5	0.7
Garlic, Olive Oil & Butter, Pizza Express*	½ Pot/17g	106	11.5	621	1.5	2.8	67.4	0.5
Garlic & Herb, Big Dipper, Morrisons*	¼ Pot/75g	278	28.1	370	1.3	6.9	37.5	0.4
Garlic & Herb, M & S*	1 Tbsp/10g	47	4.8	465	1.6	7.4	47.7	0.5
Garlic & Herb, Tesco*	¼ Pack/42.5g	260	28.1	604	0.9	3.2	65.4	0.3
Hot Salsa, Doritos, Walkers*	1 Jar/300g	87	0.6	29	0.9	5.8	0.2	1.6
Mature Cheddar Cheese & Chive, Fresh, Waitrose*	½ Pot/85g	393	40.5	462	5.8	2.4	47.7	1.7
Mexican Bean, Doritos, Walkers*	1 Tbsp/20g	18	0.7	89	2.7	12.1	3.3	2.4
Mild Salsa, Doritos, Walkers*	1 Tbsp/30g	9	0.1	30	0.8	6.0	0.3	1.5
Mustard & Honey, Fresh, Sainsbury's*	1oz/28g	100	10.2	356	2.2	5.1	36.3	0.0
Nacho Cheese, M & S*	1oz/28g	76	6.6	270	9.8	3.8	23.7	0.4
Nacho Cheese, Sainsbury's*	1 Serving/50g	244	25.1	487	4.8	3.9	50.2	0.0
Onion & Garlic, 50% Less Fat, Asda*	1oz/28g	59	4.8	209	4.5	9.0	17.2	0.0
Onion & Garlic, Classic, Tesco*	1 Serving/30g	133	13.9	442	1.7	4.6	46.3	0.2
Onion & Garlic, HL, Tesco*	1 Serving/42.5g	81	7.3	188	2.5	6.3	17.0	0.1
Pecorino, Basil & Pine Nut, Fresh, Waitrose*	½ Pot/85g	338	33.7	398	5.1	5.1	39.7	0.0
Smoked Salmon & Dill, Fresh, Waitrose*	½ Pot/85g	373	38.0	439	5.1	4.1	44.7	0.1
Sour Cream, Tesco*	1 Serving/38g	111	11.2	297	3.4	3.9	29.8	0.2

	Measure INFO/WEIGHT	per Measure KCAL	FAT	Nutrition Values per 100g / 100ml KCAL	PROT	CARB	FAT	FIBRE
DIP								
Sour Cream & Chive, Asda*	1 Pot/50.5g	150	15.0	297	3.4	3.9	29.8	0.2
Sour Cream & Chive, BGTY, Sainsbury's*	1oz/28g	46	4.1	165	4.9	3.4	14.6	0.7
Sour Cream & Chive, Doritos, Walkers*	1 Tbsp/20g	52	4.9	258	1.9	6.9	24.7	1.9
Sour Cream & Chive, Fresh, Tesco*	½ Pot/75g	305	31.8	407	2.1	4.1	42.4	0.0
Sour Cream & Chive, Primula*	1oz/28g	97	9.9	346	5.0	1.8	35.3	0.0
Sour Cream & Chive, Sainsbury's*	1 Serving/50g	141	13.8	282	3.1	5.4	27.5	0.1
Sour Cream & Chives, Mexican Style, Morrisons*	¼ Pack/25g	69	7.0	274	2.2	3.4	27.9	0.4
Soured Cream & Chive, BGTY, Sainsbury's*	1 Serving/170g	253	17.5	149	4.2	9.9	10.3	0.1
Soured Cream & Chive, Classic, Tesco*	1 Serving/25g	81	8.4	323	1.7	3.2	33.7	0.2
Soured Cream & Chive, HL, Tesco*	1 Serving/31g	45	3.3	145	3.8	7.5	10.6	0.2
Soured Cream & Chive, M & S*	1 Serving/50g	115	11.1	230	2.1	5.8	22.1	0.7
Sun Dried Tomato, Somerfield*	1oz/28g	155	16.5	552	1.0	5.0	59.0	0.0
Sweet & Zesty, Doritos, Walkers*	1 Jar/375g	150	1.9	40	1.3	8.0	0.5	1.4
Sweet Chilli, Chinese Snack Selection, Morrisons*	½ Pot/20g	64	0.0	320	0.1	79.4	0.2	0.6
DIPPER								
Broad Beans & Pea, COU, M & S*	1 Pack/130g	91	3.1	70	3.7	8.9	2.4	2.8
Carrot, Thousand Island, M & S*	1 Pack/130g	72	2.6	55	0.9	7.9	2.0	2.3
Celery, M & S*	1 Pot/130g	163	14.3	125	1.8	4.4	11.0	1.2
Cheese & Onion, Weight Watchers*	1 Pack/50g	93	1.9	186	15.2	24.8	3.8	2.0
DISCOS								
Beef, KP Snacks*	1 Pack/28g	145	8.2	518	5.1	58.7	29.3	2.4
Cheese & Onion, KP Snacks*	1 Pack/28g	146	8.2	520	5.1	59.1	29.3	2.5
Salt & Vinegar, KP Snacks*	1 Bag/31g	160	9.1	517	4.7	58.3	29.5	2.3
DOLLY MIXTURES								
M & S*	1 Pack/115g	431	1.6	375	1.8	89.2	1.4	0.0
Sainsbury's*	1 Serving/10g	40	0.2	401	1.4	94.4	1.9	0.1
SmartPrice, Asda*	1 Sweet/2.9g	11	0.0	380	0.5	91.0	1.6	0.0
Tesco*	1 Pack/100g	376	1.5	376	1.6	88.9	1.5	0.0
DOPIAZA								
Chicken, Safeway*	1 Pack/326g	450	27.4	138	10.4	5.3	8.4	1.4
Chicken, Sainsbury's*	½ Pack/200g	272	15.8	136	13.2	3.1	7.9	0.8
Chicken, Tesco*	1 Pack/350g	448	24.9	128	10.8	5.3	7.1	0.6
Chicken, with Pilau Rice, Sharwood's*	1 Pack/375g	473	17.3	126	5.3	15.8	4.6	0.8
Chicken, with Pilau Rice, Tesco*	1 Pack/400g	424	15.2	106	5.7	12.3	3.8	1.5
Mushroom, Retail	1oz/28g	19	1.6	69	1.3	3.7	5.7	1.1
Mushroom, Tesco*	1 Pack/225g	155	9.9	69	2.4	5.1	4.4	1.5
Mushroom, Waitrose*	½ Pack/150g	81	4.7	54	2.2	4.3	3.1	2.3
DORITOS								
Chargrilled BBQ, Walkers*	1 Bag/35g	170	8.8	485	5.5	59.0	25.0	3.5
Cheesy 3d's, Doritos, Walkers*	1 Pack/20g	89	3.2	445	7.0	68.0	16.0	3.0
Chilli Heatwave, Walkers*	1 Bag/35g	175	9.1	500	7.0	60.0	26.0	3.0
Cool, Ranch Chips, Walkers*	1 Package/49.6g	250	13.0	504	8.1	64.5	26.2	4.0
Cool Original, Walkers*	1 Bag/30.1g	151	8.1	500	7.5	58.0	27.0	3.0
Cool Spice 3ds, Walkers*	1 Bag/24g	108	4.3	450	8.0	64.0	18.0	4.4
Dippas, Hint of Chilli, Dipping Chips, Walkers*	1 Bag/35g	173	8.8	495	7.0	61.0	25.0	3.5
Dippas, Hint of Lime, Walkers*	1 Bag/35g	173	8.8	495	7.0	60.0	25.0	3.5
Dippas, Lightly Salted, Dipping Chips, Walkers*	1 Serving/35g	179	9.5	510	6.5	60.0	27.0	3.0
Latinos, Chargrilled BBQ, Walkers*	1 Serving/35g	170	8.8	485	5.5	59.0	25.0	3.5
Latinos, Mexican Grill, Walkers*	1 Serving/35g	170	8.8	485	6.5	59.0	25.0	3.5
Lightly Salted Dippas, Doritos, Walkers*	1 Bag/50g	255	13.5	510	6.5	60.0	27.0	3.0
Mexican Hot, Walkers*	1 Bag/40g	202	10.8	505	8.0	57.0	27.0	3.5
Tangy Cheese, Walkers*	1 Bag/40g	200	10.8	500	7.0	57.0	27.0	3.0

	Measure INFO/WEIGHT	per Measure KCAL	FAT	Nutrition Values per 100g / 100ml KCAL	PROT	CARB	FAT	FIBRE
DOUBLE DECKER								
Cadbury*	1 Bar/51g	235	9.6	460	4.4	68.4	18.9	0.6
DOUGH BALLS								
Cheese & Garlic, Occasions, Sainsbury's*	1 Ball/12g	41	2.2	341	10.3	33.4	18.5	2.1
Garlic, Tesco*	1 Serving/10g	40	2.3	400	7.0	40.0	23.0	1.0
Garlic, Waitrose*	1 Ball/11g	38	1.8	347	8.5	41.4	16.4	3.3
Garlic & Herb, Occasions, Sainsbury's*	1 Ball/12g	41	2.1	343	8.4	38.7	17.2	2.2
Sainsbury's*	1 Ball/12g	41	2.1	343	8.4	38.7	17.2	2.2
Supermarket, Pizza Express*	8 Balls/100g	363	1.7	363	14.3	72.9	1.7	3.3
with Garlic & Herb Butter, Aldi*	1 Ball/12.3g	44	2.2	365	7.7	46.7	18.2	1.8
DOUGHNUTS								
Apple & Custard, Finger, Sainsbury's*	1 Serving/65g	137	6.0	210	4.4	27.5	9.2	1.9
Apple & Fresh Cream, Sainsbury's*	1 Doughnut/79g	216	11.4	273	5.4	30.5	14.4	1.9
Baked, HL, Tesco*	1 Doughnut/67g	166	3.9	248	6.4	42.2	5.9	1.4
Chocolate, Somerfield*	1 Doughnut/57g	203	9.5	356	7.8	43.8	16.6	1.7
Cream & Jam, Tesco*	1 Doughnut/90g	288	14.1	320	5.4	39.4	15.7	2.0
Custard, Sainsbury's*	1 Doughnut/70g	172	7.5	246	5.1	32.3	10.7	2.3
Custard, Tesco*	1 Doughnut/91g	266	14.4	292	4.1	33.4	15.8	1.1
Custard Filled, Average	1 Doughnut/75g	269	14.3	358	6.2	43.3	19.0	0.0
Dairy Cream, M & S*	1oz/28g	87	3.9	310	4.9	40.8	14.1	1.3
Dairy Cream & Jam, Somerfield*	1 Doughnut/80g	296	18.5	370	4.6	35.8	23.1	1.3
Dairy Cream Finger, Safeway*	1 Doughnut/98g	342	19.7	349	5.5	36.4	20.1	1.8
Jam, American Style, Budgens*	1 Doughnut/46g	127	3.1	275	7.1	46.5	6.7	0.0
Jam, American Style, Sainsbury's*	1 Doughnut/65g	220	20.6	339	4.9	49.6	31.8	3.5
Jam, M & S*	1 Doughnut/49g	141	2.0	287	5.0	57.6	4.0	1.3
Jam, Mini, Somerfield*	1 Doughnut/45g	138	4.1	307	6.4	50.1	9.0	1.4
Jam, Somerfield*	1 Doughnut/69g	225	8.4	325	5.7	47.2	12.2	1.8
Jam Filled, Average	1 Doughnut/75g	252	10.9	336	5.7	48.8	14.5	0.0
Mini, Sainsbury's*	1 Doughnut/14g	53	2.7	379	5.2	47.9	18.9	2.1
Mini Donuts, Crunchie, Cadbury*	1oz/28g	105	4.8	375	4.8	49.8	17.0	0.0
Plain, Ring, Average	1 Doughnut/60g	238	13.0	397	6.1	47.2	21.7	0.0
Ring, Co-Op*	1 Doughnut/106g	392	21.2	370	4.0	44.0	20.0	1.0
Ring, Iced, Average	1 Doughnut/70g	268	12.3	383	4.8	55.1	17.5	0.0
Ring, Waitrose*	1 Doughnut/107g	396	21.3	370	4.2	43.5	19.9	0.7
Strawberry Jam & Cream, Sainsbury's*	1 Doughnut/80g	299	18.5	374	5.3	36.2	23.2	1.3
Toffee, Tesco*	1 Doughnut/75g	235	8.7	313	8.0	44.2	11.6	1.6
Yum Yums, Glazed, Sweet, Waitrose*	1 Donut/45g	172	10.0	382	4.0	41.6	22.2	2.0
Yum Yums, M & S*	1 Doughnut/37g	155	8.9	420	4.9	45.7	23.9	1.6
Yum Yums, Tesco*	1 Doughnut/61g	232	10.1	380	6.1	51.6	16.6	1.7
DOVER SOLE								
Raw, Average	1oz/28g	25	0.5	89	18.1	0.0	1.8	0.0
DR PEPPER*								
Coca-Cola*	1 Bottle/500ml	210	0.0	42	0.0	10.9	0.0	0.0
Zero, Coca-Cola*	1 Can/330ml	2	0.0	1	0.0	0.0	0.0	0.0
DRAMBUIE								
39% Volume	1 Pub Shot/35ml	95	0.0	272	0.0	0.0	0.0	0.0
DREAM								
Cadbury*	1 Bar/45g	250	15.0	555	4.5	59.7	33.3	0.0
Double Fudge, Cadbury*	1oz/28g	139	7.1	495	6.3	61.4	25.2	0.0
White Chocolate, Cadbury*	1 Piece/8g	44	2.7	555	4.5	59.7	33.3	0.0
DREAM TOPPING								
Dry, Bird's*	1oz/28g	193	16.4	690	6.7	32.5	58.5	0.5
Made Up, Skimmed Milk, Bird's*	1oz/28g	21	1.5	75	2.0	4.8	5.3	0.0

D

DRESSING

INFO/WEIGHT	Measure	per Measure		Nutrition Values per 100g / 100ml				
		KCAL	FAT	KCAL	PROT	CARB	FAT	FIBRE
Balsamic, Extra Virgin Olive Oil, TTD, Sainsbury's*	1 Tsp/5ml	19	1.8	376	0.5	12.8	36.0	0.4
Balsamic, Fresh Olive Co*	1 Tbsp/15g	42	0.1	282	1.5	67.8	0.5	0.6
Balsamic, M & S*	1 Tbsp/15g	74	7.2	490	0.3	9.7	48.0	0.5
Balsamic, New, Sainsbury's*	1 Tbsp/15g	58	5.2	389	0.6	18.3	34.8	0.8
Balsamic, Sainsbury's*	1 Tbsp/15ml	47	4.3	316	0.4	13.8	28.8	0.4
Balsamic, Schwartz*	2 Tbsp/30ml	23	0.6	77	0.5	14.2	2.0	0.0
Balsamic, Sweet, Finest, Tesco*	1 Serving/10ml	16	0.0	155	0.4	36.9	0.1	0.4
Balsamic, TTD, Sainsbury's*	1 Serving/15g	58	5.2	389	0.6	18.3	34.8	0.8
Balsamic Bliss, Ainsley Harriott*	1 Tbsp/15g	41	3.2	272	0.8	19.3	21.1	0.0
Balsamic Vinegar, Aged & Oregano, Waitrose*	1 Tbsp/15ml	51	5.1	340	0.0	9.3	34.0	0.0
Balsamic Vinegar, Asda*	1 Pack/44ml	121	11.9	275	0.9	7.0	27.0	0.0
Balsamic Vinegar, Morrisons*	1 Serving/15ml	17	0.2	111	0.1	22.9	1.6	0.1
Balsamic Vinegar, Olives & Herb, COU, M & S*	1 Serving/30g	23	0.6	75	0.5	14.3	2.0	0.5
Balsamic with Olive Oil, Pizza Express*	1 Serving/10g	42	4.1	421	0.3	10.3	41.2	0.0
Basil & Pesto, COU, M & S*	1 Serving/50ml	30	1.1	60	0.6	8.3	2.2	0.8
Blossom Honey & Four Mustard, Low Fat, M & S*	1 Serving/10g	11	0.1	110	1.6	22.5	1.4	0.1
Blue Cheese, HE, Tesco*	1 Tsp/5g	4	0.2	82	4.4	9.0	3.1	0.1
Blue Cheese, Hellmann's*	1 Tbsp/15g	69	7.1	459	0.7	6.3	47.2	1.1
Blue Cheese, Salad, Waitrose*	1 Serving/50g	265	25.2	530	2.1	17.3	50.3	4.1
Blue Cheese, Tesco*	1 Serving/15ml	75	7.7	500	2.5	6.9	51.4	0.2
Caesar, 95% Fat Free, Tesco*	1 Tsp/6g	5	0.2	88	4.1	8.9	3.7	0.3
Caesar, Chilled, Reduced Fat, Tesco*	1 Tsp/5ml	13	1.2	252	6.5	3.1	23.7	0.1
Caesar, Classic, Sainsbury's*	1 Tsp/5ml	22	2.3	442	2.7	4.6	45.9	0.5
Caesar, Finest, Tesco*	1 Tbsp/15ml	72	7.6	477	1.9	2.8	50.9	0.2
Caesar, Fresh, Asda*	1 Dtsp/10ml	45	4.8	454	2.4	3.2	48.0	0.0
Caesar, Fresh, M & S*	1 Tsp/6g	32	3.4	525	2.0	1.8	56.4	0.2
Caesar, HE, Tesco*	1 Tbsp/15ml	11	0.4	74	3.0	8.4	2.8	0.2
Caesar, Hellmann's*	1 Tsp/6g	30	3.1	499	2.5	4.5	51.7	0.3
Caesar, HL, Tesco*	1 Serving/125ml	93	3.5	74	3.0	8.4	2.8	0.2
Caesar, Less Than 3% Fat, BGTY, Sainsbury's*	1 Serving/20g	10	0.4	48	0.8	7.0	1.9	0.3
Caesar, Light, Kraft*	1 Serving/15g	14	0.5	95	1.7	13.0	3.6	0.2
Caesar, Low Fat, Cardini's*	2 Tbsp/28g	23	0.8	82	2.4	11.6	2.9	0.3
Caesar, Luxury, Hellmann's*	1 Tsp/4g	20	2.1	498	2.5	4.4	51.7	0.3
Caesar, M & S*	1 Tbsp/15ml	91	9.6	605	4.0	2.7	64.3	0.6
Caesar, Original, Cardini's*	1 Serving/10g	56	6.0	555	2.3	1.5	60.0	0.2
Caesar, Tesco*	1 Tbsp/15ml	71	7.5	475	4.6	2.1	49.8	0.1
Caesar, Waitrose*	1 Serving/15ml	72	7.6	479	4.5	0.9	50.8	0.2
Caesar Salad, Fresh, Sainsbury's*	1 Tbsp/15ml	72	7.5	477	3.7	3.7	49.7	1.9
Caesar Style, GFY, Asda*	1 Sachet/44ml	34	1.0	77	5.0	9.0	2.3	0.0
Caesar Style, Kraft*	1 Tbsp/15ml	15	0.5	102	2.1	15.0	3.5	0.1
Caesar Style, Low Fat, Weight Watchers*	1 Tsp/6g	4	0.2	60	1.6	5.8	3.4	0.1
Classic French, Fresh, M & S*	1 Serving/10ml	52	5.3	515	0.6	8.2	53.1	0.2
Classic Italian, Get Dressed, Kraft*	1 Serving/25ml	30	2.6	120	0.1	5.6	10.3	0.5
Cream Cheese & Chive, Creamy Ranch, Kraft*	1 Serving/15ml	31	2.6	205	1.2	11.0	17.0	0.0
Creamy Caesar, Get Dressed, Kraft*	1 Serving/66.7g	68	2.3	102	2.1	15.0	3.5	0.1
Creamy Ranch, 95% Fat Free, Kraft*	1 Tsp/6ml	7	0.3	111	1.4	14.5	5.0	0.3
Dijon Honey Mustard, Briannas*	2 Tbsp/30ml	130	12.0	433	0.0	20.0	40.0	0.0
French, BGTY, Organic, Sainsbury's*	1 Tbsp/15ml	11	0.6	71	0.2	8.3	4.1	0.5
French, BGTY, Sainsbury's*	1 Tbsp/15ml	12	0.7	79	1.1	8.8	4.4	0.5
French, Chilled, Tesco*	1 Tbsp/15ml	63	5.9	421	1.1	15.1	39.6	0.0
French, Classic, Fat Free, Kraft*	1 Tsp/5ml	2	0.0	39	0.1	8.7	0.0	0.5
French, Classic, Sainsbury's*	1 Tbsp/15ml	71	7.4	473	1.0	5.7	49.6	0.5
French, Classics, M & S*	1 Tbsp/15ml	77	8.0	516	0.6	8.2	53.1	0.2

D

DRESSING

INFO/WEIGHT	Measure	per Measure		Nutrition Values per 100g / 100ml				
		KCAL	FAT	KCAL	PROT	CARB	FAT	FIBRE
French, Fresh, HE, Tesco*	1 Tbsp/15ml	8	0.4	56	1.1	6.7	2.8	0.0
French, Fresh, Morrisons*	1 Tbsp/15ml	75	7.3	499	1.5	13.6	48.7	0.0
French, Fresh, Organic, Sainsbury's*	1 Tbsp/15ml	45	4.7	301	0.4	5.5	31.0	0.4
French, Fresh, Sainsbury's*	1 Tbsp/15ml	64	6.7	429	0.6	6.6	44.6	0.6
French, GFY, Asda*	1 Tbsp/15g	8	0.3	50	0.7	7.0	2.1	0.1
French, Good Intentions, Somerfield*	1 Serving/15ml	12	0.5	83	0.7	12.1	3.5	0.3
French, HE, Tesco*	1 Tbsp/15ml	3	0.1	23	0.8	3.1	0.8	0.0
French, HL, Tesco*	1 Serving/25ml	14	0.7	56	1.1	6.7	2.8	0.0
French, Less Than 3% Fat, M & S*	1 Tbsp/15ml	10	0.4	68	0.7	11.5	2.6	0.7
French, Oil Free, French, Waitrose*	1 Tsp/5ml	4	0.1	76	1.5	13.1	2.0	0.6
French, Oil Free, PB, Waitrose*	1 Serving/15ml	11	0.2	72	2.2	12.2	1.6	1.1
French, Organic, M & S*	1 Tbsp/15g	98	10.4	655	0.2	7.5	69.4	0.3
French, Organic, Tesco*	1 Tsp/5ml	23	2.2	451	0.6	11.0	44.9	0.2
French, Reduced Fat, M & S*	1 Tbsp/15g	11	0.4	70	0.7	11.5	2.8	0.7
French, Sainsbury's*	1 Tbsp/15ml	33	2.9	219	0.6	9.8	19.1	0.5
French, Tesco*	1 Serving/25ml	110	11.2	441	0.7	7.2	44.9	0.2
French, Virtually Fat Free, Aldi*	1 Serving/10g	3	0.0	33	0.9	6.7	0.3	1.1
French Salad, M & S*	1 Serving/25ml	156	16.8	625	0.5	3.8	67.3	0.1
French Style, Eat Smart, Safeway*	1 Serving/15ml	22	0.4	145	0.7	28.9	2.5	0.7
French Style, Oil Free, HE, Tesco*	1 Tbsp/15g	5	0.0	30	0.3	6.0	0.2	1.4
Garlic & Herb, PB, Waitrose*	1 Serving/50ml	68	0.7	135	0.6	29.9	1.4	0.8
Herb, Eat Smart, Safeway*	1 Tbsp/15ml	9	0.3	60	0.5	9.5	2.0	0.5
Herb & Garlic, Light, 5% Fat, Get Dressed, Kraft*	1 Serving/25ml	29	1.3	116	1.3	15.5	5.1	0.2
Honey, Orange & Mustard, BGTY, Sainsbury's*	1 Tbsp/15ml	16	0.4	105	1.8	18.6	2.5	1.8
Honey & Mustard, Eat Smart, Safeway*	1 Tbsp/15ml	25	0.1	165	0.8	37.5	0.9	0.3
Honey & Mustard, EPC*	1 Tbsp/15ml	17	0.2	111	2.5	21.8	1.5	1.0
Honey & Mustard, Finest, Tesco*	1 Serving/25ml	72	5.6	288	1.7	19.6	22.5	0.7
Honey & Mustard, Fresh, M & S*	1 Serving/10ml	43	4.2	430	1.7	9.7	42.4	0.5
Honey & Mustard, GFY, Asda*	1 Tbsp/15g	13	0.5	89	1.5	13.0	3.4	0.8
Honey & Mustard, HE, Tesco*	1 Tbsp/15g	12	0.4	79	1.5	12.1	2.7	0.9
Honey & Mustard, HL, Tesco*	1 Serving/15ml	12	0.4	82	1.0	13.5	2.7	0.9
Honey & Mustard, M & S*	1 Tbsp/15ml	64	6.4	427	1.7	9.7	42.4	0.6
Honey & Mustard, Sainsbury's*	1 Serving/10ml	37	3.3	366	1.0	15.4	33.0	0.1
Honey & Mustard, Tesco*	1 Serving/10ml	38	3.6	378	0.8	13.1	35.8	0.6
Hot Lime & Coconut, BGTY, Sainsbury's*	1 Tbsp/15ml	8	0.4	51	0.7	5.7	2.9	1.2
Italian, M & S*	1 Tbsp/15ml	62	6.2	415	0.9	8.9	41.5	1.0
Italian Salad, Hellmann's*	1 Serving/50g	103	8.4	206	0.7	12.8	16.7	0.0
Lemon, Feta & Oregano, M & S*	1 Tbsp/15ml	24	2.0	160	1.3	8.2	13.4	0.6
Lemon & Cracked Black Pepper, GFY, Asda*	1 Tbsp/15g	9	0.0	57	0.2	14.0	0.0	0.3
Lime & Coriander, EPC*	1 Serving/50g	29	0.2	57	0.3	13.3	0.3	0.0
Lime & Coriander, Oil Free, Waitrose*	1 Tsp/5ml	3	0.1	65	1.5	11.9	1.3	0.4
Mustard & Dill, PB, Waitrose*	1 Tbsp/15ml	24	0.5	159	1.1	31.5	3.2	1.1
Oil & Lemon	1 Tbsp/15g	97	10.6	647	0.3	2.8	70.6	0.0
Olive Oil, Pizza Express*	2 Tsp/5g	29	3.2	573	1.4	3.4	63.0	0.0
Olive Oil & Balsamic Vinegar, Sainsbury's*	1 Serving/25ml	104	10.5	415	0.9	9.4	41.8	0.2
Pesto, Finest, Tesco*	1 Serving/30ml	108	11.1	360	3.5	2.9	37.1	0.9
Ranch Style, Asda*	1 Serving/44ml	37	1.7	85	3.5	9.0	3.9	0.0
Raspberry Balsamic Vinegar, EPC*	1 Serving/50g	34	0.1	67	0.4	15.7	0.1	0.6
Red Pepper, M & S*	1 Tbsp/15ml	58	5.9	385	0.6	7.6	39.2	0.5
Roasted Red Pepper, TTD, Sainsbury's*	1 Tbsp/15ml	35	2.9	235	1.1	14.9	19.0	1.4
Salad, HE, Tesco*	1 Tbsp/15g	22	1.4	144	0.7	14.0	9.5	0.5
Salad, Honey & Mustard, Light, Kraft*	1 Tbsp/15ml	19	0.7	126	1.2	19.0	4.6	1.1
Salad, Italian, Light, Kraft*	1 Tbsp/15ml	5	0.0	31	0.1	6.8	0.0	0.6

D

	Measure INFO/WEIGHT	per Measure		Nutrition Values per 100g / 100ml				
		KCAL	FAT	KCAL	PROT	CARB	FAT	FIBRE

DRESSING

	Measure INFO/WEIGHT	KCAL	FAT	KCAL	PROT	CARB	FAT	FIBRE
Salad, Italian, Newman's Own*	1 Tbsp/10g	55	6.0	545	0.2	1.0	59.8	0.0
Salad, Kickin' Mango, Oil Free, Ainsley Harriott*	1 Tbsp/15ml	14	0.0	92	0.1	21.1	0.1	0.0
Salad, Light, Heinz*	1 Serving/9.8g	24	2.0	244	1.8	13.5	19.9	0.0
Salad, Low Fat, Weight Watchers*	1 Tbsp/10g	11	0.4	106	1.5	15.4	4.3	0.0
Salad, Pizza Express*	1 Serving/5g	29	3.2	573	1.4	3.4	63.0	0.0
Salad, Thousand Island, 95% Fat Free, Asda*	1 Tsp/6g	6	0.3	99	1.6	12.6	4.7	0.5
Salad, Thousand Island, Hellmann's*	1oz/28g	97	8.7	347	0.9	15.2	31.0	1.0
Salad, Vinaigrette Style, 95% Fat Free, Asda*	1 Tbsp/15ml	6	0.0	42	0.1	10.6	0.0	0.3
Salad Cream Style, Weight Watchers*	1 Tbsp/10g	12	0.4	115	1.5	16.2	4.4	0.0
Seafood, M & S*	1 Tsp/7g	39	4.2	555	0.9	4.9	59.3	0.9
Sweet Balsamic & Garlic, BGTY, Sainsbury's*	1 Serving/20g	10	0.1	51	0.2	11.9	0.3	0.2
Sweet Chilli, COU, M & S*	1 Tbsp/15ml	9	0.1	60	0.5	14.5	0.5	0.4
Sweetfire Pepper, HE, Tesco*	1 Serving/10ml	7	0.0	67	0.6	15.7	0.3	0.1
Thai Lime & Coriander, EPC*	1 Serving/25g	26	0.2	104	1.6	22.3	0.9	1.1
Thousand Island	1 Tsp/6g	19	1.8	323	1.1	12.5	30.2	0.4
Thousand Island, COU, M & S*	1 Serving/30g	26	0.8	85	1.4	14.2	2.6	1.1
Thousand Island, HE, Tesco*	1 Serving/25ml	47	3.8	189	2.9	10.0	15.1	0.4
Thousand Island, Original, Kraft*	1oz/28g	102	8.8	365	0.9	19.0	31.5	0.4
Thousand Island, Reduced Calorie	1 Tsp/6g	12	0.9	195	0.7	14.7	15.2	0.0
Thousand Island, Tesco*	1 Tbsp/15.3g	55	4.7	360	1.1	19.5	30.5	0.3
Tomato & Basil, HE, Tesco*	1 Serving/10ml	7	0.2	73	0.5	12.9	2.0	0.5
Tomato & Basil, HL, Tesco*	½ Pot/75ml	41	1.1	55	0.8	9.0	1.5	0.5
Tomato & Herb, Less Than 1% Fat, Asda*	1 Tbsp/15g	6	0.1	43	0.7	8.0	0.9	0.4
Tomato & Red Pepper, BGTY, Sainsbury's*	1 Serving/50ml	42	2.2	83	1.1	10.0	4.3	0.6
Tomato Basil, Light, Kraft*	1 Serving/15ml	10	0.1	68	1.0	14.5	0.4	2.5
True Blue Cheese, Briannas*	2 Tbsp/30ml	120	11.0	400	3.3	16.7	36.7	0.0
Waistline, Reduced Fat, Crosse & Blackwell*	1oz/28g	29	1.7	105	0.8	11.6	6.0	0.3
Yoghurt & Mint, GFY, Asda*	1 Tbsp/15g	11	0.3	76	2.8	11.7	2.0	0.4
Yoghurt & Mint, PB, Waitrose*	1 Serving/100ml	130	2.6	130	4.6	22.1	2.6	0.7
Yoghurt & Mint, Safeway*	1 Serving/15ml	54	5.3	360	3.3	6.7	35.3	0.0
Yoghurt Mint Cucumber, M & S*	1 Tsp/5ml	6	0.4	115	1.0	8.7	8.0	0.0

DRIED FRUIT

Exotic, Ready to Eat, Sainsbury's*	1/3 Pack/85g	241	0.1	284	0.2	70.6	0.1	2.4
Juicy Sprinkle, Nature's Harvest*	1 Serving/20g	79	2.0	397	4.9	71.9	10.0	4.2
Nut & Seed Mix, M & S*	½ Pack/35g	160	8.8	457	12.4	44.3	25.1	6.0

DRIED FRUIT & NUT MIX

Cranberries & Macadamias, Co-Op*	¼ Pack/120g	180	11.0	150	1.0	16.3	9.2	1.9
The Mix, Whitworths*	1 Pot/90g	341	13.1	379	4.1	63.1	14.6	7.3

DRIED FRUIT & SEED MIX

Sainsbury's*	1 Pack/50g	204	10.7	408	11.6	42.0	21.4	5.1

DRIED FRUIT MIX

5 Fruits, Ready to Eat, Sundora*	½ Pack/100g	233	0.4	233	1.6	58.4	0.4	6.8
Albert Heijn*	1 Serving/50g	110	0.3	220	2.1	51.0	0.5	0.0
Asda*	1 Serving/50g	153	0.3	305	2.0	74.0	0.5	0.6
Average	1 Tbsp/25g	67	0.1	268	2.3	68.1	0.4	2.2
Baby Mix, Somerfield*	1 Pack/250g	520	1.8	208	3.1	47.2	0.7	5.3
Berry, Whole Foods, Tesco*	1 Serving/25g	66	0.2	265	3.3	60.0	0.7	7.5
Exotic Mix, Sundora*	1 Sm Pack/50g	138	1.4	276	2.3	60.6	2.7	3.8
Fruit Salad, Whitworths*	1 Serving/62g	113	0.3	183	2.9	41.8	0.5	6.6
Luxury, Co-Op*	1 Serving/40g	114	0.2	285	2.0	68.0	0.6	4.0
Medley, Shapers, Boots*	1 Serving/50g	131	0.3	262	3.2	61.0	0.6	5.5
Taste of Hawaii, Extra Special, Asda*	1 Serving/100g	314	0.8	314	1.7	75.0	0.8	4.4
Taste of New England, Asda*	1 Serving/50g	158	0.6	316	2.2	74.0	1.2	5.0

D

	Measure INFO/WEIGHT	per Measure KCAL	FAT	Nutrition Values per 100g / 100ml KCAL	PROT	CARB	FAT	FIBRE
DRIED FRUIT MIX								
Tesco*	1 Tbsp/25g	71	0.1	284	2.3	67.9	0.4	2.2
Tropical, Morrisons*	1 Pack/200g	368	1.0	184	1.7	50.6	0.5	6.3
Tropical, Somerfield*	1 Bag/50g	306	3.0	611	71.1	68.4	5.9	3.7
DRIFTER								
Nestle*	1 Finger/31g	143	6.5	478	3.7	67.3	21.5	0.8
DRINK								
Elderflower, Sparkling, Co-Op*	1 Glass/250ml	75	0.0	30	0.0	7.7	0.0	0.0
DRINK MIX								
Chocolate, Flavia*	1 Serving/18g	64	0.7	368	15.6	67.2	4.0	0.0
Milk Chocolate, Instant Break, Cadbury*	4 Tsp/28g	119	3.9	425	10.9	64.2	14.0	0.0
DRINKING CHOCOLATE								
Cadbury*	1 Heaped Tbs/16g	64	0.4	402	4.4	89.3	2.4	0.0
Dry, Asda*	1 Serving/30g	111	1.8	370	6.0	73.0	6.0	0.0
Dry, Tesco*	3 Tsp/25g	92	1.5	368	6.4	72.6	5.8	4.2
Dry, Waitrose*	3 Tsp/12g	48	0.7	403	7.2	79.9	6.1	2.9
Dry Powder, Cocodirect*	1 Serving/18g	67	1.5	372	8.9	65.1	8.4	0.0
Made Up, BGTY, Sainsbury's*	1 Serving/178.1g	114	0.4	64	3.9	11.4	0.2	0.7
Made Up with Semi-Skimmed Milk, Av	1 Mug/227ml	129	4.3	57	3.5	7.0	1.9	0.2
Made Up with Skimmed Milk, Average	1 Mug/227ml	100	1.1	44	3.5	7.0	0.5	0.0
Made Up with Whole Milk, Average	1 Mug/227ml	173	9.5	76	3.4	6.8	4.2	0.2
Maxpax, Light, Suchard*	1 Cup/10.5g	39	0.6	355	20.0	56.0	5.5	9.3
Powder, Made Up with Skimmed Milk	1 Mug/227ml	134	1.4	59	3.5	10.8	0.6	0.0
Powder, Made Up with Whole Milk	1 Mug/227ml	204	9.3	90	3.4	10.6	4.1	0.0
DRIPPING								
Beef	1oz/28g	249	27.7	891	0.0	0.0	99.0	0.0
DUCK								
Breast, Meat Only, Cooked, Average	1oz/28g	48	2.0	173	25.3	1.8	7.1	0.0
Breast, Meat Only, Raw, Average	1 Serving/160g	206	6.8	129	22.6	0.1	4.3	0.2
Leg, Meat & Skin, Average	1oz/28g	80	5.6	286	17.2	9.5	20.0	0.4
Legs, in Plum Sauce, Asda*	1 Leg/200g	452	23.0	226	24.1	6.4	11.5	0.5
Raw, Meat, Fat & Skin	1oz/28g	109	10.4	388	13.1	0.0	37.3	0.0
Roasted, Meat, Fat & Skin	1oz/28g	118	10.7	423	20.0	0.0	38.1	0.0
Wings, Chinese Barbecue, Sainsbury's*	1 Serving/175g	430	25.0	246	19.4	9.7	14.3	0.0
DUCK &								
Plum Sauce, Roasted, Sainsbury's*	½ Pack/150g	174	3.8	116	6.9	16.0	2.5	1.8
DUCK A L' ORANGE								
Roast, M & S*	½ Pack/270g	554	42.1	205	12.5	4.1	15.6	0.6
DUCK AROMATIC								
Crispy, ¼, with Sauce & Pancakes, Tesco*	1 Serving/61g	153	6.5	250	12.3	25.3	10.6	2.0
Crispy, ½, with Sauce & Pancakes, Tesco*	1/6 Pack/69.8g	162	7.4	232	18.3	15.9	10.6	1.1
Crispy, Asda*	1/3 Pack/165.7g	470	24.9	283	19.0	18.0	15.0	0.8
Crispy, Half, with Hoisin Sauce & 12 Pancakes, Tesco*	1/6 Pack/69.8g	162	7.4	232	18.3	15.9	10.6	1.1
Crispy, Half, with Sauce & Pancakes, Tesco*	1/6 Pack/69.8g	162	7.4	232	18.3	15.9	10.6	1.1
Crispy, Half Duck & Pancakes, M & S*	½ Pack/310.5g	590	26.7	190	13.9	14.0	8.6	2.1
Crispy, Quarter, Sauce & Pancakes, Tesco*	1 Serving/61g	153	6.5	250	12.3	25.3	10.6	2.0
Crispy, Quarter, with Hoisin Sauce & 6 Pancakes, Tesco*	1 Serving/61g	153	6.5	250	12.3	25.3	10.6	2.0
Crispy, Somerfield*	1 Serving/265g	782	49.0	295	18.1	14.0	18.5	0.7
Crispy, Whole, & Sauce & Pancakes, Tesco*	1/9 Pack/100g	280	17.2	280	18.9	12.0	17.2	0.4
Crispy, Whole, with Hoisin Sauce & 18 Pancakes, Tesco*	1/9 Pack/100g	280	17.2	280	18.9	12.0	17.2	0.4
with a Plum Sauce, Finest, Tesco*	1 Serving/250g	400	14.0	160	16.1	11.3	5.6	4.6
with Plum Sauce, Tesco*	½ Pack/250g	350	11.5	140	9.3	15.2	4.6	0.3
DUCK CANTONESE								
Style, Roast, Tesco*	1 Pack/300g	375	6.9	125	8.2	17.9	2.3	0.5

D

	Measure INFO/WEIGHT	per Measure KCAL FAT		Nutrition Values per 100g / 100ml KCAL PROT CARB FAT FIBRE				

DUCK IN

	Measure INFO/WEIGHT	per Measure KCAL	per Measure FAT	KCAL	PROT	CARB	FAT	FIBRE
a Plum Sauce, Crispy, M & S*	1 Pack/325g	569	31.2	175	10.7	11.2	9.6	0.9
Orange Sauce, Iceland*	1 Serving/200g	336	20.8	168	11.3	7.4	10.4	1.2
Oriental Sauce, Iceland*	1 Pack/201.1g	352	22.7	175	12.0	6.3	11.3	1.5
Red Wine Sauce, Free Range Fillets, Waitrose*	½ Pack/250g	378	19.3	151	16.4	4.1	7.7	2.2
DUCK PEKING								
Crispy, Aromatic, Sainsbury's*	½ Pack/300g	1236	110.7	412	19.5	0.6	36.9	0.1
Crispy, Cherry Valley*	1 Serving/270g	702	35.9	260	17.5	17.8	13.3	0.7
DUCK WITH								
Apple & Calvados Sauce, GFY, Asda*	1 Serving/162g	144	3.6	89	13.0	4.2	2.2	1.4
Diuelection, M & S*	1 Serving/67g	194	9.0	290	7.2	34.8	13.4	2.2
Noodles, Shanghai Roast, Sainsbury's*	1 Pack/450g	581	17.1	129	5.6	18.0	3.8	1.2
Pancakes, Shredded, Iceland*	1 Pack/220g	471	5.9	214	20.4	27.0	2.7	1.5
Pancakes, with Hoisin Sauce, M & S*	1 Pack/80g	136	3.2	170	13.0	19.9	4.0	0.9
DUMPLINGS								
Average	1oz/28g	58	3.3	208	2.8	24.5	11.7	0.9
Homestyle, Baked Weight, Aunt Bessie's*	1 Dumpling/49g	188	8.6	384	9.7	44.4	17.6	2.8
Homestyle, Baked Weight, Frozen, Aunt Bessie's*	1 Dumpling/49g	188	8.6	384	9.7	44.4	17.6	2.8
Homestyle, Frozen, Baked, Aunt Bessie's*	1 Dumpling/49g	188	8.6	384	9.7	44.4	17.6	2.8
Pork & Garlic Chive, Waitrose*	1 Pack/115g	215	8.1	187	9.4	20.4	7.0	1.1
Prawn, Cantonese, Crispy, Sainsbury's*	1 Dumpling/11g	27	1.5	241	9.3	20.9	13.4	1.1
Prawn Siu Mai, Chinese, M & S*	1 Serving/170g	187	7.3	110	14.0	4.2	4.3	1.2

D

	Measure INFO/WEIGHT	per Measure KCAL	FAT	Nutrition Values per 100g / 100ml KCAL	PROT	CARB	FAT	FIBRE
EASTER EGG								
Buttons, Cadbury*	1 Pack/200g	1060	60.2	530	7.7	56.6	30.1	0.7
Kit Kat, Chunky, Nestle*	1 Pack/235g	1224	67.0	521	5.9	60.3	28.5	0.8
Milky Bar, Nestle*	1 Egg/40g	182	6.9	454	4.2	70.8	17.2	0.0
Smarties, Nestle*	½ Egg/37.5g	182	7.6	478	4.8	69.6	20.0	0.7
ECLAIR								
Chocolate, Asda*	1 Eclair/33g	144	11.0	436	6.7	27.3	33.3	4.9
Chocolate, Cream, Fresh, Mini, Tesco*	1 Eclair/39g	160	11.5	410	6.4	29.0	29.5	1.8
Chocolate, Cream, Fresh, Tesco*	1 Eclair/66.3g	285	20.5	430	6.0	31.1	30.9	1.8
Chocolate, Dairy Cream, Co-Op*	1 Eclair/59g	227	17.1	385	5.0	26.0	29.0	0.3
Chocolate, Fresh Cream, M & S*	1 Eclair/43.6g	170	12.2	390	6.3	28.4	27.9	2.0
Chocolate, Fresh Cream, Sainsbury's*	1 Eclair/59g	212	13.9	360	4.2	32.7	23.6	0.5
Chocolate, Frozen, Weight Watchers*	1 Eclair/28g	76	3.3	271	3.9	37.6	11.7	6.6
Chocolate, HL, Tesco*	1 Serving/77g	192	9.7	249	6.8	27.1	12.6	0.9
Chocolate, Mini, Iceland*	1 Eclair/13g	55	4.6	426	4.9	21.5	35.6	0.4
EEL								
Jellied, Average	1oz/28g	27	2.0	98	8.4	0.0	7.1	0.0
Raw, Average	1oz/28g	47	3.2	168	16.6	0.0	11.3	0.0
EGGS								
Dried, White, Average	1 Tbsp/14g	41	0.0	295	73.8	0.0	0.0	0.0
Dried, Whole, Average	1oz/28g	159	11.6	568	48.4	0.0	41.6	0.0
Duck, Boiled & Salted, Average	1 Egg/75g	149	11.6	198	14.6	0.0	15.5	0.0
Duck, Whole, Raw, Average	1 Egg/75g	122	8.9	163	14.3	0.0	11.8	0.0
Free Range, Large, Average	1 Egg/63g	93	6.5	143	12.6	0.8	9.9	0.0
Fried, Average	1 Med/60g	107	8.3	179	13.6	0.0	13.9	0.0
Large, Average	1 Egg/63g	92	6.8	147	12.5	0.1	10.8	0.1
Medium, Average	1 Egg/50g	72	5.0	143	12.6	0.8	9.9	0.0
Poached	1 Med/50g	74	5.4	147	12.5	0.0	10.8	0.0
Quail, Whole, Raw	1 Egg/13g	20	1.4	151	12.9	0.0	11.1	0.0
Scrambled, Average	1 Egg/68g	100	7.3	147	12.5	0.0	10.8	0.0
Scrambled with Milk, Average	2 Med Egg/120g	296	27.1	247	10.7	0.6	22.6	0.0
Turkey, Whole, Raw	1oz/28g	46	3.4	165	13.7	0.0	12.2	0.0
Very Large, Morrisons*	1 Egg/70g	106	7.8	151	12.5	0.0	11.2	0.0
Whole, Raw	1 Lge Egg/57g	84	6.2	147	12.5	0.0	10.8	0.0
Yolks, Raw	1 Av Yolk/14g	47	4.3	339	16.1	0.0	30.5	0.0
ELDERBERRIES								
Average	1oz/28g	10	0.1	35	0.7	7.4	0.5	0.0
ELICHE								
Dry Weight, Buitoni*	1 Serving/80g	282	1.5	352	11.2	72.6	1.9	0.0
ENCHILADAS								
Chicken, American, HL, Tesco*	1 Serving/240g	353	4.3	147	10.4	22.5	1.8	1.2
Chicken, Asda*	1 Serving/500g	690	30.0	138	10.0	17.0	6.0	1.0
Chicken, Diner Specials, M & S*	½ Pack/226.7g	340	12.0	150	9.9	15.4	5.3	2.0
Chicken, in a Spicy Salsa & Bean Sauce, Asda*	½ Pack/211.9g	373	17.0	176	10.0	16.0	8.0	0.0
Chicken, Morrisons*	½ Pack/274.8g	393	12.6	143	10.0	15.4	4.6	1.8
Chicken, PB, Waitrose*	1 Pack/450g	482	14.4	107	6.9	12.7	3.2	1.1
Chicken, PB, Waitrose*	1 Pack/450g	482	14.4	107	6.9	12.7	3.2	1.1
Chicken, Safeway*	1 Serving/230g	384	11.3	167	7.9	22.9	4.9	1.0
Chicken, Value, Tesco*	1 Serving/212g	297	8.3	140	7.0	19.3	3.9	1.1
Chilli Beef, Asda*	½ Pack/225g	344	11.3	153	12.0	15.0	5.0	3.5
Vegetable, GFY, Asda*	1 Pack/350g	399	15.8	114	4.4	14.0	4.5	1.3
Vegetable, Morrisons*	1 Pack/400g	468	18.4	117	4.5	14.4	4.6	1.8
Vegetable & Bean, Eat Smart, Morrisons*	1 Pack/380g	475	9.9	125	4.7	20.7	2.6	3.2

E

	Measure INFO/WEIGHT	per Measure KCAL FAT		Nutrition Values per 100g / 100ml				
				KCAL	PROT	CARB	FAT	FIBRE
ENDIVE								
Raw	1oz/28g	4	0.1	13	1.8	1.0	0.2	2.0
ENERGY DRINK								
Lemon, Active Sport, Tesco*	1 Bottle/500ml	135	0.0	27	0.0	6.5	0.0	0.0
Orange, Active Sport, Tesco*	1 Bottle/500ml	135	0.0	27	0.0	6.5	0.0	0.0
Powerade, Aqua+*	1 Bottle/500ml	80	0.0	16	0.0	3.7	0.0	0.0
V, Frucor Beverages*	1 Can/250ml	113	0.0	45	0.0	11.2	0.0	0.0

E

	Measure INFO/WEIGHT	per Measure KCAL	FAT	Nutrition Values per 100g / 100ml KCAL	PROT	CARB	FAT	FIBRE
FAGGOTS								
in Rich Gravy, Iceland*	1 Faggot/81g	116	5.2	143	6.5	15.9	6.4	1.1
Mushy Peas & Mash, Sainsbury's*	1 Pack/450g	576	19.4	128	6.0	16.3	4.3	1.6
Pork, in Rich, West Country Sauce, Mr Brains*	1 Pack/378g	484	24.9	128	5.3	11.9	6.6	0.6
FAGOTTINI								
Mushroom, Sainsbury's*	½ Pack/155g	339	11.6	219	10.2	27.7	7.5	2.7
FAJITA								
Beef, GFY, Asda*	½ Pack/208g	354	9.8	170	11.0	21.0	4.7	1.6
Chicken, American Style, Tesco*	1 Pack/275g	388	14.0	141	9.5	14.2	5.1	1.0
Chicken, Asda*	½ Pack/225g	371	10.1	165	11.0	20.0	4.5	3.5
Chicken, BGTY, Sainsbury's*	1 Pack/171.8g	256	4.3	149	10.8	20.9	2.5	1.7
Chicken, Boots*	1 Pack/223g	448	16.1	201	9.1	25.0	7.2	3.9
Chicken, Char Grilled Style, Safeway*	½ Pack/234.8g	588	5.4	250	17.2	40.5	2.3	1.9
Chicken, Co-Op*	1 Serving/230g	391	16.1	170	11.0	15.0	7.0	3.0
Chicken, COU, M & S*	1 Pack/230g	288	5.3	125	10.0	16.5	2.3	1.5
Chicken, Eat Smart, Safeway*	1 Serving/248g	290	4.2	117	10.6	14.8	1.7	1.6
Chicken, Finest, Tesco*	½ Pack/287.5g	457	19.6	159	9.9	14.4	6.8	2.1
Chicken, GFY, Asda*	½ Pack/225g	233	4.1	104	9.3	12.9	1.8	2.0
Chicken, HL, Tesco*	1 Pack/325g	374	8.5	115	9.9	12.3	2.6	2.3
Chicken, Just Cook, Sainsbury's*	½ Pack/200g	200	3.0	100	18.5	3.1	1.5	2.0
Chicken, M & S*	1 Pack/230g	345	12.2	150	8.6	17.7	5.3	1.0
Chicken, Mexican, No Mayo, Foo-Go*	1 Pack/198g	360	11.1	182	9.6	23.3	5.6	2.4
Chicken, Morrisons*	1 Serving/300g	370	15.2	123	7.4	12.2	5.1	1.9
Chicken, Sainsbury's*	½ Pack/275g	396	14.6	144	9.5	14.5	5.3	1.9
Chicken, Salt Balanced, COU, M & S*	1 Pack/230g	253	5.3	110	9.5	13.2	2.3	1.7
Chicken, Somerfield*	4 Fajitas/440g	528	18.0	120	7.8	13.2	4.1	2.8
Chicken, Tesco*	½ Pack /275g	382	14.3	139	9.2	13.9	5.2	1.9
Chicken, Value, Tesco*	1 Serving/250g	255	6.0	102	6.9	13.2	2.4	1.5
Chicken with Salsa & Sour Cream Dips, Safeway*	1 Pack/242g	390	14.8	161	9.8	16.7	6.1	1.9
Gammon Steaks, Tesco*	1 Serving/250g	368	15.5	147	17.5	5.3	6.2	0.0
Steak, M & S*	1oz/28g	53	2.5	190	8.9	17.2	9.1	0.6
Tuna, Eat Smart, Safeway*	1 Pack/263g	302	4.7	115	9.7	15.0	1.8	1.4
Tuna, Sainsbury's*	1 Pack/450g	752	24.3	167	11.4	18.2	5.4	1.6
Vegetable, Somerfield*	1 Pack/500g	640	25.0	128	3.0	17.0	5.0	0.0
Vegetable, Tesco*	1 Wrap/112g	133	5.6	119	4.2	14.3	5.0	1.1
FALAFEL								
Cauldron*	1 Falafel/25g	51	2.3	203	7.6	29.8	9.0	7.2
Fried in Vegetable Oil, Average	1 Falafel.25g	45	2.8	179	6.4	15.6	11.2	3.4
M & S*	1 Falafel/13.8g	42	3.2	305	6.8	18.2	23.0	7.0
Mini, Sainsbury's*	1 Serving/168g	499	29.6	297	8.0	26.8	17.6	3.2
Mix, Lebanese Style, Al'fez*	½ Pack/200g	470	27.6	235	7.1	26.3	13.8	0.0
Mix, Sainsbury's*	½ Pack/110g	197	6.6	179	7.7	23.5	6.0	5.2
Organic, Cauldron*	1 Falafel/25g	51	2.5	203	8.4	20.3	9.8	7.2
Vegetarian, Organic, Waitrose*	1 Felafel/25g	55	2.6	220	8.0	23.3	10.5	7.6
FANTA								
Apple, Z, Coca-Cola*	1 Can/330ml	13	0.0	4	0.0	0.6	0.0	0.0
Fruit Twist, Coca-Cola*	1 Serving/250ml	133	0.0	53	0.0	13.0	0.0	0.0
Icy Lemon, Coca-Cola*	1 Can/330mls	165	0.0	50	0.0	12.2	0.0	0.0
Icy Lemon, Zero, Coca-Cola*	1 Can/330mls	7	0.0	2	0.0	0.2	0.0	0.0
Lemon, Coca-Cola*	1 Can/330ml	165	0.0	50	0.0	12.0	0.0	0.0
Orange, Coca-Cola*	1 Serving/250ml	108	0.0	43	0.1	10.6	0.0	0.0
Orange, Z, Coca-Cola*	1 Can/330ml	10	0.0	3	0.0	0.5	0.0	0.0
FARFALLE								
Bows, Dry, Average	1 Serving/75g	265	1.4	353	11.4	72.6	1.9	1.9

F

	Measure INFO/WEIGHT	per Measure KCAL	FAT	Nutrition Values per 100g / 100ml KCAL	PROT	CARB	FAT	FIBRE
FARFALLE								
Dry, Average	1 Serving/50g	178	0.9	357	11.7	73.5	1.8	2.7
Salmon & Broccoli, Eat Smart, Safeway*	1 Pack/380g	361	9.1	95	6.4	11.6	2.4	1.1
FARFALLINE								
Bows, Mini, Tesco*	1oz/28g	93	0.6	333	13.2	65.6	2.0	2.9
FENNEL								
Florence, Boiled in Salted Water	1oz/28g	3	0.1	11	0.9	1.5	0.2	2.3
Florence, Raw, Unprepared	1 Med Serving/50g	6	0.1	12	0.9	1.8	0.2	2.4
FENUGREEK LEAVES								
Raw	1oz/28g	10	0.1	35	4.6	4.8	0.2	0.0
FETTUCINI								
Cajun Chicken, COU, M & S*	1 Pack/400g	380	8.0	95	8.0	10.8	2.0	2.9
Chicken Mushroom, GFY, Asda*	1 Pack/400g	359	7.0	90	7.3	11.3	1.8	0.7
Dry Weight, Buitoni*	1 Serving/90g	326	1.5	362	12.2	74.4	1.7	0.0
with Tomato & Mushroom, Easy Cook, Napolina*	1 Pack/120g	461	8.6	384	11.8	67.9	7.2	0.0
FIG ROLLS								
Asda*	1 Biscuit/19g	71	1.7	372	4.8	68.0	9.0	0.0
Bolands*	1 Biscuit/18g	69	1.6	382	2.9	73.5	8.8	2.9
Jacob's*	1 Biscuit/17.9g	68	1.5	380	4.0	71.4	8.5	3.3
Vitalinea, Jacob's*	1 Biscuit/18g	61	1.0	339	3.7	68.2	5.8	3.8
FIGS								
Dried, Average	1 Fig/14g	32	0.1	232	3.6	53.2	1.1	8.7
Raw, Average	1 Fig/35g	16	0.1	45	1.3	9.8	0.2	1.5
FISH								
Balls, Gefilte, M & S*	1 Pack/200g	280	7.8	140	14.1	11.9	3.9	1.0
Battered, Portion, Ross*	1 Portion/109.9g	223	11.9	203	10.4	16.1	10.8	0.8
Battered, White, Skinless & Boneless, Farmfoods*	1 Serving/122g	238	12.3	195	9.3	16.7	10.1	2.3
Breaded, Asda*	1 Serving/150g	351	21.0	234	15.0	12.0	14.0	0.5
Crumbed, Pak-N-Save*	2 Pieces/139.9g	298	17.8	213	10.8	13.9	12.7	0.0
Dried, Small, Ogura*	1 Serving/10g	32	0.3	320	69.0	0.3	3.0	0.0
Fillets, Garlic & Herb, Youngs*	1 Fillet/117.6g	262	14.9	222	11.0	16.2	12.6	1.4
Fillets, Lemon & Pepper, Youngs*	1 Fillet/130g	283	16.7	218	10.3	15.3	12.9	4.3
Fillets, White, Breaded, Tesco*	1 Piece/95g	198	10.4	208	10.6	16.9	10.9	1.0
Fillets, White, Breaded, Value, Tesco*	1 Serving/100g	192	9.7	192	10.6	15.6	9.7	2.2
Fillets, White, Natural, Tesco*	1 Fillet/100g	72	0.6	72	16.6	0.0	0.6	0.0
Goujons, Asda*	1 Serving/125g	240	8.0	192	12.8	20.8	6.4	0.2
in Batter, Light, Iceland*	1 Fillet/120g	230	12.1	192	13.6	11.6	10.1	0.7
in Batter, Morrisons*	1 Fish/140g	235	8.1	168	14.0	15.0	5.8	0.2
in Batter, Youngs*	1 Serving/100g	315	19.7	315	14.9	20.4	19.7	0.8
Medley, SteamFresh, Birds Eye*	1 Serving/170g	170	6.3	100	13.0	2.3	3.7	0.1
Nuggets, Battered, Farmfoods*	1oz/28g	60	3.3	214	10.9	16.0	11.8	0.7
Portion, Chip Shop, Youngs*	1 Portion/135g	315	19.7	233	11.0	15.1	14.6	0.6
Portions, in Oven Crisp Batter, Value, Tesco*	1 Serving/100g	209	11.0	209	11.0	16.4	11.0	2.6
Salted, Chinese, Steamed	1oz/28g	43	0.6	155	33.9	0.0	2.2	0.0
Smoked River Cobbler, Tesco*	1 Fillet/163g	181	4.7	111	20.6	0.0	2.9	0.0
Steaks, Chip Shop, Youngs*	1 Portion/100g	198	10.4	198	11.0	14.9	10.4	0.9
Steaks, Skinless & Boneless, Youngs*	1 Serving/104.7g	225	12.4	214	10.5	16.6	11.8	0.8
Tilapia, Raw, Average	100g	95	1.0	95	20.0	0.0	1.0	0.0
White, Breaded, Fillets, Ocean Pure*	1 Fillet/112.5g	276	11.5	245	20.8	16.9	10.2	1.2
White, Smoked, Average	1 Serving/100g	108	0.9	108	23.4	0.0	0.9	0.0
White, Tesco*	1 Fillet/100g	78	0.6	78	16.6	0.0	0.6	0.0
FISH & CHIPS								
Breaded, Budgens*	1 Pack/340g	544	18.0	160	8.6	19.3	5.3	1.5
Budgens*	1 Pack/284g	625	28.4	220	8.0	24.5	10.0	2.3

F

	Measure INFO/WEIGHT	per Measure KCAL	FAT	Nutrition Values per 100g / 100ml KCAL	PROT	CARB	FAT	FIBRE
FISH & CHIPS								
Cod, & Chunky Chips, Waitrose*	1 Pack/285g	470	18.0	165	7.2	18.8	6.3	2.5
Cod, Asda*	1 Serving/279.5g	451	14.0	161	8.0	21.0	5.0	1.1
Cod, HL, Tesco*	1 Pack/400g	492	7.2	123	5.3	21.4	1.8	1.7
Co-Op*	1 Pack/250g	388	15.0	155	6.0	18.0	6.0	2.0
Ross*	1 Serving/250g	415	19.0	166	6.2	18.1	7.6	1.6
Safeway*	1 Pack/249g	518	20.9	208	8.0	25.0	8.4	3.5
Somerfield*	1 Serving/283g	495	17.0	175	8.0	22.0	6.0	0.0
Tesco*	1 Serving/300g	489	18.6	163	5.5	21.2	6.2	1.6
with Mushy Peas, Kershaws*	1 Pack/315g	450	18.3	143	6.4	16.4	5.8	1.6
FISH BAKE								
Cheese & Leek, HL, Tesco*	1 Pack/400g	340	8.0	85	11.0	5.8	2.0	0.8
Cheese Pastry, Birds Eye*	1 Piece/171g	390	23.3	228	9.3	17.2	13.6	1.9
Haddock & Prawn, COU, M & S*	1 Bake/340g	289	9.5	85	7.3	7.3	2.8	0.4
Italiano, Birds Eye*	1 Pack/400g	404	16.4	101	12.0	3.9	4.1	0.4
Mediterranean, HL, Tesco*	½ Pack/200g	158	3.2	79	10.3	5.9	1.6	1.4
Mediterranean, Youngs*	½ Pack/200g	132	4.4	66	9.3	2.3	2.2	1.2
Vegetable Tuscany, Birds Eye*	1 Pack/380g	391	13.7	103	10.6	7.1	3.6	0.4
with Pasta, Cheese & Broccoli, Birds Eye*	½ Pack/185g	244	14.1	132	12.2	3.6	7.6	0.4
FISH CAKES								
Breaded, Sainsbury's*	1 Cake/42g	75	3.4	179	10.0	16.2	8.1	0.7
Bubbly Batter, Youngs*	1 Cake/44.1g	109	6.6	247	7.1	20.5	15.1	1.4
Captain's Coins, Mini, Birds Eye*	1 Cake/20g	38	1.7	188	9.5	18.7	8.3	1.1
Cod, & Pancetta, Cafe Culture, M & S*	1 Cake/85g	166	13.2	195	9.2	7.2	15.5	2.0
Cod, Asda*	1 Cake/50g	97	5.0	194	11.0	15.0	10.0	1.6
Cod, Big Time, Birds Eye*	1 Cake/114g	223	11.6	196	8.3	17.8	10.2	1.0
Cod, Birds Eye*	2 Cakes/102.2g	190	8.8	186	11.3	15.9	8.6	1.0
Cod, Chunky, Breaded, Chilled, Youngs*	1 Cake/50g	107	6.4	213	9.5	14.9	12.8	1.2
Cod, Fresh, Asda*	1 Cake/75g	164	8.3	219	7.0	23.0	11.0	1.6
Cod, Homemade, Average	1 Cake/50g	121	8.3	241	9.3	14.4	16.6	0.7
Cod, in Crunch Crumb, Birds Eye*	2 Cakes/99g	185	8.5	187	11.4	16.0	8.6	1.0
Cod, in Light Crispy Breadcrumbs, Sainsbury's*	1 Cake/90g	176	7.8	195	11.1	18.0	8.7	2.4
Cod, M & S*	1 Cake/85g	155	7.8	182	8.9	15.4	9.2	1.3
Cod, Macfisheries*	1 Cake/85.4g	163	7.0	192	7.6	22.1	8.2	1.1
Cod, Tesco*	1 Cake/49g	110	5.1	224	8.9	23.8	10.4	0.2
Cod & Parsley, Waitrose*	1 Cake/85g	147	6.5	173	9.2	16.9	7.6	1.1
Crab, & Prawn, Thai, Tesco*	1 Cake/115g	269	16.6	234	8.8	17.4	14.4	1.2
Fried in Blended Oil	1 Cake/50g	109	6.7	218	8.6	16.8	13.4	0.0
Frozen, Average	1 Cake/85g	112	3.3	132	8.6	16.7	3.9	0.0
Great Value, Iceland*	1 Cake/42.3g	74	2.7	175	9.1	20.3	6.4	1.6
Grilled, Average	1 Cake/50g	77	2.3	154	9.9	19.7	4.5	0.0
Haddock, Asda*	1 Cake/88g	181	8.8	206	8.0	21.0	10.0	1.5
Haddock, M & S*	1 Cake/85g	157	7.6	185	8.0	17.9	8.9	1.6
Haddock, Sainsbury's*	1 Cake/83.4g	166	6.8	199	11.4	20.1	8.1	1.8
Haddock, Smoked, Asda*	1 Cake/90g	185	9.0	206	10.0	19.0	10.0	1.4
Haddock, Smoked, Breaded, Asda*	1 Cake/90g	203	11.7	225	9.0	18.0	13.0	1.6
Haddock, Smoked, Frozen, Waitrose*	1 Cake/85g	186	10.3	219	9.6	17.8	12.1	0.8
Haddock, Smoked, M & S*	1 Cake/85g	153	8.0	180	10.6	13.4	9.4	2.6
Haddock, Smoked, Sainsbury's*	1 Cake/63.2g	127	6.0	201	11.0	17.8	9.5	2.1
Haddock, Smoked, Tesco*	1 Cake/90g	198	9.4	220	10.3	21.0	10.4	0.2
Haddock, Smoked, TTD, Sainsbury's*	1 Cake/115g	201	10.7	175	9.8	13.0	9.3	1.4
Halibut, TTD, Sainsbury's*	1 Cake/115g	289	17.9	251	10.0	17.6	15.6	1.3
Halibut Cod Loin, Finest, Tesco*	1 Cake/115g	213	8.3	185	8.8	21.3	7.2	1.4
M & S*	1 Cake/80g	180	10.6	225	8.0	18.0	13.3	0.0

F

	Measure INFO/WEIGHT	per Measure		Nutrition Values per 100g / 100ml				
		KCAL	FAT	KCAL	PROT	CARB	FAT	FIBRE
FISH CAKES								
Makes Sense, Somerfield*	1 Cake/42.2g	70	2.7	166	8.2	18.7	6.5	1.5
Prawn, Battered, Asda*	1 Cake/90g	182	10.0	202	10.0	15.6	11.1	1.0
Prawn, Sainsbury's*	1 Cake/83.3g	170	7.2	204	9.6	21.7	8.7	1.2
Prawn, Tesco*	1 Cake/90g	209	8.2	232	8.2	29.2	9.1	1.8
Ross*	1 Cake/52g	82	3.8	160	7.4	15.9	7.4	1.2
Salmon, & Asparagus, Finest, Tesco*	1 Cake/115g	300	17.8	261	10.7	19.6	15.5	0.4
Salmon, & Broccoli, Morrisons*	1 Cake/60g	126	7.1	210	9.8	17.2	11.9	1.3
Salmon, & Dill, COOK*	1 Cake/95g	144	5.3	152	11.3	14.2	5.6	1.5
Salmon, & Dill, Waitrose*	1 Cake/85g	206	11.9	242	11.5	17.5	14.0	1.8
Salmon, & Lemon Butter Sauce, Finest, Tesco*	1 Cake/220g	524	40.3	238	7.3	10.9	18.3	1.0
Salmon, & Tarragon, Waitrose*	1 Cake/85g	179	10.0	211	11.9	14.3	11.8	2.2
Salmon, Asda*	1 Cake/86g	215	12.0	250	8.0	23.0	14.0	1.4
Salmon, Birds Eye*	1 Cake/50g	84	4.5	168	9.5	12.2	9.0	1.4
Salmon, Breaded, Crispy, Frozen, Sainsbury's*	1 Cake/60g	140	8.7	234	12.2	13.7	14.5	1.9
Salmon, Chunky, Sainsbury's*	1 Cake/84g	192	10.5	228	13.2	15.8	12.5	2.9
Salmon, Homemade, Average	1 Cake/50g	137	9.9	273	10.4	14.4	19.7	0.7
Salmon, in Crunch Crumb, Birds Eye*	2 Cakes/99g	214	12.9	216	9.7	15.0	13.0	1.4
Salmon, M & S*	1 Cake/85.7g	180	10.9	210	9.1	15.1	12.7	1.7
Salmon, Morrisons*	1 Cake/90g	241	11.8	268	10.1	27.6	13.1	1.5
Salmon, Sainsbury's*	1 Cake/88.1g	171	7.6	194	12.6	16.5	8.6	1.6
Salmon, Tesco*	1 Cake/90g	239	13.5	266	11.4	21.3	15.0	0.0
Salmon, with Parsley Sauce, Finest, Tesco*	½ Pack/170g	350	23.6	206	8.6	11.7	13.9	1.0
SmartPrice, Asda*	1 Cake/41.5g	77	3.3	188	7.0	22.0	8.0	0.9
Thai, Finest, Tesco*	1 Cake/65g	150	8.6	230	7.5	20.3	13.2	1.6
Thai, Frozen, Sainsbury's*	1 Cake/15g	28	1.1	187	21.3	9.3	7.3	0.7
Thai, Oriental Selection, Waitrose*	1 Cake/11.2g	18	0.3	161	17.8	15.3	3.0	1.5
Thai, Tesco*	4 Cakes/88.9g	148	4.5	166	17.4	12.8	5.0	1.1
Thai Prawn, Morrisons*	1 Cake/90g	211	9.6	234	7.9	26.4	10.7	0.3
Thai Style, Sainsbury's*	1 Cake/49g	69	2.1	141	12.0	13.8	4.2	1.7
Tuna, & Red Pepper, Waitrose*	1 Cake/85g	175	10.0	206	9.5	15.4	11.8	1.6
Tuna, Asda*	1 Cake/74.9g	185	10.1	247	14.9	16.5	13.5	1.4
Tuna, Lime & Coriander, BGTY, Sainsbury's*	1 Cake/90.9g	200	10.7	220	10.7	17.7	11.8	2.6
Tuna, M & S*	1 Cake/85g	140	6.0	165	9.3	15.9	7.0	1.5
Tuna, Sainsbury's*	1 Cake/90g	183	7.5	203	13.7	18.4	8.3	2.1
Tuna, Tesco*	1 Cake/90g	222	9.5	247	12.8	25.4	10.5	0.2
Value, Tesco*	1 Cake/40g	74	3.2	183	7.1	21.2	7.8	1.2
FISH FINGERS								
Atlantis*	1 Finger/30g	52	2.3	172	12.0	14.0	7.5	0.4
Chip Shop, Youngs*	1 Finger/30g	75	4.9	251	9.3	16.6	16.4	1.2
Cod, 100% Cod Fillet, Tesco*	1 Finger/30g	53	2.3	177	12.4	14.9	7.5	1.4
Cod, Chunky, Tesco*	2 Fingers/80g	140	6.1	175	12.3	14.3	7.6	1.6
Cod, Fillet, 100%, Birds Eye*	1 Finger/31g	56	2.4	184	12.5	15.6	7.9	0.7
Cod, Fillet, Asda*	1 Finger/31g	66	3.1	214	13.0	18.0	10.0	0.0
Cod, Fillet, Chunky, M & S*	1 Finger/40g	70	2.4	175	12.0	17.3	6.0	1.0
Cod, Fillet, Iceland*	1 Finger/30g	62	2.5	205	13.0	19.5	8.3	1.4
Cod, Fillet, Waitrose*	1 Finger/30g	55	2.3	183	11.9	16.9	7.5	0.7
Cod, Fried in Blended Oil, Average	1 Finger/28g	67	3.9	238	13.2	15.5	14.1	0.6
Cod, Frozen, Average	1 Finger/28g	48	2.2	170	11.6	14.2	7.8	0.6
Cod, Grilled, Average	1 Finger/28g	56	2.5	200	14.3	16.6	8.9	0.7
Cod, Morrisons*	1 Finger/30g	54	2.3	180	11.7	16.4	7.5	1.1
Cod, Sainsbury's*	1 Finger/28g	53	2.2	190	12.5	17.7	7.7	1.0
Economy, Sainsbury's*	1 Finger/26g	51	2.2	198	12.6	17.7	8.5	1.3
Farmfoods*	1 Finger/27g	49	2.2	183	12.2	15.6	8.0	1.2

F

	INFO/WEIGHT	KCAL	FAT	KCAL	PROT	CARB	FAT	FIBRE
FISH FINGERS								
Free From, Sainsbury's*	1 Finger/30g	56	2.3	188	11.4	18.0	7.8	0.7
Haddock, Fillet, Asda*	1 Finger/30g	62	2.7	205	14.0	17.0	9.0	0.0
Haddock, in Crispy Batter, Birds Eye*	1 Finger/29g	55	2.3	188	14.3	15.1	7.8	0.7
Haddock, in Crunchy Crumb, Morrisons*	1 Finger/30g	57	2.4	190	13.1	16.3	8.0	1.1
Hoki, Fillet, Birds Eye*	1 Finger/30g	58	2.7	193	12.6	15.6	8.9	0.7
Iceland*	1 Finger/23g	44	2.0	192	11.5	17.3	8.5	1.3
in Batter, Crispy, Jumbo, Morrisons*	1 Finger/71g	146	8.9	205	11.3	12.2	12.5	0.6
Ross*	1 Finger/26g	50	2.3	193	10.7	17.7	8.8	0.8
Sainsbury's*	1 Finger/27g	52	2.3	194	13.4	16.0	8.5	0.7
SmartPrice, Asda*	1 Finger/25g	46	2.0	184	12.0	16.0	8.0	1.1
Value, Tesco*	1 Finger/25g	42	2.0	166	11.5	11.9	8.1	1.7
FISH IN								
Butter Sauce, Steaks, Ross*	1 Serving/150g	126	5.9	84	9.1	3.2	3.9	0.1
Parsley Sauce, Steaks, Ross*	1 Serving/150g	123	5.6	82	9.1	3.1	3.7	0.1
FISH WITH								
Mushrooms, Carrots & Broccoli, Parcel, Birds Eye*	1 Pack/250g	235	14.0	94	7.9	3.1	5.6	0.8
FIVE SPICE								
Powder, Sharwood's*	1 Tsp/2g	3	0.2	172	12.2	11.6	8.6	23.4
FLAKE								
Cadbury*	1 Flake/32.1g	170	9.9	530	8.1	55.6	30.8	0.7
Dipped, Cadbury*	1 Flake/40.6g	215	12.5	530	7.6	56.1	30.8	0.8
Luxury, Cadbury*	1 Bar/45g	240	13.6	533	7.3	57.8	30.2	0.0
Praline, Cadbury*	1 Bar/38g	201	12.9	535	7.7	49.5	34.3	0.0
FLAN								
Cauliflower, Cheese & Broccoli, Hot, Sainsbury's*	¼ Flan/100g	303	19.8	303	6.4	24.7	19.8	1.2
Cauliflower Cheese, Safeway*	1 Sm Flan/150g	420	24.8	280	7.3	25.0	16.5	2.0
Cheese & Onion, M & S*	1oz/28g	81	5.2	290	6.1	25.1	18.7	1.4
Cheese & Potato, Hot, Tesco*	¼ Flan/100g	282	19.7	282	6.0	20.0	19.7	2.3
Chicken & Smoked Bacon, Hot, Sainsbury's*	¼ Flan/100g	293	18.5	293	10.2	21.5	18.5	1.2
Mediterranean Vegetable, Co-Op*	¼ Flan/87.5g	189	10.6	215	4.0	22.0	12.0	3.0
Parsnip, Broccoli & Gruyere, Safeway*	½ Flan/200g	534	32.8	267	7.0	23.0	16.4	2.8
Pastry, with Fruit	1oz/28g	33	1.2	118	1.4	19.3	4.4	0.7
Potato, Cheddar & Onion, Safeway*	1 Serving/150g	420	25.1	280	6.4	25.6	16.7	2.7
Smoked Ham Cheese & Leek, Safeway*	½ Flan/200g	520	32.8	260	8.0	20.0	16.4	2.0
Sponge with Fruit	1oz/28g	31	0.4	112	2.8	23.3	1.5	0.6
FLAN CASE								
Sponge, Average	1oz/28g	90	1.5	320	7.0	62.5	5.4	0.7
FLAPJACK								
All Butter, Organic, Sainsbury's*	1 Serving/35g	156	8.1	446	5.3	54.5	23.0	2.7
All Butter, Sainsbury's*	1 Flapjack/35g	156	8.0	446	5.7	54.5	22.8	2.7
All Butter, Squares, M & S*	1 Flapjack/34g	150	7.2	441	6.2	56.2	21.2	4.4
All Butter, Waitrose*	1 Piece/34g	126	9.0	376	3.8	52.4	26.8	1.2
Apple & Sultana, Blackfriars*	1 Flapjack/110g	507	24.2	461	5.5	61.0	22.0	0.0
Apricot, The Handmade Flapjack Company*	1 Flapjack/90g	321	4.8	357	5.5	71.7	5.4	0.0
Apricot & Raisin, Waitrose*	1 Flapjack/38g	143	4.2	376	4.7	64.3	11.1	5.8
Average	1 Sm/50g	242	13.3	484	4.5	60.4	26.6	2.7
Banana, The Handmade Flapjack Company*	1 Flapjack/90g	379	13.1	421	5.3	67.2	14.6	0.0
Belgian Chocolate Dipped, Asda*	1 Serving/67g	321	16.8	477	6.0	57.0	25.0	3.2
Cappuccino, Blackfriars*	1 Flapjack/110g	481	27.5	437	5.0	61.0	25.0	0.0
Cherry & Coconut, Blackfriars*	1 Flapjack/110g	490	23.1	445	5.0	58.0	21.0	0.0
Cherry & Sultana, Cookie Coach*	1 Pack/90g	373	15.6	414	6.2	58.2	17.3	0.0
Chocolate, McVitie's*	1 Flapjack/85g	422	23.0	496	6.6	56.6	27.1	3.2
Chocolate, The Handmade Flapjack Company*	1 Flapjack/90g	392	17.6	435	6.0	58.6	19.6	0.0

F

	Measure INFO/WEIGHT	per Measure		Nutrition Values per 100g / 100ml				
		KCAL	FAT	KCAL	PROT	CARB	FAT	FIBRE
FLAPJACK								
Chocolate Dipped, M & S*	1 Flapjack/96g	442	21.5	460	6.1	61.3	22.4	3.0
Chunky Chocolate, M & S*	1 FlapJack/80g	348	15.1	435	5.8	59.9	18.9	2.2
Crazy Raizin, Fabulous Bakin' Boys*	1 Pack/90g	378	15.3	420	6.0	60.0	17.0	4.0
Fingers, Really Raspberry, Fabulous Bakin' Boys*	1 Finger/30g	137	7.0	457	6.7	60.0	23.3	3.3
Fruit, GFY, Asda*	1 Flapjack/45g	173	3.6	384	6.0	72.0	8.0	3.4
Fruit, Tesco*	1 Cake/33g	136	5.2	412	5.7	62.0	15.7	4.0
Fruity, Waitrose*	1 Serving/50g	199	6.8	398	6.1	62.9	13.5	3.9
Golden Oaty, Fingers, Fabulous Bakin' Boys*	1 Finger/28g	126	5.9	450	5.7	59.6	21.1	3.4
Hob Nobs, Milk Chocolate, McVitie's*	1 Flapjack/35g	159	7.5	454	5.7	59.4	21.4	4.0
Mighty Oat, Fabulous Bakin' Boys*	1 Bar/85g	366	17.0	430	6.0	58.0	20.0	3.0
Mini, Sainsbury's*	1 Slice/15.1g	65	2.9	431	5.6	59.3	19.0	2.7
Mixed Fruit, Organic, Evernat*	1oz/28g	136	7.4	484	4.5	60.4	26.6	0.0
Oats, Butter & Syrup, McVitie's*	1 Serving/75g	341	16.9	454	4.9	57.9	22.5	3.7
Plain, The Handmade Flapjack Company*	1 Flapjack/90g	398	19.2	442	5.4	57.1	21.3	0.0
Really Raspberry, Fabulous Bakin' Boys*	1 Flapjack/90g	378	16.2	420	6.0	60.0	18.0	0.0
Snickers, McVitie's*	1 Flapjack/65g	315	18.5	484	7.9	49.0	28.5	6.0
Sultana, Tesco*	1 Flapjack/50g	173	10.1	346	5.0	36.2	20.1	3.7
Toffee, Finest, Tesco*	1 Piece/35g	156	6.7	446	4.9	63.6	19.1	1.3
Weight Watchers*	1 Slice/30g	109	1.8	363	6.7	71.0	6.0	4.0
with Sultanas, Tesco*	1 Flapjack/49g	217	10.3	442	5.3	57.9	21.0	3.7
FLATBREAD								
BBQ Chicken, Improved, Shapers, Boots*	1 Pack/165.4g	267	3.8	162	10.0	25.0	2.3	1.2
BBQ Style Chicken, Shapers, Boots*	1 Serving/108g	187	5.0	173	10.0	23.0	4.6	2.8
Chargrilled Chicken, COU, M & S*	1 Pack/163.3g	245	3.1	150	10.8	23.0	1.9	5.2
Chicken Tikka, Shapers, Boots*	1 Flatbread/164g	269	4.1	164	11.0	24.0	2.5	1.5
Greek Style, GFY, Asda*	1 Flatbread/165g	256	7.1	155	7.0	22.0	4.3	2.1
King Prawn Tikka, Waitrose*	1 Pack/165g	257	3.3	156	9.4	25.1	2.0	1.5
Mediterranean Chicken, Ginsters*	1 Pack/167.8g	302	6.7	180	10.6	25.5	4.0	0.0
Mediterranean Tuna, Ginsters*	1 Pack/166.9g	297	6.3	178	10.3	25.6	3.8	0.0
Spicy Mexican, New, Shapers, Boots*	1 Pack/183.7g	282	5.0	153	8.0	24.0	2.7	1.9
Tomato & Chilli, BGTY, Sainsbury's*	¼ Bread/100g	155	3.1	155	7.7	24.0	3.1	1.8
Tomato & Chilli, Sainsbury's*	¼ Bread/65g	155	3.1	238	11.9	36.9	4.7	2.8
FLOUR								
Bread, Brown, Strong, Average	1 Serving/100g	311	1.8	311	14.0	61.0	1.8	6.4
Bread, White, Strong, Sainsbury's*	1/3 Pack/500g	1690	6.5	338	13.4	68.2	1.3	3.0
Bread, White, Very Strong, Allinson*	1 Serving/100g	348	1.8	348	13.9	69.0	1.8	3.2
Bread, White, Very Strong, Canadian, Waitrose*	1 Portion/100g	348	1.4	348	15.0	68.8	1.4	2.5
Bread, Wholemeal, Strong, Allinson*	1 Serving/100g	325	2.2	325	14.5	59.9	2.2	9.0
Brown, Chapati, Average	1 Tbsp/20g	67	0.2	333	11.5	73.7	1.2	0.0
Brown, Wheat	1oz/28g	90	0.5	323	12.6	68.5	1.8	6.4
Chick Pea	1oz/28g	88	1.5	313	19.7	49.6	5.4	10.7
Millet	1oz/28g	99	0.5	354	5.8	75.4	1.7	0.0
Plain, Average	1oz/28g	98	0.4	349	10.3	73.8	1.5	2.2
Potato	1oz/28g	92	0.3	328	7.4	75.6	0.9	5.7
Rice	1oz/28g	102	0.2	366	6.4	80.1	0.8	2.0
Rye, Whole	1oz/28g	94	0.6	335	8.2	75.9	2.0	11.7
Sauce, Dry, Sainsbury's*	1 Serving/20g	69	0.3	343	9.8	73.0	1.3	3.0
Soya, Full Fat, Average	1oz/28g	118	6.1	422	37.9	19.8	21.8	11.6
Soya, Low Fat, Average	1oz/28g	99	2.0	352	45.3	28.2	7.2	13.5
Speciality Gluten Free, Dove's Farm*	1 Serving/100g	353	1.8	353	4.7	85.2	1.8	2.7
Strong, Wholemeal, Average	1 Serving/100g	315	2.2	315	13.3	60.6	2.2	9.0
White, Average	1oz/28g	89	0.3	319	9.8	66.8	1.0	2.9
White, Chapati, Average	1 Tbsp/20g	67	0.1	335	9.8	77.6	0.5	0.0

F

	Measure INFO/WEIGHT	per Measure KCAL	FAT	Nutrition Values per 100g / 100ml KCAL	PROT	CARB	FAT	FIBRE
FLOUR								
White, Self Raising, Average	1oz/28g	94	0.4	336	9.9	71.8	1.3	2.9
White, Wheat, Average	1oz/28g	95	0.4	341	10.5	76.5	1.4	3.1
Wholemeal, Average	1oz/28g	87	0.6	312	12.6	61.9	2.2	9.0
Wholemeal, Self Raising, Tesco*	1oz/28g	89	0.6	317	11.5	62.9	2.2	9.0
FLYING SAUCERS								
Asda*	1 Bag/23g	82	0.6	355	0.1	83.0	2.5	0.8
Co-Op*	1 Sweet/1g	4	0.0	370	0.5	90.0	1.0	0.6
FLYTE								
Mars*	1 Bar/22.5g	99	3.2	441	3.4	74.8	14.2	0.0
Snacksize, Mars*	1 Bar/22.5g	98	3.3	436	3.8	72.5	14.5	0.0
FOOL								
Apricot, Fruit, Tesco*	1 Pot/113g	200	12.7	177	2.6	16.4	11.2	0.3
Blackcurrant, Asda*	1 Pot/114g	89	3.0	78	3.6	10.0	2.6	0.6
Gooseberry, Real Fruit, Safeway*	1 Pot/114g	215	12.9	189	2.8	19.1	11.3	0.5
Gooseberry, Sainsbury's*	1 Pot/113g	214	12.9	189	2.6	19.1	11.4	1.1
Raspberry, Fruit, Tesco*	1 Pot/113g	234	12.8	207	2.6	23.6	11.3	0.3
Rhubarb, Fruit, Somerfield*	1 Pot/114g	201	12.5	176	3.0	16.0	11.0	0.0
Rhubarb, Fruit, Waitrose*	1 Pot/114g	182	12.9	160	2.7	11.9	11.3	0.3
Rhubarb, Sainsbury's*	1 Pot/113g	180	12.9	159	2.6	11.5	11.4	0.4
Strawberry, Fruit, BGTY, Sainsbury's*	1 Pot/120g	100	3.1	83	3.7	11.1	2.6	0.8
Strawberry, Fruit, Co-Op*	1 Pot/114g	188	10.3	165	2.0	18.0	9.0	0.8
Strawberry, Real Fruit, Safeway*	1 Pot/114g	197	12.8	173	2.7	15.4	11.2	0.3
FOR MILK								
Peachy Banana, Robinson's*	1 Serving/50ml	79	0.0	158	0.0	39.0	0.0	0.0
FRANKFURTERS								
Average	1 Frank/42g	123	11.2	292	12.0	1.3	26.6	0.0
Sainsbury's*	1 Frank/35.1g	108	9.8	308	12.5	1.5	28.0	0.1
FRANKFURTERS VEGETARIAN								
Asda*	1 Frankfurter/26.9g	54	3.4	199	18.0	3.5	12.5	2.5
Tivall*	3 Sausages/90g	220	14.4	244	18.0	7.0	16.0	3.0
FRAZZLES								
Bacon, Smith's, Walkers*	1 Bag/23g	112	5.3	485	6.5	62.0	23.0	1.3
FRENCH FRIES								
Cheese & Onion, Walkers*	1 Pack/22g	95	3.5	430	5.0	66.0	16.0	5.0
Ready Salted, Walkers*	1 Bag/22g	94	3.5	425	5.0	65.0	16.0	5.0
Salt & Vinegar, Eat Smart, Safeway*	1 Bag/20g	75	0.3	375	5.1	80.9	1.6	2.3
Salt & Vinegar, Walkers*	1 Bag/22g	95	3.5	430	5.0	66.0	16.0	5.0
Worcester Sauce, Walkers*	1 Bag/22g	94	3.7	425	4.5	64.0	17.0	4.1
FRENCH TOAST								
Asda*	1 Slice/8g	30	0.4	381	10.0	74.0	5.0	4.0
Sainsbury's*	1 Serving/8g	31	0.5	382	10.0	72.0	6.6	5.0
Tesco*	1 Serving/100g	393	6.6	393	11.0	72.5	6.6	3.0
FRIES								
9/16" Straight Cut Home, Deep Fried, McCain*	1oz/28g	65	2.8	233	3.2	32.7	9.9	0.0
9/16" Straight Cut Home, Oven Baked, McCain*	1oz/28g	53	1.5	188	3.2	31.5	5.5	0.0
American, 3 Way Cook, Somerfield*	1oz/28g	43	1.4	155	3.0	25.0	5.0	0.0
American, Oven, Asda*	1 Serving/180g	432	18.0	240	3.4	34.0	10.0	3.0
American, Somerfield*	1 Serving/100g	165	5.0	165	2.1	28.0	5.0	4.6
American Style, Frozen, Thin, Tesco*	1 Serving/125g	208	10.1	166	2.2	21.1	8.1	1.9
American Style, Seasoned, Straight Cut, Morrisons*	1 Portion/130g	215	10.4	165	2.4	20.8	8.0	1.9
American Style, Slim, Iceland*	1 Serving/100g	187	6.1	187	2.4	30.6	6.1	2.4
Crispy French, Weighed Deep Fried, McCain*	1 Serving/100g	193	8.5	193	1.9	27.4	8.5	0.9
Curly, Cajun, Weighed Frozen, McCain*	1 Portion/100g	156	8.7	156	1.6	17.7	8.7	1.8

F

	Measure INFO/WEIGHT	per Measure KCAL	FAT	Nutrition Values per 100g / 100ml KCAL	PROT	CARB	FAT	FIBRE
FRIES								
Curly, Southern Style, Tesco*	1 Serving/50g	124	3.7	248	3.8	41.7	7.3	3.8
Extra Chunky, Oven Baked, Homefries, McCain*	1 Serving/200g	306	6.2	153	3.2	28.0	3.1	2.3
Oven, American Style, Asda*	1 Serving/180.1g	407	14.4	226	3.9	34.6	8.0	4.0
Oven, Straight Cut, Morrisons*	1 Serving/100g	149	4.3	149	2.8	24.6	4.3	2.6
Southern Spicy Spiral, Deep Fried, McCain*	1oz/28g	58	2.9	208	2.7	26.4	10.2	0.0
Southern Spicy Spiral, Oven Baked, McCain*	1oz/28g	46	1.8	165	1.7	24.6	6.6	0.0
FRISPS								
Ready Salted, KP Snacks*	1 Bag/28g	151	9.5	538	4.7	53.4	33.9	2.8
Tangy Salt & Vinegar, KP Snacks*	1 Bag/30g	160	10.1	532	5.0	52.6	33.5	2.9
Tasty Cheese & Onion, KP Snacks*	1 Bag/28g	166	10.4	537	5.5	53.2	33.6	3.2
FRITTERS								
Sweetcorn, with Chilli Dip, American Style, Sainsbury's*	1 Fritter/40g	97	4.5	243	4.4	31.1	11.2	2.9
Sweetcorn, with Chilli Dip, Sainsbury's*	1 Fritter/40g	97	4.5	243	4.4	31.1	11.2	2.9
FROMAGE FRAIS								
Apricot, Layered, Weight Watchers*	1 Pot/100g	58	0.1	58	5.4	8.1	0.1	1.6
Black Cherry, GFY, Asda*	1 Pot/100g	54	0.2	54	6.0	7.0	0.2	0.0
Blackberry, Layered, Weight Watchers*	1 Pot/100g	64	0.2	64	5.3	10.4	0.2	1.0
Blackcurrant, HE, Tesco*	1 Pot/100g	59	0.2	59	7.7	6.5	0.2	0.6
Blackcurrant, HL, Tesco*	1 Pot/100g	56	0.2	56	6.2	7.4	0.2	0.4
COU, M & S*	1 Pot/100g	48	0.1	48	7.8	4.5	0.1	0.5
Fabby, Loved By Kids, M & S*	1 Pot/42.9g	45	1.6	105	6.2	12.3	3.7	0.0
Fat Free, Average	1oz/28g	16	0.1	58	7.7	6.8	0.2	0.0
Fruit, Balanced Lifestyle, Aldi*	1 Pot/100g	52	0.2	52	5.4	7.1	0.2	0.7
Good Intentions, Somerfield*	1 Pot/100g	49	0.1	49	7.6	4.5	0.1	0.0
Kids, Yeo Valley*	1 Serving/90g	111	4.8	123	6.6	12.6	5.3	0.0
Lemon, Balanced Lifestyle, Aldi*	1 Pot/100g	52	0.3	52	5.6	6.6	0.3	0.6
Lemon Pie, Low Fat, Sainsbury's*	1 Pot/90g	108	2.4	120	6.7	17.3	2.7	0.2
Low Fat, Aldi*	1 Pot/100g	52	0.3	52	5.4	7.1	0.3	0.7
Mandarin, Eat Smart, Safeway*	1 Pot/100g	55	0.2	55	7.7	5.2	0.2	1.6
Mandarin & Orange, HL, Tesco*	1 Pot/100g	55	0.2	55	6.2	7.0	0.2	0.3
Munch Bunch, Nestle*	1 Pot/42g	44	1.3	105	6.7	12.6	3.0	0.0
Natural, GFY, Asda*	½ Pot/100g	52	0.3	52	7.3	5.0	0.3	0.0
Natural, HL, Tesco*	1 Serving/65g	30	0.1	46	7.8	3.3	0.2	0.0
Natural, Virtually Fat Free, Safeway*	1 Serving/50g	23	0.1	46	7.3	3.7	0.2	0.0
Normandy, Sainsbury's*	1 Serving/25g	29	2.0	116	7.7	3.4	8.1	0.0
Peach, BGTY, Sainsbury's*	1 Pot/100g	53	0.2	53	7.2	5.5	0.2	0.5
Peach, Layered, Weight Watchers*	1 Pot/100g	57	0.1	57	5.4	7.9	0.1	1.2
Plain, Average	1oz/28g	32	2.0	113	6.8	5.7	7.1	0.0
Raspberry, Layered, Weight Watchers*	1 Pot/100g	51	0.1	51	5.5	6.3	0.1	1.1
Raspberry, Little Stars, Muller*	1 Pot/60g	66	2.4	110	5.0	12.7	4.0	0.4
Raspberry, Value, Tesco*	1 Serving/60g	56	0.8	93	7.2	13.5	1.3	0.0
Safeway*	1 Serving/45g	21	0.1	46	7.3	3.7	0.2	0.0
Strawberry, 99.9% Fat Free, Onken*	1 Serving/50g	46	0.1	91	6.9	15.3	0.1	0.0
Strawberry, Balanced Lifestyle, Aldi*	1 Pot/100g	52	0.2	52	5.4	7.1	0.2	0.7
Strawberry, BGTY, Sainsbury's*	1 Pot/90g	77	0.1	86	7.0	14.1	0.1	0.1
Strawberry, HE, Tesco*	1 Pot/100g	54	0.2	54	6.2	6.8	0.2	0.1
Strawberry, Layered, Weight Watchers*	1 Pot/100g	50	0.1	50	5.4	6.2	0.1	0.8
Strawberry, Puree, Somerfield*	1 Pot/50g	60	2.0	120	7.0	14.0	4.0	0.0
Strawberry, Tesco*	1 Pot/100g	75	3.0	75	6.5	5.5	3.0	2.5
Strawberry, Value, Tesco*	1 Pot/60g	55	0.8	92	7.2	13.0	1.3	0.0
Tropical Fruits, BGTY, Sainsbury's*	1 Pot/90g	77	0.1	86	7.0	14.1	0.1	0.1
Vanilla, Danone*	1 Serving/200g	274	8.2	137	5.3	19.6	4.1	0.0
Virtually Fat Free, Safeway*	1 Pot/100g	41	0.2	41	6.7	3.2	0.2	0.0

	Measure INFO/WEIGHT	per Measure KCAL	FAT	Nutrition Values per 100g / 100ml KCAL	PROT	CARB	FAT	FIBRE
FROMAGE FRAIS								
Virtually Fat Free, Tesco*	1 Pot/100g	56	0.1	56	5.6	8.2	0.1	0.0
Wildlife, Yoplait*	1 Pot/50g	47	0.7	93	7.1	13.2	1.3	0.2
FROZEN DESSERT								
Banoffee, HL, Tesco*	1 Serving/60g	92	1.6	153	2.5	29.9	2.6	0.6
FROZEN YOGHURT								
Black Cherry, M & S*	1 Pot/125g	164	1.4	131	3.1	27.1	1.1	0.5
Cherry Garcia, Low Fat, Ben & Jerry's*	1 Serving/100g	160	3.0	160	3.8	30.0	3.0	0.0
Choc Fudge Brownie, Low Fat, Ben & Jerry's*	1 Serving/100g	180	2.5	180	5.0	34.0	2.5	0.0
Raspberry, Farmhouse, Sainsbury's*	1 Serving/100g	132	3.8	132	2.7	21.8	3.8	2.2
Strawberry, Organic, Yeo Valley*	1 Serving/100g	140	3.0	140	4.8	23.5	3.0	0.1
Strawberry, Tesco*	1 Pot/60g	82	1.3	136	2.6	26.5	2.2	0.8
Vanilla, Less Than 5% Fat, Tesco*	1 Pot/120g	179	2.9	149	8.1	23.8	2.4	0.7
FRUIT								
Berry Medley, Freshly Prepared, M & S*	1 Pack/180g	90	0.4	50	0.7	10.9	0.2	2.9
Bites, Apple & Grape, Food Explorers, Waitrose*	1 Pack/80g	44	0.1	55	0.4	13.2	0.1	1.4
Bites, Raspberry, Mini, HL, Tesco*	1 Bag/25g	88	0.7	350	4.5	76.8	2.7	4.4
Black Forest, Frozen, Tesco*	1 Serving/80g	37	0.0	46	0.8	10.5	0.0	1.8
Black Forest, Shearway*	1oz/28g	12	0.0	44	0.7	9.9	0.1	0.0
Blueberries, Shearway*	1 Serving/80g	41	0.5	51	0.4	12.2	0.6	0.0
Citrus Selection, Fresh, Sainsbury's*	1 Pack/240g	79	0.2	33	0.9	7.1	0.1	1.6
Collection, Freshly Prepared, M & S*	1 Pack/400g	180	0.8	45	0.6	10.3	0.2	1.3
Deluxe, Fresh, Rindless, Shapers, Boots*	1 Pack/168g	64	0.3	38	0.7	8.3	0.2	0.7
Exotic, M & S*	1 Pack/425g	213	1.3	50	0.7	11.8	0.3	0.0
Grapefruit & Orange Segments, Del Monte*	1 Can/411g	193	0.4	47	1.0	10.2	0.1	1.0
Melon, Kiwi, & Strawberry, Fully Prepared, Sainsbury's*	1 Pack/245g	74	0.5	30	0.8	6.3	0.2	1.3
Melon, Mango & Blueberry, Tesco*	1 Serving/200g	76	0.4	38	0.6	8.4	0.2	1.7
Mixed, Fresh, 5 a Day, Tesco*	1 Pack/400g	136	0.8	34	0.8	7.4	0.2	1.4
Mixed, Fresh, Tesco*	1 Pack/200g	70	0.4	35	0.8	7.4	0.2	1.4
Mixed, Fruitime, Pieces, Tesco*	1 Can/140g	84	0.0	60	0.4	14.0	0.0	1.0
Mixed, Pieces, in Orange Jelly, Fruitini, Del Monte*	1 Can/140g	94	0.1	67	0.3	15.8	0.1	0.0
Mixed, Tropical, Fruit Express, Del Monte*	1 Pot/185g	89	0.2	48	0.2	11.2	0.1	1.2
Mixed, Vine, Crazy Jack*	1 Serving/10g	31	0.0	309	2.8	74.0	0.3	4.7
Mixed Pieces, in Fruit Juice, Fruitini, Del Monte*	1 Pot/120g	61	0.1	51	0.4	12.0	0.1	0.5
Nut & Seed Mix, Waitrose*	1 Serving/20g	90	5.6	452	13.5	36.5	28.0	5.5
Pieces, Mixed in Fruit Juice, Fruiyini, Del Monte*	1 Serving/120g	61	0.1	51	0.4	12.0	0.1	0.5
Pineapple, Grape & Kiwi, Asda*	1 Serving/200g	98	0.6	49	0.6	11.0	0.3	1.7
Pure, Just Apple, Heinz*	1 Jar/128g	60	0.1	47	0.4	11.2	0.1	1.8
Snack, Apple & Grape, Blue Parrot Cafe, Sainsbury's*	1 Pack/80g	42	0.1	53	0.4	12.5	0.1	2.1
Snack Pack, Fresh, Sainsbury's*	1 Serving/120g	54	0.1	45	0.1	11.0	0.1	1.3
to Go, Del Monte*	1 Can/113g	80	0.0	71	0.0	17.7	0.0	0.0
Tropical, Fresh, M & S*	1 Pack/425g	191	0.9	45	0.8	10.4	0.2	2.0
Tropical, in Juice, Dole*	1 Pot/113g	59	0.0	52	0.3	14.2	0.0	1.8
Tropical, Tesco*	1 Pack/180g	85	0.4	47	0.6	10.8	0.2	1.9
FRUIT & NUT MIX								
Almond, Raisin & Berry, Sainsbury's*	1 Bag/50g	189	7.2	377	6.1	57.6	14.3	4.2
Exotic, Waitrose*	1 Serving/50g	207	8.9	414	9.0	54.6	17.7	4.6
Luxury, Asda*	1 Serving/50g	226	15.3	451	9.0	33.5	30.5	7.4
M & S*	1 Serving/28g	126	7.1	450	12.4	44.3	25.3	6.0
Organic, Waitrose*	1 Pack/100g	489	32.6	489	15.0	33.8	32.6	5.4
Papaya & Cranberry, Sainsbury's*	1 Serving/75g	300	11.0	400	4.1	63.1	14.6	7.3
TTD, Sainsbury's*	1 Bag/250g	900	39.3	360	5.1	49.5	15.7	5.9
FRUIT COCKTAIL								
Fresh & Ready, Sainsbury's*	1 Pack/300g	117	0.3	39	0.6	9.0	0.1	1.2

F

INFO/WEIGHT	Measure	per Measure		Nutrition Values per 100g / 100ml				
	INFO/WEIGHT	KCAL	FAT	KCAL	PROT	CARB	FAT	FIBRE

FRUIT COCKTAIL

in Apple Juice, Asda*	1/3 Can/80g	40	0.1	50	0.3	12.0	0.1	1.6
in Fruit Juice, Morrisons*	1 Can/140g	64	0.0	46	0.4	11.0	0.0	0.0
in Fruit Juice, Safeway*	1 Serving/220g	68	0.0	31	0.4	7.2	0.0	1.0
in Fruit Juice, Sainsbury's*	1 Serving/198g	97	0.2	49	0.3	11.9	0.1	1.3
in Fruit Juice, Waitrose*	1 Can/142g	71	0.0	50	0.4	12.0	0.0	1.0
in Grape Juice, Tesco*	1oz/28g	12	0.0	43	0.4	10.0	0.0	1.0
in Juice, Del Monte*	1 Can/415g	203	0.4	49	0.4	11.2	0.1	0.0
in Light Syrup, Makes Sense, Somerfield*	½ Can/205g	127	0.0	62	0.4	15.0	0.0	1.0
in Light Syrup, Princes*	1 Serving/206g	64	0.0	31	0.4	7.3	0.0	1.0
in Light Syrup, Sainsbury's*	½ Can/125g	73	0.1	58	0.4	14.0	0.1	1.3
in Light Syrup, Valfrutta*	1 Serving/206g	95	0.0	46	0.2	11.4	0.0	1.5
in Pear Juice, Kwik Save*	1 Can/411g	189	0.0	46	0.5	11.0	0.0	1.0
in Syrup, Del Monte*	1 Can/420g	315	0.4	75	0.4	18.0	0.1	0.0
in Syrup, Morrisons*	½ Can/205g	129	0.2	63	0.3	14.9	0.1	0.0
in Syrup, SmartPrice, Asda*	1 Tin/411g	173	0.4	42	0.3	10.0	0.1	1.6
in Syrup, Tesco*	1 Serving/135g	85	0.0	63	0.4	15.0	0.0	1.0
in Very Light Syrup, Value, Tesco*	1 Can/410g	123	0.0	30	0.4	7.3	0.0	1.0
No Added Sugar, Asda*	1 Serving/134g	67	0.1	50	0.3	12.0	0.1	1.6
Safeway*	1 Serving/205g	117	0.0	57	0.4	14.0	0.0	1.0
Tropical, Asda*	½ Can/135g	81	0.0	60	0.0	15.0	0.0	1.6
Tropical, in Juice, Morrisons*	1 Serving/100g	56	0.0	56	0.0	14.0	0.0	0.0
Tropical, in Syrup, Sainsbury's*	½ Can/130g	95	0.1	73	0.5	17.6	0.1	1.4
Tropical, Morrisons*	½ Can/212g	144	0.0	68	0.0	17.0	0.0	0.0
Tropical, Safeway*	½ Can/214g	154	0.0	72	0.5	17.6	0.0	1.4

FRUIT COMPOTE

& Vanilla Sponge, Weight Watchers*	1 Pack/140.3g	202	2.9	144	2.2	29.0	2.1	1.8
Apricot & Prune, Yeo Valley*	1 Pot/225g	207	0.2	92	0.6	22.3	0.1	1.6
Hartley's*	1 Serving/95g	63	0.1	66	0.8	15.5	0.1	2.4
HE, Tesco*	1 Pot/140g	113	0.3	81	0.9	19.1	0.2	1.6
Orchard Fruits, GFY, Asda*	1 Pot/180g	113	0.2	63	0.5	15.0	0.1	0.0
Organic, Yeo Valley*	1 Pot/225g	146	0.2	65	0.5	15.5	0.1	2.0
Spiced, Tesco*	1 Serving/112g	122	0.6	109	1.7	24.4	0.5	3.1
Strawberry & Raspberry, M & S*	1 Serving/80g	72	0.1	90	0.7	23.5	0.1	2.3
Summerfruit, M & S*	¼ Pot/125g	119	0.8	95	0.9	22.7	0.6	0.8

FRUIT DRINK

Infusion, Peach, Lime & Ginger, M & S*	1 Serving/250ml	88	0.0	35	0.0	8.5	0.0	0.0
Lemon & Lime, Diet, Carbonated, M & S*	1 Glass/250ml	5	0.0	2	0.0	0.2	0.0	0.0

FRUIT FILLING

Red Cherry, Morton*	1 Serving/70g	69	0.0	98	0.4	23.9	0.0	0.0

FRUIT FLAKES

Blackcurrant, with Yoghurt Coating, Fruit Bowl*	1 Bag/24.9g	112	5.1	449	1.7	64.2	20.6	0.0
Raisins, with Yoghurt Coating, Fruit Bowl*	1 Pack/30g	133	5.5	444	2.9	66.6	18.4	0.0
Raspberry, with Yoghurt Coating, Fruit Bowl*	1 Serving/25g	112	5.2	449	1.7	64.2	20.6	0.0
Strawberry, Fruit Bowl*	1 Pack/20g	66	0.4	330	1.0	78.0	2.0	2.0
Strawberry, with Yoghurt Coating, Fruit Bowl*	1 Serving/25g	112	5.2	449	1.7	64.2	20.6	0.0

FRUIT GUMS

Fruit Salad, Tesco*	6 Sweets/30g	101	0.2	335	8.3	73.4	0.5	0.3
Rowntree's*	1 Pack/48g	164	0.1	342	4.7	80.8	0.2	0.0
Sugar Free, Sainsbury's*	1 Serving/30g	63	0.1	209	7.7	71.3	0.2	0.1

FRUIT MEDLEY

Citrus, Somerfield*	1 Serving/80.6g	25	0.1	31	0.6	6.9	0.1	0.4
Dried, Tropical, Soft, Waitrose*	1 Serving/33g	93	0.0	283	0.2	70.6	0.0	2.5
Exotic, Co-Op*	1 Serving/120g	54	0.2	45	0.6	10.0	0.2	0.0

F

	Measure INFO/WEIGHT	per Measure KCAL	FAT	Nutrition Values per 100g / 100ml KCAL	PROT	CARB	FAT	FIBRE
FRUIT MEDLEY								
Exotic, Julian Graves*	1 Serving/50g	157	0.6	313	2.9	72.8	1.1	5.5
Exotic, Waitrose*	1 Medley/300g	126	0.6	42	0.6	9.5	0.2	1.1
in Fresh Orange Juice, Co-Op*	1 Serving/140g	49	0.0	35	0.5	9.0	0.0	0.0
Mango, Melon, Kiwi & Blueberry, M & S*	1 Pack/260g	104	0.8	40	0.7	9.1	0.3	1.6
Melon & Grape, Somerfield*	1 Serving/200g	70	0.2	35	0.5	8.0	0.1	0.7
Mixed, Fruit Harvest, Whitworths*	1 Pack/50g	166	0.4	331	1.8	79.4	0.7	4.8
Nectarine, Mango & Blueberry, Fresh, M & S*	1 Pack/245g	123	0.5	50	1.0	11.1	0.2	2.1
Pineapple, Papaya & Mango, Waitrose*	1 Pack/550g	297	0.6	54	0.6	12.8	0.1	1.1
Raisin, Fruit Harvest, Whitworths*	1 Pack/50g	158	0.7	315	1.8	74.4	1.3	4.3
Shapers, Boots*	1 Pack/140g	55	0.3	39	0.7	8.6	0.2	1.0
FRUIT MIX								
Berry, Sainsbury's*	1 Serving/20g	64	0.4	319	1.0	78.1	1.9	5.5
Luxury, Sainsbury's*	1 Serving/30g	78	0.2	261	1.8	62.3	0.5	2.7
Mango & Cranberry, Way to Five, Sainsbury's*	1 Serving/50g	166	0.4	331	1.8	79.4	0.7	4.8
Pineapple, Melon, Mango, Tesco*	1 Pack/440g	242	0.9	55	1.1	11.4	0.2	1.3
Summer Fruits, British, Frozen, Waitrose*	1 Pack/380g	99	0.8	26	1.0	5.2	0.2	5.5
Tropical, Fresh, Waitrose*	1 Pack/240g	122	0.5	51	0.6	11.6	0.2	1.9
TTD, Sainsbury's*	1 Serving/50g	69	0.2	137	0.3	36.4	0.4	1.6
FRUIT PUREE								
Apple, & Blueberry, Organix*	1 Pot/100g	54	0.6	54	0.4	11.6	0.6	2.5
Apple, & Peach, Organix*	1 Pot/100g	49	0.3	49	0.6	11.0	0.3	2.1
Banana, Apple, & Apricot, Organix*	1 Pot/100g	68	0.4	68	0.8	15.4	0.4	2.0
FRUIT SALAD								
Autumn, Fresh, M & S*	½ Pack/160g	64	0.2	40	0.7	9.4	0.1	2.9
Berry, Seasonal, Asda*	1 Pack/300g	93	0.3	31	0.6	7.0	0.1	2.1
Chunky, in Fruit Juice, Canned, Tesco*	1 Serving/135g	63	0.3	47	0.4	11.0	0.2	0.8
Citrus, Asda*	1 Serving/265g	88	0.3	33	0.9	7.2	0.1	1.5
Citrus, Fresh, M & S*	½ Pack/225g	79	0.2	35	0.9	7.7	0.1	1.5
Classic, Fresh, Sainsbury's*	1 Pack/400g	148	0.8	37	0.6	8.6	0.2	1.8
Classic, Shapers, Boots*	1 Pack/200g	75	0.2	38	0.7	8.5	0.1	1.3
Dried, M & S*	½ Pack/125g	269	0.5	215	1.8	51.4	0.4	5.9
Dried, Morrisons*	1 Serving/75g	124	0.3	165	2.8	37.3	0.4	5.6
Dried, Nature's Harvest*	1 Serving/100g	181	0.7	181	2.9	42.4	0.7	6.9
Exotic, Fresh, Tesco*	1 Serving/225g	86	0.5	38	0.7	8.4	0.2	1.5
Exotic, Fully Prepared, Sainsbury's*	1 Serving/200g	74	0.4	37	0.6	8.3	0.2	1.3
Exotic, Morrisons*	1 Serving/150g	78	0.3	52	0.6	12.2	0.2	0.0
Exotic, Prepared, Sainsbury's*	1 Serving/400g	148	0.8	37	0.6	8.3	0.2	1.3
Exotic, Somerfield*	1 Pot/350g	140	0.7	40	0.6	9.0	0.2	1.3
Exotic, Waitrose*	1 Pack/300g	126	0.6	42	0.6	9.5	0.2	1.1
Fresh, Asda*	1 Pack/200g	88	0.2	44	0.7	10.0	0.1	2.1
Fresh, Budgens*	1 Pack/250g	105	0.3	42	0.7	9.6	0.1	1.3
Fresh, Morrisons*	1 Tub/350g	151	0.4	43	0.7	9.9	0.1	0.0
Fresh, Somerfield*	1 Sm Pack/200g	94	0.2	47	0.6	11.0	0.1	2.0
Fresh, Sweet, Ripe & Moist, Tesco*	1 Serving/750g	345	0.8	46	0.7	10.6	0.1	1.6
Fresh, Tesco*	1 Serving/100g	42	0.2	42	0.7	9.3	0.1	1.5
Fresh, Washed, Ready to Eat, Tesco*	1 Pack/200g	92	0.2	46	0.7	10.6	0.1	1.6
Fresh for You, Tesco*	1 Pack/160g	59	0.3	37	0.6	8.2	0.2	1.1
Freshly Prepared, M & S*	1 Pack/350g	140	0.7	40	0.5	9.3	0.2	1.0
Fruit, Mediterranean Style, Shapers, Boots*	1 Pack/141.9g	61	0.1	43	0.6	10.0	0.1	1.5
Golden, Fresh, Asda*	1 Pot/146.8g	69	0.1	47	0.6	11.0	0.1	1.6
Grapefruit & Orange, Fresh, M & S*	1 Serving/250g	88	0.3	35	0.9	7.4	0.1	1.6
Green, M & S*	1 Bowl/400g	200	0.8	50	0.6	10.9	0.2	1.2
Homemade, Unsweetened, Average	1 Serving/140g	77	0.1	55	0.7	13.8	0.1	1.5

F

	Measure INFO/WEIGHT	per Measure KCAL	FAT	Nutrition Values per 100g / 100ml KCAL	PROT	CARB	FAT	FIBRE
FRUIT SALAD								
Layered, Rainbow, M & S*	1 Pack/350g	140	0.7	40	0.5	9.3	0.2	1.0
Luxury, Fresh, Tesco*	1 Serving/400g	164	0.8	41	0.7	9.2	0.2	1.6
Luxury, Frozen, Boylans*	1 Serving/100g	54	0.2	54	0.8	12.7	0.2	0.0
Luxury, Frozen, Tesco*	½ Pack/250g	115	0.3	46	0.7	10.7	0.1	1.3
Luxury, M & S*	1oz/28g	11	0.0	40	0.6	9.2	0.1	1.1
Luxury, Shearway*	1 Serving/625g	271	0.6	43	0.6	10.0	0.1	0.0
Mediterranean Style, Budgens*	1 Serving/250g	95	0.5	38	0.6	8.5	0.2	0.8
Melon, Kiwi, Strawbery, Way to Five, Sainsbury's*	1 Pack/245g	74	0.5	30	0.8	6.3	0.2	1.3
Melon & Red Grape, Freshly Prepared, M & S*	1 Pack/450g	158	0.5	35	0.5	8.4	0.1	0.7
Mixed, Food to Go, M & S*	1 Pack/400g	400	1.2	100	0.9	23.3	0.3	2.8
Mixed, Fresh, Sainsbury's*	½ Pack/215g	90	0.4	42	0.7	9.4	0.2	1.9
Mixed, Tesco*	1 Pack/225g	86	0.5	38	0.7	8.3	0.2	1.3
Peaches & Pears, Fruit Express, Del Monte*	1 Serving/185g	87	0.2	47	0.4	10.8	0.1	0.9
Pineapple, Mandarin & Grapefruit, Asda*	1 Serving/200g	86	0.2	43	0.6	10.0	0.1	0.0
Pineapple, Mango & Passion Fruit, M & S*	1 Pack/400g	200	0.8	50	0.7	10.8	0.2	1.8
Seasonal, Fresh, Asda*	1 Pack/125g	55	0.1	44	0.5	10.4	0.1	1.2
Seasonal, M & S*	1 Serving/200g	100	0.4	50	0.5	11.8	0.2	2.1
Shapers, Boots*	1 Pack/140g	55	0.3	39	0.7	8.6	0.2	1.0
Summer, Red, Fresh, M & S*	1 Pack/400g	160	0.8	40	0.0	10.0	0.2	1.2
Summer, Sainsbury's*	1 Pack/240g	84	0.5	35	0.7	7.8	0.2	1.3
Sunshine, Fresh, M & S*	1 Serving/200g	70	0.2	35	0.0	8.3	0.1	1.3
Tropical, Asda*	1 Serving/200g	82	0.4	41	0.7	9.0	0.2	1.8
Tropical, Australian Gold*	1 Pot/130g	92	0.1	71	0.6	17.2	0.1	0.0
Tropical, Budgens*	1 Pack/250g	128	0.5	51	0.6	11.7	0.2	1.8
Tropical, Co-Op*	1 Serving/150g	68	0.3	45	0.6	9.0	0.2	1.0
Tropical, Fresh, Asda*	1 Pack/400g	164	0.8	41	0.7	9.0	0.2	1.8
Tropical, Fresh, Sainsbury's*	1 Pack/350g	147	0.7	42	0.6	10.3	0.2	2.0
Tropical, Fruit Snacks, Frozen, Sainsbury's*	1 Serving/175g	79	0.2	45	0.7	10.4	0.1	1.6
Tropical, Tropical Harvest*	1 Serving/100g	52	0.0	52	0.3	12.8	0.0	1.4
Virgin Trains*	1 Serving/140g	56	0.1	40	0.4	10.0	0.1	0.8
Weight Watchers*	1 Serving/135g	50	0.1	37	0.2	9.0	0.1	0.7
FRUIT SELECTION								
Fresh, M & S*	1 Pack/400g	180	0.8	45	0.6	10.1	0.2	1.3
New, Shapers, Boots*	1 Pack/160g	72	0.2	45	0.6	11.0	0.1	1.8
Shapers, Boots*	1 Pack/235g	96	0.5	41	0.5	9.2	0.2	0.8
Summer, British, M & S*	1 Serving/100g	25	0.2	25	1.0	5.3	0.2	5.4
FRUIT SHOOT								
Apple & Blackcurrant, Robinson's*	1 Bottle/200ml	10	0.0	5	0.1	0.8	0.0	0.0
Orange, Pure, Robinson's*	1 Bottle/250ml	115	0.3	46	0.5	9.9	0.1	0.2
FRUIT SPREAD								
Apricot, Pure, Organic, Whole Earth*	1 Serving/20g	33	0.1	167	0.8	40.0	0.4	0.9
Blackcurrant, Carb Check, Heinz*	1 Tbsp/15g	8	0.0	54	0.5	12.8	0.1	2.7
Blackcurrant, Weight Watchers*	1 Tsp/5.7g	6	0.0	106	0.2	26.3	0.0	0.9
Cherries & Berries, Organic, Meridian Foods*	1 Tbsp/15g	16	0.0	109	0.5	26.0	0.3	1.1
High, Blueberry, St Dalfour*	1 Tsp/15g	34	0.0	228	0.5	56.0	0.2	2.2
Raspberry, Weight Watchers*	1 Tsp/6.3g	7	0.0	111	0.4	27.1	0.1	0.9
Seville Orange, Weight Watchers*	1 Serving/28g	31	0.0	111	0.2	27.5	0.0	0.3
Strawberry, Carb Check, Heinz*	1 Tbsp/15g	8	0.0	56	0.3	13.6	0.0	0.5
Strawberry, Weight Watchers*	1 Tbsp/15g	23	0.0	156	0.7	39.8	0.1	1.8
FRUIT WINDERS								
Real Fruit, Kellogg's*	1 Serving/18g	67	1.3	370	0.5	77.0	7.0	3.0
FU YUNG								
Egg, Average	1oz/28g	67	5.8	239	9.9	2.2	20.6	1.3

F

FUDGE

All Butter, Finest, Tesco*	1 Sweet/10g		43	1.5	429	1.3	73.4	14.5	0.0
All Butter, TTD, Sainsbury's*	1 Sweet/10g		43	1.5	429	1.3	73.4	14.5	0.0
Butter, Milk, Thorntons*	1 Chocolate/13g		60	2.5	462	3.7	68.5	19.2	0.0
Butter Tablet, Thorntons*	1oz/28g		116	3.1	414	0.9	77.6	11.1	0.0
Cadbury*	1 Bar/25g		110	3.8	435	2.5	72.7	14.9	0.0
Cherry & Almond, Thorntons*	1 Bag/100g		464	19.1	464	3.2	70.5	19.1	0.4
Chocolate, Average	1 Piece/30g		132	4.1	441	3.3	81.1	13.7	0.0
Chocolate, Thorntons*	1 Bag/100g		459	19.1	459	3.1	69.0	19.1	0.6
Clotted Cream, Sainsbury's*	1 Sweet/8g		35	0.9	430	1.9	81.5	10.7	0.7
Dairy, Co-Op*	1 Sweet/9g		39	1.2	430	2.0	76.0	13.0	0.0
Devon, Somerfield*	1 Pack/250g		1060	27.8	424	2.0	78.9	11.1	0.0
Maple, TTD, Sainsbury's*	1 Sweet/10g		43	1.4	426	1.3	73.0	14.3	0.0
Vanilla, Bar, M & S*	1 Bar/43g		205	10.0	476	3.7	63.0	23.3	0.4
Vanilla, Thorntons*	1 Bag/100g		465	21.9	465	1.8	65.9	21.9	0.0

FUSILLI

Carb Check, Heinz*	1 Serving/75g		219	1.7	292	52.7	15.2	2.3	20.8
Carb Options, Knorr*	1oz/28g		98	0.4	350	28.5	34.0	1.5	21.0
Cooked, Average	1 Serving/210g		248	1.4	118	4.2	23.8	0.7	1.2
Corn, Italian, Free From, Sainsbury's*	1 Serving/75g		265	1.1	353	8.0	76.8	1.5	2.0
Dry, Average	1 Serving/90g		316	1.4	352	12.3	72.0	1.6	2.2
Dry Weight, Wholewheat, Authentic, Italian, Tesco*	1 Portion/75g		244	1.9	325	12.5	62.5	2.5	9.0
Fresh, Cooked, Average	1 Serving/200g		329	3.6	165	6.4	30.7	1.8	1.8
Fresh, Dry, Average	1 Serving/75g		208	2.0	277	10.9	53.4	2.7	2.1
Microwaveable, Express, Dolmio*	1 Pack/220g		308	3.1	140	5.9	26.0	1.4	1.3
Tomato, Weight Watchers*	1 Can/388g		198	1.6	51	1.9	10.1	0.4	0.8
Tricolore, Dry, Average	1 Serving/75g		264	1.3	351	12.2	71.8	1.7	2.7
Whole Wheat, Dry Weight, Average	1 Serving/90g		290	2.1	322	13.1	62.3	2.3	9.0

F

	Measure INFO/WEIGHT	per Measure KCAL	FAT	Nutrition Values per 100g / 100ml KCAL	PROT	CARB	FAT	FIBRE
GALAXY								
Amicelli, Mars*	1 Serving/13g	66	3.5	507	6.2	59.7	27.1	0.0
Caramel, Mars*	1 Bar/49g	254	13.0	518	5.8	64.2	26.4	0.0
Caramel Crunch, Promises, Mars*	1 Sm Bar/40g	216	12.7	540	6.1	57.5	31.8	0.0
Chocolate, Milk, Mars*	1 Bar/47g	255	14.9	543	6.8	57.9	31.6	1.5
Fruit & Hazelnut, Milk, Mars*	1 Bar/47g	235	13.2	501	7.1	55.2	28.0	0.0
Hazelnut, Mars*	1 Piece/6.3g	37	2.5	582	7.8	49.4	39.2	0.0
Snack Size, Mars*	1 Serving/24.5g	135	7.9	540	6.8	57.0	31.7	0.0
GAMMON								
Breaded, Average	1oz/28g	34	0.9	120	22.5	1.0	3.1	0.0
Dry Cured, Ready to Roast, M & S*	½ Joint/255g	255	3.8	100	20.5	0.5	1.5	0.5
Honey & Mustard, Average	½ Pack/190g	294	13.5	155	19.1	3.6	7.1	0.1
Joint, Applewood Smoked, Tesco*	1 Serving/100g	152	9.0	152	17.5	0.2	9.0	0.0
Steak, & Parsley Sauce, Tesco*	½ Pack/140g	217	7.3	155	23.7	2.9	5.2	0.5
Steaks, Average	1 Steak/97.1g	157	7.1	161	23.3	0.4	7.4	0.0
Steaks, Healthy Range, Average	1 Serving/110g	107	3.5	97	18.0	0.4	3.2	0.2
Steaks, Honey Roast, Average	1 Steak/100g	142	5.3	142	21.5	2.3	5.3	0.1
Steaks, Smoked, Average	1 Steak/110g	150	5.5	137	22.7	0.1	5.0	0.1
GAMMON &								
Pineapple, Roast, Dinner, Iceland*	1 Meal/400g	360	6.4	90	6.2	12.7	1.6	1.7
GARAM MASALA								
Average	1oz/28g	106	4.2	379	15.6	45.2	15.1	0.0
GARGANELLI								
Egg, Dry, Waitrose*	1 Serving/125g	450	5.3	360	13.5	66.9	4.2	3.5
GARLIC								
Minced, Nishaan*	1 Tsp/5g	5	0.0	97	6.0	16.2	0.9	0.0
Powder	1 Tsp/3g	7	0.0	246	18.7	42.7	1.2	9.9
Raw, Average	1 Clove/3g	3	0.0	98	7.9	16.3	0.6	4.1
Very Lazy, The English Provender Co.*	1 Tsp/3g	3	0.0	111	6.0	20.9	0.4	3.0
GARLIC PUREE								
Average	1 Tbsp/18g	61	5.4	380	3.5	16.9	33.6	0.0
in Vegetable Oil, GIA*	1 Tsp/5g	20	2.1	391	3.3	1.6	41.3	0.0
with Tomato, GIA*	2 Tsp/10g	7	0.1	70	5.1	0.5	1.2	0.0
GATEAU								
Black Forest, 500g Size, Tesco*	1 Serving/55g	124	6.1	225	4.0	27.1	11.0	1.8
Black Forest, Family Size, 860g, Tesco*	1 Slice/76g	175	10.0	230	3.4	24.8	13.2	0.9
Black Forest, Mini, Tesco*	1 Serving/55g	136	5.1	247	5.7	35.3	9.2	1.0
Black Forest, Sara Lee*	1 Serving/80g	221	9.8	276	3.6	37.9	12.3	1.2
Blackforest, Sainsbury's*	1/8 Gateau/63g	163	10.8	259	3.9	27.7	17.1	3.5
Chocolate, Asda*	1 Serving/100g	176	10.0	176	2.4	19.0	10.0	0.4
Chocolate Layer, M & S*	1 Serving/86g	278	15.7	323	4.2	35.9	18.3	0.9
Coffee, Tesco*	1 Serving/100g	300	17.0	300	4.2	32.5	17.0	0.6
Double Chocolate, Tesco*	1 Serving/45g	124	6.5	276	4.4	32.1	14.4	2.2
Double Strawberry, Sara Lee*	1/8 Slice/199g	533	24.3	268	3.2	36.2	12.2	0.6
Ice Cream, Chocolate & Vanilla, Iceland*	1 Serving/130g	252	12.2	194	3.3	24.1	9.4	0.6
Orange & Lemon, Iceland*	1 Serving/90g	221	9.9	245	2.6	33.8	11.0	0.3
Profiterole, TTD, Sainsbury's*	1/6 Gateau/112g	410	30.6	365	3.9	26.2	27.2	1.1
Strawberry, Co-Op*	1 Slice/77g	222	12.9	288	5.1	29.2	16.7	1.0
Strawberry, Family Size, Tesco*	1 Serving/84g	197	11.4	235	2.9	25.2	13.6	0.6
Swiss, Cadbury*	1/6 Cake/60g	228	10.1	380	5.2	52.0	16.8	0.9
GELATINE								
Average	1oz/28g	95	0.0	338	84.4	0.0	0.0	0.0
GEMELLI								
Durum Wheat, Tesco*	1 Serving/100g	354	2.0	354	13.2	68.5	2.0	2.9

G

	Measure INFO/WEIGHT	per Measure KCAL	FAT	Nutrition Values per 100g / 100ml KCAL	PROT	CARB	FAT	FIBRE
GHEE								
Butter	1oz/28g	251	27.9	898	0.0	0.0	99.8	0.0
Palm	1oz/28g	251	27.9	897	0.0	0.0	99.7	0.0
Vegetable	1oz/28g	251	27.8	895	0.0	0.0	99.4	0.0
GHERKINS								
Pickled, Average	1 Gherkin/36g	5	0.0	14	0.9	2.6	0.1	1.2
GIGLIO								
Egg, Tesco*	1 Serving/100g	355	3.5	355	14.5	66.4	3.5	2.6
GIN								
& Tonic, Premixed, Canned, Gordons*	1 Can/250ml	213	0.0	85	0.0	6.7	0.0	0.0
37.5% Volume	1 Pub Shot/35ml	72	0.0	207	0.0	0.0	0.0	0.0
40% Volume	1 Shot/25ml	56	0.0	222	0.0	0.0	0.0	0.0
GINGER								
Chunks, Crystallized, Julian Graves*	1 Serving/10g	34	0.0	340	0.0	88.0	0.0	0.0
Lazy, Minced, The English Provender Co.*	1 Tsp/5g	1	0.0	15	0.2	3.2	0.2	1.5
Root, Raw, Pared, Average	1oz/28g	24	0.2	86	2.0	19.1	0.8	2.2
Root, Raw, Unprepared, Average	1oz/28g	22	0.2	80	1.8	17.8	0.8	2.0
Stem, in Sugar Syrup, Sainsbury's*	1oz/28g	76	0.0	271	0.2	67.3	0.1	1.4
GINGER ALE								
American, Finest, Tesco*	1 Serving/150ml	68	0.0	45	0.0	11.0	0.0	0.0
American, Low Calorie, Tesco*	1 fl oz/30ml	0	0.0	1	0.0	0.0	0.0	0.0
Dry	1 Glass/250ml	38	0.0	15	0.0	3.9	0.0	0.0
Dry, Sainsbury's*	1 Glass/250ml	95	0.3	38	0.1	9.1	0.1	0.1
GINGER BEER								
Asda*	1 Can/330ml	144	0.0	44	0.0	10.9	0.0	0.0
Classic, Schweppes*	1 Can/330ml	115	0.0	35	0.0	8.4	0.0	0.0
Jamaican, Boots*	1 Bottle/500ml	5	0.0	1	0.0	0.0	0.0	0.0
Light, Waitrose*	1 Glass/250ml	3	0.3	1	0.0	0.0	0.1	0.1
Sainsbury's*	1 Can/330ml	69	0.0	21	0.0	5.1	0.0	0.0
Tesco*	1 Serving/200ml	70	0.2	35	0.1	8.2	0.1	0.0
Traditional Style, Tesco*	1 Can/330ml	218	0.0	66	0.0	16.1	0.0	0.0
GINGERBREAD								
Average	1oz/28g	106	3.5	379	5.7	64.7	12.6	1.2
Men, Mini, Asda*	1 Biscuit/10.6g	46	1.4	433	5.0	74.0	13.0	1.8
Men, Mini, M & S*	1 Biscuit/16.6g	80	3.2	470	6.2	63.9	18.6	1.7
Men, Mini, Sainsbury's*	1 Man/12g	56	1.4	463	5.7	83.4	11.8	1.5
GLAZE								
Balsamic, A Drizzle of, Waitrose*	1 Serving/15ml	18	0.0	122	0.0	26.0	0.0	0.0
GNOCCHI								
Aldi*	1 Serving/100g	160	0.3	160	3.8	35.6	0.3	0.0
Di Patate, Buitoni*	1 Serving/250g	373	0.3	149	3.1	33.8	0.1	0.0
Di Patate, Italfresco*	½ Pack/200g	296	0.4	148	3.3	33.2	0.2	0.0
Fresh, Italian, Chilled, Sainsbury's*	¼ Pack/125g	190	0.4	152	3.8	33.6	0.3	1.4
Potato, Average	1 Serving/150g	200	0.0	133	0.0	33.2	0.0	0.0
GOAT								
Raw	1oz/28g	31	0.6	109	20.6	0.0	2.3	0.0
GOJI BERRIES								
Percy Dalton's*	1 Pack/50g	146	0.2	292	2.7	69.4	0.4	2.0
GOOSE								
Meat, Fat & Skin, Raw	1oz/28g	101	9.2	361	16.5	0.0	32.8	0.0
Meat Only, Roasted	1oz/28g	89	6.3	319	29.3	0.0	22.4	0.0
GOOSEBERRIES								
Dessert, Raw	1oz/28g	11	0.1	40	0.7	9.2	0.3	2.4

G

INFO/WEIGHT	Measure		per Measure		Nutrition Values per 100g / 100ml				
			KCAL	FAT	KCAL	PROT	CARB	FAT	FIBRE
GOULASH									
Beef, Bistro Range, Tesco*	1 Pack/450g		545	15.3	121	7.9	14.6	3.4	0.6
Beef, Finest, Tesco*	½ Pack/300g		297	9.3	99	11.6	6.2	3.1	0.6
Beef, Weight Watchers*	1 Pack/330g		241	5.6	73	4.8	9.5	1.7	0.6
Beef, with Tagliatelle, COU, M & S*	1 Pack/360g		414	8.3	115	8.5	14.5	2.3	1.0
GRAPEFRUIT									
in Juice, Average	1oz/28g		13	0.0	46	0.5	10.6	0.0	0.4
in Syrup, Average	1oz/28g		19	0.0	69	0.5	16.8	0.1	0.5
Raw, Flesh Only, Average	½ Grapefruit/160g		34	0.1	21	0.6	4.8	0.1	0.9
Ruby Red, in Juice, Average	1 Serving/135g		54	0.1	40	0.6	9.4	0.1	0.5
GRAPES									
Green, Average	1oz/28g		17	0.0	62	0.4	15.2	0.1	0.7
Red, Average	1 Serving/79g		53	0.1	67	0.5	16.5	0.1	0.8
Red & Green Selection, Average	1 Serving/80g		50	0.1	63	0.4	15.2	0.1	0.9
GRATIN									
Cauliflower, Findus*	1 Pack/400g		340	20.0	85	3.5	7.0	5.0	0.0
Dauphinoise, Budgens*	½ Pack/218g		277	15.7	127	3.0	12.5	7.2	2.5
Leek & Carrot, Findus*	1 Pack/400g		440	26.0	110	3.5	9.5	6.5	0.0
Potato, Creamy, M & S*	½ Pack/225g		360	25.0	160	2.2	11.9	11.1	0.9
Potato, HL, Tesco*	1 Serving/225g		169	5.0	75	2.3	11.4	2.2	0.6
Potato, Sainsbury's*	½ Pack/225		448	34.0	199	4.4	11.4	15.1	1.0
Potato, Somerfield*	½ Pack/225g		356	27.0	158	2.0	11.0	12.0	0.0
Spinach & Mushroom, Safeway*	1 Packet/520g		728	43.7	140	4.8	10.3	8.4	1.5
Vegetable, Somerfield*	1 Pack/300g		417	39.0	139	1.0	5.0	13.0	0.0
GRAVY									
Beef, Aunt Bessie's*	1 Serving/100g		73	5.3	73	1.0	5.3	5.3	0.5
Beef, Fresh, Sainsbury's*	1 Serving/83ml		47	2.7	56	2.4	4.5	3.2	0.6
Beef, Heat & Serve, Morrisons*	1 Serving/150g		27	0.5	18	0.3	3.9	0.3	0.5
Beef, Rich, Ready to Heat, Schwartz*	½ Pack/100g		31	1.6	31	0.8	3.4	1.6	0.5
Beef, with Winter Berry Shallot, Made Up, Oxo*	1 Serving/105ml		24	0.3	23	0.6	4.3	0.3	0.1
Chicken, Granules For, Dry Weight, Bisto*	1 Serving/20g		80	3.2	400	1.9	62.5	15.8	0.2
Chicken, Rich, Ready to Heat, Schwartz*	½ Pack/100g		27	1.2	27	0.8	3.3	1.2	0.5
Chips & Onion, Asda*	1 Pack/357.6g		329	9.3	92	2.1	15.0	2.6	1.2
for Poultry, M & S*	½ Pack/150g		75	4.1	50	3.1	3.3	2.7	0.4
Fresh, Somerfield*	1 Pack/300g		69	3.0	23	0.0	4.0	1.0	0.0
Granules, Beef, Dry, Tesco*	1 Serving/6g		29	2.1	480	5.5	36.4	34.7	1.5
Granules, Beef, Made Up, Tesco*	1 Serving/140ml		49	3.6	35	0.3	2.6	2.5	0.1
Granules, Chicken, Dry, Oxo*	1oz/28g		83	1.4	296	11.1	54.2	4.9	0.7
Granules, Chicken, Made Up, Oxo*	1 fl oz/30ml		5	0.1	18	0.7	3.3	0.3	0.0
Granules, Chicken & Hint of Sage & Onion, Oxo*	1 Serving/30g		95	1.8	316	11.1	54.2	6.1	0.7
Granules, Dry, Bisto*	1 Serving/10g		38	1.6	384	3.1	56.4	16.2	1.5
Granules, Dry, Value, Tesco*	1oz/28g		111	5.2	397	3.2	54.4	18.5	1.0
Granules, Instant, Dry	1oz/28g		129	9.1	462	4.4	40.6	32.5	0.0
Granules, Instant, Made Up	1oz/28g		10	0.7	34	0.3	3.0	2.4	0.0
Granules, Lamb, Hint of Mint, Made Up, Oxo*	1 Serving/100ml		25	0.5	25	0.7	4.3	0.5	0.0
Granules, Made Up, Bisto*	1 Serving/50ml		15	0.7	30	0.2	4.2	1.4	0.2
Granules, Made Up, Oxo*	1 Serving/150ml		29	0.5	19	0.6	3.4	0.3	0.0
Granules, Onion, Dry, Morrisons*	1 Serving/25g		124	8.7	495	3.4	44.0	34.7	0.0
Granules, Onion, Dry, Oxo*	1oz/28g		92	1.3	328	8.2	62.3	4.8	0.8
Granules, Onion, Made Up, Oxo*	1 fl oz/30ml		6	0.1	20	0.5	3.7	0.3	0.0
Granules, Original, Dry, Oxo*	1oz/28g		88	1.3	313	10.2	57.2	4.8	1.0
Granules, Vegetable, Dry, Oxo*	1oz/28g		88	1.4	316	8.4	59.5	4.9	0.9
Granules, Vegetable, Dry, Tesco*	½ Pint/20g		94	6.7	470	3.8	38.5	33.4	3.7
Granules for Chicken, Made Up, SmartPrice. Asda*	1 Serving/100ml		34	2.3	34	0.2	3.0	2.3	0.1

G

	Measure INFO/WEIGHT	per Measure KCAL	per Measure FAT	Nutrition Values per 100g / 100ml KCAL	PROT	CARB	FAT	FIBRE
GRAVY								
Granules for Meat, Made Up, Asda*	1 Serving/100ml	38	2.4	38	0.6	4.0	2.4	0.1
Granules for Meat, Made Up, Sainsbury's*	1 Serving/100ml	37	2.4	37	0.4	3.5	2.4	0.1
Granules for Vegetarian Dishes, Dry Weight, Bisto*	1 Serving/50ml	178	6.7	356	2.7	56.0	13.3	4.5
Onion, Fresh, Asda*	1/6 Pot/77g	30	1.6	39	1.7	3.3	2.1	0.4
Onion, Fresh, Somerfield*	1 Pack/300g	195	12.0	65	1.0	7.0	4.0	0.0
Onion, Granules For, Dry Weight, Bisto*	4 Tsp/20g	78	2.9	391	2.4	62.3	14.7	2.3
Onion, Granules For, Made Up, Bisto*	1 Serving/50ml	14	0.3	28	0.2	5.6	0.6	0.0
Onion, Rich, M & S*	½ Pack/150g	60	1.8	40	2.0	5.9	1.2	0.3
Onion, Rich, Ready to Heat, Schwartz*	½ Sachet/100g	24	0.6	24	0.4	4.3	0.6	0.5
Onion, TTD, Sainsbury's*	1 Serving/100g	78	5.2	78	1.3	6.6	5.2	0.8
Paste, Beef, Antony Worrall Thompson's*	1 Portion/31g	104	5.7	334	11.8	30.3	18.4	0.6
Paste, Onion, Antony Worrall Thompson's*	1 Tsp/10g	26	0.4	262	7.0	48.7	4.4	1.4
Powder, Dry, Tesco*	1 Serving/20g	57	0.3	286	7.2	61.0	1.5	2.0
Powder, Made Up, Sainsbury's*	1 Serving/100ml	15	0.1	15	0.4	3.2	0.1	0.1
Powder, Vegetarian, Organic, Marigold*	1 Serving/22g	79	1.7	361	10.6	61.5	7.7	1.3
Roast Beef, Best, in Glass Jar, Made Up, Bisto*	1 Serving/50ml	13	0.2	26	0.4	5.4	0.4	0.2
Roast Pork, Best, in Glass Jar, Dry Weight, Bisto*	4 Tsp/20g	63	0.9	314	4.3	64.1	4.5	0.0
Turkey, Granules For, Dry Weight, Bisto*	4 Tsp/20g	75	3.1	377	2.4	57.2	15.5	1.0
Turkey, Rich, Ready to Heat, Schwartz*	1 Pack/200g	62	2.4	31	1.9	3.1	1.2	0.5
Vegetable, Granules For, Dry Weight, Bisto*	1 Tsp/4g	15	0.5	380	2.1	63.0	13.3	4.5
Vegetable, Granules For, Made Up, Bisto*	1 Serving/140ml	39	0.6	28	0.2	5.6	0.4	0.2
GRAVY MIX								
Instant, Dry Weight, BFY, Morrisons*	1 Serving/25g	80	0.1	320	3.5	77.0	0.3	1.2
Instant, Made Up, BGTY, Sainsbury's*	1 fl oz/30ml	10	0.0	32	0.3	7.4	0.1	0.1
Roast Beef, Classic, Schwartz*	1 Pack/27g	83	0.8	306	11.2	58.8	2.9	3.8
Roast Chicken, Classic, Schwartz*	1 Pack/26g	49	1.5	189	10.3	23.6	5.9	2.5
Roast Lamb, Classic, Schwartz*	1 Serving/13g	44	0.6	336	10.4	63.6	4.5	0.0
Roast Pork & Sage, Classic, Schwartz*	1 Pack/25g	89	1.5	354	11.8	63.8	5.8	0.0
Roast Turkey, Classic, Schwartz*	1 Serving/6g	20	0.4	337	12.2	56.8	6.8	2.9
GREENGAGES								
Raw, Average	1 Fruit/66g	26	0.1	40	0.8	9.5	0.1	2.1
GREENS								
Spring, Boiled, Average	1 Serving/80g	16	0.6	20	1.9	1.6	0.7	2.6
Spring, Raw, Average	1 Serving/80g	26	0.8	33	3.0	3.1	1.0	3.4
GRILLS								
Bacon & Cheese, Tesco*	1 Grill/78g	222	14.7	284	15.0	13.4	18.9	1.2
Cheese & Bacon, Danepak*	1 Grill/84.9g	241	16.0	284	15.0	13.4	18.9	1.2
Vegetable, Dalepak*	1 Grill/82.9g	131	4.4	158	3.9	23.6	5.3	1.7
Vegetable, Ross*	1 Grill/114g	252	12.9	221	4.3	25.5	11.3	0.9
Vegetable, Tesco*	1 Grill/72.2g	129	7.2	179	4.2	18.0	10.0	2.2
GRITS								
Enriched White Hominy, Old Fashioned, Quaker*	1/3 Cup/41g	140	0.5	341	7.3	78.1	1.2	4.9
GROUSE								
Meat Only, Roasted	1oz/28g	36	0.6	128	27.6	0.0	2.0	0.0
GUACAMOLE								
Asda*	½ Pot/56.5g	114	11.4	200	1.8	3.3	20.0	4.0
Average	1 Tbsp/17g	22	2.2	128	1.4	2.2	12.7	2.5
Chunky, M & S*	1 Pot/170g	221	19.2	130	1.5	5.1	11.3	1.7
Chunky, Sainsbury's*	½ Pot/64.9g	120	12.0	185	1.6	3.2	18.4	3.8
Doritos, Walkers*	1 Tbsp/20g	32	3.2	159	1.2	2.6	16.0	0.1
Fresh, Waitrose*	½ Pack/100g	190	18.4	190	1.9	4.1	18.4	2.5
GFY, Asda*	1 Pack/113g	144	12.4	127	2.8	4.3	11.0	2.2
Mexican Style, Dip Selection, Morrisons*	½ Pack/50g	102	10.2	204	1.5	3.7	20.4	0.9

G

	Measure INFO/WEIGHT	per Measure KCAL	FAT	Nutrition Values per 100g / 100ml KCAL	PROT	CARB	FAT	FIBRE
GUACAMOLE								
Reduced Fat, Sainsbury's*	½ Pot/65g	87	8.2	134	1.5	3.5	12.6	4.0
Reduced Fat, Tesco*	1 Pack/170g	238	19.4	140	2.7	5.7	11.4	3.0
Reduced Fat, Waitrose*	1 Serving/25g	32	2.5	126	2.9	5.7	10.1	2.3
Somerfield*	½ Pot/85g	175	17.9	206	1.7	2.6	21.0	3.6
GUAVA								
Canned, in Syrup	1oz/28g	17	0.0	60	0.4	15.7	0.0	3.0
GUINEA FOWL								
Boned & Stuffed, Fresh, Fayrefield Foods*	1 Serving/325g	650	39.3	200	19.1	3.3	12.1	0.5
Fresh, Free Range, Waitrose*	1 Portion/192.5g	258	11.9	134	19.5	0.0	6.2	0.3
GUMBO								
Cajun Vegetable, Sainsbury's*	1 Serving/450g	266	11.3	59	1.4	7.7	2.5	1.5
Louisiana Chicken, PB, Waitrose*	1 Serving/235g	207	6.6	88	12.2	3.5	2.8	1.3
GUMS								
American, Hard, Tesco*	1 Serving/200g	646	0.0	323	0.0	80.8	0.0	0.0
American Hard, Sainsbury's*	1 Sweet/6g	22	0.0	360	0.1	90.0	0.1	0.0
Milk, Cow, Sainsbury's*	1 Sweet/3g	10	0.0	353	6.2	78.3	1.6	0.0
Milk Bottles, Bassett's*	1 Pack/25g	88	0.4	353	6.2	78.3	1.6	0.0

G

	Measure INFO/WEIGHT	per Measure KCAL	FAT	Nutrition Values per 100g / 100ml KCAL	PROT	CARB	FAT	FIBRE
HADDOCK								
Atlantic, with Cheese & Chive Sauce, Youngs*	½ Pack/180g	184	8.6	102	13.0	1.7	4.8	0.2
En Croute, Youngs*	1 Serving/170.1g	432	28.7	254	8.0	17.1	16.9	4.3
Fillet, Breaded, Scottish, with Chips, M & S*	1 Pack/340g	510	18.4	150	7.7	17.8	5.4	1.4
Fillet, Breaded, Scottish with Chunky Chips, M & S*	1 Pack/340g	510	18.4	150	7.7	17.8	5.4	1.4
Fillets, Battered, Average	1oz/28g	64	3.4	228	13.4	16.3	12.2	1.1
Fillets, in Breadcrumbs, Average	1oz/28g	57	2.8	203	13.5	14.9	9.9	1.2
Fillets, Large, Chip Shop, Youngs*	1 Fillet/104g	243	15.1	234	11.1	14.8	14.5	1.1
Fillets, Raw, Average	1oz/28g	22	0.2	80	18.0	0.2	0.9	0.0
Fillets, Smoked, Cooked, Average	1 Pack/300g	337	7.7	112	21.9	0.4	2.6	0.1
Fillets, Smoked, Raw, Average	1 Pack/227g	194	1.0	86	20.3	0.1	0.5	0.2
Flour, Fried in Blended Oil	1oz/28g	39	1.1	138	21.1	4.5	4.1	0.2
Goujons, Batter, Crispy, M & S*	1 Serving/100g	250	14.1	250	11.7	18.5	14.1	0.8
in Crispy Batter, Large, Morrisons*	1 Fish/150.2g	362	23.0	241	10.9	15.0	15.3	2.1
Lightly Dusted, Eat Well, M & S*	1 Fillet/130g	176	7.0	135	16.4	5.8	5.4	0.7
Mornay, COU, M & S*	½ Pack/194.1g	165	3.9	85	14.5	2.6	2.0	0.6
HADDOCK &								
Cauliflower Crunchies, Iceland*	1 Serving/111g	222	13.1	200	8.0	15.5	11.8	2.0
HADDOCK FLORENTINE								
Eat Smart, Safeway*	1 Serving/250g	200	4.5	80	12.0	2.5	1.8	1.3
HE, Tesco*	1 Pack/370g	303	3.7	82	8.2	10.0	1.0	0.5
HADDOCK IN								
Butter Sauce, Steaks, Youngs*	1 Portion/150g	134	5.6	89	9.9	4.0	3.7	0.5
Cheese & Chive Sauce, HL, Tesco*	1 Serving/200g	150	4.2	75	12.7	1.2	2.1	0.6
Smoked Leek & Cheese Sauce, Asda*	½ Pack/200g	232	10.0	116	14.0	3.7	5.0	1.5
Tomato Herb Sauce, Fillets, BGTY, Sainsbury's*	½ Pack/165g	150	4.6	91	12.9	3.6	2.8	0.1
Watercress Sauce, GFY, Asda*	1 Pack/400g	268	6.8	67	6.0	7.0	1.7	1.4
HADDOCK RAREBIT								
Smoked, Finest, Tesco*	1 Rarebit/180g	326	16.6	181	5.6	19.1	9.2	0.4
HADDOCK WITH								
a Rich Cheese Crust, Smoked, Sainsbury's*	1 Serving/199g	295	18.9	148	13.0	2.5	9.5	0.9
Broccoli & Cheese, Lakeland*	1 Serving/150g	281	10.5	187	10.4	20.6	7.0	0.0
Creme Fraiche & Chive Sauce, Tesco*	1 Serving/150g	155	4.7	103	16.8	2.1	3.1	0.3
HAGGIS								
Neeps & Tatties, M & S*	1 Pack/300g	330	14.4	110	3.8	12.3	4.8	0.8
Vegetarian, McSween*	1 Serving/100g	216	10.2	216	6.6	26.8	10.2	2.4
HAKE								
Fillets, in Breadcrumbs, Average	1oz/28g	66	3.7	235	12.9	16.0	13.4	1.0
Goujons, Average	1 Serving/150g	345	17.9	230	12.4	18.7	11.9	1.3
Raw, Average	1oz/28g	29	0.6	102	20.4	0.0	2.2	0.0
with Tomato & Chilli Salsa, Just Cook, Sainsbury's*	½ Pack/180g	112	1.6	62	11.4	2.2	0.9	0.0
HALIBUT								
Cooked, Average	1oz/28g	38	1.1	135	24.6	0.4	4.0	0.0
Raw	1oz/28g	29	0.5	103	21.5	0.0	1.9	0.0
HALIBUT WITH								
Roasted Pepper Sauce, Fillets, M & S*	1 Serving/145g	218	14.4	150	12.7	2.4	9.9	0.6
HALVA								
Average	1oz/28g	107	3.7	381	1.8	68.0	13.2	0.0
HAM								
Applewood Smoked, Average	1 Slice/28g	31	0.8	112	21.3	0.6	2.8	0.3
Baked, Average	1 Slice/74g	106	4.3	143	21.1	1.8	5.8	0.3
Beechwood Smoked, Morrisons*	1 Slice/20g	32	1.8	160	19.5	0.5	9.0	0.0
Boiled, Average	1 Pack/113g	154	6.5	137	20.6	0.6	5.8	0.0
Breaded, Average	1 Slice/37g	57	2.3	155	23.1	1.9	6.3	1.6

	Measure INFO/WEIGHT	per Measure KCAL	FAT	Nutrition Values per 100g / 100ml KCAL	PROT	CARB	FAT	FIBRE
HAM								
Breaded, Dry Cured, Average	1 Slice/33g	47	1.8	142	22.2	1.4	5.4	0.0
Brunswick, Average	1 Slice/20g	32	1.8	160	19.5	0.6	8.8	0.1
Cooked, Sliced, Average	1 Serving/50g	57	1.9	115	19.1	0.9	3.9	0.1
Cooked, Somerfield*	1 Slice/25.2g	30	0.7	119	22.1	1.4	2.8	0.0
Danish, Average	1 Slice/11g	14	0.6	125	18.4	1.1	5.4	0.0
Danish, Lean, Average	1 Slice/15g	14	0.3	93	17.9	1.0	1.8	0.0
Dry Cured, Average	1 Slice/18g	26	1.0	144	22.4	1.0	5.6	0.2
Dry Cured, Rosemary & Thyme, Safeway*	1 Slice/28g	37	0.9	133	24.8	1.5	3.1	0.0
Extra Lean, Average	1 Slice/11g	10	0.2	90	18.0	1.4	1.4	0.0
Gammon, Honey Roast, Average	1 Serving/60g	81	2.9	135	22.5	0.5	4.8	0.0
German Black Forest, Average	½ Pack/35g	93	6.0	267	27.2	1.3	17.0	0.5
Honey & Ginger, Roast, Waitrose*	1 Slice/16g	21	0.9	134	20.0	0.0	6.0	0.0
Honey & Mustard, Average	1oz/28g	39	1.2	140	20.8	4.6	4.3	0.0
Honey Roast, Average	1 Slice/20g	25	0.8	123	20.3	1.6	3.8	0.1
Honey Roast, Dry Cured, Average	1 Slice/33g	46	1.5	140	22.7	2.3	4.4	0.2
Honey Roast, Lean, Average	1 Serving/25g	28	0.8	111	18.2	2.7	3.1	0.0
Honey Roast, Wafer Thin, Average	1 Slice/10g	11	0.3	113	17.4	3.7	3.2	0.3
Honey Roast, Wafer Thin, Premium, Average	1 Slice/10g	15	0.6	149	22.0	1.6	6.0	0.0
Italian Rostello, Safeway*	1 Serving/60g	78	3.0	130	21.0	0.2	5.0	0.0
Joint, Easy Carve, Asda*	1oz/28g	41	1.7	146	22.8	1.2	5.9	0.6
Joint, Honey Roast, Asda*	1oz/28g	35	0.8	124	23.9	1.7	2.8	0.7
Joint, Roast, Christmas, Tesco*	1/6 Joint/167g	225	10.8	135	17.9	1.1	6.5	0.0
Lean, Average	1 Slice/18g	19	0.4	104	19.5	1.1	2.4	0.3
Maple Drycure, Asda*	1 Slice/37.1g	49	1.3	132	22.0	3.0	3.5	0.0
Oak Smoked, Average	1 Slice/20g	26	0.9	130	21.0	1.0	4.7	0.3
on the Bone, Breaded, Somerfield*	1oz/28g	45	2.5	161	21.0	0.0	9.0	0.0
Parma, Average	1 Serving/10g	21	1.1	213	29.3	0.0	10.6	0.0
Parma, Premium, Average	1 Serving/80g	206	12.9	258	27.9	0.3	16.1	0.0
Peppered, Average	1 Slice/12g	13	0.3	110	18.5	2.1	2.7	0.0
Peppered, Dry Cured, Average	1 Slice/31g	43	1.5	140	23.1	1.3	4.7	0.2
Prosciutto, Average	1 Slice/12g	27	1.5	227	28.7	0.1	12.4	0.4
San Daniele, Finest, Tesco*	2 Slices/20g	48	2.6	242	30.5	0.5	13.1	0.0
Scrumpy Cured, Tesco*	1 Slice/34g	60	2.4	176	27.2	0.9	7.1	0.0
Serrano, Spanish, The Best, Safeway*	1 Pack/70g	153	7.0	218	32.0	0.0	10.0	0.0
Smoked, Average	1 Slice/18g	21	0.7	117	19.7	0.9	3.7	0.0
Smoked, Dry Cured, Average	1 Slice/28g	38	1.2	137	23.0	1.5	4.4	0.2
Smoked, HL, Tesco*	1 Slice/22g	24	0.5	109	22.0	0.4	2.2	0.0
Smoked, Wafer Thin, Average	1 Serving/40g	41	1.2	102	17.7	1.2	2.9	0.2
Wafer Thin, Average	1 Slice/10g	10	0.3	101	17.9	1.4	2.6	0.1
Wiltshire, Average	1oz/28g	41	1.7	148	23.1	0.0	6.1	0.0
Wiltshire, Crumbed, Finest, Tesco*	1 Slice/35.1g	46	1.3	131	23.7	0.5	3.8	0.4
Wiltshire, Orange Marmalade Roasted, Finest, Tesco*	1 Slice/40g	67	2.4	167	26.0	2.0	6.1	0.3
HAM VEGETARIAN								
Cheatin', Co, Redwood*	1 Slice/10g	25	1.5	247	19.7	8.9	14.7	0.0
HARE								
Raw, Lean Only, Average	1oz/28g	35	1.0	125	23.5	0.2	3.5	0.0
Stewed, Lean Only, Average	1oz/28g	48	1.5	170	29.5	0.2	5.5	0.0
HARIBO*								
Build a Burger, Haribo*	1oz/28g	96	0.1	344	6.6	79.0	0.2	0.3
Chamallows, Haribo*	1oz/28g	92	0.0	330	2.0	80.0	0.0	0.0
Cola Bottles, Fizzy, Haribo*	1 Med Pack/175g	595	0.4	340	6.3	78.3	0.2	0.3
Cola Bottles, Haribo*	1 Sm Pack/16g	56	0.0	348	7.7	78.9	0.2	0.3
Dinosaurs, Haribo*	1oz/28g	95	0.1	340	6.3	78.3	0.2	0.5

H

	Measure INFO/WEIGHT	per Measure KCAL	FAT	Nutrition Values per 100g / 100ml KCAL	PROT	CARB	FAT	FIBRE
HARIBO*								
Dolly Mixtures, Haribo*	1 Pack/175g	719	8.4	411	1.8	90.2	4.8	0.2
Fantasy Mix, Haribo*	1 Sm Pack/100g	344	0.2	344	6.6	79.0	0.2	0.3
Fried Eggs/eggstras, Haribo*	1oz/28g	96	0.1	344	6.6	79.0	0.2	0.0
Gold Bears, Haribo*	1 Pack/100g	348	0.2	348	7.7	78.9	0.2	0.3
Horror Mix, Haribo*	1 Sm Pack/100g	344	0.2	344	6.6	79.0	0.2	0.3
Jelly Babies, Haribo*	1oz/28g	97	0.1	348	4.5	82.1	0.2	0.5
Jelly Beans, Haribo*	1 Pack/100g	379	0.2	379	0.6	93.8	0.2	0.1
Kiddies Super Mix, Haribo*	1 Pack/100g	344	0.2	344	6.6	79.0	0.2	0.3
Liquorice Cream Rock, Haribo*	1oz/28g	107	1.5	382	2.3	81.2	5.3	0.3
Liquorice Favourite, Haribo*	1oz/28g	100	0.8	357	2.8	78.8	3.0	2.3
Magic Mix, Haribo*	1oz/28g	102	0.5	366	5.4	82.0	1.9	0.3
Maoam Stripes, Haribo*	1 Chew/7g	27	0.4	384	1.2	81.7	6.1	0.3
Mega Roulette, Haribo*	1oz/28g	97	0.1	348	7.7	78.9	0.2	0.3
Mega Roulette Sour, Haribo*	1oz/28g	95	0.1	340	6.3	78.3	0.2	0.5
Micro Mix, Haribo*	1oz/28g	106	0.7	379	4.7	84.5	2.5	0.4
Milky Mix, Haribo*	1 Pack/175g	607	0.4	347	7.1	79.6	0.2	0.4
Mint Imperials, Haribo*	1 Pack/175g	695	0.9	397	0.4	98.8	0.5	0.1
Peaches, Haribo*	1oz/28g	98	0.0	350	4.3	82.1	0.0	0.0
Pontefract Cakes, Haribo*	1 Pack/200g	612	2.6	306	5.3	68.2	1.3	5.6
Shrimps, Haribo*	1oz/28g	99	0.1	352	6.1	81.5	0.2	0.1
Starmix, Haribo*	1 Pack/100g	344	0.2	344	6.6	79.0	0.2	0.3
Tangfastics, Haribo*	1 Pack/100g	359	2.3	359	6.3	78.3	2.3	0.5
Tropifruit, Haribo*	1oz/28g	97	0.1	348	4.5	82.1	0.2	0.5
HARISSA								
Moroccan Style, Al'fez*	1 Tsp/10g	19	1.1	190	4.0	18.2	11.2	3.4
HASH								
Barbecue Beef, COU, M & S*	1 Pack/400g	360	1.6	90	7.0	14.0	0.4	1.4
Chicken Salsa, HE, Tesco*	1 Pack/350g	291	9.5	83	4.1	10.6	2.7	1.1
Corned Beef, Apetito*	1 Pack/380g	423	23.6	111	3.8	10.3	6.2	1.3
Corned Beef, Asda*	1 Pack/400g	416	14.4	104	6.0	12.0	3.6	1.1
Corned Beef, Basics, Sainsbury's*	1 Pack/300g	369	10.5	123	5.3	17.6	3.5	3.0
Corned Beef, Chilled, Co-Op*	1 Pack/300g	345	18.0	115	9.0	5.0	6.0	1.0
Corned Beef, Frozen, Tesco*	1 Serving/400g	348	10.4	87	5.7	10.3	2.6	0.7
Corned Beef, M & S*	½ Pack/320.8g	385	20.2	120	8.1	7.4	6.3	1.3
Corned Beef, Somerfield*	1 Pack/300g	324	16.5	108	6.2	8.5	5.5	1.6
Corned Beef, Tesco*	1 Serving/400g	416	10.4	104	5.3	14.8	2.6	1.7
Corned Beef, Value, Tesco*	1 Pack/300g	339	12.6	113	6.7	12.2	4.2	0.9
Farmhouse, HE, Tesco*	1 Serving/300g	264	8.1	88	2.2	13.6	2.7	1.1
Vegetable & Lentil, Asda*	1 Pack/289g	254	6.1	88	3.2	14.0	2.1	0.0
HASH BROWNS								
Aldi*	1 Serving/41g	61	2.9	146	1.7	19.3	6.9	1.8
Birds Eye*	1 Serving/63g	126	7.3	200	2.0	21.9	11.6	1.6
Farmfoods*	1oz/28g	35	1.3	124	2.1	18.2	4.7	2.1
Oven Baked, Weighed Cooked, McCain*	2 Pieces/75g	161	8.6	214	2.1	25.7	11.4	2.2
Oven Baked, Weighed Frozen, McCain*	1 Hash Brown/40g	75	4.1	187	1.7	21.8	10.3	2.1
Potato, Iceland*	1 Hash Brown/33g	75	4.0	227	2.2	27.1	12.2	2.6
Ross*	1 Hash Brown/46g	84	4.0	183	2.0	23.9	8.7	2.0
Tesco*	1oz/28g	43	2.0	154	2.4	20.0	7.2	1.7
HAZELNUTS								
Whole, Average	10 Whole/10g	66	6.4	655	15.4	5.8	63.5	6.5
HEART								
Ox, Raw	1oz/28g	29	1.0	104	18.2	0.0	3.5	0.0
Ox, Stewed	1oz/28g	44	1.4	157	27.8	0.0	5.1	0.0

H

	Measure INFO/WEIGHT	per Measure		Nutrition Values per 100g / 100ml				
		KCAL	FAT	KCAL	PROT	CARB	FAT	FIBRE
HEART								
Pig, Raw	1oz/28g	27	0.9	97	17.1	0.0	3.2	0.0
Pig, Stewed	1oz/28g	45	1.9	162	25.1	0.0	6.8	0.0
HERMESETAS								
Powdered, Hermes*	1 Tsp/0.78	3	0.0	387	1.0	96.8	0.0	0.0
The Classic Sweetener, Hermes*	1 Tablet/0.5g	0	0.0	294	14.2	59.3	0.0	0.0
HEROES								
Dairy Milk, Whole Nut, Cadbury*	1 Chocolate/11g	60	3.9	545	9.1	48.2	35.2	0.0
Fudge, Cadbury*	1 Sweet/10g	44	1.5	435	2.5	72.7	14.9	0.0
HERRING								
Canned, in Tomato Sauce, Average	1oz/28g	57	4.3	204	11.9	4.1	15.5	0.1
Dried, Salted, Average	1oz/28g	47	2.1	168	25.3	0.0	7.4	0.0
Fillets, in Mustard & Dill Sauce, John West*	1 Can/190g	426	34.2	224	11.7	3.7	18.0	0.1
Fillets, in Olive Oil, Succulent, Princes*	1 Serving/50g	108	7.5	215	20.0	0.0	15.0	0.0
Fillets, Raw, Average	1 Herring/100g	185	12.6	185	18.4	0.0	12.6	0.0
Grilled, Average	1oz/28g	51	3.1	181	20.1	0.0	11.2	0.0
in Horseradish Sauce, John West*	1oz/28g	64	5.0	230	13.0	4.0	18.0	0.0
Oatmeal Breaded, Fried in Vegetable Oil, Average	1oz/28g	66	4.2	234	23.1	1.5	15.1	0.1
Pickled, in Mustard Sauce, Abba*	1 Serving/57.5g	150	10.9	260	7.0	16.0	19.0	0.0
Rollmop, with Onion, Asda*	1 Rollmop/65g	89	3.1	137	13.2	10.3	4.8	0.8
Rollmops, Tesco*	1 Rollmop/65g	111	5.5	170	12.0	10.4	8.4	0.4
Smoked, Pepper, in Oil, Glyngøre*	1 Can/130g	338	24.7	260	21.0	0.0	19.0	0.0
HIGH LIGHTS								
Caffe Latte, Made Up, Cadbury*	1 Serving/200g	40	1.4	20	1.0	2.5	0.7	0.0
Choc Mint, Made Up, Cadbury*	1 Serving/200ml	40	1.4	20	1.0	2.5	0.7	0.3
Chocolate, Dairy Fudge, Dry Weight, Cadbury*	1 Serving/11g	40	1.1	363	17.0	50.0	10.0	0.0
Chocolate Orange, Made Up, Cadbury*	1 Serving/200ml	40	1.4	20	1.0	2.3	0.7	0.3
Dark Chocolate, Cadbury*	1 Sachet/11g	35	0.9	315	23.1	37.3	8.1	0.0
Dark Chocolate, Made Up, Cadbury*	1 Serving/200ml	35	0.9	18	1.3	2.1	0.5	0.0
Espresso, Made Up, Cadbury*	1 Serving/200ml	35	0.9	18	1.3	2.0	0.5	0.0
Instant, Dry Weight, Cadbury*	1 Sachet/10g	37	1.3	365	17.1	44.7	13.0	4.6
Instant, Made Up, Cadbury*	1 Cup/200ml	40	1.4	20	1.0	2.5	0.7	0.3
Mint, Cadbury*	1 Serving/200ml	40	1.4	20	1.0	2.5	0.7	0.0
Toffee Flavour, Made Up, Cadbury*	1 Serving/200ml	40	1.4	20	1.0	2.6	0.7	0.0
HOKI								
Grilled	1oz/28g	34	0.8	121	24.1	0.0	2.7	0.0
in Breadcrumbs, Average	1 Piece/156g	298	13.8	191	14.5	13.9	8.9	1.2
Raw	1oz/28g	24	0.5	85	16.9	0.0	1.9	0.0
Steaks, in Batter, Crispy, Birds Eye*	1 Steak/123.1g	320	17.1	260	12.4	21.3	13.9	0.8
HONEY								
Acacia, Tesco*	1 Tsp/4g	12	0.0	307	0.4	76.4	0.0	0.0
Acacia Blossom, Sainsbury's*	1 Serving/24g	81	0.0	339	0.1	84.7	0.1	0.3
Australian Eucalyptus, Finest, Tesco*	1 Tsp/4g	12	0.0	307	0.4	76.4	0.0	0.0
Canadian Clover, TTD, Sainsbury's*	1 Tsp/5g	17	0.0	339	0.1	84.7	0.1	0.3
Florida Orange, Extra Special, Asda*	1 Tbsp/15g	50	0.0	334	0.5	83.0	0.0	0.0
Pure, Clear, Average	1 Tbsp/20g	63	0.0	314	0.4	79.1	0.0	0.0
Pure, Set, Average	1 Tbsp/20g	62	0.0	312	0.4	77.6	0.0	0.0
Spanish Orange Blossom, Sainsbury's*	1 Tbsp/15g	51	0.0	339	0.1	84.7	0.0	0.3
Tasmanian Leatherwood, TTD, Sainsbury's*	1 Serving/6g	20	0.0	339	0.1	84.7	0.1	0.3
HORLICKS								
Malted Drink, Light, Dry Weight, Horlicks*	1 Serving/32g	116	1.2	364	14.8	72.2	3.8	1.9
Malted Drink, Light, Made Up with Water, Horlicks*	1 Mug/200ml	116	1.2	58	2.4	11.6	0.6	0.3
Powder, Made Up with Semi-Skimmed Milk	1 Mug/227ml	184	4.3	81	4.3	12.9	1.9	0.0
Powder, Made Up with Skimmed Milk	1 Mug/227ml	159	1.1	70	4.3	12.9	0.5	0.0

H

	Measure INFO/WEIGHT	per Measure KCAL	FAT	Nutrition Values per 100g / 100ml KCAL	PROT	CARB	FAT	FIBRE
HORLICKS								
Powder, Made Up with Whole Milk	1 Mug/227ml	225	8.9	99	4.2	12.7	3.9	0.0
HORSE								
Meat, Raw, Average	1 Serving/110g	146	5.1	133	21.4	0.0	4.6	0.0
HORSERADISH								
Prepared, Average	1 Tsp/5g	3	0.0	62	4.5	11.0	0.3	6.2
HOT CHOCOLATE								
Balanced Lifestyle, Camelot*	1 Sachet/11g	40	1.6	363	18.5	40.6	14.1	0.5
Chocolate Break, Dry, Tesco*	1 Serving/21g	110	6.0	524	7.9	58.9	28.5	1.7
Cocoa, Lidl*	1 Serving/20g	77	1.2	386	6.1	74.1	6.2	0.0
Drink, Dry Organic, Green & Black's*	1 Tsp/3.5g	13	0.3	374	9.1	63.5	9.3	0.1
Dry Weight, Tassimo, Suchard*	1 Cup/27g	88	2.4	325	3.2	58.0	8.9	2.6
Galaxy, Mars*	1 Sachet/28g	115	3.4	411	7.0	68.7	12.1	0.0
Instant, Tesco*	1 Serving/32g	155	10.3	485	10.5	38.1	32.3	5.0
Instant Break, Cadbury*	1 Sachet/28g	119	3.9	425	10.9	64.2	14.0	0.0
Organic, Clipper*	1 Packet/28g	99	0.6	354	15.5	68.6	2.0	2.4
Value, Tesco*	1 Serving/32g	132	3.9	414	8.0	68.3	12.1	0.7
HOT DOG								
American Style, Hunters*	1 Hot Dog/22.9g	39	2.7	170	10.7	5.1	11.9	1.7
Feasters, Eat Well, M & S*	1 Hot Dog/140g	326	11.3	233	11.0	29.1	8.1	1.6
Sausage, American Style, Average	1 Sausage/75g	180	14.3	241	11.6	6.2	19.0	0.0
Sausage, Average	1 Sausage/23g	40	3.0	175	10.8	4.3	12.8	0.3
HOT DOG VEGETARIAN								
Meat Free, Sainsbury's*	1 Sausage/30.1g	71	4.5	237	18.0	7.6	15.0	1.0
Tesco*	1 Sausage/30g	66	4.5	220	18.0	2.7	15.0	2.0
HOT POT								
Beef, Apetito*	1 Pack/340g	303	10.4	89	5.1	10.3	3.1	1.3
Beef, Minced, Sainsbury's*	1 Pack/450g	464	22.1	103	5.3	9.5	4.9	2.2
Beef, Ross*	1 Pack/322g	254	11.3	79	2.5	9.4	3.5	0.4
Beef, Weight Watchers*	1 Pack/320g	210	6.7	66	3.6	8.1	2.1	1.3
Chicken, Co-Op*	1 Pack/340g	289	10.2	85	6.0	9.0	3.0	0.7
Chicken, From Heinz, Weight Watchers*	1 Pack/320g	271	8.8	85	4.7	10.3	2.8	0.6
Chicken, GFY, Asda*	1 Serving/400g	292	5.6	73	5.0	10.0	1.4	0.8
Chicken, Good Choice, Iceland*	1 Pack/400g	276	5.2	69	5.0	9.3	1.3	1.0
Chicken, HL, Tesco*	1 Pack/450g	315	7.3	70	4.0	9.6	1.6	1.2
Chicken, Safeway*	1 Pack/400g	292	6.0	73	4.2	10.7	1.5	1.6
Chicken, Sainsbury's*	1 Pack/400g	340	11.0	85	5.2	9.9	2.8	1.3
Chicken, Traditional, Pro Cuisine*	1 Pack/400g	208	3.6	52	5.8	5.2	0.9	0.0
Chicken & Cider, Ready Meals, Waitrose*	1 Pack/400g	500	20.4	125	6.8	12.9	5.1	1.1
Chicken & Mushroom, HL, Tesco*	1 Serving/450g	369	6.8	82	6.3	11.8	1.5	0.5
Lamb, Heinz*	1 Pack/340g	337	10.5	99	4.9	12.7	3.1	1.7
Lamb & Vegetable, Asda*	1 Pot/500g	240	2.0	48	4.0	7.0	0.4	0.0
Lancashire, Asda*	1 Pack/401g	269	5.2	67	3.8	10.0	1.3	0.9
Lancashire, Hollands*	1 Serving/250g	340	11.8	136	3.6	19.6	4.7	0.0
Lancashire, M & S*	1 Pack/454g	431	15.0	95	10.1	6.7	3.3	1.0
Lancashire, Sainsbury's*	½ Pack/225g	221	8.8	98	6.1	9.5	3.9	1.0
Lancashire, Tesco*	½ Pack/225g	205	7.0	91	6.0	9.7	3.1	0.5
Liver & Bacon, Tesco*	1 Pack/550g	693	31.4	126	6.4	12.3	5.7	1.5
Minced Beef, Asda*	1 Pack/375g	409	17.3	109	7.0	10.0	4.6	1.7
Minced Beef, Frozen, Tesco*	1 Pack/450g	338	11.3	75	4.0	9.1	2.5	1.4
Minced Beef, Iceland*	1 Pack/500g	505	15.5	101	5.5	12.7	3.1	1.3
Minced Beef, M & S*	1 Pack/220g	240	13.2	109	7.4	6.5	6.0	1.2
Minced Beef, Mini Classic, Tesco*	1 Pack/300g	232	4.5	77	3.4	12.6	1.5	1.4
Minced Beef, SmartPrice, Asda*	1 Pack/300g	199	3.9	66	3.7	10.0	1.3	0.4

H

	Measure INFO/WEIGHT	per Measure KCAL	FAT	Nutrition Values per 100g / 100ml KCAL	PROT	CARB	FAT	FIBRE
HOT POT								
Minced Beef & Vegetable, COU, M & S*	1 Pack/400g	380	6.8	95	10.3	9.0	1.7	2.4
Roast, Vegetable, with Gravy, Hometown Buffet*	1 Serving/113g	50	0.5	44	0.9	11.5	0.4	1.8
Sausage, Aunt Bessie's*	¼ Pack/200g	212	9.2	106	3.6	12.6	4.6	1.9
Sausage, SmartPrice, Asda*	1 Pack/300g	239	7.0	80	3.7	11.0	2.3	0.4
Sausage, with Baked Beans, Heinz*	1 Can/340g	354	10.9	104	4.6	14.3	3.2	2.4
Vegetable, Tesco*	1 Serving/450g	432	22.1	96	1.7	11.2	4.9	3.5
Vegetable, Vegetable Recipes, Ross*	1 Pack/300g	159	5.4	53	1.5	9.4	1.8	1.6
Vegetable, Weight Watchers*	1 Pack/335g	228	6.4	68	2.6	9.9	1.9	1.5
HOUMOUS								
30% Less Fat, Asda*	1oz/28g	73	5.3	259	9.0	13.0	19.0	3.8
Caramelised Onion, Tesco*	¼ Pack/50g	125	9.7	250	5.5	13.0	19.4	4.2
Co-Op*	¼ Pack/50g	168	14.0	335	8.0	13.0	28.0	3.0
Feta, Fresh, Sainsbury's*	1 Serving/100g	292	27.4	292	8.0	3.5	27.4	6.7
Fresh, Waitrose*	¼ Pot/74.9g	219	19.8	292	7.2	6.3	26.4	7.6
Garlic & Pesto, Asda*	1 Serving/34g	107	8.8	314	8.0	12.0	26.0	0.0
GFY, Asda*	1 Serving/50g	136	10.0	272	9.0	14.0	20.0	3.8
Greek, Somerfield*	1 Serving/50g	152	13.4	304	7.6	8.2	26.8	5.5
Lemon & Coriander, Sainsbury's*	½ Pot/85g	247	21.3	291	7.0	9.1	25.1	6.0
Lemon & Coriander, Tesco*	1 Serving/50g	170	14.5	340	7.0	12.7	29.0	2.1
Light, Morrisons*	½ Pack/85g	200	15.3	235	7.4	10.9	18.0	0.0
Mediterranean Deli, M & S*	¼ Pack/70g	203	17.7	290	7.8	8.0	25.3	6.5
Mixed Olive, Sainsbury's*	¼ Pot/50g	134	11.6	268	6.7	8.4	23.1	7.7
Morrisons*	2 Tbsp/50g	188	17.2	375	8.7	7.8	34.3	5.2
Organic, M & S*	¼ Pack/25g	83	7.4	330	6.9	9.1	29.7	3.3
Organic, Sainsbury's*	¼ Pot/43g	139	12.1	326	6.8	10.7	28.4	3.5
Organic, Tesco*	¼ Tub/42g	134	11.4	320	6.5	12.3	27.2	2.4
Reduced Fat, BGTY, Sainsbury's*	1 Serving/50g	77	4.5	153	6.6	11.7	8.9	6.1
Reduced Fat, Budgens*	1 Serving/50g	131	9.7	261	9.1	12.6	19.3	3.3
Reduced Fat, Co-Op*	1 Tbsp/25g	63	4.8	250	8.0	12.0	19.0	3.0
Reduced Fat, Eat Smart, Morrisons*	1 Mini Pot/70g	172	12.4	246	7.9	13.8	17.7	2.7
Reduced Fat, Moroccan Style, Topped, M & S*	1 Serving/100g	220	15.3	220	6.6	13.2	15.3	9.2
Reduced Fat, Morrisons*	1 Serving/50g	123	8.9	246	7.9	13.8	17.7	2.7
Reduced Fat, Somerfield*	½ Pack/100g	218	14.7	218	7.7	13.7	14.7	4.8
Reduced Fat, Tesco*	¼ Sm Pot/50g	121	8.4	241	9.2	13.3	16.8	3.6
Reduced Fat, Waitrose*	1 Pot/60g	130	8.5	216	7.4	14.7	14.2	5.8
Roasted Aubergine, M & S*	½ Pot/85g	132	10.3	155	4.9	6.9	12.1	5.1
Roasted Red Pepper, 50% Less Fat, Tesco*	½ Pot/85g	156	10.5	184	7.3	10.9	12.4	9.5
Roasted Red Pepper, BGTY, Sainsbury's*	¼ Tub/50g	85	4.8	169	6.5	14.4	9.5	6.2
Roasted Red Pepper, Sainsbury's*	½ Pot/85.2g	252	22.6	297	7.0	7.4	26.6	3.5
Roasted Red Pepper, Somerfield*	½ Pot/85g	244	21.3	287	7.1	8.1	25.1	5.2
Roasted Red Pepper, Tesco*	1 Serving/75g	255	22.3	340	7.1	11.1	29.7	2.4
Roasted Vegetable, Fresh, Sainsbury's*	¼ Pot/50.2g	144	13.6	287	5.9	4.9	27.1	7.8
Spicy Red Pepper, M & S*	1 Pack/283g	580	43.3	205	7.0	9.9	15.3	6.0
Sun Dried Tomato, Chunky, Tesco*	½ Pot/95g	322	27.0	339	6.7	14.0	28.4	3.3
Three Bean, Reduced Fat, BGTY, Sainsbury's*	¼ Tub/50g	92	6.0	183	7.3	11.4	12.0	6.0
with Extra Virgin Olive Oil, Tesco*	1 Pack/190g	564	46.2	297	7.9	11.7	24.3	5.1
Zorba Delicacies Ltd*	1 Serving/50g	157	13.3	313	7.6	10.7	26.6	3.0
HULA HOOPS								
Bacon & Ketchup Flavour, KP Snacks*	1 Bag/27g	140	8.3	517	3.4	56.3	30.9	2.0
BBQ Beef, 55% Less Saturated Fat, KP Snacks*	1 Pack/34g	174	9.7	512	3.5	60.6	28.5	1.8
Cheese & Onion 55% Less Fat, KP Snacks*	1 Bag/34g	175	9.7	515	3.6	61.0	28.5	1.9
Minis, Original, KP Snacks*	1 Tub/140g	752	48.7	537	3.0	52.9	34.8	1.7
Multigrain, KP Snacks*	1 Pack/23g	113	5.9	491	5.7	60.0	25.7	4.4

H

	Measure INFO/WEIGHT	per Measure		Nutrition Values per 100g / 100ml				
		KCAL	FAT	KCAL	PROT	CARB	FAT	FIBRE
HULA HOOPS								
Original, 55% Less Saturated Fat, KP Snacks*	1 Bag/34g	175	9.7	515	3.2	61.6	28.4	1.8
Original, KP Snacks*	1 Bag/25g	129	7.1	514	3.2	61.5	28.4	1.8
Roast Chicken, 50% Less Fat, KP Snacks*	1 Bag/25g	129	7.1	514	3.4	61.0	28.5	1.7
Salt & Vinegar, 50% Less Fat, KP Snacks*	1 Pack/25g	128	7.1	513	3.2	61.0	28.4	1.7
Sizzling Bacon, KP Snacks*	1 Bag/34g	175	9.7	514	3.4	60.9	28.5	1.7
HUNGER BREAKS								
The Full Monty, Crosse & Blackwell*	1 Can/410g	332	15.6	81	5.6	7.2	3.8	1.3

H

ICE CREAM

INFO/WEIGHT	Measure KCAL	FAT	Nutrition Values per 100g / 100ml KCAL	PROT	CARB	FAT	FIBRE
After Eight, Nestle*	1 Serving/55.1g	114	5.2	207	3.6	27.1	9.4	0.3
Almond Indulgence, Sainsbury's*	1 Serving/120g	286	18.8	238	2.8	21.4	15.7	0.6
Baileys, Haagen-Dazs*	1 Tub/500ml	1125	73.6	225	3.8	19.2	14.7	0.0
Banana, Thorntons*	1oz/28g	63	3.5	225	4.0	23.8	12.6	0.0
Banoffee, Haagen-Dazs*	1 Serving/120ml	274	15.6	228	4.0	23.0	13.0	0.0
Belgian Chocolate, Haagen-Dazs*	1oz/28g	89	5.8	318	4.6	28.4	20.7	0.0
Berry Nice, Ben & Jerry's*	1 Serving/100g	200	11.0	200	0.0	23.0	11.0	0.0
Bounty, Mars*	1oz/28g	77	5.1	274	3.3	23.8	18.3	0.0
Bourbon Biscuit, Asda*	1 Dessert/37g	120	4.5	324	5.9	48.6	12.2	1.6
Cappuccino, Thorntons*	1oz/28g	61	3.6	218	4.4	20.7	12.9	0.0
Caramel, Carte d'Or*	2 Boules/50g	106	4.4	212	2.6	30.8	8.7	0.0
Caramel Chew Chew, Ben & Jerry's*	1 Serving/100g	270	15.0	270	4.0	28.0	15.0	0.0
Caramel Craze, Organic, Tesco*	1 Serving/100g	253	15.3	253	3.3	25.5	15.3	0.0
Caramella, Tesco*	1 Scoop/60g	141	6.4	235	2.6	32.0	10.7	1.1
Cheeky Choc, Brownie, Skinny Cow*	1 Tub/500ml	590	5.5	118	3.0	23.9	1.1	4.1
Cherry Garcia, Ben & Jerry's*	1 Serving/100g	250	15.0	250	3.0	26.0	15.0	0.0
Cherrylicious, Tesco*	1 Serving/57.7g	122	3.2	210	2.8	37.0	5.6	0.2
Choc Chip, Cookie Dough, Haagen-Dazs*	1oz/28g	74	4.7	266	3.8	24.9	16.9	0.0
Choc Chip, Haagen-Dazs*	1oz/28g	80	5.2	286	4.7	24.8	18.7	0.0
Choc Chip Cookie Dough, Ben & Jerry's*	1 Serving/100g	230	14.0	230	3.0	23.0	14.0	0.0
Chocolate, COU, M & S*	1 Serving/140g	231	4.1	165	3.9	35.0	2.9	0.8
Chocolate, Dairy, The Best, Safeway*	1 Serving/82.4g	243	15.0	296	4.6	28.1	18.3	2.0
Chocolate, Haagen-Dazs*	1 Serving/120ml	269	18.0	224	4.0	19.0	15.0	0.0
Chocolate, Organic, Green & Black's*	1 Serving/125g	310	17.6	248	5.0	25.3	14.1	1.1
Chocolate, Rich, Organic, Sainsbury's*	1 Serving/100g	213	11.7	213	4.4	22.6	11.7	1.2
Chocolate, Soft Scoop, Asda*	1 Scoop/47g	84	3.8	179	3.7	23.0	8.0	0.0
Chocolate, Soft Scoop, Tesco*	1 Serving/50g	93	4.1	186	3.2	25.1	8.1	0.3
Chocolate, Swirl Pot, Skinny Cow*	1 Pot/100ml	98	0.6	98	2.9	20.2	0.6	2.7
Chocolate, Thorntons*	1oz/28g	67	3.6	238	4.6	25.1	12.9	0.0
Chocolate, Triple, Sainsbury's*	1 Serving/100g	176	8.3	176	3.5	21.7	8.3	0.5
Chocolate, Weight Watchers*	1 Serving/100ml	140	1.2	140	4.3	28.7	1.2	0.0
Chocolate & Caramel, Stick, Slim Fast*	1 Ice Cream/55g	87	2.3	159	4.1	26.3	4.2	2.2
Chocolate & Orange, Organic, Green & Black's*	1 Serving/100g	248	14.1	248	5.0	25.3	14.1	0.1
Chocolate Chip, Baskin Robbins*	1 Serving/75g	170	10.0	227	4.0	24.0	13.3	0.0
Chocolate Flavour, Soft Scoop, Sainsbury's*	1 Serving/70g	122	5.3	174	3.1	23.6	7.5	0.3
Chocolate Fudge Swirl, Haagen-Dazs*	1oz/28g	77	4.8	276	4.6	25.6	17.2	0.0
Chocolate Honeycomb, Co-Op*	¼ Pot/81g	186	10.5	230	4.0	26.0	13.0	0.3
Chocolate Honeycomb, COU, M & S*	1 Serving/100ml	150	2.6	150	3.5	31.5	2.6	0.7
Chocolate Midnight Cookies, Haagen-Dazs*	1oz/28g	81	4.8	289	4.9	28.7	17.2	0.0
Chocolate Orange, Deliciously Dairy, Co-Op*	1oz/28g	55	2.0	195	4.0	29.0	7.0	0.8
Chocolate Ripple, PB, Waitrose*	1 Serving/125ml	205	3.1	164	4.8	30.5	2.5	4.1
Chocolate Trio, Thorntons*	1 Bar/100g	310	20.6	310	3.3	28.0	20.6	1.8
Chocolatino, Tesco*	1 Serving/56g	115	3.8	205	3.4	31.4	6.8	1.8
Chunky Chocolate, Giant, M & S*	1 Lolly/89.6g	302	20.7	335	4.0	28.0	23.0	2.3
Chunky Monkey, Ben & Jerry's*	1 Serving/100g	280	17.0	280	4.0	28.0	17.0	1.0
Coconut, Carte d'Or*	1 Serving/100ml	125	7.1	125	1.8	14.0	7.1	0.5
Coffee, Finest, Tesco*	¼ Pot/93g	236	14.9	254	4.9	22.5	16.0	0.0
Coffee, Haagen-Dazs*	1 Serving/120ml	271	18.4	226	4.1	17.9	15.3	0.0
Coffee, Waitrose*	1 Serving/180ml	421	23.6	234	3.6	25.4	13.1	0.0
Completely Mintal, Skinny Cow*	1 Serving/100ml	142	1.3	142	4.1	28.4	1.3	3.4
Cookies & Cream, Haagen-Dazs*	1 Serving/102g	270	17.0	265	4.9	22.5	16.7	0.0
Cornish, Asda*	1 Serving/100ml	100	5.0	100	1.8	12.0	5.0	0.0
Cornish, Full Fat, Asda*	1 Serving/100g	204	11.6	204	3.5	21.4	11.6	0.1

ICE CREAM

Measure INFO/WEIGHT		per Measure		Nutrition Values per 100g / 100ml				
		KCAL	FAT	KCAL	PROT	CARB	FAT	FIBRE
Cornish Clotted, M & S*	1 Pot/90g	207	13.1	230	2.8	21.8	14.5	0.1
Cornish Dairy, Waitrose*	1 Serving/125ml	161	8.5	129	2.3	14.6	6.8	0.0
Crema Di Mascarpone, Carte d'Or*	1 Serving/100g	207	8.9	207	2.8	29.0	8.9	0.0
Crunchie, Blast, Cadbury*	1 Lolly/100ml	225	13.2	225	2.9	23.5	13.2	0.1
Dairy, Flavoured	1oz/28g	50	2.2	179	3.5	24.7	8.0	0.0
Dairy Cornish, Tesco*	1 Serving/49g	112	6.0	228	3.2	24.7	12.3	0.1
Dairy Milk, Orange, Cadbury*	1 Serving/120ml	259	13.9	216	3.5	26.0	11.6	0.0
Date & Almond Cream, Haagen-Dazs*	1 Serving/120ml	254	15.6	212	5.0	19.0	13.0	0.0
Demon Chocolate, M & S*	1 Serving/79g	208	8.8	263	3.7	37.1	11.1	0.6
Double Chocolate, Nestle*	1 Serving/77.5g	250	14.4	320	4.8	33.7	18.4	0.0
Dream, Cadbury*	1 Bar/120ml	264	14.3	220	3.6	26.0	11.9	0.0
Dulce De Leche, Bar, Haagen-Dazs*	1 Bar/105g	370	24.0	352	3.8	32.3	22.9	0.0
Galaxy, Mars*	1 Bar/60ml	203	13.4	339	4.7	29.7	22.4	0.0
Get Fruit, Tropical, Solero*	1 Serving/125ml	163	5.5	130	1.6	20.6	4.4	0.4
Greek Yoghurt & Honey, Carte d'Or*	1 Serving/55g	114	4.8	207	2.7	29.0	8.8	0.0
Heavenly Vanilla, Cadbury*	1 Serving/250ml	355	23.3	142	2.5	12.8	9.3	0.0
Honey, I'm Home, Ben & Jerry's*	1 Serving/100g	260	15.0	260	0.0	28.0	15.0	0.0
Honeycomb Harvest, Mackies*	1 Serving/100g	209	10.0	209	4.0	25.0	10.0	0.0
Knickerbocker Glory	1oz/28g	31	1.4	112	1.5	16.4	5.0	0.2
Lavazza, Carte d'Or*	1 Serving/55g	120	5.4	218	3.5	29.0	9.9	0.0
Lemon, Haagen-Dazs*	1 Serving/120ml	144	0.2	120	0.3	29.3	0.2	0.0
Lemon Pie, Haagen-Dazs*	1oz/28g	73	4.6	262	3.9	24.5	16.3	0.0
Less Than 5% Fat, Asda*	2 Scoops/80g	111	3.6	139	2.7	22.0	4.5	0.0
Luscious Mint Choc Chip, Morrisons*	1 Serving/50g	99	5.3	198	2.9	23.1	10.5	0.7
Macadamia Nut, Baskin Robbins*	1 Serving/113g	270	18.0	239	4.4	22.1	15.9	0.9
Madly Deeply, Skinny Cow*	1 Serving/100g	149	2.2	149	4.2	28.3	2.2	3.4
Magic Maple, M & S*	1 Ice Cream/93g	259	11.4	278	2.9	39.0	12.3	0.6
Magnum Moments, Wall's*	1 Serving/18ml	58	3.7	323	4.0	30.0	20.8	0.0
Mango, 98% Fat Free, Bulla*	1 Serving/70g	94	1.1	134	4.2	25.4	1.6	0.0
Maple & Walnut, American, Sainsbury's*	1/8 Pot/68g	121	4.9	179	3.1	25.6	7.2	0.2
Maple Brazil, Thorntons*	1oz/28g	66	3.8	236	4.1	24.4	13.6	0.0
Mint, Majestic Luxury, Iceland*	1 Serving/79.8g	270	14.6	337	3.8	39.3	18.3	1.3
Mint, Thorntons*	1oz/28g	66	3.8	237	4.0	25.0	13.4	0.0
Mint & Chocolate, Sainsbury's*	1/8 Pot/71.4g	137	6.7	192	3.4	23.5	9.4	0.4
Mint Choc Chip Soft Scoop, Asda*	1 Serving/46g	86	4.1	187	2.9	24.0	9.0	0.3
Mint Chocolate Chip, Baskin Robbins*	1 Scoop/113g	270	16.0	239	4.4	24.8	14.2	0.9
Mint Crisp, Nestle*	1 Serving/75ml	232	16.4	309	2.9	25.5	21.9	0.9
Mint Crunch, Dairy Milk, Cadbury*	1 Serving/60ml	162	13.3	270	3.0	29.0	22.2	0.0
Mocha Coffee Indulgence, Sainsbury's*	1/4 Pot/82g	178	10.6	217	3.2	22.1	12.9	0.1
Neapolitan, Brick, Tesco*	1 Serving/50g	82	3.5	163	3.3	21.9	6.9	0.4
Neapolitan, Lidl*	1 Serving/48g	108	4.8	226	4.3	29.5	10.0	0.0
Neapolitan, Soft Scoop, Asda*	1 Scoop/47g	82	3.8	175	2.8	23.0	8.0	0.2
Neapolitan, Soft Scoop, M & S*	1/8 Tub/62.5g	100	4.6	160	2.7	21.3	7.4	0.3
Neapolitan, Soft Scoop, Sainsbury's*	1 Serving/75g	124	5.2	165	2.8	22.8	6.9	0.2
Neapolitan, Soft Scoop, Somerfield*	1 Serving/75g	125	5.5	166	2.8	22.6	7.3	0.3
Neopolitian, Soft Scoop, Tesco*	1 Serving/43g	70	3.0	163	3.3	21.9	6.9	0.4
Peach Melba, Soft Scoop, M & S*	1oz/28g	46	2.1	165	2.8	21.4	7.6	0.3
Phish Food, Ben & Jerry's*	1 Serving/100g	280	13.0	280	4.0	36.0	13.0	0.0
Pistachio, Haagen-Dazs*	1 Serving/120ml	276	18.8	230	4.4	17.7	15.7	0.0
Praline, Green & Black's*	1 Sm Pot/100g	191	10.8	191	3.5	20.0	10.8	0.9
Praline & Chocolate, Thorntons*	1oz/28g	87	6.4	309	4.6	21.3	22.9	0.6
Pralines & Cream, Haagen-Dazs*	1 Pot/500ml	1210	75.5	242	3.7	22.9	15.1	0.0
Raspberries, Clotted Cream, Waitrose*	1 Tub/500ml	790	39.5	158	2.9	18.9	7.9	0.1

ICE CREAM

INFO/WEIGHT	Measure	per Measure		Nutrition Values per 100g / 100ml				
		KCAL	FAT	KCAL	PROT	CARB	FAT	FIBRE
Raspberry, Haagen-Dazs*	1 Serving/120ml	127	0.2	106	0.2	25.9	0.2	0.0
Raspberry, Swirl Pot, Skinny Cow*	1 Pot/100ml	86	0.3	86	2.5	18.4	0.3	2.2
Raspberry Ripple, Dairy, Waitrose*	1 Serving/186ml	195	10.0	105	1.9	12.3	5.4	0.0
Raspberry Ripple, Soft Scoop, Asda*	1 Scoop/46g	75	2.8	164	2.5	25.0	6.0	0.0
Raspberry Ripple, Soft Scoop, Sainsbury's*	1 Serving/75g	128	5.3	170	2.6	24.2	7.0	0.3
Raspberry Ripple, Soft Scoop, Tesco*	2 Scoops/50g	79	3.1	157	2.5	23.0	6.1	0.2
Raspberry Ripple Brick, Tesco*	1 Serving/48g	71	2.9	148	2.6	20.8	6.0	0.2
Really Creamy Chocolate, Asda*	1 Serving/100g	227	11.0	227	4.1	28.0	11.0	0.4
Really Creamy Lemon Meringue, Asda*	1 Serving/100ml	100	5.0	100	1.8	12.0	5.0	0.1
Really Creamy Toffee, Asda*	1 Serving/120ml	146	6.0	122	1.8	17.5	5.0	0.1
Rocky Road, Sainsbury's*	1/8 Pot/67g	137	4.9	205	3.8	30.9	7.3	1.0
Rolo, Nestle*	½ Tub/500ml	1180	52.5	236	3.4	31.9	10.5	0.2
Rum & Raisin, Haagen-Dazs*	1 Serving/120ml	264	17.6	220	3.4	18.6	14.7	0.0
Screwball, Asda*	1 Screwball/60.1g	122	6.0	203	3.3	25.0	10.0	1.5
Screwball, Farmfoods*	1 Lolly/72ml	101	3.5	177	3.3	27.1	6.1	0.0
Screwball, Morrisons*	1 Screwball/100ml	133	6.3	133	2.0	17.0	6.3	0.0
Screwball, Safeway*	1 Serving/65g	129	6.3	198	3.1	24.5	9.7	0.6
Screwball, Tesco*	1 Screwball/61g	116	5.2	190	2.9	25.2	8.6	0.3
Smarties, Nestle*	1 Serving/50g	125	6.0	250	3.6	32.3	11.9	0.2
Spagnola, Carte d'Or*	1 Serving/100g	187	5.7	187	2.0	32.0	5.7	0.0
Stem Ginger with Belgian Chocolate, Waitrose*	1 Lolly/109.9g	255	14.4	232	2.9	25.5	13.1	1.7
Sticky Toffee, Cream O' Galloway*	1 Serving/30g	80	4.4	266	4.7	28.7	14.7	0.0
Strawberry, Get Fruit, Solero*	1 Serving/100ml	120	4.5	120	1.5	18.8	4.5	1.3
Strawberry, Haagen-Dazs*	1oz/28g	67	4.3	241	4.0	21.5	15.5	0.0
Strawberry, Soft Scoop, Tesco*	1 Serving/45.8g	78	3.4	170	2.8	23.1	7.4	0.1
Strawberry, Thorntons*	1oz/28g	52	2.6	185	3.2	22.5	9.3	0.1
Strawberry, Weight Watchers*	1 Pot/57g	81	2.2	142	2.5	23.4	3.9	0.2
Strawberry & Cream, Mivvi, Nestle*	1 Serving/60g	118	4.6	196	2.6	29.4	7.6	0.2
Strawberry & Cream, Organic, Sainsbury's*	1 Serving/100g	193	9.8	193	3.6	22.6	9.8	0.4
Strawberry Cheesecake, Co-Op*	1/6 Pot/86g	163	6.0	190	3.0	29.0	7.0	0.2
Strawberry Cheesecake, Haagen-Dazs*	1 Scoop/104g	260	15.0	250	3.9	26.0	14.4	0.0
Tiramisu, Haagen-Dazs*	1 Serving/120ml	303	19.6	253	3.8	22.7	16.3	0.0
Toffee, Somerfield*	1 Serving/75g	172	6.9	229	3.4	33.2	9.2	0.9
Toffee, Thorntons*	1oz/28g	61	3.2	218	4.1	24.5	11.6	0.0
Toffee & Vanilla, Sainsbury's*	1 Serving/71.2g	146	6.7	205	3.1	26.7	9.5	0.1
Toffee Creme, Haagen-Dazs*	1oz/28g	74	4.4	265	4.5	26.7	15.6	0.0
Toffee Fudge, Soft Scoop, Asda*	1 Serving/50g	93	3.5	185	2.6	28.0	7.0	0.0
Toffee Ripple, Tesco*	1 Serving/100g	173	7.2	173	2.7	24.4	7.2	0.1
Totally Toffee, Safeway*	1 Serving/100ml	136	5.1	136	1.3	21.1	5.1	0.1
Triple Chocolate, Carte d'Or*	1 Serving/58g	122	5.7	210	3.7	27.0	9.8	0.0
Vanilla, Carte d'Or*	1 Serving/50g	105	4.8	210	3.0	26.0	9.5	0.0
Vanilla, COU, M & S*	¼ Pot/79g	111	2.2	140	1.7	25.9	2.8	0.8
Vanilla, Dairy, Finest, Tesco*	1 Serving/92g	227	16.0	247	4.5	18.0	17.4	0.3
Vanilla, Dairy, Organic, Yeo Valley*	1 Serving/100g	206	11.2	206	4.9	21.3	11.2	0.0
Vanilla, Dairy, Safeway*	1 Serving/64.1g	125	6.4	195	3.5	22.5	10.0	0.1
Vanilla, Haagen-Dazs*	1oz/28g	70	4.8	250	4.5	19.7	17.1	0.0
Vanilla, Light, Carte d'Or*	1 Serving/100g	136	4.4	136	2.4	22.0	4.4	4.0
Vanilla, Low Fat, Weight Watchers*	1 Scoop/125ml	75	2.1	60	1.1	9.7	1.7	0.1
Vanilla, Mackies*	1 Serving/100g	193	11.0	193	4.0	18.0	11.0	0.0
Vanilla, Non-Dairy, Average	1 Portion/60g	107	5.2	178	3.2	23.1	8.7	0.0
Vanilla, Organic, Green & Black's*	1 Sm Tub/100ml	220	13.4	220	4.7	20.1	13.4	0.1
Vanilla, Organic, Sainsbury's*	1 Serving/85g	176	10.2	207	4.3	20.5	12.0	0.1
Vanilla, Organic, Tesco*	1 Serving/100g	237	17.2	237	3.7	16.8	17.2	0.0

	Measure INFO/WEIGHT	KCAL	FAT	KCAL	PROT	CARB	FAT	FIBRE
ICE CREAM								
Vanilla, Organic, Waitrose*	1 Serving/125g	178	11.3	142	2.7	12.4	9.0	0.0
Vanilla, Pecan, Haagen-Dazs*	1 Serving/120ml	316	23.5	263	4.3	17.1	19.6	0.0
Vanilla, Pizza Express*	1 Serving/100g	119	6.8	119	0.9	13.8	6.8	0.0
Vanilla, Really Creamy, Asda*	1 Serving/50g	98	5.0	196	3.5	23.0	10.0	0.1
Vanilla, Safeway*	1 Scoop/50g	85	3.8	170	2.8	21.5	7.6	0.2
Vanilla, SmartPrice, Asda*	1 Scoop/40g	55	2.4	137	2.8	19.0	6.0	0.2
Vanilla, Soft, Non Milk Fat, Waitrose*	1 Serving/125ml	78	3.4	62	1.3	8.0	2.7	0.1
Vanilla, Soft Scoop, 25% Less Fat, Asda*	1oz/28g	42	1.4	149	2.9	23.0	5.0	0.0
Vanilla, Soft Scoop, BGTY, Sainsbury's*	1 Serving/75g	88	1.3	117	3.1	22.2	1.7	0.2
Vanilla, Soft Scoop, Light, Wall's*	1 Scoop/50ml	31	1.3	62	1.3	7.0	2.6	0.9
Vanilla, Soft Scoop, M & S*	1 Serving/30g	50	2.5	165	2.7	19.9	8.2	0.3
Vanilla, Soft Scoop, Tesco*	1oz/28g	46	2.0	164	3.1	21.8	7.1	0.1
Vanilla, Soft Slice, Wall's*	1 Serving/100ml	90	4.4	90	1.4	11.2	4.4	0.1
Vanilla, Thorntons*	1oz/28g	63	3.8	225	4.9	20.5	13.6	0.0
Vanilla, Too Good to Be True, Wall's*	1 Serving/50ml	35	0.2	70	2.0	14.9	0.4	0.1
Vanilla, Value, Tesco*	1 Serving/56g	77	3.2	137	2.8	18.7	5.7	0.2
Vanilla, Waitrose*	1 Serving/100ml	156	10.8	156	2.6	12.0	10.8	0.0
Vanilla, With Vanilla Pods, Sainsbury's*	1 Serving/100g	195	10.1	195	3.5	22.5	10.1	0.1
Vanilla & Cinnamon, Finest, Tesco*	1 Serving/50g	115	7.4	229	3.9	20.2	14.7	0.4
Vanilla & Strawberry, Weight Watchers*	1 Serving/100ml	81	2.2	81	1.4	13.3	2.2	0.1
Vanilla Bean, Purbeck*	1 Serving/100g	198	11.5	198	4.8	18.7	11.5	0.0
Vanilla Caramel Brownie, Haagen-Dazs*	1 Serving/150g	410	24.8	273	4.5	26.8	16.5	0.0
Vanilla Caramel Fudge, Ben & Jerry's*	1 Serving/100g	260	14.0	260	4.0	28.0	14.0	0.0
Vanilla Choc Fudge, Haagen-Dazs*	1oz/28g	75	4.8	267	4.3	23.5	17.2	0.0
Vanilla Flavour, Soft Scoop, Sainsbury's*	1 Serving/70g	96	3.9	136	2.9	18.8	5.5	0.2
Vanilletta, Tesco*	1 Serving/46.8g	82	3.8	175	4.0	21.6	8.1	0.0
Viennetta, Biscuit Caramel, Wall's*	1/6 Serving/58g	183	12.1	315	3.3	27.8	20.9	0.0
Viennetta, Chocolate, Wall's*	¼ Pot/80g	200	12.2	250	4.1	24.0	15.2	0.0
Viennetta, Forest Fruit, Wall's*	1 Serving/98g	265	15.9	270	3.4	27.2	16.2	0.0
Viennetta, Mint, Wall's*	1 Serving/80g	204	13.3	255	3.4	23.0	16.6	0.0
Viennetta, Selection Brownie, Wall's*	1 Serving/70g	194	11.3	277	4.2	28.5	16.2	0.0
Viennetta, Strawberry Cheesecake Biscuit, Wall's**	1 Serving/100g	305	20.7	305	3.5	28.1	20.7	0.0
Viennetta, Vanilla, Wall's*	¼ Bar/80g	204	13.4	255	3.3	23.0	16.7	0.0
Voluptuous Vanilla, COU, M & S*	1 Pot/400g	520	10.4	130	4.6	22.0	2.6	0.6
White Vanilla, Soft Scoop, Tesco*	1oz/28g	46	2.0	164	3.1	21.8	7.1	0.1
with Cherry Sauce, Tesco*	1 Serving/57.7g	122	3.2	210	2.8	37.0	5.6	0.2
Zesty Lemon Meringue, COU, M & S*	¼ Pot/73g	120	1.8	165	2.6	33.0	2.5	0.5
ICE CREAM BAR								
Bailey's, Haagen-Dazs*	1oz/28g	86	5.9	307	4.1	24.8	21.2	0.0
Bounty, 100 Ml Bar, Mars*	1 Bar/100ml	278	18.5	278	3.4	24.7	18.5	0.7
Chunky Chocolate, Co-Op*	1 Bar/60g	204	12.0	340	5.0	35.0	20.0	1.0
Dairy Milk, Caramel, Cadbury*	1 Bar/60.3ml	174	10.3	290	3.6	30.2	17.1	0.0
Dairy Milk, Fruit & Nut, Cadbury*	1 Bar/74g	178	10.8	240	2.2	25.3	14.5	0.0
Dairy Milk, Fudge, Cadbury*	1 Bar/60g	165	10.3	275	3.0	27.6	17.2	0.0
Galaxy, Mars*	1 Bar/54g	184	12.2	341	3.8	30.7	22.5	0.6
Maltesers, Mars*	1 Bar/44.8ml	113	7.0	252	2.9	25.0	15.6	0.7
Mars, Mars*	1 Bar/63g	177	10.3	283	3.6	30.1	16.4	0.0
Milky Way, Wall's*	1 Bar/32g	108	6.5	338	4.7	33.8	20.3	1.3
Racer, Aldi*	1 Bar/59g	194	11.0	328	6.0	34.2	18.6	0.0
Red Fruits, Solero*	1 Bar/80g	99	2.2	124	1.6	25.0	2.7	0.0
Snickers, Mars*	1 Bar/67g	250	15.0	373	6.0	37.3	22.4	0.0
Toffee Crisp, Nestle*	1 Bar/60ml	152	9.2	254	3.0	26.1	15.3	0.4
Twix, Mars*	1 Serving/43.5g	231	14.2	524	6.9	52.9	32.2	0.0

	Measure INFO/WEIGHT	per Measure KCAL	FAT	Nutrition Values per 100g / 100ml KCAL	PROT	CARB	FAT	FIBRE
ICE CREAM CONE								
After Eight, Nestle*	1 Cone/100ml	174	8.0	174	2.4	23.0	8.0	0.9
Arctic, Average	1 Portion/70g	140	4.6	200	4.1	33.3	6.6	0.0
Average	1 Cone/75g	140	6.4	186	3.5	25.5	8.5	0.0
Carousel Wafer Company*	1 Cone/4.8g	19	0.2	392	9.8	78.6	4.2	0.0
Choc 'n' Nut, Farmfoods*	1 Cone/120ml	183	9.2	278	5.0	33.0	14.0	1.0
Chocolate, M & S*	1oz/28g	94	6.4	335	4.0	28.0	23.0	2.3
Chocolate, Mini, Cornetto, Wall's*	1 Cone/19g	69	4.4	363	4.2	34.2	23.2	0.0
Chocolate, Vanilla & Hazelnut, Sainsbury's*	1 Cone/62g	190	10.5	306	4.5	33.9	16.9	0.6
Chocolate & Nut, Co-Op*	1 Cone/110g	307	17.1	279	3.9	31.0	15.5	0.6
Chocolate & Vanilla, Good Choice, Iceland*	1 Cone/110ml	161	7.2	146	2.7	22.9	6.5	0.8
Chocolate & Vanilla, M & S*	1oz/28g	83	4.8	295	4.2	31.8	17.0	0.7
Chocolate Flavour, Somerfield*	1 Cone/110ml	329	16.5	299	4.0	38.0	15.0	0.0
Cone, Haagen-Dazs*	1oz/28g	85	5.7	303	4.7	25.5	20.3	0.0
Cornet, Wafer Cone, Askeys*	1 Cone/3.5g	13	0.1	376	10.7	77.6	2.5	0.0
Cornetto, Classico, Mini, Wall's*	1 Cone/19g	67	4.4	353	4.2	32.6	23.2	0.0
Cornetto, Classico, Wall's*	1 Cone/98g	200	12.6	205	2.7	19.7	12.9	0.0
Cornetto, GFY, Asda*	1 Cone/67.2g	161	6.0	241	3.0	37.0	9.0	0.1
Cornetto, Mint, Wall's*	1 Cone/75g	225	13.5	300	3.7	32.0	18.0	1.1
Cornetto, Wall's*	1 Cone/75g	195	9.7	260	3.7	34.5	12.9	0.0
Cup Cornet, Wafer Cone, Askeys*	1 Cone/3.5g	15	0.1	376	10.7	77.6	2.5	0.0
Dairy Milk, Mint, Cadbury*	1 Cone/115ml	190	8.9	165	2.4	21.5	7.7	0.0
Extreme Raspberry, Cornetto, Nestle*	1 Cornetto/88g	220	8.8	250	2.5	36.0	10.0	0.2
Flake 99, Cadbury*	1 Cone/125ml	244	12.5	195	2.6	23.2	10.0	0.0
Flake 99, Strawberry, Cadbury*	1 Serving/125g	250	10.9	200	2.6	27.3	8.7	0.0
Mini, Tesco*	1 Cone/48g	152	9.3	316	4.1	31.5	19.3	0.8
Mint Choc Chip, Iceland*	1 Cone/72g	210	9.4	292	3.3	40.4	13.0	1.0
Smarties, Nestle*	1 Cone/100g	177	8.1	177	2.4	23.6	8.1	0.7
Sticky Toffee, Farmfoods*	1 Cone/120ml	177	8.3	272	3.2	36.0	12.8	2.0
Strawberry, Co-Op*	1 Cone/110g	283	13.3	257	3.5	33.6	12.1	0.5
Strawberry & Vanilla, Asda*	1 Cone/115ml	193	9.0	168	1.8	22.6	7.8	0.1
Strawberry & Vanilla, Farmfoods*	1 Cone/120ml	170	8.6	257	3.0	32.0	13.0	2.0
Strawberry & Vanilla, Iceland*	1 Serving/70g	182	7.6	260	3.3	37.5	10.8	0.7
Strawberry & Vanilla, Sainsbury's*	1 Cone/70g	171	6.8	243	3.4	35.6	9.7	1.0
Strawberry & Vanilla, Tesco*	1 Cone/70g	194	9.5	277	3.0	35.9	13.5	0.3
Tesco*	¼ Roll/57g	131	4.9	230	3.7	34.5	8.6	0.4
ICE CREAM SANDWICH								
Vanilla, Chocolate Coated, Lidl*	1 Serving/51g	145	9.5	284	1.8	21.6	18.6	0.0
Wich, Ben & Jerry's*	1 Serving/117g	350	18.0	299	3.4	38.5	15.4	0.9
ICE CREAM STICK								
Berry Blast, Smoothie, Skinny Cow*	1 Stick/110ml	71	0.1	65	0.9	15.1	0.1	1.9
Cookies 'n' Cream, Skinny Cow*	1 Stick/66.9g	89	1.0	133	4.8	25.3	1.5	3.6
Mint Double Chocolate, Skinny Cow*	1 Stick/110ml	94	1.8	85	2.7	15.1	1.6	2.4
Strawberries & Cream, Skinny Cow*	1 Stick/110ml	82	1.0	75	2.8	13.6	0.9	2.3
Toffee, Skinny Cow*	1 Stick/71.9g	87	0.4	121	3.9	25.2	0.5	4.2
Tripple Chocolate, Skinny Cow*	1 Stick/68g	87	1.5	128	4.3	22.8	2.2	2.8
ICE LOLLY								
Assorted, Farmfoods*	1 Lolly/56ml	35	0.0	62	0.0	15.6	0.0	0.0
Assorted, Iceland*	1 Lolly/51g	33	0.0	65	0.0	16.2	0.0	0.0
Assorted, Safeway*	1 Lolly/31ml	26	0.0	85	0.0	20.9	0.0	0.1
Berry Burst, Sainsbury's*	1 Lolly/90ml	93	1.6	103	1.1	20.8	1.8	0.7
Blackcurrant, Dairy Split, Sainsbury's*	1 Lolly/72.7ml	88	2.6	121	1.8	20.4	3.6	0.1
Blackcurrant, Ribena*	1 Lolly/55ml	43	0.0	79	0.0	19.2	0.0	0.0
Blackcurrant Split, Iceland*	1 Lolly/75g	61	2.4	81	1.1	12.0	3.2	0.1

ICE LOLLY

	Measure INFO/WEIGHT	per Measure KCAL	FAT	KCAL	PROT	CARB	FAT	FIBRE
Calippo, Strawberry Tropical, Wall's*	1 Calippo/105g	89	0.1	85	0.1	21.0	0.1	0.0
Chocolate, Mini Milk, Milk Time, Wall's*	1 Lolly/23g	31	0.7	135	4.3	22.0	3.1	1.0
Cider Refresher, Treats*	1 Lolly/70ml	54	0.0	77	0.0	19.2	0.0	0.0
Exotic Fruit, Tesco*	1 Lolly/31.5g	41	0.6	131	1.8	26.4	2.0	0.6
Fab, Nestle*	1 Lolly/57g	78	2.7	136	0.5	22.8	4.7	0.2
Feast, Chocolate, Mini, Wall's*	1 Lolly/52g	165	11.9	318	3.3	24.0	23.0	0.0
Feast, Ice Cream, Original, Wall's*	1 Lolly/92ml	294	21.6	320	3.2	23.8	23.5	0.0
Feast, Wall's*	1 Lolly/60g	190	13.7	317	3.3	24.7	22.8	0.0
Fruit, Assorted, Waitrose*	1 Lolly/73g	59	0.0	81	0.0	20.0	0.0	0.1
Fruit Assorted, Basics, Somerfield*	1 Lolly/56ml	32	0.0	58	0.0	15.0	0.0	0.0
Fruit Fusion, Mini, Farmfoods*	1 Lolly/45ml	36	0.0	79	0.2	19.2	0.1	0.2
Fruit Ices, Made with Orange Juice, Del Monte*	1 Lolly/75ml	79	0.0	105	0.5	25.7	0.0	0.0
Fruit Pastil-Lolly, Rowntree's, Nestle*	1 Lolly/75ml	69	0.0	92	0.2	23.1	0.0	0.0
Fruit Split, Asda*	1 Lolly/73.9g	85	2.7	115	1.7	19.0	3.6	0.0
Fruit Split, Assorted, Co-Op*	1 Lolly/73g	80	2.2	110	1.0	20.0	3.0	0.1
Fruit Splits, Assorted, Somerfield*	1 Lolly/73ml	74	2.2	102	0.0	18.0	3.0	0.0
Fruit Splits, Treats*	1 Lolly/75ml	77	3.1	103	1.4	17.6	4.1	0.0
Lemonade & Cola, Morrisons*	1 Lolly/55ml	36	0.0	65	0.0	16.2	0.0	0.0
Lemonade Sparkle, Wall's*	1 Lolly/55g	40	0.0	73	0.0	18.2	0.0	0.0
Mango & Passion Fruit, Sainsbury's*	1 Lolly/73ml	76	0.1	104	0.2	25.5	0.1	0.6
Mango & Passion Fruit Bursts, Sainsbury's*	1 Lolly/88.8ml	75	0.1	84	0.2	20.4	0.1	0.0
Milk, Blue Parrot Cafe, Sainsbury's*	1 Lolly/30ml	34	1.0	113	2.7	18.0	3.3	0.3
Mint Chocolate, Tesco*	1 Lolly/70g	234	13.9	334	3.6	35.4	19.8	1.2
Morrisons*	1 Lolly/100g	30	0.0	30	0.0	7.4	0.0	0.0
Nobbly Bobbly, Nestle*	1 Lolly/70ml	158	8.2	226	2.3	27.6	11.7	0.3
Orange, Lidl*	1 Lolly/50g	50	0.0	100	0.5	24.4	0.1	0.0
Orange, Real Fruit Juice, Sainsbury's*	1 Lolly/73ml	49	0.1	67	0.2	16.5	0.1	0.1
Orange, Ribena*	1 Lolly/110ml	95	0.0	86	0.1	21.4	0.0	0.0
Orange, Tesco*	1 Lolly/77.4g	52	0.0	68	0.2	16.8	0.0	0.3
Orange, Water, Iceland*	1 Lolly/75g	74	0.0	98	0.2	24.4	0.0	0.2
Orange & Lemon Splits, Farmfoods*	1 Lolly/56ml	56	1.9	124	1.6	19.8	4.3	0.2
Orange Juice, Asda*	1 Lolly/70g	58	0.0	83	0.7	20.0	0.0	0.0
Orange Juice, Bar, M & S*	1 Lolly/75g	65	0.0	86	0.5	21.0	0.0	0.1
Orange Juice, Co-Op*	1 Lolly/73g	51	0.1	70	0.4	17.0	0.1	0.1
Orange Juice, Farmfoods*	1 Lolly/78.7g	74	0.0	94	0.1	23.4	0.0	0.3
Orange Juice, Freshly Squeezed, Finest, Tesco*	1 Lolly/80ml	89	0.0	111	0.7	27.0	0.0	0.0
Orange Juice, Morrisons*	1 Lolly/55ml	46	0.0	84	0.0	20.0	0.0	0.0
Orange Juice, Tropicana*	1 Lolly/50g	43	0.0	85	0.5	20.7	0.0	0.0
Orange Maid, Nestle*	1 Lolly/73ml	66	0.0	91	0.5	21.6	0.0	0.0
Pineapple, Real Fruit Juice, Sainsbury's*	1 Lolly/73ml	55	0.1	76	0.1	19.0	0.1	0.1
Raspberry, Real Fruit Juice, Sainsbury's*	1 Lolly/72g	62	0.1	86	0.3	21.0	0.1	0.1
Raspberry, Rocket Split, De Roma*	1 Lolly/60ml	65	2.6	108	1.0	16.2	4.3	0.2
Raspberry & Apple, Sainsbury's*	1 Lolly/57ml	39	0.1	68	0.1	17.1	0.1	0.1
Real Fruit, Dairy Split, Sainsbury's*	1 Lolly/73ml	100	3.1	137	2.1	22.8	4.2	0.1
Rocket, Co-Op*	1 Lolly/60g	42	0.0	70	0.0	17.0	0.0	0.0
Rocket, Sainsbury's*	1 Lolly/58g	42	0.1	72	0.1	17.8	0.1	0.1
Scooby-Doo, Freezepops, Calypso*	1 Lolly/50ml	14	0.0	28	0.0	7.0	0.0	0.0
Solero, Exotic, Wall's*	1 Lolly/82g	99	2.3	121	1.6	22.0	2.8	0.5
Solero, Orange Fresh, Wall's*	1 Lolly/96g	78	0.0	81	0.2	20.0	0.0	0.0
Solero, Red Fruits, Wall's*	1 Lolly/95g	99	2.1	104	1.3	21.0	2.2	0.0
Strawberry, Dairy Split, Sainsbury's*	1 Lolly/72.9ml	86	2.6	118	1.7	19.8	3.6	0.1
Strawberry, Fruit Split, Iceland*	1 Lolly/75g	79	2.5	105	0.9	17.8	3.3	0.5
Strawberry, Mini Milk, Milk Time, Wall's*	1 Lolly/23g	30	0.7	131	4.0	22.0	2.9	0.5

	Measure INFO/WEIGHT	per Measure KCAL	FAT	Nutrition Values per 100g / 100ml KCAL	PROT	CARB	FAT	FIBRE
ICE LOLLY								
Strawberry, Orange & Pineapple, Rocket, Iceland*	1 Lolly/47g	38	0.0	81	0.0	20.2	0.0	0.1
Strawberry & Banana, Smoothies, Sainsbury's*	1 Lolly/60g	100	3.2	166	1.5	28.0	5.3	0.2
Strawberry Split, Co-Op*	1 Lolly/71ml	75	2.1	105	1.0	17.0	3.0	0.1
Tip Top, Calypso*	1 Lolly/20ml	6	0.0	30	0.1	7.1	0.1	0.0
Tropical Fruit, Starburst, Mars*	1 Lolly/93ml	94	0.1	101	0.3	24.8	0.1	0.0
Tropical Fruit Sorbet, Waitrose*	1 Lolly/109.8g	90	2.2	82	1.5	14.5	2.0	0.2
Twister, Wall's*	1 Lolly/80ml	76	1.5	95	0.6	18.4	1.9	0.0
Vanilla, Mini Milk, Milk Time, Wall's*	1 Lolly/23g	29	0.7	127	3.8	21.0	2.9	0.3
Vimto*	1 Lolly/73.0ml	84	3.0	115	1.3	18.2	4.1	0.1
Zoom, Nestle*	1 Lolly/58.1ml	54	0.4	93	0.9	20.6	0.7	0.0
ICED DESSERT								
Chocolate Mint Crisp, COU, M & S*	¼ Pot/85.2g	115	2.5	135	5.4	21.9	2.9	1.0
Vanilla, 3% Fat, M & S*	1oz/28g	40	0.8	143	3.5	25.9	2.8	0.7
Vanilla, Dairy, Sainsbury's*	1 Serving/65g	77	2.0	119	3.0	19.9	3.0	3.7
Vanilla, Non Dairy, Soft, Swedish Glace*	1 Serving/100g	200	10.0	200	2.5	25.0	10.0	1.0
INDIAN MEAL								
Banquet, for One, COU, M & S*	1 Pack/500g	400	6.0	80	6.7	10.2	1.2	3.1
for One, Asda*	1 Pack/550g	834	25.3	152	6.7	20.9	4.6	1.4
for One, Eat Smart, Safeway*	1 Serving/600g	690	15.6	115	6.5	16.2	2.6	2.0
for One, GFY, Asda*	1 Serving/495g	644	23.3	130	8.0	14.0	4.7	1.0
for One, HE, Tesco*	1 Pack/420g	437	8.8	104	7.4	14.0	2.1	1.4
for One, Vegetarian, Asda*	1 Pack/500g	789	44.9	158	3.2	16.0	9.0	1.4
for Two, Hot, Takeaway, Tesco*	1 Pack/825g	1215	60.6	147	6.6	13.6	7.4	1.9
for Two, Menu, Tesco*	1 Serving/537g	811	34.4	151	6.3	17.0	6.4	0.8
for Two, Peshwari Naan, Finest, Tesco*	½ Pack/200g	612	17.8	306	8.3	48.3	8.9	5.2
Takeaway, Meal for Two, M & S*	½ Pack/500g	775	38.5	155	5.7	16.0	7.7	1.6
INDIAN MENU								
COU, M & S*	1 Pack/550g	413	6.6	75	8.4	7.5	1.2	2.1
INDIAN SELECTION								
Snack, Safeway*	1 Serving/170g	347	16.0	204	4.0	25.8	9.4	1.9
INSTANT WHIP								
Strawberry Flavour, Dry, Bird's*	1oz/28g	112	1.5	400	2.5	85.0	5.4	0.4
IRON BRU								
Barr's*	1 Can/330ml	155	0.0	47	0.0	11.5	0.0	0.0

	Measure INFO/WEIGHT	per Measure KCAL	FAT	Nutrition Values per 100g / 100ml KCAL	PROT	CARB	FAT	FIBRE
JACKFRUIT								
Raw, Average, Flesh Only	1 Serving/162g	155	0.5	95	1.5	24.4	0.3	1.6
JALFREZI								
Chicken, & Rice, HL, Tesco*	1 Pack/450g	495	9.5	110	6.0	16.9	2.1	1.0
Chicken, & Rice, Serves 1, Tesco*	1 Serving/475g	589	38.0	124	7.4	5.7	8.0	1.6
Chicken, Asda*	1 Pack/340g	415	20.4	122	10.0	7.0	6.0	1.6
Chicken, Budgens*	1 Serving/200g	210	6.4	105	9.8	9.2	3.2	0.9
Chicken, GFY, Asda*	1 Pack/350g	238	3.2	68	9.0	6.0	0.9	1.8
Chicken, HL, Tesco*	1 Serving/450g	482	3.6	107	6.9	18.0	0.8	0.9
Chicken, Hot & Spicy, Sainsbury's*	½ Pack/200g	228	11.4	114	12.8	2.9	5.7	1.0
Chicken, Indian Style Meal for One, Morrisons*	1 Pack/350g	350	17.2	100	10.1	3.9	4.9	1.6
Chicken, Indian Takeaway, Tesco*	1 Serving/350g	245	8.7	70	7.4	4.3	2.5	1.8
Chicken, M & S*	1 Pack/350g	455	26.3	130	13.6	1.6	7.5	1.4
Chicken, Medium, GFY, Asda*	1 Pack/644g	972	27.7	151	6.0	22.0	4.3	0.9
Chicken, Somerfield*	1 Pack/350g	340	16.1	97	11.2	2.6	4.6	1.2
Chicken, Tesco*	1 Pack/350g	385	21.3	110	9.9	3.9	6.1	1.2
Chicken, with Pilau Rice, BGTY, Sainsbury's*	1 Pack/400g	337	4.4	84	7.1	11.5	1.1	1.9
Chicken, with Pilau Rice, Spar*	1 Pack/400g	472	19.2	118	6.7	12.0	4.8	1.2
Chicken, with Pilau Rice, Tesco*	1 Pack/460g	506	17.5	110	5.3	13.6	3.8	0.9
Chicken, with Rice, Morrisons*	1 Pack/400g	564	20.8	141	7.7	15.9	5.2	1.4
Chicken, with Rice, Tesco*	1 Pack/475g	632	22.8	133	5.5	17.0	4.8	1.0
Chicken & Pilau Rice, Sainsbury's*	1 Pack/500g	600	20.5	120	6.9	13.9	4.1	1.5
Chicken with Basmati Rice, Eat Smart, Safeway*	1 Pack/400g	300	4.0	75	6.8	8.5	1.0	1.7
Chicken with Basmati Rice, Weight Watchers*	1 Pack/330g	238	1.7	72	5.0	11.8	0.5	0.5
Chicken with Pilau Basmati Rice, Frozen, Patak's*	1 Pack/400g	556	18.4	139	9.8	14.7	4.6	0.9
Chicken with Pilau Rice, GFY, Asda*	1 Pack/445.9g	495	11.2	111	8.0	14.0	2.5	1.2
Chicken with Pilau Rice, PB, Waitrose*	1 Pack/400g	388	4.0	97	8.0	14.0	1.0	2.4
Chicken with Pilau Rice, Safeway*	1 Pack/424.2g	700	21.2	165	8.1	20.9	5.0	0.8
Chicken with Rice, COU, M & S*	1 Pack/400g	320	4.4	80	9.2	8.3	1.1	1.2
Meal for One, M & S*	1 Serving/500g	700	35.0	140	6.1	13.4	7.0	3.0
Vegetable, Co-Op*	1 Pack/400g	320	16.0	80	1.0	9.0	4.0	2.0
Vegetable, Eastern Indian, Sainsbury's*	1 Pack/400g	208	13.6	52	3.4	2.0	3.4	1.7
Vegetable, Take Away Menu, BGTY, Sainsbury's*	1 Pack/148g	43	0.0	29	1.8	5.4	0.0	2.3
Vegetable, Waitrose*	1 Pack/400g	256	16.0	64	2.2	4.7	4.0	3.7
Vegetable, with Rice, Birds Eye*	1 Pack/350g	354	3.9	101	2.5	20.2	1.1	1.0
JAM								
Apricot, Average	1 Tbsp/15g	37	0.0	248	0.2	61.6	0.0	1.5
Apricot, Reduced Sugar, Average	1 Serving/20g	37	0.1	187	0.5	46.0	0.3	0.4
Black Cherry, Average	2 Tbsp/30g	74	0.1	247	0.4	61.2	0.3	0.4
Blackcurrant, Average	1 Tbsp/15g	38	0.0	250	0.2	62.3	0.0	1.0
Blackcurrant, Reduced Sugar, Average	1 Tsp/5.7g	11	0.0	178	0.5	44.4	0.2	1.0
Blueberry, Best, Hartley's*	1 Tsp/20g	49	0.0	244	0.3	60.6	0.1	0.0
Blueberry, St Dalfour*	1 Serving/20g	46	0.0	228	0.5	56.0	0.2	2.2
Damson, Extra Fruit, Best, Hartley's*	1 Tsp/5g	12	0.0	244	0.2	60.8	0.0	0.0
Golden Peach, Rhapsodie De Fruit, St Dalfour*	2 Tsp/20g	45	0.0	227	0.5	56.0	0.1	1.3
Kiwi & Goosberry, 66% Fruit, Asda*	1 Serving/30g	56	0.2	187	0.5	45.0	0.5	0.0
Mixed Fruit, Average	1 Tbsp/15g	38	0.0	253	0.3	63.5	0.0	0.5
Plum, Tesco*	1 Serving/50g	131	0.0	261	0.2	64.4	0.0	0.6
Rasberry, Reduced Sugar, Average	1 Tsp/6.3g	10	0.0	160	0.5	39.3	0.2	0.6
Raspberry, Average	1 Tbsp/15.1g	36	0.0	239	0.6	58.7	0.1	0.9
Raspberry, Seedless, Average	1 Tsp/10g	26	0.0	257	0.5	63.6	0.0	0.3
Strawberry, Average	1 Tsp/10g	25	0.0	253	0.3	62.8	0.0	0.6
Strawberry, Reduced Sugar, Average	1 Tbsp/15g	28	0.0	187	0.4	45.8	0.3	0.2

J

	Measure INFO/WEIGHT	per Measure KCAL	FAT	Nutrition Values per 100g / 100ml KCAL	PROT	CARB	FAT	FIBRE
JAMBALAYA								
American, HE, Tesco*	1 Pack/450g	477	9.0	106	6.4	15.5	2.0	0.9
American Style, Tesco*	1 Serving/275g	432	19.3	157	7.7	16.0	7.0	0.5
Cajun Chicken, BGTY, Sainsbury's*	1 Pack/400g	364	5.6	91	7.7	11.9	1.4	1.1
Chicken, Spicy, Eat Smart, Morrisons*	1 Pack/400g	384	4.8	96	7.4	13.9	1.2	2.7
COU, M & S*	1 Pack/400g	340	8.0	85	6.5	10.8	2.0	0.9
GFY, Asda*	1 Pack/450g	387	3.2	86	6.0	14.0	0.7	2.7
M & S*	1 Pack/480g	552	16.8	115	5.8	14.6	3.5	1.2
Tesco*	1 Pack/550g	765	36.3	139	6.9	13.1	6.6	1.1
JELLY								
Blackcurrant, Made Up, Rowntree's*	¼ Jelly/140ml	100	0.1	71	1.4	16.4	0.1	0.0
Blackcurrant, Made Up, Sainsbury's*	¼ Jelly/150g	98	0.0	65	1.2	15.1	0.0	0.0
Blackcurrant, Sugar Free, Unprepared, Rowntree's*	1 Pack/24g	73	0.0	305	50.0	25.0	0.0	25.0
Bramble, Tesco*	1 Serving/100g	257	0.1	257	0.3	63.7	0.1	1.3
Crystals, Orange, Sugar Free, Bird's*	1 Sachet/11½g	39	0.1	335	62.5	6.4	0.9	0.0
Crystals, Strawberry, Made Up, Tesco*	1 Serving/145g	9	0.0	6	1.3	0.3	0.0	0.0
Exotic Fruit, M & S*	1 Pot/175g	140	0.4	80	0.1	18.9	0.2	0.9
Fresh Fruit, M & S*	1 Pot/175g	131	0.2	75	0.2	18.4	0.1	0.3
Fruitini, Del Monte*	1 Serving/120g	78	0.1	65	0.3	15.3	0.1	0.5
Lemon & Lime, Sugar Free, Unprepared, Rowntree's*	1oz/28g	85	0.0	305	4.5	60.7	0.0	0.0
Lime, Made Up, Rowntree's*	¼ Jelly/140ml	100	0.1	71	1.4	16.4	0.1	0.0
Made Up with Water, Average	1oz/28g	17	0.0	61	1.2	15.1	0.0	0.0
Mixed Berry, Sainsbury's*	1 Serving/160g	112	0.3	70	0.7	16.3	0.2	1.5
Orange, Sugar Free, Made Up, Hartley's*	1 Pint/560ml	32	0.0	6	1.4	0.1	0.0	0.0
Orange, Sugar Free, Rowntree's*	1 Serving/140ml	8	0.0	6	1.4	0.1	0.0	0.0
Pineapple, with Pineapple Pieces, Tesco*	1 Serving/120g	96	0.1	80	1.2	18.6	0.1	0.7
Raspberry Flavour, Sugar Free, Made Up, Rowntree's*	1 Portion/140ml	9	0.0	6	1.4	0.1	0.0	0.0
Raspberry Flavour, Tesco*	1 Serving/34g	22	0.0	64	1.0	15.0	0.0	0.1
Raspberry Flavoured, with Raspberries, M & S*	1 Sm Pot/175g	105	0.5	60	0.2	14.0	0.3	1.5
Redcurrant, Average	1oz/28g	70	0.0	250	0.2	64.4	0.0	0.0
Strawberry, No Added Sugar, Hartley's*	1 Pot/115g	3	0.0	3	0.0	0.4	0.0	0.3
Strawberry, Sugar Free, Crystals, Dry Weight, Hartley's*	1 Sachet/14g	39	0.0	280	56.8	13.1	0.0	0.0
Strawberry Flavour, Sugar Free, Made Up, Rowntree's*	1 Serving/140ml	10	0.0	7	1.5	0.1	0.0	0.0
Sugar Free, Dry, Tesco*	1 Pack/12.5g	36	0.0	285	55.4	15.6	0.0	0.2
Tangerine, Unprepared, Rowntree's*	1 Serving/33g	99	0.1	300	5.6	67.3	0.4	0.0
JELLY BABIES								
Bassett's*	1 Baby/6g	20	0.0	335	4.0	79.5	0.0	0.0
M & S*	1 Pack/125g	418	0.0	334	5.2	78.0	0.0	0.0
Mini, Rowntree's*	1 Sm Bag/35g	128	0.0	366	4.6	86.9	0.0	0.0
Sainsbury's*	1 Serving/70g	247	0.5	353	4.1	82.5	0.7	0.3
Somerfield*	1 Sweet/6g	21	0.0	343	4.7	80.7	0.0	0.0
Tesco*	1 Baby/6g	21	0.0	344	5.3	80.7	0.0	0.0
JELLY BEANS								
Asda*	1 Bag/100g	364	0.4	364	0.1	90.0	0.4	0.2
Jelly Belly*	35 Beans/40g	140	0.0	350	0.0	90.0	0.0	0.0
M & S*	1 Bag/113g	407	0.0	360	0.1	89.6	0.0	0.0
No Added Sugar, Jelly Belly*	1 Serving/40g	80	0.0	200	0.0	50.0	0.0	20.0
Rowntree's*	1 Pack/35g	128	0.0	367	0.0	91.8	0.0	0.0
JELLY TOTS								
Rowntree's*	1 Pack/42g	145	0.0	346	0.1	86.5	0.0	0.0
JERKY								
Beef, Peppered, Jack Link's*	1 Serving/28g	80	0.5	286	53.6	14.3	1.8	0.0
JUICE								
100% Vegetable, V8*	1 Bottle/354ml	57	0.0	16	0.7	3.3	0.0	0.8

J

JUICE

	Measure	per Measure KCAL	per Measure FAT	KCAL	PROT	CARB	FAT	FIBRE
Apple, Concentrate, Average	1 Tbsp/15ml	45	0.0	302	0.1	73.6	0.2	0.0
Apple, English, Copella*	1 Bottle/250ml	118	0.0	47	0.0	11.6	0.0	0.4
Apple, English with Cherry, Cawston Vale*	1 Can/250ml	118	0.3	47	0.4	11.6	0.1	0.0
Apple, Pure, Average	1 Glass/100ml	47	0.0	47	0.1	11.2	0.0	0.0
Apple, Pure, Organic, Average	1 Serving/200ml	93	0.1	46	0.1	11.2	0.1	0.1
Apple, Raspberry, & Grape, Pressed, Sainsbury's*	1 Serving/200ml	92	0.2	46	0.3	11.2	0.1	0.5
Apple, with Calcium, Juice Plus, Tesco*	1 Serving/250ml	118	0.0	47	0.1	11.2	0.0	0.0
Apple, with Mango Puree, Safeway*	1 Glass/150ml	80	0.0	53	0.3	12.6	0.0	0.0
Apple & Elderflower, Copella*	1 Glass/250ml	108	0.3	43	0.4	10.2	0.1	0.0
Apple & Mango, Average	1 Glass/200ml	108	0.1	54	0.3	12.6	0.0	0.1
Apple & Orange, Fresh Up*	1 Serving/250ml	105	0.0	42	0.0	10.3	0.0	0.0
Apple & Pomegranate, Pommy, Sparky*	1 Serving/250ml	124	0.5	50	0.4	10.0	0.2	0.5
Apple & Raspberry, Average	1 Serving/200ml	89	0.1	45	0.5	10.2	0.1	0.2
Apple & Rhubarb, Caxton Vale*	1 Glass/250mls	115	1.0	46	0.2	9.7	0.4	0.0
Breakfast, Sainsbury's*	1 Serving/200ml	94	0.2	47	0.7	11.3	0.1	0.3
Carrot, Average	1 Glass/200ml	46	0.0	23	0.6	5.2	0.0	0.1
Citrus Fruit & Veg, V8*	1 Serving/150ml	56	0.3	37	0.3	8.4	0.2	0.0
Clementine, Morrisons*	1 Serving/100ml	48	0.1	48	0.5	10.9	0.1	0.1
Cranberry, Average	1 Bottle/250ml	139	0.2	56	0.1	13.4	0.1	0.3
Cranberry, Iceland*	1 Glass/200ml	92	0.0	46	0.0	11.1	0.0	0.0
Cranberry & Apple, No Added Sugar, Sainsbury's*	1 Glass/250ml	15	0.0	6	0.0	1.5	0.0	0.0
Cranberry & Pomegranate, Ocean Spray*	1 Glass/200ml	100	0.2	50	0.1	11.8	0.1	0.1
Cranberry & Raspberry, Low Sugar, Sainsbury's*	1 Glass/250ml	10	0.3	4	0.1	0.7	0.1	0.1
Exotic Fruit, Pure, Del Monte*	1 Glass/200ml	96	0.0	48	0.3	11.3	0.0	0.0
Exotic Fruit, Waitrose*	1 Glass/175ml	88	0.0	50	0.4	11.6	0.0	0.0
Fibre, Tropicana*	1 Serving/200ml	130	0.0	65	0.4	15.8	0.0	3.4
Froot Refresh, Orange & Passion Fruit, Minute Maid*	1 Bottle/330ml	79	0.0	24	0.0	6.0	0.0	0.0
Froot Refresh, Red Grape & Raspberry, Minute Maid*	1 Bottle/330ml	99	0.0	30	0.0	7.3	0.0	0.0
Go!, Tropicana*	1 Bottle/200ml	80	0.0	40	0.3	9.7	0.0	0.0
Gold Pineapple & Mango, Del Monte*	1 Serving/200ml	104	0.0	52	0.4	12.0	0.0	0.0
Grape, Purple, Welch's*	1 Serving/200ml	136	0.0	68	0.1	16.5	0.0	0.0
Grape, Red, Average	1 Serving/100ml	62	0.0	62	0.2	15.2	0.0	0.0
Grape, White, Average	1 Can/160ml	95	0.1	60	0.2	14.3	0.1	0.1
Grape & Peach, Don Simon*	1 Serving/200ml	94	0.0	47	0.4	11.3	0.0	0.0
Grape & Raspberry, Pressed, M & S*	1 Carton/330ml	182	0.3	55	0.4	12.9	0.1	0.1
Grapefruit, Low Calorie, Natreen*	1 Sm Glass/100ml	18	0.5	18	0.5	3.3	0.5	0.0
Grapefruit, Pink, Average	1 Glass/200ml	81	0.1	41	0.6	9.0	0.1	0.2
Grapefruit, Pure, Average	1 Glass/200ml	77	0.2	38	0.5	8.5	0.1	0.1
Lemon, Fresh, Average	1 Fruit/36ml	2	0.0	7	0.3	1.6	0.0	0.1
Lemon, Made with Concentrated Lemon Juice, Tesco*	1 Serving/100ml	10	0.0	10	0.4	2.0	0.0	0.0
Lime, Fresh, Average	1 Tsp/5ml	0	0.0	9	0.4	1.6	0.1	0.1
Lime, Tesco*	1 Tbsp/12g	3	0.0	22	0.3	1.0	0.1	0.2
Mango, Canned	1 Glass/200ml	78	0.4	39	0.1	9.8	0.2	0.0
Mango & Apple, Copella*	1 Serving/200ml	92	0.0	46	0.0	11.6	0.0	1.0
Multivitamin, Fruit, Vitafit*	1 Glass/200ml	106	0.0	53	1.0	12.0	0.0	0.5
Orange, 100% Pure Squeezed, Waitrose*	1 Glass/200ml	92	0.0	46	0.4	10.6	0.0	0.3
Orange, Apple & Mango, Calypso*	1 Carton/200ml	92	0.4	46	0.0	11.0	0.2	0.1
Orange, Pure, Smooth, Average	1 Glass/200ml	88	0.1	44	0.7	9.8	0.0	0.2
Orange, Pure, with Bits, Average	1 Glass/200ml	90	0.1	45	0.7	10.2	0.1	0.1
Orange, Red, Average	1 Glass/250ml	115	0.1	46	0.4	10.7	0.0	0.2
Orange, Valencia, 100% Pure Squeezed, Sainsbury's*	1 Glass/200ml	84	0.2	42	0.5	9.1	0.1	0.1
Orange & Banana, Sainsbury's*	1 Glass/200ml	108	0.2	54	0.7	12.5	0.1	0.3
Orange & Grapefruit, Average	1 Serving/200g	85	0.2	42	0.8	9.3	0.1	0.4

J

JUICE

Measure INFO/WEIGHT	per Measure KCAL	per Measure FAT	Nutrition Values per 100g / 100ml KCAL	PROT	CARB	FAT	FIBRE
JUICE							
Orange & Kiwi Fruit, Tropicana*	1 Serving/175ml	90	0.0	51	0.5	12.0	0.0	0.0
Orange & Pineapple, Average	1 Glass/120ml	56	0.6	47	0.5	10.5	0.5	0.5
Orange & Raspberry, Average	1 fl oz/30ml	15	0.0	50	0.6	11.4	0.1	0.2
Orange & Strawberry, Average	1 Serving/125ml	64	0.5	51	0.6	10.9	0.4	0.8
Orange Banana & Grapefruit, M & S*	1 Serving/250ml	125	0.5	50	0.8	11.5	0.2	0.3
Orange with Carrot Puree, M & S*	1 Bottle/500ml	200	1.5	40	0.6	8.0	0.3	0.3
Orange with Cranberry Juice, M & S*	1 Bottle/250ml	138	1.3	55	0.5	14.0	0.5	1.0
Passion Fruit, Average	1 Glass/200ml	94	0.2	47	0.8	10.7	0.1	0.0
Pear, Concentrate, Meridian Foods*	1 Serving/45ml	134	0.0	298	0.0	74.6	0.0	0.0
Pear, Pure, Heinz*	1 Serving/100ml	41	0.1	41	0.1	9.8	0.1	0.0
Pear, with a Hint of Ginger, Pressed, M & S*	1 Glass/250ml	125	0.3	50	0.3	11.7	0.1	0.0
Pineapple, Average	1 Glass/200ml	100	0.1	50	0.3	11.7	0.1	0.2
Pineapple & Coconut, Sainsbury's*	1 Glass/250ml	153	3.5	61	0.5	11.6	1.4	0.1
Pineapple & Coconut, Tesco*	1 Serving/250ml	138	1.0	55	0.4	11.3	0.4	0.0
Pineapple & Coconut, Waitrose*	1 Serving/250ml	125	0.8	50	0.2	11.5	0.3	0.2
Pineapple Mango Crush, Just Juice*	1 Glass/250ml	108	0.0	43	0.0	10.6	0.0	0.0
Pink Grapefruit, 100% Pure Squeezed, Sainsbury's*	1 Serving/150ml	59	0.2	39	0.5	9.2	0.1	0.3
Pomegranate, Pomegreat*	1 Glass/200ml	88	0.0	44	0.1	11.1	0.0	0.0
Pressed Apple, Strawberry & Lychee, M & S*	1 Serving/250ml	113	0.8	45	0.3	9.7	0.3	0.3
Pressed Apple & Rhubarb, Cawston Vale*	1 Glass/200ml	92	0.8	46	0.2	9.7	0.4	0.0
Prune, Average	1 Serving/200ml	123	0.1	61	0.6	15.3	0.1	1.8
Raspberry Cooler, with Mint, Sainsbury's*	1 Serving/250ml	63	0.3	25	0.1	6.0	0.1	0.1
Sweet Carrot & Orange, Shapers, Boots*	1 Serving/250ml	100	0.4	40	0.9	8.8	0.2	0.4
Tomato, Average	1 Glass/200ml	40	0.1	20	0.8	4.0	0.1	0.5
Tomato, M & S*	1 Serving/266.7ml	40	0.3	15	0.7	3.2	0.1	1.0
Tropical, Fruit & Vegetable, V8*	1 fl oz/30ml	11	0.0	35	0.4	8.1	0.1	1.1
Tropical, Pure, Sainsbury's*	1 Glass/200ml	104	0.2	52	0.5	12.0	0.1	0.1
Tropical, Tropics, Tropicana*	1 Serving/250ml	113	0.0	45	0.4	11.0	0.0	0.0
Tropical Fruit, Plenty*	1 Glass/200ml	120	0.2	60	0.5	13.7	0.1	0.0
JUICE DRINK							
Apple, Cranberry, & Blueberry, Waitrose*	1 Serving/150ml	75	0.0	50	0.1	11.9	0.0	0.1
Apple & Blueberry, The Feel Good Drinks Co*	1 Serving/375ml	163	0.4	44	0.1	10.6	0.1	0.0
Apple & Elderflower, Tesco*	1 Serving/200ml	76	0.0	38	0.0	9.4	0.0	0.0
Apple & Raspberry, Sainsbury's*	1 Serving/200ml	112	0.2	56	0.1	13.8	0.1	0.1
Apple & Raspberry, Tesco*	1 Serving/300ml	138	0.0	46	0.0	11.2	0.0	0.0
Apple & Strawberry, Sainsbury's*	1 Serving/250ml	13	0.1	5	0.0	1.0	0.0	0.0
Berry & Elderberry, Fusion, Oasis*	1 Bottle/375ml	11	0.0	3	0.0	0.4	0.0	0.0
Berry Blast, 5 Alive*	1 Glass/250ml	63	0.0	25	0.0	6.1	0.0	0.0
Blackcurrant, 45% High, No Added Sugar, Asda*	1 Serving/25ml	2	0.0	7	0.0	1.4	0.0	0.0
Blackcurrant, CVit*	1 Glass/200ml	4	0.0	2	0.0	0.2	0.0	0.0
Blackcurrant, Kids, Tesco*	1 Serving/250ml	128	0.0	51	0.0	12.4	0.0	0.0
Blackcurrant, Purity*	1 Bottle/500ml	265	0.0	53	0.0	13.2	0.0	0.0
Blackcurrant & Apple, Oasis*	1 Serving/500ml	140	0.0	28	0.0	6.8	0.0	0.0
Blueberry, BGTY, Sainsbury's*	1 Serving/250ml	15	0.0	6	0.1	1.0	0.0	0.0
Cherry, No Added Sugar, Sainsbury's*	1 Carton/250ml	25	0.1	10	0.2	1.9	0.0	0.0
Citrus, Co-Op*	1 Serving/150ml	68	0.0	45	0.2	11.0	0.0	0.0
Citrus, Sainsbury's*	1 Serving/200ml	102	0.2	51	0.3	12.3	0.1	0.2
Cranberry, Classic, Ocean Spray*	1 Bottle/500ml	245	0.5	49	0.1	11.7	0.1	0.1
Cranberry, Concentrated, Ocean Spray*	1 Serving/15ml	27	0.0	183	0.2	44.1	0.0	0.0
Cranberry, Grape & Apple, Ocean Spray*	1 Glass/200ml	108	0.0	54	0.1	12.9	0.0	0.0
Cranberry, Juice Burst, Purity*	1 Bottle/500ml	245	0.0	49	0.0	12.0	0.0	0.0
Cranberry, Morrisons*	1 Glass/200ml	92	0.0	46	0.0	11.6	0.0	0.0
Cranberry, No Added Sugar, HL, Tesco*	1 Glass/200ml	8	0.0	4	0.0	1.1	0.0	0.0

JUICE DRINK

	Measure INFO/WEIGHT	per Measure KCAL	FAT	Nutrition Values per 100g / 100ml KCAL	PROT	CARB	FAT	FIBRE
Cranberry, Organic, Sainsbury's*	1 Serving/200ml	100	0.0	50	0.0	11.9	0.0	0.1
Cranberry, Tesco*	1 Serving/330ml	152	0.0	46	0.0	11.1	0.0	0.0
Cranberry, Tropical, Ocean Spray*	1 Glass/200ml	96	0.0	48	0.1	11.5	0.0	0.0
Cranberry, Waitrose*	1 Serving/250ml	145	0.0	58	0.1	13.9	0.0	0.1
Cranberry & Apple, Ocean Spray*	1 Glass/200ml	92	0.0	46	0.0	11.1	0.0	0.0
Cranberry & Blackberry, Ocean Spray*	1 Glass/250ml	120	0.3	48	0.1	11.3	0.1	0.2
Cranberry & Blackcurrant, Ocean Spray*	1 Bottle/500ml	265	0.0	53	0.2	12.7	0.0	0.0
Cranberry & Blueberry, Ocean Spray*	1 Serving/100ml	48	0.0	48	0.0	11.6	0.0	0.0
Cranberry & Orange, HE, Tesco*	1 Glass/200ml	10	0.0	5	0.0	0.8	0.0	0.0
Cranberry & Raspberry, Asda*	1 Glass/250ml	125	0.0	50	0.2	12.0	0.0	0.0
Cranberry & Raspberry, BGTY, Sainsbury's*	1 Glass/250ml	10	0.3	4	0.1	0.7	0.1	0.1
Cranberry & Raspberry, Ocean Spray*	1 Glass/200ml	104	0.0	52	0.0	12.6	0.0	0.0
Cranberry & Raspberry, Sainsbury's*	1 Serving/250ml	105	0.0	42	0.1	9.9	0.0	0.0
Cranberry & Raspberry, Tesco*	1 Serving/200ml	96	0.0	48	0.0	11.6	0.0	0.0
Exotic, Tesco*	1 Serving/250ml	128	0.0	51	0.1	12.3	0.0	0.0
Fruit Cocktail, Sainsbury's*	1 Glass/200ml	90	0.0	45	0.2	10.6	0.0	0.1
Grape, Apple & Raspberry, Asda*	1 Glass/200ml	90	0.0	45	0.2	11.0	0.0	0.0
Grape, Apple & Raspberry, Co-Op*	1 Serving/150ml	75	0.0	50	0.4	12.0	0.0	0.1
Grapefruit & Cranberry, M & S*	1 Serving/250ml	125	0.3	50	0.2	11.9	0.1	0.0
Guava Exotic, Rubicon*	1 Carton/288ml	150	0.3	52	0.2	12.8	0.1	0.0
J20, Apple & Mango, Britvic*	1 Bottle/275ml	132	0.2	48	0.1	11.3	0.1	0.0
J20, Apple & Raspberry, Britvic*	1 Bottle/275ml	146	0.3	53	0.1	12.0	0.1	0.0
J20, Orange & Passion Fruit, Britvic*	1 Bottle/275ml	132	0.2	48	0.1	11.3	0.1	0.0
Lemon, The Feel Good Drinks Co*	1 Bottle/171.4ml	78	0.2	46	0.1	10.8	0.1	0.0
Lemon & Lime, Light, Oasis*	1 Bottle/250ml	7	0.0	3	0.0	0.2	0.0	0.0
Lemonade, Asda*	1 Glass/200ml	88	0.0	44	0.1	11.0	0.0	0.0
Mango, Rubicon*	1 Serving/100ml	54	0.1	54	0.1	13.1	0.1	0.0
Mango, Sparkling, Rubicon*	1 Can/330ml	172	0.0	52	0.0	12.8	0.0	0.0
Mega Green, Smucker's*	1 Serving/473ml	237	0.0	50	0.0	12.5	0.0	0.0
Orange, Caprisun*	1 Pouch/200ml	89	0.0	45	0.0	10.8	0.0	0.0
Orange, Carrot & Lemon, Pago*	1 Serving/200g	90	0.2	45	0.2	10.5	0.1	0.0
Orange, Fruitish, Spar*	1 Carton/330ml	13	0.3	4	0.1	0.8	0.1	0.0
Orange, HE, Tesco*	1 Glass/200ml	56	0.2	28	0.3	6.1	0.1	0.0
Orange, Juice Burst, Purity*	1 Bottle/500ml	220	0.0	44	1.0	10.2	0.0	0.0
Orange, Morrisons*	1 Serving/250ml	13	0.3	5	0.1	0.9	0.1	0.1
Orange, No Added Sugar, Tesco*	1 fl oz/30ml	1	0.0	4	0.0	0.7	0.0	0.0
Orange, Sainsbury's*	1 Serving/250ml	18	0.3	7	0.1	1.4	0.1	0.1
Orange, Value, Tesco*	1 Glass/250ml	33	0.0	13	0.0	3.3	0.0	0.0
Orange & Banana, Pure, Average	1 Glass/150ml	79	0.1	53	0.7	12.1	0.1	0.2
Orange & Mango, Average	1 Bottle/375ml	176	0.4	47	0.5	10.7	0.1	0.3
Passion Fruit, Exotic, Rubicon*	1 Serving/200ml	110	0.0	55	0.1	13.6	0.0	0.0
Peach, Fruit Float, Frubob*	1 Can/250ml	150	0.0	60	0.2	14.8	0.0	0.0
Peach & Passionfruit Fruit, Sunmagic*	1 Serving/330ml	172	0.0	52	0.3	13.0	0.0	0.1
Pink Grapefruit, Juice Burst, Purity*	1 Bottle/500ml	210	0.0	42	0.4	10.0	0.0	0.0
Pomegranate & Blueberry, Weight Watchers*	1 Bottle/500ml	15	0.0	3	0.0	0.5	0.0	0.0
Pomegranate & Raspberry, Shapers, Boots*	1 Bottle/500ml	45	0.0	9	0.0	2.0	0.0	0.0
Raspberry & Pear, Tesco*	1 Serving/250ml	118	0.0	47	0.0	11.3	0.0	0.0
Spirit, Lemon & Grapefruit, Tropicana*	1 Bottle/400ml	184	0.0	46	0.3	10.4	0.0	0.6
Summer Fruits, Fresh, Tesco*	1 Glass/250ml	113	0.3	45	0.1	10.8	0.1	0.3
Summer Fruits, Oasis*	1 Bottle/500ml	90	0.0	18	0.0	4.2	0.0	0.0
Tropical, Be Light, Aldi*	1 Glass/250mls	63	0.3	25	0.2	5.4	0.1	0.2
Tropical Fruit, Safeway*	1 Glass/250ml	118	0.0	47	0.2	11.2	0.0	0.0
Tropical Fruit, Tesco*	1 Glass/250ml	118	0.0	47	0.0	11.4	0.0	0.0

J

	Measure INFO/WEIGHT	per Measure KCAL	per Measure FAT	Nutrition Values per 100g / 100ml KCAL	PROT	CARB	FAT	FIBRE
JUICE DRINK								
Tropical Fruit, Waitrose*	1 Glass/250ml	118	0.0	47	0.2	11.2	0.0	0.0
Tropical Hit, 5 Alive*	1 Carton/250ml	93	0.0	37	0.0	9.3	0.0	0.0
White Cranberry & Grape, Oceanspay*	1 Serving/100ml	48	0.0	48	0.0	11.6	0.0	0.0
White Cranberry & Lychee, Ocean Spray*	1 Glass/200ml	86	0.0	43	0.0	11.5	0.0	0.0
White Grape & Peach, Sainsbury's*	1 Glass/250ml	95	0.3	38	0.2	9.0	0.1	0.1

J

	Measure INFO/WEIGHT	per Measure KCAL	per Measure FAT	Nutrition Values per 100g / 100ml KCAL	PROT	CARB	FAT	FIBRE
KALE								
Curly, Boiled in Salted Water, Average	1 Sm Serving/60g	14	0.7	24	2.4	1.0	1.1	2.8
Curly, Raw, Average	1 Med Serving/90g	30	1.4	33	3.4	1.4	1.6	3.1
KEBAB								
Barbecue Chicken Tikka, Mini, Somerfield*	1oz/28g	38	1.1	134	21.0	4.0	4.0	0.0
BBQ Pork, Sainsbury's*	1 Serving/90g	65	2.2	72	11.0	1.4	2.4	0.9
Beef & Pepper Kofta, Waitrose*	1 Kebab/138g	223	13.9	162	14.8	2.9	10.1	0.6
Beef with Onion, Dulano, Lidl*	1 Serving/100g	224	16.0	224	18.0	2.0	16.0	0.0
Cajun Salmon, Tesco*	1 Kebab/75g	100	3.2	133	19.8	3.9	4.2	1.3
Chicken, Barbecue, Sainsbury's*	1 Pack/200g	238	3.4	119	24.4	1.5	1.7	1.8
Chicken, Breast, Mediterranean, Sainsbury's*	1 Kebab/65g	73	2.1	113	16.5	4.6	3.2	0.6
Chicken, Breast, Salsa, Sainsbury's*	1 Kebab/80g	94	0.9	118	20.1	6.5	1.1	0.6
Chicken, Breast, Sweet, Oriental, COU, M & S*	½ Pack/200g	220	2.0	110	20.8	4.3	1.0	0.1
Chicken, Caribbean, Iceland*	1 Kebab/44g	36	0.1	82	12.0	8.0	0.2	0.5
Chicken, Chilli & Lime, Breast Fillet, Sainsbury's*	1 Kebab/77g	120	0.7	156	29.9	6.2	0.9	0.3
Chicken, Chinese, Mini, M & S*	1 Kebab/11g	24	1.4	215	19.5	5.1	12.9	0.6
Chicken, Citrus Tikka, Mini, Sainsbury's*	1 Serving/50g	72	1.1	151	30.3	2.7	2.3	0.2
Chicken, Honey & Mustard, M & S*	1oz/28g	41	1.3	145	16.7	8.2	4.8	1.0
Chicken, Indian Style, M & S*	½ Pack/125g	169	3.3	135	27.2	0.9	2.6	0.8
Chicken, Mini Fillet, M & S*	1 Serving/150g	210	8.7	140	20.2	2.0	5.8	0.3
Chicken, Red Pepper, Mini, Sainsbury's*	1 Kebab/52g	79	1.0	152	30.1	3.5	2.0	0.2
Chicken, Sweet Chilli, PB, Waitrose*	1 Kebab/81.5g	110	0.9	135	28.6	1.7	1.1	0.5
Chicken, Thigh, Sticky Barbecue, M & S*	1 Kebab/100g	160	7.5	160	15.6	7.4	7.5	0.8
Chicken, Thin Sliced, Heat 'n' Eat, Asda*	½ Pack/50g	92	6.0	184	15.0	3.9	12.0	1.1
Chicken, with Sweet Chilli Sauce, M & S*	1 Serving/165g	228	1.3	138	17.9	14.7	0.8	1.2
Chicken & Pineapple, Aldi*	1 Kebab/85g	89	2.6	105	13.9	5.3	3.1	0.0
Chicken & Pineapple, Caribbean Style, Iceland*	1 Kebab/44.1g	41	0.6	93	11.6	8.7	1.4	1.4
Chicken & Sausage, with Teriyaki Sauce, Asda*	1 Serving/110g	257	15.4	234	17.0	10.0	14.0	1.0
Chicken Tikka, Breast, Safeway*	1 Kebab/88g	127	0.9	145	23.8	9.8	1.0	0.7
Chicken with Sweet Chilli Sauce, Finest, Tesco*	½ Pack/175g	242	1.4	138	17.9	14.7	0.8	1.2
Chinese Salmon, Iceland*	1 Kebab/75g	115	3.5	153	23.8	4.1	4.6	1.6
Citrus Tikka Chicken Breast, Sainsbury's*	1 Kebab/61g	79	0.3	129	25.6	5.4	0.5	0.9
Doner, Heat 'n' Eat Thin Sliced, Asda*	1 Pack/100g	196	10.6	196	16.7	8.4	10.6	1.7
Doner, Iceland*	1 Serving/152.3g	268	7.1	176	9.2	24.4	4.7	2.4
Doner, Lidl*	1 Kebab/170g	509	31.3	300	14.7	15.3	18.4	0.0
Green Thai Chicken, Waitrose*	1 Serving/180g	223	7.2	124	20.5	1.4	4.0	1.4
Halloumi & Vegetable, Waitrose*	1 Kebab/127g	235	21.6	185	5.6	2.2	17.0	2.4
Honey & Mustard Chicken, Sainsbury's*	1 Serving/50g	66	0.9	131	24.5	4.3	1.8	0.0
Lamb, Greek Style, Lakeland*	1 Serving/100g	196	15.6	196	11.8	1.9	15.6	0.0
Lamb, Greek Style, Sainsbury's*	1 Serving/70g	196	15.3	282	16.1	4.9	22.0	1.8
Lamb, Kofta, Citrus Tikka, Sainsbury's*	1 Kebab/84g	199	11.6	235	18.1	9.8	13.7	2.6
Lamb, Kofta Kleftico, TTD, Sainsbury's*	1 Pack/400g	652	38.8	163	13.5	5.5	9.7	0.5
Lamb, Shish, M & S*	2 Skewers/170g	330	19.9	194	17.1	4.8	11.7	0.6
Lamb, Shish, Sainsbury's*	1 Kebab/85g	179	11.3	210	19.7	2.8	13.3	0.7
Lamb, Shish, Waitrose*	1 Kebab/56.2g	114	7.1	203	15.3	6.8	12.7	1.1
Lamb, Shoulder, M & S*	½ Pack/250g	313	10.8	125	20.4	0.9	4.3	1.7
Lamb, with Halloumi Cheese & Olives, Waitrose*	2 Kebabs/150g	246	12.5	164	20.0	2.4	8.3	0.2
Lamb, with Mint, Tesco*	1 Serving/80g	192	13.4	240	16.0	5.5	16.7	0.4
Lamb Kofta, Indian Style, Waitrose*	1 Kebab/125g	266	19.8	213	12.3	5.5	15.8	1.6
Lamb Kofta, Safeway*	1 Pack/227g	465	30.4	205	14.3	5.8	13.4	1.0
Lamb Kofta with a Mint & Coriander Raita, Safeway*	1 Pack/290g	632	37.7	218	16.9	8.4	13.0	1.2
Lamb Shami with a Mint Raita Dip, M & S*	½ Pack/90g	189	12.1	210	12.8	9.7	13.4	3.5
Mango & Lime Chicken, PB, Waitrose*	2 Kebabs/165g	206	2.6	125	26.0	1.2	1.6	1.1
Mango Salsa Chicken Breast, Sainsbury's*	1 Kebab/60g	85	1.0	142	26.3	5.5	1.6	0.6

K

	Measure	per Measure		Nutrition Values per 100g / 100ml				
	INFO/WEIGHT	KCAL	FAT	KCAL	PROT	CARB	FAT	FIBRE
KEBAB								
Pork & Pepper, BBQ, Sainsbury's*	1 Kebab/41g	65	2.2	158	24.1	3.1	5.4	1.9
Pork & Pepper, Co-Op*	1 Kebab/74g	78	3.0	105	17.0	1.0	4.0	0.5
Pork Sausage, Mini, Grilled, Safeway*	1 Serving/100g	175	13.5	175	9.1	3.4	13.5	1.1
Salmon, Hot & Spicy, Tesco*	1 Kebab/75g	89	2.2	118	22.0	1.1	2.9	0.0
Shish in Pitta Bread with Salad	1oz/28g	43	1.1	155	13.5	17.2	4.1	1.0
Shish with Onions & Peppers	1oz/28g	59	4.5	212	12.9	3.9	16.2	1.2
Spicy Tomato Creole King Prawn, M & S*	1 Pack/240g	240	7.9	100	14.3	2.9	3.3	0.7
Sweetcorn, Tesco*	1 Kebab/130g	74	1.3	57	2.0	9.9	1.0	0.9
Tandoori, M & S*	1oz/28g	34	0.7	120	23.3	1.0	2.5	0.0
Thai Style Chicken, Eat Smart, Safeway*	1 Kebab/85g	85	1.1	100	15.3	6.4	1.3	1.4
Tiger Prawn, Asda*	1oz/28g	17	0.0	59	14.6	0.0	0.1	0.0
Tikka, Mini, M & S*	1 Kebab/11g	23	1.4	205	18.4	4.0	12.7	0.6
Tikka Chicken, Mini, Somerfield*	1oz/28g	38	1.1	134	21.0	4.0	4.0	0.0
Tomato & Basil Chicken, Eat Smart, Safeway*	1 Kebab/71.5g	82	1.5	115	18.0	5.0	2.1	1.5
Turkey, Wth Chinese Style Dressing, Sainsbury's*	1 Kebab/5g	84	2.7	157	21.4	6.4	5.1	1.7
Vegeatable, Mini, Sainsbury's*	1 Kebab/36g	22	0.8	61	2.5	7.4	2.3	2.4
Vegetable, Asda*	1 Kebab/40g	25	1.7	63	1.8	4.5	4.3	2.4
Vegetable, Sainsbury's*	1 Kebab/100g	36	0.5	36	1.5	6.4	0.5	1.2
Vegetable, Tesco*	1 Kebab/120g	47	0.7	39	1.7	6.8	0.6	1.1
KEDGEREE								
Average	1oz/28g	48	2.4	171	15.9	7.8	8.7	0.1
COU, M & S*	1 Pack/370g	389	8.1	105	7.6	13.7	2.2	2.1
Seafood Masala, PB, Waitrose*	1 Pack/400g	380	4.0	95	7.5	13.9	1.0	0.6
Smoked Haddock, Big Dish, M & S*	1 Pack/450g	585	22.5	130	8.5	13.0	5.0	1.9
KETCHUP								
Barbeque, Asda*	1 Tbsp/15g	20	0.0	136	0.9	33.0	0.0	0.0
BBQ, Heinz*	1 Serving/10g	14	0.0	137	1.3	31.3	0.3	0.3
Tomato, Average	1 Tsp/5g	6	0.0	120	1.5	28.1	0.2	0.8
Tomato, Ketchup, Light, Linessa, Lidl*	1 Serving/30g	11	0.0	35	1.7	5.9	0.1	0.0
Tomato, Original, Heinz*	1 Tbsp/15g	15.3	0.0	102	0.9	23.9	0.1	0.6
Tomato, Reduced Sugar, Average	1 Tbsp/10g	9	0.1	87	2.0	16.9	1.2	0.9
Tomato, Reduced Sugar & Salt, Sainsbury's*	1 Serving/5g	5	0.0	92	1.5	20.3	0.1	0.4
Tomato, Value, Tesco*	1 Serving/10g	14	0.0	139	2.3	32.2	0.1	1.4
KIDNEY								
Lamb, Raw, Average	1oz/28g	44	2.2	156	21.5	0.0	7.7	0.0
Ox, Raw	1oz/28g	25	0.6	88	17.2	0.0	2.1	0.0
Ox, Stewed	1oz/28g	39	1.2	138	24.5	0.0	4.4	0.0
Pig, Fried	1oz/28g	57	2.7	202	29.2	0.0	9.5	0.0
Pig, Raw	1oz/28g	24	0.8	86	15.5	0.0	2.7	0.0
Pig, Stewed	1oz/28g	43	1.7	153	24.4	0.0	6.1	0.0
KIEV								
Cheese, Smoked Ham & Chicken, Sainsbury's*	1 Kiev/132g	305	17.6	231	13.0	14.8	13.3	1.2
Cheese & Ham, Tesco*	1 Kiev/142.9g	300	13.7	210	19.2	10.7	9.6	0.4
Cheese & Herb, Mini, Bernard Matthews*	1 Kiev/23g	46	2.3	199	15.7	12.1	9.8	0.0
Cheese & Mushroom Chicken, Somerfield*	½ Pack/142g	294	15.6	207	14.0	15.0	11.0	0.0
Chicken, Bernard Matthews*	1 Kiev/125g	374	27.9	299	10.6	13.9	22.3	2.7
Chicken, BFY, Morrisons*	1 Kiev/134g	304	17.4	227	16.1	11.5	13.0	1.0
Chicken, Breaded, Mini, Family, Bernard Matthews*	1 Kiev/23g	46	2.3	199	15.7	12.1	9.8	0.0
Chicken, Breast, Hand Filled, Birds Eye*	1 Kiev/172g	330	17.2	192	15.5	9.9	10.0	2.0
Chicken, Cheesy Bean, Asda*	1 Kiev/94.0g	202	10.3	215	12.0	17.0	11.0	1.9
Chicken, COU, M & S*	1 Kiev/150g	188	2.7	125	15.8	10.8	1.8	0.5
Chicken, Creamy Garlic, Chilled, Tesco*	½ Pack/142.5g	285	17.1	200	12.9	9.7	12.0	1.3
Chicken, Creamy Pepper, Safeway*	1 Kiev/133g	306	20.5	230	11.9	11.1	15.4	1.1

K

	Measure INFO/WEIGHT	per Measure KCAL	per Measure FAT	Nutrition Values per 100g / 100ml KCAL	PROT	CARB	FAT	FIBRE
KIEV								
Chicken, Creamy Peppercorn, Sun Valley*	1 Kiev/140g	382	25.9	273	13.3	13.5	18.5	0.0
Chicken, Creamy Peppercorn, Tesco*	1 Kiev/142.5g	278	16.1	195	13.7	9.4	11.3	1.4
Chicken, Finest, Tesco*	1 Kiev/237.5g	456	25.9	192	15.8	7.7	10.9	1.5
Chicken, Garlic, Asda*	1 Kiev/125g	299	18.8	239	13.0	13.0	15.0	1.0
Chicken, Garlic, Fresh, Reduced Fat, Morrisons*	1 Kiev/141g	350	25.5	248	13.2	8.0	18.1	0.7
Chicken, Garlic, M & S*	1 Kiev/150g	370	24.8	247	15.6	8.2	16.5	2.9
Chicken, Garlic, Morrisons*	1 Kiev/122g	289	19.2	237	14.3	9.8	15.7	0.0
Chicken, Garlic, Safeway*	1 Kiev/147g	413	30.1	281	12.9	11.2	20.5	0.9
Chicken, Garlic & Herb, Reduced Fat, Safeway*	1 Kiev/125g	270	16.5	216	13.0	11.4	13.2	1.0
Chicken, Garlic & Herb, Reduced Fat, Sainsbury's*	1 Kiev/142g	317	18.0	223	15.1	12.1	12.7	0.6
Chicken, Garlic & Herb, Sainsbury's*	1 Kiev/133.5g	318	19.6	239	15.0	11.7	14.7	1.3
Chicken, Garlic & Mushroom, Sainsbury's*	1 Kiev/142.4g	345	19.0	243	16.2	14.5	13.4	1.4
Chicken, Garlic & Parsley, BGTY, Sainsbury's*	1 Kiev/123g	276	15.8	224	13.6	13.5	12.8	0.6
Chicken, Garlic & Parsley, Sainsbury's*	1 Kiev/120.1g	365	25.6	304	11.1	17.1	21.3	0.8
Chicken, Garlic Butter, HL, Tesco*	1 Kiev/142.5g	285	16.4	200	14.3	9.9	11.5	0.6
Chicken, Garlic Butter, Safeway*	1 Kiev/115g	316	22.0	275	13.3	12.5	19.1	1.1
Chicken, Garlic Butter, Somerfield*	1 Kiev/142g	425	33.9	299	12.6	8.5	23.9	1.2
Chicken, Good Choice, Iceland*	1 Kiev/120g	366	27.2	305	12.7	12.6	22.7	0.8
Chicken, Ham, & Cheese, Tesco*	1 Serving/142.5g	306	18.5	215	14.4	9.3	13.0	1.3
Chicken, in Crispy Breadcrumbs, Sainsbury's*	1 Kiev/116.5g	311	22.5	266	12.8	10.6	19.2	1.1
Chicken, Italian Style, Sainsbury's*	1 Kiev/134.8g	342	21.7	253	14.3	12.8	16.1	1.3
Chicken, Maitre Jean-Pierre*	1 Kiev/140g	385	26.7	275	13.3	12.7	19.1	0.8
Chicken, Tesco*	1oz/28g	86	7.2	307	11.4	7.6	25.7	1.6
Chicken, Tomato & Mozzerella, Tesco*	1 Kiev/142.5g	285	17.4	200	13.4	9.0	12.2	1.4
Chicken, Value, Tesco*	1 Serving/125g	355	27.1	284	10.4	11.7	21.7	1.8
Chicken, White Wine & Mushroom, Tesco*	1 Serving/145g	281	13.8	194	16.7	10.3	9.5	0.5
Chicken Breast, Garlic, Frozen, Tesco*	1 Kiev/141g	430	34.7	305	13.0	6.9	24.6	1.3
Chicken Breast, Garlic Butter, Sun Valley*	1 Kiev/141g	436	32.7	309	13.2	11.8	23.2	0.9
Cod & Parsley, Safeway*	1 Kiev/160g	310	14.7	194	10.6	17.0	9.2	0.0
Garlic & Parsley, TTD, Sainsbury's*	1 Kiev/150g	371	23.4	247	15.7	11.1	15.6	0.8
Ham & Cheese Chicken, Somerfield*	½ Pack/142g	294	15.6	207	14.0	14.0	11.0	0.0
Lemon Butter Chicken, Somerfield*	½ Pack/142g	409	29.8	288	12.0	12.0	21.0	0.0
Mushroom & Cheese, Oven Baked, Safeway*	1 Kiev/100g	305	17.3	305	22.6	14.8	17.3	1.9
Salmon, Fillet, Tesco*	1 Kiev/160g	376	19.5	235	13.3	18.0	12.2	2.5
Tikka, Safeway*	1 Kiev/132g	327	23.1	248	11.9	10.5	17.5	1.0
Tikka Chicken, Asda*	1 Kiev/133.7g	274	14.8	205	12.8	13.5	11.1	0.6
Turkey, Mini, Baked, Bernard Matthews*	1 Kiev/22.5g	50	2.7	221	17.5	11.2	11.8	1.1
KIEV VEGETARIAN								
Cheesy Garlic, Meat Free, Sainsbury's*	1 Kiev/123g	263	14.0	214	17.3	10.6	11.4	3.0
Garlic Butter, Tivall*	1 Kiev/125g	366	26.3	293	15.1	10.8	21.0	2.6
Meat Free, Garlic Butter, Tesco*	1 Kiev/125g	256	13.8	205	17.0	9.0	11.0	3.0
Vegetable, M & S*	1 Kiev/155g	326	20.8	210	4.6	17.8	13.4	2.5
KIPPER								
Baked, Average	1oz/28g	57	3.2	205	25.5	0.0	11.4	0.0
Fillets, in Brine, John West*	1 Can/140g	269	16.8	192	21.0	0.0	12.0	0.0
Fillets, in Sunflower Oil, John West*	1 Can/140g	321	23.8	229	19.0	0.0	17.0	0.0
Fillets, Raw, Average	1 Serving/200g	451	34.3	226	17.0	0.0	17.1	0.0
Fillets, Smoked, Fresh, TTD, Sainsbury's*	1 Fillet/140g	357	27.2	255	20.1	0.1	19.4	0.0
Fillets, Smoked, with Butter, Boil in Bag, Tesco*	1 Serving/200g	450	34.4	225	17.0	0.0	17.2	0.0
Fillets, with Butter, Farmfoods*	1oz/28g	64	5.0	229	17.5	0.0	17.7	0.0
Fillets, with Butter, Scottish, M & S*	1 Pack/200g	382	27.6	191	16.7	0.0	13.8	0.0
Fillets, with Butter, Scottish, Somerfield*	1 Serving/100g	178	12.4	178	16.5	0.0	12.4	0.0
Grilled, Average	1oz/28g	71	5.4	255	20.1	0.0	19.4	0.0

K

	Measure INFO/WEIGHT	per Measure KCAL	FAT	Nutrition Values per 100g / 100ml KCAL	PROT	CARB	FAT	FIBRE
KIPPER								
Raw, Average	1oz/28g	64	5.0	229	17.5	0.0	17.7	0.0
Smoked, Average	1 Serving/150g	322	23.0	215	18.9	0.0	15.4	0.0
KIT KAT								
2 Finger, Nestle*	2 Fingers/21g	106	5.5	507	5.9	62.0	26.1	0.0
4 Fingers, Nestle*	4 Fingers/45.5g	233	12.2	512	5.5	62.0	26.8	1.1
Caramac, 4 Finger, Nestle*	4 Fingers/48.7g	261	14.2	532	5.9	61.9	29.0	0.6
Chunky, Nestle*	1 Bar/55g	283	15.1	514	5.6	61.3	27.4	1.0
Chunky, Peanut, Nestle*	1 Bar/50g	269	15.8	537	8.4	54.9	31.5	0.0
Chunky, Snack Size, Nestle*	1 Bar/26g	133	7.1	513	6.6	60.4	27.2	1.1
Low Carb, 4 Finger, Nestle*	1 Finger/11g	46	3.3	438	9.2	28.3	31.3	1.3
Mini, Nestle*	1 Bar/15g	75	3.9	502	7.5	59.4	26.0	0.0
Mint, Nestle*	4 Fingers/48g	244	12.7	508	6.0	61.5	26.4	1.1
Orange, 2 Finger, Nestle*	1 Bar/21.1g	107	5.6	507	5.5	61.7	26.5	0.0
Senses, Nestle*	1 Bar/31g	165	9.5	532	7.4	56.5	30.7	0.0
White, Chunky, Nestle*	1 Bar/53g	276	14.6	521	8.3	60.3	27.5	0.7
KIWI FRUIT								
Fresh, Raw, Average	1oz/28g	14	0.1	49	1.1	10.6	0.5	1.9
Weighed with Skin, Average	1 Kiwi/60g	25	0.2	42	1.0	9.1	0.4	1.6
KOHLRABI								
Boiled in Salted Water	1oz/28g	5	0.1	18	1.2	3.1	0.2	1.9
Raw	1oz/28g	6	0.1	23	1.6	3.7	0.2	2.2
KORMA								
Chicken, & Basmati Rice, Tesco*	1 Pot/350g	588	32.6	168	4.3	16.9	9.3	2.3
Chicken, & Pilau Rice, BGTY, Sainsbury's*	1 Pack/400g	404	5.2	101	8.0	14.3	1.3	0.6
Chicken, & Pilau Rice, GFY, Asda*	1 Pack/400g	600	24.0	150	8.0	16.0	6.0	1.3
Chicken, & Pilau Rice, Good Intentions, Somerfield*	1 Pack/400g	472	11.6	118	7.7	15.3	2.9	0.8
Chicken, & Pilau Rice, Morrisons*	1 Pack/450g	889	48.2	198	9.4	15.9	10.7	1.4
Chicken, & Pilau Rice, Somerfield*	1 Pack/340g	687	37.4	202	9.0	16.0	11.0	0.0
Chicken, & Pilau Rice, Tesco*	1 Serving/460g	722	45.1	157	5.6	11.5	9.8	1.3
Chicken, & Rice, 95% Fat Free, Birds Eye*	1 Pack/370g	444	7.0	120	6.2	19.6	1.9	1.1
Chicken, & Rice, Good Choice, Iceland*	1 Pack/400g	464	8.4	116	5.8	18.4	2.1	0.8
Chicken, & Rice, HL, Co-Op*	1 Pack/400g	480	8.0	120	8.0	17.0	2.0	1.0
Chicken, & Rice, HL, Tesco*	1 Pack/450g	487	9.9	108	6.8	15.3	2.2	0.8
Chicken, & Rice, Indian Meal for Two, Sainsbury's*	1 Pack/501g	787	40.6	157	6.8	14.3	8.1	3.1
Chicken, & Rice, Organic, Tesco*	1 Pack/450g	923	47.7	205	6.0	21.5	10.6	0.4
Chicken, & Rice, World Flavours*	1 Pack/500g	705	23.5	141	8.7	16.0	4.7	0.0
Chicken, & White Rice, BGTY, Frozen, Sainsbury's*	1 Pack/375g	341	3.8	91	5.6	14.9	1.0	0.5
Chicken, Curry & Rice, Tesco*	1 Pack/450g	495	10.8	110	7.1	15.2	2.4	1.4
Chicken, Fresh, Chilled, Tesco*	1 Pack/350g	819	60.9	234	13.1	6.3	17.4	2.3
Chicken, HL, Tesco*	1 Pack/350g	371	4.2	106	7.7	15.9	1.2	0.8
Chicken, Indian, Take Away, Tesco*	½ Pack/175g	222	13.5	127	9.0	5.5	7.7	1.8
Chicken, Indian Meal for 2, Finest, Tesco*	½ Pack/200g	348	24.0	174	10.3	6.2	12.0	2.5
Chicken, Indian Takeaway, Iceland*	1 Pack/400g	656	44.0	164	11.0	4.5	11.0	1.4
Chicken, Indian Takeaway for One, Sainsbury's*	1 Serving/300g	498	30.9	166	13.0	5.3	10.3	1.6
Chicken, Less Than 3% Fat, Birds Eye*	1 Pack/358g	440	6.8	123	6.5	20.4	1.9	0.8
Chicken, Morrisons*	1 Pack/350g	707	46.6	202	13.6	7.0	13.3	0.7
Chicken, Plumrose*	1 Can/392g	431	22.0	110	8.0	6.9	5.6	0.0
Chicken, Rich & Creamy, Sainsbury's*	½ Pack/200g	356	24.2	178	14.4	2.8	12.1	2.6
Chicken, Safeway*	1 Pack/350g	648	37.1	185	14.1	8.4	10.6	2.0
Chicken, Tesco*	1 Pack/350g	620	41.3	177	10.8	6.8	11.8	0.6
Chicken, Tinned, Asda*	½ Can/196.9g	321	21.7	163	8.0	8.0	11.0	2.3
Chicken, Waitrose*	1 Pack/399.4g	678	46.7	170	13.7	2.4	11.7	1.9
Chicken, with Basmati Rice, Eat Smart, Safeway*	1 Pack/380g	399	7.2	105	7.0	13.8	1.9	1.5

K

	Measure INFO/WEIGHT	per Measure		Nutrition Values per 100g / 100ml				
		KCAL	FAT	KCAL	PROT	CARB	FAT	FIBRE
KORMA								
Chicken, with Coriander & Rice, Slim Fast*	1 Pack/375g	394	3.4	105	5.7	18.6	0.9	0.7
Chicken, with Peshwari Coriander Rice, Finest, Tesco*	1 Pack/550g	908	48.4	165	7.5	13.9	8.8	0.9
Chicken, with Pilau Rice, Asda*	1 Serving/350g	735	49.0	210	12.0	9.0	14.0	2.0
Chicken, with Pilau Rice, PB, Waitrose*	1 Pack/400g	452	6.8	113	8.9	15.4	1.7	1.3
Chicken, with Pilau Rice, Safeway*	1 Pack/400g	784	43.6	196	7.6	16.9	10.9	2.4
Chicken, with Pilau Rice, Sharwood's*	1 Pack/375g	566	26.3	151	6.7	15.4	7.0	0.9
Creamy, with Pilau Rice, Safeway*	1 Pack/400g	560	22.8	140	5.2	15.8	5.7	2.3
Vegetable, Ready to Cook, Fresh, Sainsbury's*	½ Pack/255g	263	17.3	103	2.8	7.7	6.8	2.1
Vegetable, Sainsbury's*	1 Serving/200g	302	25.2	151	2.7	6.6	12.6	2.2
Vegetable & Rice, Tesco*	1 Pack/450g	621	26.6	138	2.9	18.3	5.9	1.6
Vegetable with Rice, Eat Smart, Safeway*	1 Pack/400g	412	9.2	103	3.1	17.5	2.3	1.6
KRISPROLLS								
Cracked Wheat, Original, Pagen*	2 Rolls/25g	95	1.8	380	12.0	67.0	7.0	9.0
Golden, Swedish Toasts, Pagen*	1 Krisproll/12g	48	1.0	400	11.0	69.0	8.5	5.0
KULFI								
Average	1oz/28g	119	11.2	424	5.4	11.8	39.9	0.6
KUMQUATS								
Canned, in Syrup	1oz/28g	39	0.1	138	0.4	35.4	0.5	1.7
Raw	1oz/28g	12	0.1	43	0.9	9.3	0.5	3.8

	Measure INFO/WEIGHT	per Measure KCAL	FAT	Nutrition Values per 100g / 100ml KCAL	PROT	CARB	FAT	FIBRE
LACES								
Apple Flavour, Tesco*	5 Laces/15g	52	0.5	347	3.6	74.8	3.2	2.1
Strawberry, Fizzy, Somerfield*	1 Pack/100g	380	2.0	380	3.0	86.0	2.0	0.0
Strawberry, Sainsbury's*	1 Serving/25g	94	1.2	377	3.3	76.3	4.6	0.1
Strawberry, Tesco*	1 Serving/75g	260	2.4	347	3.6	74.8	3.2	2.1
LAGER								
Alcohol Free, Becks*	1 Serving/275ml	55	0.0	20	0.7	5.0	0.0	0.0
Amstel, Heinekin 'n' V*	1 Pint/568ml	227	0.0	40	0.5	3.0	0.0	0.0
Average	1 Pint/568ml	233	0.0	41	0.3	3.1	0.0	0.0
Becks*	1 Can/275ml	113	0.0	41	0.0	3.0	0.0	0.0
Blanc, Kronenbourg*	1 Serving/250ml	105	0.0	42	0.0	3.3	0.0	0.0
C2, Carling*	½ Pint/284ml	80	0.0	28	0.0	3.5	0.0	0.0
Draught, Carling*	1 Pint/568ml	189	0.0	33	0.0	1.4	0.0	0.0
Export, Carlsberg*	1 Can/440ml	189	0.0	43	0.4	4.0	0.0	0.4
Export, Foster's*	1 Pint/568ml	210	0.0	37	0.0	2.2	0.0	0.0
Foster's*	1 Pint/568ml	227	0.0	40	0.0	3.1	0.0	0.0
German, Low Alcohol, Sainsbury's*	1 Bottle/330ml	92	0.3	28	0.4	5.9	0.1	0.1
Grolsch*	1 Sm Can/330ml	145	0.0	44	0.0	2.2	0.0	0.0
Heineken, Heineken 'n' V*	1 Pint/568ml	256	0.0	45	0.5	3.0	0.0	0.0
Heineken*, 5%	1 Bottle/250ml	110	0.0	44	0.4	3.4	0.0	0.0
Kaliber, Guinness*	1 Can/440ml	79	0.0	18	0.0	3.8	0.0	0.0
Light, Coors*	1 Pint/500ml	204	0.0	41	0.0	0.0	0.0	0.0
Light, Corona*	1 Bottle/330ml	105	0.0	32	1.5	0.0	0.0	0.0
Light, Michelob*	1 Serving/340ml	113	0.0	33	0.3	2.0	0.0	0.0
Low Alcohol	1 Can/440ml	44	0.0	10	0.2	1.5	0.0	0.0
Organic, Tesco*	1 Bottle/500ml	215	0.0	43	0.2	3.5	0.0	0.0
Pills, Holsten*	1 Can/440ml	167	0.0	38	0.3	2.4	0.0	0.0
Premier, Kronenbourg*	1 Serving/100ml	48	0.0	48	0.0	0.0	0.0	0.0
Premium	1 Can/440ml	260	0.0	59	0.3	2.4	0.0	0.0
Premium, Co-Op*	1 Can/440ml	132	0.4	30	0.4	0.9	0.1	0.0
Premium, French, Biere Speciale, Tesco*	1 Serving/250ml	105	0.0	42	0.3	3.3	0.0	0.0
Premium, Tesco*	1 Can/440	229	0.0	52	0.4	4.0	0.0	0.0
Shandy, Traditional Style, Asda*	1 Serving/200ml	44	0.0	22	0.0	4.6	0.0	0.0
Ultra Low Carb, Michelob*	1 Bottle/275ml	88	0.0	32	0.2	0.9	0.0	0.0
Value, Tesco*	1 Can/440ml	75	0.0	17	0.2	1.2	0.0	0.0
LAKSA								
Chicken, COU, M & S*	1 Pack/450g	360	9.9	80	7.5	7.0	2.2	1.1
Thai Noodle, with Chicken, M & S*	1 Pack/400g	460	21.6	115	7.0	9.8	5.4	1.1
LAMB								
Braised, Shanks with Chunky Vegetables, M & S*	½ Pack/425g	808	38.3	190	24.7	2.0	9.0	0.7
Chops, Average	1oz/28g	65	4.6	231	20.6	0.4	16.4	0.0
Chops, Leg, with Mint Gravy, Tesco*	1 Serving/175g	214	9.8	122	15.0	3.2	5.6	1.7
Chops, Minted, Average	1 Chop/100g	260	15.1	260	25.9	5.1	15.1	0.3
Chops, Shoulder, Mango & Mint, Waitrose*	1 Chop/250g	555	40.5	222	16.7	2.3	16.2	0.5
Cutlets, Neck, Raw, Lean & Fat, Weighed with Bone	1 Pack 210g	485	42.8	231	11.9	0.0	20.4	0.0
Diced, From Supermarket, Healthy Range, Average	½ Pack/200g	277	8.9	138	24.6	0.1	4.5	0.0
Escalope, Asda*	1 Serving/100g	173	5.0	173	32.0	0.0	5.0	0.0
Escalope, British, HL, Tesco*	1 Piece/95g	105	3.1	110	20.1	0.0	3.3	0.0
Grill Steak, Average	1oz/28g	70	4.7	251	20.2	4.4	16.9	0.4
Grill Steak, Minted, Sainsbury's*	1 Serving/138g	313	17.3	227	24.6	4.0	12.5	1.0
Grill Steak, Prime, Average	1 Steak/63g	197	16.1	312	18.5	2.1	25.5	0.1
Grill Steak, Rosemary & Mint, Tesco*	1 Steak/62g	172	10.9	277	24.4	5.6	17.6	1.8
Joint, with a Sticky Plum & Orange Glaze, Waitrose*	1 Serving/100g	164	7.9	164	13.4	9.8	7.9	3.1
Joint, with Gravy, Tesco*	1 Serving/225g	277	13.1	123	14.9	2.8	5.8	0.0

L

	Measure INFO/WEIGHT	per Measure KCAL	FAT	Nutrition Values per 100g / 100ml KCAL	PROT	CARB	FAT	FIBRE
LAMB								
Joint, with Mango & Mint Sauce, Boneless, Asda*	1 Serving/100g	302	22.0	302	26.0	0.0	22.0	1.4
Joint, with Mint Gravy, Tesco*	1 Serving/100g	88	1.7	88	16.6	1.8	1.7	0.1
Joint, with Rosemary, Tesco*	1 Serving/125g	250	17.6	200	17.5	0.8	14.1	0.5
Joint, with Sweet Mint Dressing, Tesco*	1 Serving/50g	97	5.9	193	19.9	1.8	11.8	0.6
Leg, Butterflied, COOK!, M & S*	1 Serving/156g	304	18.4	195	14.7	7.6	11.8	0.5
Leg, Chops, with Mint, Morrisons*	2 Chops/350g	858	45.2	245	29.4	2.4	12.9	0.9
Leg, Joint, Raw, Average	1 Joint/510g	858	45.5	168	20.9	1.4	8.9	0.2
Leg, Roasted, Lean, Average	1oz/28g	58	2.7	206	29.9	0.0	9.6	0.0
Leg, Roasted, Lean & Fat, Average	1oz/28g	66	3.8	237	28.6	0.0	13.6	0.0
Mince, Average	1oz/28g	58	4.2	207	17.7	0.5	14.9	0.1
Mince, Extra Lean, Sainsbury's*	1 Serving/225g	324	11.9	144	24.1	0.0	5.3	0.1
Rack, Raw, Lean & Fat	1oz/28g	79	6.7	283	17.3	0.0	23.8	0.0
Rack, Roasted, Lean	1oz/28g	63	3.6	225	27.1	0.0	13.0	0.0
Rack, Roasted, Lean & Fat	1oz/28g	102	8.4	363	23.0	0.0	30.1	0.0
Roast, Bernard Matthews*	1 Serving/200g	434	31.0	217	19.3	0.1	15.5	0.0
Shank, in Rich Minted Gravy, Morrisons*	1 Pack/400g	612	26.4	153	18.8	5.2	6.6	0.0
Shank, Mediterranean, Finest, Tesco*	1 Serving/404g	671	35.6	166	15.0	6.6	8.8	2.0
Shank, Roasted with Vegetables, M & S*	½ Pack/420g	660	30.6	157	14.9	8.3	7.3	0.7
Shank, Tesco*	1 Serving/350g	721	46.2	206	20.1	1.6	13.2	0.7
Shank, Tuscan, Somerfield*	½ Shank/200g	350	17.4	175	19.0	5.2	8.7	1.5
Shank, with Rosemary Gravy, Sainsbury's*	1 Serving/200g	204	8.2	102	13.2	3.1	4.1	0.3
Shoulder, Cooked, Lean & Fat	1oz/28g	84	6.3	301	24.4	0.0	22.5	0.0
Shoulder, Raw, Average	1oz/28g	70	5.7	249	16.8	0.0	20.2	0.0
Steak, Leg, Raw, Average	1 Steak/150g	169	5.5	113	20.1	0.0	3.7	0.0
Steak, Minted, Average	1 Steak/125g	212	9.0	170	22.7	3.4	7.2	0.9
Steak, Raw, Average	1 Steak/140g	190	7.6	136	21.7	0.2	5.4	0.0
Steaks, with Mint Butter, Leg, Waitrose*	1 Serving/155g	270	16.3	174	19.6	0.4	10.5	0.1
Stewing, Raw, Lean & Fat	1oz/28g	57	3.5	203	22.5	0.0	12.6	0.0
Stewing, Stewed, Lean	1oz/28g	67	4.1	240	26.6	0.0	14.8	0.0
Stewing, Stewed, Lean & Fat	1oz/28g	78	5.6	279	24.4	0.0	20.1	0.0
Tagine, Moroccan Style, with Couscous, COU, M & S*	1 Pack/400g	340	5.6	85	8.9	8.3	1.4	1.6
LAMB BRAISED								
& Mash, Tesco*	1 Serving/450g	413	12.2	92	6.1	10.7	2.7	0.8
LAMB DINNER								
Roast, Birds Eye*	1 Dinner/340g	370	14.0	109	5.9	12.1	4.1	1.5
LAMB IN								
a Pot, Sainsbury's*	1 Pack/450g	554	17.1	123	7.6	14.6	3.8	0.7
a Rich Balsamic Sauce, Shank, Safeway*	½ Pack/705g	1304	77.6	185	18.0	3.1	11.0	0.9
Gravy, Minted, Roast, M & S*	1 Pack/200g	140	3.0	70	6.8	6.6	1.5	0.9
Gravy, Roast, Birds Eye*	1 Pack/239g	160	5.3	67	8.1	3.8	2.2	0.1
Mint Gravy, Sliced, Sainsbury's*	1 Pack/125g	134	4.8	107	15.3	2.9	3.8	0.8
Minted Gravy, Shank, Iceland*	1 Shank/284.5g	569	35.6	200	19.4	2.4	12.5	0.5
LAMB MEAL								
Roast, M & S*	1 Meal/360g	560	23.4	156	7.4	16.6	6.5	1.2
LAMB MOROCCAN								
with Cous Cous, PB, Waitrose*	1 Pack/400g	390	5.2	98	7.7	13.6	1.3	2.2
with Cous Cous, PB, Waitrose*	1 Pack/400g	390	5.2	98	7.7	13.6	1.3	2.2
LAMB WITH								
Carrot & Swede Mash, Braised, Eat Smart, Morrisons*	1 Pack/400g	304	9.2	76	5.2	8.2	2.3	1.5
Cous Cous, Morrocan Style, Tesco*	1 Pack/550g	710	14.9	129	6.6	19.6	2.7	1.3
Rosemary, Ready to Roast, M & S*	1 Serving/100g	165	10.5	165	17.7	1.4	10.5	0.2
LARD								
Average	1oz/28g	249	27.7	891	0.0	0.0	99.0	0.0

L

	Measure INFO/WEIGHT	per Measure KCAL	per Measure FAT	Nutrition Values per 100g / 100ml KCAL	PROT	CARB	FAT	FIBRE

LASAGNE

	Measure INFO/WEIGHT	KCAL	FAT	KCAL	PROT	CARB	FAT	FIBRE
Al Forno, Beef, M & S*	1 Pack/400g	640	38.0	160	8.2	10.7	9.5	2.8
Asda*	1 Pack/398.4g	502	23.9	126	7.3	10.6	6.0	1.1
Asparagus, M & S*	1 Pack/360g	432	22.0	120	4.3	11.9	6.1	1.1
Balsamic Onion & Chicken, M & S*	1 Pack/375g	563	25.1	150	9.5	12.5	6.7	1.5
Basics, Sainsbury's*	1 Pack/300g	330	12.9	110	4.8	13.1	4.3	1.2
Beef, 3% Less Fat, Eat Smart, Safeway*	1 Pack/380g	342	8.7	90	5.9	11.1	2.3	1.3
Beef, Asda*	1 Pack/400g	372	14.4	93	4.2	11.0	3.6	0.6
Beef, BGTY, Sainsbury's*	1 Pack/400g	352	8.0	88	7.8	9.8	2.0	1.4
Beef, Chilled, Safeway*	½ Pack/325g	452	19.2	139	7.5	11.8	5.9	1.2
Beef, Eat Smart, Safeway*	1 Pack/380g	380	10.3	100	7.6	10.9	2.7	1.3
Beef, Frozen, Co-Op*	1 Pack/340g	388	15.6	114	7.5	10.7	4.6	1.4
Beef, Frozen, Eat Smart, Morrisons*	1 Pack/380g	331	10.3	87	6.1	9.5	2.7	1.3
Beef, Frozen, GFY, Asda*	1 Pack/400g	380	10.4	95	6.0	12.0	2.6	0.7
Beef, Frozen, Heinz, Weight Watchers*	1 Pack/300g	259	8.3	86	5.3	10.0	2.8	0.3
Beef, Frozen, Morrisons*	1 Serving/250g	373	21.0	149	6.3	12.0	8.4	0.3
Beef, Frozen, Tesco*	1 Pack/450g	608	25.2	135	7.5	12.6	5.6	0.8
Beef, GFY, Asda*	1 Pack/350g	385	7.0	110	9.0	14.0	2.0	1.0
Beef, HL, Tesco*	1 Pack/450g	450	10.4	100	6.7	12.6	2.3	1.4
Beef, Less Than 5% Fat, Asda*	1 Pack/400g	460	17.2	115	5.0	14.0	4.3	0.6
Beef, Low Saturated Fat, Waitrose*	1 Pack/400g	312	6.0	78	4.7	11.4	1.5	0.4
Beef, Ready Meals, Waitrose*	1 Pack/325g	361	16.7	111	5.8	10.4	5.1	0.8
Beef, Taste of Italy, Somerfield*	½ Pack/300g	270	8.1	90	5.1	11.3	2.7	1.0
Beef, TTD, Sainsbury's*	1 Pack/400g	632	28.4	158	9.7	13.7	7.1	0.6
Beef, with Fresh Pasta, Birds Eye*	1 Pack/400g	396	9.2	99	7.3	12.2	2.3	0.5
Beef & Chunky Vegetable, HL, Tesco*	1 Pack/340g	354	9.5	104	5.9	13.8	2.8	1.2
BFY, Morrisons*	1 Pack/350g	340	14.0	97	7.1	8.6	4.0	0.2
Bolognese, Co-Op*	1 Pack/500g	758	35.5	152	8.1	13.8	7.1	0.0
Bolognese, Lidl*	1 Serving/200g	336	18.0	168	8.0	13.7	9.0	0.0
Bolognese, Trattorie Alfredo*	1 Serving/125g	204	11.3	163	9.0	13.0	9.0	0.0
Chicken, HL, Tesco*	1 Pack/400g	388	7.2	97	9.9	10.3	1.8	1.2
Chicken, Italian, Sainsbury's*	1 Pack/450g	549	18.9	122	8.4	12.6	4.2	0.5
Chicken, Italiano, Tesco*	1 Serving/450g	491	13.5	109	8.6	12.0	3.0	0.6
Chicken, Mushroom & Asparagus, Finest, Tesco*	½ Pack/300g	360	16.2	120	7.6	10.2	5.4	0.8
Chicken, Ready Meals, Waitrose*	1 Pack/300g	411	19.8	137	6.3	13.0	6.6	0.9
Chicken, Safeway*	1 Pack/400g	420	18.4	105	7.2	8.6	4.6	1.1
Chilled, Somerfield*	1 Pack/300g	312	9.3	104	6.8	12.2	3.1	1.3
Classic, Deep Filled, M & S*	1 Pack/400g	760	47.6	190	10.0	11.2	11.9	0.6
Extra Special, Asda*	½ Pack/290.9g	416	20.4	143	7.0	13.0	7.0	0.3
Family, M & S*	¼ Pack/225g	281	14.0	125	10.3	6.9	6.2	1.1
Finest, Tesco*	½ Pack/310g	425	22.3	137	7.4	10.7	7.2	0.8
Fresh, Findus*	1 Pack/350g	403	15.8	115	6.2	11.7	4.5	1.0
Frozen, Safeway*	1 Serving/400g	455	18.4	114	6.0	11.8	4.6	0.2
GFY, Asda*	1 Pack/410g	344	8.2	84	5.5	11.0	2.0	0.3
Good Choice, Iceland*	1 Pack/400g	444	15.2	111	7.7	11.6	3.8	0.2
HL, Tesco*	1 Pack/430g	426	11.2	99	6.4	12.5	2.6	0.7
Iceland*	1 Pack/400g	548	22.0	137	7.5	14.3	5.5	0.9
Italian, Family, Asda*	¼ Pack/184.6	306	18.5	166	8.0	11.0	10.0	1.7
Italian, Fresh, Chilled, Sainsbury's*	1 Pack/400g	480	22.0	120	10.1	7.5	5.5	1.4
Italian, Tesco*	1 Pack/400g	540	28.8	135	6.3	11.1	7.2	1.5
Layered, Asda*	1 Pack/300g	444	24.0	148	5.0	14.0	8.0	0.3
Less Than 5% Fat, BFY, Morrisons*	½ Pack/350g	227	8.8	65	5.9	8.2	2.5	0.7
Low Fat, Co-Op*	1 Pack/300g	255	9.0	85	6.0	10.0	3.0	1.0
M & S*	1/3 Pack/333g	466	24.6	140	8.5	10.4	7.4	0.9

L

	Measure INFO/WEIGHT	per Measure KCAL	FAT	KCAL	PROT	CARB	FAT	FIBRE
LASAGNE								
Made with Scottish Beef, TTD, Sainsbury's*	1 Pack/400g	596	31.2	149	10.1	9.6	7.8	2.2
Meat, Somerfield*	1 Pack/600g	768	36.0	128	6.0	12.0	6.0	0.0
Mediterranean Vegetable, COU, M & S*	1 Pack/360g	306	9.7	85	3.4	11.5	2.7	1.4
Mega, Value, Tesco*	1 Pack/600g	726	35.4	121	4.7	12.2	5.9	0.5
Minced Beef, Great Stuff, Asda*	1 Pack/300g	333	13.2	111	6.2	11.7	4.4	1.3
Pepperoni, Chicago Town*	1 Serving/500g	865	44.0	173	4.0	17.4	8.8	0.0
Pizza Express*	1 Serving/350g	514	24.3	147	6.2	14.9	6.9	1.4
Primana, Aldi*	1 Serving/250g	423	22.5	169	8.0	14.0	9.0	0.0
Roasted Mushrooms, Safeway*	1 Serving/400g	440	20.0	110	3.9	11.2	5.0	1.4
Roasted Vegetable, GFY, Asda*	1 Pack/425g	306	7.2	72	3.3	10.9	1.7	1.6
Safeway*	1 Pack/300g	354	16.5	118	5.7	11.5	5.5	0.5
Sheets, Boiled, Average	1oz/28g	28	0.2	100	3.0	22.0	0.6	0.9
Sheets, Cooked, Safeway*	1 Serving/125g	184	1.8	147	5.5	28.3	1.4	1.8
Sheets, Dry, Average	1 Sheet/20g	70	0.3	349	11.9	72.1	1.5	2.9
Sheets, Dry, Trufree*	1 Serving/75g	263	1.5	350	8.0	75.0	2.0	2.0
Sheets, Fresh, Dry, Average	1 Sheet/21g	56	0.4	271	10.9	52.7	2.1	1.9
Sheets, Verdi, Dry, Average	1 Serving/50g	178	1.1	356	12.7	71.1	2.3	2.8
Smoked Salmon & Asparagus, Sainsbury's*	1 Pack/350g	665	37.5	190	7.9	15.6	10.7	0.7
Spinach & Cheese, Italian, Sainsbury's*	1 Pack/450g	666	30.6	148	6.0	15.5	6.8	0.5
Spinach & Ricotta, Asda*	1 Pack/400g	488	24.0	122	4.9	12.0	6.0	1.5
Spinach & Ricotta, Finest, Tesco*	1 Pack/350g	585	37.1	167	6.1	11.7	10.6	1.2
Traditional, Finest, Tesco*	½ Pack/500g	720	31.0	144	7.4	14.7	6.2	1.2
Triangles with Chicken, COU, M & S*	1 Pack/360g	324	6.5	90	7.8	11.9	1.8	1.0
Value, Tesco*	1 Pack/300g	330	15.0	110	3.3	12.9	5.0	0.8
Vegetable, Average	1oz/28g	29	1.2	102	4.1	12.4	4.4	1.0
Vegetable, BGTY, Sainsbury's*	1 Pack/400g	320	8.0	80	4.6	11.0	2.0	3.1
Vegetable, Chilled, BGTY, Sainsbury's*	1 Pack/400g	288	6.4	72	4.8	9.5	1.6	1.4
Vegetable, Findus*	1 Pack/330g	314	8.3	95	4.0	13.0	2.5	0.0
Vegetable, Italian, Frozen, Cooked, Sainsbury's*	1 Pack/378g	442	18.9	117	4.6	13.5	5.0	1.1
Vegetable, Italian Roasted, Asda*	1 Serving/200g	234	14.0	117	2.6	11.0	7.0	0.7
Vegetable, Italian Three Layer, Sainsbury's*	1 Pack/450g	554	23.4	123	4.8	14.3	5.2	0.5
Vegetable, Italiano, Tesco*	1 Pack/410g	369	13.5	90	2.7	11.7	3.3	1.2
Vegetable, Less Than 3% Fat, BGTY, Sainsbury's*	1 Pack/400g	277	6.9	69	5.0	9.5	1.7	2.7
Vegetable, Low Fat, Co-Op*	1 Pack/300g	195	6.0	65	4.0	10.0	2.0	1.0
Vegetable, Luxury Roasted, Safeway*	1 Pack/400g	492	20.4	123	3.4	15.8	5.1	1.1
Vegetable, Mediterranean Style, Eat Smart, Safeway*	1 Pack/380g	228	3.0	60	3.0	10.1	0.8	1.5
Vegetable, Morrisons*	1 Pack/400g	464	22.8	116	3.8	12.3	5.7	0.7
Vegetable, Ross*	1 Pack/300g	270	8.4	90	2.9	13.3	2.8	1.2
Vegetable, Value, Tesco*	1 Pack/500g	410	15.0	82	4.1	9.7	3.0	2.3
Vegetable, Waitrose*	1 Pack/351g	386	20.4	110	3.2	11.3	5.8	1.2
Vegetable, Weight Watchers*	1 Pack/330g	251	5.6	76	3.6	11.8	1.7	0.7
LASAGNE VEGETARIAN								
Linda McCartney*	1 Pack/360g	451	20.2	125	6.3	12.4	5.6	1.4
Tesco*	1 Pack/450g	630	34.7	140	6.0	11.6	7.7	1.6
Vegetable, Eat Smart, Safeway*	1 Pack/380g	266	13.3	70	3.5	10.8	1.3	1.4
LAVERBREAD								
Average	1oz/28g	15	1.0	52	3.2	1.6	3.7	0.0
LEEKS								
Boiled, Average	1oz/28g	6	0.2	21	1.2	2.6	0.7	1.7
Creamed, Frozen, Waitrose*	1 Serving/225g	115	5.4	51	1.8	5.5	2.4	0.0
Raw, Unprepared, Average	1oz/28g	7	0.1	25	1.7	3.7	0.4	2.4
LEMON								
Fresh, Raw, Average	1 Slice/5g	0	0.0	7	0.3	1.6	0.0	1.7

L

	Measure INFO/WEIGHT	per Measure KCAL	FAT	Nutrition Values per 100g / 100ml KCAL	PROT	CARB	FAT	FIBRE
LEMON CURD								
Average	1 Tbsp/15g	44	0.7	294	0.7	62.9	4.7	0.1
Luxury, Average	1 Tsp/7g	23	0.6	326	2.8	59.7	8.4	0.1
M & S*	1 Tsp/7g	21.3	0.2	304	2.4	58.8	6.6	0.0
LEMON SOLE								
Breaded, Goujons, Lightly Dusted, M & S*	½ Pack/100g	195	9.7	195	14.0	14.0	9.7	0.8
Fillets, Raw, Average	1 Serving/220g	180	2.8	82	17.3	0.2	1.3	0.3
Goujons, & Lemon Mayonnaise, Finest, Tesco*	1 Pack/200g	620	45.6	310	10.6	15.6	22.8	1.0
Goujons, Average	1 Serving/150g	359	18.3	239	13.9	18.5	12.2	1.0
in Breadcrumbs, Average	1 Fillet/142g	322	17.4	228	13.7	15.7	12.3	1.0
in White Wine, & Herb Butter, Fillets, M & S*	1 Pack/220g	385	27.7	175	15.1	0.1	12.6	0.0
LEMONADE								
7-Up, Light, Britvic*	1 Can/330ml	4	0.0	1	0.1	0.2	0.0	0.0
7up, Zero, Britvic*	1 Can/330mls	6	0.0	2	0.1	0.1	0.0	0.0
Asda*	1 Glass/250ml	83	0.0	33	0.0	8.0	0.0	0.0
Average	1 Glass/250ml	53	0.3	21	0.1	5.0	0.1	0.1
Cloudy, Diet, Sainsbury's*	1 Can/330ml	7	0.3	2	0.1	0.2	0.1	0.3
Cloudy, Diet, Tesco*	1 Serving/200ml	6	0.0	3	0.0	0.8	0.0	0.0
Cloudy, Sainsbury's*	1 Glass/250ml	118	0.3	47	0.1	12.0	0.1	0.1
Cloudy, Waitrose*	1 Glass/250g	125	0.0	50	0.0	12.2	0.0	0.0
Diet, Amerista*	1 Glass/200ml	3	0.0	2	0.1	0.2	0.0	0.0
Diet, Traditional Style, Tesco*	1 Glass/200ml	6	0.0	3	0.0	0.8	0.0	0.0
Lime, Safeway*	1 Can/144ml	63	0.0	44	0.0	10.6	0.0	0.0
Low Calorie, SmartPrice, Asda*	1 Glass/250ml	1	0.0	0	0.0	0.1	0.0	0.0
Organic, Tesco*	1 Can/142ml	61	0.0	43	0.0	10.6	0.0	0.0
R White*	1 Glass/250ml	65	0.1	26	0.1	6.2	0.0	0.0
Sainsbury's*	1 Serving/250ml	53	0.3	21	0.1	4.9	0.1	0.1
Schweppes*	1 Glass/250ml	45	0.0	18	0.0	4.2	0.0	0.0
Sparkling, Morrisons*	1 Glass/250ml	63	0.0	25	0.0	6.1	0.0	0.0
Sparkling, with Spanish Lemon Juice, Waitrose*	1 Serving/250ml	85	0.0	34	0.0	8.3	0.0	0.0
Sprite*	1 Bottle/500ml	215	0.0	43	0.0	10.5	0.0	0.0
Still, Freshly Squeezed, M & S*	½ Bottle/250ml	100	0.5	40	0.1	9.0	0.2	0.5
Tesco*	1 Glass/200ml	30	0.0	15	0.0	3.6	0.0	0.0
Traditional Style, Tesco*	1 Glass/200ml	100	0.0	50	0.0	12.3	0.0	0.0
LENTILS								
Green & Brown, Dried, Boiled in Salted Water, Av	1 Tbsp/30g	32	0.2	105	8.8	16.9	0.7	3.8
Green Or Brown, Dried, Average	1 Serving/50g	151	0.8	301	22.8	49.8	1.5	9.6
Green Or Brown, in Water, Tinned, Average	½ Can/132g	131	0.8	99	8.1	15.4	0.6	3.8
Red, Boiled in Unsalted Water, Average	1oz/28g	28	0.1	102	7.6	17.5	0.4	2.6
Red, Dried, Average	1oz/28g	88	0.4	315	23.8	53.8	1.3	4.9
LETTUCE								
Cos, Sweet, Baby, Somerfield*	1 Pack/600g	90	3.0	15	0.8	1.7	0.5	0.9
Crest, Sainsbury's*	1/3 Lettuce/33g	5	0.2	14	0.8	1.7	0.5	0.0
Curly Leaf, Sainsbury's*	1 Serving/20g	3	0.1	14	0.8	1.7	0.5	0.0
Iceberg, Average	1 Serving/100g	13	0.3	13	0.8	1.8	0.3	0.5
Lamb's, Average	1 Serving/25g	4	0.1	15	1.4	1.6	0.3	1.0
Leafy, Tesco*	1 Serving/20g	3	0.1	14	1.2	1.5	0.4	1.9
Romaine, Average	1 Serving/80g	12	0.4	15	0.9	1.7	0.5	0.7
LILT								
Fruit Crush, Coca-Cola*	1 Can/330ml	66	0.0	20	0.0	4.6	0.0	0.0
Fruit Crush, Zero, Coca-Cola*	1 Can/330mls	12	0.0	4	0.0	0.3	0.0	0.0
Z, Coca-Cola*	1 Can/330ml	10	0.0	3	0.0	0.4	0.0	0.0
LIME								
Peel, Raw	1 Tbsp/6g	3	0.0	47	1.5	16.0	0.3	10.6

L

	Measure INFO/WEIGHT	per Measure KCAL	FAT	Nutrition Values per 100g / 100ml KCAL	PROT	CARB	FAT	FIBRE
LIME								
Raw, Flesh Only, Average	1 Lime/71g	18	0.1	25	0.6	8.9	0.2	2.4
Raw, Weighed with Peel & Seeds, Average	1 Lime/85g	26	0.2	30	0.7	10.5	0.2	2.8
LINGUINI								
Asparagas & Ricotta, Sainsbury's*	1 Serving/400g	524	23.2	131	3.8	15.8	5.8	2.5
Asparagus & Ricotta, Sainsbury's*	1 Serving/400g	524	23.2	131	3.8	15.8	5.8	2.5
Dry, Average	1 Serving/100g	352	2.2	352	13.1	70.0	2.2	2.8
Fresh, Dry, Average	1 Pack/250g	681	6.5	273	12.3	51.7	2.6	4.0
King Prawn, Meal for One, M & S*	1 Pack/400g	380	6.8	95	6.6	13.1	1.7	2.2
Pomodoro, M & S*	1 Pack/300g	360	10.5	120	4.1	17.6	3.5	1.2
Smoked Salmon, Sainsbury's*	1 Serving/400g	586	28.8	147	6.2	14.2	7.2	1.2
Sun Dried Tomato & Chicken, PB, Waitrose*	1 Serving/400g	316	7.6	79	7.5	8.0	1.9	3.5
Sun Dried Tomato & Egg, Asda*	1 Serving/200g	324	4.8	162	7.0	28.0	2.4	3.9
Tomato & Mushroom, PB, Waitrose*	1 Pack/350g	294	13.3	84	2.2	10.6	3.8	1.0
Vegetable & Ham, BGTY, Sainsbury's*	1 Pack/450g	410	13.5	91	4.4	11.7	3.0	0.9
with Prawns & Scallops, BGTY, Sainsbury's*	1 Pack/400g	320	2.0	80	6.2	12.7	0.5	0.8
LINSEEDS								
Average	1 Serving/5g	23	1.7	464	21.7	18.5	33.5	26.3
LION BAR								
Mini, Nestle*	1 Bar/16g	80	3.6	486	4.6	67.7	21.7	0.0
Nestle*	1 Bar/43.1g	206	9.3	478	6.5	64.6	21.6	0.0
Peanut, Nestle*	1 Bar/49g	256	14.5	522	7.1	56.9	29.6	0.0
LIQUEURS								
Amaretto, Average	1 Serving/50ml	194	0.0	388	0.0	60.0	0.0	0.0
Cream, Average	1 Shot/25ml	81	4.0	325	0.0	22.8	16.1	0.0
Grand Marnier*	1 Serving/100ml	268	0.0	268	0.0	22.9	0.0	0.0
High Strength, Average	1 Shot/25ml	79	0.0	314	0.0	24.4	0.0	0.0
LIQUORICE								
Allsorts, Average	1 Sm Bag/56g	195	2.9	349	3.7	76.7	5.2	2.0
Allsorts, Bassett's*	1 Pack/225g	792	10.1	352	2.3	75.5	4.5	1.6
Assorted, Filled, Panda*	1 Licorice/4g	15	0.4	385	3.7	68.0	11.0	0.0
Bars, Panda*	1 Bar/32g	100	0.1	314	3.7	73.0	0.4	0.0
Catherine Wheels, Barratt*	1 Wheel/22.4g	65	0.1	290	3.8	67.2	0.3	0.7
Catherine Wheels, Sainsbury's*	1 Wheel/17g	49	0.1	286	3.8	67.2	0.3	0.7
Organic, Laidback Liquorice*	1 Bar/28g	90	0.3	320	4.7	75.0	1.0	3.0
Panda*	1 Bar/32g	109	0.2	340	3.8	78.0	0.5	0.0
Shapes, Average	1oz/28g	78	0.4	278	5.5	65.0	1.4	1.9
Soft Eating, Australia, Darrell Lea*	1 Piece/20g	68	0.4	338	2.8	76.1	1.9	0.0
Sweets, Blackcurrant, Tesco*	1 Sweet/8g	32	0.3	410	0.0	92.3	3.8	0.0
Twists, Tesco*	1 Serving/63g	186	0.2	297	2.7	71.0	0.3	0.7
LIVER								
Calves, Fried	1oz/28g	49	2.7	176	22.3	0.0	9.6	0.0
Calves, Raw	1oz/28g	29	1.0	104	18.3	0.0	3.4	0.0
Calves, with Fresh Sage Butter, M & S*	1 Serving/116.7g	211	12.5	180	12.8	10.1	10.7	1.5
Calves, with Garlic Butter, M & S*	1oz/28g	56	3.8	200	13.3	7.3	13.5	0.4
Chicken, Fried, Average	1oz/28g	47	2.5	169	22.1	0.0	8.9	0.0
Chicken, Raw, Average	1oz/28g	26	0.6	92	17.7	0.0	2.3	0.0
Lamb's, Fried, Average	1oz/28g	66	3.6	237	30.1	0.1	12.9	0.1
Lamb's, Raw, Average	1 Serving/125g	171	7.8	137	20.3	0.0	6.2	0.0
Lamb's with Onions, M & S*	1oz/28g	52	3.2	185	14.1	6.8	11.3	0.1
Ox, Raw	1oz/28g	43	2.2	155	21.1	0.0	7.8	0.0
Ox, Stewed	1oz/28g	55	2.7	198	24.8	3.6	9.5	0.0
Pig's, Raw	1oz/28g	32	0.9	113	21.3	0.0	3.1	0.0
Pig's, Stewed	1 Serving/70g	132	5.7	189	25.6	3.6	8.1	0.0

L

	Measure INFO/WEIGHT	per Measure KCAL	FAT	Nutrition Values per 100g / 100ml KCAL	PROT	CARB	FAT	FIBRE
LIVER & BACON								
in Rich Onion Gravy, Chilled, Sainsbury's*	½ Pack/250g	303	12.3	121	10.9	8.3	4.9	0.4
Meal for One, M & S*	1 Pack/452.2g	430	16.7	95	7.0	8.0	3.7	1.2
with Creamy Mash, GFY, Asda*	1 Pack/385.9g	324	8.5	84	6.0	10.0	2.2	1.5
with Fresh Mashed Potato, Waitrose*	1 Pack/400g	416	17.2	104	7.3	9.0	4.3	1.3
with Mash, British Classics, Tesco*	1 Pack/500g	575	23.5	115	6.6	10.6	4.7	1.0
LIVER & ONIONS								
British Classics, Tesco*	1 Pack/250g	265	12.0	106	9.7	5.9	4.8	0.5
Finest, Tesco*	½ Pack/225g	349	18.7	155	15.6	3.7	8.3	1.6
M & S*	1 Serving/200g	250	12.0	125	7.6	10.5	6.0	0.9
LIVER SAUSAGE								
Average	1 Slice/10g	22	1.5	216	15.3	4.5	15.2	0.2
LOBSTER								
Boiled, Average	1oz/28g	29	0.4	103	22.1	0.0	1.6	0.0
Breaded, Mini, Sainsbury's*	1 Serving/100g	204	10.1	204	8.7	18.8	10.1	1.4
Breaded Squat, & Lemon Mayo Dip, Finest, Tesco*	1 Pack/210g	380	19.1	181	6.3	18.4	9.1	0.1
Dressed, M & S*	1oz/28g	76	6.6	273	14.3	0.8	23.6	0.1
Half, M & S*	1oz/28g	66	5.5	235	12.1	2.4	19.6	0.2
Squat, Tails, Youngs*	½ Pack/125g	246	10.8	197	9.8	20.1	8.6	1.1
Thermidor, M & S*	1 Serving/140g	287	19.2	205	10.7	9.7	13.7	0.0
LOGANBERRIES								
Raw	1oz/28g	5	0.0	17	1.1	3.4	0.0	2.5
LOLLIPOPS								
Assorted, Co-Op*	1 Lolly/10g	40	0.0	400	0.0	97.0	0.0	0.0
Assorted Flavours, Asda*	1 Lolly/7g	27	0.0	380	0.0	95.0	0.0	0.0
Chocolate Lolly, M & S*	1 Lolly/45g	248	15.8	550	6.8	54.0	35.1	2.7
Chupa Chups*	1 Lolly/18g	44	0.2	247	0.0	96.5	1.3	0.0
Cremosa, Sugar Free, Chupa Chups*	1 Lolly/10g	28	0.5	275	0.2	92.5	5.4	0.0
Cuore Di Frutta, Chupa Chups*	1 Lolly/10g	25	0.1	247	0.0	96.5	1.3	0.0
Drumstick, Matlow's*	1 Pack/40g	163.6	0.2	409	0.4	88.3	5.5	0.0
Refreshers, Bassett's*	1 Lolly/6g	25	0.0	417	0.0	108.3	0.0	0.0
LONGANS								
Canned, in Syrup, Drained	1oz/28g	19	0.1	67	0.4	17.1	0.3	0.0
LOQUATS								
Raw	1oz/28g	8	0.1	28	0.7	6.3	0.2	0.0
LOZENGES								
Original, Victory V*	1 Lozenge/3g	9	0.0	350	0.0	91.0	0.0	0.0
LUCOZADE*								
Citrus Clear, Energy Drink	1 Bottle/380ml	266	0.0	70	0.1	17.0	0.0	0.0
Orange Energy Drink	1 Bottle/500ml	350	0.0	70	0.0	17.2	0.0	0.0
Original, Energy Drink	1 Bottle/345ml	252	0.0	73	0.0	17.9	0.0	0.0
LUNCHEON MEAT								
Pork, Average	1oz/28g	81	6.8	288	13.3	4.0	24.3	0.0
Pork, Sainsbury's*	1 Slice/15g	35.4	2.8	236	18.5	2.8	16.8	0.3
Pork, Tesco*	1 Slice/14g	40.2	2.0	287	14.0	4.0	23.9	0.0
LYCHEES								
Fresh, Raw	1oz/28g	16	0.0	58	0.9	14.3	0.1	0.7
in Juice, Amoy*	1oz/28g	13	0.0	46	0.4	10.9	0.0	0.0
in Syrup, Average	1oz/28g	19	0.0	69	0.4	17.7	0.0	0.4
Raw, Weighed with Skin & Stone	1oz/28g	10	0.0	36	0.5	8.9	0.1	0.4

L

	Measure INFO/WEIGHT	per Measure KCAL	FAT	Nutrition Values per 100g / 100ml KCAL	PROT	CARB	FAT	FIBRE
M&M'S								
Mini, Mars*	1 Sm Pack/36g	176	8.4	489	6.3	63.6	23.2	0.0
Peanut, Mars*	1 Pack/45g	234	12.0	520	9.8	60.2	26.7	2.7
Peanut Butter, Mars*	1 Candy/1.8g	10	0.5	548	9.5	57.1	28.6	4.8
Plain, Mars*	1 Pack/48g	235	10.3	490	5.1	69.4	21.4	2.8
MACADAMIA NUTS								
Plain, Average	1 Pack/100g	750	77.6	750	7.9	4.8	77.6	5.3
Roasted, Salted, Average	6 Nuts/10g	75	7.8	748	7.9	4.8	77.6	5.3
MACARONI								
Dry, Average	1oz/28g	99	0.5	354	11.9	73.5	1.7	2.6
MACARONI CHEESE								
Average	1 Serving/300g	534	32.4	178	7.3	13.6	10.8	0.5
Bettabuy, Morrisons*	1 Serving/205g	229	11.7	112	4.3	10.8	5.7	0.4
Birds Eye*	1 Pack/300g	470	15.0	157	5.7	22.3	5.0	0.8
Canned	1oz/28g	39	1.8	138	4.5	16.4	6.5	0.4
Canned, Sainsbury's*	1 Can/400g	480	24.0	120	4.4	12.0	6.0	0.3
Chilled, BGTY, Sainsbury's*	1 Pack/375g	480	10.1	128	6.0	19.7	2.7	1.4
Chilled, GFY, Asda*	1 Pack/442.5g	469	12.8	106	6.0	14.0	2.9	1.6
Combino, Lidl*	1 Can/410g	472	25.8	115	4.5	10.1	6.3	0.3
Dinner, Original, Kraft*	½ Pack/140g	580	12.0	414	12.9	68.6	8.6	1.4
Eat Smart, Safeway*	1 Pack/315g	394	6.6	125	6.5	19.2	2.1	0.8
Findus*	1 Pack/360g	576	30.6	160	6.3	14.3	8.5	0.0
Finest, Tesco*	1 Serving/500g	1055	53.0	211	8.3	20.6	10.6	0.7
HE, Tesco*	1 Pack/340g	252	8.5	74	6.6	6.2	2.5	0.6
HL, Tesco*	I Serving/385g	443	4.6	115	9.3	15.9	1.2	1.0
Italian, Sainsbury's*	½ Pack/225g	360	15.8	160	6.9	17.3	7.0	1.5
Italian, Tesco*	1 Pack/420g	830	40.7	198	9.2	18.2	9.7	1.2
Kids, Sainsbury's*	1 Pack/300g	336	7.2	112	4.6	17.9	2.4	1.7
M & S*	1 Pack/400g	680	39.6	170	6.9	12.8	9.9	0.6
Morrisons, Canned, Morrisons*	1 Can/410g	279	5.7	68	5.1	8.8	1.4	1.0
Red Leicester, Heinz*	1 Can/400g	332	10.8	83	3.5	11.1	2.7	0.3
Ross*	1 Pack/300g	327	9.3	109	4.2	16.2	3.1	1.3
Tesco*	1 Can/410g	513	25.8	125	4.5	10.1	6.3	0.3
Value, Tesco*	1 Pack/300g	507	24.3	169	5.7	18.3	8.1	0.5
Waitrose*	1 Pack/350g	466	32.9	133	6.8	5.2	9.4	0.0
MACAROONS								
Butterscotch, Picard*	1 Macaroon/20g	85	3.6	424	9.7	55.1	18.2	0.0
Coconut, Sainsbury's*	1 Macaroon/33g	146	6.1	441	4.7	63.7	18.6	0.8
Coconut, Tesco*	1 Macaroon/33g	140	6.1	425	4.4	59.0	18.6	5.7
MACKEREL								
Atlantic, Raw, Average	1 Fillet/75g	154	10.4	205	18.6	0.0	13.9	0.0
Fillets, Honey Roast Smoked, Sainsbury's*	1 Serving/100g	349	27.3	349	21.5	4.5	27.3	12.4
Fillets, Hot Smoked, Arbroath, M & S*	1 Pack/135g	466	39.3	345	20.4	0.1	29.1	0.5
Fillets, in a Hot Chilli Dressing, Princes*	1 Pack/125g	370	33.8	296	13.3	0.0	27.0	0.0
Fillets, in Brine, Average	1 Can/88g	206	15.3	234	19.4	0.0	17.4	0.0
Fillets, in Curry Sauce, John West*	1 Can/125g	275	20.8	220	14.2	3.5	16.6	0.2
Fillets, in Green Peppercorn Sauce, John West*	1 Can/125g	329	26.3	263	14.0	4.5	21.0	0.1
Fillets, in Mustard Sauce, Average	1 Can/125g	274	19.4	219	14.1	5.4	15.5	0.1
Fillets, in Olive Oil, Average	1 Serving/50g	149	12.2	298	18.5	1.0	24.4	0.1
Fillets, in Spicy Tomato Sauce, Average	1oz/28g	56	3.9	199	14.3	3.9	14.1	0.0
Fillets, in Sunflower Oil, Average	1 Can/94g	262	20.6	279	20.2	0.2	21.9	0.2
Fillets, in Tomato Sauce, Average	1 Can/125g	251	18.3	200	14.3	2.7	14.7	0.0
Fillets, in White Wine & Spices, Connetable*	1 Can/120g	169	9.8	141	15.5	1.2	8.2	0.0
Fillets, Red Pepper & Onion, Smoked, Asda*	1 Serving/90g	319	27.9	354	18.0	0.8	31.0	1.2

	Measure	per Measure		Nutrition Values per 100g / 100ml				
	INFO/WEIGHT	KCAL	FAT	KCAL	PROT	CARB	FAT	FIBRE
MACKEREL								
Fillets, Smoked, Average	1oz/28g	94	7.9	335	19.8	0.5	28.2	0.3
Fried in Blended Oil	1oz/28g	76	5.5	272	24.0	0.0	19.5	0.0
Hot Smoked, Peppered, Arbroath, M & S*	1 Portion/100g	305	24.7	305	19.7	0.1	24.7	0.5
Raw, with Skin, Weighed with Bone, Average	1oz/28g	67	4.9	238	19.9	0.0	17.6	0.0
Smoked, Lemon & Parsley, Morrisons*	½ Pack/100g	282	20.0	282	20.9	4.6	20.0	1.0
Smoked, Peppered, Average	1oz/28g	87	7.0	310	20.4	0.3	25.2	0.2
Whole, Tesco*	1 Fish/200g	440	32.2	220	18.7	0.0	16.1	0.0
MADRAS								
Beef, Canned, BGTY, Sainsbury's*	1 Can/400g	344	14.4	86	9.5	4.0	3.6	0.9
Beef, Tesco*	1 Pack/460g	616	37.7	134	10.6	4.5	8.2	1.2
Chicken, & Pilau Rice, Somerfield*	1 Pack/340g	496	23.8	146	7.0	14.0	7.0	0.0
Chicken, & Rice, Hot & Spicy, Sainsbury's*	1 Pack/500g	670	25.5	134	7.1	14.9	5.1	2.2
Chicken, Asda*	1 Serving/350g	431	31.5	123	7.0	3.6	9.0	2.3
Chicken, Budgens*	1 Pack/350g	553	38.9	158	10.7	3.9	11.1	1.8
Chicken, Iceland*	1 Pack/400g	376	19.2	94	7.7	4.9	4.8	1.1
Chicken, Indian, Tesco*	1 Pack/350g	518	31.2	148	11.3	5.6	8.9	1.9
Chicken, Indian Take Away, Tesco*	1 Serving/175g	254	17.7	145	8.2	4.8	10.1	1.7
Chicken, Morrisons*	1 Pack/350g	448	30.5	128	9.6	2.8	8.7	2.4
Chicken, Safeway*	1 Pack/350g	469	25.2	134	13.4	4.0	7.2	1.8
Chicken, Sainsbury's*	1 Pack/400g	468	27.2	117	11.7	2.2	6.8	2.8
Chicken, Tesco*	1 Pack/350g	326	14.4	93	10.6	3.6	4.1	0.6
Chicken, Vite Fait*	1 Pack/300g	372	18.0	124	14.0	3.5	6.0	0.0
Chicken, Waitrose*	1oz/28g	47	2.9	168	14.6	3.7	10.5	1.8
Chicken & Pilau Rice, Asda*	1 Pack/400g	588	28.0	147	8.0	13.0	7.0	1.7
MAGNUM								
Almond, Wall's*	1 Bar/86g	271	16.3	315	5.1	31.0	19.0	0.0
Caramel & Nuts Bar, Wall's*	1 Bar/60g	132	9.0	220	4.0	19.0	15.0	0.0
Classic, Wall's*	1 Magnum/86.1g	261	16.4	303	3.8	29.0	19.0	0.0
Greed, Wall's*	1 Bar/110ml	307	18.0	279	3.6	29.1	16.4	0.0
White, Wall's*	1 Serving/86.5g	255	14.6	296	3.8	32.0	17.0	0.0
MAKHANI								
Chicken, Sainsbury's*	½ Pack/199.4g	312	21.3	157	12.2	2.9	10.7	2.5
Chicken Tikka, BGTY, Sainsbury's*	1 Pack/251.4g	186	4.8	74	11.3	3.0	1.9	1.7
Chicken Tikka, Waitrose*	1 Pack/400g	560	30.4	140	14.0	3.8	7.6	2.1
Chicken Tikka & Pilau Rice, BGTY, Sainsbury's*	1 Pack/400g	448	4.0	112	8.3	17.5	1.0	1.9
King Prawn & Rice, Sainsbury's*	½ Pack/250g	355	20.0	142	5.4	12.1	8.0	1.6
Paneer, Ashoka*	½ Pouch/150g	283	23.0	189	4.7	8.0	15.3	1.0
MALABAR								
Chicken with Pilau Rice, Waitrose*	1 Pack/450g	540	12.6	120	7.6	16.1	2.8	1.5
MALTESERS								
Mars*	1 Bag/21.5g	109	5.3	505	7.9	62.8	24.7	0.9
White Chocolate, Mars*	1 Pack/37g	186	9.4	504	7.9	61.0	25.4	0.0
MANDARIN ORANGES								
in Juice, Average	1oz/28g	11	0.0	39	0.7	9.0	0.0	0.5
in Light Syrup, Average	1 Can/298g	201	0.1	68	0.6	16.0	0.1	0.1
in Orange Gel, Del Monte*	1 Can/128g	60	0.0	47	0.0	10.9	0.0	0.0
Weighed with Peel, Average	1 Sm/50g	18	0.1	37	0.9	8.4	0.1	1.3
MANGE TOUT								
& Sugar Snap Peas, Tesco*	1 Pack/150g	102	0.6	68	7.0	9.2	0.4	3.8
Boiled in Salted Water	1oz/28g	7	0.0	26	3.2	3.3	0.1	2.2
Raw, Average	1 Serving/80g	26	0.2	33	3.6	4.2	0.2	1.2
Stir-Fried in Blended Oil	1oz/28g	20	1.3	71	3.8	3.5	4.8	2.4

	Measure INFO/WEIGHT	per Measure KCAL	FAT	Nutrition Values per 100g / 100ml KCAL	PROT	CARB	FAT	FIBRE
MANGO								
Dried, Average	1 Serving/50g	174	0.5	347	1.4	83.1	1.0	4.9
Fresh, Prepared, Slices, Eat Well, M & S*	1 Pack/100g	60	0.2	60	0.7	14.1	0.2	2.6
Fresh, Tesco*	1 Pack/200g	116	0.4	58	0.7	13.4	0.2	1.8
in Syrup, Average	1oz/28g	22	0.0	80	0.3	20.5	0.0	0.9
MANGOSTEEN								
Canned, in Syrup, Drained, Average	1 Cup/196g	143	1.1	73	0.4	17.9	0.6	1.8
Raw, Fresh, Average	1 Serving/80g	50	0.5	63	0.6	15.6	0.6	5.1
MARGARINE								
Average	1 Thin Spread/7g	51	5.7	727	0.1	0.5	81.0	0.0
Butter Style, Average	1 Thin Spread/7g	44	4.8	627	0.7	1.1	68.9	0.0
Buttery Taste, Flora*	1 Serving/28g	178	19.6	634	0.4	0.6	70.0	0.5
Diet, Flora*	1 Serving/7.5g	17	1.7	227	3.5	1.6	23.0	0.0
for Baking, Average	1 Serving/8g	49	5.4	607	0.2	0.4	67.2	0.0
Light, Flora*	1 Spread/8g	28	3.0	354	0.1	2.8	38.0	0.0
No Salt, Flora*	1 Serving/10g	53	5.9	531	0.0	0.0	59.0	0.0
Omega 3 Plus, Flora*	1 Spread/10g	35	3.8	350	0.1	3.0	38.0	0.0
Original, Flora*	1 Serving/8g	42	4.7	531	0.0	0.0	59.0	0.0
Pro Activ, Extra Light, Flora*	1 Tsp/15g	33	3.5	218	0.1	2.9	23.0	0.2
Pro Activ, Light, Flora*	2 Tsp/10g	33	3.5	331	0.1	4.0	35.0	0.2
Pro Activ, with Olive Oil, Flora*	1 Tsp/8g	26	2.8	331	0.1	4.0	35.0	0.0
Reduced Fat, Average	1 Thin Spread/7g	25	2.7	356	0.6	3.0	38.0	0.0
Soft, Tub, Stork*	1 Thin Spread/7g	37	4.1	531	0.0	0.0	59.0	0.0
Soya, Granose*	1 Thin Spread/7g	52	5.7	745	0.1	0.1	82.0	0.0
White, Flora*	1 Thin Spread/7g	60	6.7	855	0.0	0.0	95.0	0.0
MARINADE								
Cajun Spice, EPC*	1 Serving/50g	94	6.7	187	1.3	15.3	13.4	1.6
Hot & Spicy Barbecue, M & S*	1 Serving/18g	23	0.1	130	1.0	31.1	0.3	0.8
Lemon & Rosemary, Nando's*	1 Serving/18g	26	2.3	147	1.0	11.8	13.0	0.2
Sticky Barbecue, Tesco*	¼ Jar/69.6g	80	0.1	115	0.7	26.7	0.2	0.6
Thai Coconut, Coriander & Lime, Lea & Perrins*	1oz/28g	45	1.7	159	1.3	25.7	6.1	0.0
Tomato & Herb, Lea & Perrins*	1oz/28g	28	0.1	100	1.2	24.1	0.5	0.0
MARLIN								
Smoked, H. Forman & Son*	1 Pack/200g	240	0.2	120	29.8	0.0	0.1	0.0
Steaks, Chargrilled, Sainsbury's*	1 Serving/240g	367	14.6	153	23.6	0.8	6.1	0.6
Steaks, Raw, Sainsbury's*	1 Steak/110g	109	0.2	99	24.3	0.0	0.2	0.0
MARMALADE								
Blood Orange, Grandessa*	1 Serving/15g	36	0.0	240	0.4	59.0	0.1	0.7
Christmas Orange & Whisky, M & S*	1oz/28g	67	0.1	240	0.3	59.5	0.2	1.9
Lemon, with Shred, Average	1 Serving/20g	50	0.0	248	0.2	61.6	0.1	0.6
Lemon & Lime, Average	1 Tbsp/20g	53	0.0	267	0.2	66.4	0.1	0.4
Lime, with Shred, Average	1 Tbsp/15g	39	0.0	261	0.2	65.0	0.1	0.4
Onion, Organic, Antony Worrall Thompson's*	1 Serving/10.5g	19	0.1	191	1.1	44.9	0.8	1.8
Orange, with Drambuie, Finest, Tesco*	1 Serving/10g	33	0.0	329	0.3	82.0	0.0	0.7
Orange, with Shred, Average	1 Tbsp/15g	39	0.0	263	0.2	65.2	0.0	0.3
Orange & Ginger, Average	1 Tbsp/15g	40	0.0	264	0.2	65.7	0.1	0.3
Pink Grapefruit, Thin Cut, Waitrose*	1 Serving/10g	26	0.0	261	0.2	65.0	0.0	0.4
MARMITE								
Yeast Extract, Marmite*	1 Tsp/9g	20	0.0	219	38.4	19.2	0.1	3.1
MARROW								
Boiled, Average	1oz/28g	3	0.1	9	0.4	1.6	0.2	0.6
Raw	1oz/28g	3	0.1	12	0.5	2.2	0.2	0.5
MARS								
Bar, 5 Little Ones, Mars*	1 Piece/8g	38	1.5	477	4.5	73.6	18.3	0.0

	Measure INFO/WEIGHT	per Measure KCAL	FAT	Nutrition Values per 100g / 100ml KCAL	PROT	CARB	FAT	FIBRE
MARS								
Bar, Duo, Mars*	1 Bar/42g	193	7.5	455	4.1	69.7	17.7	1.3
Bar, Fun Size, Mars*	1 Bar/20g	89	3.4	444	3.7	69.7	16.8	1.1
Bar, Mars*	1 Bar/62.5	281	10.9	449	4.2	69.0	17.4	1.2
Delight, Mars*	1 Bar/19.9g	110	6.7	552	4.5	57.8	33.6	1.3
MARSHMALLOWS								
Average	1 Mallow/5g	16	0.0	327	3.9	83.1	0.0	0.0
Fat Free, Tesco*	4 Mallows/28g	95	0.1	339	3.4	80.8	0.2	0.5
Haribo*	1 Sweet/5g	17	0.0	330	3.0	80.0	0.0	0.0
Mushy, Mini, Safeway*	1 Serving/30g	98	0.0	325	5.5	75.5	0.0	0.0
Pascall*	1 Mallow/4.5g	17	0.0	335	2.6	80.0	0.0	0.0
Pink & White, Co-Op*	1 Sweet/7g	24	0.0	340	3.0	82.0	0.0	0.0
Raspberry & Cream, Sainsbury's*	1 Sweet/7g	23	0.0	330	4.1	78.5	0.0	0.5
Sainsbury's*	1 Mallow/7g	23	0.0	330	4.1	78.5	0.0	0.5
MARZIPAN								
Bar, Chocolate, Plain, Thorntons*	1 Bar/46g	206	8.0	448	5.2	69.1	17.4	2.0
Plain, Average	1oz/28g	115	4.0	412	5.9	67.5	14.2	1.7
MASALA								
Chicken, Tandoori, M & S*	½ Pack/175g	210	11.6	120	11.3	4.3	6.6	4.5
Prawn, & Rice, Tesco*	1 Pack/475g	656	24.7	138	5.2	17.9	5.2	1.2
Prawn, King, Waitrose*	1 Pack/350g	385	25.9	110	7.1	3.8	7.4	1.8
Vegetable, Sainsbury's*	1 Pack/400g	388	30.0	97	2.1	5.2	7.5	2.5
Vegetable, Somerfield*	1 Pack/350g	406	23.8	116	2.7	11.0	6.8	3.0
Vegetable, Waitrose*	1 Serving/400g	288	19.2	72	2.2	4.9	4.8	2.5
Vegetable, with Rice, Feeling Great, Findus*	1 Pack/350g	350	7.0	100	3.0	18.0	2.0	1.7
MASALA DAL								
Waitrose*	½ Pack/300g	414	14.1	138	6.5	17.3	4.7	4.5
MASH								
Root, Asda*	½ Pack/200g	142	8.0	71	0.7	8.0	4.0	3.1
Winter Root, Sainsbury's*	1 Serving/140g	157	2.1	112	2.7	22.0	1.5	0.9
MATZO								
Crackers, Rakusen's*	1 Matzo/4.9g	18	0.1	369	10.5	82.9	1.1	3.6
MAYONNAISE								
50% Less Fat, GFY, Asda*	1 Tbsp/10g	32	3.1	322	0.8	10.0	31.0	0.0
60% Less Fat, BGTY, Sainsbury's*	1 Tbsp/15ml	42	4.1	277	0.4	7.3	27.3	0.0
Aioli, Finest, Tesco*	1 Tsp/5g	20	2.1	408	0.8	8.5	41.2	0.0
Average	1 Tsp/11g	80	8.7	724	1.9	0.2	79.3	0.0
Dressing, Weight Watchers*	1 Serving/15g	44	4.5	290	1.2	6.9	29.7	2.5
Egg, Reduced Fat, Safeway*	½ Pot/85g	136	10.4	160	10.2	1.4	12.2	1.6
Egg, Safeway*	1 Serving/50g	121	11.0	241	10.4	0.4	22.0	1.0
Extra Light, Now Only 3% Fat, Hellmann's*	1 Serving/16g	12	0.5	73	0.6	11.0	3.0	0.6
Extra Light, Weight Watchers*	1 Serving/15g	15	0.9	97	1.1	9.6	5.9	3.2
Finest, Tesco*	1 Dtsp/22g	155	16.9	703	1.1	1.5	77.0	0.0
French, Light, Sainsbury's*	1 Serving/15ml	46	4.7	307	0.4	6.1	31.1	0.2
French Style, BGTY, Sainsbury's*	1 Tbsp/15ml	55	5.5	366	0.6	7.5	36.9	0.0
Garlic, Classic, Asda*	1 Tsp/5g	33	3.6	658	1.2	3.6	71.0	0.5
Garlic, Morrisons*	1 Tbsp/15ml	55	5.4	365	0.7	8.8	36.0	0.0
Garlic, Waitrose*	1 Tsp/6g	21	2.1	346	0.6	8.6	34.3	0.0
Garlic & Herb, M & S*	1 Tsp/6g	43	4.6	712	3.4	2.4	76.9	0.9
Garlic & Herb, Reduced Calorie, Hellmann's*	1 Serving/25ml	58	4.8	233	0.7	13.1	19.3	0.4
Garlic Flavoured, Frank Cooper*	1 Tsp/6g	28	2.8	460	2.2	8.8	46.2	0.1
Good Intentions, Somerfield*	1 Serving/30g	93	9.2	309	0.5	7.4	30.8	0.0
Half Fat, Healthy Choice, Safeway*	1 Tsp/11g	35	3.3	319	0.8	10.8	30.3	0.0
Lemon, Waitrose*	1 Tsp/8ml	56	6.1	694	1.2	1.3	76.0	5.4

	Measure INFO/WEIGHT	per Measure		Nutrition Values per 100g / 100ml				
		KCAL	FAT	KCAL	PROT	CARB	FAT	FIBRE
MAYONNAISE								
Light, BGTY, Sainsbury's*	1 Tsp/11g	33	3.2	296	0.5	7.2	29.3	0.0
Light, Hellmann's*	1 Serving/10g	30	3.0	298	0.7	6.5	29.8	0.1
Light, Kraft*	1 Serving/25g	61	5.0	245	0.6	15.0	20.0	0.0
Light, Morrisons*	1 Tsp/11g	32	3.0	287	1.4	8.5	27.5	0.0
Light, Organic, Simply Delicious*	1 Tbsp/14g	46	4.2	328	0.8	13.0	30.3	0.4
Light, Squeezable, Hellmann's*	1 Tbsp/15g	44	4.4	293	0.7	6.4	29.4	0.0
Light Dijon, Benedicta*	1 Tbsp/15g	44	4.4	292	0.7	6.7	29.2	0.0
Low Fat, Belolive*	1 Serving/15ml	45	4.4	298	0.8	11.1	29.0	0.0
Made with Free Range Eggs, M & S*	1 Tbsp/15g	108	11.8	720	1.1	1.2	78.5	0.0
Mild Dijon Mustard, Frank Cooper*	1 Pot/28g	114	11.1	406	3.3	9.3	39.5	0.1
Olive Oil, Hellmann's*	1 Serving/15g	108	11.9	722	1.1	1.3	79.1	0.0
Organic, Tesco*	1 Tbsp/15g	121	13.1	805	1.2	2.2	87.4	0.0
Organic, Whole Foods*	1 Tbsp/14g	100	11.0	714	0.0	7.1	78.6	0.0
Real, Asda*	1 Serving/10g	72	7.9	721	1.3	1.2	79.0	0.1
Real, Hellmann's*	1 Tsp/11g	79	8.7	722	1.1	1.3	79.1	0.0
Real, The Big Squeeze, Hellmann's*	1 Tbsp/15ml	101	11.1	676	1.0	1.2	74.0	0.0
Reduced Calorie	1 Tsp/11g	32	3.1	288	1.0	8.2	28.1	0.0
Reduced Calorie, Tesco*	1 Tbsp/15g	49	4.7	326	0.8	9.8	31.5	0.0
Reduced Calorie, Waitrose*	1 Tsp/11g	32	3.0	287	1.4	8.5	27.5	0.0
Reduced Fat, Tesco*	1 Tbsp/15ml	44	4.3	292	0.8	7.9	28.6	0.0
Sainsbury's*	1 Tsp/11g	75	8.3	686	0.4	1.2	75.4	0.0
Tesco*	1 Tbsp/15ml	113	12.3	750	0.6	1.4	82.2	0.0
Value, Tesco*	1 Tbsp/15g	73	7.7	488	0.8	5.4	51.4	0.0
Waitrose*	1 Tbsp/15ml	106	11.7	709	1.3	0.8	77.8	0.0
with Dijon Mustard, Hellmann's*	1 Tbsp/15ml	32	3.0	210	2.9	5.1	19.7	0.0
MEAL REPLACEMENT								
Ny-Tro Pro-40, Cool Vanilla, AST Sports Science*	1 Sachet/72g	250	1.5	347	55.6	30.6	2.1	2.8
Ny-Tro Pro-40, Creamy Strawberry, AST Sports Science*	1 Sachet/72g	250	1.5	347	55.6	30.6	2.1	2.8
Ultra Slim, Ready to Drink, Strawberry, Tesco*	1 Carton/330ml	231	3.0	70	4.2	10.5	0.9	1.5
Ultra Slim, Ready to Drink, Vanilla, Tesco*	1 Carton/330ml	224	3.0	68	4.2	10.5	0.9	1.5
Ultra-Slim, Ready to Drink, Chocolate, Tesco*	1 Carton/330ml	215	3.6	65	3.9	9.8	1.1	1.3
MEAT LOAF								
Beef & Pork, Co-Op*	¼ Loaf/114g	314	25.1	275	13.0	7.0	22.0	1.0
Iceland*	1 Serving/150g	332	23.6	221	10.8	9.3	15.7	0.9
Somerfield*	1 Pack/454g	867	59.0	191	10.0	8.0	13.0	0.0
Turkey & Bacon, Tesco*	1 Serving/225g	401	22.3	178	14.7	7.4	9.9	1.1
MEATBALLS								
& Mashed Potato, Tesco*	1 Pack/450g	527	29.7	117	4.0	10.4	6.6	1.0
& Pasta, Sainsbury's*	1 Serving/300g	333	9.3	111	5.3	15.5	3.1	1.9
& Pasta in Tomato Sauce, Wayfayrer*	1 Pack/300g	375	17.4	125	9.0	9.2	5.8	1.0
Aberdeen Angus, & Herb Potatoes, Finest, Tesco*	1 Serving/392.5g	472	23.6	120	6.0	9.1	6.0	2.0
Aberdeen Angus, Fresh, Chilled, Waitrose*	1 Meatball/36g	92	7.1	256	18.0	1.5	19.8	0.0
Aberdeen Angus, with Herb Potatoes, Finest, Tesco*	1 Serving/392.5g	472	23.6	120	6.0	9.1	6.0	2.0
Aberdeen Angus in Sauce, PB, Waitrose*	½ Pack/240g	228	7.2	95	10.5	6.5	3.0	1.1
Al Forno, Safeway*	1 Pack/450g	684	30.6	152	6.0	16.8	6.8	0.4
Beanz & Lamb, Heinz*	½ Can/207g	213	8.9	103	5.2	10.9	4.3	2.8
Beef, Asda*	2 Balls/69.3g	140	7.1	202	18.4	9.0	10.3	0.0
Beef, Tesco*	1 Pack/336g	806	60.5	240	15.0	3.7	18.0	0.1
Chicken, in Tomato Sauce, Average	1 Can/392g	580	32.9	148	7.7	10.4	8.4	0.0
Cumberland, Pub Specials, Birds Eye*	1 Pack/450g	365	11.3	81	3.7	11.8	2.5	1.9
Galician Style, Cafe Culture, M & S*	½ Pack/500g	675	33.5	135	5.9	13.2	6.7	1.1
Greek, M & S*	1 Serving/350g	403	18.9	115	7.7	9.1	5.4	1.5
in Bolognese Sauce, Somerfield*	1 Pack/454g	704	49.9	155	7.0	7.0	11.0	0.0

MEATBALLS

INFO/WEIGHT	Measure	per Measure		Nutrition Values per 100g / 100ml				
		KCAL	FAT	KCAL	PROT	CARB	FAT	FIBRE
MEATBALLS								
in Gravy, Campbell's*	½ Can/205g	164	5.3	80	5.6	8.6	2.6	0.0
in Rich Gravy, Westlers*	½ Can/200g	170	6.8	85	4.1	9.5	3.4	0.4
in Sherry Sauce, Tapas, Waitrose*	1 Serving/185g	272	7.4	147	18.8	5.9	4.0	1.2
in Tomato Sauce, Canned, Average	1 Can/410g	387	15.1	95	5.6	9.9	3.7	0.0
in Tomato Sauce, Tapas, Waitrose*	1 Pack/185g	285	16.8	154	10.8	7.2	9.1	1.3
Italian Pork, Al Forno, Sainsbury's*	1 Pack/450g	644	23.9	143	6.1	17.6	5.3	1.4
Lemon Chicken, with Rice, BGTY, Sainsbury's*	1 Pack/400g	388	8.4	97	6.8	12.8	2.1	1.4
Lion's Head, M & S*	1 Serving/300g	435	27.9	145	10.4	5.1	9.3	1.0
M & S*	1oz/28g	58	3.8	208	10.9	10.7	13.5	2.4
Manhattan Style & Spaghetti, Spicy, Safeway*	1 Pack/450g	540	21.6	120	5.7	13.2	4.8	2.0
Mighty, in Tomato Sauce, Westlers*	1 Tin/400g	424	19.0	106	5.8	10.2	4.8	0.0
Roman-Style with Basil Mash, COU, M & S*	1 Pack/430g	344	9.5	80	3.7	10.9	2.2	1.9
Spaghetti, Tesco*	1 Pack/385g	377	16.0	98	5.4	9.8	4.2	1.2
Spicy, Deli Melt, Sainsbury's*	1 Pack/200g	338	21.4	169	12.7	5.5	10.7	2.9
Spicy, M & S*	1 Pack/400g	540	24.0	135	8.8	12.0	6.0	1.4
Swedish, Average	¼ Pack/88g	198	13.8	225	14.0	7.4	15.7	1.3
Turkey, GFY, Asda*	½ Pack/330g	333	12.2	101	10.0	7.0	3.7	0.0
with Spicy Tomato Sauce, Just Cook, Sainsbury's*	½ Pack/169.7g	246	11.9	145	14.8	5.7	7.0	0.9
MEATBALLS VEGETARIAN								
Swedish Style, Sainsbury's*	1 Ball/27g	53	2.6	194	21.5	5.5	9.5	4.0
MEDLAR								
Raw, Flesh Only	1 Fruit/28g	11	0.1	40	0.5	10.6	0.4	10.0
MELBA TOAST								
Asda*	1 Slice/3.3g	13	0.2	395	12.0	76.0	4.8	4.6
Average	1 Serving/3.3g	12	0.1	396	12.0	76.0	4.9	4.6
Buitoni*	1 Serving/33g	130	1.6	395	12.1	75.5	4.9	4.6
Co-Op*	1 Slice/3g	13	0.1	430	13.3	83.3	3.3	6.7
Dutch, HL, Tesco*	1 Pack/20g	75	0.5	375	13.1	75.0	2.4	4.6
Organic, Trimlyne*	6 Toasts/20g	81	1.4	407	13.7	71.6	6.8	5.3
Original, Van Der Meulen*	1 Slice/3g	12	0.1	399	12.8	80.5	2.9	3.9
MELON								
Cantaloupe, Flesh Only, Average	½ Melon/255g	44	0.3	17	0.4	4.2	0.1	0.5
Cantaloupe, Weighed with Rind, Average	1 Slice/100g	35	0.3	35	0.8	8.3	0.3	0.8
Galia, Average	1 Serving/240g	60	0.1	25	0.8	5.8	0.1	0.2
Honeydew, Raw, Flesh Only, Average	1oz/28g	8	0.0	30	0.7	7.0	0.1	0.5
Pineapple & Strawberry, Fully Prepared, Sainsbury's*	1 Serving/245g	86	0.2	35	0.6	7.8	0.1	0.9
MELON & GRAPES								
Fresh, Sainsbury's*	½ Pack/200g	58	0.2	29	0.6	6.4	0.1	0.8
Fresh, Shapers, Boots*	1 Pack/220g	75	0.2	34	0.6	7.7	0.1	0.8
Fresh, Tesco*	1 Lge Pack/400g	132	0.8	33	0.5	7.3	0.2	0.6
MELON MEDLEY								
Average	1 Pack/240g	66	0.3	27	0.6	6.0	0.1	0.5
MELT								
Cheese, Chilli, Fresh, Asda*	1 Melt/29g	87	4.9	301	6.0	31.0	17.0	0.0
Cheesy Fish, Youngs*	1 Pack/340g	418	22.4	123	7.6	8.3	6.6	0.9
Chilli with Spicy Potato Wedges, Asda*	1 Pack/450g	540	19.8	120	8.0	12.0	4.4	1.2
Mushroom & Broccoli Potato Wedge, Weight Watchers*	1 Pack/310g	285	9.3	92	3.1	13.3	3.0	1.0
Salmon & Broccoli Wedge, From Heinz, Weight Watchers*	1 Pack/320g	298	10.6	93	5.1	10.6	3.3	1.1
Salmon & Broccoli Wedge, Weight Watchers*	1 Pack/320g	298	10.6	93	5.1	10.6	3.3	1.1
Sausage & Bean, Iceland*	1 Pack/400g	588	23.2	147	6.5	17.1	5.8	1.6
Tuna, Go Large, Asda*	1 Melt/175g	509	26.3	291	12.0	27.0	15.0	0.0
Tuna, Iceland*	1 Pack/400g	424	16.8	106	6.0	11.3	4.2	0.7
Tuna, M & S*	1 Pack/218g	621	37.1	285	13.0	20.1	17.0	1.0

	Measure INFO/WEIGHT	per Measure KCAL	per Measure FAT	Nutrition Values per 100g / 100ml KCAL	PROT	CARB	FAT	FIBRE
MELT								
Vegetable & Potato, Asda*	1 Serving/100g	451	23.0	451	17.0	44.0	23.0	6.2
MERINGUE								
Average	1 Portion/8g	30	0.0	379	5.3	95.4	0.0	0.0
Chocolate, Waitrose*	1 Meringue/76.8g	342	11.3	444	2.6	75.3	14.7	0.5
Cream, Fresh, Sainsbury's*	1 Meringue/35g	142	5.1	407	3.5	65.4	14.6	0.5
Cream, M & S*	1 Meringue/34g	145	7.6	425	4.1	52.6	22.2	1.4
Mini, M & S*	1 Meringue/3.8g	15	0.0	395	6.1	91.6	0.0	0.2
Nests, Asda*	1 Nest/15g	59	0.0	394	5.0	93.0	0.2	0.5
Nests, M & S*	1 Nest/12g	47	0.0	390	6.1	91.6	0.0	0.0
Nests, Mini, Tesco*	1 Nest/4g	14	0.0	387	3.9	92.8	0.0	0.0
Nests, Sainsbury's*	1 Nest/13.3g	52	0.0	392	4.2	93.6	0.1	0.1
Raspberry, M & S*	1 Serving/105g	215	13.8	205	1.8	20.6	13.1	3.1
Shells, Mini, Asda*	1 Shell/3.8g	15	0.0	392	4.2	93.6	0.1	0.0
Shells, Sainsbury's*	2 Shells/24g	93	0.0	387	3.9	92.8	0.0	0.0
Strawberry, COU, M & S*	1 Meringue/5.2g	19	0.0	385	6.4	90.0	0.1	1.4
Strawberry, Mini, Extra Special, Asda*	1 Meringue/3.9g	15	0.0	387	5.0	91.0	0.3	0.5
Summer Fruits, 90% Fat Free, Sara Lee*	1 Meringue/135g	308	11.5	228	2.5	35.7	8.5	2.2
Tropical, M & S*	1 Serving/53g	212	14.3	400	3.1	37.0	26.9	0.0
MESSICANI								
Egg, M & S*	1 Serving/100g	355	2.8	355	13.9	68.5	2.8	3.0
MIDGET GEMS								
M & S*	1 Bag/113g	367	0.1	325	6.3	75.1	0.1	0.0
SmartPrice, Asda*	1 Pack/178g	586	0.2	329	6.0	76.0	0.1	0.0
MILK								
Channel Island, Finest, Tesco*	1 Glass/200ml	160	10.4	80	3.7	4.7	5.2	0.0
Colombian Coffee Flavoured, Waitrose*	1 Serving/250ml	233	9.5	93	4.3	10.5	3.8	0.0
Condensed, Semi Skimmed, Sweetened	1oz/28g	75	0.1	267	10.0	60.0	0.2	0.0
Condensed, Skimmed, Unsweetened, Average	1 Sm Can/205g	221	8.2	108	7.5	10.5	4.0	0.0
Condensed, Whole, Sweetened, Average	1oz/28g	93	2.8	333	8.5	55.5	10.1	0.0
Dried, Skimmed, Average	1oz/28g	99	0.3	355	35.4	52.3	0.9	0.0
Dried, Whole, Average	1oz/28g	137	7.4	490	26.3	39.4	26.3	0.0
Evaporated, Average	1 Serving/85g	136	7.7	160	8.2	11.6	9.0	0.0
Evaporated, Reduced Fat, Average	1oz/28g	33	1.5	118	7.4	10.5	5.2	0.0
Goats, Pasteurised	1 fl oz/30ml	18	1.1	60	3.1	4.4	3.5	0.0
Goats, Semi-Skimmed, St Helen's Farm*	1 Serving/250ml	109	4.0	44	3.0	4.3	1.6	0.0
Low Fat, Calcia Extra Calcium, Unigate*	1 fl oz/30ml	14	0.2	45	4.3	6.3	0.5	0.0
Semi Skimmed, Advance, with Omega 3, St Ivel*	1 Glass/250ml	123	4.3	49	3.4	5.0	1.7	0.0
Semi Skimmed, Average	1 fl oz/30ml	15	0.5	49	3.4	5.0	1.7	0.0
Semi Skimmed, Fresh Pasteurised, Lidl*	1 Serving/100ml	47	1.7	47	3.4	4.9	1.7	0.0
Semi Skimmed, Long Average, Life*	1 fl oz/30ml	15	0.5	49	3.4	5.0	1.7	0.0
Semi Skimmed, Low Lactose, Arla*	1 Glass/125ml	56	1.9	45	3.4	5.0	1.5	0.0
Semi Skimmed, M & S*	1 Pint/568ml	278	9.7	49	3.4	5.0	1.7	0.0
Semi Skimmed, Pasteurised, Tesco*	1 Serving/100ml	50	1.8	50	3.6	4.8	1.8	0.0
Semi Skimmed, Spar*	1 Serving/50ml	25	0.9	49	3.4	5.0	1.7	0.0
Skimmed, Average	1fl oz/28ml	10	0.0	34	3.3	5.0	0.1	0.0
Skimmed, Uht, Average	1 fl oz/30ml	10	0.0	34	3.4	5.0	0.1	0.0
Strawberry Flavoured, Tesco*	1 Serving/500ml	370	8.0	74	4.4	10.4	1.6	0.3
The One, 1% Fat, Robert Wiseman Dairies*	1 Serving/50ml	20	0.5	40	3.1	4.6	1.0	0.0
Whole, Average	1 Serving/200ml	134	7.8	67	3.3	4.7	3.9	0.0
Whole, with Vitamin D, Oak Farms*	1 Container/236ml	150	8.0	64	3.4	4.7	3.4	0.0
MILK DRINK								
Chocolate, Break Time, Arla*	1 Bottle/500ml	290	1.5	58	3.6	10.2	0.3	0.0
Chocolate, Skimmed, Happy Shopper*	1 Bottle/500ml	295	1.5	59	3.6	10.4	0.3	0.0

M

	Measure INFO/WEIGHT	per Measure KCAL	FAT	Nutrition Values per 100g / 100ml KCAL	PROT	CARB	FAT	FIBRE
MILK DRINK								
Chocolate, Spar*	1 Serving/500ml	290	1.5	58	3.6	10.2	0.3	0.0
Extra Choc, Mars*	1 Bottle/330g	281	6.6	85	3.1	13.7	2.0	0.0
Family Fuel, Mars*	1 Serving/200ml	172	4.0	86	3.1	13.7	2.0	0.0
Mocalatte, Cafe Met*	1 Bottle/290ml	160	3.8	55	2.9	8.0	1.3	0.0
Original, Mars*	1 Serving/330g	284	6.9	86	3.1	13.7	2.1	0.0
MILK SHAKE								
Banana, Yazoo, Campina*	1 Bottle/200ml	130	2.6	65	3.1	10.3	1.3	0.0
Banana Flavour, Frijj*	1 Bottle/500ml	310	4.0	62	3.4	10.1	0.8	0.0
Banana Flavour, Shapers, Boots*	1 Bottle/250ml	201	1.9	80	5.6	12.8	0.8	1.9
Chocolate, Asda*	1 Serving/250ml	198	9.3	79	4.4	7.0	3.7	0.4
Chocolate, Extreme, Frijj*	1 Bottle/500g	425	10.5	85	3.9	12.7	2.1	0.0
Chocolate Flavoured, Fresh, Thick, Frijj*	1 Bottle/500ml	350	5.0	70	3.5	11.7	1.0	0.0
Measure Up, Asda*	1 Glass/250ml	200	2.4	80	6.0	12.0	1.0	2.4
Powder, Made Up with Semi-Skimmed Milk	1 Serving/250ml	173	4.0	69	3.2	11.3	1.6	0.0
Powder, Made Up with Whole Milk	1 Serving/250ml	218	9.3	87	3.1	11.1	3.7	0.0
Strawberry, Yazoo, Campina*	1 Bottle/500ml	325	6.0	65	3.1	10.3	1.2	0.0
Strawberry Flavour, Thick, Low Fat, Frijj*	1 Bottle/250ml	155	2.0	62	3.4	10.1	0.8	0.0
Vanilla, Frijj*	1 Bottle/500ml	320	4.0	64	3.4	10.7	0.8	0.0
MILKY BAR								
Buttons, Nestle*	1 Pack/30g	164	9.5	547	7.3	58.4	31.7	0.0
Choo, Nestle*	1 Bar/25g	116	4.3	464	4.2	73.1	17.2	0.0
Chunky, Nestle*	¼ Bar/37.8g	207	12.0	547	7.3	58.4	31.7	0.0
Crunchies, Nestle*	1 Pack/30g	168	10.4	560	7.0	54.9	34.7	0.0
Munchies, Nestle*	1 Serving/70g	392	24.3	560	7.0	54.9	34.7	0.1
Nestle*	1 Bar/12g	66	3.8	547	7.3	58.4	31.7	0.0
MILKY WAY								
Fun Size, Mars*	1 Bar/16.7g	76	2.8	447	3.8	71.6	16.2	0.0
Magic Stars, Mars*	1 Bag/33g	184	11.5	559	6.3	55.3	34.7	0.0
Mars*	1 Bar/26g	114	3.7	440	3.4	74.8	14.1	0.0
MILO								
Energy Drink, Powder, Dry Weight, Nestle*	1 Serving/20g	75	1.2	373	7.8	71.9	6.0	5.4
MINCEMEAT								
Average	1oz/28g	77	1.2	274	0.6	62.1	4.3	1.3
Organic, Waitrose*	1oz/28g	81	0.7	290	0.9	65.8	2.6	2.0
Tesco*	1 Serving/20g	58	0.7	292	0.8	64.2	3.5	1.6
Traditional, Robertson*	1 Tbsp/7g	49	0.6	286	0.6	62.5	3.4	2.5
Traditional, Sainsbury's*	1 Tbsp/23g	65	0.7	282	0.9	62.4	3.2	1.4
with Cherries, Almonds & Brandy, Tesco*	¼ Jar/103g	295	5.0	287	1.4	58.8	4.9	1.4
MINI BITES								
Blueberry & Yoghurt Clusters, M & S*	1 Mini Bite/12.9g	60	2.7	465	5.0	64.4	20.7	4.7
Chocolate Caramel, M & S*	1 Bite/20.7g	97	5.2	460	5.6	53.5	24.6	1.6
Chocolate Cornflake, M & S*	1 Bite/11.8g	55	2.4	470	6.2	66.3	20.1	3.6
Chocolate Orange, M & S*	1 Bite/22g	95	4.8	430	5.5	54.6	21.6	1.8
Extremely Chocolatey, M & S*	1 Bite/20g	90	4.9	450	5.7	52.4	24.6	1.6
Flapjack, M & S*	1 Bite/14g	70	3.5	500	6.4	62.1	25.0	3.6
Oat, Cranberry & Yoghurt Clusters, M & S*	1 Mini Bite/13.2g	60	2.4	455	5.5	66.4	18.5	2.7
Shortbread, All Butter, M & S*	1 Biscuit/9.8g	50	2.7	510	5.7	58.9	27.8	2.3
MINSTRELS								
Galaxy, Mars*	1 Serving/100g	503	22.2	503	5.1	70.5	22.2	1.1
MINT								
Dried	1oz/28g	78	1.3	279	24.8	34.6	4.6	0.0
Fresh, Average	2 Tbsp/3.2g	1	0.0	43	3.8	5.3	0.7	0.0

M

MINTOES

	Measure INFO/WEIGHT	KCAL	FAT	KCAL	PROT	CARB	FAT	FIBRE
Morrisons*	1 Sweet/8.1g	33	0.6	411	0.1	84.4	8.1	0.0

MINTS

	Measure INFO/WEIGHT	KCAL	FAT	KCAL	PROT	CARB	FAT	FIBRE
After Dinner, Dark, Elizabeth Shaw*	1 Chocolate/9g	42	2.1	469	2.8	62.5	23.1	0.0
After Dinner, Sainsbury's*	1 Mint/7g	32	1.5	456	4.1	62.1	21.2	4.1
After Eight, Dark Chocolate, Nestle*	1 Mint/8g	37	1.0	461	5.0	63.0	12.9	2.0
After Eight, Orange, Nestle*	1 Sweet/7g	29	0.9	417	2.5	72.6	12.9	1.1
Butter Mintoes, M & S*	1 Sweet/9g	35	0.6	391	0.0	84.0	6.8	0.0
Butter Mintoes, Tesco*	1 Sweet/7g	24	0.5	349	0.0	71.3	7.1	0.0
Clear, Co-Op*	1 Sweet/6g	24	0.0	395	0.0	98.0	0.0	0.0
Cream, Luxury, Thorntons*	1 Chocolate/13g	62	3.1	477	4.2	62.3	23.8	2.3
Creams, Bassett's*	1 Sweet/11g	40	0.0	365	0.0	91.8	0.0	0.0
Curiously Strong, M & S*	1 Sweet/1g	4	0.0	390	0.4	97.5	0.0	0.0
Everton, Co-Op*	1 Sweet/6g	25	0.2	410	0.6	92.0	4.0	0.0
Extra, Wrigleys*	1 Sweet/1.1g	3	0.0	240	0.0	64.0	1.0	0.0
Extra Strong, Peppermint, Trebor*	1 Pack/45g	180	0.1	395	0.4	98.1	0.2	0.0
Extra Strong, Spearmint, Trebor*	1 Pack/44g	174	0.0	395	0.4	98.7	0.0	0.0
Extra Strong, Trebor*	1 Pack/45.5g	180	0.3	396	0.3	98.7	0.0	0.0
Glacier, Fox's*	1 Mint/5g	19	0.0	386	0.0	96.4	0.0	0.0
Humbugs, Classic Favourites, Asda*	1 Sweet/8.6g	32	0.4	373	0.5	81.3	5.1	0.0
Humbugs, Co-Op*	1 Sweet/8g	34	0.6	425	0.6	89.9	7.0	0.0
Humbugs, M & S*	1 Sweet/9g	37	0.4	407	0.6	91.1	4.4	0.0
Humbugs, Thorntons*	1 Sweet/9g	31	0.4	340	1.0	87.8	4.4	0.0
Imperials, Co-Op*	1 Sweet/3g	12	0.0	395	0.3	98.0	0.2	0.0
Imperials, Sainsbury's*	1 Mint/2g	11	0.0	374	0.0	92.1	0.0	0.0
Imperials, Tesco*	1 Mint/3g	12	0.0	397	0.6	98.7	0.0	0.0
Mento, Sugar Free, Mentos*	1 Sweet/2g	5	0.1	260	1.0	87.0	5.5	0.0
Mint Assortment, M & S*	1 Sweet/7g	29	0.5	414	0.7	85.4	7.7	0.0
Mint Favourites, Bassett's*	1 Sweet/6g	22	0.4	367	0.9	77.4	5.9	0.0
Soft, Trebor*	1 Pack/48g	182	0.0	380	0.0	94.9	0.0	0.0
Softmints, Peppermint, Trebor*	1 Pack/45g	160	0.0	355	0.0	88.9	0.0	0.0
Softmints, Spearmint, Trebor*	1 Pack/45g	170	0.0	375	0.0	94.3	0.0	0.0

MISO

	Measure INFO/WEIGHT	KCAL	FAT	KCAL	PROT	CARB	FAT	FIBRE
Average	1oz/28g	57	1.7	203	13.3	23.5	6.2	0.0

MIXED HERBS

	Measure INFO/WEIGHT	KCAL	FAT	KCAL	PROT	CARB	FAT	FIBRE
Average	1 Tsp/5g	13	0.4	260	13.0	37.5	8.5	6.7

MIXED SPICE

	Measure INFO/WEIGHT	KCAL	FAT	KCAL	PROT	CARB	FAT	FIBRE
Schwartz*	1 Tsp/2g	8	0.2	390	10.4	65.8	9.5	2.0

MIXED VEGETABLES

	Measure INFO/WEIGHT	KCAL	FAT	KCAL	PROT	CARB	FAT	FIBRE
Baby, Iceland*	1 Serving/100g	20	0.0	20	1.2	3.9	0.0	2.7
Baby, Steam, Fresh, Tesco*	1 Pack/160g	72	1.3	45	2.7	6.7	0.8	3.8
Bag, M & S*	1 Serving/200g	70	0.4	35	2.9	5.6	0.2	0.0
Canned, Drained, Co-Op*	½ Can/100g	45	0.1	45	2.0	9.0	0.1	2.0
Canned, Drained, Sainsbury's*	1 Can/200g	114	0.6	57	3.0	10.6	0.3	2.3
Canned, Re-Heated, Drained	1oz/28g	11	0.2	38	1.9	6.1	0.8	1.7
Casserole, Co-Op*	1 Serving/100g	40	0.3	40	1.2	7.5	0.3	2.1
Casserole, Frozen, Morrisons*	1 Serving/150g	21	0.3	14	0.5	2.8	0.2	1.5
Casserole, Frozen, Tesco*	1 Serving/100g	26	0.4	26	0.8	4.8	0.4	2.0
Casserole, Ready to Cook, Sainsbury's*	½ Pack/240g	74	0.7	31	0.9	6.2	0.3	1.4
Casserole, Tesco*	1 Pack/440g	176	1.3	40	1.2	8.0	0.3	2.3
Chinese, Stir Fry, Amoy*	1 Serving/110g	27	0.3	25	1.8	3.7	0.3	0.0
Chunky, Frozen, Sainsbury's*	1 Serving/85g	31	0.6	37	2.9	4.7	0.7	3.1
Crunchy, Tesco*	1 Pack/210g	63	0.8	30	1.7	5.0	0.4	2.4
Farmhouse, Four Seasons*	1 Serving/100g	26	0.7	26	2.2	2.7	0.7	0.0

M

MIXED VEGETABLES

INFO/WEIGHT	Measure KCAL	FAT	KCAL	PROT	CARB	FAT	FIBRE
Farmhouse, Frozen, Four Seasons, Aldi*	1oz/28g	10	0.2	34	2.8	4.3	0.7	0.0
Farmhouse, Frozen, Waitrose*	1 Serving/90g	23	0.5	25	1.9	3.1	0.6	2.4
Fresh, Asda*	1oz/28g	7	0.2	26	1.9	3.0	0.7	1.0
Freshly Frozen, Iceland*	1 Serving/100g	52	0.9	52	3.4	8.3	0.9	3.4
Frozen, Aldi*	1 Serving/100g	34	0.7	34	2.8	4.3	0.7	0.0
Frozen, Boiled in Salted Water	1oz/28g	12	0.1	42	3.3	6.6	0.5	0.0
Frozen, Safeway*	1 Serving/120g	70	1.1	58	3.0	9.4	0.9	3.4
Frozen, Sainsbury's*	1 Serving/90g	49	0.9	54	2.8	8.4	1.0	3.1
Frozen, SuperValu*	1 Serving/70g	22	0.3	31	1.7	5.1	0.4	0.7
Frozen, Waitrose*	1 Portion/80g	44	0.8	55	3.3	8.2	1.0	3.7
Green, Microwave, Aldi*	1 Serving/300g	189	9.0	63	3.5	5.6	3.0	4.1
in Salt Water, Tesco*	1/3 Can/65g	34	0.4	53	2.6	9.2	0.6	2.7
in Salted Water, Canned, Asda*	1 Serving/65g	31	0.1	48	2.6	9.0	0.2	1.7
in Salted Water, Nisa Heritage*	1 Serving/100g	39	0.8	39	1.9	6.1	0.8	1.7
Layered, Classics, M & S*	½ Pack/160g	112	6.2	70	1.2	7.3	3.9	1.2
Organic, Waitrose*	1oz/28g	19	0.4	69	4.4	10.0	1.3	2.7
Oriental, M & S*	1 Serving/250g	50	0.8	20	1.6	3.4	0.3	1.6
Potatoes, Broad Beans & Peas, M & S*	1 Pack/245g	147	3.2	60	2.9	12.9	1.3	3.4
Premium, Frozen, Somerfield*	1 Serving/100g	53	1.0	53	3.2	7.9	1.0	2.7
Ready to Roast, Asda*	½ Pack/362g	315	11.6	87	1.6	13.0	3.2	2.4
Red Peppers & Courgette, Tesco*	1 Pack/250g	68	1.3	27	1.7	3.8	0.5	2.0
Roast, Four Seasons*	1 Serving/187g	79	0.4	42	1.2	8.8	0.2	0.0
Sainsbury's*	1 Serving/230g	55	1.4	24	2.1	2.5	0.6	0.0
Seasonal Selection, Tesco*	1 Serving/100g	37	0.4	37	1.1	7.2	0.4	2.2
Special, Freshly Frozen, Morrisons*	1 Serving/100g	48	0.8	48	3.2	7.2	0.8	0.0
Special, Frozen, Sainsbury's*	1 Serving/80g	46	0.8	57	3.2	8.9	1.0	2.9
Special, Sainsbury's*	1 Serving/120g	68	1.2	57	3.2	8.9	1.0	2.9
Supreme, Frozen, Somerfield*	1 Serving/90g	23	0.0	25	1.9	4.3	0.0	3.1

MOLASSES

INFO/WEIGHT	Measure KCAL	FAT	KCAL	PROT	CARB	FAT	FIBRE
Average	1 Tbsp/20g	53	0.0	266	0.0	68.8	0.1	0.0

MONKEY NUTS

INFO/WEIGHT	Measure KCAL	FAT	KCAL	PROT	CARB	FAT	FIBRE
Average	1oz/28g	158	13.4	565	25.6	8.2	48.0	6.3

MONKFISH

INFO/WEIGHT	Measure KCAL	FAT	KCAL	PROT	CARB	FAT	FIBRE
Fillets, Fresh, Cornish, M & S*	1 Serving/100g	65	0.4	65	15.7	0.0	0.4	0.0
Grilled	1oz/28g	27	0.2	96	22.7	0.0	0.6	0.0
Raw	1oz/28g	18	0.1	66	15.7	0.0	0.4	0.0

MONSTER MUNCH

INFO/WEIGHT	Measure KCAL	FAT	KCAL	PROT	CARB	FAT	FIBRE
Flamin' Hot, Walkers*	1 Bag/25g	123	6.3	490	7.0	59.0	25.0	1.5
Pickled Onion, Walkers*	1 Pack/22g	108	5.5	490	6.0	60.0	25.0	1.7
Roast Beef, Walkers*	1 Pack/25g	123	6.3	490	7.0	59.0	25.0	1.7
Spicy, Walkers*	1 Bag/25g	125	7.3	500	5.0	55.0	29.0	1.3

MORNAY

INFO/WEIGHT	Measure KCAL	FAT	KCAL	PROT	CARB	FAT	FIBRE
Beef, BGTY, Sainsbury's*	1 Pack/400g	300	10.4	75	6.1	6.8	2.6	1.2
Beef, GFY, Asda*	1 Pack/400g	300	8.4	75	7.0	7.0	2.1	0.7
Beef, Good Intentions, Somerfield*	1 Pack/400g	364	14.8	91	7.1	7.2	3.7	3.3
Beef, HL, Tesco*	1 Pack/450g	396	12.2	88	5.0	10.9	2.7	0.4
Broccoli, Somerfield*	1 Pack/400g	372	24.8	93	3.5	5.9	6.2	0.5
Cafe Culture, M & S*	1 Serving/375g	619	39.4	165	9.2	7.8	10.5	0.8
Cod, Fillets, Sainsbury's*	1 Serving/153g	236	14.4	154	15.2	2.2	9.4	0.9
Cod, Sainsbury's*	1 Serving/180g	277	16.9	154	15.2	2.2	9.4	0.9
COU, M & S*	1 Pack/340g	272	9.9	80	5.3	8.5	2.9	1.4
Eat Smart, Safeway*	1 Pack/400g	380	10.4	95	5.2	12.6	2.6	1.2
Haddock, PB, Waitrose*	1 Pack/360g	310	5.4	86	16.6	1.6	1.5	0.5

	Measure INFO/WEIGHT	per Measure		Nutrition Values per 100g / 100ml				
		KCAL	FAT	KCAL	PROT	CARB	FAT	FIBRE
MORNAY								
Haddock, with Leek Mash, Eat Smart, Safeway*	1 Pack/369.9g	307	9.3	83	7.1	7.9	2.5	1.0
Haddock, Youngs*	½ Pack/190g	236	14.8	124	12.1	1.3	7.8	0.6
Lamb, Eat Smart, Safeway*	1 Pack/380g	304	10.3	80	6.8	6.4	2.7	1.3
Lamb, Finest, Tesco*	1 Pack/350g	510	38.1	146	5.8	6.2	10.9	3.4
Lamb, Sainsbury's*	1 Pack/329.1g	497	32.2	151	8.4	7.2	9.8	1.0
Lamb, Tesco*	1 Serving/460g	442	15.2	96	3.4	13.2	3.3	0.5
Ready Meals, Waitrose*	1 Pack/300g	492	29.1	164	8.2	10.9	9.7	1.7
Salmon, with Broccoli, Weight Watchers*	1 Pack/290g	261	4.9	90	9.6	9.0	1.7	0.7
Spinach, Waitrose*	½ Pack/125g	113	8.6	90	3.3	3.6	6.9	1.6
Vegetable, Ready Meals, Waitrose*	1oz/28g	38	2.2	134	3.7	12.3	7.8	2.3
Vegetable, Roasted, Safeway*	1 Pack/365g	365	20.8	100	3.7	7.9	5.7	2.9
Vegetable, Vegetarian, M & S*	1 Pack/300g	345	23.1	115	3.3	7.8	7.7	3.1
Vegetarian, Tesco*	1 Pack/300g	489	31.2	163	6.4	11.0	10.4	0.9
MOUSSE								
Aero Chocolate, Nestle*	1 Pot/58g	101	3.0	174	4.8	27.3	5.1	1.1
Aero Mint, Nestle*	1 Pot/100g	218	11.9	218	4.1	23.6	11.9	0.0
Aero Twist Cappuccino & Chocolate, Nestle*	1 Pot/75g	135	8.1	180	4.2	16.8	10.8	0.2
Banoffee, COU, M & S*	1 Pot/70g	102	1.5	145	2.9	28.8	2.1	1.5
Belgian Chocolate & Vanilla, Weight Watchers*	1 Pot/80g	106	2.2	132	4.4	22.2	2.8	0.9
Cadbury's Light Chocolate, St Ivel*	1 Pot/64g	79	2.0	123	6.2	17.3	3.2	0.0
Chocolate	1 Pot/60g	83	3.2	139	4.0	19.9	5.4	0.0
Chocolate, Asda*	1 Pot/61g	134	6.1	219	3.7	26.0	10.0	1.0
Chocolate, BGTY, Sainsbury's*	1 Pot/62.5g	82	1.8	133	4.9	21.8	2.9	0.5
Chocolate, Cadbury*	1 Pot/55g	107	4.5	195	6.1	24.6	8.2	0.0
Chocolate, COU, M & S*	1 Pot/70.4g	95	1.7	135	4.6	22.9	2.4	1.6
Chocolate, Eat Smart, Safeway*	1 Pot/62g	81	1.7	130	4.1	21.5	2.7	1.1
Chocolate, Finest, Tesco*	1 Pot/82g	321	26.4	391	3.7	21.7	32.2	0.0
Chocolate, GFY, Asda*	1 Pot/60g	70	1.7	117	4.8	17.9	2.9	3.5
Chocolate, Healthy Selection, Low Fat, Somerfield*	1 Pot/60g	81	2.8	135	5.3	18.2	4.6	0.0
Chocolate, HL, Tesco*	1 Serving/63g	84	1.6	135	4.8	23.3	2.5	3.2
Chocolate, Iceland*	1 Pot/62g	113	4.3	183	4.0	26.3	6.9	0.0
Chocolate, Light, Cadbury*	1 Pot/55g	61	1.9	110	4.6	14.2	3.4	0.0
Chocolate, Low Fat, Danette, Danone*	1 Pot/60g	73	1.1	121	5.1	20.8	1.9	1.5
Chocolate, Sainsbury's*	1 Pot/62g	118	5.3	190	4.7	23.8	8.5	1.0
Chocolate, Somerfield*	1 Pot/60g	115	5.1	192	4.3	24.5	8.5	0.0
Chocolate, Tesco*	1 Pot/60g	120	5.0	200	3.6	27.6	8.4	0.9
Chocolate, with Chunks of Dairy Milk, Cadbury*	1 Pot/100g	215	9.9	215	6.1	25.7	9.9	0.0
Chocolate & Hazelnut, Onken*	1 Pot/125g	171	7.5	137	3.3	17.8	6.0	0.0
Chocolate & Mint, COU, M & S*	1 Pot/70g	84	1.8	120	6.2	18.7	2.5	1.0
Lemon, Classic, Onken*	1 Pot/150g	210	9.5	140	5.1	15.8	6.3	0.1
Lemon, COU, M & S*	1 Pot/70g	81	2.5	115	2.9	19.4	3.5	3.5
Lemon, Less Than 3% Fat, HE, Tesco*	1 Pot/60g	57	1.6	95	3.4	14.3	2.7	0.7
Lemon, Lite, Onken*	1 Pot/150g	156	2.3	104	4.6	17.2	1.5	0.2
Lemon, Low Fat, Morrisons*	1 Pot/62.5g	99	5.8	158	3.7	15.4	9.3	0.3
Lemon, Somerfield*	1 Pot/62.5g	114	5.9	181	3.5	20.7	9.4	0.6
Orange, Mango & Lime, Onken*	1 Pot/150g	207	9.5	138	5.1	15.3	6.3	0.1
Peach, Onken*	1 Pot/150g	204	9.5	136	5.1	15.1	6.3	0.2
Peach & Passion Fruit, PB, Waitrose*	1 Pot/95g	118	2.7	124	3.5	21.2	2.8	0.5
Plain Chocolate, Low Fat, Nestle*	1 Pot/120g	71	0.9	59	2.4	10.4	0.8	0.0
Raspberry, Berrylicious, COU, M & S*	1 Tub/120g	156	2.4	130	3.0	24.5	2.0	3.0
Raspberry Ripple, Value, Tesco*	1 Mousse/47g	70	2.9	149	2.1	21.3	6.1	0.1
Strawberry, Asda*	1 Pot/64g	107	5.8	167	3.5	18.0	9.0	0.2
Strawberry, HL, Tesco*	1 Pot/114g	90	3.0	79	3.8	10.2	2.6	0.8

MOUSSE

INFO/WEIGHT	Measure KCAL	FAT	Nutrition Values per 100g / 100ml KCAL	PROT	CARB	FAT	FIBRE
Strawberry, Light, Muller*	1 Pot/150g	147	0.6	98	4.3	19.4	0.4	0.0
Strawberry, Lite, Onken*	1 Pot/150g	152	2.3	101	4.6	17.2	1.5	0.2
Strawberry, Morrisons*	1 Pot/62.5g	107	6.0	170	3.5	17.6	9.5	0.2
Strawberry, Onken*	1 Pot/150g	213	10.1	142	5.6	14.9	6.7	0.0
Strawberry, Tesco*	1 Pot/63g	106	5.8	169	3.5	17.9	9.3	0.2
Strawberry & Vanilla, Weight Watchers*	1 Pot/80g	87	1.9	109	3.8	18.1	2.4	0.4
White Chocolate, Finest, Tesco*	1 Pot/92g	436	34.5	474	3.9	30.2	37.5	0.0

MOZZARELLA STICKS

INFO/WEIGHT	Measure KCAL	FAT	Nutrition Values per 100g / 100ml KCAL	PROT	CARB	FAT	FIBRE
Breaded, with Tomato Dip, D'esir*	1 Pack/200g	462	22.0	231	12.0	21.0	11.0	0.0

MUFFIN

INFO/WEIGHT	Measure KCAL	FAT	Nutrition Values per 100g / 100ml KCAL	PROT	CARB	FAT	FIBRE
Berry Burst, Asda*	1 Muffin/60g	139	1.4	232	6.2	46.7	2.3	1.7
Blueberry, & Redcurrant, BGTY, Sainsbury's*	1 Muffin/65g	159	1.6	245	5.0	50.0	2.5	3.1
Blueberry, American Style, Aldi*	1 Muffin/85g	344	17.3	405	4.3	51.2	20.3	0.0
Blueberry, American Style, Sainsbury's*	1 Muffin/85g	302	15.5	355	5.1	42.7	18.2	1.9
Blueberry, Asda*	1 Muffin/77.3g	272	13.1	353	5.0	45.0	17.0	1.3
Blueberry, Big, Asda*	1 Muffin/105g	342	11.2	326	7.5	49.8	10.7	2.3
Blueberry, GFY, Asda*	1 Muffin/58.6g	147	1.4	249	6.0	51.0	2.3	3.0
Blueberry, Low Fat, David Powell*	1 Muffin/100g	246	3.8	246	6.0	47.9	3.8	0.0
Blueberry, M & S*	1 Muffin/75g	255	12.6	340	4.9	41.9	16.8	1.3
Blueberry, Mini, Sainsbury's*	1 Serving/28g	82	2.3	293	6.3	48.9	8.1	1.9
Blueberry, Mini, Tesco*	1 Muffin/28g	104	5.4	370	5.6	43.5	19.3	1.2
Blueberry, PB, Waitrose*	1 Muffin/100g	225	2.2	225	4.6	46.5	2.2	1.8
Blueberry, Tesco*	1 Muffin/73g	248	12.5	340	4.7	41.0	17.1	1.9
Blueberry, The Handmade Flapjack Company*	1 Muffin/135g	479	26.6	355	4.7	39.9	19.7	0.0
Blueberry, Waitrose*	1 Muffin/65g	239	9.2	367	4.7	55.2	14.2	1.7
Blueberry, Weight Watchers*	1 Muffin/65g	172	3.7	265	6.4	46.9	5.7	2.6
Blueberry, Wild Canadian, Fabulous Bakin' Boys*	1 Muffin/40g	140	8.0	349	4.0	39.0	20.0	1.0
Blueberry Buster, McVitie's*	1 Muffin/95g	408	22.4	429	4.3	49.9	23.6	1.1
Bran, Average	1 Muffin/57g	155	4.4	272	7.8	45.6	7.7	7.7
Carrot, Asda*	1 Muffin/59.2g	137	1.4	233	6.0	47.0	2.3	1.6
Carrot Cake, Entenmann's*	1 Muffin/105g	344	15.9	328	5.1	45.8	15.1	3.0
Cheese, Tesco*	1 Muffin/67g	150	1.9	224	13.0	36.4	2.9	3.0
Cheese & Black Pepper, TTD, Sainsbury's*	1 Muffin/70.1g	213	7.4	304	13.1	39.1	10.6	3.0
Cherry, Cheeky, Fabulous Bakin' Boys*	1 Muffin/118g	446	21.0	378	5.5	51.0	17.8	0.7
Cherry, The Handmade Flapjack Company*	1 Muffin/135g	500	26.6	370	4.6	43.8	19.7	0.0
Cherry Mega, The Handmade Flapjack Company*	1 Muffin/135g	506	26.7	375	4.4	44.8	19.8	0.0
Choc Chip, Mini, Weight Watchers*	1 Muffin/15g	47	1.3	312	6.6	52.1	8.6	3.1
Chocolate, Dairy Cream, Safeway*	1 Muffin/109.7g	430	28.7	391	7.3	31.9	26.1	3.1
Chocolate, Dessert, COU, M & S*	1 Serving/110g	127	2.5	115	6.2	16.8	2.3	1.4
Chocolate, Dessert, Light Choices, Tesco*	1 Pot/107.7g	140	2.4	130	4.3	22.6	2.2	1.3
Chocolate, Galaxy, McVitie's*	1 Muffin/87.6g	320	17.2	364	5.0	44.5	19.5	0.0
Chocolate, HL, Tesco*	1 Muffin/71g	204	6.2	288	5.5	46.9	8.7	5.5
Chocolate, The Handmade Flapjack Company*	1 Muffin/135g	527	30.8	390	5.3	41.5	22.8	0.0
Chocolate Chip, American Style, Sainsbury's*	1 Muffin/72g	284	14.4	395	5.0	48.8	20.0	2.1
Chocolate Chip, BGTY, Sainsbury's*	1 Muffin/75g	282	12.3	376	5.2	51.8	16.4	1.6
Chocolate Chip, Mini, Asda*	1 Muffin/22g	77	2.9	349	7.0	51.0	13.0	2.1
Chocolate Chip, Mini, BGTY, Sainsbury's*	1 Muffin/28g	91	2.4	324	6.5	55.1	8.7	1.6
Chocolate Chip, Plain, Tesco*	1 Muffin/72g	270	12.7	375	5.0	48.1	17.6	1.4
Chocolate Indulgence, McVitie's*	1 Muffin/75g	254	6.9	338	5.8	57.9	9.2	1.3
Chunky Choc 'n' Orange, Fabulous Bakin' Boys*	1 Muffin/40g	154	8.8	384	5.0	42.0	22.0	1.0
Cranberry & White Chocolate, Sainsbury's*	1 Muffin/72g	253	13.3	352	5.7	40.7	18.5	1.5
Double Chocolate, Chocolate Chip, Mini, Tesco*	1 Muffin/28g	116	6.4	414	6.3	45.7	23.0	1.4
Double Chocolate, Free From, Tesco*	1 Muffin/70g	281	12.7	402	4.7	54.8	18.2	1.7

	Measure INFO/WEIGHT	per Measure KCAL	per Measure FAT	Nutrition Values per 100g / 100ml KCAL	PROT	CARB	FAT	FIBRE
MUFFIN								
Double Chocolate, M & S*	1 Muffin/70g	277	14.8	395	4.8	46.1	21.2	2.8
Double Chocolate, Mini, M & S*	1 Muffin/32g	133	6.9	416	5.4	49.8	21.7	1.1
Double Chocolate Chip, American Style, Sainsbury's*	1 Muffin/71.9g	276	14.6	384	5.2	45.0	20.3	2.9
Double Chocolate Chip, Co-Op*	1 Muffin/60g	246	12.6	410	6.0	49.0	21.0	3.0
Double Chocolate Chip, Mini, Asda*	1 Muffin/19g	76	3.7	400	7.4	48.5	19.6	2.7
Double Chocolate Chip, Tesco*	1 Muffin/72g	259	12.9	360	6.1	44.9	17.9	5.4
English, Butter, Tesco*	1 Muffin/67.2g	170	3.6	253	11.2	39.8	5.4	2.0
English, Kingsmill*	1 Muffin/75g	168	1.3	224	9.8	42.3	1.7	2.2
English, M & S*	1 Muffin/60g	135	1.1	225	11.2	43.7	1.9	2.9
English, Tesco*	1 Muffin/72g	171	2.3	238	11.3	41.7	3.2	2.8
Lemon, Boots*	1 Muffin/110g	424	20.9	385	3.6	50.0	19.0	1.3
Lemon & Blueberry, Tesco*	1 Muffin/110g	411	23.0	374	4.0	42.4	20.9	1.1
Lemon & Poppy Seed, Entenmann's*	1 Muffin/105g	417	20.3	397	5.6	52.8	19.3	2.5
Lemon & Poppy Seed, M & S*	1 Muffin/72g	281	14.3	390	6.3	46.1	19.8	1.5
Mini, Tesco*	1 Muffin/28g	120	6.3	428	6.4	50.0	22.6	1.2
Mixed Fruit, Low Fat, Abbey Bakery*	1 Muffin/35g	93	1.6	267	4.5	55.6	4.5	1.4
Oven Bottom, Aldi*	1 Muffin/68g	173	1.0	255	10.0	50.4	1.5	2.2
Oven Bottom, Tesco*	1 Muffin/68g	173	1.0	255	10.0	50.4	1.5	2.2
Oven Bottom, Warburton's*	1 Muffin/69g	175	2.0	253	10.9	45.8	2.9	0.0
Plain, Co-Op*	1 Muffin/60g	150	1.0	250	13.3	45.0	1.7	1.7
Plain, Morrisons*	1 Muffin/70g	140	0.8	200	8.0	41.4	1.1	0.0
Raspberry, PB, Waitrose*	1 Muffin/101g	220	2.1	219	4.7	45.4	2.1	3.7
Raspberry Cream, Sainsbury's*	1 Muffin/90g	314	19.8	349	3.9	33.8	22.0	1.3
Spiced Fruit, TTD, Sainsbury's*	1 Muffin/70g	181	3.6	259	10.1	43.1	5.1	2.3
Toffee & Pecan, Finest, Tesco*	1 Muffin/127g	551	29.0	434	5.4	51.8	22.8	0.9
Toffee Mega, The Handmade Flapjack Company*	1 Muffin/135g	567	34.7	420	4.5	43.2	25.7	0.0
Vanilla & Choc Chip, GFY, Asda*	1 Muffin/58.5g	151	1.3	260	7.0	53.0	2.2	1.6
White, All Butter, Sainsbury's*	1 Muffin/67g	173	4.2	258	10.6	39.6	6.3	3.6
White, Asda*	1 Muffin/66.7g	148	1.3	222	11.0	40.0	2.0	2.5
White, Tesco*	1 Muffin/60g	144	1.9	240	11.3	41.6	3.2	2.8
White, Waitrose*	1 Muffin/66.9g	174	4.3	260	11.0	39.3	6.5	3.1
White Chocolate Chunk Lemon, Mini, M & S*	1 Muffin/28g	130	6.7	464	6.4	55.4	23.9	2.1
Wholegrain, Organic, Waitrose*	1 Muffin/68.2g	165	2.5	242	11.7	40.8	3.6	6.3
Wholemeal, Tesco*	1 Muffin/65g	130	1.3	200	12.6	32.9	2.0	5.7
MUFFIN MIX								
Banana Nut, Betty Crocker*	1 Serving/30g	130	5.0	433	6.7	70.0	16.7	0.0
MULBERRIES								
Raw	1oz/28g	10	0.0	36	1.3	8.1	0.0	0.0
MULLET								
Grey, Grilled	1oz/28g	42	1.5	150	25.7	0.0	5.2	0.0
Grey, Raw	1oz/28g	32	1.1	115	19.8	0.0	4.0	0.0
Red, Grilled	1oz/28g	34	1.2	121	20.4	0.0	4.4	0.0
Red, Raw, Weighed Whole	1oz/28g	31	1.1	109	18.7	0.0	3.8	0.0
MUNCHIES								
Mint, Nestle*	1 Pack/61g	267	10.2	432	3.8	67.5	16.4	0.0
Original, Tube, Nestle*	1 Tube/54.7g	272	13.3	498	4.1	65.6	24.4	0.5
MUSHROOMS								
Breaded, Average	1oz/28g	42	1.6	152	4.3	20.8	5.7	0.7
Breaded, Garlic, Average	1 Serving/50.3g	91	4.8	183	5.2	18.7	9.7	1.7
Buna Shimeji, Livesey Brothers*	½ Pack/75g	29	0.3	39	2.7	5.9	0.4	1.2
Button, Average	1 Serving/50g	7	0.2	15	2.3	0.5	0.4	1.2
Cheesey, Stuffed, Asda*	1 Serving/290g	322	17.4	111	4.3	10.0	6.0	0.0
Chestnut, Average	1 Mushroom/63g	8	0.3	13	1.8	0.4	0.5	0.6

MUSHROOMS

INFO/WEIGHT	Measure	per Measure		Nutrition Values per 100g / 100ml				
		KCAL	FAT	KCAL	PROT	CARB	FAT	FIBRE
Chinese, Dried, Raw	1oz/28g	80	0.5	284	10.0	59.9	1.8	0.0
Closed Cup, Average	1oz/28g	5	0.1	18	2.9	0.5	0.5	0.6
Common, Boiled in Salted Water, Average	1oz/28g	3	0.1	11	1.8	0.4	0.3	1.1
Common, Fried, Average	1oz/28g	44	4.5	157	2.4	0.3	16.2	1.5
Common, Raw, Average	1oz/28g	4	0.1	13	1.9	0.3	0.5	1.1
Creamed, Average	1oz/28g	23	1.5	82	1.3	6.8	5.5	0.5
Dried	1oz/28g	45	1.7	159	21.8	4.8	6.0	13.3
Flat, Large, Average	1 Mushroom/52g	10	0.3	20	3.3	0.5	0.5	0.7
Garlic, Average	½ Pack/150g	159	14.0	106	2.1	3.7	9.3	1.7
Giant, with Tomatoes & Mozzarella, M & S*	1 Serving/145g	218	15.8	150	6.3	7.1	10.9	5.5
Hon Shimeji, Sainsbury's*	1 Serving/80g	18	0.4	23	4.0	3.9	0.5	1.1
Oyster, Average	1oz/28g	4	0.1	15	1.6	1.7	0.3	1.3
Porcini, Wild, Dried, Merchant Gourmet*	1 Pack/25g	85	0.6	340	27.6	52.0	2.4	0.0
Shiitake, Cooked	1oz/28g	15	0.1	55	1.6	12.3	0.2	0.0
Shiitake, Dried, Raw	1oz/28g	83	0.3	296	9.6	63.9	1.0	0.0
Sliced, Average	1oz/28g	3	0.1	12	1.8	0.4	0.3	1.1
Straw, Canned, Drained	1oz/28g	4	0.1	15	2.1	1.2	0.2	0.0
Stuffed, Finest, Tesco*	1 Mushroom/130g	211	17.2	162	3.9	6.7	13.2	1.1
Stuffed, Ready to Roast, Waitrose*	1 Serving/125g	94	4.6	75	3.9	6.5	3.7	1.5

MUSSELS

Boiled, Average	1 Mussel/7g	7	0.2	104	16.7	3.5	2.7	0.0
Fresh, with Tomato & Garlic, M & S*	1 Serving/650g	455	10.4	70	7.9	6.5	1.6	0.1
Greenshell, New Zealand, Sainsbury's*	1 Serving/60g	74	1.4	123	19.2	4.3	2.3	0.1
in a Creamy Garlic Butter Sauce, Bantry Bay*	1 Serving/225g	198	7.9	88	9.0	5.2	3.5	0.6
in a Seasoned White Wine Sauce, Bantry Bay*	1 Serving/450g	270	9.0	60	6.3	4.1	2.0	0.1
in a White Wine Sauce, Sainsbury's*	½ Pack/250g	221	9.3	89	8.0	5.8	3.7	0.0
in Garlic Butter Sauce, Average	½ Pack/225g	179	11.5	80	6.4	2.0	5.1	0.2
in Thai Sauce, Scottish, Waitrose*	1 Serving/250g	135	6.3	54	5.4	2.6	2.5	0.6
Pickled, Drained, Average	1oz/28g	32	0.6	113	20.0	1.5	2.3	0.0
Raw, Average	1oz/28g	24	0.7	87	12.7	3.6	2.5	0.2
Smoked, in Sunflower Oil, Drained, John West*	1 Can/75g	149	9.1	199	13.9	8.7	12.1	0.0
Thai Fragrant, M & S*	½ Pack/325g	358	18.5	110	10.6	4.5	5.7	0.1

MUSTARD

American, French's*	1 Tbsp/15g	27	1.8	180	6.0	16.0	12.0	0.0
Cajun, Colman's*	1 Tsp/6g	11	0.4	187	7.0	23.0	6.5	2.7
Coarse Grain, Frank Cooper*	1 Tsp/6g	12	0.7	206	8.9	17.0	11.4	0.0
Coarse Grain, Organic, Simply Delicious*	1 Tbsp/5g	9	0.5	170	8.7	11.5	9.1	2.6
Dijon, Asda*	1 Tsp/7g	11	0.8	163	7.7	6.6	11.1	0.0
Dijon, French, Sainsbury's*	1 Tsp/5g	7	0.5	139	7.5	3.5	10.5	0.0
Dijon, M & S*	1 Tsp/6g	9	0.6	153	10.0	7.2	9.5	1.0
Dijon, Tesco*	1 Serving/10g	14	0.8	141	8.4	6.4	8.2	0.0
English, Asda*	½ Tsp/5g	7	0.2	144	6.0	22.0	3.6	1.9
English, Colman's*	1 Tsp/10ml	19	0.9	188	7.0	19.0	9.3	1.6
English, M & S*	1 Tsp/6g	14	1.0	226	12.6	8.7	15.9	1.0
English, Powder, Colman's*	1 Tsp/5g	26	1.7	518	29.0	24.0	34.0	6.2
English, Safeway*	1 Tsp/6g	10	0.4	163	6.1	18.3	6.7	0.0
English, Somerfield*	1 Tsp/5g	8	0.3	158	6.1	18.3	6.7	0.2
English, Tesco*	1 Serving/10g	17	0.6	171	7.0	20.2	6.4	0.4
French, Dark, Sainsbury's*	1 Tsp/5g	4	0.2	76	5.1	3.7	4.5	0.0
Honey, Colman's*	1 Tsp/6g	12	0.5	208	7.4	24.0	8.2	0.0
Whole Grain, Average	1 Tsp/8g	11	0.8	140	8.2	4.2	10.2	4.9
Whole Grain, Colman's*	1 Tsp/6g	9	0.5	157	8.4	12.0	8.4	6.6
Whole Grain, Safeway*	1 Tbsp/15g	27	1.4	183	8.0	15.2	9.1	0.0

	Measure INFO/WEIGHT	per Measure		Nutrition Values per 100g / 100ml				
		KCAL	FAT	KCAL	PROT	CARB	FAT	FIBRE
MUSTARD								
Whole Grain, Sainsbury's*	1 Tsp/5g	7	0.5	137	6.5	4.2	10.5	0.0
Whole Grain, Tesco*	1 Tsp/6g	9	0.6	153	8.2	8.7	9.5	5.8
Wholegrain, Maille*	1 Serving/10g	15	1.0	150	7.0	8.0	10.0	9.0
MUSTARD CRESS								
Raw	1oz/28g	4	0.2	13	1.6	0.4	0.6	1.1

	Measure INFO/WEIGHT	per Measure		Nutrition Values per 100g / 100ml				
		KCAL	FAT	KCAL	PROT	CARB	FAT	FIBRE
NACHOS								
American Chilli Beef, Asda*	1 Serving/200g	208	10.0	104	10.0	4.7	5.0	0.8
Cheesy, with Salsa & Soured Cream, Sainsbury's*	½ Pack/170g	449	26.9	264	8.8	21.5	15.8	1.4
Chicken, Safeway*	½ Pack/170g	352	19.4	207	10.3	15.7	11.4	1.8
Chilli, Sainsbury's*	½ Pack/250g	695	32.3	278	10.9	29.5	12.9	1.3
Kit, Old El Paso*	½ Pack/260g	598	26.0	230	4.0	31.0	10.0	0.0
NASI GORENG								
Indonesian, Asda*	1 Pack/360g	778	22.7	216	7.4	32.3	6.3	1.3
NECTARINES								
Weighed with Stone, Fresh, Raw, Average	1 Med/140g	53	0.1	38	1.3	8.5	0.1	1.2
NESQUIK								
Chocolate, Dry Weight, Nesquik, Nestle*	1 Serving/15g	56	0.5	372	3.0	82.9	3.1	6.5
Strawberry, Dry Weight, Nesquik, Nestle*	1 Serving/15g	59	0.0	393	0.0	98.1	0.0	0.0
Strawberry Milk, Fresh, Nesquik, Nestle*	1 Glass/250g	175	4.0	70	3.3	10.4	1.6	0.3
NIBBLES								
Cheese & Ham, Sainsbury's*	½ Pack/50g	257	13.6	514	13.1	54.8	27.1	2.6
NIK NAKS								
Cream 'n' Cheesy, Golden Wonder*	1 Bag/34g	196	13.0	575	5.2	52.7	38.1	0.2
Nice 'n' Spicy, Golden Wonder*	1 Bag/34g	191	13.0	561	4.7	49.6	38.3	3.0
Rib 'n' Saucy, Golden Wonder*	1 Bag/34g	194	12.8	571	4.5	53.7	37.6	0.5
Scampi 'n' Lemon, Golden Wonder*	1 Bag/34g	195	12.8	573	4.9	53.1	37.5	0.1
NOODLE BOWL								
Chilli Beef, HL, Tesco*	1 Bowl/400g	368	5.6	92	4.5	15.4	1.4	1.1
Chilli Beef, Tesco*	1 Serving/475g	456	7.6	96	7.2	13.2	1.6	1.1
Chow Mein, Chicken, Uncle Ben's*	1 Pack/330g	307	4.6	93	6.1	13.5	1.4	0.0
Szechuan Style Prawn, Tesco*	1 Bowl/400g	376	1.2	94	5.5	17.3	0.3	0.9
NOODLE BOX								
Cantonese Chow Mein, Sharwood's*	1 Pack/350g	466	10.2	133	3.8	22.9	2.9	1.5
Hong Kong Sweet & Sour, Sharwood's*	1 Box/350g	410	4.6	117	3.7	22.6	1.3	1.8
Thai Red Curry, Sharwood's*	1 Pack/350g	445	10.9	127	3.9	20.9	3.1	1.6
NOODLE SNACK								
Spicy Curry Flavour, Made Up, Asda*	1 Pot/250g	335	10.3	134	3.3	21.0	4.1	1.1
NOODLES								
Barbecue Beef, Instant, Asda*	1 Pack/333g	420	16.0	126	2.6	18.0	4.8	0.0
Beef Flavour, Instant, Prepared, Heinz*	1 Pack/384g	257	0.4	67	2.1	14.4	0.1	0.6
Buckwheat, Cold, Famima*	1 Package/295g	163	3.0	55	4.8	9.5	1.0	0.7
Char Sui, Cantonese, Sainsbury's*	1 Pack/450g	378	7.2	84	6.8	10.5	1.6	1.5
Chicken, Chinese, Asda*	1 Pot/302g	305	4.2	101	6.0	16.0	1.4	0.8
Chicken, Chinese Style, GFY, Asda*	1 Pack/393g	295	6.7	75	6.0	9.0	1.7	0.6
Chicken, Dry Weight, Heinz*	1 Pack/85g	257	0.3	302	9.5	65.3	0.4	2.7
Chicken, Instant, Jade*	1 Pack/108g	161	7.3	149	4.1	17.9	6.8	2.7
Chicken & Red Thai, Easy Steam, Tesco*	1 Serving/400g	556	28.4	139	10.3	8.6	7.1	1.1
Chicken Curry, Instant, Made Up, Sainsbury's*	1 Pack/335g	657	24.5	196	4.6	27.9	7.3	0.8
Chicken Flavour, 3 Minute, Dry, Blue Dragon*	1 Pack/85g	403	18.2	475	9.3	61.2	21.4	0.0
Chicken Flavour, Dry, Eldorado*	1 Pack/85g	360	12.8	423	14.0	61.0	15.0	0.0
Chicken Flavour, Dry, Princes*	1 Pack/85g	395	16.0	465	10.0	63.8	18.8	0.0
Chicken Flavour, Instant, Made Up, Tesco*	½ Pack/168g	285	10.6	170	4.1	23.7	6.3	1.5
Chicken Flavour, Instant, Sainsbury's*	1 Pack/335g	549	21.4	164	4.4	22.3	6.4	1.3
Chilli Beef, Finest, Tesco*	1 Pack/450g	486	8.6	108	7.7	15.2	1.9	0.9
Chilli Chicken, GFY, Asda*	1 Pack/415g	461	3.3	111	6.0	20.0	0.8	1.0
Chilli Chicken, Sweet, Sainsbury's*	1 Pack/200g	202	2.8	101	6.6	15.5	1.4	0.8
Chilli Infused, Blue Dragon*	1 Serving/150g	287	1.1	191	6.1	33.6	0.7	0.3
Chinese, Stir Fry, Sainsbury's*	1 Serving/100g	185	4.8	185	6.0	29.5	4.8	1.5
Chow Mein, Dry, Snack in a Pot, HL, Tesco*	1 Pot/56g	202	0.8	360	13.4	72.2	1.4	5.0

NOODLES

	Measure INFO/WEIGHT	per Measure KCAL	FAT	Nutrition Values per 100g / 100ml KCAL	PROT	CARB	FAT	FIBRE
Chow Mein, Instant, Made Up, Tesco*	1 Pack/167.5g	255	8.4	152	3.8	23.0	5.0	1.2
Chow Mein, Sainsbury's*	1 Pack/125g	136	2.3	109	3.9	19.2	1.8	0.8
Chow Mein, Snack in a Pot, HL, Tesco*	1 Pot/56g	202	0.8	360	13.4	72.2	1.4	5.0
Chow Mein, Stir Fry, Tesco*	1 Serving/200g	116	2.4	58	2.1	9.7	1.2	1.0
Chow Mein Flavour, Dry, Princes*	1 Pack/85g	396	15.8	466	10.1	64.6	18.6	0.0
Chow Mein Flavour, Instant, Morrisons*	1 Pack/85g	162	5.5	191	4.8	29.9	6.5	1.6
Crab Flavour, Dry, 3 Minute, Blue Dragon*	1 Pack/85g	393	16.3	463	9.9	62.6	19.2	0.0
Crispy, Dry, Blue Dragon*	1 Box/125g	438	0.6	350	2.4	84.0	0.5	0.0
Curry, Instant Weight, Dry, Heinz*	1 Serving/85g	261	0.3	307	9.5	66.4	0.4	2.7
Curry Flavour, Instant, Dry, Asda*	1 Serving/65g	415	11.0	638	20.0	101.5	16.9	0.9
Curry Flavour, Instant, Sainsbury's*	1 Pack/335g	412	15.4	123	2.6	17.8	4.6	0.1
Curry Flavour, Instant, Value, Made Up, Tesco*	1 Pack/65g	83	2.4	127	3.1	20.3	3.7	0.8
Curry Flavour, Instant, Weight Watchers*	1 Pack/385g	266	0.4	69	2.2	14.8	0.1	0.6
Egg, & Bean Sprouts, Cooked, Tesco*	1 Pack/250g	238	5.3	95	4.4	14.6	2.1	1.5
Egg, Boiled	1oz/28g	17	0.1	62	2.2	13.0	0.5	0.6
Egg, Dry	1oz/28g	109	2.3	391	12.1	71.7	8.2	2.9
Egg, Fine, Blue Dragon*	1 Serving/100g	171	1.0	171	5.5	35.0	1.0	0.0
Egg, Fine, Dry Weight, Sharwood's*	1 Block/62.5g	216	1.3	346	12.0	70.0	2.1	2.5
Egg, Fine, Fresh, M & S*	1 Pack/275g	330	6.1	120	4.4	20.7	2.2	1.5
Egg, Fine Thread, Dry, M & S*	1 Serving/63g	221	0.6	350	14.3	71.6	0.9	5.1
Egg, Fresh, Tesco*	1 Serving/150g	102	2.0	68	2.8	11.8	1.3	0.6
Egg, M & S*	½ Pack/110g	165	1.9	150	4.9	28.3	1.7	2.8
Egg, Medium, Asda*	1 Layer/190g	289	1.5	152	4.8	31.0	0.8	1.3
Egg, Medium, Dry, Blue Dragon*	1 Sheet/81g	279	1.5	345	12.0	70.0	1.9	2.5
Egg, Medium, Dry, Sharwood's*	1 Block/62.5g	216	1.3	346	12.0	70.0	2.1	2.5
Egg, Medium, Sainsbury's*	1 Serving/122.1g	168	1.0	138	5.7	26.9	0.8	1.0
Egg, Stir Fry, Fresh, Tesco*	½ Pack/205g	287	3.9	140	4.9	25.3	1.9	2.0
Egg, Thick, Dry Weight, Sharwood's*	1 Block/62.5g	214	1.1	342	10.8	71.0	1.7	2.5
Egg, Thread, Cooked Weight, Sharwood's*	1oz/28g	30	0.2	107	3.6	21.8	0.6	1.1
Egg, Tossed in Sesame Oil, Asda*	½ Pack/150g	174	10.5	116	2.3	11.0	7.0	0.6
Egg Fried, Cantonese, Safeway*	1oz/28g	29	1.5	104	3.4	10.7	5.3	1.1
Fried, Average	1oz/28g	43	3.2	153	1.9	11.3	11.5	0.5
Instant, Dry, Sainsbury's*	1 Pack/100g	392	14.0	392	9.4	57.0	14.0	0.2
Instant, Express, Dry, Blue Dragon*	1 Serving/75g	338	12.8	450	10.0	65.0	17.0	2.0
Instant, Fat Free, Koka*	1 Piece/80g	143	0.0	179	6.2	38.5	0.0	1.0
Japanese Udon, Sainsbury's*	1 Serving/150g	210	2.7	140	3.9	27.1	1.8	1.2
Oriental, Chinese, Tesco*	1 Pack/200g	184	5.0	92	2.8	14.7	2.5	1.0
Oriental, Snack Pot, Dry, HL, Tesco*	1 Pot/57g	210	1.0	369	14.0	74.4	1.7	2.0
Pasta, 100% Hard Durum Wheat, Dry, Goody*	1 Serving/100g	362	1.7	362	12.5	73.0	1.7	0.0
Peking Duck, Shapers, Boots*	1 Pack/280g	395	3.9	141	7.2	25.0	1.4	1.8
Plain, Boiled	1oz/28g	17	0.1	62	2.4	13.0	0.4	0.7
Plain, Dry	1oz/28g	109	1.7	388	11.7	76.1	6.2	2.9
Prawn, Instant, Made Up, Tesco*	1 Serving/168g	251	8.7	150	3.8	21.9	5.2	1.3
Prawn Satay, Safeway*	1 Serving/400g	460	18.4	115	5.3	12.4	4.6	1.8
Ramen, with Chilli Beef, M & S*	1 Pack/484g	532	17.4	110	8.1	11.9	3.6	0.8
Rice, Cooked, Sharwood's*	1 Serving/200g	239	0.6	120	2.1	27.2	0.3	0.8
Rice, Dry, Amoy*	1oz/28g	101	0.3	361	6.5	86.6	1.0	0.0
Rice, Dry, Blue Dragon*	1 Serving/30g	113	0.0	376	7.0	84.0	0.0	0.0
Rice, Medium, Blue Dragon*	1 Serving/62.5g	237	0.0	376	7.0	84.0	0.0	0.0
Rice, Oriental, Thai, Stir Fry, Dry, Sharwood's*	1 Serving/62.5g	227	0.6	361	6.5	86.8	1.0	2.4
Rice, Thick, Thai, Dry, M & S*	1 Serving/100g	355	0.7	355	6.0	80.6	0.7	1.4
Savoury Vegetable, COU, M & S*	1 Pack/450g	270	2.7	60	2.9	11.5	0.6	1.2
Shanghai Beef, COU, M & S*	1 Pack/400g	380	6.4	95	6.8	13.1	1.6	1.5

N

NOODLES

	Measure INFO/WEIGHT	per Measure KCAL	FAT	Nutrition Values per 100g / 100ml KCAL	PROT	CARB	FAT	FIBRE
Singapore, M & S*	½ Pack/200g	320	14.4	160	6.0	17.1	7.2	0.8
Singapore, Morrisons*	1 Serving/400g	480	26.8	120	4.8	11.6	6.7	1.6
Singapore, Oriental, Sainsbury's*	1 Pack/400g	432	15.6	108	6.4	11.7	3.9	2.8
Singapore, Somerfield*	1 Pot/300g	261	3.0	87	5.0	15.0	1.0	0.0
Singapore, Tesco*	1 Pack/350g	389	7.4	111	6.3	16.8	2.1	0.7
Singapore, Waitrose*	1 Pack/400g	476	17.6	119	7.3	12.6	4.4	2.1
Singapore Spicy, Safeway*	1 Serving/225g	270	9.7	120	6.0	14.2	4.3	1.7
Singapore Style, Asda*	1 Pack/400g	688	32.0	172	7.0	18.0	8.0	1.0
Special, Chinese Takeaway, Iceland*	1 Pack/340g	422	10.9	124	6.5	17.2	3.2	0.6
Spicy, Sainsbury's*	1 Serving/180g	182	8.3	101	10.4	4.5	4.6	0.9
Spicy Curry Flavour, Dry, Princes*	1 Pack/85g	395	16.0	465	9.6	64.1	18.8	0.0
Spicy Thai, Instant, Heinz*	1 Pack/385g	262	0.4	68	2.1	14.6	0.1	0.6
Stir Fry, Tesco*	1 Serving/150g	203	3.6	135	5.3	23.0	2.4	1.5
Straight to Wok, Medium, Amoy*	1 Pack/150g	240	2.3	160	5.8	31.7	1.5	0.0
Straight to Wok, Rice, Amoy*	1 Pack/150g	174	0.2	116	1.6	27.4	0.1	0.0
Straight to Wok, Singapore, Amoy*	1 Serving/150g	233	4.2	155	4.8	28.4	2.8	0.0
Straight to Wok, Thread, Fine, Amoy*	1 Pack/150g	237	3.9	158	5.0	28.7	2.6	0.0
Straight to Wok, Udon, Amoy*	1 Pack/150g	212	2.0	141	4.4	28.8	1.3	0.0
Super, Bacon Flavour, Dry Weight, Batchelors*	1 Packet/100g	526	23.6	526	9.4	69.2	23.6	1.6
Super, BBQ Beef, Made Up, Batchelors*	1 Serving/100g	156	6.7	156	3.2	20.9	6.7	1.1
Super, BBQ Beef, to Go, 98% Fat Free, Batchelors*	1 Pack/380g	308	0.6	81	2.4	17.6	0.2	0.6
Super, Cheese & Ham, Made Up, Batchelors*	1 Serving/100g	171	7.3	171	3.4	22.9	7.3	0.6
Super, Chicken & Ham, Dry Weight, Batchelors*	1 Pack/100g	472	20.2	472	9.4	63.2	20.2	1.5
Super, Chicken & Herb, Low Fat, Dry, Batchelors*	½ Pack/42.5g	161	0.8	379	12.2	78.4	1.9	2.4
Super, Chicken Flavour, Dry Weight, Batchelors*	1 Serving/100g	449	19.2	449	8.7	60.3	19.2	2.5
Super, Chicken Flavour, Made Up, Batchelors*	1 Serving/100g	170	7.3	170	3.3	22.9	7.3	0.9
Super, Chow Mein Flavour, Made Up, Batchelors*	½ Pack/149.7g	262	11.8	175	3.0	23.0	7.9	0.4
Super, Mild Curry, Dry Weight, Batchelors*	½ Pack/50g	260	11.7	520	9.4	67.8	23.4	1.4
Super, Mild Curry Flavour, Made Up, Batchelors*	1 Serving/100g	157	6.7	157	3.2	20.9	6.7	1.0
Super, Mushroom Flavour, Made Up, Batchelors*	1 Serving/100g	157	6.8	157	3.2	20.9	6.8	1.0
Super, Spicy Balti, Made Up, Batchelors*	1 Serving/100g	166	7.5	166	3.0	21.5	7.5	1.1
Super, Spicy Salsa, Dry Weight, Batchelors*	1 Pack/105g	474	19.5	451	7.0	63.8	18.6	1.7
Super, Sweet Thai Chilli, Dry Weight, Batchelors*	1 Pack/85g	292	1.0	343	10.6	72.5	1.2	3.0
Sweet & Sour, BGTY, Sainsbury's*	1 Serving/100g	112	3.1	112	2.3	18.6	3.1	0.0
Sweet Chilli, Wok, Findus*	1 Pack/300g	300	1.5	100	3.0	20.0	0.5	0.0
Szechuan Beef Flavour, Dry, Blue Dragon*	½ Pack/100g	350	1.2	350	10.5	72.3	1.2	0.0
Thai, Spicy, Stir Fry, HL, Tesco*	½ Pack/250g	220	5.5	88	4.1	12.9	2.2	1.7
Thai, Waitrose*	1 Pack/300g	357	6.3	119	6.8	18.4	2.1	1.7
Thai Chicken, Takeaway, Somerfield*	1 Pack/300g	426	16.8	142	7.8	16.0	5.6	0.8
Thai Style, Asda*	1 Pot/237.9g	226	0.7	95	3.0	20.0	0.3	0.8
Thai Style, Sainsbury's*	1 Pack/340g	381	7.8	112	3.3	19.4	2.3	0.7
Tiger Prawn, Stir Fry, Tesco*	1 Pack/400g	596	14.8	149	6.0	23.0	3.7	2.7
Tom Yum Flavour, Cup Noodles, Tiger Tiger*	1 Pack/90g	406	15.2	451	9.2	65.4	16.9	5.0
Udon Japanese, & Dashi Soup Stock, Yutaka*	1 Pack/230g	290	1.2	126	3.0	26.8	0.5	0.0
Whole Wheat, Dry, Blue Dragon*	1 Serving/65g	208	1.3	320	12.5	63.0	2.0	8.0
with Sweet Chilli Chicken, COU, M & S*	1 Serving/300g	360	8.1	120	6.6	17.8	2.7	1.3
Yaki Udan, Chicken & Prawn, M & S*	1 Pack/395g	435	14.2	110	8.1	11.9	3.6	0.8

NOUGAT

	Measure INFO/WEIGHT	per Measure KCAL	FAT	Nutrition Values per 100g / 100ml KCAL	PROT	CARB	FAT	FIBRE
Average	1 Sm Bar/28g	108	2.4	384	4.4	77.3	8.5	0.9
Bassetts & Beyond, Cadbury*	1oz/28g	105	1.1	375	4.0	82.0	4.0	0.0
Soft, Bar, Bassett's*	1 Serving/25g	94	1.0	375	4.0	82.0	4.0	0.0

NUT ROAST

	Measure INFO/WEIGHT	per Measure KCAL	FAT	Nutrition Values per 100g / 100ml KCAL	PROT	CARB	FAT	FIBRE
Average	1 Serving/200g	704	51.4	352	13.3	18.3	25.7	4.2

	Measure INFO/WEIGHT	per Measure KCAL	per Measure FAT	Nutrition Values per 100g / 100ml KCAL	PROT	CARB	FAT	FIBRE
NUT ROAST								
Courgette & Spiced Tomato, Cauldron*	1 Serving/100g	208	12.3	208	11.7	12.5	12.3	4.9
Lentil, Average	1oz/28g	62	3.4	222	10.6	18.8	12.1	3.8
Vegetarian, Tesco*	½ Pack/200g	340	17.0	170	5.1	17.2	8.5	2.7
NUTMEG								
Ground, Average	1 Tsp/3g	16	1.1	525	5.8	45.3	36.3	0.0
NUTS								
Lemon & Chilli Flavour, Mix, TTD, Sainsbury's*	1 Serving/50g	321	28.7	641	20.0	11.2	57.3	5.7
Luxury Assortment, Tesco*	1 Serving/10g	68	6.5	676	17.5	6.1	64.6	5.0
Mixed	1 Pack/40g	243	21.6	607	22.9	7.9	54.1	6.0
Mixed, Chopped, Safeway*	1 Serving/2g	12	1.0	588	22.0	10.3	51.0	5.9
Mixed, Chopped, Sainsbury's*	1 Serving/100g	605	50.9	605	27.1	9.6	50.9	6.0
Mixed, Chopped, Tesco*	1 Serving/25g	149	12.7	595	23.5	10.5	50.6	6.0
Mixed, Honey Roasted, Waitrose*	1 Serving/50g	292	22.5	583	17.1	27.5	45.0	5.3
Mixed, M & S*	1 Pack/70g	462	44.8	660	16.0	4.8	64.0	5.4
Mixed, Nature's Harvest*	1 Serving/25g	145	13.4	581	17.5	7.7	53.4	6.3
Mixed, Roasted, Salted, Waitrose*	1 Pack/200g	1252	116.8	626	13.7	11.3	58.4	4.4
Mixed, Roasted, Waitrose*	1 Serving/25g	166	16.0	662	15.2	6.2	64.0	8.2
Mixed, Sainsbury's*	1 Serving/20g	124	11.3	622	20.2	7.8	56.7	5.6
Mixed, Unsalted, Sainsbury's*	1 Serving/50g	311	28.9	622	18.5	7.2	57.7	8.7
Natural, Mixed, Waitrose*	1 Serving/50g	324	30.6	648	17.7	6.8	61.1	8.2
Natural Assortment, Tesco*	1 Serving/50g	338	32.3	676	17.5	6.1	64.6	5.0
Oak Smoke Flavour Selection, Finest, Tesco*	1 Serving/25g	158	14.0	633	21.4	11.2	55.8	6.3
Peanuts & Cashews, Honey Roast, Tesco*	1 Serving/25g	145	10.7	579	21.6	26.6	42.9	4.2
Pine, Tesco*	1 Pack/100g	699	68.6	699	16.5	4.0	68.6	1.9
Roast Salted, Luxury, KP Snacks*	1oz/28g	181	16.1	646	21.9	10.1	57.6	5.9
Roasted, Salted, Assortment, Luxury, Tesco*	1 Serving/25g	161	14.5	643	21.1	9.4	57.9	8.1
Salted, Selection, Sainsbury's*	1 Serving/30g	190	17.1	634	20.6	9.7	56.9	8.2
Salted, Selection, TTD, Sainsbury's*	1 Pack/75g	509	48.2	678	16.3	8.9	64.2	7.2
Soya, Dry Roasted, The Food Doctor*	1 Serving/50g	203	10.7	406	37.5	15.9	21.4	16.1
Unsalted, Selection, Sainsbury's*	1 Serving/75g	491	48.0	655	14.7	5.0	64.0	6.7
NUTS & RAISINS								
Mixed, Average	1 Serving/40g	192	13.6	481	14.1	31.5	34.1	4.5
Peanuts, Mixed, Average	1 Pack/40g	174	10.4	435	15.3	37.5	26.0	4.4
Yoghurt Coated, Waitrose*	1 Serving/50g	264	18.4	527	10.9	38.2	36.7	3.0

N

	Measure INFO/WEIGHT	per Measure KCAL	FAT	KCAL	PROT	CARB	FAT	FIBRE
OAT CAKES								
Bran, Paterson's*	1 Cake/12.5g	50	1.9	416	10.0	58.5	15.8	9.5
Cheese, Nairn's*	1 Oatcake/8.9g	42	2.3	472	12.9	46.7	26.0	7.1
Fine Milled, Nairn's*	1 Cake/7g	31	1.5	448	10.8	53.7	21.8	8.2
Highland, Organic, Sainsbury's*	1 Cake/12.5g	59	2.5	456	10.2	59.8	19.5	5.5
Highland, Walkers Shortbread*	1 Cake/12g	54	2.5	451	10.3	56.0	20.6	6.7
Organic, The Village Bakery*	1 Cake/12.5g	59	2.8	452	10.9	54.5	21.3	5.6
Retail, Average	1 Cake/13g	57	2.4	441	10.0	63.0	18.3	0.0
Rough, Nairn's*	1 Cake/10.7g	45	1.9	419	11.2	53.2	17.9	10.7
Rough, Sainsbury's*	1 Cake/10.6g	47	1.9	426	11.7	65.2	16.9	8.6
Rough, Scottish, Tesco*	1 Cake/11g	48	2.0	434	12.3	54.8	18.4	6.6
Rough, with Olive Oil, Paterson's*	1 Cake/12.5g	54	2.2	431	10.6	58.4	17.2	8.1
Rough Scottish, Sainsbury's*	1 Cake/11g	51	2.1	462	12.3	59.9	19.3	6.5
Scottish, M & S*	1oz/28g	116	3.5	413	9.1	70.0	12.6	8.5
Scottish, Organic, Waitrose*	1 Cake/13g	58	2.5	447	11.2	57.0	19.4	6.6
OAT DRINK								
Healthy Oat, Enriched, Oatly*	1 Serving/100ml	45	1.5	45	1.0	6.5	1.5	0.8
Healthy Oat, Organic, Oatly*	1 Serving/150ml	53	1.1	35	1.0	6.5	0.7	0.8
OATMEAL								
Raw	1oz/28g	112	2.4	401	12.4	72.8	8.7	6.8
OATS								
Easy, Original, Sainsbury's*	1 Serving/27g	97	2.2	359	11.0	60.4	8.1	8.5
Jumbo, Organic, Evernat*	1oz/28g	117	2.7	418	13.0	69.0	9.6	7.4
OCEAN								
Prawnies, Mini, Asda*	1 Prawnie/11g	9	0.1	84	11.0	8.0	0.9	0.5
Snacks, Sainsbury's*	1 Stick/16g	18	0.0	113	7.0	21.0	0.1	0.1
Sticks, Average	1 Stick/16g	17	0.0	109	7.1	19.9	0.2	0.2
OCTOPUS								
Raw	1oz/28g	23	0.4	83	17.9	0.0	1.3	0.0
OIL								
Again & Again, No Cholesterol, Anglia*	1 Tbsp/15ml	124	13.8	828	0.0	0.0	92.0	0.0
Avocado, Olivado*	1 Tsp/5ml	40	4.4	802	0.0	0.0	88.0	0.0
Black Truffle, Grapeseed, Cuisine Perel*	1 Tsp/5ml	43	5.0	857	0.0	7.1	100.0	0.0
Chilli, Average	1 Tsp/5ml	41	4.6	824	0.0	0.0	91.5	0.0
Chinese Stir Fry, Asda*	1 Tbsp/15ml	123	13.7	823	0.0	0.0	91.4	0.0
Coconut, Average	1 Tsp/5ml	45	5.0	899	0.0	0.0	99.9	0.0
Corn, Average	1 Tsp/5ml	43	4.8	865	0.0	0.0	96.0	0.0
Dipping, Herb, Italian Style, Finest, Tesco*	1 Serving/5g	44	4.8	877	0.4	0.9	96.9	0.4
Dipping, with Balsamic Vinegar, Finest, Tesco*	1 Tsp/5ml	33	3.6	668	0.0	4.4	71.7	0.0
Fry Light, Bodyline*	4 Sprays/0.8ml	5	0.6	522	0.0	0.0	55.2	0.0
Groundnut, Average	1 Serving/25ml	206	23.0	824	0.0	0.0	91.8	0.0
Hazelnut, Average	1 Tsp/5ml	45	5.0	899	0.0	0.0	99.9	0.0
Linseed, Organic, Biona*	1 Serving/10ml	84	9.3	837	0.0	0.0	93.0	0.0
Macadamia Nut, Oz Tukka*	1 Tsp/5ml	40	4.6	805	0.0	0.0	91.0	0.0
Olive, Average	1 Tsp/5ml	43	4.7	855	0.0	0.0	94.9	0.0
Olive, Basil Infused, Tesco*	1 Serving/20ml	180	20.0	900	0.0	0.0	100.0	0.0
Olive, Extra Virgin, Average	1 Tsp/5ml	42	4.7	848	0.0	0.0	94.5	0.0
Olive, Extra Virgin, Mist Spray, Belolive*	1 Serving/5ml	25	2.8	500	0.0	0.0	55.0	0.0
Olive, Extra Virgin, Only 1 Cal, Spray, Fry Light*	1 Spray/0.2ml	1	0.1	498	0.0	0.0	55.2	0.0
Olive, Garlic, Average	1 Tbsp/15ml	127	14.1	848	0.0	0.0	94.3	0.0
Olive, Lemon Flavoured, Sainsbury's*	1 Tbsp/15ml	123	13.7	823	0.1	0.0	91.4	0.1
Olive, Mild, Average	1 Tbsp/15mll	129	14.4	862	0.1	0.0	95.7	0.0
Olive, Spray, Fry Light*	5 Sprays/1ml	5	0.6	498	0.0	0.0	55.2	0.0
Palm, Average	1 Tsp/5ml	45	5.0	899	0.0	0.0	99.9	0.0

	Measure INFO/WEIGHT	per Measure KCAL	FAT	Nutrition Values per 100g / 100ml KCAL	PROT	CARB	FAT	FIBRE
OIL								
Peanut, Average	1 Tsp/5ml	45	5.0	899	0.0	0.0	99.9	0.0
Rapeseed, Average	1 Tbsp/15ml	130	14.4	864	0.0	0.0	96.0	0.0
Red Palm & Canola, Carotino*	1 Tsp/5ml	41	4.6	812	0.0	0.0	92.0	0.0
Safflower, Average	1 Tsp/5ml	45	5.0	899	0.0	0.0	99.9	0.0
Sesame, Average	1 Tsp/5ml	45	5.0	892	0.1	0.0	99.9	0.0
Soya, Average	1 Tsp/5ml	45	5.0	899	0.0	0.0	99.9	0.0
Stir Fry, Sharwood's*	1 fl oz/30ml	269	29.9	897	0.0	0.0	99.7	0.0
Sunflower, Average	1 Tsp/5ml	43	4.8	869	0.0	0.0	96.6	0.0
Sunflower, Spray, Fry Light*	1 Spray/0.2ml	1	0.1	522	0.0	0.0	55.2	0.0
Vegetable, Average	1 Tbsp/15ml	129	14.3	858	0.0	0.0	95.3	0.0
Walnut, Average	1 Tsp/5ml	45	5.0	899	0.0	0.0	99.9	0.0
Wheatgerm, Average	1 Tsp/5ml	45	5.0	899	0.0	0.0	99.9	0.0
OKRA								
Boiled in Unsalted Water, Average	1 Serving/60g	17	0.5	28	2.5	2.7	0.9	3.6
Canned, Drained, Average	1 Serving/60g	13	0.4	21	1.4	2.5	0.7	2.6
Raw, Average	10 Med Okra/50g	16	0.5	31	2.8	3.0	1.0	4.0
Stir-Fried in Corn Oil, Average	1 Serving/60g	161	15.7	269	4.3	4.4	26.1	6.3
OLIVES								
Black, Pitted, Average	½ Jar/82g	135	13.3	164	1.0	3.5	16.2	3.1
Green, Garlic Stuffed, Asda*	1 Olive/3.4g	5	0.5	174	1.8	3.5	17.0	0.0
Green, Pimiento Stuffed, Somerfield*	1 Olive/3g	4	0.4	126	1.0	4.0	12.0	0.0
Green, Pitted, Average	1 Olive/3g	4	0.4	130	1.1	0.9	13.3	2.5
Green, Pitted, Minced Pimiento Stuffed, Sainsbury's*	3 Olives/15.6g	23	2.2	147	1.2	3.9	14.1	2.0
Green, Pitted, Stuffed with Anchovies, Sainsbury's*	1 Serving/50g	78	8.1	155	1.8	0.6	16.1	3.2
Green, Queen, Sainsbury's*	1 Olive/8g	12	0.8	145	1.3	11.0	10.6	2.5
Green, Stuffed with Almonds, Pitted, Waitrose*	1 Serving/50g	90	8.5	180	3.8	3.2	16.9	2.5
Green, Stuffed with Anchovy, Waitrose*	½ Can/40g	38	3.1	94	1.5	4.7	7.7	2.3
Kalamata, Gaea*	1 Serving/50g	54	4.9	107	0.0	3.8	9.8	3.4
Kalamata, Greek, Whole, Waitrose*	1 Serving/28g	30	2.7	107	1.0	3.8	9.8	3.4
Marinated, Mixed, Anti Pasti, Asda*	1 Serving/100g	215	22.0	215	1.8	0.7	22.0	3.1
Marinated, Mixed, M & S*	1 Serving/20g	33	3.0	165	1.6	6.5	14.9	3.0
Marinated, Mixed, with Feta & Red Peppers, Asda*	1 Pot/120g	233	21.6	194	5.8	2.2	18.0	1.7
Marinated, Selection, M & S*	4 Olives/19.6g	45	4.5	225	1.4	3.9	22.6	2.1
Pimento Stuffed, in Brine, Tesco*	1 Serving/25g	38	4.1	153	0.8	0.1	16.4	2.1
Pitted, with Anchovy Paste, Safeway*	1/3 Can/50g	70	7.1	139	2.7	0.1	14.2	2.0
OMELETTE								
Cheese, 2 Egg, Average	1 Omelette/180g	479	40.7	266	15.9	0.0	22.6	0.0
Cheese, Asda*	1 Omelette/119g	270	22.8	225	12.0	1.5	19.0	0.0
Cheese, Findus*	1 Serving/200g	400	26.0	200	9.5	14.0	13.0	0.0
Cheese, Tesco*	1 Omelette/120g	258	20.9	215	11.6	2.8	17.4	0.6
Cheese & Mushroom, Apetito*	1 Serving/320g	486	25.0	152	6.2	14.4	7.8	1.9
Cheese & Mushroom, Chef's Fastfood*	1 Omelette/100g	180	14.1	180	9.6	3.9	14.1	0.0
Ham & Mushroom, Farmfoods*	1 Omelette/120g	200	16.7	167	8.7	1.8	13.9	0.1
Mushroom & Cheese, Tesco*	1 Omelette/120g	248	21.5	207	9.8	1.6	17.9	0.2
Plain, 2 Egg	1 Omelette/120g	229	19.7	191	10.9	0.0	16.4	0.0
Spanish	1oz/28g	34	2.3	120	5.7	6.2	8.3	1.4
ONION RINGS								
Battered, Asda*	1 Serving/100g	343	22.7	343	3.8	31.0	22.7	1.7
Battered, Oven Baked, Tesco*	1 Serving/50g	110	5.0	219	3.9	28.4	10.0	3.5
Battered, Sainsbury's*	1 Ring/12g	26	1.2	219	3.9	28.4	10.0	3.5
Breadcrumbs, Tesco*	1 Serving/100g	294	15.6	294	4.3	34.1	15.6	2.3
Breaded, Asda*	1 Serving/10g	29	1.5	289	4.4	34.0	15.0	2.7
Breaded, Iceland*	4 Rings/45g	132	6.9	293	4.4	34.2	15.4	2.7

	Measure INFO/WEIGHT	per Measure KCAL	FAT	Nutrition Values per 100g / 100ml KCAL	PROT	CARB	FAT	FIBRE
ONION RINGS								
Breaded, Sainsbury's*	1 Serving/100g	280	12.4	280	4.6	37.6	12.4	4.1
Oven Crisp Batter, Tesco*	1 Ring/17g	40	2.3	236	4.2	24.8	13.3	2.5
ONIONS								
Baked	1oz/28g	29	0.2	103	3.5	22.3	0.6	3.9
Boiled in Unsalted Water	1oz/28g	5	0.0	17	0.6	3.7	0.1	0.7
Borettane, Char-Grilled, Sacla*	1 Serving/100g	90	5.6	90	0.9	8.9	5.6	2.5
Dried, Raw	1oz/28g	88	0.5	313	10.2	68.6	1.7	12.1
Fried, Average	1oz/28g	46	3.1	164	2.3	14.1	11.2	3.1
Organic, Tesco*	1 Onion/120g	46	0.2	38	1.2	7.9	0.2	1.4
Pickled, Average	1oz/28g	6	0.0	23	0.8	4.9	0.1	0.7
Raw, Average	1 Med/180g	55	0.3	31	1.3	6.0	0.2	1.4
Red, Raw, Average	1 Med/180g	66	0.4	37	1.2	7.9	0.2	1.5
OPTIONS								
Belgian Chocolate Drink, Ovaltine*	1 Sachet/11g	37	0.9	336	11.8	52.7	8.2	0.0
Carribbean Coconut, Ovaltine*	1 Sachet/11g	33	0.8	300	11.8	46.4	7.3	0.0
Choca Mocha Drink, Ovaltine*	1 Sachet/11g	39	1.3	359	14.1	50.1	11.4	7.0
Chocolate Au Lait, Ovaltine*	1 Sachet/11g	36	1.0	355	11.8	54.5	10.0	7.3
Cracking Hazelnut, Ovaltine*	1 Sachet/11g	40	1.2	361	16.0	57.0	11.0	0.0
Irish Cream, Ovaltine*	1 Sachet/11g	39	1.2	357	13.9	50.0	11.3	8.1
Mint Madness, Ovaltine*	1 Serving/11g	40	1.3	365	15.0	50.6	11.4	0.0
Outrageous Orange, Ovaltine*	1 Serving/11g	40	1.3	367	15.3	50.8	11.4	0.0
Tempting Toffee, Ovaltine*	1 Sachet/11g	43	1.0	391	13.6	66.4	9.1	0.0
Turkish Delight, Ovaltine*	1 Serving/11.1g	34	0.9	305	11.8	46.9	7.8	18.0
Wicked White Chocolate, Ovaltine*	1 Sachet/11g	43	1.2	391	9.5	63.0	10.5	0.0
ORANGE DRINK								
Sparkling, Diet, Tesco*	1 Glass/250ml	8	0.3	3	0.1	0.5	0.1	0.0
Sparkling, Florida, M & S*	1 Serving/500ml	250	0.0	50	0.0	12.5	0.0	0.0
Sugar Free, Tesco*	1 Glass/250ml	3	0.0	1	0.0	0.0	0.0	0.0
ORANGES								
Blood	1 Orange/140g	82	0.0	58	0.8	13.3	0.0	2.5
Fresh, Weighed with Peel, Average	1 Med/185g	115	0.5	62	1.0	15.6	0.3	3.2
Fresh, without Peel, Average	1 Med/145g	90	0.4	62	1.0	15.6	0.3	3.2
OREGANO								
Dried, Ground	1 Tsp/1g	3	0.1	306	11.0	49.5	10.3	0.0
Fresh	1oz/28g	18	0.6	66	2.2	9.7	2.0	0.0
OVALTINE*								
Hi Malt, Light, Instant Drink, Dry, Ovaltine*	1 Sachet/20g	72	1.2	358	9.1	67.1	5.9	2.8
Made with Semi-Skimmed Milk, Ovaltine*	1 Mug/227ml	179	3.9	79	3.9	13.0	1.7	0.0
Made with Whole Milk, Ovaltine*	1 Mug/227ml	220	8.6	97	3.8	12.9	3.8	0.0
OXTAIL								
Raw	1oz/28g	48	2.8	171	20.0	0.0	10.1	0.0
Stewed	1oz/28g	68	3.8	243	30.5	0.0	13.4	0.0
OYSTERS								
in Vegetable Oil, Smoked, John West*	1oz/28g	64	3.9	230	16.0	10.0	14.0	0.0
Raw	1oz/28g	18	0.4	65	10.8	2.7	1.3	0.0

O

	Measure INFO/WEIGHT	per Measure KCAL	FAT	Nutrition Values per 100g / 100ml KCAL	PROT	CARB	FAT	FIBRE
PAELLA								
Bistro, Waitrose*	1 Serving/300g	534	19.8	178	7.4	22.2	6.6	0.7
Chicken, HE, Tesco*	1 Pack/400g	416	3.2	104	8.9	15.4	0.8	2.2
Chicken, HL, Tesco*	1 Pack/400g	432	2.0	108	6.7	19.2	0.5	1.7
Chicken, Steam Pack, HE, Tesco*	1 Pack/350g	291	1.4	83	8.1	11.8	0.4	7.0
Chicken, Tesco*	1 Serving/475g	575	14.3	121	7.9	15.7	3.0	1.6
Chicken & Chorizo, Asda*	1 Pack/390g	484	8.6	124	10.0	16.0	2.2	2.6
Chicken & Chorizo, Big Dish, M & S*	1 Pack/450g	630	17.6	140	7.9	18.4	3.9	1.6
Chicken & Vegetable, HL, Tesco*	1 Pack/450g	441	5.9	98	9.7	11.8	1.3	1.1
Enjoy, Birds Eye*	1 Pack/500g	620	16.0	124	7.7	16.2	3.2	0.6
Seafood, Finest, Tesco*	1 Pack/400g	756	23.6	189	6.8	27.2	5.9	1.0
Seafood, M & S*	1 Pack/450g	518	17.1	115	6.4	13.7	3.8	3.2
Seafood, Sainsbury's*	1 Pack/400g	504	5.2	126	8.3	20.3	1.3	0.6
Spanish, TTD, Sainsbury's*	½ Pack/350g	448	12.6	128	7.9	15.9	3.6	0.2
Tesco*	1 Serving/460g	584	17.0	127	4.6	18.9	3.7	1.0
Vegetable, Waitrose*	1 Serving/174g	202	3.1	116	2.2	22.7	1.8	1.5
PANCAKE								
HL, Tesco*	1 Pancake/25g	60	0.5	240	5.8	48.8	2.0	1.9
Maple & Raisin, M & S*	1 Pancake/32.7g	89	1.8	269	6.5	49.7	5.4	2.2
Mini, for, Kids, Tesco*	1 Pancake/16g	45	0.9	283	6.6	51.7	5.5	1.3
Mini, Scotch, Tesco*	1 Pancake/16g	44	0.9	277	6.7	50.0	5.6	1.4
Morrisons*	1 Pancake/60g	133	3.0	221	8.4	37.3	5.0	1.5
Perfect, Kingsmill*	1 Pancake/26.9g	71	1.2	264	6.2	49.7	4.5	1.2
Plain, Sainsbury's*	2 Pancakes/92g	203	4.9	221	6.9	36.1	5.3	1.2
Raisin & Lemon, Asda*	1 Serving/30g	92	2.4	304	6.0	52.0	8.0	1.4
Savoury, Made with Skimmed Milk, Average	1 6"/77g	192	11.3	249	6.4	24.1	14.7	0.8
Savoury, Made with Whole Milk, Average	1 6"/77g	210	13.5	273	6.3	24.0	17.5	0.8
Scotch	1 Pancake/50g	146	5.9	292	5.8	43.6	11.7	1.4
Scotch, M & S*	1 Pancake/34g	95	1.4	280	6.5	54.5	4.0	1.6
Scotch, Sainsbury's*	1 Pancake/30g	81	2.1	280	6.3	47.6	7.2	1.7
Scotch, SmartPrice, Asda*	1 Pancake/35g	107	3.2	305	7.0	49.0	9.0	1.4
Sweet, Made with Skimmed Milk	1oz/28g	78	3.9	280	6.0	35.1	13.8	0.8
Sweet, Made with Whole Milk	1oz/28g	84	4.5	301	5.9	35.0	16.2	0.8
Syrup, Tesco*	1 Pancake/30g	80	2.5	265	4.7	42.1	8.2	1.5
Traditional, Aunt Bessie's*	1 Pancake/60g	90	1.9	150	6.1	24.6	3.1	1.1
Traditional, Tesco*	1 Pancake/62g	137	3.1	221	8.4	35.6	5.0	1.5
Vegetable Roll	1 Roll/85g	185	10.6	218	6.6	21.0	12.5	0.0
Warburton's*	1 Pancake/35g	84	2.2	239	7.6	37.7	6.4	2.4
with Syrup, American Style, Lge, Tesco*	2 Pancakes/76g	204	2.6	268	5.1	54.2	3.4	0.9
PANCAKE MIX								
Fresh, M & S*	1 Pancake/38.3g	89	5.0	235	7.5	22.4	13.1	0.5
Glutano*	3 Tbs/45g	170	1.0	378	8.9	75.6	2.2	0.0
Traditional, Asda*	1 Pack/256g	545	23.0	213	6.0	27.0	9.0	1.8
PANCETTA								
Average	½ Pack/65g	212	18.7	327	17.0	0.1	28.7	0.1
PANINI								
Mozzarella & Tomato, M & S*	1 Serving/176g	484	28.5	275	11.3	21.3	16.2	2.1
Tuna & Sweetcorn, Tesco*	1 Serving/250g	559	16.4	224	12.0	29.3	6.6	1.4
Tuna Melt, Tesco*	1 Serving/230.8g	464	7.4	201	13.6	32.9	3.2	0.9
PANNA COTTA								
Sainsbury's*	1 Pot/100g	304	15.7	304	3.0	41.5	15.7	4.0
PAPAYA								
Dried, Pieces, Nature's Harvest*	1 Serving/50g	178	0.0	355	0.2	85.4	0.0	2.6
Dried, Strips, Tropical Wholefoods*	1 Strip/10g	310	0.9	310	3.9	71.4	0.9	1.5

P

	Measure INFO/WEIGHT	per Measure KCAL	FAT	Nutrition Values per 100g / 100ml KCAL	PROT	CARB	FAT	FIBRE
PAPAYA								
Dried, Sweetened, Tesco*	4 Pieces/25g	59	0.2	235	0.4	56.3	0.9	2.9
Raw, Flesh Only, Average	1 Serving/140g	37	0.1	26	0.4	6.6	0.1	1.2
Raw, Weighed with Seeds & Skin	1 Med/304g	119	0.4	39	0.6	9.8	0.1	1.8
Unripe, Raw, Weighed with Seeds & Skin	1oz/28g	8	0.0	27	0.9	5.5	0.1	1.5
PAPPADS								
Green Chilli & Garlic, Sharwood's*	1 Pappad/14g	38	0.3	268	23.2	39.4	1.9	14.6
PAPPARDELLE								
All'uovo, The Best, Morrisons*	1 Serving/75g	261	2.2	348	13.2	67.3	2.9	2.9
Basil, Fresh, Sainsbury's*	1 Serving/240g	281	3.4	117	5.0	21.2	1.4	2.0
Buitoni*	1 Serving/65g	242	3.1	373	15.0	67.5	4.8	0.0
Chilli, Fresh, Sainsbury's*	1 Serving/250g	303	4.3	121	5.7	20.7	1.7	2.0
Egg, Fresh, Waitrose*	¼ Pack/125g	350	3.4	280	12.9	51.0	2.7	1.9
Roasted Vegetable & Goats Cheese, M & S*	1 Pack/400g	400	18.8	100	3.5	11.2	4.7	2.2
Saffron, Eat Well, M & S*	Serving/100g	360	2.5	360	14.0	69.0	2.5	3.2
Salmon, COU, M & S*	1 Pack/358g	340	6.8	95	6.3	13.0	1.9	0.8
The Best Fresh, The Best, Morrisons*	¼ Pack/240g	353	3.8	147	6.3	26.9	1.6	1.9
with Salmon, COU, M & S*	1 Pack/358g	340	6.8	95	6.3	13.0	1.9	0.8
PAPRIKA								
Average	1 Tsp/2g	6	0.3	289	14.8	34.9	13.0	0.0
PARATHA								
Average	1 Paratha/80g	258	11.4	322	8.0	43.2	14.3	4.0
Roti, Plain, Crown Farms*	1 Slice/80g	250	10.0	313	5.0	46.3	12.5	1.3
PARCELS								
Basil & Parmesan, Fresh, Sainsbury's*	1 Pack/250g	550	20.8	220	10.0	26.4	8.3	3.3
Beef Steak, Sainsbury's*	½ Pack/226g	488	35.3	216	12.2	6.6	15.6	1.0
Cheese & Ham, Sainsbury's*	1 Pack/250g	445	19.0	178	7.4	19.9	7.6	1.5
Chilli Beef, Tex Mex Feast, Asda*	1 Parcel/25g	68	3.5	270	9.0	27.0	14.0	2.1
Filo, Brie & Cranberry, Tesco*	1 Parcel/22g	82	5.3	373	9.5	29.3	24.2	1.5
Filo, Mushroom, Savoury, Creamy, Somerfield*	1oz/28g	86	5.9	308	5.0	24.0	21.0	0.0
Filo, Mushroom Leek & Gruyere, Finest, Tesco*	1 Serving/160g	440	33.6	275	6.9	20.5	21.0	1.5
Salmon, in Lemon Sauce, M & S*	1 Serving/185g	350	27.9	189	12.1	1.4	15.1	0.5
Salmon, Smoked, Scottish, M & S*	1 Parcel/65g	146	10.9	225	16.6	2.3	16.7	0.8
Smoked Salmon, Sainsbury's*	1 Pack/115g	269	20.2	234	15.8	3.5	17.6	0.2
Smoked Salmon, with Soft Cheese & Herb, Waitrose*	1 Serving/57g	140	11.5	246	14.6	1.2	20.2	0.0
Turkey Breast, with Cheddar Cheese & Chive, Asda*	1 Parcel/140g	242	9.8	173	23.0	4.6	7.0	0.9
with Cheese & Sweet Pepper Sauce, Egg, Somerfield*	½ Pack/125g	349	14.8	279	12.4	30.7	11.8	2.2
PARSLEY								
Dried	1 Tsp/1.3g	2	0.1	181	15.8	14.5	7.0	26.9
Fresh, Average	1 Tbsp/3.8g	1	0.0	34	3.0	2.7	1.3	5.0
PARSNIP								
Boiled, Average	1oz/28g	18	0.3	66	1.6	12.9	1.2	4.7
Fragrant, Tesco*	1 Serving/50g	34	0.6	67	1.8	12.5	1.1	4.6
Honey Roasted, Tesco*	1 Serving/125g	203	10.3	162	1.9	20.0	8.2	2.2
Raw, Unprepared, Average	1oz/28g	19	0.3	66	1.8	12.5	1.1	4.6
PARTRIDGE								
Meat Only, Roasted	1oz/28g	59	2.0	212	36.7	0.0	7.2	0.0
PASANDA								
Chicken, M & S*	½ Pack/150g	240	16.4	160	11.3	3.8	10.9	1.3
Chicken, Sainsbury's*	1 Serving/200g	368	24.8	184	14.7	3.4	12.4	2.3
Chicken, Waitrose*	1oz/28g	52	3.4	185	14.8	3.8	12.3	1.1
Chicken, with Pilau Rice, HL, Tesco*	1 Pack/440g	466	11.0	106	5.7	15.2	2.5	0.9
PASSATA								
Basil, Del Monte*	1 Jar/500g	160	1.0	32	1.4	5.9	0.2	0.0

	Measure INFO/WEIGHT	per Measure KCAL	per Measure FAT	Nutrition Values per 100g / 100ml KCAL	PROT	CARB	FAT	FIBRE
PASSATA								
Classic Italian with Onion & Garlic, Sainsbury's*	1oz/28g	10	0.0	37	1.4	7.7	0.1	1.3
Italian, Sainsbury's*	1 Jar/700g	259	0.7	37	1.4	7.7	0.1	1.3
Morrisons*	1 Carton/500g	110	0.0	22	1.3	4.1	0.0	0.4
Napolina*	1 Bottle/690g	173	0.7	25	1.4	4.5	0.1	0.0
Sieved Tomato, Valfrutta*	1 Pack/500g	110	0.5	22	1.2	4.0	0.1	0.0
SmartPrice, Asda*	1 Serving/15g	4	0.0	25	1.4	4.5	0.1	0.2
with Fresh Leaf Basil, Waitrose*	¼ Jar/170g	44	0.2	26	1.0	5.2	0.1	0.8
with Garlic & Herbs, Roughly Chopped, Tesco*	1 Serving/200g	56	0.0	28	1.4	5.5	0.0	1.0
with Garlic & Italian Herbs, Tesco*	1 Serving/165g	53	0.3	32	1.2	6.4	0.2	1.1
PASSION FRUIT								
Raw, Fresh	1 Fruit/15g	5	0.1	36	2.6	5.8	0.4	3.3
Weighed with Skin	1oz/28g	6	0.1	22	1.7	3.5	0.2	2.0
PASTA								
& Chargrilled Mushrooms, Finest, Tesco*	1 Pack/200g	410	22.4	205	6.1	19.6	11.2	1.4
& Flame Grilled Chicken, M & S*	1 Pack/180g	414	25.2	230	8.2	17.5	14.0	0.8
& Roasted Vegetables, Waitrose*	1oz/28g	43	2.7	154	2.4	14.2	9.7	1.0
Amori, Waitrose*	1 Serving/75g	256	1.0	341	11.5	70.7	1.3	3.7
Arrabbiata Nodini, Asda*	1 Serving/150g	302	8.7	201	7.8	29.3	5.8	2.7
Bean & Tuna, BGTY, Sainsbury's*	1 Serving/200g	176	1.8	88	7.3	12.6	0.9	2.8
Blue Cheese, Bacon & Spinach, M & S*	1 Pack/400g	640	34.0	160	6.5	13.8	8.5	0.7
Boccoletti, Dried, Sainsbury's*	1 Serving/125g	446	2.1	357	12.3	73.1	1.7	2.5
Cajun Chicken, GFY, Asda*	1 Serving/297g	312	8.3	105	8.0	12.0	2.8	2.1
Carbonara, with Cheese & Bacon, Slim Fast*	1 Serving/70g	240	4.4	343	22.7	48.9	6.3	5.7
Chargrilled Chicken, Asda*	1 Serving/250g	538	27.5	215	7.0	22.0	11.0	1.7
Chargrilled Chicken Salsa, HE, Tesco*	1 Pack/450g	396	5.9	88	7.3	11.7	1.3	1.0
Cheese, Tomato, & Pesto, Boots*	1 Pack/250g	355	11.0	142	5.9	20.0	4.4	2.0
Cheese & Broccoli, Pasta Pronto, Safeway*	1 Serving/208g	352	13.5	169	5.4	22.2	6.5	0.6
Cheese & Broccoli, Tubes, Tesco*	1 Serving/202g	319	13.9	158	5.0	19.1	6.9	2.3
Cheese & Ham, Shapers, Boots*	1 Pack/76g	220	4.9	289	23.7	34.2	6.5	6.5
Cheesy Spirals, Curly Whirly, Asda*	1/3 Pack/200g	214	5.2	107	6.0	15.0	2.6	0.5
Chicken, Tomato, & Basil, Asda*	1 Pack/400g	474	10.0	119	6.5	17.5	2.5	1.2
Chicken, Tomato, & Mascarpone, Italiano, Tesco*	1 Pack/400g	572	24.8	143	7.4	14.3	6.2	1.3
Chicken, Tomato & Basil, HL, Tesco*	1 Pack/400g	264	2.0	66	7.9	7.5	0.5	1.1
Chicken, Tomato & Herb, Easy Steam, Tesco*	1 Serving/400g	528	24.8	132	8.9	10.2	6.2	1.3
Chicken, Tomato & Mascarpone, Easy Steam, Tesco*	1 Pack/400g	468	16.4	117	9.7	10.3	4.1	0.9
Chicken, Tomato & Mascarpone, Heathly Living, Tesco*	1 Pack/450g	504	11.3	112	7.5	14.8	2.5	1.1
Chicken & Asparagus, GFY, Asda*	1 Pack/400g	388	8.8	97	10.9	8.5	2.2	1.5
Chicken & Green Pesto, HL, Tesco*	1 Serving/376g	440	4.5	117	8.3	18.5	1.2	1.4
Chicken & Ham, Easy Steam, Tesco*	1 Pack/400g	572	26.4	143	9.8	11.2	6.6	0.6
Chicken & Mushroom, Pasta & Sauce, Dry, Tesco*	1 Pack/120g	427	4.3	356	16.0	65.0	3.6	3.9
Chicken & Pineapple, Shapers, Boots*	1 Pack/221g	210	1.8	95	5.4	15.0	1.5	0.9
Chicken & Roasted Tomato, HL, Tesco*	1 Serving/374g	426	7.1	114	7.4	16.7	1.9	1.3
Chicken & Tomato, Classic, Mini, Tesco*	1 Pack/300g	165	7.2	55	6.6	1.7	2.4	1.7
Chicken & Vegetable, Mediterranean, Waitrose*	1 Serving/400g	375	9.2	94	7.5	10.5	2.3	2.2
Creamy Garlic Mushroom, HL, Tesco*	1 Serving/100g	106	3.7	106	3.6	14.6	3.7	1.1
Creamy Mushroom, Sainsbury's*	1 Serving/63g	148	9.1	237	4.5	21.7	14.6	1.2
Creamy Tomato & Chicken, Great Stuff, Asda*	1 Pack/300g	351	11.7	117	7.0	13.5	3.9	2.3
Creamy Vegetable, Meal in 5, Ainsley Harriott*	1 Pot/386.9g	414	10.1	107	2.8	18.1	2.6	0.8
Elicoidali, Waitrose*	1 Serving/200g	682	2.6	341	11.5	70.7	1.3	3.7
Fagottini, Wild Mushroom, Sainsbury's*	½ Pack/125g	274	9.4	219	10.2	27.7	7.5	2.7
Fiorelli, Egg, M & S*	1 Serving/100g	355	2.8	355	13.9	68.5	2.8	3.0
Fiorelli, Mozzarella, Tomato & Basil, Waitrose*	1 Serving/125g	353	11.6	282	10.8	38.9	9.3	1.7
Florentina, with Broccoli & Spinach, Slim Fast*	1 Serving/71g	239	3.3	336	23.0	50.5	4.6	5.8

PASTA

	Measure INFO/WEIGHT	per Measure KCAL	FAT	Nutrition Values per 100g / 100ml KCAL	PROT	CARB	FAT	FIBRE
Garlic Mushroom Filled, Extra Special, Asda*	1 Serving/125g	224	8.8	179	8.0	21.0	7.0	2.5
Green & White, Duetto, Pasta Reale*	1oz/28g	79	1.7	281	10.9	49.4	6.0	3.6
Honey & Mustard Chicken, Somerfield*	1 Serving/200g	280	7.4	140	8.5	18.0	3.7	1.0
Linguine, Dry, De Cecco*	1 Serving/100g	350	1.5	350	13.0	71.0	1.5	2.9
Lumache, Tesco*	1 Serving/100g	345	2.0	345	13.2	68.5	2.0	2.9
Macaroni Cheese, Meal in 5, Ainsley Harriott*	1 Pot/386.9g	467	16.0	121	3.8	17.3	4.1	1.0
Meat Feast, Italian, Sainsbury's*	1 Pack/450g	509	18.0	113	7.4	11.8	4.0	0.6
Medaglioni, Bolognese, Rich Red Wine, Waitrose*	½ Pack/125g	266	7.0	213	12.5	28.1	5.6	2.6
Parcels, Basil & Parmesan, Fresh, Sainsbury's*	1 Serving/162g	357	13.5	220	10.0	26.4	8.3	3.3
Penne, Creamy Mushroom, Prepared, Tesco*	½ Pack/200g	288	12.8	144	4.5	17.4	6.4	3.3
Penne, Mediterranean, HL, Tesco*	1 Pack/400g	296	10.8	74	2.9	9.6	2.7	1.5
Pepper & Tomato, Asda*	1 Serving/250g	340	17.5	136	3.2	15.0	7.0	2.4
Pomodoro, with Tomato & Herbs, Slim Fast*	1 Serving/71g	235	3.1	331	21.5	51.5	4.3	6.0
Raviolini, Gorgonzola & Walnut, M & S*	½ Pack/125g	381	16.5	305	12.6	33.6	13.2	2.0
Riccioli, Dry Weight, Buitoni*	1 Serving/75g	264	1.4	352	11.2	72.6	1.9	0.0
Sausage & Tomato, Italiano, Tesco*	1 Serving/450g	680	26.6	151	5.7	18.8	5.9	1.6
Seafood, Retail	1oz/28g	31	1.3	110	8.9	7.6	4.8	0.4
Spicy Tomato, Meal in 5, Ainsley Harriott*	1 Pot/386.9g	369	2.1	95	2.6	20.0	0.5	1.5
Stuffed Mushroom & Emmental, Sainsbury's*	1 Pack/250g	650	23.0	260	11.3	33.5	9.2	3.7
Sundried Tomato, Sainsbury's*	1 Serving/50g	197	17.9	393	4.5	13.4	35.7	6.2
Tomato & Bacon, Value, Tesco*	1 Pack/300g	300	4.2	100	4.0	17.8	1.4	1.1
Tomato & Basil Chicken, Boots*	1 Serving/320g	621	28.8	194	9.0	19.0	9.0	1.4
Tomato & Mascarpone, GFY, Asda*	½ Can/200g	128	4.4	64	2.1	9.0	2.2	0.0
Tomato & Mascarpone, Tesco*	1 Pack/400g	468	16.4	117	9.7	10.3	4.1	0.9
Tomato & Onion, Shells, Tesco*	1 Serving/193g	643	3.1	333	12.5	67.1	1.6	6.3
Tomato & Pepper, GFY, Asda*	1 Pack/400g	344	7.6	86	3.1	14.0	1.9	1.1
Tuna & Sweetcorn, Sainsbury's*	1 Pack/380g	562	14.4	148	6.4	22.0	3.8	2.4
Twists, Quick Cook, Morrisons*	1 Serving/75g	265	1.5	353	12.0	72.0	2.0	3.1
Twists, Tuna & Tomato, Canned, Be Light, Aldi*	1 Can/400g	264	6.8	66	4.8	7.8	1.7	1.7
Twists, with Tuna, Italian, Weight Watchers*	1 Can/385g	239	5.4	62	4.3	8.2	1.4	0.6
Vegetable, Creamy, BGTY, Sainsbury's*	1 Pack/400g	348	6.0	87	4.0	14.3	1.5	1.9
Wheat Free, Delverde*	1 Serving/63g	229	1.2	366	0.5	86.9	1.9	1.2

PASTA 'N' SAUCE

	Measure INFO/WEIGHT	per Measure KCAL	FAT	Nutrition Values per 100g / 100ml KCAL	PROT	CARB	FAT	FIBRE
Bolognese Flavour, Dry, Batchelors*	½ Pack/64.6g	228	1.7	353	15.1	67.2	2.6	3.9
Carbonara Flavour, Dry, Batchelors*	1 Pack/120g	463	6.0	386	14.3	71.0	5.0	3.1
Cheese, Leek & Ham, Batchelors*	1 Pack/120g	454	6.1	378	16.1	67.0	5.1	2.0
Cheese & Broccoli, Made Up, Sainsbury's*	1 Pack/120g	164	6.8	137	4.2	17.2	5.7	1.1
Chicken & Mushroom, Batchelors*	½ Pack/63g	227	1.1	361	14.1	72.3	1.7	2.8
Chicken & Mushroom, Made Up, Morrisons*	1 Pack/110g	166	6.2	151	5.0	20.3	5.6	2.1
Chicken & Roasted Garlic, Dry, Batchelors*	½ Pack/60g	223	1.7	372	12.6	73.8	2.9	3.4
Creamy Tikka Masala, Dry, Batchelors*	1 Pack/122.1g	426	2.7	349	12.7	69.5	2.2	4.4
Creamy Tomato & Mushroom, Batchelors*	1 Pack/125g	458	4.1	366	13.0	71.0	3.3	3.2
Macaroni Cheese, Batchelors*	1 Pack/108g	402	5.1	372	17.2	65.2	4.7	2.7
Mild Cheese & Broccoli, Batchelors*	½ Pack/61g	221	2.4	363	15.0	67.0	3.9	4.0
Mushroom & Wine, Batchelors*	½ Pack/50.1g	242	2.8	483	18.5	89.9	5.5	4.4
Mushroom & Wine, Dry, Batchelors*	1 Pack/132g	498	6.5	377	12.0	71.3	4.9	2.5
Tomato, Onion & Herb, Made Up, Morrisons*	1 Serving/110g	141	5.0	128	3.2	18.7	4.5	2.3
Tomato & Bacon Flavour, Dry, Batchelors*	1 Pack/134g	476	3.5	355	13.0	70.0	2.6	3.0
Tomato & Mascarpone, BGTY, Sainsbury's*	1 Pack/380g	555	7.2	146	6.6	25.6	1.9	1.3
Tomato & Mushroom, Dry, Batchelors*	1 Pack/125g	458	4.1	366	13.0	71.0	3.3	3.2

PASTA ALFREDO

	Measure INFO/WEIGHT	per Measure KCAL	FAT	Nutrition Values per 100g / 100ml KCAL	PROT	CARB	FAT	FIBRE
Tesco*	1 Pack/450g	621	18.0	138	10.5	14.9	4.0	0.6

PASTA BAKE

	Measure INFO/WEIGHT	per Measure KCAL	FAT	Nutrition Values per 100g / 100ml KCAL	PROT	CARB	FAT	FIBRE
Aberdeen Angus Meatball, Waitrose*	½ Pack/350.3g	501	28.0	143	5.2	12.5	8.0	0.9
Bacon & Leek, Sainsbury's*	1 Pack/400g	660	27.6	165	7.3	18.5	6.9	1.8
Bacon & Leek, Tesco*	1 Pack/450g	774	37.4	172	8.1	16.1	8.3	2.0
Bolognese, Finest, Tesco*	1 Serving/250g	375	15.8	150	7.3	16.1	6.3	1.1
Bolognese, HL, Tesco*	1 Pack/450g	495	9.5	110	7.8	14.4	2.1	1.3
Bolognese, Italiano, Tesco*	1/3 Pack/284g	409	14.5	144	8.7	15.7	5.1	2.3
Bolognese, Penne, HL, Tesco*	1 Pack/450g	495	9.5	110	7.8	14.4	2.1	1.3
Cheese & Bacon, Asda*	1 Serving/120g	168	14.4	140	3.0	5.2	12.0	0.3
Cheese & Bacon, Fresh Italian, Asda*	1 Serving/250g	265	20.0	106	6.0	2.6	8.0	0.5
Cheese & Tomato, Italiano, Tesco*	1 Bake/300g	354	12.6	118	3.9	16.1	4.2	1.0
Cheese & Tomato, Tesco*	1 Pack/400g	388	5.6	97	3.4	17.8	1.4	1.2
Chicken, BGTY, Sainsbury's*	1 Pack/400g	348	8.0	87	9.7	7.5	2.0	0.8
Chicken, Italiano, Tesco*	1 Serving/190g	219	7.8	115	8.4	11.2	4.1	3.1
Chicken, Morrisons*	1 Pack/401.9g	442	14.5	110	4.6	14.8	3.6	0.9
Chicken, Mushroom & Leek, HE, Tesco*	1 Pack/450g	468	11.3	104	8.6	11.9	2.5	1.4
Chicken, Somerfield*	1 Pack/300g	351	18.0	117	8.0	8.0	6.0	0.0
Chicken, Tesco*	1 Serving/400g	376	5.2	94	8.2	12.4	1.3	0.9
Chicken, Tomato, & Mascarpone, Tesco*	1 Serving/400g	448	8.4	112	8.0	15.2	2.1	1.7
Chicken & Bacon, Asda*	¼ Pack/374.2g	610	26.2	163	9.0	16.0	7.0	4.1
Chicken & Bacon, Creamy Cheese Sauce, Tesco*	½ Pack/400g	620	23.2	155	9.0	15.6	5.8	1.1
Chicken & Bacon, Italian, Chilled, Tesco*	½ Pack/400g	620	23.2	155	9.0	15.6	5.8	1.1
Chicken & Broccoli, Morrisons*	1 Pack/400g	452	16.0	113	6.1	13.3	4.0	0.6
Chicken & Broccoli, Pasta Presto, Findus*	1 Pack/321g	449	22.5	140	7.5	12.0	7.0	0.0
Chicken & Broccoli, Safeway*	1 Pack/340g	405	15.0	119	8.1	11.7	4.4	1.3
Chicken & Broccoli, Weight Watchers*	1 Bake/305g	290	4.6	95	6.0	14.2	1.5	0.9
Chicken & Courgette, Asda*	½ Pack/387.3g	519	23.2	134	6.0	14.0	6.0	0.6
Chicken & Leek, HL, Tesco*	1 Pack/400g	460	7.6	115	10.8	13.1	1.9	1.6
Chicken & Mushroom, Waitrose*	1 Pack/400g	532	30.8	133	6.7	9.1	7.7	0.8
Chicken & Roast Mushroom, HL, Tesco*	1 Pack/390g	413	0.4	106	8.6	17.6	0.1	1.3
Chicken & Spinach, GFY, Asda*	1 Pack/400g	374	6.0	94	5.0	15.0	1.5	1.2
Chicken & Spinach, Morrisons*	1 Serving/500g	766	36.1	153	6.6	15.5	7.2	1.4
Chicken & Spinach, Safeway*	1 Serving/383g	440	15.3	115	6.9	12.0	4.0	1.2
Chicken & Spinach, Sainsbury's*	1 Pack/340g	286	9.2	84	4.9	10.0	2.7	0.6
Chicken & Sweetcorn, Eat Smart, Safeway*	1 Pack/400g	380	7.2	95	6.5	13.0	1.8	1.8
Chilli & Cheese, American Style, Tesco*	1 Pack/425g	638	16.6	150	6.8	21.8	3.9	1.5
Creamy Mushroom, Dolmio*	½ Jar/245g	267	22.5	109	1.1	5.5	9.2	0.0
Creamy Tomato, Dolmio*	1 Serving/125g	141	9.0	113	2.3	8.4	7.2	0.0
Creamy Tomato, Safeway*	1 Serving/250g	350	27.8	140	1.6	7.9	11.1	3.8
Findus*	1 Pack/320g	448	22.4	140	7.5	12.0	7.0	0.0
Ham & Broccoli, Asda*	1 Pack/340g	309	13.9	91	3.4	10.0	4.1	0.5
Ham & Mushroom, Italiano, Tesco*	1 Pack/425g	646	20.4	152	5.8	21.3	4.8	1.7
Italian Creamy Tomato & Bacon, Asda*	1 Serving/125g	131	11.3	105	2.0	3.9	9.0	0.6
Leek & Bacon, Morrisons*	1 Pack/400.7g	553	36.1	138	4.8	9.9	9.0	0.2
Meatball, Tesco*	1 Pack/400g	576	19.2	144	5.9	19.3	4.8	0.5
Meatfeast, Italian, Tesco*	1 Serving/500g	675	19.0	135	6.4	17.8	3.8	2.3
Mediterranean Style, Tesco*	1 Pack/450g	423	1.8	94	2.9	19.6	0.4	2.0
Mix, Tuna, Colman's*	1 Sachet/45g	145	2.3	323	9.2	60.0	5.2	4.7
Mushroom, Creamy, Asda*	¼ Jar/118g	204	20.1	173	1.8	3.3	17.0	0.5
Penne, with Tomato & Mozzarella, Sainsbury's*	1 Pack/400g	536	18.8	134	5.4	17.6	4.7	2.8
Penne Mozzarella, Tesco*	1 Pack/340g	408	8.5	120	4.7	19.7	2.5	0.6
Pepperoni & Ham, Tesco*	½ Pack/425g	502	2.6	118	8.9	19.3	0.6	2.5
Roast Vegetable, Eat Smart, Safeway*	1 Pack/330g	380	6.3	115	3.8	19.6	1.9	1.3
Spicy Tomato & Pepperoni, Asda*	1 Pack/440g	431	26.4	98	1.1	10.0	6.0	1.2

P

	Measure INFO/WEIGHT	per Measure KCAL	per Measure FAT	Nutrition Values per 100g / 100ml KCAL	PROT	CARB	FAT	FIBRE
PASTA BAKE								
Three Bean, Asda*	¼ Jar/124.7g	188	15.0	150	2.4	8.0	12.0	1.3
Tomato & Cheese, Dolmio*	1 Serving/125g	69	1.5	55	2.2	8.8	1.2	0.0
Tomato & Herb, Asda*	1 Jar/436g	715	56.7	164	1.8	10.0	13.0	1.2
Tomato & Mozzarella, HL, Tesco*	1 Pack/385g	360	8.9	94	4.3	13.7	2.3	1.8
Tomato & Mozzarella, Italiano, Tesco*	1 Pack/340g	398	8.5	117	4.8	18.9	2.5	1.7
Tuna, BGTY, Sainsbury's*	1 Pack/400g	365	6.4	91	7.2	12.0	1.6	1.7
Tuna, Co-Op*	1 Serving/340g	306	6.8	90	7.0	12.0	2.0	1.0
Tuna, COU, M & S*	1 Pack/360g	378	7.6	105	7.6	12.9	2.1	2.3
Tuna, Eat Smart, Safeway*	1 Serving/400g	340	6.8	85	5.6	11.6	1.7	1.2
Tuna, Good Intentions, Somerfield*	1 Serving/400g	400	8.4	100	5.9	14.5	2.1	1.2
Tuna, HE, Tesco*	1 Pack/340g	258	2.7	76	5.4	11.9	0.8	0.5
Tuna, HL, Tesco*	1 Serving/400g	360	6.0	90	8.3	10.7	1.5	0.9
Tuna, Italian, HL, Tesco*	1 Pack/500g	475	7.0	95	7.1	13.5	1.4	1.5
Tuna, Lean Cuisine*	1 Pack/345.5g	380	8.6	110	5.0	16.0	2.5	1.5
Tuna, Safeway*	1 Pack/400g	620	31.6	155	8.9	12.0	7.9	1.1
Tuna, Somerfield*	1 Bake/300g	411	21.0	137	9.0	10.0	7.0	0.0
Tuna, Tesco*	1oz/28g	36	1.7	129	6.9	11.7	6.1	0.9
Tuna & Sweetcorn, Asda*	1 Serving/250g	333	22.5	133	5.0	8.0	9.0	0.9
Tuna & Tomato, BGTY, Sainsbury's*	1 Pack/450g	554	18.9	123	8.7	12.6	4.2	0.4
Tuna Conchiglie, M & S*	1 Pack/400g	360	13.2	90	8.4	6.7	3.3	1.0
Vegetable, Asda*	1 Serving/300g	231	10.5	77	2.4	9.0	3.5	0.8
Vegetable, Findus*	1 Pack/330.8g	430	21.5	130	6.0	13.0	6.5	0.0
Vegetable, M & S*	1 Pack/350g	455	20.0	130	4.8	14.6	5.7	1.6
Vegetable, Mediterranean, HL, Tesco*	1 Serving/450g	374	3.6	83	2.9	16.0	0.8	1.5
Vegetable, Mediterranean, Tesco*	1 Serving/450g	495	20.7	110	4.3	12.9	4.6	1.3
Vegetable, Ready Meals, Waitrose*	1oz/28g	44	2.4	157	5.9	14.4	8.6	1.0
Vegetable, Tesco*	1 Pack/380g	467	21.3	123	5.6	12.6	5.6	1.6
PASTA BREAK								
Chicken & Herb, Prepared, Knorr*	1 Pot/347g	382	11.5	110	3.7	16.5	3.3	0.9
PASTA IN								
a Rich Tomato & Mushroom Sauce, Spirals, Tesco*	1 Serving/217g	326	13.7	150	4.6	18.8	6.3	2.5
Chicken, Garlic & Wine Sauce, Dry, Tesco*	1 Pack/120g	438	5.2	365	14.2	66.8	4.3	5.0
Garlic & Herb, Asda*	1 Serving/120g	487	12.0	406	10.0	69.0	10.0	2.3
Herb Sauce, Sainsbury's*	1 Pack/420g	441	0.8	105	3.5	22.4	0.2	0.8
PASTA MEAL								
Tomato & Basil, Shapers, Boots*	1 Serving/76g	214	3.3	282	22.4	38.2	4.3	6.8
PASTA QUILLS								
Dry, Average	1 Serving/75g	257	0.9	342	12.0	72.3	1.2	2.0
Gluten Free, Salute*	1 Serving/75g	269	1.4	359	7.5	78.1	1.9	0.0
Tomato, Onion & Herbs, Batchelors*	1 Pack/128g	445	2.6	348	13.8	68.8	2.0	4.0
Whole Wheat, Morrisons*	1 Serving/75g	251	2.0	335	11.5	65.7	2.6	7.6
PASTA SALAD								
& Mixed Leaf, with Basil Pesto Dressing, Tesco*	1 Pack/220g	528	37.6	240	4.7	16.9	17.1	0.7
Bacon, Budgens*	1 Salad/200g	570	47.8	285	5.1	12.6	23.9	0.7
Basil & Parmesan, Tesco*	1 Serving/50g	65	1.8	130	4.3	20.2	3.6	0.6
BBQ Bean, Tesco*	1 Pack/850g	1139	43.4	134	3.6	18.5	5.1	1.8
BBQ Chicken, Scottish Slimmers*	1 Serving/239.8g	223	4.3	93	6.4	14.0	1.8	1.3
Caesar, Chicken, Shapers, Boots*	1 Pack/218g	288	8.3	132	6.7	18.0	3.8	1.8
Caesar & Santa Tomatoes, M & S*	1 Serving/220g	495	33.7	225	5.2	15.9	15.3	0.8
Carbonara, Waitrose*	1oz/28g	72	6.3	257	5.4	8.1	22.6	0.5
Chargrilled Chicken, Italian Style, Asda*	1 Pack/200g	318	14.0	159	7.0	17.0	7.0	0.4
Chargrilled Chicken, M & S*	1 Serving/190g	285	5.5	150	9.6	23.6	2.9	1.6
Chargrilled Chicken & Pesto Pasta, Sainsbury's*	1 Pack/240g	454	22.1	189	7.2	19.4	9.2	0.0

P

PASTA SALAD

	Measure INFO/WEIGHT	per Measure KCAL	FAT	Nutrition Values per 100g / 100ml KCAL	PROT	CARB	FAT	FIBRE
Chargrilled Vegetables & Tomato, Shapers, Boots*	1 Pack/175g	187	5.4	107	2.8	17.0	3.1	1.5
Cheddar Cheese, Tesco*	1 Pot/215g	546	43.9	254	5.7	12.0	20.4	0.8
Cheese, Asda*	1 Serving/40g	118	9.0	296	6.5	16.6	22.6	0.5
Cheese, Morrisons*	½ Pot/125g	341	26.6	273	5.7	14.7	21.3	1.0
Cheese, with Mayo & Vinaigrette, Sainsbury's*	¼ Pot/50g	125	8.7	249	6.1	17.0	17.3	1.7
Cherry Tomato & Rocket, HE, Tesco*	1 Salad/225g	223	5.6	99	3.2	15.8	2.5	1.0
Chicken, Asda*	1 Pot/250g	323	12.3	129	5.8	15.5	4.9	1.3
Chicken & Smoked Bacon, M & S*	1 Salad/380g	817	46.7	215	7.5	19.0	12.3	1.9
Chicken & Sweetcorn, Eat Smart, Safeway*	1 Serving/200g	230	3.6	115	7.5	16.3	1.8	1.0
Chicken Caesar, Asda*	1 Pack/297g	683	41.3	230	9.6	16.6	13.9	2.5
Chicken Caesar, Ginsters*	1 Pack/220g	504	35.4	229	7.5	13.6	16.1	0.0
Chilli & Cheese, Sainsbury's*	1 Serving/300g	384	16.8	128	4.3	15.5	5.6	0.3
Crayfish, Rocket & Lemon, Finest, Tesco*	1 Serving/250g	728	39.8	291	8.9	28.0	15.9	4.2
Crayfish, Shapers, Boots*	1 Pack/280.2g	269	6.4	96	6.0	13.0	2.3	0.7
Fire Roasted Tomato, So Good, Somerfield*	½ Pack/100g	199	10.6	199	4.4	21.6	10.6	1.5
Garlic Mushroom, Salad Bar, Asda*	1oz/28g	59	4.7	212	2.5	12.5	16.9	0.8
Goats Cheese, & Mixed Pepper, Sainsbury's*	1 Pack/200g	366	18.8	183	6.4	18.2	9.4	1.5
Ham, Sainsbury's*	1 Pot/250g	610	48.3	244	4.1	13.4	19.3	0.8
Ham & Pineapple, Salad Bar, Asda*	1oz/28g	62	4.5	221	3.3	15.6	16.2	1.4
Honey & Mustard Chicken, BGTY, Sainsbury's*	1 Pack/200g	270	5.8	135	9.4	17.8	2.9	1.1
Honey & Mustard Chicken, M & S*	1 Serving/190g	304	4.8	160	8.7	26.7	2.5	1.5
Honey & Mustard Chicken, Sainsbury's*	1 Pack/190.1g	344	16.9	181	7.1	18.0	8.9	0.0
Honey & Mustard Chicken, Shapers, Boots*	1 Serving/252g	350	5.5	139	8.4	22.0	2.2	2.8
Italian, Bowl, Sainsbury's*	1 Serving/210g	309	15.5	147	3.1	16.9	7.4	1.9
Italian Style, Iceland*	1 Serving/75g	97	4.5	129	2.6	16.2	6.0	1.6
Italian Style, Safeway*	1 Serving/225g	234	5.9	104	2.9	17.2	2.6	0.6
Italian Style, Sainsbury's*	1/3 Pot/84g	129	5.3	153	3.5	20.5	6.3	1.4
Italian Style, Snack, Asda*	1 Pack/150g	141	6.0	94	3.4	11.0	4.0	4.1
Kraft*	½ Cup/68g	183	11.0	269	4.0	26.5	16.2	0.0
Lime & Coriander Chicken, M & S*	1 Serving/190g	371	23.2	195	7.6	14.4	12.2	0.6
Mediterranean, Good Intentions, Somerfield*	1 Pack/250g	290	7.0	116	2.8	19.8	2.8	1.1
Mediterranean, Tesco*	1oz/28g	24	1.3	87	2.1	9.6	4.5	1.4
Mediterranean Chicken, Waitrose*	1 Serving/200g	314	13.6	157	7.0	16.9	6.8	2.1
Mediterranean Style, Layered, Waitrose*	1 Pot/275g	190	3.6	69	2.6	11.8	1.3	1.0
Mediterranean Tuna, Shapers, Boots*	1 Serving/239g	232	3.1	97	6.2	15.0	1.3	0.9
Mozzarella & Plum Tomatoes, COU, M & S*	1 Bowl/255g	204	4.1	80	4.6	11.5	1.6	1.7
Mozzarella & Roasted Tomato, TTD, Sainsbury's*	1 Serving/50g	78	3.8	156	5.7	16.3	7.6	0.0
Mozzarella & Sun Dried Tomato, Waitrose*	1 Serving/150g	312	18.3	208	5.8	18.8	12.2	1.3
Oven Roasted Tomato & Olive, TTD, Sainsbury's*	1 Serving/50g	88	3.7	176	5.2	22.1	7.4	0.0
Pepper, HE, Tesco*	1 Salad/210g	139	0.8	66	2.4	13.3	0.4	1.0
Pepper, Side, Tesco*	1 Serving/46g	56	3.0	122	2.4	13.0	6.5	1.3
Pepper & Tomato, Fire Roasted, Finest, Tesco*	1 Pack/200g	260	8.2	130	3.7	19.4	4.1	2.5
Poached Salmon, M & S*	1 Serving/200g	340	16.8	170	7.8	16.2	8.4	1.4
Poached Salmon, Sainsbury's*	1 Serving/200g	472	30.6	236	6.7	17.9	15.3	12.0
Prawn, Shapers, Boots*	1 Pot/250g	250	7.8	100	4.1	14.0	3.1	0.4
Prawn Cocktail, Shapers, Boots*	1 Pack/248g	255	6.7	103	5.0	15.0	2.7	1.6
Prawns, King, & Tomatoes, COU, M & S*	1 Serving/270g	257	4.1	95	5.1	16.4	1.5	0.9
Ready to Eat, Somerfield*	½ Pack/123g	175	8.5	142	2.8	17.1	6.9	1.6
Roast Garlic Mushroom, TTD, Sainsbury's*	1 Pot/200g	358	17.6	179	5.1	19.8	8.8	0.0
Roasted Mushroom, Spinach & Tarragon, Tesco*	1 Pot/200g	216	4.8	108	4.3	17.2	2.4	0.8
Roasted Vegetable, Waitrose*	1 Pack/190g	270	8.7	142	6.8	18.2	4.6	1.1
Sainsbury's*	½ Pack/160g	235	9.6	147	3.2	20.0	6.0	1.5
Salmon, M & S*	1 Serving/380g	817	57.8	215	6.8	12.7	15.2	0.7

	Measure INFO/WEIGHT	per Measure		Nutrition Values per 100g / 100ml				
		KCAL	FAT	KCAL	PROT	CARB	FAT	FIBRE
PASTA SALAD								
Spicy Chicken, Budgens*	1 Serving/213g	452	22.2	212	5.1	24.5	10.4	4.4
Spicy Chicken, Geo Adams*	1 Pack/230g	580	43.9	252	5.1	14.9	19.1	2.9
Spicy Chilli Pesto, Sainsbury's*	¼ Pot/62.5g	171	12.3	272	3.8	20.1	19.6	1.6
Spinach, Pine Nuts & Pesto Dressing, M & S*	1 Pack/191g	440	19.9	230	6.7	27.5	10.4	2.2
Sun Dried Tomato Dressing, Sainsbury's*	1 Pack/320g	442	14.1	138	3.7	20.8	4.4	3.6
Sweetcorn, M & S*	½ Pack/100g	95	0.8	95	2.9	18.8	0.8	2.7
Sweetcorn, Waitrose*	1oz/28g	31	0.3	112	6.4	18.9	1.2	1.1
Sweetcorn & Pepper, GFY, Asda*	1 Serving/175g	68	0.7	39	1.9	7.0	0.4	0.0
Three Cheese, Tesco*	1 Serving/300g	633	41.1	211	7.5	14.4	13.7	2.8
Tiger Prawn, Waitrose*	1 Serving/225g	545	38.5	242	5.4	16.7	17.1	0.4
Tiger Prawn & Tomato, GFY, Asda*	1 Serving/200g	250	5.8	125	4.6	20.0	2.9	2.0
Tomato, Aldi*	1 Serving/50g	59	1.8	117	3.9	18.6	3.6	0.0
Tomato, Bacon & Cheese, Ginsters*	1 Pack/220g	381	19.8	173	7.4	15.6	9.0	0.0
Tomato & Basil, M & S*	1 Pot/225g	484	35.8	215	2.9	15.0	15.9	1.2
Tomato & Basil, PB, Waitrose*	1 Serving/100g	97	1.7	97	3.7	16.8	1.7	0.0
Tomato & Basil, Pot, HL, Tesco*	1 Pot/200g	242	5.4	121	2.0	22.1	2.7	2.2
Tomato & Basil, Red & Green Pepper, Sainsbury's*	¼ Pot/63g	89	4.3	141	3.2	16.4	6.9	3.8
Tomato & Basil, Sainsbury's*	1 Serving/62g	87	4.3	141	3.2	16.4	6.9	3.8
Tomato & Basil Chicken, M & S*	1 Serving/279g	446	22.0	160	7.0	14.8	7.9	1.8
Tomato & Chargrilled Vegetable, Tesco*	1 Serving/200g	248	7.8	124	3.7	18.6	3.9	1.4
Tomato & Mozzarella, Leaf, Shapers, Boots*	1 Pack/185g	356	22.3	192	5.1	16.0	12.0	2.5
Tomato & Mozzarella, Sainsbury's*	1 Pack/200g	440	22.6	220	7.5	22.2	11.3	1.3
Tomato & Mozzarella, Waitrose*	1 Pack/225g	380	27.9	169	4.3	10.0	12.4	0.6
Tomato & Pepper, HL, Tesco*	1 Serving/200g	162	3.2	81	2.6	13.9	1.6	1.4
Tomato & Tuna, Snack, Sainsbury's*	1 Serving/200g	238	2.4	119	5.3	21.7	1.2	0.0
Tuna, Arrabiatta, BGTY, Sainsbury's*	1 Serving/200g	196	2.6	98	6.8	14.7	1.3	0.0
Tuna, GFY, Asda*	1 Pack/250g	325	12.8	130	6.3	14.7	5.1	2.7
Tuna, Mediterranean, Johnsons*	1 Serving/225g	148	6.2	66	2.8	7.5	2.8	0.9
Tuna, PB, Waitrose*	1 Tub/190g	181	4.4	95	7.0	11.5	2.3	1.1
Tuna, Tesco*	1 Pot/300g	399	21.9	133	6.2	10.5	7.3	0.0
Tuna & Spinach, COU, M & S*	1 Pack/270g	257	4.9	95	6.8	14.3	1.8	3.8
Tuna & Sweetcorn, COU, M & S*	1 Pack/200g	210	1.8	105	7.1	18.3	0.9	1.2
Tuna & Sweetcorn, HE, Tesco*	1 Pot/200g	230	5.4	115	5.7	17.0	2.7	1.3
Tuna & Sweetcorn, Sainsbury's*	1 Serving/100g	111	1.2	111	7.1	18.3	1.2	1.2
Tuna Crunch, Shapers, Boots*	1 Pack/250g	353	6.8	141	9.8	19.0	2.7	2.8
Tuna Nicoise, Waitrose*	1 Pot/190g	306	17.1	161	5.1	14.9	9.0	1.1
Vegetable, Healthy Selection, Somerfield*	1 Pot/200g	180	0.0	90	2.8	19.6	0.0	0.7
Vegetable, Somerfield*	1 Salad/200g	288	12.0	144	3.0	20.0	6.0	0.0
Wild Mushroom, TTD, Sainsbury's*	1 Serving/259g	464	27.2	179	4.6	16.6	10.5	1.5
with Avocado & Cherry Tomatoes, M & S*	1 Pack/185g	259	14.8	140	2.9	13.9	8.0	1.2
with Italian Style Chicken, Weight Watchers*	1 Pack/185g	237	2.0	128	6.7	22.9	1.1	0.7
PASTA SAUCE								
Amatriciana, Fresh, Sainsbury's*	½ Pot/175g	98	3.9	56	3.6	5.6	2.2	0.5
Amatriciana, Italiano, Tesco*	½ Pot/175g	124	6.7	71	4.1	5.3	3.8	0.9
Amatriciana, M & S*	1 Jar/340g	425	32.3	125	3.4	6.3	9.5	2.9
Amatriciana, Morrisons*	1 Tub/350g	158	5.6	45	3.7	4.6	1.6	0.5
Amatriciana, Tesco*	1 Serving/175g	109	7.2	62	2.3	4.0	4.1	0.7
Arrabbiata, Barilla*	1 Serving/100g	47	3.0	47	1.5	3.5	3.0	0.0
Arrabbiata, Fresh, Budgens*	1 Serving/150g	83	5.1	55	1.1	5.0	3.4	1.4
Arrabbiata, Fresh, Co-Op*	½ Pot/150g	83	4.5	55	1.0	5.0	3.0	1.0
Arrabbiata, Fresh, Morrisons*	1 Pot/350g	139	5.3	40	1.9	5.4	1.5	0.0
Arrabbiata, GFY, Asda*	1 Serving/350g	133	3.9	38	1.1	6.0	1.1	0.0
Arrabbiata, Italian, Waitrose*	1 Jar/320g	115	3.2	36	1.5	6.7	1.0	1.4

PASTA SAUCE

INFO/WEIGHT	Measure	per Measure KCAL	FAT	Nutrition Values per 100g / 100ml KCAL	PROT	CARB	FAT	FIBRE
Arrabbiata, M & S*	1 Jar/320g	240	17.0	75	1.2	6.2	5.3	0.8
Arrabbiata, Red Pepper, Sainsbury's*	½ Pot/175g	79	5.1	45	1.4	3.3	2.9	1.6
Arrabiata, Morrisons*	½ Pot/175g	148	9.0	85	2.5	7.1	5.1	1.6
Aubergine & Pepper, Sacla*	½ Pot/95g	238	23.3	250	1.8	5.6	24.5	0.0
Basil & Oregano, Ragu, Knorr*	1 Serving/200g	86	0.0	43	1.3	9.4	0.0	1.1
Beef Bolognese, Fresh, Asda*	1 Pot/300g	207	12.0	69	5.4	2.9	4.0	1.8
Bolognese, Bottled, M & S*	½ Jar/165g	149	6.6	90	6.9	6.2	4.0	1.3
Bolognese, Dolmio*	1 Serving/100g	56	1.5	56	1.5	9.4	1.5	1.1
Bolognese, Finest, Tesco*	1 Serving/175g	170	10.7	97	7.0	3.8	6.1	0.5
Bolognese, Fresh, Sainsbury's*	½ Pot/150g	120	6.2	80	6.0	4.7	4.1	1.2
Bolognese, Italiano, Tesco*	1 Serving/175g	194	13.1	111	5.9	4.8	7.5	0.8
Bolognese, Light, Original, Ragu, Knorr*	1 Jar/515g	196	0.5	38	1.4	8.2	0.1	1.2
Bolognese, Original, Asda*	1 Serving/157.5g	73	2.2	46	1.4	7.0	1.4	0.8
Bolognese, Original, Light, Dolmio*	1 Serving/125g	44	0.4	35	1.5	6.7	0.3	0.9
Bolognese, Original, Sainsbury's*	¼ Jar/136g	90	2.9	66	1.9	9.9	2.1	1.3
Bolognese, SmartPrice, Asda*	½ Jar/226g	88	1.8	39	0.9	7.0	0.8	0.6
Bolognese, Somerfield*	1 Pack/300g	243	12.0	81	3.0	8.0	4.0	0.0
Bolognese, Spicy, Ragu, Knorr*	1/3 Jar/166g	73	0.2	44	1.3	9.6	0.1	1.1
Bolognese, Tesco*	1 Serving/175g	100	4.6	57	4.2	4.0	2.6	0.8
Bolognese, Traditional, Ragu, Knorr*	1 Jar/320g	157	5.4	49	1.3	7.1	1.7	1.2
Bolognese with Beef, Tesco*	½ Can/213g	179	10.0	84	4.9	5.5	4.7	0.0
Carbonara, 50% Less Fat, Asda*	½ Pot/175g	170	10.5	97	4.8	6.0	6.0	0.6
Carbonara, Co-Op*	½ Pot/150g	270	25.5	180	3.0	4.0	17.0	0.1
Carbonara, Creamy, Stir in Sauce, Dolmio*	1 Serving/75g	136	11.9	181	5.5	4.3	15.8	0.0
Carbonara, Fresh, BGTY, Sainsbury's*	1 Tub/300g	255	10.8	85	5.4	7.8	3.6	0.5
Carbonara, Fresh, Budgens*	1 Serving/300g	534	50.4	178	3.1	3.7	16.8	0.1
Carbonara, Fresh, Chilled, Finest, Tesco*	½ Tub/175g	298	24.9	170	5.5	4.2	14.2	0.0
Carbonara, Fresh, Chilled, Italiano, Tesco*	½ Tub/175g	201	11.4	115	6.1	7.2	6.5	0.1
Carbonara, Fresh, TTD, Sainsbury's*	1 Tub/300g	606	51.9	202	7.4	4.1	17.3	0.5
Carbonara, Italian, Asda*	½ Pack/175g	359	29.8	205	7.0	6.0	17.0	0.1
Carbonara, Italian, Fresh, Sainsbury's*	½ Pot/175g	209	16.3	119	5.4	3.4	9.3	0.9
Carbonara, Morrisons*	1 Pot/350g	749	64.4	214	6.2	5.8	18.4	1.1
Carbonara with Pancetta, Loyd Grossman*	½ Pack/170g	209	15.5	123	2.8	7.5	9.1	0.1
Cheery Tomato & Roasted Pepper, Asda*	1 Jar/171.7g	91	5.2	53	1.5	5.0	3.0	2.4
Cherry Tomato & Basil, Sacla*	1 Serving/96g	90	7.1	94	1.2	5.3	7.4	0.0
Chunky Vegetable, Asda*	1 Serving/250g	123	4.3	49	1.4	7.0	1.7	1.2
Chunky Vegetable, Somerfield*	1 Jar/525g	226	5.3	43	2.0	7.0	1.0	0.0
Cream & Mushroom, M & S*	1oz/28g	45	4.0	160	1.5	6.6	14.3	0.6
Creamy Mushroom, Dolmio*	1 Pack/150g	167	15.0	111	1.3	3.7	10.0	0.0
Creamy Mushroom, Express, Dolmio*	1 Serving/150g	161	14.4	107	1.4	3.8	9.6	0.0
Five Cheese, Italiano, Tesco*	½ Tub/175g	271	20.1	155	6.8	6.0	11.5	0.0
for Bolognese, Extra Mushrooms, Dolmio*	1 Jar/500g	240	6.5	48	1.7	7.6	1.3	1.1
for Bolognese, Extra Onion & Garlic, Dolmio*	1 Serving/125g	66	1.3	53	1.7	9.0	1.0	0.8
for Bolognese, Extra Spicy, Dolmio*	1 Jar/500g	260	5.5	52	1.7	8.8	1.1	0.8
for Lasagne, Tomato, Red, Ragu, Knorr*	1 Jar/515g	221	0.0	43	1.1	9.7	0.0	1.1
for Lasagne, White, Light, Ragu, Knorr*	¼ Jar/122g	88	6.1	72	0.5	5.0	5.0	0.2
for Lasagne, White, Ragu, Knorr*	¼ Jar/123g	196	18.7	159	0.5	5.1	15.2	0.3
Four Cheese, Asda*	½ Jar/155g	242	21.7	156	3.5	3.9	14.0	0.1
Four Cheese, BGTY, Sainsbury's*	1 Serving/150g	104	6.0	69	2.9	5.5	4.0	0.1
Four Cheese, Fresh, Asda*	½ Pot/162g	309	28.8	191	5.4	2.2	17.8	0.5
Four Cheese, GFY, Asda*	½ Pot/175g	144	8.0	82	4.0	6.3	4.6	0.5
Four Cheese, Sainsbury's*	1 Serving/150g	296	25.5	197	6.6	4.5	17.0	0.8
Hot Mixed Peppers Bolognese, Sainsbury's*	1oz/28g	18	0.6	66	2.0	9.7	2.1	1.5

PASTA SAUCE

INFO/WEIGHT	Measure	per Measure		Nutrition Values per 100g / 100ml				
		KCAL	FAT	KCAL	PROT	CARB	FAT	FIBRE
Italian, Vongole, Waitrose*	1 Serving/175g	116	5.6	66	4.2	5.2	3.2	0.7
Italian, with Tomato & Herbs, Somerfield*	1 Jar/340g	153	3.7	45	1.2	7.7	1.1	0.9
Italian Cheese, Finest, Tesco*	½ Pot/175g	172	8.9	98	4.8	8.4	5.1	0.0
Italian Mushroom, Sainsbury's*	1 Serving/85g	56	1.8	66	2.0	9.8	2.1	1.7
Mediterranean, BGTY, Sainsbury's*	1oz/28g	23	1.2	82	1.9	9.0	4.3	1.4
Mediterranean, Fresh, Waitrose*	1 Pot/350g	214	13.7	61	1.4	5.0	3.9	2.4
Mediterranean Tomato, Asda*	1 Jar/500g	285	6.0	57	1.5	10.0	1.2	0.0
Mediterranean Vegetable, Rustico, Bertolli*	½ Jar/160g	141	11.5	88	1.7	4.1	7.2	0.7
Mushroom, Co-Op*	¼ Jar/125g	75	2.5	60	2.0	9.0	2.0	1.0
Mushroom, Fresh, Waitrose*	1 Serving/175g	142	10.0	81	1.6	5.7	5.7	0.5
Mushroom, Morrisons*	1 Serving/128g	76	2.9	59	1.6	7.9	2.3	1.1
Mushroom, Tesco*	¼ Jar/188g	90	3.2	48	1.4	6.8	1.7	1.0
Mushroom & Marsala Wine, Sacla*	½ Pot/85g	165	16.0	194	2.2	3.9	18.8	0.0
Mushroom & Mascarpone, HE, Tesco*	½ Jar/175g	86	3.9	49	2.1	5.3	2.2	0.3
Napoletana, BGTY, Sainsbury's*	½ Pot/151g	71	3.8	47	1.2	5.0	2.5	1.3
Napoletana, Buitoni*	½ Jar/200g	146	8.2	73	1.6	7.3	4.1	2.2
Napoletana, Fresh, Asda*	1 Pot/330g	149	7.3	45	1.4	5.0	2.2	2.8
Napoletana, Fresh, Waitrose*	1 Serving/175g	82	3.0	47	1.3	6.6	1.7	1.0
Napoletana, Morrisons*	1 Serving/175g	82	2.6	47	2.6	6.7	1.5	0.0
Napoletana, Sainsbury's*	½ Pot/150g	126	8.4	84	1.9	6.6	5.6	0.9
Olive & Tomato, Sacla*	1 Serving/95g	87	7.6	92	1.3	3.6	8.0	0.0
Onion & Garlic, Co-Op*	1 Serving/125g	106	3.8	85	2.0	12.0	3.0	0.7
Onion & Garlic, Tesco*	¼ Jar/125g	35	0.1	28	1.2	5.6	0.1	2.6
Original, Tesco*	1 Jar/300g	123	4.2	41	1.0	6.1	1.4	2.3
Oven Roasted Vegetables, Stir in, Dolmio*	1 Pack/150g	201	15.5	134	1.5	8.8	10.3	1.0
Primavera, Fresh, Morrisons*	½ Pot/175g	152	10.3	87	2.4	6.1	5.9	0.0
Primavera, Loyd Grossman*	1 Jar/350g	343	25.9	98	1.4	6.3	7.4	0.9
Puttanesca, Italian, Waitrose*	1 Jar/350g	195	9.8	56	1.5	6.1	2.8	1.3
Puttanesca, Loyd Grossman*	1 Jar/350g	315	21.7	90	1.7	6.8	6.2	0.9
Puttanesca, M & S*	1 Jar/320g	256	17.6	80	1.5	6.2	5.5	1.9
Puttanesca, Sainsbury's*	1 Serving/110g	132	9.7	120	2.0	8.1	8.8	0.0
Red Wine & Shallots, Bertolli*	1 Serving/80g	36	1.4	45	1.5	6.0	1.7	1.0
Roasted Red Pepper & Tomato, Finest, Tesco*	1 Serving/145g	117	7.8	81	1.2	6.8	5.4	2.2
Roasted Vegetable, GFY, Asda*	½ Pot/175g	84	2.8	48	1.3	7.0	1.6	0.5
Roasted Vegetable, Microwaveable, Dolmio*	½ Pack/190g	103	3.8	54	1.4	7.6	2.0	0.0
Roasted Vegetable, Sainsbury's*	½ Pot/151g	103	5.9	68	1.6	6.7	3.9	0.4
Roasted Vegetable, Tesco*	1 Pack/175g	114	5.3	65	1.5	8.0	3.0	0.8
Rustico Sweet Chilli & Red Onion, Bertolli*	½ Jar/160g	146	11.5	91	1.7	4.9	7.2	0.7
Siciliana, Sainsbury's*	1/3 Jar/113g	168	14.7	149	1.8	6.2	13.0	0.0
Smoky Bacon, Loyd Grossman*	1 Jar/350g	343	25.2	98	3.1	5.4	7.2	0.7
Spicy Italian Chilli, Express, Dolmio*	1 Serving/170g	87	2.7	51	1.5	7.5	1.6	0.0
Spicy Pepper, Tesco*	1 Jar/500g	245	5.0	49	1.7	8.4	1.0	1.0
Spicy Red Pepper & Roasted Vegetable, Asda*	1 Serving/175g	140	7.7	80	1.2	9.0	4.4	1.0
Spicy Tomato, Asda*	1 Serving/155g	76	1.9	49	1.5	8.0	1.2	1.0
Spicy with Peppers, Tesco*	1 Jar/455g	177	1.4	39	1.2	7.9	0.3	1.1
Spinach & Ricotta, Asda*	½ Pot/175g	175	12.3	100	3.2	6.0	7.0	0.5
Sun Dried Tomato, Asda*	½ Jar/158.7g	165	12.7	104	1.9	6.0	8.0	1.5
Sun Dried Tomato, Stir In, Light, Dolmio*	1 Serving/75g	62	3.5	83	1.7	9.8	4.7	0.0
Sun Dried Tomato & Garlic, Sacla*	1 Serving/95g	177	14.0	186	3.0	10.3	14.7	0.0
Sun Ripened Tomato & Basil, Dolmio*	1 Serving/150g	117	6.9	78	1.3	7.9	4.6	0.0
Sun Ripened Tomato & Basil, Express, Dolmio*	1 Pouch/170g	88	2.7	52	1.5	7.9	1.6	0.0
Sundried Tomato, Chilli & Red Wine, Morrisons*	½ Pot/175g	72	2.3	41	1.5	5.9	1.3	1.3
Sundried Tomato & Garlic, M & S*	½ Jar/95g	147	13.0	155	2.9	4.4	13.7	0.8

P

PASTA SAUCE

	Measure INFO/WEIGHT	per Measure KCAL	FAT	Nutrition Values per 100g / 100ml KCAL	PROT	CARB	FAT	FIBRE
Sweet Red Pepper, Loyd Grossman*	1 Jar/350g	305	19.6	87	1.7	7.3	5.6	1.2
Three Cheeses, Co-Op*	1 Pack/300g	405	27.0	135	6.0	6.0	9.0	0.1
Tomato, Bacon & Mushroom, Asda*	½ Pot/50g	33	1.8	66	2.5	6.0	3.6	0.0
Tomato, Black Olive, Caper, Finest, Tesco*	1 Serving/145g	146	11.2	101	1.5	6.4	7.7	3.3
Tomato, Garlic & Chilli, Finest, Tesco*	1 Serving/145g	199	16.2	137	2.0	7.1	11.2	3.4
Tomato & Basil, Bertolli*	1 Jar/500g	215	5.0	43	1.2	7.3	1.0	0.4
Tomato & Basil, Classic, Sacla*	1 Serving/100g	137	11.1	137	2.0	7.2	11.1	2.8
Tomato & Basil, Dolmio*	1 Serving/170g	95	3.6	56	1.4	7.9	2.1	0.0
Tomato & Basil, Loyd Grossman*	½ Jar/175g	158	10.0	90	1.7	7.9	5.7	0.8
Tomato & Basil, Morrisons*	1 Serving/175g	63	1.1	36	2.0	5.6	0.6	1.0
Tomato & Basil, Organic, Seeds of Change*	1 Serving/125g	75	2.5	60	1.3	8.9	2.0	1.1
Tomato & Basil, Organic, Simply Organic*	1 Pot/300g	183	12.9	61	1.5	4.2	4.3	0.6
Tomato & Black Olive, Carb Control, Tesco*	1 Serving/110g	74	4.7	67	1.3	6.0	4.3	2.3
Tomato & Chilli, Loyd Grossman*	½ Jar/175g	154	10.0	88	1.7	7.3	5.7	0.9
Tomato & Chilli, Pour Over, M & S*	1 Jar/330g	231	12.5	70	1.3	7.6	3.8	1.8
Tomato & Chunky Vegetable, Asda*	¼ Jar/140g	71	2.1	51	1.4	7.9	1.5	1.2
Tomato & Herb, Co-Op*	1 Serving/125g	75	2.5	60	1.0	9.0	2.0	1.0
Tomato & Herb, M & S*	1 Jar/500g	400	15.5	80	2.6	10.1	3.1	1.7
Tomato & Herb, Organic, Meridian Foods*	½ Jar/220g	141	6.2	64	1.6	8.1	2.8	1.1
Tomato & Herb, Organic, Sainsbury's*	1 Serving/75g	38	1.5	51	1.2	6.6	2.0	0.5
Tomato & Mascarpone, Asda*	1 Serving/40g	57	4.8	142	2.4	6.0	12.0	1.0
Tomato & Mascarpone, BGTY, Sainsbury's*	½ Pot/150g	75	4.5	50	2.0	3.6	3.0	3.6
Tomato & Mascarpone, Finest, Tesco*	1 Serving/175g	135	8.8	77	2.7	5.4	5.0	0.8
Tomato & Mascarpone, Fresh, Sainsbury's*	1 Serving/150g	177	15.5	118	2.2	4.2	10.3	1.1
Tomato & Mascarpone, Italiano, Tesco*	½ Pot/175g	168	12.3	96	2.8	5.5	7.0	0.7
Tomato & Mascarpone, Pasta Reale*	1 Pack/300g	318	23.7	106	2.9	5.9	7.9	0.5
Tomato & Mascarpone, Sacla*	½ Jar/95g	161	14.3	169	2.2	6.2	15.0	0.0
Tomato & Mascarpone, Sainsbury's*	½ Pot/150g	137	9.9	91	2.1	5.9	6.6	1.2
Tomato & Mascarpone, Tesco*	1 Serving/175g	194	15.2	111	2.8	5.4	8.7	0.6
Tomato & Mascarpone, Waitrose*	½ Pot/175g	184	14.7	105	1.9	5.5	8.4	1.1
Tomato & Mushroom, Asda*	¼ Jar/137.7g	73	2.2	53	1.6	8.0	1.6	0.9
Tomato & Mushroom, Organic, Sainsbury's*	1 Serving/150g	87	3.9	58	1.6	7.1	2.6	1.5
Tomato & Olives, La Doria*	1 Jar/90g	76	5.9	84	1.2	5.0	6.6	0.0
Tomato & Parmesan, Seeds of Change*	1 Serving/150g	101	4.4	67	2.5	7.8	2.9	1.1
Tomato & Ricotta, Italian, Sainsbury's*	1 Pack/390g	238	11.7	61	2.5	6.1	3.0	1.2
Tomato & Roasted Garlic, Loyd Grossman*	½ Jar/175g	161	9.6	92	2.0	8.8	5.5	0.8
Tomato & Smokey Bacon, Dolmio*	1 Pot/150g	240	19.7	160	5.5	5.8	13.1	0.0
Tomato & Wild Mushroom, Loyd Grossman*	½ Jar/175g	154	9.8	88	2.1	7.4	5.6	1.5
Tomato Bacon, Stir & Serve, Homepride*	1 Serving/96g	81	4.3	84	2.7	8.1	4.5	0.0
Tomato with Herbs & Garlic, Italian, Safeway*	1 Serving/120g	73	2.5	61	1.9	8.7	2.1	1.3
Traditional, Healthy Choice, Safeway*	1 Jar/475g	257	7.6	54	1.8	8.2	1.6	1.3
Vegetable, Chunky, Tesco*	1 Jar/455g	223	5.9	49	0.7	8.6	1.3	1.1
with Tomatoes & Black Olives, Fit For Fun*	1 Serving/50g	30	1.9	60	1.3	5.3	3.7	0.0

PASTA SHAPES

	Measure INFO/WEIGHT	per Measure KCAL	FAT	Nutrition Values per 100g / 100ml KCAL	PROT	CARB	FAT	FIBRE
Cooked, Tesco*	1 Serving/260g	356	2.1	137	5.1	26.3	0.8	1.1
Dried, Tesco*	1 Serving/100g	345	2.0	345	13.2	68.5	2.0	2.9
Durum Wheat, Dry, Basics, Sainsbury's*	1 Serving/75g	260	1.5	346	12.0	70.0	2.0	4.0
Funky Fish, Heinz*	1 Serving/200g	108	0.6	54	1.4	11.6	0.3	0.4
in a Cheese & Broccoli Sauce, Tesco*	1 Serving/84g	317	5.5	377	13.1	66.2	6.6	4.1
Postman Pat, HP*	1 Can/410g	279	1.6	68	1.8	14.3	0.4	0.7
Scooby Doo, HP*	1 Can/410g	279	1.6	68	1.8	14.3	0.4	0.7
Teletubbies, Heinz*	1 Can/400g	244	1.6	61	2.0	12.3	0.4	0.6

P

	Measure INFO/WEIGHT	per Measure KCAL	FAT	Nutrition Values per 100g / 100ml KCAL	PROT	CARB	FAT	FIBRE
PASTA SHELLS								
Dry, Average	1 Serving/75g	265	1.5	353	11.1	71.8	2.0	2.0
Egg, Fresh, Average	1 Serving/125g	344	3.6	275	11.5	49.8	2.9	3.5
Wholewheat, HL, Co-Op*	1 Serving/75g	233	0.8	310	11.0	64.0	1.0	12.0
PASTA SNACK								
Cheese & Ham, Pot, Tesco*	1 Serving/208g	254	8.5	122	3.4	17.9	4.1	1.5
Cheese & Ham, Tubes, Made Up, Tesco*	1 Serving/214g	312	11.6	146	4.9	19.5	5.4	2.6
Chicken, Morrisons*	1 Pack/250g	285	6.8	114	3.3	19.3	2.7	0.0
Chicken, Sweetcorn & Mushroom, Pot, Tesco*	1 Pot/216g	238	5.8	110	3.0	18.5	2.7	0.7
Chicken & Smoked Bacon, Sainsbury's*	1 Pack/190g	490	36.5	258	7.2	14.1	19.2	0.0
Creamy Cheese, Mug Shot, Asda*	1 Serving/250g	273	6.3	109	2.5	19.0	2.5	1.8
Ham & Mushroom, Tesco*	1 Pack/300g	618	42.9	206	4.2	15.0	14.3	1.1
Tomato & Herb, in a Pot, Dry, Tesco*	1 Pot/59g	207	1.4	352	11.8	70.7	2.4	2.6
Tomato & Herb, Morrisons*	1 Pot/247g	247	2.7	100	3.1	19.5	1.1	0.0
PASTA SPIRALS								
Co-Op*	1 Serving/100g	350	1.0	350	12.0	73.0	1.0	3.0
Glutenfree, Glutano*	1oz/28g	100	0.3	357	4.0	83.0	1.0	0.0
PASTA TWIRLS								
Dry, Asda*	1 Serving/50g	173	0.8	346	12.0	71.0	1.5	3.0
Tri-Colour, Sainsbury's*	1 Serving/75g	268	1.3	357	12.3	73.1	1.7	2.5
PASTA TWISTS								
Dry, Average	1oz/28g	99	0.4	354	12.3	71.8	1.5	2.2
Wheat & Gluten Free, Glutafin*	1 Serving/75g	263	1.5	350	8.0	75.0	2.0	0.1
PASTA WITH								
Cheese & Tomato, Al Forno, Sainsbury's*	½ Pack/499g	749	29.0	150	5.5	18.9	5.8	1.8
Feta Cheese & Slow Roasted Tomatoes, M & S*	1 Pack/190g	352	13.7	185	6.8	22.8	7.2	2.0
Honey Mustard Chicken, COU, M & S*	1 Pack/300g	360	7.2	120	8.4	16.2	2.4	1.9
Meatballs, Puglian Style, M & S*	½ Pack/500g	600	26.5	120	5.5	12.5	5.3	1.2
Meatballs, Sainsbury's*	1 Can/300g	339	14.7	113	6.6	10.6	4.9	1.6
Salmon & Broccoli, Lemon Dressed, Sainsbury's*	1 Serving/300g	486	17.7	162	6.9	20.4	5.9	2.1
Spicy Chicken, Sainsbury's*	1 Pot/300g	489	18.3	163	7.1	20.1	6.1	2.3
Tomato & Basil Chicken, BGTY, Sainsbury's*	1 Pack/190g	250	2.1	132	9.2	21.2	1.1	2.7
Tuna & Roasted Peppers, M & S*	1 Serving/220g	308	8.6	140	9.1	17.7	3.9	0.9
PASTE								
Beef, Asda*	1 Serving/37g	72	5.2	194	17.0	0.1	14.0	0.0
Beef, Princes*	1 Serving/18g	40	2.8	220	14.4	5.2	15.8	0.0
Beef, Sainsbury's*	1 Jar/75g	142	9.9	189	16.0	1.5	13.2	1.4
Chicken, Asda*	1 Thin Spread/7g	13	0.9	184	16.0	0.8	13.0	0.0
Chicken, Princes*	1 Thin Spread/9g	22	1.7	240	12.6	5.6	18.5	0.0
Chicken, Tesco*	1 Serving/12g	30	2.4	248	14.8	2.3	20.0	0.1
Chicken & Ham, Asda*	½ Jar/38g	82	6.5	217	14.0	2.1	17.0	0.0
Chicken & Ham, Tesco*	1 Serving/19g	44	3.7	231	12.5	1.4	19.5	0.0
Chicken & Stuffing, Asda*	½ Jar/35g	71	4.9	203	16.0	3.3	14.0	0.0
Chicken & Stuffing, Princes*	1 Jar/100g	229	17.0	229	15.7	3.3	17.0	0.0
Crab, Princes*	1 Pot/35g	36	1.2	104	13.4	4.8	3.5	0.0
Crab, Sainsbury's*	1 Thick Spread/5g	6	0.2	115	16.5	1.7	4.7	0.5
Crab, Tesco*	1 Jar/75g	89	3.8	119	14.0	4.6	5.0	0.1
Salmon, Asda*	1 Serving/53g	76	3.7	143	15.0	5.0	7.0	0.0
Salmon, Princes*	1 Serving/30g	59	3.8	195	13.5	6.5	12.8	0.0
Salmon, Value, Tesco*	1 Serving/10g	17	1.0	165	14.0	4.6	10.1	0.8
Salmon & Shrimp, Tesco*	1 Jar/75g	83	2.6	111	15.1	5.0	3.4	0.1
Sardine & Tomato, Asda*	1 Thin Spread/9g	11	0.5	123	14.0	3.3	6.0	0.0
Sardine & Tomato, Princes*	1 Jar/75g	110	5.4	146	15.4	5.0	7.2	0.0
Sardine & Tomato, Sainsbury's*	1 Pot/35g	60	3.8	170	16.9	1.2	10.8	1.3

INFO/WEIGHT	Measure	per Measure KCAL	FAT	Nutrition Values per 100g / 100ml KCAL	PROT	CARB	FAT	FIBRE

PASTE
Sardine & Tomato, Tesco*	1 Jar/75g	98	4.4	130	14.6	4.8	5.8	0.1
Tuna & Mayonnaise, Asda*	1 Jar/75g	165	12.0	220	17.0	2.1	16.0	0.6
Tuna & Mayonnaise, Princes*	1 Pot/75g	86	12.3	115	16.8	3.8	16.4	0.0
Tuna & Mayonnaise, Sainsbury's*	1 Tbsp/17g	41	3.1	242	19.2	0.6	18.1	1.6
Tuna & Mayonnaise, Somerfield*	1 Thin Spread/9g	19	1.4	209	15.0	2.0	16.0	0.0
Tuna & Mayonnaise, Tesco*	1 Serving/15g	31	2.4	209	14.9	2.1	15.7	0.1

PASTILLES
Blackcurrant, Rowntree's*	1 Tube/53.3g	188	0.0	353	4.4	84.0	0.0	0.0
Fruit, Average	1 Tube/33g	108	0.0	327	2.8	84.2	0.0	0.0
Fruit, Co-Op*	1 Sweet/6g	20	0.0	337	2.8	81.5	0.0	0.0
Fruit, Rowntree's*	1 Tube/53g	186	0.0	351	4.4	83.7	0.0	0.0
Wine, Maynards*	1 Pack/52g	161	0.0	310	3.9	72.1	0.0	0.0

PASTRAMI
American Style, Morrisons*	1 Slice/10g	11	0.2	114	22.2	2.5	1.7	0.8
Asda*	1 Serving/10g	10	0.1	105	24.0	0.3	0.9	0.0
Beef, Average	1 Serving/40g	51	1.4	128	23.1	1.1	3.6	0.2
British, Waitrose*	1 Pack/80g	92	2.2	115	21.8	0.9	2.7	0.0
Turkey, Average	½ Packet/35g	38	0.5	107	21.8	1.7	1.5	0.5

PASTRY
Bacon & Cheese Slices, Savoury, Somerfield*	1 Slice/165g	490	33.5	297	7.4	21.2	20.3	1.5
Bacon & Cheese Slices, Tesco*	1 Slice/165g	480	32.0	291	7.4	21.7	19.4	1.0
Cheese, Potato & Onion Slices, Taste!*	1 Serving/155g	501	30.4	323	8.6	28.1	19.6	0.0
Cheese & Ham Slice, Sainsbury's*	1 Slice/118g	352	23.2	298	7.8	22.5	19.7	1.8
Cheese & Ham Slice, Savoury, Somerfield*	1 Slice/150g	399	24.0	266	7.0	23.0	16.0	0.0
Cheese & Onion Slices, Savoury, Somerfield*	1 Slice/165g	518	34.5	314	7.4	24.0	20.9	0.6
Cheese & Onion Slices, Tesco*	1 Slice/150g	503	37.1	335	8.0	20.1	24.7	1.4
Chicken Breast, Bacon & Cheese Slices, Tesco*	1 Serving/150g	237	11.7	158	20.7	1.2	7.8	0.5
Custard Slice, Tesco*	1 Slice/108g	275	11.1	255	2.8	37.2	10.3	1.3
Fillo, Fresh, Raw, Cypressa*	1 Sheet/14g	43	0.5	305	10.8	57.4	3.6	1.9
Filo, Average	1 Sheet/45g	137	1.2	304	9.0	61.4	2.7	0.9
Filo, Frozen, Jus-Rol*	1 Sheet/45g	105	1.2	234	8.1	52.1	2.7	2.1
Greek, Average	1oz/28g	90	4.8	322	4.7	40.0	17.0	0.0
Ham & Cheese Slices, Ginsters*	1 Slice/155g	625	43.7	403	9.8	31.9	28.2	4.2
Puff, Blocks, Frozen, Farmfoods*	1 Block/340g	1329	68.0	391	5.6	32.1	20.0	1.9
Puff, Fresh, Sainsbury's*	½ Pack/250g	1113	85.8	445	5.4	28.8	34.3	1.3
Puff, Frozen, Average	1 Shell/47g	188	12.0	401	5.1	29.2	25.6	0.0
Puff, Individual Rounds, Jus-Rol*	1 Round/53g	212	14.7	400	5.8	31.7	27.7	1.4
Shortcrust, Cooked, Average	1oz/28g	146	9.0	521	6.6	54.2	32.3	2.2
Shortcrust, Raw, Average	1oz/28g	127	8.1	453	5.6	44.0	29.1	1.3
Spring Roll Wrapper, TYJ Food*	1 Sheet/18g	54	0.0	300	0.0	73.0	0.0	0.0
Steak & Onion, Slices, M & S*	1 Slice/165g	479	30.2	290	11.1	20.4	18.3	4.2

PASTRY MIX
Short Crust, Somerfield*	1oz/28g	134	7.8	479	7.0	49.0	28.0	0.0

PASTY
Beef, Port Royal*	1 Pasty/130g	299	13.3	230	10.2	24.4	10.2	0.0
Bite Size Pasties, Food to Go, Sainsbury's*	1 Serving/60g	226	14.6	377	8.2	31.2	24.4	1.5
Cheddar & Onion, Hand Crimped, Waitrose*	1 Pasty/70g	191	14.8	273	8.8	22.5	21.1	2.2
Cheese & Onion, Co-Op*	1 Pasty/75g	235	14.9	313	9.2	24.5	19.8	1.7
Cheese & Onion, Farmfoods*	1 Pasty/191g	485	26.7	254	6.6	25.5	14.0	2.0
Cheese & Onion, Freshbake*	1 Pastry/135g	368	22.5	272	5.6	25.5	16.6	1.1
Cheese & Onion, Geo Adams*	1 Pasty/150g	420	23.4	280	6.9	27.9	15.6	1.1
Cheese & Onion, Safeway*	1 Pasty/165g	482	31.1	292	6.5	24.1	18.8	1.0
Cheese & Onion, Sainsbury's*	1 Serving/150g	486	32.7	324	7.4	24.5	21.8	1.3

	Measure INFO/WEIGHT	per Measure KCAL FAT		Nutrition Values per 100g / 100ml KCAL PROT CARB FAT FIBRE				

PASTY

	Measure INFO/WEIGHT	KCAL	FAT	KCAL	PROT	CARB	FAT	FIBRE
Cheese & Onion, Somerfield*	1 Pasty/145g	419	26.1	289	7.0	24.0	18.0	0.0
Cheese & Onion, Tesco*	1 Pasty/150g	416	26.4	277	5.9	23.7	17.6	2.2
Chicken, Port Royal*	1 Pasty/130g	289	10.9	222	5.5	31.2	8.4	0.0
Chicken & Vegetable, Proper Cornish Ltd*	1 Pasty/255g	671	34.7	263	7.4	30.2	13.6	2.4
Cornish, BGTY, Sainsbury's*	1 Pasty/135g	308	12.7	228	7.7	28.2	9.4	1.6
Cornish, Cheese & Onion, Ginsters*	1 Pasty/130g	511	33.0	393	10.4	30.7	25.4	2.3
Cornish, Chicken & Bacon, Ginsters*	1 Pasty/227g	574	34.5	253	6.9	22.2	15.2	0.8
Cornish, Co-Op*	1 Pasty/75g	200	12.3	267	6.4	23.4	16.4	1.6
Cornish, M & S*	1 Pasty/300g	780	46.2	260	7.1	23.4	15.4	2.8
Cornish, Mini, Iceland*	1 Pasty/70.3g	214	14.8	306	7.0	22.1	21.1	1.2
Cornish, Mini, M & S*	1 Pasty/75g	244	17.6	325	7.3	21.9	23.4	1.8
Cornish, Mini, Sainsbury's*	1 Pasty/70g	280	20.1	400	7.3	28.1	28.7	1.5
Cornish, Mini, Tesco*	1 Pasty/24g	66	4.2	274	5.6	23.2	17.7	0.5
Cornish, Morrisons*	1 Pasty/200g	626	37.0	313	7.5	29.1	18.5	0.0
Cornish, Original, Ginsters*	1 Pasty/227g	1317	79.7	580	14.0	49.0	35.1	4.3
Cornish, Pork Farms*	1 Pasty/250g	673	40.8	269	7.7	22.8	16.3	0.0
Cornish, Safeway*	1 Pasty/170g	490	31.6	288	7.5	22.6	18.6	1.5
Cornish, Sainsbury's*	1 Pasty/150g	489	32.1	326	6.7	26.6	21.4	2.0
Cornish, SmartPrice, Asda*	1 Pasty/94g	286	15.0	304	8.0	32.0	16.0	1.7
Cornish, Tesco*	1 Pasty/150g	467	32.7	311	6.8	21.9	21.8	1.6
Cornish, Traditional Style, Geo Adams*	1 Pasty/165g	488	30.4	296	7.1	25.4	18.4	1.3
Cornish, Value, Tesco*	1 Pasty/150g	425	26.6	283	6.7	24.2	17.7	2.2
Cornish Roaster, Ginsters*	1 Pasty/130g	417	24.2	321	8.5	29.9	18.6	1.3
Lamb, Port Royal*	1 Pasty/130g	352	17.4	271	7.2	30.5	13.4	0.0
Olive & Cheese, Tapas, Waitrose*	1 Pack/130g	455	25.2	350	8.1	35.8	19.4	1.3
Salt Fish, Port Royal*	1 Pasty/130g	300	13.4	231	6.8	27.8	10.3	0.0
Tandoori & Vegetable, Holland & Barrett*	1 Pack/110g	232	9.4	211	4.3	29.4	8.5	1.8
Vegetable	1oz/28g	77	4.2	274	4.1	33.3	14.9	1.9
Vegetable, Hand Crimped, Waitrose*	1 Pasty/200g	454	22.6	227	4.5	26.8	11.3	2.2
Vegetarian, Country Slice, Linda McCartney*	1 Pasty/150g	373	20.2	249	5.6	26.5	13.5	2.9
Vegetarian, Port Royal*	1 Pattie/130g	315	13.8	242	12.5	24.1	10.6	0.0

PATE

	Measure INFO/WEIGHT	KCAL	FAT	KCAL	PROT	CARB	FAT	FIBRE
Ardennes, Asda*	1 Serving/50g	143	12.0	286	13.9	3.6	24.0	1.3
Ardennes, BGTY, Sainsbury's*	¼ Pack/50g	90	5.7	180	16.6	2.9	11.4	0.0
Ardennes, Healthy Choice, Somerfield*	1 Pack/175g	341	23.1	195	16.4	2.6	13.2	1.6
Ardennes, HL, Tesco*	1 Serving/50g	88	6.3	176	12.1	3.6	12.6	1.8
Ardennes, Iceland*	1 Serving/70g	223	20.0	318	12.0	3.4	28.5	0.5
Ardennes, Medium Coarse, Sainsbury's*	1/6 Pack/28.2g	77	6.4	273	15.2	2.1	22.6	0.1
Ardennes, Reduced Fat, Safeway*	1 Serving/50g	97	6.0	194	18.5	3.1	11.9	0.1
Ardennes, Reduced Fat, Waitrose*	¼ Pack/42g	94	7.1	224	15.4	2.6	16.9	0.5
Ardennes, Safeway*	1 Serving/50g	166	14.2	331	12.8	6.0	28.4	0.8
Ardennes, Tesco*	1 Tbsp/15g	53	5.0	354	13.3	0.5	33.2	1.2
Ardennes, with Bacon, Tesco*	½ Pack/85g	241	20.6	284	11.4	5.1	24.2	1.1
Breton, Country, with Apricots, Coarse, Sainsbury's*	1 Serving/21g	60	4.7	285	13.5	7.0	22.5	0.5
Brie & Cranberry, M & S*	1 Serving/55g	193	18.3	350	6.0	7.3	33.3	1.5
Brussels, & Garlic, Reduced Fat, Tesco*	1 Serving/65g	135	8.0	208	16.2	8.1	12.3	0.6
Brussels, 25% Less Fat, Morrisons*	¼ Pack/42.5g	107	8.9	249	14.2	0.7	20.6	0.0
Brussels, 30% Less Fat, GFY, Asda*	1 Serving/50g	79	5.2	158	14.3	1.9	10.4	3.7
Brussels, BGTY, 50% Less Fat, Sainsbury's*	1 Serving/100g	223	16.0	223	14.6	5.1	16.0	0.1
Brussels, Co-Op*	1 Serving/15g	51	4.7	340	11.0	4.0	31.0	2.0
Brussels, Fat Reduced, Somerfield*	1 Serving/50g	96	7.0	192	14.0	2.0	14.0	0.0
Brussels, GFY, Asda*	¼ Pack/42.5g	108	8.5	254	16.0	2.4	20.0	0.0
Brussels, HL, Tesco*	1 Serving/29g	66	4.4	229	14.4	8.4	15.3	1.8

PATE

	Measure INFO/WEIGHT	KCAL	FAT	KCAL	PROT	CARB	FAT	FIBRE
Brussels, M & S*	1 Pot/170g	519	45.2	305	13.3	2.8	26.6	1.0
Brussels, Reduced Fat, Waitrose*	1 Serving/40g	92	7.4	229	13.2	2.4	18.5	0.5
Brussels, Sainsbury's*	1 Pack/170g	663	64.9	390	10.6	1.1	38.2	0.1
Brussels, Smooth, Safeway*	1 Pack/170g	553	49.8	325	11.5	3.9	29.3	1.6
Brussels, Smooth, Spreadable, Sainsbury's*	1 Serving/30g	97	8.7	323	10.7	4.7	29.0	0.0
Brussels, Tesco*	1 Serving/28g	92	8.5	330	11.0	3.0	30.5	1.1
Brussels, with Forest Mushroom, Co-Op*	1 Serving/57g	180	16.5	315	12.0	2.0	29.0	1.0
Brussels, with Garlic, Asda*	1 Serving/50g	170	15.7	340	10.7	4.0	31.3	2.5
Brussels, with Herbs, Tesco*	1 Serving/25g	87	8.2	347	8.4	6.4	32.6	1.5
Carrot, Ginger & Spring Onion, M & S*	1 Serving/50g	73	5.5	145	1.5	9.6	11.0	0.9
Chargrilled Vegetable, BGTY, Sainsbury's*	½ Pot/57.3g	43	0.7	75	4.9	10.8	1.3	2.7
Chicken & Brandy, Morrisons*	1 Serving/44g	133	11.8	303	10.8	4.3	26.9	0.8
Chicken Liver, Asda*	1 Serving/65g	131	10.4	202	13.0	4.0	16.0	0.8
Chicken Liver, BGTY, Sainsbury's*	1 Serving/30g	64	4.8	214	11.5	6.0	16.0	0.5
Chicken Liver, M & S*	1oz/28g	79	6.7	281	14.0	1.9	24.1	0.1
Chicken Liver, Organic, Waitrose*	½ Tub/87.5g	205	16.2	233	12.6	1.8	18.4	1.4
Chicken Liver, with Madeira, Sainsbury's*	1 Serving/30g	84	7.3	279	13.1	1.9	24.3	0.0
Chicken Liver & Brandy, Asda*	1 Serving/50g	177	16.4	353	9.0	5.5	32.8	3.2
Chicken Liver & Garlic, Smooth, Asda*	1 Serving/30.7g	120	11.2	388	9.0	7.0	36.0	3.2
Chicken Liver Parfait, TTD, Sainsbury's*	1 Serving/20g	72	7.0	359	8.0	2.0	35.0	0.5
Chicken Liver with Brandy, Tesco*	1oz/28g	82	7.2	293	11.8	3.5	25.8	1.4
Chickpea, Moroccan, Organic, Cauldron*	1 Tsp/15g	31	2.1	207	6.8	16.3	13.7	4.9
Coarse Farmhouse, Organic, Sainsbury's*	1 Serving/56g	138	11.0	246	13.3	3.7	19.7	0.8
Crab, M & S*	1oz/28g	63	4.8	225	12.1	5.9	17.3	0.0
Crab, Waitrose*	1oz/28g	59	4.6	209	14.5	0.5	16.6	0.0
De Campagne, Sainsbury's*	1 Serving/55g	129	10.0	235	16.3	1.4	18.2	0.0
Duck & Champagne, Luxury, M & S*	1oz/28g	106	9.9	380	8.3	8.3	35.2	7.8
Duck & Orange, Asda*	1 Serving/40g	94	7.2	235	16.0	2.2	18.0	0.0
Duck & Orange, M & S*	½ Pot/65g	189	16.7	290	10.5	3.9	25.7	1.1
Duck & Orange, Smooth, Tesco*	1 Serving/50g	189	17.7	377	10.5	4.0	35.4	0.5
Duck Liver, Champagne & Truffles, TTD, Sainsbury's*	1 Serving/50g	212	21.1	423	8.2	2.5	42.2	0.0
Farmhouse Mushroom, Asda*	1 Serving/50g	126	10.0	252	13.0	5.0	20.0	0.7
Farmhouse Style, Finest, Tesco*	1 Serving/28g	83	7.3	295	11.9	3.6	25.9	1.0
Farmhouse Style, M & S*	¼ Pack/42g	90	7.1	215	14.4	1.9	16.9	1.2
Farmhouse Style, Weight Watchers*	1 Serving/36.8g	49	2.1	133	14.8	5.5	5.7	0.5
Farmhouse with Mushrooms & Garlic, Tesco*	1 Serving/90g	257	22.8	285	13.8	0.6	25.3	1.3
Forestiere, M & S*	1 Serving/20g	61	5.3	305	11.5	4.2	26.6	1.4
Isle of Skye Smoked Salmon, TTD, Sainsbury's*	½ Pot/58g	161	13.4	277	16.5	0.8	23.1	0.1
Kipper, Waitrose*	¼ Tub/28g	105	9.2	370	16.8	2.0	32.7	0.6
Liver, Value, Tesco*	1 Serving/50g	151	13.0	302	13.0	4.1	26.0	0.5
Liver & Bacon, Tesco*	1 Serving/10g	28	2.3	276	12.9	4.3	23.0	0.4
Luxury Orkney Crab, Castle MacLellan*	1 Serving/15g	27	1.6	178	11.1	9.2	10.7	0.8
Mackerel, Smoked	1oz/28g	103	9.6	368	13.4	1.3	34.4	0.0
Mackerel, Tesco*	1 Serving/29g	102	9.5	353	14.3	0.5	32.6	0.0
Mediterranean Roast Vegetable, Tesco*	1 Serving/28g	31	2.6	112	2.4	4.3	9.4	1.2
Mushroom, BGTY, Sainsbury's*	½ Pot/58g	29	0.3	50	4.6	6.7	0.5	3.0
Mushroom, M & S*	1 Pot/115g	224	20.1	195	4.2	4.8	17.5	1.5
Mushroom, Organic, Cauldron*	1 Pot/113g	170	15.0	150	2.9	6.2	13.3	1.5
Mushroom, Roast, Tesco*	1 Serving/25g	36	3.2	145	3.6	3.6	12.9	4.5
Mushroom, Sainsbury's*	½ Pot/57.2g	79	6.3	138	3.7	6.1	11.0	2.2
Mushroom, Tesco*	1oz/28g	39	2.7	138	3.3	9.8	9.5	1.0
Mushroom & Tarragon, Waitrose*	1 Serving/30g	47	4.1	155	2.8	5.5	13.5	1.4
Pheasant, TTD, Sainsbury's*	1/6 Pack/28g	59	4.2	212	15.4	3.9	15.0	0.8

P

PATE

	Measure INFO/WEIGHT	per Measure KCAL	per Measure FAT	KCAL	PROT	CARB	FAT	FIBRE
Poached Salmon & Watercress, Tesco*	1 Serving/25g	60	4.4	238	19.2	0.4	17.7	0.2
Pork, with Apple & Cider, Sainsbury's*	1 Serving/50g	152	12.7	303	12.5	6.3	25.3	1.1
Pork, with Peppercorns, Tesco*	1 Serving/28g	84	7.5	300	12.9	1.4	26.8	0.7
Red Pepper, M & S*	1oz/28g	52	4.5	185	3.0	6.6	16.2	0.9
Ricotta, Subdried Tomato & Basil, Princes*	1 Jar/110g	343	31.6	312	5.2	8.3	28.7	0.0
Roasted Parsnip & Carrot, Organic, Cauldron*	1 Serving/60g	69	4.0	115	3.5	10.2	6.7	4.9
Roasted Red Pepper, Oven Roasted, Castle MacLellan*	1oz/28g	46	3.8	163	3.3	8.2	13.5	0.8
Roasted Vegetable & Feta, Cauldron*	1 Pot/115g	148	8.2	129	4.3	10.0	7.1	2.1
Salmon, Organic, M & S*	1oz/28g	76	6.3	270	16.9	0.0	22.5	0.0
Salmon, Smoked, M & S*	1oz/28g	74	6.2	265	16.9	0.0	22.0	0.0
Salmon Dill, Princes*	1 Serving/70g	124	7.8	177	15.4	4.0	11.1	0.5
Scottish Smoked Salmon, Castle MacLellan*	¼ Tub/28g	62	4.5	220	13.5	5.6	16.0	0.0
Scottish Smoked Salmon, M & S*	1 Serving/30g	81	6.7	270	17.0	0.2	22.3	0.0
Smoked Duck, with Cranberry Coulis, TTD, Sainsbury's*	1 Serving/62g	174	13.8	280	10.7	9.3	22.2	1.0
Smoked Mackerel, M & S*	1oz/28g	104	9.7	370	13.4	0.7	34.7	0.3
Smoked Mackerel, Sainsbury's*	½ Pot/57g	215	20.1	378	14.2	0.8	35.3	0.0
Smoked Mackerel, Scottish, M & S*	½ Pot/57.5g	160	13.5	275	15.9	0.6	23.2	0.1
Smoked Salmon, Luxury, Morrisons*	½ Pot/56.5g	152	12.5	266	16.0	0.9	22.0	0.5
Smoked Salmon, Organic, Waitrose*	1oz/28g	83	7.2	296	13.9	2.4	25.6	0.0
Smoked Salmon, Tesco*	1 Pack/115g	282	22.0	245	15.0	3.0	19.1	1.0
Smoked Salmon, Waitrose*	½ Pot/56.5g	120	8.9	212	17.1	0.5	15.7	0.6
Smoked Trout, Waitrose*	½ Pot/56g	130	10.3	232	15.8	0.9	18.4	0.6
Spicy Bean, BGTY, Sainsbury's*	½ Pot/58g	56	1.1	97	5.0	15.1	1.9	5.4
Spicy Bean, Princes*	½ Pot/55g	46	0.2	84	3.6	16.7	0.3	0.0
Spinach & Soft Cheese, Organic, Cauldron*	1 Pot/115g	206	16.3	179	7.7	5.1	14.2	3.2
Sun-Dried Tomato & Basil, Cauldron*	1 Pot/115g	189	11.7	164	6.9	11.1	10.2	4.6
Tofu, Spicy Mexican, Organic, GranoVita*	1 Serving/50g	108	10.0	216	6.0	3.0	20.0	0.0
Tomato, Lentil & Basil, Cauldron*	1 Pack/113g	158	7.7	140	6.8	14.0	6.8	3.2
Tomato, Organic, GranoVita*	1 Tsp/5g	11	1.0	215	5.0	6.0	19.0	0.0
Tuna, M & S*	1oz/28g	99	8.8	355	18.0	0.0	31.3	0.0
Tuna, Tesco*	1 Pack/115g	332	26.7	289	19.8	0.3	23.2	0.2
Tuna with Butter & Lemon Juice, Sainsbury's*	½ Pot/58g	209	18.3	360	19.0	0.1	31.6	0.3
Yeast, Garlic & Herb, Tartex*	1 Serving/30g	69	5.4	230	7.0	10.0	18.0	0.0
Yeast, Pateole, GranoVita*	1 Portion/30g	66	5.3	219	10.2	4.5	17.8	0.0
Yeast with Mushrooms, Organic, Tartex*	1 Serving/50g	120	9.5	239	7.0	10.0	19.0	0.0

PAVLOVA

	Measure INFO/WEIGHT	per Measure KCAL	per Measure FAT	KCAL	PROT	CARB	FAT	FIBRE
Raspberry, Co-Op*	1/6 Pavlova/49g	147	5.9	300	3.2	44.8	12.0	1.1
Raspberry, Individual, M & S*	1 Pavlova/65g	133	1.6	205	4.0	41.8	2.4	0.2
Raspberry, M & S*	1 Serving/84g	193	8.1	230	2.3	33.3	9.6	0.3
Raspberry, Mini, Co-Op*	1 Pavlova/19g	61	1.7	320	3.0	56.0	9.0	0.6
Raspberry, Mini, Iceland*	1 Pavlova/21.2g	57	2.9	273	2.3	35.1	13.7	2.6
Raspberry, Safeway*	1 Serving/53g	163	6.9	307	2.9	44.6	13.0	0.5
Raspberry, Sara Lee*	1/6 Slice/55.4g	167	8.4	303	2.7	38.5	15.3	1.1
Raspberry, Tesco*	1 Serving/65g	191	8.4	294	2.7	41.8	12.9	1.1
Strawberry, Co-Op*	1 Serving/52g	177	7.3	340	3.0	50.0	14.0	0.4
Strawberry, COU, M & S*	1 Pot/95g	147	2.3	155	2.4	30.5	2.4	0.8
Strawberry, Farmfoods*	1/6 Cake/52g	152	7.8	292	2.3	36.9	15.0	2.2
Toffee Pecan, M & S*	1oz/28g	118	7.4	420	3.9	41.5	26.6	0.4

PAW-PAW

	Measure INFO/WEIGHT	per Measure KCAL	per Measure FAT	KCAL	PROT	CARB	FAT	FIBRE
Raw, Fresh	1oz/28g	10	0.0	36	0.5	8.8	0.1	2.2
Raw, Weighed with Skin & Pips	1oz/28g	8	0.0	27	0.4	6.6	0.1	1.7

PEACH

	Measure INFO/WEIGHT	per Measure KCAL	per Measure FAT	KCAL	PROT	CARB	FAT	FIBRE
Dried, Average	1 Pack/250g	473	1.6	189	2.6	45.0	0.7	6.9

	Measure INFO/WEIGHT	per Measure KCAL	FAT	Nutrition Values per 100g / 100ml KCAL	PROT	CARB	FAT	FIBRE
PEACH								
in Fruit Juice, Average	1oz/28g	13	0.0	47	0.5	11.3	0.0	0.7
in Syrup, Average	1oz/28g	19	0.0	67	0.4	16.3	0.1	0.4
Pieces in Strawberry Jelly, Fruitini, Del Monte*	1 Can/140g	91	0.1	65	0.3	15.3	0.1	0.0
Raw, Average	1 Peach/125g	39	0.1	32	1.0	7.2	0.1	1.4
PEANUT BRITTLE								
Thorntons*	2 Pieces/32g	163	8.6	509	12.4	54.3	26.9	2.6
PEANUT BUTTER								
Creamy, Smooth, Sun Pat*	1 Serving/15g	93	7.5	620	24.0	17.5	50.2	6.1
Crunchy, Asda*	1 Serving/10g	61	5.1	611	28.0	12.0	51.0	6.0
Crunchy, Bettabuy, Morrisons*	1 Serving/10g	61	5.2	606	22.5	17.3	52.2	5.7
Crunchy, Harvest Spread*	1 Serving/25g	148	12.4	592	23.6	12.5	49.7	6.9
Crunchy, Organic, Evernat*	1 Tsp/10g	64	5.3	641	29.0	13.0	53.0	7.0
Crunchy, Organic, Tesco*	1 Serving/25g	149	12.4	595	23.6	12.5	49.7	6.9
Crunchy, Original, Sun Pat*	1 Serving/10g	60	4.8	600	27.0	14.5	48.2	6.8
Crunchy, Original Style, Whole Earth*	1 Serving/20g	118	10.0	592	24.9	10.1	50.2	7.3
Crunchy, Route 66*	1 Serving/10g	65	5.8	648	20.0	13.0	58.0	5.4
Crunchy, Sainsbury's*	1 Serving/10g	59	5.0	594	23.2	12.4	50.2	6.7
Crunchy, Somerfield*	1 Tsp/10g	59	4.9	586	24.4	11.8	49.0	7.1
Crunchy, Tesco*	1 Tsp/4g	25	2.0	614	27.8	12.0	50.5	6.5
Crunchy, Value, Tesco*	1 Serving/20g	123	10.7	615	21.5	11.7	53.6	5.4
Extra Crunchy, Sun Pat*	1 Serving/20g	119	10.2	597	21.9	12.6	51.0	7.3
GFY, Asda*	1 Serving/15g	80	5.3	531	28.0	31.0	35.0	0.0
Organic, Rapunzel*	1 Serving/5g	31	2.7	613	29.0	4.5	53.0	0.0
SmartPrice, Asda*	1 Serving/15g	87	7.5	582	23.0	10.0	50.0	6.0
Smooth, 25% Less Fat, Tesco*	1 Serving/15g	85	5.9	555	20.5	31.0	38.7	5.5
Smooth, 30% Reduced Fat, Duerr's*	1 Tsp/6g	32	2.1	533	22.6	31.7	35.1	6.7
Smooth, 33% Less Fat, BGTY, Sainsbury's*	1 Serving/10g	53	3.5	533	22.6	31.7	35.1	6.7
Smooth, Average	1 Serving/20g	125	10.7	623	22.6	13.1	53.7	5.4
Smooth, Kernel King, Duerr's*	1 Serving/15g	89	7.5	596	23.3	12.4	50.3	6.8
Smooth, Kraft*	1 Serving/20g	127	10.7	636	23.1	17.6	53.5	0.0
Smooth, Light, Kraft*	1 Serving/20g	114	7.7	571	16.3	40.1	38.6	0.0
Smooth, Morrisons*	1 Serving/10g	60	5.0	596	23.3	12.4	50.3	0.0
Smooth, Organic, Essential*	1 Serving/20g	125	10.2	623	28.0	13.0	51.0	0.0
Smooth, Organic, Meridian Foods*	1 Serving/10g	61	4.9	612	31.2	12.2	48.7	6.5
Smooth, Organic, Tesco*	1 Serving/15g	90	7.5	600	23.3	12.4	50.3	6.5
Smooth, Organic, Waitrose*	1 Serving/12g	71	6.1	595	24.6	9.9	50.8	7.1
Smooth, Somerfield*	1 Tsp/10g	59	5.0	592	24.0	11.0	50.0	0.0
Smooth, Sun Pat*	1 Serving/20g	116	9.9	581	24.0	10.1	49.4	8.0
Smooth, Tesco*	1 Tsp/16.3g	100	8.2	614	27.8	12.0	50.5	6.5
Stripy, Sun Pat*	1 Tsp/10g	62	4.7	617	13.0	35.0	47.0	3.0
Whole Nut, Crunchy, Average	1 Tsp/10g	61	5.3	606	24.9	7.7	53.1	6.0
Wholenut, Sainsbury's*	1 Serving/15g	90	7.7	598	24.2	9.8	51.3	7.0
Wholenut, Tesco*	1 Tbsp/15.3g	95	8.0	620	24.0	12.9	52.1	6.9
PEANUT SHOOTS								
Cooked with Oil, Sainsbury's*	1 Pack/80g	177	13.5	221	10.6	4.1	16.9	2.5
PEANUTS								
Chilli, Average	½ Pack/50g	303	25.3	605	28.2	9.3	50.6	6.8
Dry Roasted, Average	1 Serving/20g	117	9.8	587	25.7	11.5	48.8	6.5
Honey Roasted, Average	1oz/28g	169	13.2	605	26.9	23.6	47.1	5.5
Plain, Average	10 Whole/10g	59	5.0	592	24.7	11.0	50.0	6.3
Roast, Salted, Average	10 Nuts/12g	74	6.3	614	27.8	7.9	52.4	4.9
Salted, Average	10 Peanuts/6g	37	3.1	609	27.0	8.3	52.1	5.4

	Measure INFO/WEIGHT	per Measure KCAL	FAT	Nutrition Values per 100g / 100ml KCAL	PROT	CARB	FAT	FIBRE
PEARL BARLEY								
Boiled	1oz/28g	34	0.2	120	2.7	27.6	0.6	0.0
Raw, Average	1oz/28g	99	0.3	352	9.9	77.7	1.2	15.6
PEARS								
Abate Fetel, Average	1 Pear/133g	48	0.1	36	0.4	8.3	0.1	2.2
Asian, Nashi, Raw, Average	1 Lge/209g	88	0.5	42	0.5	10.7	0.2	3.6
Comice, Raw, Weighed with Core	1 Med/170g	56	0.0	33	0.3	8.5	0.0	2.0
Conference, Average	1 Lge/209g	102	0.4	49	0.3	11.6	0.2	2.3
Dried, Average	1 Pear Half/16g	33	0.1	204	1.9	48.4	0.5	9.7
in Fruit Juice, Average	1 Serving/225g	102	0.1	45	0.3	10.9	0.0	1.2
in Syrup, Average	1oz/28g	16	0.0	58	0.3	14.4	0.1	1.4
Prickly, Raw, Fresh	1oz/28g	14	0.1	49	0.7	11.5	0.3	0.0
Raw, Weighed with Core, Average	1 Lge/209g	78	0.2	38	0.3	9.1	0.1	1.4
William, Raw, Average	1 Med/170g	58	0.2	34	0.4	8.3	0.1	2.2
PEAS								
Dried, Boiled in Unsalted Water, Average	1oz/28g	31	0.2	109	6.9	19.9	0.8	5.5
Dried, Raw, Average	1oz/28g	85	0.7	303	21.6	52.0	2.4	13.0
Frozen, Average	1 Serving/85g	55	0.7	64	5.4	9.0	0.8	4.9
Frozen, Boiled, Average	1 Serving/75g	51	0.7	68	6.0	9.4	0.9	5.1
Garden, Canned, No Sugar Or Salt, Average	1 Can/80g	36	0.3	45	4.4	6.0	0.4	2.8
Garden, Canned, with Sugar & Salt, Average	1 Serving/90g	59	0.6	66	5.3	9.3	0.7	5.1
Garden, Frozen, Average	1 Serving/90g	66	1.0	74	6.3	9.8	1.1	3.3
Garden, Minted, Average	1 Serving/113g	84	1.2	74	6.3	9.7	1.1	5.9
Hand Shelled, & Baby Leeks, Sainsbury's*	1 Serving/120g	59	1.4	49	4.0	5.8	1.2	3.3
Marrowfat, Average	1 Sm Can/160g	140	0.9	88	6.4	14.3	0.6	3.9
Mushy, Average	1 Can/200g	173	1.0	86	6.2	14.4	0.5	2.2
Processed, Canned, Average	1 Sm Can/220g	176	1.8	80	6.1	12.3	0.8	3.7
Sugar Snap, Average	1oz/28g	10	0.1	34	3.3	4.9	0.2	1.4
PEASE PUDDING								
Canned, Re-Heated, Drained	1oz/28g	26	0.2	93	6.8	16.1	0.6	1.8
PECAN NUTS								
Average	3 Nuts/18g	125	12.6	693	10.1	5.7	70.1	4.7
PECORINO ROMANO								
Tesco*	1 Serving/100g	366	28.0	366	28.5	0.0	28.0	0.0
PENNE								
Arrabbiata, BGTY, Sainsbury's*	1 Pack/450g	414	7.2	92	2.9	16.5	1.6	1.9
Chicken & Red Wine, Italiana, Weight Watchers*	1 Pack/395g	249	2.8	63	3.7	10.1	0.7	0.6
Chicken & Tomato, Italian, Sainsbury's*	½ Pack/350g	473	11.2	135	7.6	19.0	3.2	1.6
Chilli & Garlic, Asda*	1 Serving/75g	260	1.1	346	12.0	71.0	1.5	3.0
Cooked, Average	1 Serving/185g	244	1.3	132	4.7	26.7	0.7	1.1
Corn, Free From, Dry Weight, Sainsbury's*	1 Serving/100g	348	2.3	348	7.6	74.2	2.3	5.2
Creamy Sun Dried Tomato & Mascarpone, Somerfield*	1 Pack/500g	775	30.0	155	5.0	21.0	6.0	0.0
Dry, Average	1 Serving/100g	352	1.9	352	12.4	71.3	1.9	2.7
Dry, Trufree*	1 Serving/75g	263	1.5	350	8.0	75.0	2.0	0.0
Egg, Fresh, Average	1 Serving/125g	353	4.0	282	11.1	52.2	3.2	2.0
Free From, Tesco*	1 Serving/100g	340	2.0	340	8.0	72.5	2.0	2.5
Fresh, Dry, Average	1 Serving/125g	223	2.4	178	7.3	32.2	1.9	1.6
Hickory Steak, American, Sainsbury's*	1 Pack/450g	545	8.1	121	6.5	19.8	1.8	1.5
Hickory Steak, COU, M & S*	1 Pack/400g	320	4.0	80	5.6	11.9	1.0	1.3
Hickory Steak, M & S*	1 Pack/400g	540	12.4	135	6.9	19.3	3.1	1.3
in Tomato & Basil Sauce, Sainsbury's*	½ Pack/110g	118	0.7	107	3.6	21.8	0.6	1.1
Leek & Bacon, Al Forno, Asda*	½ Pack/300g	531	39.0	177	5.0	10.0	13.0	0.5
Mozzarella, Safeway*	1 Serving/400g	480	15.2	120	5.2	16.3	3.8	1.5
Napoletana Chicken, BFY, Morrisons*	1 Pack/350g	252	5.6	72	6.4	7.2	1.6	0.2

P

	Measure INFO/WEIGHT	per Measure KCAL	FAT	Nutrition Values per 100g / 100ml KCAL	PROT	CARB	FAT	FIBRE
PENNE								
Organic, Dry, Average	1 Serving/100g	352	1.8	352	12.4	71.6	1.8	1.9
Rigate, Dry Weight, Average	1 Serving/90g	318	1.6	353	12.3	72.1	1.8	1.8
Roasted Red Pepper, GFY, Asda*	1 Pack/400g	212	2.4	53	1.9	10.0	0.6	0.8
Tomato & Basil Sauce, Asda*	½ Pack/314g	185	11.0	59	0.8	6.0	3.5	2.0
Tomato & Vegetable, Heinz*	1 Serving/300g	135	1.8	45	1.7	8.3	0.6	0.7
Tuna, Tomato & Olive, Asda*	1 Pack/340g	173	6.5	51	4.2	4.2	1.9	0.6
with Chicken & Vegetables, Eat Positive, Birds Eye*	1 Meal/396.3g	325	5.2	82	7.7	9.8	1.3	1.2
with Chilli & Red Peppers, Asda*	1 Can/400g	224	4.8	56	1.3	10.0	1.2	0.6
with Roasted Vegetables, Waitrose*	1 Pack/400g	424	15.6	106	2.8	15.0	3.9	0.8
PENNETTE								
Tricolore, Sainsbury's*	1 Serving/100g	357	1.7	357	12.3	73.1	1.7	2.5
PEPERAMI*								
Firestick, Peperami*	1 Stick/25g	127	11.0	508	24.5	3.5	44.0	1.2
Hot, Peperami*	1oz/28g	156	14.6	556	19.2	2.4	52.0	1.2
Mini, 30% Less Fat, Peperami*	1 Stick/10g	38	3.0	379	25.0	1.5	30.0	3.0
Original, Peperami*	1oz/28g	150	13.7	536	22.0	1.7	49.0	0.1
PEPPER								
Black, Freshly Groound, Average	1 Tsp/2g	5.1	0.1	255	11.0	64.8	3.3	26.5
Cayenne, Ground	1 Tsp/1.8g	6	0.3	318	12.0	31.7	17.3	0.0
PEPPERONATA								
Salmon, BGTY, Sainsbury's*	1 Pack/380g	300	8.7	79	5.8	8.8	2.3	0.9
PEPPERS								
Capsicum, Green, Boiled in Salted Water	1oz/28g	5	0.1	18	1.0	2.6	0.5	1.8
Capsicum, Green, Raw, Unprepared, Average	1 Med/160g	24	0.5	15	0.8	2.6	0.3	1.6
Capsicum, Red, Boiled in Salted Water	1oz/28g	10	0.1	34	1.1	7.0	0.4	1.7
Capsicum, Red, Raw, Unprepared, Average	1 Med/160g	51	0.6	32	1.0	6.4	0.4	1.6
Capsicum, Sweet, Raw, Average	1 Serving/100g	16	0.3	16	0.8	2.6	0.3	1.6
Capsicum, Yellow, Raw, Unprepared, Average	1 Med/160g	42	0.3	26	1.2	5.3	0.2	1.7
Chilli, Green, Very Lazy, EPC*	1 Serving/10g	11	0.4	114	4.2	15.3	4.0	0.5
Chilli, Mixed, Raw, Tesco*	1 Chili/13g	3	0.0	27	1.8	4.2	0.3	1.6
Flame Seared, with Greek Feta, M & S*	½ Tub/85g	106	8.2	125	3.6	5.4	9.7	1.8
Italian Style, Sainsbury's*	1 Serving/150g	161	7.5	107	3.5	14.1	5.0	2.1
Jalapeno, Co-Op*	1oz/28g	74	3.6	265	5.0	31.0	13.0	0.9
Jalapeno, Flamin' Hot, Kitchen Range Foods*	1oz/28g	62	3.6	223	4.6	22.9	12.7	0.0
Mixed Bag, From Supermarket, Average	1oz/28g	7	0.1	25	1.0	4.5	0.4	1.7
Pickled, Hot, Turkish, Melis	1 Serving/25g	9	0.0	35	1.0	7.9	0.0	1.0
Ramiro, Red, Sainsbury's*	1 Pepper/100g	30	0.3	30	1.6	5.1	0.3	2.2
Red, Filled, Halves, Vegetarian, M & S*	½ Pack/145g	116	4.8	80	2.8	12.1	3.3	1.8
Red, Filled with Feta, COU, M & S*	1 Pepper/153.8g	200	11.1	130	4.1	12.4	7.2	0.6
Roasted Red & Yellow, in Oil, M & S*	1 Serving/100g	57	4.6	57	0.8	3.0	4.6	2.8
PERNOD*								
19% Volume, Pernod*	1 Pub Shot/35ml	46	0.0	130	0.0	0.0	0.0	0.0
PESTO								
Black Olive, Sacla*	1oz/28g	115	11.8	409	2.9	4.3	42.2	0.0
Chargrilled Aubergine, Sacla*	1 Serving/30g	102	10.5	339	2.4	3.8	34.9	0.0
Coriander, Sacla*	1 Tsp/10g	42	4.3	415	4.4	1.6	43.4	2.2
Green, Alla Genovese, Finest, Tesco*	1 Serving/65g	189	25.7	290	5.7	1.5	39.6	2.8
Green, Asda*	2 Dtsp/25g	94	9.8	374	5.0	0.8	39.0	5.0
Green, Classic, Sacla*	1 Serving/40g	185	18.6	462	5.2	7.6	46.5	0.0
Green, Verde, Bertolli*	¼ Jar/46.25g	270	28.0	575	5.7	4.3	59.5	0.0
Red, Fresh, Sainsbury's*	1 Pack/150g	702	66.8	468	7.2	9.6	44.5	0.8
Red, Rosso, Bertolli*	1 Jar/185g	703	64.8	380	6.8	9.5	35.0	2.0
Red, Sainsbury's*	1 Jar/190g	671	64.6	353	4.8	7.0	34.0	1.6

P

	Measure INFO/WEIGHT	per Measure KCAL	FAT	Nutrition Values per 100g / 100ml KCAL	PROT	CARB	FAT	FIBRE
PESTO								
Roasted Red Pepper, Sacla*	1 Serving/30g	72	6.8	241	4.3	4.6	22.8	5.3
Sun Dried Tomato, Sacla*	1 Serving/10g	29	2.8	289	4.2	5.2	27.9	0.0
Tomato, Organic, Sacla*	1 Serving/30g	95	9.5	317	3.9	4.3	31.6	0.0
Wild Rocket, Sacla*	1 Serving/30g	128	13.1	425	5.2	3.2	43.5	4.5
PETIT POIS								
& Baby Carrots, Safeway*	1 Can/138g	57	0.0	41	2.5	7.4	0.0	1.0
Average	1 Serving/65g	34	0.5	53	5.0	6.8	0.7	3.5
Freshly Frozen, Boiled, Asda*	1 Serving/50g	25	0.5	49	5.0	5.5	0.9	4.5
Frozen, M & S*	1 Serving/80g	56	0.7	70	5.0	5.5	0.9	4.5
PHEASANT								
Meat Only, Roasted	1oz/28g	62	3.4	220	27.9	0.0	12.0	0.0
Meat Only, Roasted, Weighed with Bone	1oz/28g	32	1.7	114	14.5	0.0	6.2	0.0
Stuffed, Easy Carve, Finest, Tesco*	1 Serving/200g	540	37.4	270	23.2	2.2	18.7	0.9
PICCALILLI								
Haywards*	1 Serving/28g	18	0.1	66	1.4	13.9	0.5	0.0
Heinz*	1 Serving/10g	11	0.1	107	1.7	21.6	0.7	0.6
M & S*	1 Serving/25g	29	0.4	115	1.3	23.9	1.4	1.4
Sainsbury's*	1 Dtsp/15g	9	0.1	60	1.8	11.9	0.6	0.7
Sandwich, Tesco*	1 Serving/20g	16	0.0	80	0.4	18.5	0.0	1.6
Sweet, Asda*	1 Tbsp/15g	17	0.0	112	0.5	27.0	0.2	0.6
Tesco*	1 Serving/50g	51	1.8	102	0.5	17.8	3.6	2.0
Three Mustard, Finest, Tesco*	1 Serving/30g	40	0.2	134	1.3	30.7	0.7	1.0
PICKLE								
Branston, Crosse & Blackwell*	1 Tsp/10g	11	0.0	109	0.8	26.1	0.2	1.1
Brinjal, Patak's*	1 Tsp/16g	59	3.9	367	2.2	34.6	24.4	0.9
Chilli, Branston*	1 Tsp/16g	21	0.1	130	0.7	30.0	0.7	1.5
Chilli, Patak's*	1 Tsp/16g	52	5.4	325	4.3	1.3	33.7	0.0
Dill, Cucumbers, Safeway*	1oz/28g	5	0.1	19	0.9	3.5	0.2	0.0
Garlic, Patak's*	1 Tsp/16g	42	3.0	261	3.6	20.0	18.5	1.6
Lime, Hot, Asda*	1 Dtsp/10g	12	1.0	123	2.2	6.0	10.0	1.0
Lime, Hot, Patak's*	1 Tsp/16g	31	3.0	194	2.2	4.0	18.7	0.4
Lime, Oily	1oz/28g	50	4.3	178	1.9	8.3	15.5	0.0
Lime, Sharwood's*	1 Tsp/16g	24	1.5	152	2.2	15.0	9.3	2.9
Mango, Hot, Patak's*	1 Tsp/16g	43	4.1	270	2.3	7.4	25.7	1.9
Mild Mustard, Heinz*	1 Tbsp/10g	13	0.1	129	2.2	25.7	1.3	0.9
Mixed, Haywards*	½ Jar/120g	22	0.4	18	1.4	2.4	0.3	0.0
Mixed, Patak's*	1 Serving/30g	78	7.7	259	2.3	4.7	25.7	0.8
Sandwich, Branston*	1 Tsp/10g	14	0.0	140	0.7	34.2	0.3	1.3
Sandwich, Tesco*	1 Serving/5g	7	0.0	138	1.0	33.1	0.2	1.0
Small Chunk, Branston*	1 Serving/20g	22	0.0	109	0.8	26.1	0.2	1.1
Smooth, Branston*	1 Serving/20g	25	0.0	125	0.9	29.8	0.2	1.1
Spicy, Branston*	1 Heaped Tsp/15g	21	0.0	140	0.7	34.7	0.3	1.3
Sweet	1 Tsp/10g	14	0.0	141	0.6	36.0	0.1	1.2
Sweet, Branston*	1 Serving/30g	33	0.1	109	0.8	26.1	0.2	1.1
Sweet, Country, Morrisons*	1 Tbsp/15g	20	0.0	130	0.9	31.1	0.2	0.0
Sweet, Low Price, Sainsbury's*	1 Serving/23g	23	0.1	98	0.7	23.2	0.3	0.7
Sweet, Value, Tesco*	1 Serving/10g	10	0.0	96	0.6	23.0	0.2	0.7
Tomato, Tangy, Heinz*	1 Tsp/10g	10	0.0	102	2.0	22.0	0.3	1.5
PICKLES								
Cornichons, in Sweet & Sour Vinegar, Waitrose*	1 Serving/10g	3	0.0	28	0.6	6.1	0.1	0.6
Mixed, Salad Bar, Asda*	1oz/28g	11	0.0	40	0.5	9.2	0.1	0.0
PICNIC								
Cadbury*	1 Bar/48g	228	11.3	475	7.5	58.3	23.6	0.0

PIE

	Measure INFO/WEIGHT	per Measure KCAL	FAT	Nutrition Values per 100g / 100ml KCAL	PROT	CARB	FAT	FIBRE
Admiral, Frozen, Youngs*	1 Pie/340g	357	16.7	105	4.6	10.7	4.9	0.7
Admiral's, Ross*	1 Pie/340g	357	15.6	105	4.8	10.9	4.6	0.7
Apple, & Blackberry, Fruit, Finest, Tesco*	1 Pie/95g	265	11.3	279	13.7	29.3	11.9	2.8
Apple, American, Iceland*	1 Portion/92g	258	10.7	280	4.8	39.2	11.6	2.2
Apple, Asda*	¼ Pack/106.7g	288	11.8	269	3.6	39.0	11.0	1.7
Apple, Bramley, Aunt Bessie's*	¼ Pie/138g	351	15.1	255	2.8	36.2	11.0	1.2
Apple, Bramley, Free From, Tesco*	1 Pie/60g	185	5.2	309	2.5	55.4	8.6	1.4
Apple, Bramley, Individual, Sainsbury's*	1 Pie/53.7g	166	5.0	307	3.6	52.2	9.3	1.3
Apple, Bramley, Individual, Tesco*	1 Pie/61g	210	7.9	344	3.4	53.1	13.0	1.5
Apple, Bramley, Large, Tesco*	1/8 Slice/87g	311	13.1	358	3.9	51.9	15.0	1.9
Apple, Bramley, Tesco*	1 Serving/106g	284	11.6	268	3.6	38.8	10.9	1.7
Apple, Deep Filled, Iceland*	1 Portion/116g	332	15.3	286	2.5	39.2	13.2	1.1
Apple, Deep Filled, Sainsbury's*	¼ Pie/137g	374	17.5	273	3.8	35.6	12.8	1.6
Apple, Family, Asda*	1/6 Pie/118.5g	314	13.0	265	3.6	38.0	11.0	2.9
Apple, Family, Morrisons*	1/6 Pie/116g	326	14.0	281	3.1	39.9	12.1	3.1
Apple, Individual, Somerfield*	1 Pie/47.2g	178	7.9	379	3.5	53.2	16.9	1.3
Apple, Lattice, Tesco*	1 Serving/145g	325	13.3	224	2.2	33.2	9.2	1.4
Apple, McVitie's*	1 Slice/117g	316	12.9	270	3.0	39.0	11.0	2.0
Apple, Pastry Top & Bottom	1oz/28g	74	3.7	266	2.9	35.8	13.3	1.7
Apple, Puff Pastry, M & S*	1 Pie/135g	338	17.1	250	2.4	31.3	12.7	1.0
Apple, Ready to Bake, TTD, Sainsbury's*	1/6 Pie/125g	353	16.1	282	3.2	38.2	12.9	0.7
Apple, Sainsbury's*	1/6/118g	314	13.6	266	3.4	37.1	11.5	0.6
Apple, SmartPrice, Asda*	1 Serving/47g	178	8.0	379	3.5	53.0	17.0	1.3
Apple, Tesco*	1 Pie/47g	191	8.1	406	3.3	59.4	17.2	1.5
Apple, Value, Tesco*	1 Pie/47g	133	6.8	284	4.0	34.3	14.5	0.9
Apple & Blackberry, Co-Op*	1 Serving/138g	338	15.2	245	3.0	33.0	11.0	2.0
Apple & Blackberry, Lattice Topped, BGTY, Sainsbury's*	¼ Serving/100g	256	7.5	256	2.8	44.4	7.5	3.1
Apple & Blackberry, Shortcrust, M & S*	1 Serving/142g	469	17.8	330	4.3	50.2	12.5	1.1
Apple & Blackberry, Tesco*	1 Serving/106g	287	11.9	271	4.2	38.4	11.2	1.7
Apple & Blackcurrant, Mr Kipling*	1 Pie/66g	211	8.4	320	3.3	47.9	12.8	1.2
Apricot Fruit, GFY, Asda*	1 Serving/52g	162	5.2	311	3.3	52.0	10.0	0.0
Banoffee, Individual, Sainsbury's*	1 Pie/104g	365	21.0	351	3.2	39.2	20.2	2.2
Banoffee, Tesco*	1/6 Pie/93.3g	365	19.7	390	3.9	45.8	21.1	1.5
Banoffee Cream, American Dream, Heinz*	1/6 Pie/70g	239	15.0	342	3.7	33.7	21.4	3.9
Beef, Lean, BGTY, Sainsbury's*	1 Serving/212g	280	12.7	132	7.3	12.2	6.0	1.5
Beef, Minced, Aberdeen Angus, Shortcrust, M & S*	1 Pie/170.6g	435	26.6	255	9.3	19.3	15.6	3.0
Beef, Sainsbury's*	1 Pie/209.8g	536	30.0	255	10.3	21.2	14.3	2.0
Beef & Vegetable, Macdougalls, McDougalls*	¼ Pie/114g	292	19.3	256	5.3	20.6	16.9	0.3
Beef Steak, Aberdeen Angus, Top Crust, Waitrose*	½ Pie/280g	476	24.1	170	10.0	13.4	8.6	4.1
Blackcurrant, Deep Filled, Sainsbury's*	1 Slice/137g	440	19.3	321	5.8	42.6	14.1	2.2
Bramley Apple, Co-Op*	1 Slice/68g	177	7.5	260	4.0	36.0	11.0	3.0
Bramley Apple, Deep Filled, Sainsbury's*	1/6 Pie/120g	329	14.3	274	3.7	38.0	11.9	1.9
Bramley Apple, Individual, Mr Kipling*	1 Pie/66g	228	8.6	346	3.4	53.8	13.0	1.4
Bramley Apple, M & S*	1 Pie/55g	184	6.4	335	2.9	57.6	11.7	1.6
Bramley Apple, Somerfield*	1/6 Pie/70.2g	193	9.0	275	3.5	34.0	12.8	2.4
Bramley Apple & Blackberry, M & S*	¼ Pie/146g	380	14.5	260	3.4	39.8	9.9	1.3
Bramley Apple & Custard, Lattice Topped, Mr Kipling*	1 Pie/64g	236	9.9	369	3.8	53.7	15.4	1.1
Cheese & Onion, Hollands*	1 Pie/200g	516	24.4	258	6.3	30.9	12.2	0.0
Cheese & Potato	1oz/28g	39	2.3	139	4.8	12.6	8.1	0.7
Cheese & Potato, Aunt Bessie's*	¼ Portion/200g	288	18.8	144	4.6	11.7	9.4	1.5
Cherry, Asda*	1/6 Pie/116.7g	337	14.5	289	3.1	41.2	12.4	1.8
Cherry, Deep Filled, Somerfield*	1/6 Pie/90g	259	10.8	288	3.0	41.0	12.0	0.0
Cherry, Sainsbury's*	1 Serving/117g	325	13.6	278	3.9	39.6	11.6	1.7

P

PIE

INFO/WEIGHT	Measure		per Measure		Nutrition Values per 100g / 100ml				
			KCAL	FAT	KCAL	PROT	CARB	FAT	FIBRE
Cherry, Shortcrust, M & S*	¼ Pie/135.6g		305	3.3	225	3.3	47.3	2.4	2.9
Cherry, Tesco*	1 Serving/106g		294	12.7	277	4.0	38.3	12.0	1.8
Chicken, Aunt Bessie's*	¼ Pie/200g		474	24.2	237	10.6	21.4	12.1	2.1
Chicken, Bacon & Cheddar Cheese, Lattice, Birds Eye*	1 Lattice/157g		460	27.2	293	13.4	21.0	17.3	1.5
Chicken, Broccoli & White Wine, Waitrose*	1 Serving/200g		605	40.5	303	12.6	17.7	20.3	2.3
Chicken, Cheese & Bacon, HL, Tesco*	1 Pack/450g		383	9.9	85	5.9	9.4	2.2	1.6
Chicken, Cheese & Broccoli Lattice, Birds Eye*	1 Lattice/134g		385	21.8	288	12.6	22.7	16.3	1.1
Chicken, Cheese & Leek Lattice, Sun Valley*	1 Lattice/125g		315	21.9	252	15.2	8.6	17.5	1.0
Chicken, Cottage, Frozen, Tesco*	1 Pack/450g		293	2.3	65	2.8	11.7	0.5	1.0
Chicken, Deep Filled, Puff Pastry, Sainsbury's*	1 Pie/210g		538	31.9	256	10.0	19.9	15.2	3.1
Chicken, Eat Smart, Safeway*	1 Pack/400g		340	6.8	85	8.2	9.0	1.7	1.2
Chicken, Finest, Tesco*	1 Pie/250g		615	32.3	246	10.7	21.9	12.9	1.2
Chicken, Individual, Made with 100% Breast, Birds Eye*	1 Pie/153.7g		455	28.1	296	7.9	25.0	18.3	1.0
Chicken, Individual Shortcrust, Asda*	1 Pie/175g		534	29.8	305	10.0	28.0	17.0	1.0
Chicken, Leek & Ham, Morrisons*	1 Serving/113g		305	16.6	270	8.8	25.7	14.7	1.1
Chicken, Newgate*	1 Pie/142g		358	23.6	252	6.1	23.1	16.6	1.0
Chicken, Puff Pastry, Tesco*	¼ Pie/114g		250	12.7	220	8.6	21.3	11.2	1.4
Chicken, Roast, Puff Pastry, Deep Fill, Asda*	½ Pie/259g		739	44.1	285	10.0	23.0	17.0	0.8
Chicken, Short Crust, M & S*	1 Pie/170g		510	29.6	300	9.7	26.2	17.4	1.7
Chicken, Tomato & Basil Lattice, Birds Eye*	1 Serving/155g		340	19.6	220	10.8	15.7	12.7	1.4
Chicken & Asparagus, Lattice, Waitrose*	1 Serving/100g		295	19.6	295	7.4	22.3	19.6	1.8
Chicken & Asparagus, McDougalls*	1 Serving/170g		394	21.9	232	7.4	21.6	12.9	1.5
Chicken & Asparagus, Puff Pasty, John Bullers*	1 Pie/174g		477	29.6	274	11.0	19.0	17.0	2.0
Chicken & Asparagus, Tesco*	1 Serving/170g		468	28.7	275	8.3	22.4	16.9	0.8
Chicken & Bacon, Filo Pastry, Finest, Tesco*	1 Serving/160g		362	18.7	226	11.3	18.9	11.7	1.7
Chicken & Bacon, Puff Pastry, Deep Fill, Sainsbury's*	1/3 Pie/200g		532	34.0	266	9.1	19.1	17.0	1.3
Chicken & Bacon, with Cheese Sauce, Tesco*	1 Serving/200g		540	33.6	270	12.0	17.6	16.8	0.8
Chicken & Basil, M & S*	1oz/28g		59	3.3	210	8.9	17.0	11.9	1.1
Chicken & Broccoli, BGTY, Sainsbury's*	1 Pack/450g		297	3.6	66	5.9	8.9	0.8	1.8
Chicken & Broccoli, COU, M & S*	1 Serving/320g		272	6.1	85	8.1	8.8	1.9	1.3
Chicken & Broccoli, Eat Smart, Safeway*	1 Pack/400g		320	8.0	80	6.9	8.5	2.0	1.2
Chicken & Broccoli, Good Intentions, Somerfield*	1 Pack/450g		383	8.1	85	6.8	10.5	1.8	0.5
Chicken & Broccoli, Lattice, Tesco*	½ Pie/200g		496	30.8	248	8.5	18.9	15.4	2.1
Chicken & Broccoli Lattice, Sainsbury's*	½ Pie/192g		520	30.7	271	9.3	22.4	16.0	0.9
Chicken & Broccoli Potato, Top, Asda*	1 Pack/400g		319	7.0	80	5.3	10.8	1.8	0.7
Chicken & Gravy, Deep Fill, Asda*	1 Serving/130g		371	22.1	285	10.0	23.0	17.0	0.8
Chicken & Gravy, HL, Tesco*	1 Serving/450g		338	6.3	75	6.2	9.1	1.4	1.8
Chicken & Gravy, Puff Pastry, Deep Fill, Sainsbury's*	1 Pie/250g		575	30.8	230	9.1	20.9	12.3	1.9
Chicken & Gravy, Shortcrust Pastry, Large, Tesco*	1 Pie/600g		1578	91.2	263	8.2	23.4	15.2	1.0
Chicken & Gravy, Shortcrust Pastry, Sainsbury's*	1 Serving/250g		638	35.3	255	8.0	24.1	14.1	1.0
Chicken & Gravy, Shortcrust Pastry, Tesco*	1 Pie/250g		618	34.5	247	6.8	23.9	13.8	1.0
Chicken & Ham, Deep Filled, Sainsbury's*	1 Pie/210g		594	37.2	283	8.0	23.0	17.7	1.0
Chicken & Ham, Deep Filled, Somerfield*	¼ Pie/138g		348	19.3	252	11.0	21.0	14.0	0.0
Chicken & Ham, Morrisons*	¼ Pie/115.1g		267	13.7	232	8.7	22.5	11.9	0.8
Chicken & Ham, Safeway*	1 Pie/134.7g		385	23.5	285	9.2	23.0	17.4	1.3
Chicken & Ham, Sainsbury's*	1 Pie/128g		461	28.7	360	11.0	28.5	22.4	2.0
Chicken & Ham, Tesco*	1 Serving/113g		293	17.6	259	9.4	20.2	15.6	1.2
Chicken & Leek, Deep Filled, Puff Pastry, Sainsbury's*	1/3 Pie/451g		1109	65.4	246	10.1	18.7	14.5	1.5
Chicken & Leek, M & S*	1oz/28g		70	4.2	250	10.1	18.8	15.1	1.1
Chicken & Mushroom, Asda*	1 Pie/ 150g		384	24.0	256	9.0	19.0	16.0	1.0
Chicken & Mushroom, Co-Op*	1 Pie/150g		443	27.0	295	8.0	27.0	18.0	0.8
Chicken & Mushroom, Deep Filled, Frozen, Tesco*	¼ Pie/197.9g		465	22.2	235	9.0	23.8	11.2	1.2
Chicken & Mushroom, Farmfoods*	1 Pie/110g		271	16.4	246	5.6	22.4	14.9	0.9

	Measure INFO/WEIGHT	per Measure KCAL	FAT	Nutrition Values per 100g / 100ml KCAL	PROT	CARB	FAT	FIBRE
PIE								
Chicken & Mushroom, Favourites, Morrisons*	¼ Pie/352g	989	61.2	281	7.2	23.8	17.4	0.9
Chicken & Mushroom, Finest, Tesco*	1 Pie/250g	743	46.8	297	9.3	21.1	18.7	0.9
Chicken & Mushroom, Fray Bentos*	1 Pie/425g	684	40.4	161	6.7	11.5	9.5	0.0
Chicken & Mushroom, Individual, Co-Op*	1 Pie/149g	465	29.7	312	8.6	24.5	19.9	1.2
Chicken & Mushroom, Individual, Frozen, Tesco*	1 Pie/150g	368	18.9	245	8.9	23.5	12.6	1.2
Chicken & Mushroom, Luxury, M & S*	½ Pie/275g	880	61.9	320	9.9	20.0	22.5	1.0
Chicken & Mushroom, Morrisons*	1 Serving/100g	261	15.4	261	7.6	22.9	15.4	0.9
Chicken & Mushroom, Puff Pastry, Birds Eye*	1 Pie/152.0g	415	21.3	273	11.9	24.9	14.0	1.6
Chicken & Mushroom, Puff Pastry, Sainsbury's*	1 Pie/150g	450	25.1	300	7.8	29.6	16.7	0.9
Chicken & Mushroom, Shortcrust, Somerfield*	¼ Pie/125g	410	28.4	328	6.2	24.7	22.7	1.2
Chicken & Vegetable, Asda*	1 Pie/138.2g	380	19.2	275	9.6	27.9	13.9	2.2
Chicken & Vegetable, Farmfoods*	1 Pie/128g	384	24.1	300	7.2	25.4	18.8	1.4
Chicken & Vegetable, Freshbake*	1 Pie/125g	319	19.6	255	6.5	21.8	15.7	2.7
Chicken & Vegetable, Individual, Somerfield*	1 Pie/142g	382	22.0	269	7.6	24.8	15.5	1.3
Chicken & Vegetable, Kids, Tesco*	1 Serving/235g	235	10.6	100	5.9	9.1	4.5	0.7
Chicken & Vegetable, Microbake, Freshbake*	1 Pie/100g	348	16.1	348	10.2	40.8	16.1	1.8
Chicken & Vegetable, PB, Waitrose*	1 Serving/375g	285	5.3	76	5.1	10.8	1.4	1.3
Chicken & Vegetable, Potato Topped, Somerfield*	1 Pack/350g	270	10.5	77	3.7	8.8	3.0	2.0
Chicken & Vegetable, Value, Tesco*	1 Pie/150g	378	22.1	252	8.0	21.9	14.7	1.3
Chicken & Wiltshire Ham, Finest, Tesco*	1 Pie/220g	605	32.8	275	11.6	22.7	14.9	1.1
Chicken Curry, Iceland*	1 Pie/156g	440	23.7	282	10.2	26.2	15.2	2.0
Chocolate, Mini, Waitrose*	1 Pie/24.0g	109	6.1	455	5.3	51.4	25.3	1.7
Cod & Prawn, M & S*	1oz/28g	43	2.5	155	10.6	8.7	8.9	0.7
Cod & Smoked Haddock, COU, M & S*	1 Serving/300g	240	7.2	80	6.1	9.0	2.4	1.2
Cottage, Aberdeen Angus, Waitrose*	1 Pie/350g	340	12.3	97	5.3	11.0	3.5	0.9
Cottage, Aldi*	1 Pack/440g	484	27.3	110	4.1	9.5	6.2	0.2
Cottage, Asda*	1 Pie/300g	324	12.6	108	7.0	9.0	4.2	0.7
Cottage, Aunt Bessie's*	1 Pack/350g	413	18.2	118	4.8	12.1	5.2	1.0
Cottage, British Pies, Chilled, Tesco*	1 Pack/500g	450	14.0	90	4.6	10.3	2.8	1.5
Cottage, Budgens*	1 Pie/400g	404	18.0	101	5.6	9.6	4.5	1.0
Cottage, Chilled, HL, Tesco*	1 Pack/500g	475	13.0	95	5.6	11.5	2.6	1.0
Cottage, Classic British, Sainsbury's*	1 Pack/450g	500	20.7	111	6.3	11.1	4.6	0.6
Cottage, Classics, Asda*	½ Pack/450g	531	27.0	118	7.0	9.0	6.0	1.0
Cottage, Fresh, M & S*	1 Pie/400g	460	22.4	115	6.8	9.9	5.6	0.6
Cottage, Frozen, Asda*	1 Serving/121g	146	7.3	121	4.8	12.0	6.0	0.6
Cottage, GFY, Asda*	1 Pack/400g	312	5.2	78	6.0	10.5	1.3	0.5
Cottage, HL, Co-Op*	1 Pack/400g	320	6.4	80	5.0	11.0	1.6	2.0
Cottage, Iceland*	1 Pack/400g	468	18.8	117	5.1	13.6	4.7	0.7
Cottage, Individual, SmartPrice, Asda*	1 Pie/159g	149	5.9	94	3.1	12.0	3.7	0.7
Cottage, Luxury, M & S*	½ Pack/310g	403	21.7	130	7.9	8.3	7.0	1.8
Cottage, Mini Classics, Morrisons*	1 Pack/300g	220	7.8	73	4.4	8.2	2.6	2.3
Cottage, Ross*	1 Pack/320g	240	7.0	75	3.0	10.9	2.2	0.3
Cottage, Safeway*	1 Serving/400g	1000	17.2	250	13.6	38.8	4.3	7.8
Cottage, Sainsbury's*	1 Pack/300g	297	10.2	99	6.4	10.7	3.4	1.1
Cottage, Simply Value, Somerfield*	1 Pack/300g	198	3.9	66	3.9	9.7	1.3	1.6
Cottage, Vegetarian, Sainsbury's*	1 Pack/450g	329	9.9	73	3.0	10.2	2.2	1.8
Cottage, Vegetarian, Tesco*	1 Pack/450g	345	13.4	77	3.6	8.9	3.0	1.9
Cottage, Weight Watchers*	1 Pack/320g	230	3.8	72	3.8	11.3	1.2	1.6
Cottage Meal for One, M & S*	1 Pack/437.5g	350	15.8	80	5.4	6.2	3.6	1.7
Country, Vegetarian, Tesco*	1 Pie/142g	381	21.6	268	5.6	27.3	15.2	1.2
Cumberland, Beef, HL, Tesco*	1 Pack/500g	460	13.5	92	5.0	11.8	2.7	0.9
Cumberland, BGTY, Sainsbury's*	1 Pack/450g	360	9.0	80	5.3	10.1	2.0	1.6
Cumberland, British Pies, Tesco*	1 Pack/400g	470	24.4	118	3.9	11.6	6.1	0.8

PIE

	Measure INFO/WEIGHT	per Measure KCAL	FAT	Nutrition Values per 100g / 100ml KCAL	PROT	CARB	FAT	FIBRE
Cumberland, Fish, HL, Tesco*	1 Pack/450g	428	12.2	95	5.6	11.0	2.7	1.3
Cumberland, GFY, Asda*	1 Pack/450.7g	469	9.9	104	11.4	11.4	2.2	2.1
Cumberland, HL, Tesco*	1 Pie/500g	430	13.5	86	4.5	10.8	2.7	1.2
Cumberland, M & S*	1 Pie/195g	312	20.3	160	6.9	10.1	10.4	1.1
Cumberland, Safeway*	1 Pie/450g	608	32.4	135	5.9	11.4	7.2	1.3
Fish	1 Serving/250g	263	7.5	105	8.0	12.3	3.0	0.7
Fish, Asda*	1 Pack/338g	426	20.3	126	5.0	13.0	6.0	1.1
Fish, BFY, Morrisons*	1 Pack/350g	301	10.2	86	5.0	10.0	2.9	0.9
Fish, Co-Op*	1 Pack/400g	380	16.0	95	4.0	12.0	4.0	0.9
Fish, Creamy, Finest, Tesco*	½ /342.9g	480	31.2	140	8.6	5.1	9.1	1.3
Fish, Cumberland, BGTY, Sainsbury's*	1 Pack/450g	342	8.6	76	7.3	7.3	1.9	1.8
Fish, Frozen, Asda*	1 Pie/400g	504	24.0	126	5.0	13.0	6.0	1.1
Fish, Good Intentions, Somerfield*	1 Pack/400g	300	5.2	75	5.6	10.3	1.3	0.5
Fish, HL, Tesco*	1 Pack/400g	316	8.8	79	4.0	10.8	2.2	1.7
Fish, Luxury, Cafe Culture, M & S*	1 Pack/660g	627	26.4	95	7.1	7.8	4.0	1.1
Fish, Luxury, M & S*	1 Pack/300g	330	16.8	110	7.3	7.6	5.6	1.5
Fish, Mariner's, Frozen, Youngs*	1 Pack/360g	382	16.2	106	5.3	11.0	4.5	1.0
Fish, Mashed Potato Topped, Asda*	¼ Pie/257g	306	18.0	119	6.0	8.0	7.0	0.5
Fish, Spar*	1 Pack/400g	460	18.4	115	5.4	12.9	4.6	1.5
Fish, Topped with Potato, 3% Less Fat, GFY, Asda*	1 Pie/450g	379	11.8	84	6.4	8.7	2.6	1.3
Fish, with Grated Cheddar, Asda*	¼ Pie/250g	263	12.5	105	7.0	8.0	5.0	1.0
Fish & Prawn, PB, Waitrose*	1 Serving/375g	379	13.5	101	6.8	10.4	3.6	0.7
Fish with Cheese, Ross*	1 Pack/300g	321	13.5	107	4.7	12.0	4.5	0.8
Fish with Vegetables, Ross*	1 Pack/300g	255	8.7	85	4.4	10.2	2.9	1.3
Fisherman's, Asda*	1 Serving/300g	429	21.0	143	7.0	13.0	7.0	0.0
Fisherman's, Chilled, Co-Op*	1 Pie/300g	345	18.0	115	4.0	11.0	6.0	0.7
Fisherman's, Famous, Chilled, Youngs*	1 Pack/400g	448	22.8	112	7.6	7.6	5.7	0.9
Fisherman's, HE, Tesco*	1 Pie/400g	308	8.8	77	5.1	9.2	2.2	1.3
Fisherman's, Healthy Options, Asda*	1 Pie/406g	337	10.2	83	5.0	10.0	2.5	0.9
Fisherman's, M & S*	1 Pie/248g	335	15.9	135	9.3	9.8	6.4	0.3
Fisherman's, Morrisons*	1 Serving/300g	246	9.9	82	3.8	9.5	3.3	1.0
Fisherman's, Nisa Heritage*	1 Serving/550g	589	30.8	107	5.2	9.0	5.6	0.2
Fisherman's, Sainsbury's*	1 Pack/300g	195	3.6	65	3.9	9.7	1.2	1.2
Fisherman's, Tesco*	1 Pie/400g	400	19.6	100	4.2	9.8	4.9	1.1
Fishermans, British Recipe, Waitrose*	1 Pack/400g	408	16.4	102	7.7	8.5	4.1	1.2
Fishermans, PB, Waitrose*	1 Serving/400g	436	11.2	109	8.1	12.8	2.8	0.9
Fruit, Pastry Top & Bottom	1oz/28g	73	3.7	260	3.0	34.0	13.3	1.8
Fruit, Selection, Mr Kipling*	1 Pie/66.4g	231	9.0	350	3.5	53.5	13.6	1.3
Gala, Tesco*	1 Serving/70g	241	17.6	344	10.6	24.5	25.2	0.0
Haddock, Eat Smart, Safeway*	1 Pack/400g	300	5.6	75	5.2	10.0	1.4	1.0
Haddock & Broccoli, M & S*	1 Serving/250g	263	10.0	105	8.1	9.3	4.0	0.5
Haddock Cumberland, M & S*	1 Pie/300g	305	11.4	102	7.9	8.8	3.8	1.2
Key Lime, Sainsbury's*	¼ Pie/80g	280	11.2	350	4.2	51.8	14.0	0.7
Lamb & Mint, Shortcrust Pasty, Tesco*	¼ Pack/150g	413	26.1	275	5.9	23.6	17.4	1.6
Lemon Meringue	1oz/28g	89	4.0	319	4.5	45.9	14.4	0.7
Lemon Meringue, Lyons*	1 Serving/100g	310	14.4	310	0.0	45.9	14.4	0.0
Lemon Meringue, M & S*	1/6 Pie/80.3g	265	10.6	330	3.4	49.7	13.2	0.9
Lemon Meringue, Ready to Bake, Aunt Bessie's*	¼ Pie/106g	305	8.7	288	3.8	49.8	8.2	2.0
Lemon Meringue, Sainsbury's*	¼ Pie/110g	351	9.9	319	2.3	57.3	9.0	0.5
Lemon Meringue, Sara Lee*	1oz/28g	77	2.6	276	2.6	46.6	9.2	0.9
Lemon Meringue, Tesco*	1 Pie/385g	989	28.1	257	4.0	43.7	7.3	0.5
Macaroni Cheese, Countryside*	1 Serving/143.9g	282	10.1	196	4.9	28.3	7.0	1.2
Mariner's, Ross*	1 Pie/340g	435	20.1	128	5.0	13.9	5.9	1.0

	Measure INFO/WEIGHT	per Measure KCAL	per Measure FAT	Nutrition Values per 100g / 100ml KCAL	PROT	CARB	FAT	FIBRE
Mashed Potato Topped Cumberland, M & S*	1/3 Pack/300g	360	17.7	120	5.8	9.6	5.9	1.0
Meat, Freshbake*	1 Pie/48.6g	153	10.6	313	6.6	23.2	21.6	1.0
Meat & Potato, Hollands*	1 Pie/175g	410	19.3	234	6.1	27.5	11.0	0.0
Meat & Potato, Shortcrust, Co-Op*	¼ Pie/137g	403	26.2	294	7.3	23.3	19.1	1.4
Meat & Potato, Tesco*	1 Serving/150g	414	26.9	276	5.1	23.6	17.9	1.6
Meat & Potato, Value, Tesco*	1 Pie/95g	274	17.5	288	6.9	23.8	18.4	3.5
Mediteranean Vegetable, Cheesy, COU, M & S*	1 Pack/400g	280	8.4	70	2.1	10.6	2.1	2.1
Mince, Asda*	1 Pie/53.4g	202	8.0	382	3.8	58.0	15.0	1.5
Mince, Individual, Average	1 Pie/48g	203	9.8	423	4.3	59.0	20.4	2.1
Mince, Somerfield*	1oz/28g	111	4.8	398	4.0	56.0	17.0	0.0
Mince Puff, Tesco*	1 Cake/25g	105	4.4	420	3.3	62.0	17.6	2.0
Minced Beef, Plate, M & S*	1oz/28g	71	4.5	253	7.6	20.7	16.0	2.0
Minced Beef & Onion, Aberdeen Angus, Somerfield*	1 Serving/240g	732	44.6	305	8.6	25.8	18.6	1.0
Minced Beef & Onion, Birds Eye*	1 Pie/145g	419	25.1	289	7.1	26.3	17.3	0.7
Minced Beef & Onion, Denny*	1 Sm Pie/140g	288	19.7	206	6.1	17.3	14.1	0.0
Minced Beef & Onion, Farmfoods*	1 Pie/128g	378	23.9	295	7.3	24.4	18.7	1.0
Minced Beef & Onion, Tesco*	1 Pie/150g	455	28.5	303	5.7	27.4	19.0	1.7
Minced Beef & Vegetable, Pot, M & S*	1/3 Pie/183g	366	26.5	200	7.8	9.1	14.5	7.1
Minced Steak & Onion, Puff Pastry, Sainsbury's*	1 Pie/150g	477	29.1	318	8.9	27.0	19.4	0.9
Mississippi Mud, Tesco*	1 Serving/104g	399	26.6	384	5.3	33.1	25.6	1.8
Mushroom & Parsley Potato, Waitrose*	1 Pack/350g	347	17.5	99	2.5	10.9	5.0	1.2
Ocean, Basics, Sainsbury's*	1 Serving/302g	196	3.6	65	3.9	9.7	1.2	1.2
Ocean, BGTY, Sainsbury's*	1 Pack/350g	285	4.7	81	6.3	11.1	1.3	0.8
Ocean, From Heinz, Weight Watchers*	1 Pack/300g	209	4.4	70	4.5	9.6	1.5	0.2
Ocean, Frozen, BGTY, Sainsbury's*	1 Pack/350g	319	5.3	91	7.0	12.4	1.5	0.9
Ocean, M & S*	1 Pie/650g	532	19.6	95	8.2	7.6	3.5	0.9
Ocean, Original, Frozen, Youngs*	1 Pie/373.7g	419	21.3	112	7.6	7.6	5.7	0.9
Pork, & Egg, M & S*	¼ Pie/108g	379	28.0	351	9.7	19.8	25.9	0.8
Pork, & Pickle, Bowyers*	1 Pie/150g	576	41.0	384	10.0	26.3	27.3	0.0
Pork, Buffet, Bowyers*	1 Pie/60g	217	14.7	362	10.4	24.9	24.5	0.0
Pork, Buffet, Farmfoods*	1 Pie/65g	252	17.4	388	8.8	28.2	26.7	1.0
Pork, Buffet, Mini, Somerfield*	1 Pie/70g	292	19.9	418	10.8	29.5	28.5	0.2
Pork, Cheese & Pickle, Mini, Tesco*	1 Pie/49g	191	12.8	389	9.2	29.3	26.1	1.2
Pork, Crusty Bake, Mini, Sainsbury's*	1 Pie/43g	165	11.2	384	11.5	26.0	26.0	1.5
Pork, Crusty Bake, Sainsbury's*	1 Pie/75g	293	20.0	390	10.5	27.0	26.7	1.0
Pork, Geo Adams*	1 Pie/125g	488	34.8	390	11.8	23.1	27.8	0.9
Pork, Medium, Pork Farms*	1 Pie/200g	744	53.0	372	9.5	23.6	26.5	1.7
Pork, Melton, Mini, Pork Farms*	1 Pie/50g	200	14.6	399	8.9	26.2	29.2	0.0
Pork, Melton Mowbray, Cured, M & S*	1 Pie/290g	1044	71.1	360	10.1	25.9	24.5	1.0
Pork, Melton Mowbray, Cured, Mini, M & S*	1 Pie/50g	193	12.2	385	9.8	32.6	24.4	1.0
Pork, Melton Mowbray, Ginsters*	1 Pie/75g	317	22.7	423	12.3	25.2	30.3	0.9
Pork, Melton Mowbray, Individual, Sainsbury's*	1 Pie/75g	296	20.8	395	10.2	26.1	27.7	2.4
Pork, Melton Mowbray, Large, Co-Op*	¼ Pie/110g	418	35.2	380	11.0	12.0	32.0	5.0
Pork, Melton Mowbray, Lattice, Sainsbury's*	1 Serving/100g	342	23.6	342	10.8	21.7	23.6	1.2
Pork, Melton Mowbray, Medium, Somerfield*	¼ Pie/70g	275	18.9	393	11.0	27.0	27.0	0.0
Pork, Melton Mowbray, Mini, Co-Op*	1 Pie/49g	189	13.2	385	11.0	24.0	27.0	2.0
Pork, Melton Mowbray, Mini, Finest, Tesco*	1 Pie/50g	180	11.4	359	12.1	26.6	22.7	0.9
Pork, Melton Mowbray, Mini, Morrisons*	1 Pie/50g	197	12.5	393	10.9	31.3	24.9	0.9
Pork, Melton Mowbray, Mini, Tesco*	1 Pie/50g	196	14.4	392	12.6	20.8	28.7	2.9
Pork, Melton Mowbray, Safeway*	1 Pie/50g	197	12.5	393	10.9	31.3	24.9	0.9
Pork, Melton Mowbray, Small, Somerfield*	½ Pie/64g	237	14.7	371	12.0	30.0	23.0	0.0
Pork, Melton Mowbray, Snack, Tesco*	1 Pie/75g	289	19.4	385	10.1	27.0	25.9	2.7
Pork, Melton Mowbray, Tesco*	1 Pie/148g	679	49.9	459	10.0	29.0	33.7	1.3

PIE

INFO/WEIGHT	Measure	per Measure KCAL	FAT	Nutrition Values per 100g / 100ml KCAL	PROT	CARB	FAT	FIBRE
Pork, Melton Mowbray, Uncured, Small, Tesco*	1 Pie/140g	465	29.5	332	11.2	24.4	21.1	2.4
Pork, Mini, Christmas, Tesco*	1 Pie/50g	195	13.4	389	10.7	26.3	26.8	2.3
Pork, Mini, Tesco*	1 Pie/45g	162	10.7	359	10.2	25.9	23.8	1.0
Pork, Somerfield*	1 Pie/110g	442	31.9	402	11.0	24.0	29.0	0.0
Pork, with Cheese & Pickle, Waitrose*	1 Pack/150g	569	36.9	379	10.3	29.1	24.6	2.7
Potato & Meat, Farmfoods*	1 Pie/158g	416	26.9	263	5.4	22.0	17.0	1.0
Rhubarb, Sara Lee*	1 Serving/89.6g	225	12.4	250	2.9	28.7	13.8	1.3
Roast Chicken, COU, M & S*	1 Pack/320g	272	3.2	85	9.4	9.7	1.0	0.8
Roast Chicken, M & S*	½ Pie/175.5g	465	27.4	265	9.5	22.2	15.6	1.8
Roast Chicken, Sainsbury's*	1/3 Pie/173g	535	30.6	311	10.5	27.2	17.8	0.9
Roast Chicken, Shortcrust, Sainsbury's*	1 Pie/200g	1012	56.0	506	19.2	44.4	28.0	2.4
Roast Chicken & Vegetable, Pot, M & S*	1/3 Pie/183g	366	22.9	200	7.7	13.5	12.5	4.5
Salmon, Value, Tesco*	1 Pack/300g	312	13.5	104	4.5	11.3	4.5	1.0
Salmon & Broccoli, Birds Eye*	1 Pie/351g	449	21.8	128	6.6	11.4	6.2	0.7
Salmon & Broccoli, Filo Pastry, Finest, Tesco*	1 Pie/170g	386	22.6	227	7.9	18.9	13.3	2.1
Salmon & Broccoli, HL, Tesco*	1 Pack/450g	270	5.0	60	6.0	6.5	1.1	1.2
Salmon & Broccoli, Premium, Tesco*	1 Serving/170g	425	29.2	250	6.1	17.7	17.2	0.7
Salmon & Broccoli Lattice, M & S*	½ Pack/175.5g	465	32.5	265	8.7	15.6	18.5	3.2
Salmon & Broccoli Lattice Bar, Asda*	1/3 Bar/133g	360	20.0	271	6.0	28.0	15.0	0.8
Salmon Cottage, Sainsbury's*	1 Serving/298.6g	218	4.2	73	4.6	10.4	1.4	1.3
Sausage & Onion, Lattice, Puff Pastry, Tesco*	1/3 Pie/133g	480	22.5	361	9.1	20.6	16.9	4.6
Sausage & Onion, Tesco*	1 Pack/300g	333	18.3	111	2.3	11.7	6.1	0.5
Scotch, Co-Op*	1 Pie/132g	408	24.9	309	7.3	27.3	18.9	1.5
Scotch, Farmfoods*	1 Pie/151g	430	24.6	285	7.8	26.8	16.3	1.2
Shepherd's, Asda*	1 Pie/153g	193	9.2	126	5.0	13.0	6.0	0.8
Shepherd's, Average	1oz/28g	31	1.7	112	6.0	9.3	5.9	0.7
Shepherd's, Baked Bean Cuisine, Heinz*	1 Pie/340g	299	9.5	88	4.1	11.6	2.8	1.5
Shepherd's, BGTY, Sainsbury's*	1 Pack/300g	225	6.6	75	3.6	10.2	2.2	1.7
Shepherd's, British Classics, Chilled, Tesco*	1 Pack/500g	500	20.5	100	4.8	10.6	4.1	1.2
Shepherd's, Chilled, Finest, Tesco*	1 Pack/350g	403	14.4	115	6.9	8.0	4.1	1.9
Shepherd's, Classic British, Sainsbury's*	1 Pack/450g	500	20.7	111	6.6	10.8	4.6	0.7
Shepherd's, COU, M & S*	1 Pack/300g	210	3.9	70	5.2	8.6	1.3	1.6
Shepherd's, Frozen, Tesco*	1 Pack/400g	508	28.4	127	4.2	11.7	7.1	1.0
Shepherd's, Good Intentions, Somerfield*	1 Pack/450g	405	14.4	90	4.1	10.9	3.2	1.6
Shepherd's, Great Value, Asda*	1 Pack/400g	376	12.0	94	4.7	12.0	3.0	0.6
Shepherd's, Iceland*	1 Serving/170g	224	9.5	132	5.4	14.7	5.6	0.8
Shepherd's, M & S*	1 Pie/190g	190	8.6	100	5.4	9.6	4.5	1.2
Shepherd's, Safeway*	1 Serving/200g	200	5.8	100	6.5	11.4	2.9	1.1
Shepherd's, Sainsbury's*	1 Pie/300g	225	6.6	75	3.6	10.2	2.2	1.7
Shepherd's, Weight Watchers*	1 Pack/400g	300	6.8	75	2.4	12.5	1.7	0.9
Shepherd's, Welsh Hill Lamb, Gastropub, M & S*	½ Pack/330g	314	11.6	95	5.4	10.2	3.5	1.5
Shepherds, Classics, Asda*	1 Pack/455g	459	22.7	101	5.0	9.0	5.0	1.1
Smoked Haddock, Eat Smart, Safeway*	1 Pack/400g	376	9.6	94	8.1	10.1	2.4	1.2
Steak, Au Gratin, Tesco*	1 Pack/450g	594	27.0	132	8.7	10.7	6.0	1.1
Steak, Braised, Shortcrust Pastry, Asda*	½ Pack/260g	785	46.8	302	9.0	26.0	18.0	0.9
Steak, in Rich Gravy, Aunt Bessie's*	¼ Pie/200g	440	20.6	220	9.6	22.0	10.3	1.5
Steak, in Rich Gravy, Shortcrust Pastry, Sainsbury's*	1/3 Pie/200g	528	30.4	264	12.0	19.6	15.2	3.6
Steak, Individual, British Classics, Tesco*	1 Pie/150g	450	27.6	300	9.1	23.3	18.4	2.5
Steak, Large, Glenfell*	¼ Pie/170g	445	27.9	262	6.8	21.8	16.4	1.0
Steak, M & S*	1oz/28g	64	3.6	230	10.0	19.0	12.7	1.2
Steak, Mini, Asda*	1 Serving/67g	117	5.3	176	9.0	17.0	8.0	0.9
Steak, Mushroom & Ale, Topcrust, Waitrose*	1 Pie/250g	500	29.5	200	11.1	12.2	11.8	1.1
Steak, Puff Pastry, Deep Filled, Sainsbury's*	1 Pie/210g	536	30.0	255	10.3	21.2	14.3	2.0

P

PIE

INFO/WEIGHT	KCAL	FAT	KCAL	PROT	CARB	FAT	FIBRE
Steak, Puff Pastry, Deep Filled, Somerfield*	½ Pie/275g	715	38.2	260	10.0	23.7	13.9	0.8
Steak, Safeway*	¼ Pie/130g	381	21.1	293	9.4	27.4	16.2	1.1
Steak, Scotch, Bell's Bakery*	1 Serving/150g	378	20.3	252	13.6	18.6	13.5	0.7
Steak, Short Crust, Sainsbury's*	¼ Pie/131g	392	22.0	299	9.9	27.1	16.8	0.9
Steak, Shortcrust Pastry, Finest, Tesco*	1 Pie/250g	660	37.8	264	10.9	21.2	15.1	0.8
Steak, Shortcrust Pastry, Tesco*	¼ Pie/148.1g	385	20.4	260	10.5	22.6	13.8	3.0
Steak, Tesco*	1 Serving/205g	556	33.8	271	7.2	23.3	16.5	1.4
Steak, Topcrust Puff Pastry, Individual, Scottish, M & S*	1 Pie/170g	375	19.3	220	15.4	13.8	11.3	2.8
Steak & Ale, Budgens*	1 Pack/225g	583	38.0	259	7.2	19.5	16.9	0.9
Steak & Ale, Deep Filled, Somerfield*	1 Pie/200g	550	32.0	275	12.0	22.0	16.0	0.0
Steak & Ale, Fray Bentos*	1 Pie/425g	697	38.7	164	7.6	13.0	9.1	0.0
Steak & Ale, Pub Style, Co-Op*	1 Pie/250g	538	30.0	215	9.0	17.0	12.0	2.0
Steak & Ale, Sainsbury's*	1 Serving/190g	445	23.4	234	8.3	22.6	12.3	0.9
Steak & Guinness, Sainsbury's*	¼ Pie/137g	399	25.5	291	8.7	22.2	18.6	1.0
Steak & Kidney, Birds Eye*	1 Pie/146g	447	28.5	306	9.0	23.7	19.5	2.3
Steak & Kidney, Deep Fill, Sainsbury's*	½ Pie/125g	314	18.7	251	8.4	21.0	14.9	2.0
Steak & Kidney, Family, Co-Op*	1/6 Pie/87g	278	17.4	320	9.0	26.0	20.0	0.9
Steak & Kidney, Family, Iceland*	1/3 Pie/225g	502	29.3	223	10.2	16.3	13.0	2.1
Steak & Kidney, Individual	1 Pie/200g	646	42.4	323	9.1	25.6	21.2	0.9
Steak & Kidney, Individual, Morrisons*	1 Pie/141.9g	393	23.3	277	9.3	23.0	16.4	1.3
Steak & Kidney, Premium, Tesco*	1 Serving/170g	428	26.4	252	9.9	18.3	15.5	1.2
Steak & Kidney, Princes*	½ Pack/212g	379	19.9	179	8.8	14.8	9.4	0.0
Steak & Kidney, Puff Pastry, Sainsbury's*	1 Pie/150g	423	23.6	282	8.2	26.9	15.7	0.9
Steak & Kidney, Tesco*	1 Pie/250g	638	37.3	255	8.7	21.5	14.9	1.0
Steak & Kidney, Tinned, Fray Bentos*	½ Pie/212g	346	18.7	163	8.2	12.9	8.8	0.0
Steak & Kidney Shortcrust Pastry, Individual, M & S*	1 Pie/195g	545	33.5	279	8.1	23.8	17.2	2.2
Steak & Mushroom, Asda*	1 Pie/129.6g	351	18.2	270	9.0	27.0	14.0	1.4
Steak & Mushroom, Co-Op*	1 Pie/454g	1158	68.1	255	9.0	20.0	15.0	1.0
Steak & Mushroom, Deep Fill, Asda*	1/3 Pie/175g	476	28.0	272	11.0	21.0	16.0	1.1
Steak & Mushroom, Family, Iceland*	¼ Pie/164g	366	21.8	223	10.5	15.4	13.3	2.9
Steak & Mushroom, Finest, Tesco*	1 Pie/250g	640	36.5	256	9.2	21.9	14.6	1.1
Steak & Mushroom, HE, Tesco*	1 Serving/200g	380	11.4	190	10.5	24.2	5.7	1.9
Steak & Mushroom, Individual, Birds Eye*	1 Pie/142g	389	24.1	274	7.5	22.7	17.0	2.0
Steak & Mushroom, McDougalls*	1 Pack/340g	779	57.8	229	9.0	10.0	17.0	1.0
Steak & Mushroom, Sainsbury's*	¼ Pie/130g	372	21.3	286	8.6	26.0	16.4	1.0
Steak & Mushroom, Tesco*	1 Pie/142g	410	26.8	289	7.1	22.5	18.9	1.2
Steak & Onion, Farmfoods*	1 Pie/127g	382	24.3	301	6.0	26.4	19.1	1.0
Steak & Onion, Minced, Aberdeen Angus, Tesco*	½ Pie/300g	897	57.6	299	9.4	22.1	19.2	0.7
Steak & Potato, Asda*	1/3 Pie/173g	442	26.0	255	6.9	23.1	15.0	0.9
Steak & Red Wine, Puff Pastry, Pub, Sainsbury's*	1 Pie/240g	497	29.5	207	7.2	16.8	12.3	2.1
Summer Fruits, Orchard Tree*	1/8 Pie/75g	242	10.4	323	3.0	46.6	13.8	1.2
Teviot, Minced Beef, Morrisons*	½ Pie/250g	383	17.3	153	8.0	14.5	6.9	1.6
Tuna & Sweetcorn, HL, Tesco*	1 Pack/450g	392	12.2	87	7.1	8.6	2.7	2.0
Turkey & Ham, Shortcrust, M & S*	1/3 Pie/183g	494	29.1	270	11.9	19.5	15.9	1.0
Vegetable	1oz/28g	42	2.1	151	3.0	18.9	7.6	1.5
Vegetable, HE, Tesco*	1 Pack/450g	360	12.2	80	2.7	11.1	2.7	0.8
Vegetable & Cheddar Cheese, Waitrose*	1 Pie/210g	475	31.5	226	4.9	17.8	15.0	1.2
Vegetable & Cheese, Asda*	1 Pie/141g	330	16.2	234	5.8	26.9	11.5	1.0
Vegetable & Cheese, Safeway*	1 Pie/142g	373	22.2	263	5.1	25.4	15.6	1.5
Vegetarian, Deep Country, Linda McCartney*	1 Pie/166.1g	412	22.8	248	5.1	26.1	13.7	1.4
Vegetarian, Shepherd's, Linda McCartney*	1 Pack/340g	286	7.5	84	3.7	12.3	2.2	2.3
Vegetarian, Vegetable Cumberland, M & S*	½ Pack/211.1g	190	5.5	90	2.8	13.4	2.6	1.6
Welsh Lamb, Sainsbury's*	¼ Pie/120g	290	17.2	242	9.1	19.2	14.3	0.8

P

	Measure INFO/WEIGHT	per Measure KCAL	per Measure FAT	Nutrition Values per 100g / 100ml KCAL	PROT	CARB	FAT	FIBRE
PIE								
West Country Chicken, Sainsbury's*	1 Serving/240g	614	37.4	256	11.9	17.1	15.6	2.1
PIE FILLING								
Black Cherry, Fruit, Sainsbury's*	1 Serving/100g	73	0.1	73	0.3	17.7	0.1	0.3
Lemon, Sainsbury's*	1 Sachet/280g	218	1.1	78	0.1	18.6	0.4	0.0
PIGEON								
Meat Only, Roasted, Average	1 Pigeon/115g	215	9.1	187	29.0	0.0	7.9	0.0
Meat Only, Roasted, Weighed with Bone, Average	1oz/28g	25	1.0	88	13.6	0.0	3.7	0.0
PIKELETS								
Classics, M & S*	1 Pikelet/35g	70	0.5	200	7.3	39.1	1.3	1.6
Tesco*	1 Pikelet/35g	68	0.2	193	5.8	40.9	0.7	1.7
PILAF								
Bulgar Wheat, Sainsbury's*	1 Pack/381.3g	347	11.1	91	3.9	12.3	2.9	6.3
Forest Mushroom & Pine Nut, Bistro, Waitrose*	1 Serving/225g	338	14.6	150	7.0	15.8	6.5	1.5
with Tomato, Average	1oz/28g	40	0.9	144	2.5	28.0	3.3	0.4
PILCHARDS								
Fillets, in Tomato Sauce, Average	1 Can/120g	158	7.8	132	16.2	2.2	6.5	0.1
Fillets, in Virgin Olive Oil, Glenryck*	1 Serving/92g	223	14.4	242	23.3	2.0	15.7	0.0
in Brine, Average	½ Can/77g	114	5.6	148	20.8	0.0	7.3	0.0
PIMMS*								
& Lemonade, Premixed, Canned, Pimms*	1 Can/250ml	167	0.0	67	0.0	9.4	0.0	0.0
25% Volume, Pimms*	1 Serving/25ml	40	0.0	160	0.0	5.0	0.0	0.0
PINE NUTS								
Average	1oz/28g	195	19.2	695	15.7	3.9	68.6	1.9
PINEAPPLE								
& Papaya, Dried, Garden Gang, Asda*	1 Pack/50g	142	0.9	283	2.8	64.0	1.7	8.0
Dried, Sweetened, Ready to Eat, Tesco*	1/5 Pack/50g	118	1.0	235	0.4	52.9	1.9	1.7
Dried, Tropical Wholefoods*	1 Slice/10g	355	1.2	355	1.8	84.2	1.2	8.6
Dried, Unsweetened, Sainsbury's*	1 Bag/75g	255	1.5	340	1.7	84.7	2.0	6.0
in Juice, Average	1 Can/106g	57	0.0	53	0.3	12.9	0.0	0.6
in Syrup, Average	1 Can/240g	158	0.0	66	0.3	16.1	0.0	0.8
Pieces, Yoghurt Coated, Holland & Barrett*	1 Pack/100g	344	19.3	344	2.1	46.8	19.3	0.6
Raw, Average	1 Pineapple/472g	233	0.7	49	0.4	11.6	0.2	0.9
PINK GRAPEFRUIT								
in Natural Juice, Waitrose*	1 Serving/100g	32	0.0	32	0.6	7.3	0.0	0.4
Segments, Waitrose*	¼ Can/134ml	43	0.0	32	0.6	7.3	0.0	0.4
PISTACHIO NUTS								
Roasted & Salted, Average	1 Serving/25g	152	13.6	608	19.6	9.9	54.5	6.1
PIZZA								
American Hot, 12 Inch, Pizza Express*	½ Pizza/140.7g	300	10.6	213	10.5	25.9	7.5	2.6
American Hot, Chicago Town*	1 Pizza/170g	445	20.1	262	8.2	30.8	11.8	0.9
American Hot, Pizza Express*	1 Pizza/536g	1142	40.2	213	10.5	25.9	7.5	2.6
Bacon, Mushroom & Tomato, Deep Pan, Loaded, Tesco*	½ Pizza/219g	464	12.7	212	9.3	30.6	5.8	1.5
Bacon, Mushroom & Tomato, HL, Tesco*	1 Pizza/231g	395	6.2	171	10.6	25.9	2.7	1.5
Bacon, Mushroom & Tomato, Stonebaked, Tesco*	1 Serving/173g	351	12.8	203	9.9	24.1	7.4	2.0
Bacon & Mushroom, Deeply Delicious, Goodfella's*	1 Serving/200g	456	18.6	228	9.8	26.3	9.3	2.8
Bacon & Mushroom, Stone Bake, M & S*	1 Pizza/375g	750	24.0	200	9.9	27.2	6.4	1.6
Bacon & Mushroom, Stonebaked, Tesco*	1 Serving/157g	352	14.8	224	10.5	24.3	9.4	3.3
Bacon & Mushroom, Thin & Crispy, Sainsbury's*	½ Pizza/150g	396	15.9	264	12.9	29.2	10.6	1.7
Bacon & Mushroom, Thin & Crispy, Somerfield*	¼ Pizza/81g	189	8.1	233	11.0	24.0	10.0	0.0
Bacon & Mushroom, Thin Crust, Tesco*	½ Pizza/162.5g	380	14.3	234	11.1	27.5	8.8	1.8
Bacon & Mushroom Pizzeria, Sainsbury's*	1 Pizza/355g	880	24.9	248	11.7	34.5	7.0	3.7
Balsamic Roast Vegetable & Mozzarella, Sainsbury's*	½ Pizza/200g	444	15.6	222	8.5	29.4	7.8	2.4
BBQ Chicken, M & S*	½ Pizza/210g	431	11.8	205	11.6	27.5	5.6	1.8

PIZZA

INFO/WEIGHT	Measure	per Measure		Nutrition Values per 100g / 100ml				
		KCAL	FAT	KCAL	PROT	CARB	FAT	FIBRE
BBQ Chicken, Stonebaked, Tesco*	½ Pizza/158g	285	9.5	180	10.5	20.9	6.0	3.9
BBQ Chicken, Thin & Crispy, Sainsbury's*	½ Pizza/147g	384	12.1	261	13.8	33.1	8.2	1.6
BBQ Chicken, Thin & Crispy, Tesco*	1 Serving/165g	355	7.4	215	11.9	31.6	4.5	1.2
BBQ Chicken, Weight Watchers*	1 Pizza/224g	412	7.8	184	11.5	26.5	3.5	2.7
BBQ Chicken Stuffed Crust, Asda*	½ Pizza/245g	613	24.5	250	13.0	27.0	10.0	2.7
Bianca, Bistro, Waitrose*	½ Pizza/207g	618	32.6	298	12.9	26.2	15.7	2.3
Big American, Dr Oetker*	1 Serving/225g	572	24.8	254	9.7	28.9	11.0	0.0
Bistro Caramelised Onion, Feta & Rosemary, Waitrose*	½ Pizza/229.9g	607	32.0	264	8.6	26.1	13.9	2.4
Bistro Salami & Pepperoni, Waitrose*	½ Pizza/190g	492	19.4	259	12.9	28.8	10.2	1.5
Buffalo Mozzarella, Rustic Tomato, Finest, Tesco*	½ Pizza/172g	354	11.4	206	6.8	29.8	6.6	1.9
Cajun Chicken, BGTY, Sainsbury's*	½ Pizza/165g	363	5.9	220	11.0	36.0	3.6	1.7
Cajun Chicken, Pizzatilla, M & S*	½ Pizza/240g	636	36.2	265	10.5	21.8	15.1	1.3
Cajun Chicken, Sainsbury's*	½ Pizza/146g	285	2.6	195	12.9	31.8	1.8	2.6
Cajun Style Chicken, Stonebaked, Tesco*	1 Pizza/561g	1318	55.0	235	11.9	24.8	9.8	1.4
Calzone Speciale, Ristorante, Dr Oetker*	½ Pizza/145g	378	23.2	261	11.5	22.1	16.0	0.0
Capricciosa, Pizza Express*	1 Serving/300g	753	29.3	251	13.6	29.1	9.8	0.0
Caprina, Pizza Express*	1 Pizza/300g	635	22.0	212	8.0	31.0	7.3	0.0
Charged Up Chilli Beef, Goodfella's*	½ Pizza/357g	857	32.8	240	12.8	26.4	9.2	1.6
Chargrilled Chicken, Iceland*	1 Pizza/381g	804	25.5	211	12.3	25.4	6.7	2.0
Chargrilled Chicken, Thin & Crispy, Asda*	1 Pizza/373g	780	18.7	209	9.0	32.0	5.0	1.6
Chargrilled Chicken & Vegetable, GFY, Asda*	½ Pizza/166g	355	3.3	214	13.0	36.0	2.0	2.0
Chargrilled Chicken & Vegetable, Low Fat, Bertorelli*	1 Pizza/180g	439	7.9	244	14.2	39.3	4.4	2.3
Chargrilled Vegetable, Eat Smart, Safeway*	1 Pizza/206g	361	4.3	175	10.2	27.6	2.1	2.6
Chargrilled Vegetable, Frozen, BGTY, Sainsbury's*	1 Pizza/290g	548	13.3	189	10.2	26.7	4.6	3.0
Chargrilled Vegetable, HE, Tesco*	½ Pizza/143g	320	3.9	224	10.4	39.6	2.7	1.1
Chargrilled Vegetable, Thin & Crispy, GFY, Asda*	1 Serving/188.3g	290	3.8	154	6.0	28.0	2.0	3.1
Cheese, Deep Pan, Tesco*	½ Pizza/455g	990	26.4	218	11.4	29.8	5.8	3.1
Cheese, Onion & Garlic, Pizzeria, Waitrose*	½ Pizza/245.2g	684	28.9	279	10.8	29.8	11.8	2.5
Cheese, Stuffed, Crust, Sainsbury's*	1 Pizza/525g	1428	52.5	272	14.0	31.5	10.0	2.0
Cheese, Thin & Crispy, Goodfella's*	1 Serving/275g	729	27.8	265	15.7	27.6	10.1	1.8
Cheese, Three, Slice, Microwaveable, Tesco*	1 Slice/160g	486	18.7	304	13.3	36.7	11.7	1.6
Cheese & Onion, Tesco*	1 Serving/22g	56	2.0	255	10.5	32.7	9.1	2.7
Cheese & Tomato, Average	1 Serving/300g	711	35.4	237	9.1	25.2	11.8	1.4
Cheese & Tomato, Basics, Somerfield*	1 Serving/80g	194	5.6	242	9.7	35.1	7.0	1.9
Cheese & Tomato, Big Value, Ross*	1 Pizza/716g	1446	33.7	202	7.8	32.2	4.7	2.7
Cheese & Tomato, Bistro, Waitrose*	½ Pizza/205g	488	19.9	238	10.0	27.6	9.7	1.2
Cheese & Tomato, Blue Parrot Cafe, Sainsbury's*	¼ Pizza/87.5g	218	7.7	248	12.7	29.5	8.8	1.2
Cheese & Tomato, Deep & Crispy, Safeway*	1 Pizza/510g	1214	36.2	238	10.2	33.3	7.1	1.5
Cheese & Tomato, Deep & Crispy, Tesco*	1oz/28g	65	1.9	231	10.8	31.7	6.8	1.2
Cheese & Tomato, Deep Pan, Co-Op*	½ Pizza/200g	476	14.2	235	12.0	32.0	7.0	1.0
Cheese & Tomato, Deep Pan, Goodfella's*	¼ Pizza/102.4g	258	10.7	253	11.5	29.6	10.5	3.7
Cheese & Tomato, Deep Pan, Sainsbury's*	1 Pizza/182g	470	15.8	258	11.7	33.1	8.7	1.9
Cheese & Tomato, Eat Smart, Safeway*	1 Pizza/165g	355	1.2	215	11.5	40.1	0.7	1.9
Cheese & Tomato, Economy, Sainsbury's*	1 Pizza/60g	142	3.7	237	11.2	34.1	6.2	1.8
Cheese & Tomato, French Bread, Co-Op*	1 Pizza/135g	270	8.1	200	9.0	27.0	6.0	2.0
Cheese & Tomato, Frozen, Sainsbury's*	1 Serving/122g	300	10.7	246	13.7	28.0	8.8	3.0
Cheese & Tomato, HE, Tesco*	1 Serving/100g	211	2.4	211	11.9	35.5	2.4	1.6
Cheese & Tomato, Kids, Tesco*	1 Pizza/95g	219	5.2	231	11.5	33.9	5.5	1.9
Cheese & Tomato, Kids Crew, Iceland*	1 Pizza/89.9g	204	5.9	227	9.6	32.4	6.5	1.2
Cheese & Tomato, Micro, McCain*	1 Pizza/121.8g	319	12.2	262	13.4	29.7	10.0	2.4
Cheese & Tomato, Mini, Bruschetta, Iceland*	1 Pizza/33.5g	64	2.4	188	8.0	23.0	7.0	2.1
Cheese & Tomato, Mini, M & S*	1 Pizza/95g	233	5.5	245	10.0	38.7	5.8	1.6
Cheese & Tomato, Piccadella, Tesco*	1 Pizza/295g	684	31.4	232	9.1	24.8	10.6	1.5

PIZZA

INFO/WEIGHT	Measure per Measure			Nutrition Values per 100g / 100ml				
	Measure	KCAL	FAT	KCAL	PROT	CARB	FAT	FIBRE
Cheese & Tomato, Retail, Frozen, Average	1oz/28g	70	3.0	250	7.5	32.9	10.7	1.4
Cheese & Tomato, Sainsbury's*	1 Pizza/247g	706	24.5	286	13.7	35.4	9.9	2.4
Cheese & Tomato, Small, Tesco*	1 Pizza/102g	226	6.4	222	9.5	31.9	6.3	1.2
Cheese & Tomato, SmartPrice, Asda*	1 Pizza/125g	325	6.3	260	4.7	27.0	5.0	1.6
Cheese & Tomato, Square, Sainsbury's*	1 Square/160g	435	11.7	272	14.0	37.6	7.3	2.1
Cheese & Tomato, Stonebaked, Co-Op*	1 Pizza/325g	699	26.0	215	10.0	26.0	8.0	3.0
Cheese & Tomato, Stonebaked, Organic, Co-Op*	1 Pizza/330g	677	23.1	205	9.0	26.0	7.0	4.0
Cheese & Tomato, Stonebaked, Safeway*	½ Pizza/190g	437	11.2	230	12.0	32.3	5.9	1.5
Cheese & Tomato, Stonebaked, Thin & Crispy, Tesco*	½ Pizza/161g	388	13.8	241	11.6	29.4	8.6	2.1
Cheese & Tomato, Thin & Crispy, Asda*	1 Pizza/366g	827	36.6	226	11.0	23.0	10.0	2.0
Cheese & Tomato, Thin & Crispy, Carlos*	1 Pizza/155g	405	13.0	261	11.4	35.0	8.4	1.2
Cheese & Tomato, Thin & Crispy, Morrisons*	1 Pizza/335g	734	23.8	219	11.2	27.7	7.1	3.1
Cheese & Tomato, Thin & Crispy, Organic, Tesco*	½ Pizza/147g	369	14.4	251	10.6	30.1	9.8	1.3
Cheese & Tomato, Thin & Crispy, Safeway*	1 Serving/365g	949	25.6	260	11.7	37.2	7.0	4.7
Cheese & Tomato, Thin & Crispy, Sainsbury's*	1 Serving/135g	344	10.0	255	14.9	32.2	7.4	5.0
Cheese & Tomato, Thin & Crispy, Stonebaked, Tesco*	1/3 Pizza/212g	509	19.5	240	10.1	29.2	9.2	1.4
Cheese & Tomato, Thin & Crispy, SuperValu*	1 Slice/75.8g	182	6.5	240	11.4	30.0	8.6	2.7
Cheese & Tomato, Thin & Crispy, Waitrose*	½ Pizza/152.6g	359	15.4	235	12.3	23.6	10.1	2.3
Cheese & Tomato, Value, Tesco*	1 Serving/140g	388	13.6	277	11.4	36.0	9.7	1.8
Cheese & Tomato French Bread, Findus*	1 Piece/143g	322	11.6	225	9.4	29.0	8.1	0.0
Cheese & Tomato Range, Italiano, Tesco*	1 Pizza/380g	969	35.0	255	11.4	31.7	9.2	3.3
Cheese & Tomato Slice, Ross*	1 Slice/77g	148	6.6	192	6.5	22.2	8.6	2.0
Cheese & Tomato Thin & Crispy, Stonebaked, Tesco*	1 Pizza/155g	355	12.1	229	11.6	28.1	7.8	1.3
Cheese Feast, Big Fill, Somerfield*	1 Pizza/430g	1135	47.3	264	13.0	28.0	11.0	0.0
Cheese Feast, Deep Pan, Asda*	½ Pizza/210g	422	18.9	201	13.0	17.0	9.0	2.3
Cheese Feast, Thin Crust, Chilled, Tesco*	½ Pizza/157.5g	421	20.2	267	14.7	23.4	12.8	2.5
Cheese Suprema, Freschetta, Schwan's*	½ Pizza/150g	392	14.0	261	12.4	32.4	9.3	1.8
Cheese Supreme, New Recipe, Goodfella's*	¼ Pizza/102g	269	10.2	264	12.3	31.2	10.0	2.2
Cheese Triple, Chicago Town*	1 Pizza/164.7g	486	23.6	295	11.9	29.7	14.3	1.8
Cheesefeast, Deep & Crispy 12", Takeaway, Iceland*	1 Slice/132g	342	11.1	259	13.1	32.8	8.4	1.5
Chicken & Bacon, Loaded, Tesco*	1 Serving/258g	622	25.3	241	12.8	25.4	9.8	1.9
Chicken & Bacon, Pizzeria, Italian, Sainsbury's*	½ Pizza/169.5g	509	24.1	300	13.6	29.4	14.2	2.7
Chicken & Bacon Carbonara, Thin Crust, Italian, Asda*	1 Pizza/492g	1156	34.4	235	12.0	31.0	7.0	3.4
Chicken & Maple Bacon Carbonara, Asda*	½ Pizza/195g	484	15.6	248	11.0	33.0	8.0	2.2
Chicken & Pesto, Californian Style, Asda*	½ Pizza/234.8g	533	16.5	227	10.0	31.0	7.0	2.0
Chicken & Pesto, with Red Peppers, Italian, Sainsbury's*	½ Pizza/192.2g	471	18.6	245	12.0	27.3	9.7	2.7
Chicken & Red Pepper, HE, Tesco*	1 Pizza/260g	608	6.5	234	12.7	40.1	2.5	0.7
Chicken & Spinach, Eat Smart, Safeway*	1 Pizza/165g	322	3.5	195	19.0	24.0	2.1	2.5
Chicken & Sweetcorn, Stonebaked, Tesco*	1 Serving/177g	354	9.6	200	11.9	26.0	5.4	2.0
Chicken & Sweetfire Red Pepper, GFY, Asda*	½ Pizza/167g	363	7.7	217	10.0	34.0	4.6	1.6
Chicken & Vegetable, Chargrill, Italiano, Tesco*	½ Pizza/184g	383	14.7	208	10.6	23.3	8.0	2.4
Chicken & Vegetable, Stone Baked, GFY, Asda*	½ Pizza/160.8g	349	3.7	217	13.0	36.0	2.3	1.7
Chicken Alfredo, Chicago Town*	1 Pizza/265g	583	24.9	220	11.9	21.9	9.4	1.8
Chicken Arrabbiata, M & S*	1 Pizza/325g	618	13.7	190	11.6	26.5	4.2	1.1
Chicken Arrabiata, Sainsbury's*	½ Pizza/191.4g	443	12.2	232	12.1	31.4	6.4	1.7
Chicken Provencal, Goodfella's*	½ Pizza/142.5g	389	18.0	272	13.7	25.9	12.6	2.1
Chicken Salsa, HE, Tesco*	½ Pizza/169g	313	2.2	185	13.0	30.3	1.3	1.5
Chicken Salsa, Healthy Choice, Safeway*	½ Pizza/177g	437	5.7	246	13.3	40.9	3.2	1.6
Chicken Salsa, HL, Tesco*	½ Pizza/169g	269	3.5	159	11.1	24.0	2.1	2.2
Chicken Salsa, Thin Crust, Budgens*	½ Pizza/163g	295	3.1	181	10.5	30.5	1.9	1.4
Chicken Tikka, Stonebaked, Tesco*	1 Serving/153g	326	10.4	213	10.7	27.3	6.8	1.3
Chilli Beef, Stone Bake, M & S*	1 Pizza/395g	790	22.9	200	9.6	26.7	5.8	1.9
Chorizo & Cherrybell Peppers, TTD, Sainsbury's*	½ Pizza/194.7g	589	25.0	302	13.8	33.0	12.8	2.2

PIZZA

	Measure INFO/WEIGHT	per Measure KCAL	per Measure FAT	Nutrition Values per 100g / 100ml KCAL	PROT	CARB	FAT	FIBRE
Chorizo & Sweet Pepper, Stonebaked, Safeway*	1 Serving/190g	466	12.9	245	9.9	35.5	6.8	3.8
Cream Cheese & Pepperonata, Calzone, Waitrose*	½ Pizza/165g	383	15.8	232	7.0	29.4	9.6	1.5
Deep South, Chicago Town*	1 Pizza/171g	363	12.1	212	6.9	30.0	7.1	0.0
Delicata Four Season Ultra Thin, TTD, Sainsbury's*	½ Pizza/168g	445	21.7	265	13.3	24.3	12.9	2.3
Diavolo, Pizza Express*	½ Pizza/163.5g	322	11.0	197	9.4	24.6	6.7	2.1
Double Cheese, Chicago Town*	1 Pizza/405g	932	27.1	230	11.7	30.6	6.7	0.0
Double Cheese, Square Snacks, Waitrose*	1 Pizza/145.5g	415	10.9	286	12.4	40.2	7.5	1.9
Easy Cheesy, Deep Pan, Chicago Town*	½ Pizza/547g	1455	59.1	266	11.4	30.9	10.8	1.7
Fajita Chicken, COU, M & S*	1 Pizza/255g	434	6.1	170	9.9	25.5	2.4	1.2
Fajita Vegetable, BGTY, Sainsbury's*	1 Pizza/214g	366	3.0	171	8.9	30.8	1.4	2.9
Farmhouse, Tesco*	½ Pizza/190g	353	14.1	186	9.7	20.3	7.4	2.7
Fingers, Oven Baked, McCain*	1 Finger/30g	78	2.4	261	12.6	34.8	7.9	2.4
Fingers & Curly Fries, M & S*	1 Pack/211.8g	360	10.4	170	7.9	22.9	4.9	1.6
Fire Roasted Pepper, Sainsbury's*	1 Pizza/344g	605	5.2	176	5.3	35.3	1.5	1.6
Fire Roasted Peppers & Vegetables, Waitrose*	½ Pizza/235g	442	16.7	188	9.8	21.3	7.1	2.7
Five Cheese & Pepperoni, Deep & Crispy, Waitrose*	1/3 Pizza/200g	560	23.2	280	11.7	32.3	11.6	1.3
Flamed Chicken & Vegetables, BGTY, Sainsbury's*	1 Pizza/260g	660	11.4	254	14.2	39.3	4.4	2.3
Flamin' Hot, Deep Dish, Chicago Town*	1 Pizza/170g	454	20.4	267	8.6	31.1	12.0	0.0
Focaccia Tomato & Black Olive, TTD, Sainsbury's*	½ Pizza/222g	515	19.8	232	9.3	28.7	8.9	2.9
Four Cheese, Finest, Tesco*	½ Pizza/230g	575	21.2	250	12.1	29.8	9.2	1.3
Four Cheese, Freschetta, Schwan's*	¼ Slice/75g	205	7.4	273	11.3	34.8	9.8	1.4
Four Cheese, Italian, Somerfield*	½ Pizza/175g	488	13.3	279	13.5	39.1	7.6	2.2
Four Cheese, M & S*	1oz/28g	67	2.1	240	13.2	30.3	7.5	1.2
Four Cheese, Thin & Crispy, Sainsbury's*	1 Pizza/265g	729	32.6	275	11.8	29.3	12.3	3.5
Four Cheese, Thin Crust, Tesco*	½ Pizza/142g	386	13.6	272	14.5	31.8	9.6	1.8
Four Cheese, Weight Watchers*	1 Pizza/186g	400	7.0	215	10.8	34.9	3.8	1.6
Four Cheese & Tomato, Pizzatilla, M & S*	1 Serving/69.3g	224	13.7	324	10.5	26.0	19.9	1.5
Four Cheese & Tomato, Safeway*	1 Serving/125g	318	7.6	254	12.8	36.8	6.1	1.7
French Bread, Blue Parrot Cafe, Sainsbury's*	1 Pizza/132g	271	5.7	205	10.7	30.8	4.3	1.3
Frutti Di Mare, Express, Pizza Express*	1 Pizza/373g	500	9.5	134	9.1	20.1	2.6	0.0
Funghi, Pizzaroma, Safeway*	½ Pizza/205g	506	19.7	247	10.8	29.3	9.6	2.9
Funghi, Ristorante, Dr Oetker*	1 Pizza/365g	865	43.4	237	7.9	22.5	11.9	0.0
Garden Style, Hot Stuff*	1 Slice/188g	370	21.0	197	0.0	21.3	11.2	1.6
Garlic & Mushroom, Asda*	½ Pizza/241g	696	41.0	289	10.0	24.0	17.0	1.6
Garlic & Mushroom, Thin & Crispy, Sainsbury's*	1 Pizza/260g	829	43.2	319	11.1	31.2	16.6	1.7
Garlic Bread, Stonebaked, Italiono, Tesco*	1 Serving/116.5g	405	18.3	346	7.8	43.6	15.6	1.5
Garlic Chicken, Deep Pan, Sainsbury's*	½ Pizza/214g	464	13.9	217	11.2	28.3	6.5	3.3
Garlic Chicken, Thin & Crispy, Somerfield*	1 Pizza/365g	876	32.9	240	10.0	29.1	9.0	1.6
Garlic Chicken, Thin & Crispy, Stonebake, Sainsbury's*	½ Pizza/160g	386	17.3	241	10.7	25.2	10.8	3.5
Garlic Chicken & Spinach, PB, Waitrose*	½ Pizza/172g	351	5.3	204	13.3	30.8	3.1	2.3
Garlic Mushroom, BGTY, Sainsbury's*	½ Pizza/123g	262	2.5	213	11.6	37.2	2.0	2.7
Garlic Mushroom, Ciabatta Style, Goodfella's*	½ Pizza/186.6g	475	23.0	254	10.0	27.9	12.3	2.2
Garlic Mushroom, Classico, Tesco*	½ Pizza/207.5g	415	13.9	200	10.0	24.9	6.7	2.6
Garlic Mushroom, Italian Style, Somerfield*	½ Pizza/175g	460	17.5	263	9.0	33.0	10.0	0.0
Garlic Mushroom, Safeway*	½ Pizza/155g	482	20.0	311	9.4	39.2	12.9	1.7
Garlic Mushroom, Tesco*	1 Pizza/425g	829	34.0	195	9.3	21.6	8.0	5.3
Garlic Mushroom, Thin & Crispy, Chicago Town*	1 Pizza/115g	283	13.3	246	9.0	26.4	11.6	1.9
Garlic Mushroom, Thin & Crispy, Weight Watchers*	1 Pizza/220g	376	2.9	171	11.2	28.8	1.3	3.0
Garlic Mushroom, Thin Crust, Tesco*	½ Pizza/163g	340	14.6	209	11.0	21.1	9.0	3.6
Giardiniera, From Supermarket, Pizza Express*	½ Pizza/144g	291	10.5	202	8.6	25.5	7.3	2.1
Grilled Pepper, Weight Watchers*	1 Pizza/220g	392	5.1	178	10.0	29.3	2.3	1.8
Ham, Mushroom & Gruyere, Sainsbury's*	¼ Pizza/169.0g	404	13.7	239	10.2	31.3	8.1	3.7
Ham, Mushroom & Tomato, BGTY, Sainsbury's*	½ Pizza/150g	307	6.1	206	11.8	30.4	4.1	1.2

P

PIZZA

INFO/WEIGHT	Measure	per Measure KCAL	FAT	Nutrition Values per 100g / 100ml KCAL	PROT	CARB	FAT	FIBRE
Ham, Pepperoni & Milano, M & S*	1 Pizza/290g	696	28.4	240	14.0	23.3	9.8	1.1
Ham, Roasted Mushrooms, Mascarpone, Finest, Tesco*	½ Pizza/250g	538	27.0	215	11.3	18.2	10.8	3.2
Ham & Cheese, Chunky, Asda*	1 Serving/90g	211	3.0	234	12.0	39.0	3.3	4.7
Ham & Cheese, Mini, Tesco*	1 Pizza/95g	214	5.5	225	10.3	33.0	5.8	2.6
Ham & Cheese, Ultra Thin, Sodebo*	1 Pizza/200g	400	8.6	200	11.3	29.1	4.3	0.0
Ham & Mushroom, BGTY, Sainsbury's*	½ Pizza/158g	291	6.6	184	10.2	26.4	4.2	2.9
Ham & Mushroom, Deep & Crispy, Somerfield*	½ Pizza/210g	491	15.1	234	10.4	31.9	7.2	1.6
Ham & Mushroom, Deep & Crispy, Tesco*	1 Serving/210g	420	10.3	200	9.7	29.2	4.9	1.1
Ham & Mushroom, Deep Pan, Asda*	½ Pizza/223g	444	15.6	199	9.0	25.0	7.0	1.2
Ham & Mushroom, Deep Pan, Waitrose*	½ Pizza/219.9g	453	13.6	206	10.9	26.6	6.2	1.0
Ham & Mushroom, Finest, Tesco*	½ Pizza/240g	576	26.4	240	9.5	25.9	11.0	2.2
Ham & Mushroom, Guiseppe Taverna*	1 Pizza/350g	662	17.5	189	10.0	26.0	5.0	0.0
Ham & Mushroom, HE, Tesco*	1 Pizza/252g	491	3.0	195	10.4	35.6	1.2	2.0
Ham & Mushroom, New, BGTY, Sainsbury's*	1 Pizza/248g	526	3.5	212	12.1	37.8	1.4	2.9
Ham & Mushroom, Stone Baked, Goodfella's*	½ Pizza/175g	439	20.0	251	9.6	27.6	11.4	1.2
Ham & Mushroom, Stonebaked, Stateside Foods*	¼ Pizza/101g	225	6.3	223	9.9	31.9	6.2	1.4
Ham & Mushroom, Tesco*	1/6 /57g	132	4.4	232	11.2	29.2	7.8	1.9
Ham & Mushroom, Thin & Crispy, Asda*	1 Pizza/360g	760	25.2	211	11.0	26.0	7.0	2.4
Ham & Mushroom, Thin & Crispy, Somerfield*	½ Pizza/170g	357	13.4	210	10.8	24.0	7.9	1.0
Ham & Mushroom, Thin & Crispy, Tesco*	1 Serving/166g	349	11.5	210	13.0	23.9	6.9	2.4
Ham & Mushroom Calzone, Waitrose*	½ Pizza/145g	363	13.5	250	10.0	31.6	9.3	1.6
Ham & Mushroom Slices, Farmfoods*	1 Slice/89g	170	2.3	191	8.0	34.0	2.6	0.9
Ham & Onion, Tesco*	1 Serving/181g	453	17.4	250	11.8	29.0	9.6	2.2
Ham & Pineapple, American Deep Pan, Sainsbury's*	1 Pizza/412g	1001	32.1	243	10.5	32.6	7.8	1.7
Ham & Pineapple, Chicago Town*	1 Pizza/435g	866	19.6	199	10.0	29.7	4.5	0.0
Ham & Pineapple, Deep Dish, Chicago Town*	1 Pizza/170g	434	17.9	255	9.4	30.6	10.5	1.9
Ham & Pineapple, Deep Pan, Ciabatta, Iceland*	½ Pizza/185g	440	14.4	238	11.6	30.3	7.8	0.8
Ham & Pineapple, Deep Pan, Tesco*	1 Pizza/237g	437	6.9	184	9.8	29.8	2.9	1.9
Ham & Pineapple, Eat Smart, Safeway*	1 Serving/151g	279	3.6	185	13.6	27.2	2.4	2.5
Ham & Pineapple, HE, Tesco*	1 Serving/169g	343	2.5	203	11.9	35.4	1.5	1.3
Ham & Pineapple, HL, Tesco*	¼ Pizza/105g	170	2.2	162	10.0	25.9	2.1	2.4
Ham & Pineapple, Loaded, Tesco*	½ Pizza/265g	557	14.6	210	11.3	28.7	5.5	1.4
Ham & Pineapple, Pizzerai, Simply Italian, Sainsbury's*	½ Pizza/178g	434	15.1	244	11.5	30.4	8.5	2.4
Ham & Pineapple, Stone Bake, M & S*	1 Pizza/345g	690	19.7	200	10.1	28.3	5.7	1.6
Ham & Pineapple, Stonebaked, Tesco*	1 Pizza/161g	293	9.2	182	9.2	23.5	5.7	3.5
Ham & Pineapple, Tesco*	1/6 Pizza/56g	134	4.6	240	10.4	30.9	8.3	2.1
Ham & Pineapple, Thin & Crispy, Goodfella's*	1 Serving/163g	333	12.7	204	10.6	22.8	7.8	2.4
Ham & Pineapple, Thin & Crispy, Iceland*	1 Serving/110g	285	12.5	259	9.9	29.2	11.4	1.3
Ham & Pineapple, Thin & Crispy, Safeway*	½ Pizza/182g	455	14.4	250	13.6	29.9	7.9	4.0
Ham & Pineapple, Thin & Crispy, Sainsbury's*	1 Pizza/163g	417	13.2	256	13.8	32.0	8.1	1.7
Ham & Pineapple, Thin & Crispy, Sainsbury's*	1 Pizza/330g	719	21.1	218	10.8	29.4	6.4	2.4
Ham & Pineapple, Thin & Crispy, Somerfield*	½ Pizza/156g	348	10.6	223	12.3	28.2	6.8	3.0
Ham & Pineapple, Thin & Crispy, Waitrose*	1 Pizza/220g	616	21.1	280	12.8	33.3	9.6	2.2
Ham & Pineapple, Thin & Crispy Italian, Morrisons*	1 Pizza/375g	746	22.9	199	10.2	24.9	6.1	0.0
Ham & Roast Onion, Classico, Italiano, Tesco*	1 Serving/181.5g	471	19.1	259	12.1	29.1	10.5	1.6
Hawaiian, San Marco*	¼ Pizza/90g	208	8.3	231	8.9	29.7	9.2	1.5
Hickory Steak, M & S*	1 Pizza/400g	820	26.8	205	9.9	25.7	6.7	1.4
Honey Roast Salmon & Broccoli, BGTY, Sainsbury's*	1 Serving/280g	613	12.6	219	10.2	34.4	4.5	3.5
Hot & Spicy, Deep Dish, Chicago Town*	1 Pizza/177g	434	17.5	245	8.6	30.4	9.9	0.9
Hot & Spicy, Deep Dish, Schwan's*	1 Pizza/170g	423	19.4	249	9.1	27.6	11.4	0.0
Hot & Spicy, Deep Pan, Tesco*	1 Serving/221g	423	7.3	191	10.5	30.0	3.3	2.1
Hot & Spicy, Pizzeria Style, Sainsbury's*	1 Pizza/376g	986	46.3	262	12.5	25.5	12.3	2.4
Hot & Spicy, Thin & Crispy, Morrisons*	½ Pizza/170g	393	15.8	231	10.5	26.5	9.3	3.2

PIZZA

INFO/WEIGHT	Measure	per Measure KCAL	FAT	Nutrition Values per 100g / 100ml KCAL	PROT	CARB	FAT	FIBRE
Hot & Spicy, Thin & Crispy, Somerfield*	1 Pizza/305g	918	51.9	301	12.0	25.0	17.0	0.0
Hot & Spicy Chicken, Deep Pan, Morrisons*	½ Pizza/232.5g	521	13.0	224	10.5	32.9	5.6	1.0
Hot & Spicy Chicken, Deep Pan, Tesco*	½ Pizza/222g	423	7.3	191	10.5	30.0	3.3	2.1
Hot Chicken, Stone Bake, M & S*	1 Pizza/380g	798	25.8	210	11.5	25.1	6.8	1.3
Hot Dog, Kids, Tesco*	1 Pizza/95g	233	6.3	245	9.8	36.6	6.6	2.0
Italian Cheese & Ham, The Little Big Food Company*	1 Pizza/95g	236	6.2	248	11.0	36.3	6.6	1.0
Italian Meat, So Good, Somerfield*	½ Pizza/200g	468	10.8	234	14.0	32.4	5.4	2.4
Italian Meat Feast, Thin & Crispy, Waitrose*	1 Pizza/182g	477	22.9	262	10.7	26.5	12.6	1.8
Italian Meats, Finest, Tesco*	½ Pizza/217g	449	8.5	207	13.6	29.4	3.9	1.3
Italian Meats, TTD, Sainsbury's*	½ Pizza/223.7g	587	26.9	262	12.8	25.6	12.0	2.4
Italian Mozzarella & Black Forest Ham, Asda*	¼ Pizza/110g	227	6.6	206	10.0	28.0	6.0	2.7
Italian Sausage & Roasted Peppers, Finest, Tesco*	1 Pizza/325g	650	13.7	200	7.8	31.7	4.2	1.9
Kids Smart, Morrisons*	1 Pizza/91g	203	4.0	223	8.8	36.9	4.4	3.1
Le Reine, 8 Inch, Supermarket, Pizza Express*	½ Pizza/155.2g	300	9.0	193	10.2	25.0	5.8	2.7
Loaded Cheese, Goodfella's*	1 Pizza/410g	1115	49.6	272	11.4	29.4	12.1	1.7
Margherita, 12 Inch, Supermarket, Pizza Express*	½ Pizza/243.2g	505	14.6	208	10.1	28.5	6.0	2.4
Margherita, 12", Finest, Tesco*	½ Pizza/254.5g	434	9.2	170	8.1	26.4	3.6	2.7
Margherita, Classico, Tesco*	1 Serving/150g	342	11.4	228	11.3	28.5	7.6	1.8
Margherita, Finest, Tesco*	1 Serving/207g	441	10.8	213	11.0	30.5	5.2	1.2
Margherita, HL, Tesco*	½ Pizza/125g	222	2.5	178	10.8	29.3	2.0	2.5
Margherita, Italian Stone Baked, Somerfield*	1 Pizza/290g	554	20.3	191	10.0	22.0	7.0	0.0
Margherita, Italian Stonebaked, Asda*	¼ Pizza/134.6g	323	10.8	240	11.0	31.0	8.0	1.8
Margherita, Italian Style, Somerfield*	½ Pizza/190g	424	11.4	223	10.0	32.0	6.0	0.0
Margherita, Italiano, Tesco*	1 Serving/172.5g	415	20.9	240	11.4	21.0	12.1	2.0
Margherita, Morrisons*	½ Pizza/163g	416	18.0	256	12.9	26.1	11.1	2.3
Margherita, Pizzeria, Italian, Sainsbury's*	½ Pizza/168.5g	426	17.4	253	12.2	27.9	10.3	2.5
Margherita, So Good, Somerfield*	½ Pizza/220.2g	513	18.5	233	9.9	29.5	8.4	2.2
Margherita, Stone Baked, GFY, Asda*	¼ Pizza/73g	158	1.4	217	11.0	39.0	1.9	1.8
Margherita, Stone Baked, Goodfella's*	1 Slice/36g	95	4.1	263	10.9	31.9	11.4	7.6
Margherita, Stonebaked Ciabatta, Goodfella's*	½ Pizza/149.5g	405	17.3	270	11.3	32.8	11.5	2.6
Margherita, Thin & Crispy, Iceland*	½ Pizza/170g	391	14.5	230	12.7	25.9	8.5	2.8
Margherita, Thin Crust, Tesco*	1 Serving/170g	354	13.4	208	10.1	24.1	7.9	3.6
Margherita Cheese & Tomato, San Marco*	½ Pizza/200g	454	14.4	227	10.7	29.8	7.2	1.2
Margherita Classico, Italiano, Tesco*	½ Pizza/191g	414	11.8	217	11.2	29.1	6.2	2.5
Marinated Tomato & Mascarpone, Piccadella, Tesco*	1 Pizza/260g	634	26.5	244	6.4	31.6	10.2	2.2
Massive on Meat, Deep Pan, Goodfella's*	1 Serving/106g	259	9.4	244	10.4	30.6	8.9	3.0
Meat, Mediterranean Style, Pizzeria, Waitrose*	¼ Pizza/174g	395	15.3	227	11.1	25.8	8.8	2.0
Meat Feast, American Style, Sainsbury's*	½ Pizza/263g	642	26.0	244	12.6	26.2	9.9	2.9
Meat Feast, Big Fill, Somerfield*	1 Pizza/455g	1019	36.4	224	11.0	26.0	8.0	0.0
Meat Feast, Deep & Crispy, Iceland*	1/6 Pizza/136g	345	11.3	254	11.2	33.7	8.3	2.0
Meat Feast, Deep & Loaded, Sainsbury's*	½ Pizza/297.5g	817	30.0	275	13.2	32.7	10.1	2.6
Meat Feast, Deep Pan, Co-Op*	1 Pizza/450g	1103	45.0	245	11.0	28.0	10.0	2.0
Meat Feast, Hot & Spicy, Thin & Crispy, Sainsbury's*	½ Pizza/170g	462	21.6	272	13.0	26.5	12.7	3.2
Meat Feast, Large, Tesco*	1 Pizza/735g	1904	69.1	259	10.9	32.6	9.4	2.0
Meat Feast, Loaded, Deep Pan, Large, Tesco*	½ Pizza/282g	776	38.4	275	12.0	26.1	13.6	1.9
Meat Feast, Thin & Crispy, Asda*	½ Pizza/183g	410	14.6	224	11.0	27.0	8.0	1.4
Meat Feast, Thin & Crispy, Safeway*	½ Pizza/179.2g	430	16.5	240	12.0	27.2	9.2	4.8
Meat Feast, Thin & Crispy, Somerfield*	½ Pizza/164.8g	413	17.8	250	12.4	25.7	10.8	3.2
Meat Feast, Thin Crust, Tesco*	½ Pizza/178g	430	20.2	242	13.6	21.3	11.4	2.3
Meat Feast Ultimate, Sainsbury's*	1 Pizza/465g	1302	47.9	280	13.5	35.1	10.3	1.7
Meat Mayhem, Goodfella's*	1 Pizza/436.5g	1100	41.9	252	10.6	30.9	9.6	2.5
Mediterranean, Delicia, Goodfella's*	½ Pizza/150.2g	371	18.3	247	9.1	25.3	12.2	2.1
Mediterranean Madness, Goodfella's*	¼ Pizza/108.8g	235	8.7	216	9.1	27.0	8.0	3.9

PIZZA

INFO/WEIGHT	Measure	per Measure KCAL	FAT	Nutrition Values per 100g / 100ml KCAL	PROT	CARB	FAT	FIBRE
Mediterranean Style Vegetable, Waitrose*	¼ Pizza/174.9g	327	9.8	187	7.6	26.6	5.6	2.1
Mediterranean Vegetable, Pizzeria, Sainsbury's*	1 Serving/211.3g	397	13.5	188	8.0	24.7	6.4	3.2
Mediterranean Vegetable, Stonebaked, Sainsbury's*	½ Pizza/260g	622	16.4	239	9.8	35.7	6.3	3.1
Mexican Style, Morrisons*	½ Pizza/180g	437	16.9	243	13.7	26.0	9.4	2.0
Mini, Party, Tesco*	1 Pizza/11g	26	1.1	248	11.4	28.6	10.5	1.9
Mozarella & Tomato, Asda*	1 Pizza/360g	824	32.4	229	12.0	25.0	9.0	2.4
Mozarella & Tomato, Gluten Free, Dietary Specials*	1 Pizza/320g	646	15.0	202	6.7	33.1	4.7	1.3
Mozzarella E Provolone, la Bottega, Goodfella's*	½ Pizza/156g	372	15.0	238	10.1	27.9	9.6	2.4
Mozzarella, Giuseppe Taverna*	½ Pizza/175g	383	15.8	219	10.0	24.4	9.0	0.0
Mozzarella & Black Forest Ham, Asda*	¼ Pizza/110g	227	6.6	206	10.0	28.0	6.0	2.7
Mozzarella & Cherry Tomato, Stonebaked, Safeway*	½ Pizza/262.5g	618	20.5	235	10.6	30.3	7.8	3.5
Mushroom & Ham, COU, M & S*	1 Pizza/245g	355	4.4	145	8.8	24.0	1.8	2.2
Mushroom & Roasted Onion, Waitrose*	½ Pizza/187.4g	402	12.5	215	9.8	28.9	6.7	1.3
Napoletana, Sainsbury's*	½ Pizza/186g	424	14.3	228	9.7	29.9	7.7	3.1
Napoletana, TTD, Sainsbury's*	1 Pizza/374g	1070	45.6	286	11.1	28.5	12.2	2.0
Napoli, Tesco*	½ Pizza/183.5g	432	11.6	235	11.9	32.6	6.3	1.4
Napoli Ham & Mushroom, San Marco*	½ Pizza/219g	449	13.4	205	10.0	27.5	6.1	2.8
Pasta, Ristorante, Dr Oetker*	½ Pizza/205.02g	449	18.2	219	8.0	26.6	8.9	0.0
Pepper Steak, Deep Dish, Chicago Town*	1 Pack/365g	372	9.9	102	6.1	13.4	2.7	0.0
Pepperonata, Delicata, Sainsbury's*	1 Pizza/330g	917	47.5	278	12.9	24.3	14.4	2.6
Pepperoni, Aldi*	1 Serving/55g	123	4.3	224	8.7	29.5	7.9	1.4
Pepperoni, American Style Deep Pan, Co-Op*	1 Pizza/395g	988	39.5	250	12.0	28.0	10.0	1.0
Pepperoni, Asda*	½ Pizza/150g	386	13.5	257	10.0	34.0	9.0	2.7
Pepperoni, Chicago Town*	1 Sm Pizza/170g	471	21.9	277	11.5	28.8	12.9	0.0
Pepperoni, Deep & Crispy, Iceland*	1 Serving/175g	490	21.0	280	11.9	31.1	12.0	1.8
Pepperoni, Deep & Crispy, Somerfield*	¼ Slice/101g	236	7.3	234	10.7	31.6	7.2	1.6
Pepperoni, Deep Filled, Chicago Town*	1 Serving/202.3g	620	33.5	307	11.5	28.0	16.6	1.3
Pepperoni, Deep Pan, Farmfoods*	½ Pizza/202g	491	21.2	243	8.3	28.8	10.5	2.0
Pepperoni, Deep Pan, Frozen, Tesco*	½ Pizza/215g	527	17.4	245	11.9	31.1	8.1	2.6
Pepperoni, Deep Pan, Goodfella's*	¼ Slice/109g	294	12.6	270	12.7	28.9	11.6	1.6
Pepperoni, Deep Pan, Morrisons*	1 Pizza/382g	955	36.3	250	10.1	31.0	9.5	3.2
Pepperoni, Deep Pan, Safeway*	½ Pizza/198g	558	24.4	283	13.9	28.9	12.4	2.5
Pepperoni, Deep Pan, Sainsbury's*	½ Pizza/191g	478	20.6	250	9.9	28.3	10.8	3.2
Pepperoni, Deluxe, American Deep Pan, Sainsbury's*	1 Pizza/424g	1077	40.3	254	13.3	28.7	9.5	2.7
Pepperoni, Deluxe, Deep Pan, Sainsbury's*	1 Pizza/424g	1077	40.3	254	13.3	28.7	9.5	2.7
Pepperoni, Double, Italian, Chilled, Tesco*	½ Pizza/159.6g	455	23.3	285	12.4	25.6	14.6	2.4
Pepperoni, Extra, Chicago Town*	1 Pizza/460g	994	34.0	216	9.6	27.7	7.4	0.0
Pepperoni, Feast, Deep Dish, Schwan's*	1 Pizza/435g	1188	61.8	273	9.9	26.3	14.2	0.0
Pepperoni, Freschetta, Schwan's*	1 Pizza/310g	846	35.7	273	10.8	31.6	11.5	0.0
Pepperoni, Goodfella's*	1 Pizza/337g	900	43.5	267	13.2	26.3	12.9	1.7
Pepperoni, Hot & Spicy, Stuffed Crust, Asda*	1 Pizza/245g	666	30.0	272	13.9	26.5	12.2	2.4
Pepperoni, Hot & Spicy, Thin Crust, Chilled, Tesco*	½ Pizza/173.5g	486	25.5	280	12.4	24.0	14.7	2.2
Pepperoni, Individual, Chicago Town*	1 Pizza/170g	532	27.9	313	11.3	30.0	16.4	1.9
Pepperoni, Italian Stonebaked, Asda*	¼ Pizza/131.6g	329	13.2	250	12.0	28.0	10.0	2.8
Pepperoni, Italian Style, Somerfield*	1 Pizza/380g	920	30.4	242	11.0	32.0	8.0	0.0
Pepperoni, Micro, McCain*	1 Serving/135g	405	21.9	300	12.1	26.5	16.2	0.0
Pepperoni, Mini, Tesco*	1 Serving/22g	71	3.7	323	11.8	30.5	16.8	2.7
Pepperoni, Oven Rising, Safeway*	1 Serving/95g	259	8.6	273	8.2	39.9	9.0	1.9
Pepperoni, Pizzeria, Sainsbury's*	½ Pizza/197g	559	25.8	284	13.4	28.3	13.1	2.4
Pepperoni, Pizzeria Style, Sainsbury's*	½ Pizza/183g	515	23.3	281	13.5	28.0	12.7	2.2
Pepperoni, Speciale, Sainsbury's*	½ Pizza/179g	448	19.5	250	11.9	26.6	10.9	2.3
Pepperoni, Stone Baked, Carlos*	1 Pizza/330g	832	39.6	252	13.0	23.0	12.0	0.0
Pepperoni, Stone Baked, Pizzaroma, Safeway*	½ Pizza/178.4g	479	18.9	269	12.9	30.6	10.6	2.2

PIZZA

	Measure INFO/WEIGHT	per Measure		Nutrition Values per 100g / 100ml				
		KCAL	FAT	KCAL	PROT	CARB	FAT	FIBRE
Pepperoni, Stonebake, 10", Asda*	½ Pizza/170g	435	19.0	256	12.9	25.9	11.2	2.5
Pepperoni, Stonebaked, American Hot, Sainsbury's*	½ Pizza/276g	674	30.9	244	11.6	24.1	11.2	2.9
Pepperoni, Stonebaked, GFY, Asda*	1 Pizza/314g	760	18.8	242	11.0	36.0	6.0	1.6
Pepperoni, Stonebaked, Pizzaroma, Safeway*	½ Pizza/178.4g	479	18.9	269	12.9	30.6	10.6	2.2
Pepperoni, Stonebaked, Stateside Foods*	½ Pizza/167.7g	437	18.0	260	11.8	29.0	10.7	2.1
Pepperoni, Stonebaked Ciabatta, Goodfella's*	½ Pizza/181g	503	26.1	278	11.9	27.4	14.4	2.4
Pepperoni, Thin & Crispy, Co-Op*	1 Pizza/270g	689	29.7	255	11.0	26.0	11.0	1.0
Pepperoni, Thin & Crispy, Goodfella's*	1 Pizza/593g	1595	70.0	269	13.8	26.9	11.8	2.3
Pepperoni, Thin & Crispy, Morrisons*	½ Pizza/144g	426	17.1	296	13.3	33.8	11.9	2.0
Pepperoni, Thin & Crispy, Safeway*	½ Pizza/133.1g	394	16.8	296	11.8	33.9	12.6	1.5
Pepperoni, Thin & Crispy, Sainsbury's*	½ Pizza/132g	405	18.9	307	13.9	30.7	14.3	2.6
Pepperoni, Thin & Crispy, Somerfield*	½ Pizza/169.1g	470	20.4	278	13.5	28.7	12.1	2.7
Pepperoni, Thin Crust, Chilled, Tesco*	½ Pizza/163g	479	24.4	295	13.5	25.4	15.0	1.8
Pepperoni, TTD, Sainsbury's*	1/3 Pizza/171g	461	18.3	270	14.2	29.3	10.7	2.3
Pepperoni, XXX Hot, Deep & Crispy, Chilled, Tesco*	½ Pizza/119.9g	300	12.3	250	9.1	30.1	10.3	2.0
Pepperoni, Zingy, Asda*	1 Serving/90g	255	6.3	283	12.0	43.0	7.0	4.0
Pepperoni & Cheese, Asda*	½ Pizza/150g	386	13.5	257	10.0	34.0	9.0	2.7
Pepperoni & Jalapeno Chill, Asda*	1 Pizza/277g	742	22.2	268	10.0	39.0	8.0	1.8
Pepperoni & Onion, 9", Sainsbury's*	½ Pizza/207g	615	26.9	297	13.4	31.7	13.0	1.9
Pepperoni Bacon, Primo*	½ Pizza/111g	360	14.5	324	10.5	42.5	13.1	0.0
Pleasure with Fire Roasted Vegetables, Heinz*	½ Pizza/200g	418	16.0	209	9.5	24.8	8.0	2.4
Pollo, Ristorante, Dr Oetker*	½ Pizza/177.55g	384	16.9	216	8.9	23.4	9.5	0.0
Pollo Ad Astra, Pizza Express*	1 Pizza/317g	602	14.9	190	11.6	25.2	4.7	2.7
Prosciutto, Classico, Tesco*	½ Pizza/205g	461	10.0	225	11.7	33.6	4.9	2.5
Prosciutto, Italian Style, Co-Op*	½ Pizza/183g	421	12.8	230	13.0	29.0	7.0	3.0
Prosciutto, Pizzaria, Sainsbury's*	1 Pizza/325g	806	23.1	248	11.4	34.7	7.1	3.2
Prosciutto, Ristorante, Dr Oetker*	1 Pizza/330g	752	32.3	228	10.3	24.6	9.8	0.0
Prosciutto & Fresh Rocket, TTD, Sainsbury's*	½ Pizza/164.2g	541	22.3	330	11.9	39.9	13.6	2.5
Prosciutto & Mascarpone, Safeway*	½ Pizza/200g	522	20.6	261	12.3	29.8	10.3	2.2
Quattro Formaggi, 8", Supermarket, Pizza Express*	1 Pizza/492g	1196	48.2	243	12.1	26.5	9.8	2.3
Quattro Formaggi, Ristorante, Dr Oetker*	½ Pizza/175g	473	25.0	270	11.4	23.9	14.3	0.0
Quattro Formaggi, Supermarket, Pizza Express*	1 Pizza/492g	1196	48.2	243	12.1	26.5	9.8	2.3
Quattro Formaggi Pizzeria, Sainsbury's*	½ Pizza/175g	490	21.2	280	12.8	30.8	12.1	2.5
Quattro Formaggio, Tesco*	½ Pizza/219.2g	583	27.4	266	13.3	25.1	12.5	1.8
Roasted Mushroom & Bacon, Thin Crust, M & S*	½ Pizza/111.1g	300	14.0	270	10.4	28.5	12.6	1.8
Roasted Tomato & Mozzarella, BGTY, Sainsbury's*	1 Pizza/204g	526	16.4	258	17.8	28.6	8.0	6.0
Roasted Vegetable, for One, GFY, Asda*	1 Pizza/96.0g	190	3.6	198	9.0	32.0	3.8	1.5
Roasted Vegetable, Wood Fired, Pizzaroma, Safeway*	½ Pizza/175g	350	11.0	200	7.9	27.0	6.3	5.1
Salame, Ristorante, Dr Oetker*	½ Pizza/159.82g	456	24.5	285	10.4	26.3	15.3	0.0
Salami, Lidl*	1 Pizza/350g	854	32.2	244	8.1	29.4	9.2	0.0
Salami, Ultra Thin Italian, Tesco*	1 Serving/263g	692	25.5	263	12.0	31.9	9.7	1.0
Salami & Ham, Pizzeria, Waitrose*	½ Pizza/205g	443	13.7	216	10.1	28.7	6.7	1.8
Salami & Pepperoni, Waitrose*	½ Pizza/190g	578	30.8	304	13.4	23.9	16.2	2.1
Salami Con Mozarella, Lidl*	½ Pizza/200g	534	22.4	267	9.9	31.5	11.2	0.0
Sicilian, Premium, Co-Op*	1 Pizza/600g	1320	48.0	220	9.0	27.0	8.0	2.0
Siciliana, Frozen, Finest, Tesco*	1 Serving/247.5g	432	14.4	174	8.5	21.9	5.8	3.2
Simply Cheese, Goodfella's*	¼ Pizza/81.9g	226	11.0	276	16.3	22.5	13.4	1.9
Slice Selection, M & S*	1 Serving/52g	120	4.1	230	9.4	30.3	7.8	1.9
Sloppy Giuseppe, 12", Supermarket, Pizza Express*	½ Pizza/182g	349	12.0	192	9.4	23.6	6.6	2.3
Sloppy Giuseppe, 8", Supermarket, Pizza Express*	½ Pizza/152.5g	291	9.6	191	9.4	24.1	6.3	2.5
Sloppy Giuseppe, Supermarket, Pizza Express*	½ Pizza/152.5g	291	9.6	191	9.4	24.1	6.3	2.5
Smoked Ham & Mushroom, Thin & Crispy, Co-Op*	1 Pizza/400g	792	18.0	198	9.0	30.3	4.5	1.7
Smoked Ham & Peppers, HL, Tesco*	1 Serving/282g	386	5.6	137	8.7	21.1	2.0	1.8

P

PIZZA

INFO/WEIGHT	Measure	per Measure KCAL	FAT	Nutrition Values per 100g / 100ml KCAL	PROT	CARB	FAT	FIBRE
Smoked Ham & Pineapple, Deep Pan, Co-Op*	1 Pizza/395g	1142	41.9	289	11.6	36.7	10.6	1.7
Smoked Ham & Pineapple, Weight Watchers*	1 Pizza/241g	429	7.0	178	10.3	27.6	2.9	1.5
Spicy Beef, Goodfella's*	½ Pizza/147.5g	392	17.9	265	12.4	26.5	12.1	2.2
Spicy Chicken, Foccacia, Sainsbury's*	½ Pizza/245g	581	18.6	237	12.0	30.3	7.6	2.5
Spicy Chicken, HL, Tesco*	1 Serving/252g	418	4.0	166	10.9	27.1	1.6	2.7
Spicy Chicken, Iceland*	1 Pizza/345g	797	22.8	231	13.4	29.9	6.6	1.5
Spicy Chicken, Micro, McCain*	1 Pizza/133g	388	20.0	292	12.4	26.9	15.0	0.0
Spicy Chicken, Somerfield*	1 Serving/132.5g	305	8.3	229	13.4	29.7	6.3	0.0
Spicy Chorizo, Red Pepper & Chilli, Classico, Tesco*	1 Serving/218g	474	17.4	218	10.3	26.4	8.0	2.5
Spicy Vegetable, Low Fat, Bertorelli*	1 Pizza/180g	243	4.3	135	6.0	23.4	2.4	1.9
Spicy Vegetable Nacho, GFY, Asda*	1 Pizza/282.7g	637	12.7	225	10.0	36.0	4.5	3.3
Spinach & Bacon, Thin & Crispy, M & S*	1 Pizza/290g	740	35.1	255	10.6	26.8	12.1	1.0
Spinach & Ricotta, 50% Less Fat, Italian, Sainsbury's*	1 Pizza/345g	759	16.2	220	12.8	31.6	4.7	3.4
Spinach & Ricotta, BGTY, Sainsbury's*	1 Pizza/265g	535	6.6	202	10.4	34.4	2.5	2.6
Spinach & Ricotta, Extra Special, Asda*	1 Pizza/400g	940	28.0	235	9.0	34.0	7.0	1.9
Spinach & Ricotta, GFY, Asda*	1 Pizza/160g	375	7.0	234	8.8	40.0	4.4	1.8
Spinach & Ricotta, Italian, Chilled, Sainsbury's*	1 Pizza/361g	859	34.7	238	9.3	28.7	9.6	2.3
Spinach & Ricotta, Italian, Somerfield*	1 Pizza/370g	918	37.0	248	10.3	29.2	10.0	2.2
Spinach & Ricotta, PB, Waitrose*	½ Pizza/165g	272	2.8	165	9.7	27.7	1.7	2.6
Spinach & Ricotta, Pizzaria, Waitrose*	½ Pizza/238g	501	21.1	211	10.7	21.9	8.9	2.6
Spinach & Ricotta, Pizzaroma, Safeway*	1 Pizza/420g	1042	37.0	248	10.9	31.4	8.8	3.6
Spinach & Ricotta, Thin Crust, Italian, Tesco*	½ Pizza/190g	365	16.7	192	9.6	18.7	8.8	1.9
Spinach with Bacon & Mushroom, GFY, Asda*	1 Serving/270g	618	12.2	229	13.0	34.0	4.5	2.6
Steak, Stone Bake, M & S*	1 Pizza/400g	820	26.8	205	9.9	25.7	6.7	1.4
Sunblushed Tomato & Mascarpone, Pizzadella, Tesco*	1 Serving/275g	894	44.0	325	8.5	36.7	16.0	1.5
Super Supreme, Family, Chicago Town*	¼ Pizza/225g	527	24.3	234	9.6	24.5	10.8	0.0
Supreme, Deep Dish, Individual, Chicago Town*	1 Pizza/170g	456	20.4	268	9.2	30.8	12.0	1.0
Supreme, Deep Pan, Safeway*	1 Serving/189g	450	18.1	238	10.8	27.0	9.6	4.7
Supreme, McCain*	1 Serving/125g	267	8.6	214	10.9	27.0	6.9	0.0
Supreme, Square to Share, Farmfoods*	1 Serving/93g	196	8.0	211	10.7	22.9	8.6	1.1
Sweet & Sour Chicken, Thin Crust, Tesco*	½ Pizza/186g	366	12.8	197	11.9	21.9	6.9	2.3
Sweet Chilli Chicken, BGTY, Sainsbury's*	½ Pizza/138g	276	2.3	200	13.0	33.2	1.7	2.1
Sweet Chilli Chicken, Stonebaked, Goodfella's*	½ Pizza/170g	423	20.6	249	12.9	22.3	12.1	3.0
The Big Cheese, Deep Pan, Goodfella's*	1/6 Pizza/118g	295	12.7	250	12.2	25.9	10.8	1.1
The Big Eat Meat X-Treme, Deep Pan, Goodfella's*	½ Pizza/352g	806	28.9	229	11.6	27.1	8.2	3.6
Three Cheese, Ultra Thin, Sodebo*	1 Pizza/180g	450	18.4	250	10.9	28.5	10.2	1.8
Three Cheese Calzone, Waitrose*	1 Calzone/265g	747	31.8	282	10.4	33.0	12.0	1.4
Three Cheeses & Tomato, Stonebaked, Co-Op*	1 Pizza/415g	888	33.6	214	10.0	25.2	8.1	1.5
Three Meat, Thin & Crispy, Sainsbury's*	½ Pizza/147g	344	15.7	234	12.5	23.4	10.7	1.3
Tomato, Aubergine & Spinach, Pizzeria, Waitrose*	½ Pizza/193g	403	7.7	209	7.8	35.4	4.0	3.6
Tomato, Basil & Garlic, Weight Watchers*	1 Serving/85g	169	2.9	199	12.3	29.8	3.4	1.6
Tomato, Mushroom & Bacon, Deep Pan, Co-Op*	1 Pizza/420g	882	33.6	210	9.0	25.0	8.0	2.0
Tomato & Cheese, Ross*	1 Pizza/81g	181	6.2	224	7.4	31.5	7.6	2.5
Tomato & Cheese, Savers, Safeway*	1 Pizza/140g	371	11.3	265	9.5	38.4	8.1	3.0
Tomato & Cheese, Stone Bake, M & S*	1 Pizza/340g	782	28.6	230	10.8	30.1	8.4	1.6
Tomato & Cheese, Thin & Crispy, M & S*	1 Pizza/300g	705	28.2	235	11.0	27.7	9.4	1.2
Tomato & Mascarpone Piccadella, Tesco*	½ Pizza/128g	281	9.7	220	8.4	29.8	7.6	1.5
Tomato & Pesto, Tesco*	1 Serving/176g	449	23.2	256	8.4	25.9	13.2	1.1
Tomato & Red Pepper, PB, Waitrose*	½ Pizza/163g	313	2.4	192	6.6	38.1	1.5	1.9
Tomato & Ricotta, Waitrose*	½ Pizza/207.5g	443	18.4	214	7.8	25.7	8.9	2.2
Triple Cheese, Deep Dish, Chicago Town*	1 Serving/170g	418	18.2	246	9.9	27.6	10.7	0.0
Triple Cheese, Deep Pan, Morrisons*	1/6 Pizza/74.7g	199	9.2	265	10.4	28.2	12.3	1.9
Tuna & Caramelised Red Onion, COU, M & S*	1 Pizza/245g	429	5.6	175	9.6	26.7	2.3	1.2

	Measure INFO/WEIGHT	per Measure KCAL	FAT	Nutrition Values per 100g / 100ml KCAL	PROT	CARB	FAT	FIBRE
PIZZA								
Tuna Sweetcorn, BGTY, Sainsbury's*	1 Pizza/304g	602	5.8	198	13.5	31.7	1.9	2.7
Tuscan Vegetable & Mozzarella, WTF, Sainsbury's*	1 Pizza/317g	552	15.9	174	5.7	26.6	5.0	2.3
Tuscana, Finest, Tesco*	1 Serving/255g	643	35.7	252	13.2	18.4	14.0	5.9
Vegetable, Asda*	1 Pizza/485g	1020	44.0	210	7.0	25.2	9.1	3.3
Vegetable, COU, M & S*	1 Pizza/294g	397	7.1	135	6.4	23.2	2.4	1.9
Vegetable, Deep & Crispy, Somerfield*	½ Pizza/212g	477	16.3	225	9.7	29.2	7.7	1.5
Vegetable, Deep Pan, Co-Op*	1 Pizza/425g	829	29.8	195	8.0	25.0	7.0	2.0
Vegetable, Frozen, HL, Tesco*	1 Pizza/400g	604	10.8	151	8.1	23.5	2.7	4.4
Vegetable, GFY, Asda*	¼ Pizza/94g	141	2.7	150	7.0	24.0	2.9	3.7
Vegetable, HL, Tesco*	1 Serving/200g	302	5.4	151	8.1	23.5	2.7	4.4
Vegetable, Stone Bake, M & S*	1 Serving/465g	837	26.0	180	7.8	25.0	5.6	1.5
Vegetable, Thin & Crispy, Iceland*	½ Pizza/200g	442	21.2	221	8.3	23.2	10.6	1.7
Vegetable Feast, Thin & Crispy, Iceland*	1 Slice/63g	148	6.9	237	7.8	26.5	11.1	1.8
Vegetable Supreme, Safeway*	¼ Pizza/170g	352	11.7	207	10.4	25.9	6.9	2.9
Vegetale, Ristorante, Dr Oetker*	½ Pizza/184.93g	387	16.6	209	8.1	23.9	9.0	0.0
Verona, Frozen, Finest, Tesco*	1 Serving/237.5g	543	23.3	228	11.6	23.2	9.8	2.7
PIZZA BASE								
Authentic Italian, Napolina*	½ Base/75g	218	2.3	291	7.9	58.0	3.0	0.2
Garlic Bread, Sainsbury's*	¼ Base/58.7g	109	4.2	186	5.1	25.4	7.1	1.8
Gluten & Wheat Free, Glutafin*	1 Base/110g	309	5.5	281	3.0	56.0	5.0	6.0
Italian, Classic, Sainsbury's*	1 Base/150g	452	7.2	301	7.6	57.0	4.8	1.5
Light & Crispy, Napolina*	1 Base/150g	437	4.5	291	7.9	58.0	3.0	0.2
Mini, Napolina*	1 Base/75g	218	2.3	291	7.9	58.0	3.0	0.2
Thin & Crispy, Morrisons*	1 Base/130g	355	7.4	273	8.3	47.1	5.7	4.3
Thin & Crispy, Sainsbury's*	1 Base/135g	338	4.2	251	8.4	47.3	3.1	4.4
PIZZA POCKET								
Chargrilled Chicken & Veg, HE, Tesco*	1 Pack/190g	304	4.6	160	11.4	23.1	2.4	2.8
PLAICE								
& Prawns, in Breadcrumbs, Aldi*	1 Serving/100g	212	8.4	212	8.6	25.4	8.4	0.0
Filled with Mushrooms, Somerfield*	1 Plaice/169.8g	338	18.0	199	10.2	15.7	10.6	1.2
Filled with Prawns & Garlic, Somerfield*	1 Plaice/171g	366	20.3	214	12.0	14.8	11.9	0.7
Fillets, in Breadcrumbs, Average	1 Serving/150g	331	17.9	221	12.8	15.5	11.9	0.8
Fillets, Lightly Dusted, Average	1 Fillet/113g	188	9.2	166	12.9	10.5	8.2	0.6
Fillets, Raw, Average	1oz/28g	24	0.4	87	18.3	0.0	1.5	0.0
Fillets, with Prawns, Asda*	1oz/28g	24	1.3	86	11.0	0.4	4.5	0.7
Goujons, Baked	1oz/28g	85	5.1	304	8.8	27.7	18.3	0.0
Goujons, Fried in Blended Oil	1oz/28g	119	9.0	426	8.5	27.0	32.3	0.0
in Batter, Fried in Blended Oil	1oz/28g	72	4.7	257	15.2	12.0	16.8	0.5
PLAICE WITH								
Mushrooms & Prawns, Sainsbury's*	1 Serving/170g	354	18.2	208	12.0	15.9	10.7	1.7
Spinach & Cheddar Cheese, Fillets, Sainsbury's*	1 Serving/154g	222	13.3	144	13.6	3.1	8.6	0.8
Spinach & Ricotta Cheese, Whole, Sainsbury's*	1 Fillet/159g	334	16.7	210	11.6	17.2	10.5	0.8
PLANTAIN								
Boiled in Unsalted Water	1oz/28g	31	0.1	112	0.8	28.5	0.2	1.2
Raw	1oz/28g	33	0.1	117	1.1	29.4	0.3	1.3
Ripe, Fried in Vegetable Oil	1oz/28g	75	2.6	267	1.5	47.5	9.2	2.3
PLUMS								
Average, Stewed without Sugar	1oz/28g	8	0.0	30	0.5	7.3	0.1	1.3
Dried, Soft, Blue Parrot Cafe, Sainsbury's*	1 Pack/50g	119	0.3	237	2.6	55.6	0.5	7.1
Weighed with Stone, Average	1 Plum/90g	32	0.1	36	0.6	8.6	0.1	1.6
Yellow, Waitrose*	1 Plum/50g	20	0.1	39	0.6	8.8	0.1	1.5
POLENTA								
Merchant Gourmet*	1 Serving/65g	232	0.9	357	7.4	78.8	1.4	1.3

P

INFO/WEIGHT	Measure	per Measure		Nutrition Values per 100g / 100ml				
		KCAL	FAT	KCAL	PROT	CARB	FAT	FIBRE
POLENTA								
Organic, Kallo*	1 Serving/150g	543	2.7	362	8.5	78.0	1.8	0.0
POLLOCK								
Breaded, Asda*	1 Portion/97g	200	9.7	206	12.0	17.0	10.0	1.0
POLO								
Fruits, Nestle*	1 Tube/37g	142	0.0	383	0.0	96.0	0.0	0.0
Mints, Clear Ice, Nestle*	1 Polo/4g	16	0.0	390	0.0	97.5	0.0	0.0
Mints, Original, Nestle*	1 Mint/2g	8	0.0	404	0.0	98.9	1.1	0.0
Spearmint, Nestle*	1 Tube/35g	141	0.4	402	0.0	98.2	1.1	0.0
POMEGRANATE								
Freshly Prepared, M & S*	1 Serving/110g	61	0.2	55	1.3	11.8	0.2	3.4
POP TARTS								
Strawberry Sensation, Kellogg's*	1 Pop Tart/50g	198	5.5	395	4.0	70.0	11.0	2.0
POPCORN								
94% Fat Free, Orville Redenbacher's*	1 Bag/76g	220	0.0	289	13.2	65.8	0.0	0.0
Butter, 6% Fat, Orville Redenbacher's*	1 Portion/21g	86	1.2	410	11.9	77.6	5.7	14.3
Butter, Microwave, 94% Fat Free, Act II*	½ Bag/41g	130	2.5	317	9.8	68.3	6.1	12.2
Butter, Microwave, Act II*	1 Bag/90g	425	16.2	472	9.0	69.0	18.0	9.0
Butter Flavour, Microwave, Popz*	1 Serving/100g	504	30.0	504	7.0	51.5	30.0	9.2
Butter Toffee, Asda*	1 Serving/100g	364	8.0	364	2.1	71.0	8.0	4.1
Butter Toffee, Snack-A-Jacks, Quaker*	1 Std Bag/35g	149	3.2	425	3.5	86.0	9.0	4.5
Butter Toffee, Tesco*	1 Pack/350g	1418	27.0	405	2.2	81.7	7.7	4.3
Butter Toffee, Yummy*	1 Serving/50g	228	6.4	455	2.5	82.4	12.8	3.1
Lightly Salted, Snack-A-Jack, Quaker*	1 Bag/15g	56	1.5	370	12.1	58.0	9.9	14.6
Plain, Oil Popped, Average	1 Av Sm/74g	439	31.7	593	6.2	48.7	42.8	0.0
Ready Salted, Microwave, Popz*	1 Serving/20g	101	6.0	504	7.0	51.5	30.0	9.2
Salted, Blockbuster*	1 Bowl/25g	99	2.9	397	10.6	62.2	11.7	8.6
Salted, Bop, Microwave, Zanuy*	1 Serving/25g	119	5.8	477	10.7	56.9	23.0	0.0
Salted, Light, Microwave, Act II*	1 Pack/85g	336	6.5	395	10.6	71.0	7.6	15.8
Salted, Microwave, 93% Fat Free, Act II*	1 Pack/85g	345	6.0	406	10.0	76.0	7.0	13.0
Salted, Sold At Cinema, Playtime Popcorn*	1 Av Sm/74g	384	24.9	519	8.3	45.9	33.6	0.0
Sea Salt, Sainsbury's*	1 Portion/30g	138	5.9	460	10.2	60.2	19.8	5.7
Sweet, Best-In*	1 Serving/34g	161	5.8	473	7.3	72.6	17.0	0.0
Sweet, Blockbuster*	1 Bag/120g	540	26.2	450	5.9	57.5	21.8	11.1
Sweet, Butterkist, Butterkist*	1 Pack/120g	612	29.8	510	2.8	68.5	24.8	5.6
Sweet, Microwave, Cinema, Popz*	1 Bag/85g	420	21.7	494	6.0	60.0	25.5	8.2
Toffee, 90% Fat Free, Butterkist*	1 Pack/35g	142	3.3	406	2.8	77.7	9.3	0.0
Toffee, Best-In*	1 Bag/90g	356	3.2	396	5.0	85.9	3.6	0.0
Toffee, Blockbuster*	¼ Pack/25g	111	3.4	442	2.1	80.2	13.5	4.3
Toffee, Butterkist*	1 Serving/35g	135	2.8	385	1.8	76.4	8.0	3.5
Toffee, Chicago Joes*	1 Serving/10g	31	0.5	314	3.1	84.6	4.8	0.0
Toffee, Milk Chocolate Coated, Sainsbury's*	¼ Bag/25g	130	6.6	520	6.5	64.1	26.4	1.3
Toffee, Sainsbury's*	1 Serving/50g	208	6.4	415	1.8	73.8	12.7	3.3
POPPADOMS								
Fried in Vegetable Oil, Average	1 Poppadom/10g	37	1.7	369	17.5	39.1	16.9	0.0
M & S*	1 Poppadom/8g	35	1.8	438	18.8	40.0	22.5	8.8
Mercifully Mild, Phileas Fogg*	1 Serving/30g	150	9.8	499	14.8	36.8	32.6	6.0
Mini, Sainsbury's*	½ Pack/50g	249	16.2	498	14.9	36.9	32.3	7.6
Plain, Asda*	1 Poppadom/9g	44	2.5	484	18.0	40.0	28.0	0.0
Plain, Indian to Go, Sainsbury's*	1 Poppadom/9g	32	1.4	405	18.4	43.4	17.5	9.0
Plain, Tesco*	1 Serving/9.4	41	2.0	439	17.8	44.4	21.1	4.6
Plain, Waitrose*	1 Serving/9g	37	1.7	408	21.0	39.3	18.6	9.1
Spicy, COU, M & S*	1 Pack/26g	85	0.6	325	23.5	51.9	2.4	8.1

P

	Measure INFO/WEIGHT	per Measure KCAL	FAT	Nutrition Values per 100g / 100ml KCAL	PROT	CARB	FAT	FIBRE
POPPETS*								
Chocolate Raisins, Poppets*	1 Pack/37.9g	152	5.0	401	4.9	65.4	13.3	0.0
Mint Cream, Poppets*	1oz/28g	119	3.6	424	2.0	75.0	13.0	0.0
Toffee, Milk Chocolate, Poppets*	1 Box/100g	491	23.0	491	5.3	68.0	23.0	0.0
PORK								
& Ham, Chopped, Tinned, BGTY, Sainsbury's*	1 Serving/50g	50	1.1	100	19.1	0.1	2.2	0.0
Chop, Lean & Fat, Raw, Average	1oz/28g	67	3.8	240	29.2	0.0	13.7	0.0
Diced, Lean, Average	1oz/28g	31	0.5	109	22.1	0.0	1.8	0.0
Escalope, Average	1 Escalope/75g	108	1.7	145	31.1	0.0	2.3	0.0
Escalope, Lean, Healthy Range, Average	1 Escalope/75g	80	1.5	107	22.0	0.0	2.1	0.0
Joint, Ready to Roast, Average	½ Joint/254.2g	375	18.0	148	19.3	2.3	7.1	0.2
Joint, Stuffed, Apricot & Orange, Sainsbury's*	¼ Joint/200g	566	36.2	283	29.0	0.9	18.1	1.4
Joint, Stuffed, Leek & Cheese Stuffing, Sainsbury's*	1 Serving/100g	231	10.5	231	31.0	3.0	10.5	1.1
Joint, Stuffed, Sage, Onion & Lemon, Sainsbury's*	1 Serving/260g	699	43.4	269	27.4	2.2	16.7	1.4
Leg, Joint, Healthy Range, Average	1 Serving/200g	206	4.4	103	20.1	0.6	2.2	0.0
Lemon & Thyme, TTD, Sainsbury's*	1 Serving/67g	159	10.2	238	19.8	5.6	15.2	0.3
Loin, Joint, Roast, Lean	1oz/28g	51	1.9	182	30.1	0.0	6.8	0.0
Loin, Joint, Roasted, Lean & Fat	1oz/28g	71	4.3	253	26.3	0.0	15.3	0.0
Loin, Oak Smoked, Sainsbury's*	1 Slice/13g	20	0.9	163	24.0	0.9	7.0	0.1
Loin, Roasted, with Rosemary, Arista, Sainsbury's*	1 Slice/17g	24	1.2	144	20.8	0.1	6.8	0.7
Loin, Smoked, Cured, M & S*	1oz/28g	43	2.5	155	18.1	0.0	9.1	0.0
Loin, Steak, Fried, Lean	1oz/28g	53	2.0	191	31.5	0.0	7.2	0.0
Loin, Steak, Fried, Lean & Fat	1oz/28g	77	5.2	276	27.5	0.0	18.4	0.0
Loin, Stuffed, Roast, M & S*	1 Slice/12g	22	0.9	180	24.4	2.4	7.9	0.0
Loin Steaks, with Tomato & Apricot Sauce, Sainsbury's*	½ Pack/110g	216	10.6	196	24.4	3.1	9.6	0.6
Medallions, Average	1 Pack/220g	179	2.8	163	35.1	0.1	2.5	0.5
Mince, Lean, Healthy Range, Average	1 Pack/400g	504	20.2	126	19.8	0.4	5.1	0.3
Mince, Raw	1oz/28g	46	2.7	164	19.2	0.0	9.7	0.0
Mince, Stewed	1oz/28g	53	2.9	191	24.4	0.0	10.4	0.0
Raw, Lean, Average	1oz/28g	42	1.2	151	28.6	0.0	4.1	0.0
Rib Roast, Outdoor Reared, TTD, Sainsbury's*	1 Serving/138g	206	5.2	150	27.6	1.2	3.8	1.2
Roast, Lean Only, Average	1oz/28g	34	0.9	121	22.7	0.3	3.3	0.0
Roast, Slices, Average	1 Slice/30g	40	1.4	134	22.7	0.5	4.5	0.0
Roll, Haslet, Slices, Tesco*	1 Slice/15.5g	34	2.3	220	13.2	8.3	14.6	0.0
Shoulder, Leek & Bacon Stuffing, Roast, Sainsbury's*	1 Serving/150g	237	12.5	158	18.8	2.4	8.3	0.5
Shoulder, Slices, Cured	1oz/28g	29	1.0	103	16.9	0.9	3.6	0.0
Sliced, Chinese, M & S*	1 Serving/140g	224	4.3	160	26.4	6.1	3.1	0.0
Steak, Lean, Stewed	1oz/28g	49	1.3	176	33.6	0.0	4.6	0.0
Steak, Lean & Fat, Average	1oz/28g	61	3.8	219	23.8	0.0	13.7	0.1
Stir Fry Strips, Lean, Healthy Range, Average	¼ Pack/113g	118	2.3	104	21.3	0.0	2.0	0.0
Tenderloin, Roulade, Waitrose*	1 Pack/171g	282	12.8	165	18.4	5.9	7.5	1.8
PORK &								
Apricots, Aromatic, Cafe Culture, M & S*	½ Pack/420g	672	31.1	160	10.3	12.5	7.4	2.1
Chestnut Stuffing, M & S*	1oz/28g	64	4.8	230	5.3	12.6	17.1	3.7
PORK CHAR SUI								
Chinese, Tesco*	1 Pack/400g	521	17.2	130	7.2	15.7	4.3	0.6
in Cantonese Sauce, Asda*	1 Pack/360g	623	7.9	173	9.8	28.4	2.2	0.5
Takeaway, Iceland*	1 Pack/400g	412	9.6	103	7.9	12.5	2.4	1.2
with Chicken, & Egg Fried Rice, Tesco*	1 Serving/450g	602	16.2	134	7.1	18.3	3.6	0.9
PORK CHINESE								
Style, GFY, Asda*	1 Serving/170g	286	6.0	168	18.8	15.3	3.5	0.4
with Noodles, Tesco*	1 Serving/450g	612	25.7	136	7.0	14.2	5.7	1.1
PORK DINNER								
Roast, Birds Eye*	1 Pack/340g	410	12.0	121	7.7	14.7	3.5	1.6

P

	Measure INFO/WEIGHT	per Measure KCAL	FAT	Nutrition Values per 100g / 100ml KCAL	PROT	CARB	FAT	FIBRE
PORK IN								
Light Mustard Sauce, Fillet, COU, M & S*	1 Pack/390g	312	9.4	80	10.9	3.5	2.4	0.7
Mustard & Cream, Chops	1oz/28g	73	6.0	261	14.5	2.4	21.6	0.3
Rich Sage & Onion Gravy, Steaks, Tesco*	1 Serving/160g	218	10.4	136	16.0	3.2	6.5	1.5
PORK SCRATCHINGS								
Crunch, Mr Porky*	1 Pack/30g	159	9.6	531	60.4	0.5	31.9	4.6
KP Snacks*	1 Pack/20g	125	9.6	624	47.3	0.5	48.1	0.5
Pub Original, Freshers Foods Ltd*	1 Pack/50g	311	24.7	621	46.6	0.1	49.3	0.6
Tavern Snacks*	1 Pack/30g	187	14.4	624	47.3	0.5	48.1	0.5
PORK WITH								
Cheese & Pineapple, Loin Steaks, M & S*	1 Steak/141g	240	14.0	170	14.0	6.3	9.9	0.0
Herbes De Provence, Joint, Sainsbury's*	¼ Joint/200g	302	16.4	151	19.2	0.1	8.2	0.6
Honey & Mustard Sauce, Steaks, Tesco*	½ Pack/160g	258	11.8	161	16.3	8.7	7.4	1.4
Honey & Soy, Sainsbury's*	1 Serving/260g	260	7.5	100	12.3	6.2	2.9	0.3
Maple & BBQ Sauce, Loin Steaks, Somerfield*	½ Pack/160g	336	16.0	210	20.4	9.2	10.0	0.0
Medallions, with Bramley Apple, M & S*	1 Serving/380g	418	12.9	110	17.7	2.5	3.4	0.5
Noodles, Chinese, Tesco*	1 Serving/450g	464	13.5	103	5.3	13.7	3.0	1.4
Peppers, Marinated, Tapas, Waitrose*	1 Serving/105g	181	6.7	172	26.3	2.2	6.4	0.3
Sage & Onion Stuffing, Joint, Tesco*	1 Serving/200g	208	5.6	104	17.1	2.7	2.8	0.0
Thai Style Butter, Steaks, Asda*	4 Steaks/300g	810	54.0	270	26.0	1.0	18.0	0.0
PORT								
Average	1 Serving/50ml	79	0.0	157	0.1	12.0	0.0	0.0
POT NOODLE*								
Balti Curry, Made Up, Pot Noodle*	1 Pot/301.1g	268	1.5	89	3.1	17.8	0.5	0.5
Beef & Tomato, Made Up, Pot Noodle*	1 Pot/300g	378	14.1	126	3.1	18.1	4.7	1.1
Beef & Tomato, Mini, Pot Noodle*	1 Pot/190g	254	9.5	134	3.5	18.7	5.0	1.7
Bombay Bad Boy, Made Up, Pot Noodle*	1 Pot/320g	416	15.4	130	3.3	18.4	4.8	1.1
Chicken & Mushroom, King, Pot Noodle*	1 Pack/401g	513	19.2	128	3.2	18.1	4.8	1.1
Chicken & Mushroom, Made Up, Pot Noodle*	1 Pot/300g	384	14.1	128	3.2	18.0	4.7	1.1
Chicken Curry, Hot, Made Up, Pot Noodle*	1 Pot/300g	384	14.1	128	2.8	18.7	4.7	1.1
Chow Mein, Chinese, Pot Noodle*	1 Pot/320g	395	14.8	123	2.9	17.5	4.6	1.2
Hot, Made Up, Pot Noodle*	1 Pot/300g	378	15.6	126	3.0	16.9	5.2	1.1
Hot Dog & Ketchup, Made Up, Pot Noodle*	1 Pot/189.8g	243	8.6	128	3.6	18.3	4.5	1.5
Korma Curry, Made Up, Pot Noodle*	1 Pot/300g	273	3.3	91	2.9	17.4	1.1	0.4
Nice & Spicy, Made Up, Pot Noodle*	1 Pot/300g	381	14.1	127	2.8	18.3	4.7	1.1
Seedy Sanchez, Made Up, Pot Noodle*	1 Pot/300g	396	14.4	132	3.1	19.1	4.8	1.1
Spicy Chilli, Posh, Made Up, Pot Noodle*	1 Pot/300.9g	328	17.8	109	2.5	11.7	5.9	1.0
Spicy Curry, Made Up, Pot Noodle*	1 Pot/300g	393	14.4	131	2.9	19.1	4.8	1.1
Sweet & Sour, Dry, Pot Noodle*	1 Pot/86g	376	13.8	437	12.1	60.9	16.1	3.1
Sweet & Sour, King, Dry, Pot Noodle*	1 Serving/105g	473	20.1	450	8.8	60.0	19.1	4.8
Sweet & Sour, Oriental, Posh, Pot Noodle*	1 Serving/300g	375	13.8	125	1.7	19.2	4.6	0.5
POTATO BITES								
Crispy, Morrisons*	1 Serving/115g	240	8.3	209	3.5	32.6	7.2	2.2
POTATO BOMBAY								
Average	1oz/28g	33	1.9	117	2.0	13.7	6.8	1.2
Canned, Tesco*	1 Can/400g	380	11.6	95	2.5	13.5	2.9	2.3
Chilled, Tesco*	1 Pack/300g	240	12.6	80	1.3	9.3	4.2	2.1
Curry Pot, Asda*	1 Pack/354.5g	358	21.3	101	1.7	10.0	6.0	3.1
Eat Smart, Safeway*	1 Serving/225g	124	4.3	55	1.3	7.3	1.9	2.3
Flavours of India, Canned, Sainsbury's*	½ Can/200g	160	3.8	80	2.4	13.3	1.9	1.8
Indian Meal for Two, Sainsbury's*	½ Pack/151g	154	8.5	102	1.6	11.4	5.6	3.1
Indian Takeaway for 1, Sainsbury's*	1 Serving/200g	202	10.4	101	1.8	11.8	5.2	1.7
M & S*	1 Pack/300g	300	14.4	100	1.5	12.1	4.8	1.6
Meal Solutions, Co-Op*	1 Pack/300g	210	12.0	70	1.0	8.0	4.0	2.0

P

	Measure INFO/WEIGHT	per Measure KCAL	FAT	Nutrition Values per 100g / 100ml KCAL	PROT	CARB	FAT	FIBRE
POTATO BOMBAY								
Morrisons*	1 Serving/175g	180	8.8	103	1.5	13.0	5.0	1.7
Safeway*	1 Pack/300g	205	10.8	68	1.5	7.2	3.6	2.3
Sainsbury's*	1 Pack/300g	285	14.7	95	1.8	10.8	4.9	2.5
Waitrose*	1 Pack/300g	246	12.9	82	1.6	9.3	4.3	2.2
POTATO CAKES								
Average	1 Cake/70.4g	126	1.2	180	3.9	37.5	1.7	2.4
Fried, Average	1oz/28g	66	2.5	237	4.9	35.0	9.1	0.8
POTATO CHIPS								
Hand Fried Mature Cheddar, Burts*	1 Serving/40g	202	11.1	504	6.4	57.4	27.7	0.0
Ready Salted, Sainsbury's*	¼ Pack/33g	174	10.9	526	5.6	51.7	33.0	3.8
POTATO CREAMED								
with Cabbage, Asda*	1 Pack/350g	256	9.1	73	1.3	11.0	2.6	0.0
POTATO FRIED								
Crispy, M & S*	1 Pack/400g	660	28.4	165	2.0	22.6	7.1	1.4
POTATO FRITTERS								
Crispy, Oven Baked, Birds Eye*	1 Fritter/20g	29	1.6	145	2.0	16.3	8.0	1.2
with Sweetcorn, M & S*	1 Pack/135g	304	17.0	225	4.4	24.1	12.6	2.3
POTATO MASH								
Bacon & Cheese, Tesco*	1 Serving/200g	252	12.8	126	3.1	13.9	6.4	1.3
Bacon & Spring Onion, Finest, Tesco*	½ Pack/200g	214	10.4	107	4.3	10.8	5.2	1.6
Cabbage & Spring Onion, COU, M & S*	1 Pack/450g	320	8.2	71	1.7	11.4	1.8	1.9
Cheddar, Irish, Finest, Tesco*	½ Pack/215g	301	17.0	140	6.3	10.2	7.9	1.4
Cheese & Chive, Snack in a Pot, Tesco*	1 Pot/230g	304	21.6	132	2.2	9.6	9.4	0.9
Cheese & Onion, Eat Smart, Morrisons*	1 Pack/400g	340	6.4	85	4.4	13.2	1.6	1.3
Cheese & Onion, Tesco*	1 Serving/200g	210	9.4	105	3.2	12.6	4.7	1.0
Leek & Bacon, Tesco*	1 Serving/400g	356	14.4	89	3.0	11.1	3.6	1.9
Leek & Cheese, COU, M & S*	½ Pack/225g	180	4.7	80	3.0	12.0	2.1	1.3
Mustard, & Caramelised Onions, Finest, Tesco*	1 Serving/200g	232	9.2	116	2.6	16.0	4.6	1.8
Roast Onion, Snack in a Pot, Tesco*	1 Pot/218g	257	12.9	118	1.6	14.7	5.9	0.6
Savoy Cabbage & Spring Onion, M & S*	1 Serving/225g	250	15.5	111	2.0	10.2	6.9	1.3
Sun Dried Tomato & Basil, COU, M & S*	1 Serving/170g	128	2.6	75	1.0	14.4	1.5	1.2
with Sweetcorn & Flaked Tuna, Sainsbury's*	1 Pot/224g	240	9.2	107	2.4	15.0	4.1	2.1
with Vegetables, GFY, Asda*	1 Pack/290g	186	3.2	64	1.6	12.0	1.1	2.3
with Vegetables, Sainsbury's*	½ Pack/229.0g	142	2.3	62	1.8	11.4	1.0	3.1
POTATO RINGS								
Ready Salted, M & S*	1 Serving/75g	375	21.1	500	3.5	58.9	28.1	2.6
Ready Salted, Sainsbury's*	1 Serving/50g	257	14.2	514	3.2	61.5	28.4	1.8
POTATO SAUTE								
with Onion, & Bacon, Waitrose*	¼ Pack/100g	112	4.3	112	1.9	16.4	4.3	1.3
POTATO SKINS								
¼ Cut, Deep Fried, McCain*	1oz/28g	52	1.7	186	3.0	30.1	6.0	0.0
¼ Cut, Oven Baked, McCain*	1oz/28g	53	1.3	190	3.7	33.1	4.8	0.0
American Style, Loaded, Asda*	1 Serving/78.4g	293	17.9	375	15.0	27.0	23.0	2.4
American Style, Loaded, Tesco*	1 Serving/340g	388	8.2	114	6.8	16.3	2.4	3.3
Cheese & Bacon, Loaded, Asda*	½ Pack/125g	275	15.0	220	13.0	15.0	12.0	3.3
Cheese & Bacon, Sainsbury's*	1 Serving/140g	349	21.6	249	10.3	17.3	15.4	2.5
Cheese & Bacon, Waitrose*	1 Serving/75g	146	9.4	195	7.3	13.1	12.6	3.5
Cheese & Chive, Sainsbury's*	2 Skins/150g	287	17.9	191	7.7	13.3	11.9	2.8
Loaded, HE, Tesco*	1 Serving/340g	425	8.5	125	7.7	17.9	2.5	0.6
Soured Cream, Loaded, M & S*	½ Pack/150g	308	17.9	205	9.1	15.8	11.9	0.9
POTATO SMILES								
Weighed Baked, McCain*	1 Serving/100g	237	10.1	237	3.4	33.4	10.1	3.1
Weighed Frozen, McCain*	1 Serving/100g	191	8.0	191	2.6	27.0	8.0	2.7

P

	Measure INFO/WEIGHT	per Measure KCAL	FAT	Nutrition Values per 100g / 100ml KCAL	PROT	CARB	FAT	FIBRE
POTATO SUMTHINGS								
Weighed Baked, McCain*	1 Serving/100g	220	9.0	220	3.4	31.3	9.0	2.8
Weighed Frozen, McCain*	1 Serving/100g	187	7.9	187	2.9	26.2	7.9	2.4
POTATO TWIRLS								
Sainsbury's*	1 Serving/50g	218	7.3	435	3.0	72.8	14.6	3.1
POTATO WAFFLES								
Asda*	1 Waffle/55.2g	106	5.4	192	1.6	24.7	9.8	2.4
Birds Eye*	1 Waffle/56g	94	4.8	167	2.0	20.7	8.5	1.5
Frozen, Cooked	1oz/28g	56	2.3	200	3.2	30.3	8.2	2.3
Frozen, Grilled, Asda*	1 Waffle/57g	104	5.8	183	2.0	21.0	10.1	1.7
Mini, Farmfoods*	1oz/28g	41	1.6	145	1.9	21.6	5.7	1.7
Mini, Sainsbury's*	1 Waffle/11g	27	1.8	242	2.8	20.1	16.7	1.0
Oven Baked, Mini, McCain*	1oz/28g	62	2.4	221	3.9	32.0	8.6	0.0
Sainsbury's*	1 Waffle/55.7g	109	5.7	194	2.9	22.8	10.1	1.1
Southern Fried, Asda*	1 Waffle/51g	107	5.1	209	2.8	27.0	10.0	2.1
Tesco*	1 Waffle/56.7g	122	8.6	215	1.9	17.7	15.1	3.6
POTATO WEDGES								
& Dip, M & S*	1 Pack/450g	698	33.3	155	2.5	20.4	7.4	1.8
Aldi*	1 Serving/100g	150	6.8	150	2.1	20.2	6.8	0.0
Asda*	1 Wedge/40g	57	2.0	142	3.4	21.0	4.9	1.7
Baked, GFY, Asda*	1 Pack/450g	617	11.7	137	3.4	25.0	2.6	3.4
BBQ Flavour, Asda*	1 Serving/100g	185	9.0	185	2.9	23.0	9.0	1.7
BGTY, Sainsbury's*	½ Pack/190g	179	3.4	94	3.0	16.4	1.8	3.4
Bombay, & Yoghurt & Mint Dip, HL, Tesco*	1 Serving/170g	139	3.6	82	1.3	14.5	2.1	0.9
Co-Op*	1oz/28g	38	1.7	135	2.0	20.0	6.0	2.0
Crispy, M & S*	1 Serving/200g	340	14.2	170	1.3	25.3	7.1	1.7
Four Cheese & Red Onion, Chicago Town*	1 Serving/150g	210	8.0	140	2.1	21.0	5.3	2.4
Garlic & Herb, COU, M & S*	1 Pack/300g	300	7.8	100	2.3	16.4	2.6	3.2
Garlic & Herb, Kitchen Range Foods*	1oz/28g	42	2.2	151	1.6	18.5	7.8	0.0
Garlic & Herb Crusted, Chicago Town*	1 Serving/150g	216	6.5	144	1.9	24.4	4.3	2.2
Micro, Tesco*	1 Pack/100g	170	6.8	170	2.6	24.5	6.8	2.3
New York Style, HL, Tesco*	1 Serving/125.2g	129	3.0	103	2.0	18.3	2.4	2.3
Only 5% Fat, Weighed Baked, McCain*	1 Serving/100g	173	4.3	173	3.3	30.2	4.3	2.8
Only 5% Fat, Weighed Frozen, McCain*	10 Wedges/175g	215	5.3	123	2.2	21.8	3.0	1.9
Oven Baked, Waitrose*	1oz/28g	46	1.2	165	2.4	29.2	4.3	2.1
Savoury, Waitrose*	1/3 Bag/250g	350	10.8	140	2.3	22.9	4.3	1.9
Sour Cream & Chives, McCain*	1 Serving/100g	132	4.1	132	2.4	24.0	4.1	0.0
Southern Fried, Asda*	1 Serving/100g	157	4.5	157	3.0	26.0	4.5	3.5
Southern Fried Flavour, Champion*	1oz/28g	41	1.7	147	2.1	20.8	6.2	2.8
Southern Fried Style, Tesco*	1 Serving/155g	233	14.1	150	3.0	14.1	9.1	2.0
Spicy, Asda*	1 Serving/100g	145	5.7	145	1.8	21.8	5.7	2.1
Spicy, Deep Fried, McCain*	1oz/28g	52	2.3	187	3.6	27.3	8.1	0.0
Spicy, M & S*	½ Pack/225g	349	14.6	155	2.4	21.8	6.5	1.3
Spicy, Occasions, Sainsbury's*	1 Serving/100g	144	4.3	144	2.5	23.7	4.3	0.4
Spicy, Simple Solutions, Tesco*	1 Serving/150g	141	4.5	94	4.6	12.2	3.0	1.4
Weighed Frozen, Tesco*	1 Serving/150g	188	6.0	125	1.9	20.3	4.0	1.1
with Chilli, COU, M & S*	1 Pack/400g	380	10.8	95	5.2	13.7	2.7	2.3
POTATOES								
Alphabites, Captain Birds Eye, Birds Eye*	9 Bites/56g	75	3.0	134	2.0	19.5	5.3	1.4
Anya, Boiled in Unsalted Water, TTD, Sainsbury's*	1 Serving/80g	60	0.2	75	1.5	17.8	0.3	1.1
Baby, Dressed with Garlic & Rosemary, M & S*	1 Serving/185g	130	5.2	70	2.0	9.0	2.8	2.4
Baby, Garlic & Sea Salt Roasted, Finest, Tesco*	1 Serving/200g	192	6.6	96	3.1	13.5	3.3	1.0
Baby, Oven Bake, Aunt Bessie's*	1 Serving/120g	103	1.7	86	2.2	16.3	1.4	3.0
Baby, with Butter & Herbs, Sainsbury's*	¼ Pack/142.7g	107	1.7	75	1.3	14.7	1.2	2.1

POTATOES

INFO/WEIGHT	Measure	per Measure KCAL	per Measure FAT	KCAL	PROT	CARB	FAT	FIBRE
Baby, with Herb Butter, Safeway*	1 Serving/200g	158	2.4	79	1.4	15.6	1.2	1.4
Baked, Flesh & Skin, Average	1 Potato/200g	218	0.2	109	2.3	25.2	0.1	2.4
Baked, Flesh Only, Weighed with Skin, Average	1oz/28g	26	0.0	93	2.0	21.6	0.1	1.5
Baked, in Microwave, Flesh & Skin, Average	1oz/28g	29	0.0	105	2.4	24.1	0.1	2.3
Baked, in Microwave, Flesh Only, Average	1oz/28g	28	0.0	100	2.1	23.3	0.1	1.6
Baked, in Microwave, Skin Only, Average	1oz/28g	37	0.0	132	4.4	29.6	0.1	5.5
Baked, Jacket, Beef Chilli, Mini, Classic, Asda*	1 Pack/300g	233	2.4	78	3.9	13.7	0.8	1.5
Baked, Jacket, Beef Chilli Filled, GFY, Asda*	1 Serving/300g	261	1.5	87	4.6	16.0	0.5	3.2
Baked, Jacket, Cheese, M & S*	1oz/28g	24	0.7	85	4.5	11.1	2.5	1.6
Baked, Jacket, Cheese & Beans, Somerfield*	1 Pack/338.9g	305	6.8	90	4.1	13.8	2.0	2.2
Baked, Jacket, Cheese Filled, Farmfoods*	2 Halves/255g	349	9.7	137	4.7	21.0	3.8	1.9
Baked, Jacket, Cheesy, GFY, Asda*	1 Serving/155g	129	1.6	83	2.6	16.0	1.0	2.1
Baked, Jacket, Chicken Tikka, COU, M & S*	1 Serving/300g	240	4.8	80	5.4	10.9	1.6	1.3
Baked, Jacket, Chicken Tikka, Spar*	1 Serving/300g	309	3.1	103	5.5	19.2	1.0	5.0
Baked, Jacket, Chilli, BGTY, Sainsbury's*	1 Pack/350g	319	4.9	91	5.3	14.3	1.4	1.2
Baked, Jacket, Chilli Con Carne, COU, M & S*	1 Pack/300g	270	6.3	90	6.0	11.1	2.1	1.2
Baked, Jacket, Chilli Con Carne, Eat Smart, Safeway*	1 Pack/300g	225	3.9	75	6.1	8.9	1.3	1.9
Baked, Jacket, Chilli Con Carne, Somerfield*	1 Pack/340g	319	11.6	94	5.5	10.3	3.4	1.2
Baked, Jacket, Creamy Mushroom, Asda*	1 Serving/100g	124	2.4	124	3.5	22.0	2.4	1.7
Baked, Jacket, Garlic, Mini, Asda*	1 Serving/65g	59	2.1	91	2.2	13.0	3.3	0.0
Baked, Jacket, Garlic Butter Filling, Morrisons*	1 Potato/210g	239	12.4	114	1.7	13.6	5.9	0.9
Baked, Jacket, Garlic Mushrooms, BGTY, Sainsbury's*	1 Pack/350g	263	3.2	75	2.3	14.4	0.9	1.2
Baked, Jacket, Garlic Mushrooms, Eat Smart, Safeway*	1 Pack/300g	210	8.1	70	2.7	8.1	2.7	1.6
Baked, Jacket, Halves, M & S*	1 Serving/250g	188	2.8	75	2.0	14.2	1.1	1.7
Baked, Jacket, Ham & Cheddar Cheese, Asda*	1 Pack/300g	435	11.1	145	7.0	21.0	3.7	1.6
Baked, Jacket, Herb & Rock Salt, M & S*	1 Pack/500g	375	5.5	75	2.0	14.2	1.1	1.7
Baked, Jacket, Herb & Rock Salt Seasoning, M & S*	1 Pack/500g	375	5.5	75	2.0	14.2	1.1	1.7
Baked, Jacket, Leek & Cheese, M & S*	1 Serving/206g	206	6.4	100	3.8	13.4	3.1	3.2
Baked, Jacket, Mature Cheddar Cheese, Finest, Tesco*	1 Potato/245g	360	18.4	147	5.4	14.6	7.5	2.3
Baked, Jacket, Mature Chedder Cheese, Morrisons*	1 Serving/400g	520	20.4	130	4.4	16.6	5.1	1.5
Baked, Jacket, Spicy Chilli Con Carne, Spar*	1 Pack/340g	265	5.4	78	3.4	12.4	1.6	1.5
Baked, Jacket, Stuffed, Garlic & Herb Butter, Tesco*	1 Pack/435g	570	32.6	131	1.3	14.6	7.5	1.0
Baked, Jacket, Tuna & Sweetcorn, Average	1 Serving/300g	273	6.8	91	5.0	12.6	2.3	0.9
Baked, Jacket, Tuna & Sweetcorn, BGTY, Sainsbury's*	1 Pack/350g	361	9.5	103	6.5	13.2	2.7	1.3
Baked, Jacket, Tuna & Sweetcorn, COU, M & S*	1 Pack/300g	270	5.4	90	5.1	12.8	1.8	1.4
Baked, Jacket, Tuna & Sweetcorn, Morrisons*	1 Serving/300g	243	2.1	81	5.1	13.5	0.7	0.0
Baked, Jacket, Tuna & Sweetcorn, Somerfield*	1 Pack/340g	333	13.3	98	3.2	12.5	3.9	1.0
Baked, Jacket, with Baked Bean & Sausage, Asda*	1 Pack/300g	447	9.6	149	5.0	25.0	3.2	2.7
Baked, Jacket, with Baked Bean Toppers, Safeway*	1 Topper/91.7g	166	7.2	180	5.0	22.1	7.8	4.5
Baked, Jacket, with Beef Chilli, Asda*	1 Pack/300g	381	7.8	127	5.0	21.0	2.6	2.0
Baked, Jacket, with Beef Chilli, M & S*	1 Pack/360g	288	7.2	80	5.9	9.6	2.0	0.9
Baked, Jacket, with Cheese, Favourites, Morrisons*	1 Pack/300g	312	10.8	104	3.4	14.4	3.6	1.3
Baked, Jacket, with Cheese, Fresh, Tesco*	½ Pack/215g	151	3.0	70	3.9	9.7	1.4	2.8
Baked, Jacket, with Cheese, HL, Tesco*	1 Potato/225g	203	5.0	90	4.5	13.0	2.2	1.8
Baked, Jacket, with Cheese, Safeway*	1 Potato/200g	165	1.7	83	2.1	16.3	0.9	2.1
Baked, Jacket, with Cheese & Bacon, Finest, Tesco*	1 Potato/245g	360	19.6	147	6.0	12.7	8.0	2.5
Baked, Jacket, with Cheese & Butter, Tesco*	1 Potato/224.8g	263	11.2	117	3.1	14.9	5.0	2.3
Baked, Jacket, with Cheese & Veggie Bacon, Tesco*	½ Pack/225g	279	10.8	124	4.7	15.5	4.8	1.3
Baked, Jacket, with Cheese Mash, GFY, Asda*	1 Potato/200g	192	5.6	96	4.8	13.0	2.8	2.2
Baked, Jacket, with Chicken Tikka, Tesco*	1 Potato/246.7g	185	2.2	75	3.4	12.6	0.9	1.3
Baked, Jacket, with Smoked Bacon, Finest, Tesco*	½ Pack/200g	200	8.0	100	3.5	12.1	4.0	2.5
Baked, Skin Only, Average	1oz/28g	55	0.0	198	4.3	46.1	0.1	7.9
Baked, with Cheddar Cheese, Farmfoods*	1 Potato/143g	196	5.4	137	4.7	21.0	3.8	1.9

POTATOES

INFO/WEIGHT	Measure	per Measure KCAL	FAT	KCAL	PROT	CARB	FAT	FIBRE
Baking, Raw, Average	1 Med Size/250g	198	0.3	79	2.1	18.0	0.1	1.6
Boiled, Average	1 Serving/120g	86	0.1	72	1.8	17.0	0.1	1.2
Boulangere, M & S*	½ Pack/225g	180	2.0	80	2.8	15.9	0.9	0.9
Charlotte, Average	1 Serving/184g	139	0.5	76	1.6	17.4	0.3	3.3
Crispy Bites, Weighed Frozen, McCain*	1 Serving/100g	141	4.4	141	2.5	20.4	4.4	1.5
Crispy Slices, Weighed Baked, McCain*	1 Serving/100g	240	11.0	240	3.2	32.1	11.0	2.1
Crispy Slices, Weighed Frozen, McCain*	1 Portion/100g	163	7.4	163	2.1	21.9	7.4	1.4
Frites, Fries, Golden, Crunchy, M & S*	½ Pack/100g	175	7.8	175	2.1	24.4	7.8	1.8
Garlic, Tapas Selection, Sainsbury's*	1 Serving/22g	49	4.2	224	2.6	10.4	19.1	0.7
Hasselback, Average	1 Serving/175g	182	1.6	104	1.9	22.0	0.9	2.9
Italian Style, & Vegetables, Waitrose*	1 Serving/126g	138	3.5	110	2.0	19.2	2.8	3.4
Jersey Royal, Canned, Average	1 Can/186g	116	0.2	62	1.4	14.0	0.1	1.2
Jersey Royal, New, Raw, Average	1oz/28g	21	0.1	75	1.7	17.2	0.2	1.5
Juliette, Sainsbury's*	1 Serving/250g	200	0.3	80	1.4	19.7	0.1	1.0
King Edward, Tesco*	1 Serving/100g	77	0.2	77	2.1	16.8	0.2	1.3
Lemon & Rosemary, Finest, Tesco*	½ Pack/200g	200	7.4	100	2.1	14.7	3.7	2.0
Maris Piper, Average	1 Serving/250g	180	0.3	72	1.8	17.0	0.1	1.2
Maris Piper, in Salted Water, Asda*	1 Serving/95g	67	0.1	70	1.5	15.0	0.1	0.8
Mashed, Colcannon, HL, Tesco*	1 Pack/500g	415	12.5	83	1.9	13.1	2.5	2.0
Mashed, Colcannon, Sainsbury's*	½ Pack/300g	192	12.0	64	0.4	6.7	4.0	1.4
Mashed, Colcannon, Tesco*	1 Serving/250g	225	13.5	90	1.6	8.4	5.4	1.8
Mashed, Colcannon, Waitrose*	½ Pack/150g	138	5.7	92	1.7	12.8	3.8	1.4
Mashed, From Supermarket, Average	½ Pack/200g	197	8.1	98	1.8	13.3	4.1	1.5
Mashed, From Supermarket, Healthy Range, Average	1 Serving/200g	160	3.1	80	1.8	14.6	1.6	1.3
Mashed, From Supermarket, Premium, Average	1 Serving/225g	305	17.8	136	1.7	14.4	7.9	1.1
Mashed, Vintage Cheddar Cheese, M & S*	½ Pack/225g	248	11.9	110	4.6	12.6	5.3	1.0
Mashed, with Carrot & Swede, COU, M & S*	1oz/28g	20	0.6	70	1.1	12.1	2.1	2.9
Mashed, with Carrot & Swede, M & S*	1 Serving/225g	214	14.4	95	1.6	8.3	6.4	1.4
Mashed, with Carrot & Swede, Morrisons*	1 Serving/100g	71	1.6	71	1.5	12.6	1.6	2.2
Mashed, with Carrot & Swede, Sainsbury's*	½ Pack/225.5g	230	12.0	102	1.9	11.7	5.3	1.5
Mashed, with Leeks, Creamy, Birds Eye*	1 Pack/300g	300	21.0	100	2.0	7.3	7.0	0.8
New, Baby, Average	1 Serving/180g	135	0.5	75	1.7	17.1	0.3	1.6
New, Baby, Canned, Average	1 Can/120g	70	0.2	59	1.4	13.2	0.2	1.4
New, Baby, with Mint Butter, The Best, Safeway*	½ Pack/190g	162	3.4	85	1.2	15.4	1.8	2.2
New, with Herbs & Butter, Asda*	½ Pack/169.8g	146	2.9	86	1.7	16.0	1.7	1.5
New, with Herbs & Butter, Waitrose*	1 Serving/385g	443	22.7	115	1.7	13.8	5.9	1.2
New, with Parsley Butter, TTD, Sainsbury's*	1 Serving/150g	126	3.6	84	2.2	13.3	2.4	1.0
New, with Sunblush Tomato, M & S*	1 Pack/385g	347	6.9	90	1.6	17.2	1.8	1.3
Parmentier, with Shallot Butter, M & S*	¼ Pack/125g	200	8.9	160	2.5	21.1	7.1	4.0
Red, Flesh Only, Average	1 Serving/300g	218	0.5	73	2.0	16.4	0.2	1.3
Roast, Basted in Beef Dripping, Waitrose*	1 Serving/165g	213	8.9	129	2.2	18.0	5.4	1.9
Roast, Frozen, Average	1 Av Roastie/70g	105	3.5	149	2.6	23.5	5.0	1.4
Roast, Frozen, Healthy Range, Average	1 Av Roastie/70g	70	1.7	100	2.6	18.2	2.4	2.1
Roast, Garlic, Sainsbury's*	½ Pack/225g	358	21.8	159	3.2	14.6	9.7	1.4
Roast, in Lard, Average	1oz/28g	42	1.3	149	2.9	25.9	4.5	1.8
Roast, in Oil, Average	1oz/28g	42	1.3	149	2.9	25.9	4.5	1.8
Roast, Seasoned, Butter Basted, Tesco*	½ Pack/200g	300	11.4	150	2.3	21.9	5.7	2.4
Roast, with Caramelised Onions, Finest, Tesco*	½ Pack/200g	500	16.4	250	5.5	38.6	8.2	2.9
Roast, with Garlic & Rosemary, Waitrose*	½ Pack/200g	194	6.2	97	2.4	14.9	3.1	3.7
Roasting, Average	1 Serving/150g	203	5.3	135	2.5	23.4	3.5	1.7
Saute, Deep Fried, McCain*	1oz/28g	47	2.0	167	2.6	23.3	7.0	0.0
Saute, Oven Baked, McCain*	1oz/28g	56	1.1	199	4.4	36.9	3.8	0.0
Slices, Garlic & Herb, Heinz*	1oz/28g	23	1.1	82	1.7	10.2	3.9	0.7

P

	Measure INFO/WEIGHT	per Measure KCAL	per Measure FAT	Nutrition Values per 100g / 100ml KCAL	PROT	CARB	FAT	FIBRE
POTATOES								
Slices, Ready to Roast, Crispy, M & S*	1 Pack/475g	689	24.7	145	2.9	22.2	5.2	1.9
Slices, Spicy Coated, Safeway*	½ Pack/150g	305	18.6	203	2.5	19.7	12.4	2.5
Spicy, with Chorizo, Tapas, Waitrose*	1 Serving/260g	512	35.6	197	6.7	11.8	13.7	1.1
Vivaldi, Boiled in Unsalted Water, Sainsbury's*	1 Serving/200g	144	0.2	72	1.8	17.0	0.1	1.2
White, Raw, Weighed with Skin, Flesh Only, Average	1 Potato/300g	225	0.5	75	2.0	16.8	0.2	1.3
with Seafood & Seasoned Butter, Tapas, Waitrose*	1 Pack/170g	330	19.4	194	6.2	16.7	11.4	2.1
POTATOES INSTANT								
Mashed, Made Up with Water, Average	1 Serving/180g	118	0.3	66	1.7	14.5	0.2	1.3
Mashed, Original, Dry Weight, Smash*	1 Serving/30g	107	1.4	358	10.7	68.1	4.8	3.4
Mashed, with Fried Onion, Smash*	½ Pack/269g	191	3.5	71	1.6	13.4	1.3	0.7
Mashed, with Smoked Bacon, Smash*	1 Serving/169g	137	3.7	81	1.7	13.6	2.2	0.6
POUSSIN								
Meat & Skin, Raw, Average	1oz/28g	57	3.9	202	19.1	0.0	13.9	0.0
Spatchcock, British, Waitrose*	½ Poussin/225g	365	20.3	162	19.0	1.2	9.0	0.0
Spatchcock, with Garlic & Herbs, Finest, Tesco*	½ Poussin/235g	348	17.2	148	19.7	1.0	7.3	0.5
POWERADE								
Berry & Tropical Fruit, Coca-Cola*	1 Bottle/500ml	120	0.0	24	0.0	5.6	0.0	0.0
Citrus Charge, Coca-Cola*	1 Bottle/500ml	120	0.0	24	0.0	6.0	0.0	0.0
Gold Rush, Coca-Cola*	1 Bottle/500ml	120	0.0	24	0.0	6.0	0.0	0.0
Ice Storm, Coca-Cola*	1 Bottle/500ml	120	0.0	24	0.0	6.0	0.0	0.0
Isotonic, Sports Drink, Coca-Cola*	1 Bottle/500ml	120	0.0	24	0.0	5.6	0.0	0.0
Lemon & Grapefruit, Coca-Cola*	1 Bottle/500ml	120	0.0	24	0.0	6.0	0.0	0.0
PRAWN COCKTAIL								
20% More Prawns, M & S*	½ Pack/100g	330	31.6	330	8.9	2.2	31.6	0.2
Asda*	1oz/28g	124	12.2	443	8.6	3.3	43.6	0.0
BFY, Morrisons*	1 Serving/100g	149	10.3	149	4.7	9.7	10.3	0.1
BGTY, Sainsbury's*	1oz/28g	46	3.2	165	10.1	5.1	11.6	0.5
Delicious, Boots*	1 Pack/250g	285	6.5	114	5.5	17.0	2.6	1.2
Half Fat, Safeway*	1 Serving/200g	362	27.6	181	8.0	6.4	13.8	0.6
HL, Tesco*	1 Serving/200g	276	22.6	138	6.8	2.3	11.3	0.6
Light, Asda*	1oz/28g	45	3.1	160	9.9	4.8	11.2	0.0
M & S*	1 Serving/100g	320	29.8	320	11.2	2.0	29.8	0.6
Reduced Fat, M & S*	1 Pack/200g	260	15.0	130	11.9	3.2	7.5	0.7
Reduced Fat, Tesco*	1 Serving/200g	304	21.2	152	7.6	6.5	10.6	0.4
Reduced Fat, Waitrose*	1 Serving/200g	242	15.8	121	9.1	3.4	7.9	1.3
Safeway*	½ Pot/100g	373	36.5	373	7.6	3.4	36.5	0.2
Sainsbury's*	1 Serving/200g	706	69.0	353	7.9	2.7	34.5	0.5
Tesco*	1 Tub/200g	834	83.0	417	7.3	3.5	41.5	0.1
PRAWN CRACKERS								
Asda*	1 Serving/25g	134	8.8	535	2.0	53.0	35.0	0.0
Cooked in Sunflower Oil, Sharwood's*	5 Crackers/10g	48	2.3	479	0.7	68.3	22.6	0.8
Food to Go, Sainsbury's*	1 Bag/40g	214	12.5	534	2.9	60.2	31.3	0.4
Green Thai Curry, M & S*	1 Pack/50g	250	12.9	500	3.2	62.2	25.8	1.6
M & S*	1 Pack/15g	83	4.8	550	3.0	62.3	32.0	0.0
Ready to Eat, Sharwood's*	1 Bag/60g	316	18.5	527	0.5	62.0	30.8	1.2
Sainsbury's*	1 Cracker/3g	16	1.0	537	2.4	60.4	31.7	0.8
Tesco*	1/3 Pack/20g	114	7.4	570	2.5	56.5	37.1	0.9
Waitrose*	1 Pack/50g	267	16.1	533	2.4	58.6	32.1	1.6
PRAWN PINWHEEL								
Oriental Style, BGTY, Sainsbury's*	1 Pack/189.0g	274	2.1	145	6.0	26.7	1.1	0.0
PRAWN TOAST								
Chinese Selection, Tesco*	1 Toast/9.9g	36	2.7	362	8.2	20.7	27.5	1.7
Chinese Snack Selection, Morrisons*	1 Toast/12.5g	41	2.7	328	11.3	23.1	21.2	6.6

P

	Measure INFO/WEIGHT	per Measure KCAL	FAT	Nutrition Values per 100g / 100ml KCAL	PROT	CARB	FAT	FIBRE
PRAWN TOAST								
Dim Sum Selection, Sainsbury's*	1 Toast/8g	23	1.5	283	9.9	19.2	18.5	2.0
Mini, Oriental Selection, Party, Iceland*	1 Toast/15.1g	52	3.6	345	10.5	22.0	23.9	2.1
Oriental Selection, Waitrose*	1 Toast/14g	38	2.4	272	11.1	18.3	17.2	2.1
Sesame, Occasions, Sainsbury's*	1 Toast/12g	34	2.2	283	9.9	19.2	18.5	2.0
Sesame, Oriental Snack Selection, Sainsbury's*	1 Toast/12g	40	2.7	335	9.3	23.0	22.9	5.1
Sesame Prawn, Toasted Triangles, M & S*	1 Pack/220g	616	39.6	280	12.4	17.3	18.0	2.0
Waitrose*	1 Toast/21g	47	3.6	223	9.7	7.4	17.2	5.8
PRAWNS								
Batter Crisp, Lyons*	1 Pack/160g	350	20.3	219	8.0	18.2	12.7	1.1
Boiled	1 Prawn/3g	3	0.0	99	22.6	0.0	0.9	0.0
Brine, John West*	½ Can/60g	58	0.6	97	21.0	1.0	1.0	0.0
Chilli, Battered, M & S*	1oz/28g	63	3.2	225	7.2	23.8	11.5	0.5
Chilli, M & S*	1oz/28g	22	0.1	79	17.9	0.6	0.5	0.6
Cooked & Peeled, Average	1oz/28g	21	0.2	77	17.6	0.2	0.6	0.0
Cooked & Peeled, Chilled, Tesco*	1 Pack/190g	143	1.1	75	15.6	1.0	0.6	0.1
Crevettes, Asda*	1oz/28g	11	0.2	41	8.6	0.0	0.7	0.0
Crispy, with Dipping Sauce, Sweet Chilli, M & S*	1 Pack/240g	515	27.8	215	7.5	19.9	11.6	2.3
Dried, Average	1 Prawn/3g	8	0.1	281	62.4	0.0	3.5	0.0
Filo Wrapped & Breaded, M & S*	1 Serving/19g	45	2.5	235	9.5	20.4	13.0	1.4
Frozen, Extra Large, Atlantic, TTD, Sainsbury's*	¼ Pack/100g	57	0.2	57	13.9	0.0	0.2	0.0
Honduran, & Cocktail Sauce Dipper, M & S*	1 Pack/120g	258	21.6	215	13.6	0.0	18.0	1.1
Hot & Spicy, Average	1 Serving/170g	461	26.9	271	9.4	22.9	15.8	2.2
Icelandic, Raw, Average	1oz/28g	30	0.4	106	22.7	0.0	1.6	0.0
King, Chilli, Cantonese, Battered, Sainsbury's*	1 Pack/300g	570	23.1	190	10.0	20.2	7.7	0.8
King, Chilli & Coriander, Honduran, M & S*	½ Pack/70g	70	2.2	100	17.2	0.1	3.2	0.4
King, Chilli & Coriander, Sainsbury's*	1 Pack/140g	133	5.9	95	13.8	0.5	4.2	0.5
King, Crevettes, Sainsbury's*	1 Pack/225g	205	1.1	91	21.8	0.1	0.5	0.3
King, Farmed in Vietnam, Asda*	½ Pack/88.5g	69	0.9	78	17.2	0.0	1.0	0.0
King, Fresh, Youngs*	1 Pack/188g	128	0.8	68	16.1	0.1	0.4	0.1
King, in Filo, Finest, Tesco*	1 Prawn/20g	38	0.6	189	13.0	27.8	2.9	1.6
King, Japanese, Noodle Box, M & S*	1 Pack/300g	330	8.1	110	5.8	16.0	2.7	1.6
King, Lemon & Pepper, Honduran, M & S*	1 Pack/140g	133	3.6	95	17.4	0.4	2.6	0.7
King, Raw, Average	1 Bag/200g	145	1.9	72	15.8	0.2	1.0	0.1
King, Tandoori, Average	6 Prawns/354g	195	3.9	55	5.7	5.9	1.1	0.7
King, Thai Sweet Chilli, Sainsbury's*	1 Serving/150g	177	6.2	118	6.4	13.9	4.1	1.9
King, with Chilli, Coriander & Lime, Waitrose*	1 Pack/140g	143	3.2	102	19.9	0.5	2.3	0.6
King, with Garlic Butter, M & S*	1 Serving/100g	165	9.0	165	12.5	9.1	9.0	0.5
King, with Ginger & Spring Onion, Waitrose*	1 Pack/300g	130	2.1	43	5.3	3.6	0.7	0.8
North Atlantic, Peeled, Cooked, Average	1oz/28g	22	0.3	80	17.5	0.0	1.1	0.0
North Atlantic, Raw, Average	1oz/28g	17	0.1	62	14.4	0.0	0.4	0.0
Raw, Average	¼ Pack/112g	88	0.8	79	17.8	0.2	0.7	0.0
Spirals, Shapers, Boots*	1 Pack/100g	468	22.0	468	3.1	64.0	22.0	2.8
Thai, M & S*	1oz/28g	29	0.9	103	5.2	13.6	3.1	1.3
Tiger, Cooked & Peeled, Average	1 Pack/180g	151	2.0	84	18.4	0.1	1.1	0.0
Tiger, Jumbo, Average	1 Serving/50g	39	0.3	78	18.3	0.3	0.5	0.0
Tiger, Raw, Average	1oz/28g	18	0.2	64	14.2	0.1	0.7	0.0
Tiger, Wrapped, M & S*	1 Pack/190g	477	25.8	251	11.3	20.7	13.6	1.3
PRAWNS CHILLI								
with Spicy Chilli Dip, King, Sainsbury's*	½ Pack/150g	282	10.8	188	8.6	22.2	7.2	1.0
PRAWNS CREOLE								
GFY, Asda*	1 Serving/300g	222	3.0	74	3.2	13.0	1.0	1.4
Spicy, BGTY, Sainsbury's*	1 Pack/350g	357	8.4	102	4.8	15.6	2.4	0.4
with Rice, PB, Waitrose*	1 Serving/404g	275	4.4	68	4.2	10.3	1.1	2.9

P

	Measure INFO/WEIGHT	per Measure KCAL	FAT	Nutrition Values per 100g / 100ml KCAL	PROT	CARB	FAT	FIBRE
PRAWNS CREOLE								
with Vegetable Rice, King, COU, M & S*	1 Pack/400g	300	2.4	75	4.5	13.3	0.6	0.7
PRAWNS GULNARI								
with Rice, COU, M & S*	1 Pack/400g	400	3.2	100	4.0	18.7	0.8	1.6
PRAWNS IN								
Creamy Garlic Sauce, Youngs*	1 Serving/158g	261	22.9	165	8.5	0.3	14.5	0.0
Sweet Chilli Sauce, Asda*	1 Pack/360g	500	24.8	139	4.1	15.0	6.9	0.3
PRAWNS ORIENTAL								
M & S*	1 Pack/200g	440	23.4	220	11.9	16.9	11.7	0.9
PRAWNS SZECHUAN								
Spicy, COU, M & S*	1 Pack/400g	380	3.6	95	4.5	16.9	0.9	1.5
PRAWNS WITH								
a Spicy Cajun Dip, King, Sainsbury's*	1 Pack/240g	254	4.3	106	14.8	9.1	1.8	1.4
Caribbean Style Sauce, GFY, Asda*	1 Serving/400g	408	6.8	102	4.7	17.0	1.7	2.1
Garlic & Herb Butter, King, Fresh, M & S*	1 Serving/200g	330	18.0	165	12.5	9.1	9.0	0.5
Ginger & Spring Onion, King, Budgens*	1 Pack/350g	151	4.2	43	5.9	2.1	1.2	0.7
Ginger & Spring Onion, Sainsbury's*	1 Pack/300g	198	9.3	66	4.7	4.7	3.1	0.3
Green Thai Sauce, Tiger, Waitrose*	½ Pack/117g	108	2.7	92	16.1	0.8	2.3	0.1
Rice, Sweet Chilli, Tesco*	1 Pack/460g	488	10.1	106	2.4	19.2	2.2	0.5
with Creamy Lime Dip, King, Waitrose*	1 Pot/230g	518	40.7	225	15.8	0.8	17.7	0.2
PRETZELS								
American Style, Salted, Sainsbury's*	1 Serving/50g	202	2.3	403	10.8	79.7	4.5	1.8
Cheddar Cheese, Penn State Pretzels*	1 Sm Bag/30g	124	2.8	412	10.0	71.6	9.3	3.8
Jumbo, Tesco*	1 Serving/50g	194	3.4	388	9.7	71.9	6.8	5.4
Lightly Salted, Tesco*	1 Serving/25g	99	1.8	395	9.3	73.4	7.1	5.5
Mini, M & S*	1 Pack/45g	194	6.0	430	10.4	66.6	13.4	4.9
New York Style, Salted, Mini, Shapers, Boots*	1 Bag/25g	94	0.5	375	10.0	79.0	2.1	4.2
Salt & Cracked Black Pepper, COU, M & S*	1 Pack/25g	95	0.6	380	9.7	83.3	2.4	2.7
Salted, Mini, M & S*	1 Pack/25g	94	0.5	375	10.0	79.0	2.1	4.2
Salted, Sainsbury's*	1 Serving/50g	201	1.8	401	9.8	82.4	3.6	3.4
Sea Salt, Eat Smart, Morrisons*	1 Bag/25g	87	0.6	347	10.0	71.3	2.4	4.8
Sea Salt & Black Pepper, Tesco*	1 Serving/50g	190	1.3	379	10.0	79.0	2.6	4.1
Snacks, Fabulous Bakin' Boys*	1 Pack/24g	96	1.2	401	9.0	79.5	4.9	2.5
Soft, Garlic, Auntie Anne's*	1 Pretzel/74g	320	1.0	432	12.2	89.2	1.4	2.7
Soft, Glazin' Raisin, Auntie Anne's*	1 Pretzel/74g	470	0.5	635	14.9	140.5	0.7	4.1
Soft, Salted, Original, Auntie Anne's*	1 Pretzel/74g	340	1.0	459	13.5	97.3	1.4	4.1
Soft, Sesame, Auntie Anne's*	1 Pretzel/74g	350	6.0	473	14.9	85.1	8.1	4.1
Sour Cream & Chive, Mini, HL, Tesco*	1 Pack/25g	92	0.6	369	10.9	76.3	2.2	4.6
Sour Cream & Chive, Penn State Pretzels*	1 Serving/25g	103	2.2	410	9.8	72.8	8.8	3.9
Sour Cream & Chive, Sainsbury's*	1 Serving/25g	103	2.2	410	9.9	73.0	8.7	5.0
Sour Cream & Onion, M & S*	1 Serving/30g	137	4.4	455	11.0	70.9	14.5	0.7
Sour Cream & Onion, Tesco*	1 Serving/25g	114	4.3	457	8.4	67.7	17.0	2.3
Spicy Salsa, Penn State Pretzels*	1 Serving/25g	105	2.6	420	9.5	72.4	10.4	1.3
Sweet Thai Chilli Twists, Penn State Pretzels*	1 Serving/25g	98	2.1	393	9.8	70.1	8.2	6.8
Wheat, Gluten Free, Trufree*	1 Bag/60g	282	12.0	470	2.4	70.0	20.0	1.0
with Sea Salt, Giant, M & S*	1 Pretzel/8g	31	0.5	390	9.7	77.3	6.8	5.4
PRINGLES*								
Barbecue, Pringles*	1 Serving/50g	267	18.0	533	4.9	48.0	36.0	5.1
BBQ Spare Rib, Rice Infusions, Pringles*	1 Pack/23g	108	5.3	469	5.1	60.0	23.0	2.6
Cheese & Onion, Pringles*	1 Serving/50g	264	17.0	528	4.1	50.0	34.0	3.4
Hot & Spicy, Pringles*	1 Serving/50g	265	17.0	530	4.6	49.0	34.0	3.7
Light, Original, Pringles*	1 Serving/25g	121	6.3	484	4.3	59.0	25.0	3.6
Light, Sour Cream & Onion, Pringles*	1 Serving/25g	122	6.3	487	4.7	57.0	25.0	3.6
Minis, Original, Pringles*	1 Pack/23g	118	6.9	514	5.1	55.0	30.0	3.7

P

	Measure INFO/WEIGHT	per Measure KCAL	FAT	Nutrition Values per 100g / 100ml KCAL	PROT	CARB	FAT	FIBRE
PRINGLES*								
Minis, Salt & Vinegar, Pringles*	1 Pack/23g	115	6.4	502	4.5	55.0	28.0	3.6
Minis, Sour Cream & Onion, Pringles*	1 Pack/23g	118	6.7	511	5.2	56.0	29.0	3.5
Minis, Texas BBQ Sauce, Pringles*	1 Pack/23g	116	6.4	504	5.0	56.0	28.0	3.8
Original, Pringles*	1 Serving/25g	135	9.0	540	4.1	49.0	36.0	3.6
Paprika, Pringles*	1 Serving/50g	265	17.0	529	4.9	49.0	34.0	6.5
Salt & Vinegar, Pringles*	1 Serving/50g	264	17.0	527	3.9	50.0	34.0	3.4
Sour Cream & Onion, Pringles*	1 Serving/25g	133	8.8	531	4.5	49.0	35.0	3.6
PROBIOTIC DRINK								
Yoghurt, Original, Tesco*	1 Bottle/100g	68	1.0	68	1.7	13.1	1.0	1.4
PROFITEROLES								
Asda*	1 Serving/64g	218	17.2	343	5.0	20.0	27.0	0.0
Chocolate, 8 Pack, Co-Op*	¼ Pack/112g	330	17.9	295	6.0	31.0	16.0	2.0
Chocolate, Co-Op*	1 Pot/91g	260	13.7	285	6.0	33.0	15.0	3.0
Chocolate, Stack, Sainsbury's*	¼ Pack/76g	311	19.5	409	5.3	39.3	25.6	2.0
Chocolate, Tesco*	1 Serving/76g	293	21.8	386	5.1	26.9	28.7	0.5
Chocolate Covered, Tesco*	1 Serving/72g	295	21.2	410	5.7	29.3	29.5	2.0
Choux & Chocolate Sauce, Tesco*	1 Serving/76.5g	297	22.1	386	5.1	26.9	28.7	0.5
Classic French, Sainsbury's*	1 Serving/90g	284	15.5	316	6.6	33.7	17.2	0.1
Filled with Cream, Stack, Fresh, M & S*	1 Serving/75g	281	21.4	375	5.3	23.6	28.5	1.9
in a Pot, Waitrose*	1 Pot/80g	207	11.3	259	6.3	25.6	14.1	2.9
Waitrose*	4 Profiteroles/75g	269	17.9	359	4.8	31.1	23.9	0.7
PROVENCALE								
Cabillaud à la, Weight Watchers*	1 Pack/380g	327	10.3	86	5.1	10.3	2.7	0.0
Chicken, M & S*	1 Pack/430g	366	11.6	85	13.2	2.3	2.7	0.6
Chicken, Steam Cuisine, M & S*	1oz/28g	34	1.1	120	9.6	12.7	3.8	1.4
King Prawn & Mushroom, M & S*	½ Pack/185g	120	4.6	65	7.2	3.9	2.5	0.9
Mushroom, Fresh, COU, M & S*	½ Pack/150g	60	2.3	40	2.6	4.1	1.5	1.8
Prawn & Mushroom with Pasta, COU, M & S*	1 Pack/400g	360	2.0	90	5.9	15.7	0.5	0.0
Raratouille, Asda*	½ Can/195g	98	3.9	50	1.0	7.0	2.0	1.0
Ratatouille, Tesco*	1 Can/390g	152	7.8	39	1.1	4.2	2.0	1.9
Ratatouille, Waitrose*	½ Can/195g	107	4.1	55	1.3	7.8	2.1	0.8
PRUNES								
Dried, Average	1 Serving/50g	79	0.2	158	2.5	36.4	0.4	5.8
in Apple Juice, Average	1 Serving/90g	76	0.1	84	0.8	19.8	0.1	1.4
in Fruit Juice, Average	1oz/28g	25	0.0	88	0.9	21.4	0.2	3.0
in Syrup, Average	1oz/28g	26	0.0	92	1.0	22.1	0.2	2.6
Stewed with Sugar	1oz/28g	29	0.1	103	1.3	25.5	0.2	3.1
Stewed without Sugar	1oz/28g	23	0.1	81	1.4	19.5	0.3	3.3
PUDDING								
Cherry Cobbler, GFY, Asda*	1 Cobbler/100g	158	2.0	158	2.1	33.0	2.0	0.9
Chocolate, Gu*	1 Pack/240g	780	27.4	325	3.9	51.8	11.4	1.6
Chocolate, Melting Middle, M & S*	1 Pudding/154.5g	510	27.8	330	5.8	36.2	18.0	3.1
Chocolate, Tesco*	1 Serving/110g	348	21.0	316	3.1	32.9	19.1	1.9
Chocolate with Chocolate Sauce, Heinz*	¼ Can/77g	221	7.2	287	3.1	47.7	9.3	1.4
Creamed Sago, Ambrosia*	1 Serving/200g	158	3.2	79	2.5	13.6	1.6	0.2
Eve's, Average	1oz/28g	67	3.7	241	3.5	28.9	13.1	1.4
Jam Roly Poly & Custard, Co-Op*	1 Serving/105g	263	7.4	250	3.0	44.0	7.0	0.8
Lemon, BGTY, Sainsbury's*	1 Serving/100g	151	1.9	151	2.9	31.0	1.9	0.5
Pear & Almond, Finest, Tesco*	1 Slice/70g	170	8.1	243	3.0	31.9	11.5	1.0
Queen of Puddings	1oz/28g	60	2.2	213	4.8	33.1	7.8	0.2
Sticky Toffee, Co-Op*	¼ Pudding/100g	355	20.0	355	3.0	40.0	20.0	0.7
Sticky Toffee, Extra Special, Asda*	¼ Pudding/100g	378	18.0	378	1.9	52.0	18.0	1.8
Sticky Toffee, M & S*	1 Pudding/105g	345	13.5	330	3.3	45.8	12.9	1.7

P

	Measure INFO/WEIGHT	per Measure KCAL	FAT	Nutrition Values per 100g / 100ml KCAL	PROT	CARB	FAT	FIBRE
PUDDING								
Sticky Toffee, Tesco*	1 Serving/110g	287	14.7	261	3.3	31.8	13.4	0.7
Sticky Toffee, with Custard, Somerfield*	1 Pack/245g	576	19.6	235	3.0	38.0	8.0	0.0
Summer Fruits, HE, Tesco*	1 Serving/100g	72	0.2	72	1.3	16.3	0.2	2.9
Summer Fruits, M & S*	Pudding/150g	180	1.1	120	1.5	27.1	0.7	2.5
Summer Pudding, BGTY, Sainsbury's*	1 Pot/110g	223	5.1	203	3.2	40.9	4.6	2.4
Summer Pudding, Safeway*	1 Pudding/135g	196	0.5	145	2.5	32.9	0.4	3.1
Summer Pudding, Waitrose*	1 Pot/120g	125	0.5	104	2.0	23.1	0.4	1.4
PULSES								
Mixed, in Water, Sainsbury's*	½ Can/120g	131	2.6	109	8.7	13.6	2.2	4.6
PUMPKIN								
Boiled in Salted Water	1oz/28g	4	0.1	13	0.6	2.1	0.3	1.1
Kabocha, Tesco*	1 Serving 50g	20	0.1	39	1.1	8.3	0.1	1.6
Solid Pack, 100% Pure, Canned, Libby's*	1 Can/425g	139	1.7	33	1.6	7.4	0.4	4.1
PUPPODUMS								
Black Pepper, Ready to Eat, Sharwood's*	1 Puppodum/9g	41	2.4	461	16.7	37.2	27.3	7.3
Extra Large, Cook to Eat, Sharwood's*	1oz/28g	78	0.5	279	21.3	44.7	1.7	10.3
Garlic & Coriander, Ready to Eat, Sharwood's*	1 Puppodum/9g	39	1.9	438	18.4	43.0	21.4	6.5
Plain, Cook to Eat, Sharwood's*	1 Puppodum/12g	32	0.1	273	21.9	45.7	1.0	10.1
Plain, Ready to Eat, Sharwood's*	1 Puppodum/9g	41	2.3	461	17.0	40.6	25.6	0.0
Spicy, Cook to Eat, Sharwood's*	1 Puppodum/12g	31	0.1	257	20.2	43.0	0.5	13.0

P

	Measure INFO/WEIGHT	per Measure KCAL	FAT	Nutrition Values per 100g / 100ml KCAL	PROT	CARB	FAT	FIBRE
QUADRELLI								
Organic, M & S*	1 Serving/75g	263	1.1	350	13.4	71.1	1.4	3.0
QUAVERS								
Cheese, Walkers*	1 Bag/20g	106	6.0	530	2.5	62.0	30.0	1.1
Prawn Cocktail, Walkers*	1 Pack/16g	88	5.1	550	1.9	63.8	31.9	1.3
Salt & Vinegar, Walkers*	1 Bag/16.4g	86	4.9	525	1.9	62.0	30.0	1.2
QUICHE								
Asparagus & Cheese, Safeway*	¼ Quiche/100g	260	17.4	260	7.5	18.2	17.4	1.4
Asparagus & Mushroom, Tesco*	½ Quiche/200g	474	32.8	237	5.1	17.2	16.4	1.2
Baby Spinach & Gruyere, Sainsbury's*	¼ Quiche/93g	228	16.0	245	7.4	15.1	17.2	1.0
Bacon, Cheese & Leek, Weight Watchers*	1 Quiche/165g	307	13.4	186	7.4	21.0	8.1	1.8
Bacon, Leek & Mushroom, M & S*	¼ Quiche/100g	245	16.4	245	6.9	17.2	16.4	1.3
Bacon, Mushroom & Tomato, Somerfield*	¼ Quiche/100g	264	17.2	264	7.6	19.6	17.2	1.0
Bacon, Sausage & Tomato, Tesco*	¼ Pack/100g	240	15.1	240	6.7	18.4	15.1	0.7
Bacon & Cheese, Pork Farms*	1 Pack/120g	378	24.0	315	11.1	20.8	20.0	0.0
Bacon & Cheese, Sainsbury's*	¼ Quiche/100g	237	15.0	237	7.0	18.6	15.0	0.7
Bacon & Leek, Asda*	¼ Quiche/100g	245	16.2	245	7.3	17.4	16.2	1.9
Bacon & Leek, Individual, Tesco*	1 Quiche/175g	485	32.4	277	8.3	19.4	18.5	0.9
Bacon & Leek, Tesco*	¼ Quiche/100g	260	18.0	260	6.9	17.5	18.0	1.2
Bacon & Tomato, Asda*	1 Serving/106.9g	201	8.6	188	8.0	21.0	8.0	1.1
Bacon & Tomato, Good Intentions, Somerfield*	1 Serving/145g	255	21.5	176	5.7	5.1	14.8	0.1
Bacon & Tomato, Safeway*	¼ Quiche/100g	287	19.0	287	8.6	20.3	19.0	1.4
Brie & Smoked Bacon, Asda*	¼ Quiche/90g	249	17.0	277	8.9	17.8	18.9	1.0
Broccoli, Budgens*	1 Serving/88g	213	15.5	243	6.3	14.8	17.7	1.0
Broccoli, Extra, Value, Tesco*	1 Serving/125g	341	24.0	273	10.0	15.1	19.2	0.8
Broccoli, HE, Tesco*	1 Quiche/175g	308	12.3	176	6.7	21.5	7.0	1.4
Broccoli, Tesco*	1 Serving/100g	249	17.2	249	6.0	17.6	17.2	1.4
Broccoli, Tomato & Cheese, BGTY, Sainsbury's*	1 Quiche/390g	632	32.0	162	6.4	15.7	8.2	1.3
Broccoli, Tomato & Cheese, Deep Filled, Sainsbury's*	¼ Quiche/100g	203	12.9	203	5.2	16.9	12.9	2.3
Broccoli & Cheddar Cheese, Safeway*	1 Pack/300g	813	53.7	271	7.7	19.8	17.9	1.9
Broccoli & Gruyere Cheese, Waitrose*	1 Serving/100g	241	17.8	241	7.3	13.0	17.8	2.9
Broccoli & Stilton, Mini, Sainsbury's*	1 Quiche/14g	52	3.0	369	8.8	35.2	21.4	3.3
Brocolli & Tomato, M & S*	1 Quiche/169.8g	365	23.6	215	6.3	16.0	13.9	1.7
Cheddar Cheese, & Onion, Safeway*	¼ Quiche/100g	293	19.3	293	8.3	21.6	19.3	1.5
Cheese, Broccoli & Tomato, Nisa Heritage*	1 Serving/85g	234	16.6	275	7.3	17.5	19.5	1.4
Cheese, Onion & Chive, HE, Tesco*	1 Slice/100g	202	8.2	202	10.9	21.2	8.2	1.3
Cheese, Onion & Chive, SmartPrice, Asda*	¼ Quiche/83g	213	14.1	257	6.0	20.0	17.0	0.7
Cheese, Onion & Chive, Somerfield*	1oz/28g	87	6.4	310	9.0	16.0	23.0	0.0
Cheese, Onion & Chive, Tesco*	1oz/28g	90	6.7	320	10.6	15.5	24.0	0.6
Cheese & Bacon, HE, Tesco*	1 Serving/155g	307	14.1	198	9.1	19.9	9.1	1.4
Cheese & Bacon, SmartPrice, Asda*	¼ Quiche/82g	208	13.8	257	6.0	20.0	17.0	0.7
Cheese & Bacon, Tesco*	¼ Quiche/100g	255	16.3	255	8.1	17.9	16.3	0.7
Cheese & Broccoli, Good Intentions, Somerfield*	1 Quiche/145g	409	23.1	282	6.9	27.7	15.9	1.8
Cheese & Broccoli, Morrisons*	1/3 Quiche/134g	338	22.4	253	7.1	18.4	16.8	1.7
Cheese & Chive, HE, Tesco*	1 Serving/86g	169	6.4	197	10.4	22.1	7.4	1.2
Cheese & Egg	1oz/28g	88	6.2	314	12.5	17.3	22.2	0.6
Cheese & Ham, Basics, Somerfield*	¼ Quiche/81g	187	11.0	231	7.0	20.1	13.6	0.7
Cheese & Ham, Sainsbury's*	1 Serving/100g	266	19.0	266	9.3	14.4	19.0	1.2
Cheese & Ham, Somerfield*	1 Quiche/325g	835	58.5	257	7.0	18.0	18.0	0.0
Cheese & Mushroom, Budgens*	½ Quiche/170g	474	32.8	279	7.8	18.4	19.3	1.4
Cheese & Onion, 25% Reduced Fat, Asda*	½ Quiche/78g	163	7.0	209	11.0	21.0	9.0	2.4
Cheese & Onion, Co-Op*	¼ Quiche/87.5g	264	19.4	300	10.0	17.0	22.0	1.0
Cheese & Onion, Deep Filled, Sainsbury's*	¼ Quiche/100g	254	17.2	254	7.3	17.2	17.2	2.2
Cheese & Onion, Finest, Tesco*	1 Serving/130g	346	24.3	266	9.1	15.3	18.7	2.5

QUICHE

	Measure INFO/WEIGHT	per Measure KCAL	FAT	Nutrition Values per 100g / 100ml KCAL	PROT	CARB	FAT	FIBRE
Cheese & Onion, HL, Tesco*	1 Quarter/100g	180	7.8	180	9.4	17.6	7.8	1.8
Cheese & Onion, Individual, Sainsbury's*	1 Quiche/180g	542	34.9	301	9.9	21.6	19.4	1.5
Cheese & Onion, M & S*	1 Slice/100g	250	17.2	250	8.2	16.1	17.2	1.5
Cheese & Onion, Mini, Iceland*	1 Quiche/13.9g	50	3.1	359	9.3	30.6	22.1	2.1
Cheese & Onion, Mini, Somerfield*	1oz/28g	110	7.8	394	9.0	27.0	28.0	0.0
Cheese & Onion, Morrisons*	1 Serving/100g	300	21.8	300	8.8	17.2	21.8	1.4
Cheese & Onion, Reduced Fat, Eat Smart, Morrisons*	1 Quiche/400g	824	36.8	206	7.7	16.9	9.2	0.7
Cheese & Onion, Reduced Fat, Safeway*	¼ Flan/100g	212	10.0	212	9.6	20.8	10.0	1.5
Cheese & Onion, Safeway*	1 Serving/310g	797	44.0	257	7.2	25.2	14.2	0.0
Cheese & Onion, Shell*	1 Slice/150g	362	23.1	241	7.9	16.1	15.4	0.0
Cheese & Onion, Somerfield*	1 Quiche/300g	696	48.0	232	8.0	14.0	16.0	0.0
Cheese & Onion, Tesco*	1/4 Quiche/100g	285	19.8	285	7.7	17.9	19.8	1.3
Cheese & Onion, Value, Tesco*	½ Quiche/200g	526	36.4	263	8.6	16.1	18.2	0.7
Cheese & Onion, Weight Watchers*	1 Quiche/165g	325	15.3	197	7.0	21.2	9.3	1.6
Cheese & Tomato, Asda*	¼ Quiche/105g	274	17.9	261	8.0	19.0	17.0	0.9
Cheese & Tomato, M & S*	1 Serving/100g	230	15.6	230	7.7	15.1	15.6	1.6
Cheese & Tomato, Morrisons*	½ Quiche/64g	195	13.1	304	7.3	22.8	20.5	1.0
Cheese & Tomato, Somerfield*	1 Quiche/135g	416	25.7	308	10.0	23.0	19.0	0.0
Cheese & Tomato, Tesco*	¼ Quiche/100g	255	17.3	255	5.8	18.1	17.3	1.2
Cheese Potato & Onion, Safeway*	1/3 Quiche/115g	361	23.3	314	8.8	24.1	20.3	1.5
Cherry Tomato, Mozzarella & Pesto, TTD, Sainsbury's*	1 Quiche/475g	1112	77.0	234	5.5	16.5	16.2	2.1
Chicken, Bacon & Mushroom, Asda*	½ Quiche/200g	376	24.8	188	7.8	11.3	12.4	3.7
Chicken, Garlic & Herb, Asda*	1/8 Quiche/52g	137	8.3	264	10.0	20.0	16.0	1.2
Chicken & Basil, Finest, Tesco*	1 Serving/134g	381	24.9	284	9.3	19.8	18.6	1.3
Chicken & Mushroom, Somerfield*	1oz/28g	90	5.9	320	12.0	22.0	21.0	0.0
Cumberland Sausage & Onion, Sainsbury's*	1 Serving/180g	486	33.3	270	7.0	18.8	18.5	1.3
Davidstow Cheddar Cheese & Caramelised Onion, Asda*	1/3 Quiche/117g	367	26.8	315	7.0	20.0	23.0	1.0
Egg, Bacon & Cheese, Iceland*	¼ Quiche/90g	258	15.6	286	8.8	24.0	17.3	1.9
Farmhouse Cheddar & Onion, Waitrose*	¼ Quiche/100g	257	18.1	257	8.1	15.4	18.1	1.3
Gammon, Leek & Cheddar Cheese, Somerfield*	¼ Quiche/95g	251	16.2	264	7.6	19.9	17.1	0.9
Garlic Mushroom, Asda*	¼ Quiche/105g	273	16.8	260	7.0	22.0	16.0	0.7
Goats Cheese & Red Pepper, Finest, Tesco*	1 Serving/200g	600	45.0	300	5.9	18.5	22.5	1.5
Ham, Cheese & Chive, GFY, Asda*	1 Serving/78g	173	7.8	222	9.0	24.0	10.0	1.5
Ham & Mustard, GFY, Asda*	1 Quiche/155g	327	17.1	211	9.0	19.0	11.0	3.9
Ham & Soft Cheese, Tesco*	¼ Quiche/100g	280	20.1	280	7.4	17.5	20.1	1.9
Ham & Tomato, M & S*	½ Pack/200g	440	31.0	220	8.1	12.4	15.5	2.9
Leek, Cheese & Chive, Sainsbury's*	1/3 Quiche/125g	293	20.3	234	7.1	14.9	16.2	1.3
Leek & Sweet Potato, Waitrose*	½ Quiche/200g	440	29.0	220	5.3	17.0	14.5	2.3
Lorraine, Asda*	¼ Quiche/100g	246	16.2	246	6.6	18.5	16.2	4.2
Lorraine, Average	1oz/28g	109	7.9	391	16.1	19.8	28.1	0.7
Lorraine, BGTY, Sainsbury's*	1 Serving/128g	273	14.0	213	10.9	17.7	10.9	0.7
Lorraine, Budgens*	1 Pack/180g	520	30.8	289	8.2	25.6	17.1	0.8
Lorraine, Co-Op*	1/3 Quiche/108g	313	22.7	290	11.0	20.0	21.0	3.0
Lorraine, Extra Special, Asda*	¼ Quiche/100g	270	18.0	270	8.0	19.0	18.0	2.3
Lorraine, Finest, Tesco*	1 Serving/100g	330	25.1	330	8.4	17.5	25.1	1.5
Lorraine, Half Fat, Waitrose*	¼ Quiche/100g	189	8.9	189	8.1	19.0	8.9	1.4
Lorraine, HL, Tesco*	¼ Serving/100g	190	8.0	190	12.2	16.9	8.0	1.8
Lorraine, Mini, M & S*	1oz/28g	95	6.6	340	11.6	21.0	23.6	1.6
Lorraine, Morrisons*	¼ Quiche/100g	258	17.0	258	9.2	17.1	17.0	2.8
Lorraine, Quiche Selection, M & S*	1 Slice/56g	160	11.5	285	12.8	12.3	20.6	2.1
Lorraine, Reduced Fat, Eat Smart, Morrisons*	¼ Quiche/100g	209	9.8	209	9.4	17.8	9.8	0.5
Lorraine, Reduced Fat, Safeway*	¼ Quiche/100g	231	12.4	231	11.0	18.9	12.4	1.4
Lorraine, Sainsbury's*	½ Quiche/200g	598	42.4	299	10.6	16.3	21.2	0.9

Q

QUICHE

	Measure INFO/WEIGHT	per Measure KCAL	FAT	Nutrition Values per 100g / 100ml KCAL	PROT	CARB	FAT	FIBRE
Lorraine, Small, Waitrose*	1 Pack/170g	507	35.0	298	9.8	18.4	20.6	2.3
Lorraine, Smoked Bacon & Cheese, M & S*	¼ Quiche/100g	270	18.4	270	9.7	16.4	18.4	1.6
Lorraine, Snack, Morrisons*	1 Serving/50g	143	9.4	285	10.2	19.0	18.7	2.0
Lorraine, Somerfield*	¼ Quiche/87g	260	18.4	299	10.1	17.1	21.1	0.7
Lorraine, Spar*	1 Quiche/340g	979	65.6	288	10.6	17.9	19.3	0.8
Lorraine, Tesco*	1 Serving/81g	215	13.4	265	8.9	20.0	16.6	0.8
Lorraine, TTD, Sainsbury's*	1/3 Pie/158g	482	35.9	305	10.2	15.1	22.7	0.9
Lorraine, with a Creamy Filling, Safeway*	1 Quiche/485g	1576	110.1	325	9.8	19.4	22.7	1.2
Mature Cheddar & Onion, Deep Fill, Somerfield*	¼ Quiche/100g	280	17.6	280	8.4	22.1	17.6	1.1
Mediterranean, GFY, Asda*	1 Serving/25g	54	2.3	217	9.0	25.0	9.0	2.4
Mediterranean, M & S*	1oz/28g	64	4.3	230	6.6	16.6	15.3	0.9
Mediterranean Pepper, Good Intentions, Somerfield*	1/3 Quiche/130g	264	12.0	203	7.9	22.2	9.2	1.3
Mediterranean Vegetable, BGTY, Sainsbury's*	½ Quiche/90g	160	7.2	178	7.3	19.2	8.0	1.7
Mediterranean Vegetable, Mini, M & S*	1oz/28g	78	4.9	280	6.8	23.9	17.5	1.6
Mediterranean Vegetable, Sainsbury's*	¼ Quiche/100g	207	12.3	207	4.3	19.8	12.3	1.4
Mushroom	1oz/28g	80	5.5	284	10.0	18.3	19.5	0.9
Mushroom, M & S*	¼ Quiche/100g	235	16.7	235	6.1	14.6	16.7	2.8
Mushroom, Somerfield*	¼ Quiche/82g	212	13.1	258	9.0	20.0	16.0	0.0
Mushroom, Tesco*	¼ Quiche/100g	250	17.5	250	5.6	17.4	17.5	1.0
Mushroom Medley, Waitrose*	¼ Quiche/100g	222	15.2	222	6.4	15.0	15.2	2.9
Mushroom Medley & Gruyere, TTD, Sainsbury's*	1/3 Quiche/158g	426	30.2	269	6.3	18.0	19.1	1.4
Red Pepper, Goats Cheese & Spinach, Waitrose*	1 Serving/100g	218	14.3	218	6.5	15.8	14.3	2.6
Red Pepper, Rocket & Parmesan, Waitrose*	1 Serving/100g	236	16.9	236	6.1	14.8	16.9	1.9
Roast Sweet Potato, Carrot & Coriander, Asda*	½ Quiche/208g	523	33.2	252	7.0	20.0	16.0	1.0
Salmon & Asparagus, HE, Tesco*	1 Quiche/345g	621	26.6	180	7.5	20.2	7.7	1.2
Salmon & Broccoli, Asda*	¼ Quiche/106g	289	18.0	273	10.0	20.0	17.0	2.6
Salmon & Broccoli, Budgens*	½ Quiche/187g	539	35.7	288	11.2	17.7	19.1	0.6
Salmon & Broccoli, Sainsbury's*	1 Serving	346	22.8	260	7.9	18.5	17.1	0.8
Salmon & Broccoli, Tesco*	1 Serving/133g	311	20.1	234	7.9	16.6	15.1	0.9
Salmon & Spinach, Sainsbury's*	1/3 Quiche/125g	318	21.9	254	8.2	15.9	17.5	1.0
Sausage & Onion, Sainsbury's*	1 Serving/100g	287	20.0	287	7.1	19.7	20.0	1.2
Spinach, Ricotta & Gruyere Slice, Somerfield*	1 Slice/130g	348	26.0	268	7.0	15.0	20.0	0.0
Spinach & Gruyere, Mini, Somerfield*	1oz/28g	108	7.6	384	11.0	25.0	27.0	0.0
Spinach & Gruyere, Sainsbury's*	¼ Quiche/100g	258	19.1	258	7.7	13.9	19.1	1.0
Spinach & Ricotta, M & S*	1oz/28g	73	5.3	260	8.0	14.9	18.8	1.7
Spinach & Ricotta, Safeway*	¼ Quiche/85g	193	9.9	227	7.9	22.6	11.7	1.7
Spinach & Ricotta, Tesco*	¼ Quiche/100g	237	14.9	237	5.8	19.9	14.9	1.0
Spinach Ricotta Cheese & Red Pepper, Safeway*	1 Serving/120g	304	19.7	253	6.2	20.2	16.4	1.2
Summer Vegetable, M & S*	¼ Quiche/100g	215	14.0	215	5.1	17.2	14.0	1.7
Sunblush Tomato, Basil & Mozzarella, Somerfield*	¼ Quiche/88g	221	14.5	251	7.7	17.9	16.5	1.0
Sweet Cherry Pepper & Fontal Cheese, Finest, Tesco*	¼ Slice/100g	293	22.1	293	6.7	16.9	22.1	0.9
Sweetfire Pepper, Feta & Olive, Waitrose*	¼ Quiche/100g	238	16.9	238	5.7	15.7	16.9	1.4
Three Cheese & Onion, GFY, Asda*	1 Serving/73g	188	10.2	258	10.0	23.0	14.0	3.1
Tomato, Cheese & Courgette, Asda*	1 Quiche/100g	333	17.0	333	11.0	34.0	17.0	5.0
Tomato, GFY, Asda*	¼ Quiche/50g	94	4.0	188	8.0	21.0	8.0	0.8
Tomato, Mushroom & Bacon, Sainsbury's*	1 Serving/187g	447	30.9	239	7.5	15.2	16.5	1.1
Tomato & Cheese, Sainsbury's*	1/3 Quiche/133g	374	24.5	281	7.9	20.9	18.4	1.5
Tomato Cheese & Courgette, GFY, Asda*	1 Serving/155g	333	17.1	215	7.0	22.0	11.0	3.3
Tomato Mozzarella & Basil, Deep Filled, Sainsbury's*	¼ Quiche/100g	215	14.1	215	5.8	16.3	14.1	2.2
Tuna, Tomato & Basil, Asda*	1 Serving/125g	305	20.0	244	9.0	16.0	16.0	1.5
Vegetable, Tesco*	1 Serving/100g	257	17.7	257	6.9	17.5	17.7	1.5

QUICK SNACK

	Measure INFO/WEIGHT	per Measure KCAL	FAT	Nutrition Values per 100g / 100ml KCAL	PROT	CARB	FAT	FIBRE
Chicken & Mushroom Flavour, Value, Tesco*	1 Pot/76g	325	11.2	428	11.1	61.4	14.7	3.9

	Measure INFO/WEIGHT	per Measure KCAL	FAT	Nutrition Values per 100g / 100ml KCAL	PROT	CARB	FAT	FIBRE
QUICK SNACK								
Mash, Roasted Onion, Sainsbury's*	1 Pot/58g	75	4.1	130	1.8	14.8	7.1	0.0
Rice, Chilli, Sainsbury's*	1 Pack/280g	241	0.6	86	2.5	18.6	0.2	0.0
Rice, Sweet & Sour, Sainsbury's*	1 Serving/237g	230	1.2	97	2.5	20.5	0.5	0.0
QUINCE								
Average	1oz/28g	7	0.0	26	0.3	6.3	0.1	0.0
QUINOA								
Boiled, Average	1 Serving/100g	77	1.3	77	3.5	13.9	1.3	2.2
QUORN*								
Bacon Style, Rashers, Streaky, Frozen, Quorn*	1 Rasher/18.6g	37	2.9	198	11.0	3.5	15.5	5.0
Bacon Style, Slices, Smoky, Frozen, Quorn*	¼ Pack/37.5g	75	5.8	199	11.8	3.0	15.5	5.0
Bacon Style Rashers, Deli, Quorn*	1 Rasher/30g	42	1.8	141	13.5	8.1	6.1	4.2
Balls, Swedish Style, Quorn*	1 Pack/300g	354	6.0	118	17.0	8.0	2.0	2.0
Beef Style Pieces, in Red Wine Sauce, Quorn*	1 Pack/275g	165	4.1	60	5.0	6.5	1.5	1.7
Beef Style Pieces, Quorn*	½ Pack/75g	69	1.7	92	13.5	4.5	2.2	5.0
Bites, Quorn*	½ Pack/70g	77	1.8	110	13.8	8.0	2.5	5.0
Burgers, Chicken Style, Quorn*	1 Burger/70g	136	6.7	194	11.0	16.0	9.6	4.6
Burgers, Minted Lamb Style, Quorn*	1 Burger/80g	86	3.2	108	12.0	6.0	4.0	4.0
Burgers, Original, Quorn*	1 Burger/50g	73	2.4	146	18.9	6.7	4.8	3.0
Burgers, Premium, Quorn*	1 Burger/82g	88	3.3	107	11.3	6.5	4.0	3.5
Burgers, Quarter Pounder, Mexican Style, Quorn*	1 Burger/113g	180	6.3	159	18.3	8.9	5.6	3.8
Burgers, Quarter Pounder, Quorn*	1 Burger/113.5g	158	5.1	139	18.0	6.5	4.5	4.5
Burgers, Sizzling, Quorn*	1 Burger/130g	212	9.1	163	15.0	10.0	7.0	0.0
Burgers, Southern Style, Quorn*	1 Burger/63g	119	6.2	189	10.7	14.5	9.8	3.1
Chicken Style Dippers, Quorn*	1 Dipper/19.2g	32	2.0	167	11.0	7.2	10.5	4.0
Chicken Style Pieces, Frozen Or Chilled, Quorn*	1 Serving/175g	180	4.6	103	14.0	5.8	2.6	5.5
Chilli, Quorn*	1oz/28g	23	1.2	81	4.7	6.9	4.2	2.5
Chilli, Vegetarian, Tesco*	1 Pack/400g	340	3.2	85	4.4	15.0	0.8	2.1
Cottage Pie, Quorn*	1 Serving/300g	177	4.2	59	2.5	9.0	1.4	2.6
Curry, Red Thai, Quorn*	1 Pack/400g	464	15.6	116	4.6	15.5	3.9	4.0
Curry & Rice, Quorn*	1 Pack/400g	412	8.0	103	3.8	17.5	2.0	1.5
Eggs, Picnic, Quorn*	1 Egg/20g	50	2.3	248	15.0	21.0	11.5	4.6
Escalopes, Creamy Garlic & Mushroom, Quorn*	1 Escalope/120g	266	15.0	222	7.9	19.4	12.5	3.1
Escalopes, Creamy Peppercorn, Quorn*	1 Escalope/120g	252	15.2	210	7.8	16.0	12.7	4.0
Escalopes, Garlic & Herb, Quorn*	1 Escalope/140g	293	16.5	209	8.9	16.9	11.8	3.8
Escalopes, Gruyere Cheese, Quorn*	1 Escalope/110g	262	15.4	238	10.0	18.0	14.0	2.6
Escalopes, Lemon & Black Pepper, Quorn*	1 Escalope/110g	249	12.9	226	9.6	20.5	11.7	2.1
Escalopes, Mature Cheddar & Broccoli, Quorn*	1 Serving/120g	244	13.7	203	8.7	16.5	11.4	2.9
Escalopes, Spinach & Soft Cheese, Quorn*	2 Escalopes/240g	473	26.4	197	8.5	16.1	11.0	2.9
Escalopes, Wensleydale & Blueberry, Quorn*	1 Escalope/120.1g	281	16.8	234	10.0	17.0	14.0	4.0
Fajita, Strips, Quorn*	½ Pack/75g	74	1.8	99	14.0	5.4	2.4	5.6
Fillets, Crispy, Quorn*	1 Fillet/100g	197	9.8	197	13.0	14.2	9.8	4.0
Fillets, Garlic & Herb, Quorn*	1 Fillet/100g	208	9.8	208	13.9	16.1	9.8	4.1
Fillets, Lemon & Pepper, Quorn*	1 Fillet/100g	195	8.5	195	13.3	16.2	8.5	3.5
Fillets, Plain, Quorn*	2 Fillets/102g	92	1.8	90	12.6	5.9	1.8	4.7
Fillets, Thai, Quorn*	1 Serving/79.4g	96	3.6	121	11.0	9.0	4.5	4.0
Goujons, Quorn*	1 Goujon/30.5g	56	2.9	187	10.2	15.0	9.6	4.5
Grills, Lamb Style, Quorn*	1 Grill/89.0g	97	3.3	109	11.2	7.6	3.7	4.3
Lasagne, Quorn*	1 Pack/300g	252	7.5	84	4.8	10.6	2.5	1.8
Mince, Frozen Or Chilled, Quorn*	1 Serving/87g	82	1.7	94	14.5	4.5	2.0	5.5
Nuggets, Chicken Style, Quorn*	1 Nugget/20g	41	2.2	207	10.3	16.7	11.0	3.8
Nuggets, Crispy Chicken Style, Quorn*	1 Nugget/16g	29	1.7	182	12.0	9.9	10.5	4.0
Pie, Creamy Mushroom, Quorn*	1 Pie/141.4g	357	20.4	253	4.5	26.0	14.5	2.0
Pie, Mince & Onion, Quorn*	1 Pie/141g	358	19.7	254	5.0	27.0	14.0	1.5

Q

QUORN*

	Measure INFO/WEIGHT	per Measure KCAL	per Measure FAT	Nutrition Values per 100g / 100ml KCAL	PROT	CARB	FAT	FIBRE
Pie, Quorn & Mushroom, Tesco*	1 Pie/141g	378	23.7	268	5.3	23.8	16.8	1.3
Roast, Chicken Style, Quorn*	1/5 Roast/90.8g	87	1.8	96	15.0	4.5	2.0	4.9
Sausage & Mash, Sainsbury's*	1 Pack/394g	339	11.8	86	3.8	11.0	3.0	0.7
Sausage Rolls, Quorn*	1 Roll/50g	155	11.0	310	9.0	19.0	22.0	3.0
Sausages, Bangers, Quorn*	1 Sausage/50g	58	2.4	116	11.7	6.6	4.8	3.0
Sausages, Bangers, Sizzling, Quorn*	1 Sausage/50g	88	5.5	175	9.0	10.0	11.0	15.0
Sausages, Cumberland, Quorn*	1 Sausage/50g	60	2.2	120	13.1	7.0	4.4	2.4
Sausages, Frozen, Quorn*	2 Sausages/100g	113	3.7	113	14.9	4.9	3.7	3.3
Sausages, Leek & Pork Style, Quorn*	1 Sausage/44g	56	2.2	127	15.1	5.5	4.9	4.3
Sausages, Pork & Apple Style, Quorn*	1 Sausage/50.4g	59	2.3	117	11.5	7.5	4.6	3.0
Sausages, Sizzlers, BBQ, Quorn*	1 Sausage/50.3g	86	5.5	171	10.0	8.0	11.0	3.0
Sausages, Spinach & Cheese, Quorn*	1 Sausage/50g	60	2.0	120	15.1	6.0	4.0	2.8
Sausages, Sweet Chilli, Quorn*	1 Sausage/50g	63	2.3	125	14.0	7.0	4.5	3.0
Sausages, Tomato & Basil, Quorn*	1 Sausage/50g	51	1.2	102	14.3	6.0	2.3	2.8
Slices, Chicken Style, Deli, Quorn*	3 Slices/33g	35	0.9	107	16.3	4.5	2.6	6.0
Slices, Chicken Style, Wafer Thin, Deli, Quorn*	1 Serving/28g	30	0.7	107	16.3	4.5	2.6	5.9
Slices, Ham Style, Deli, Quorn*	½ Pack/50g	55	1.1	110	16.0	6.5	2.2	5.8
Slices, Ham Style, Smoky, Quorn*	½ Pack/50g	55	1.2	110	16.5	5.7	2.4	5.0
Slices, Ham Style, Wafer Thin, Deli, Quorn*	1 Serving/18g	20	0.4	110	16.0	6.5	2.2	5.8
Slices, Peppered Beef Style, Quorn*	½ Pack/50g	54	1.1	107	14.5	7.6	2.1	4.0
Slices, Roast Chicken Style, Quorn*	¼ Pack/70g	76	1.5	109	16.0	6.4	2.2	5.6
Slices, Turkey Style, with Stuffing, Deli, Quorn*	1 Slice/13g	14	0.3	107	14.9	6.6	2.3	4.7
Slices, Turkey Style & Cranberry, Quorn*	2 Slices/28g	32	0.7	113	14.5	8.0	2.5	4.0
Spaghetti Bolognese, Quorn*	1 Pack/400g	240	3.6	60	3.7	9.2	0.9	1.6
Spaghetti Bolognese, Sainsbury's*	1 Pack/450g	347	5.0	77	4.9	11.9	1.1	1.8
Steaks, Peppered, Quorn*	1 Steak/98g	107	3.7	109	11.4	7.4	3.8	4.0
Tandoori Pieces, Quorn*	½ Pack/69g	93	3.1	133	12.0	11.0	4.5	5.0

Q

	Measure INFO/WEIGHT	per Measure KCAL	FAT	Nutrition Values per 100g / 100ml KCAL	PROT	CARB	FAT	FIBRE
RABBIT								
Meat Only, Raw	1oz/28g	38	1.5	137	21.9	0.0	5.5	0.0
Meat Only, Stewed	1oz/28g	32	0.9	114	21.2	0.0	3.2	0.0
Meat Only, Stewed, Weighed with Bone	1oz/28g	19	0.5	68	12.7	0.0	1.9	0.0
RADDICCIO								
Raw	1oz/28g	4	0.1	14	1.4	1.7	0.2	1.8
RADISH								
Red, Unprepared, Average	1oz/28g	3	0.1	12	0.7	1.9	0.2	0.9
White, Mooli, Raw	1oz/28g	4	0.0	15	0.8	2.9	0.1	0.0
RAINBOW TROUT								
Fillets, with Thyme & Lemon Butter, Asda*	1 Serving/147g	210	10.3	143	20.0	0.9	7.0	0.5
Grilled, Average	1 Serving/120g	162	6.5	135	21.5	0.0	5.4	0.0
Raw, Average	1oz/28g	36	1.4	127	20.5	0.0	5.1	0.0
Smoked, Average	1 Pack/135g	190	7.6	141	21.7	0.8	5.7	0.0
RAISINS								
& Cranberries, Waitrose*	1 Serving/30g	94	0.1	312	1.5	75.7	0.3	3.4
& Sultanas, Jumbo, M & S*	1 Portion/80g	212	0.4	265	2.4	62.4	0.5	2.6
& Sultanas, Jumbo, Safeway*	1 Pack/250g	773	2.0	309	2.4	73.1	0.8	5.7
California, Natural, Sun-Maid*	1 Pack/42.5g	129.2	1.3	304	3.0	71.4	0.7	5.8
Mini, Lunchbox, Garden Gang, Asda*	1 Box/14g	39.8	0.3	284	2.1	69.0	0.0	4.0
Organic, Waitrose*	1 Serving/35g	101.2	0.7	289	2.1	69.3	0.4	5.3
Seedless, Average	1 Serving/75g	215	0.4	287	2.2	68.5	0.5	3.2
RAITA								
Cucumber & Mint, Patak's*	1oz/28g	18	0.5	64	3.4	8.4	1.8	0.0
Plain	1oz/28g	46	4.3	166	2.6	5.5	15.3	0.0
RASPBERRIES								
Fresh, Raw, Average	1oz/28g	7	0.1	26	1.3	4.7	0.3	6.5
in Fruit Juice, Average	1oz/28g	9	0.0	32	0.9	6.7	0.2	1.7
in Syrup, Canned	1oz/28g	25	0.0	88	0.6	22.5	0.1	1.5
RATATOUILLE								
Average	1oz/28g	23	2.0	82	1.3	3.8	7.0	1.8
Chicken, Finest, Tesco*	1 Pack/550g	407	11.6	74	7.8	5.9	2.1	0.0
Princes*	1 Can/360g	86	1.4	24	1.0	4.2	0.4	0.0
Roasted Vegetable, Sainsbury's*	1 Pack/300g	134	3.0	45	1.4	7.5	1.0	2.3
Safeway*	1 Serving/200g	78	5.0	39	1.0	3.0	2.5	1.6
Sainsbury's*	1 Pack/300g	99	1.8	33	1.5	5.5	0.6	1.6
Vegetable, M & S*	1 Pack/300g	135	6.3	45	1.3	4.8	2.1	1.5
RAVIOLI								
Amatriciana, TTD, Sainsbury's*	1 Serving/125g	390	15.6	312	16.6	33.3	12.5	3.5
Asparagus, Waitrose*	1 Serving/150g	303	9.0	202	10.5	26.4	6.0	2.0
Asparagus & Ham, HE, Tesco*	½ Pack/125g	203	3.3	162	8.2	26.5	2.6	0.6
Basil & Parmesan, Organic, Sainsbury's*	½ Pack/192g	290	10.0	151	7.4	21.1	5.2	2.1
Beef, Chef Boyardee*	1 Can/100g	190	5.0	190	6.0	31.0	5.0	2.0
Beef, Fresh, Safeway*	1 Serving/137g	352	9.0	257	10.0	39.4	6.6	3.0
Beef, Italian, Asda*	1 Serving/100g	219	9.2	219	7.9	26.2	9.2	1.6
Beef, Tesco*	1 Serving/194g	175	5.0	90	4.3	12.3	2.6	1.5
Beef & Red Wine, Italian, Tesco*	½ Pack/150g	435	13.2	290	10.4	41.5	8.8	2.4
Beef & Shiraz, Finest, Tesco*	½ Pack/200g	358	9.0	179	8.4	26.1	4.5	1.8
Beef in Tomato Sauce, Canned, Asda*	1 Can/400g	352	8.0	88	3.6	14.0	2.0	3.0
Blue Cheese & Bacon, Safeway*	½ Pack/125g	288	12.0	230	10.5	24.9	9.6	1.6
Cheese, Garlic, & Herb, Fresh, Organic, Tesco*	1 Serving/125g	383	19.5	306	11.3	30.1	15.6	0.9
Cheese, Garlic, & Herb, Safeway*	½ Pack/125g	263	9.5	210	9.1	26.5	7.6	2.0
Cheese, Tomato & Basil, Italiano, Tesco*	½ Pack/125g	309	11.0	247	13.1	28.5	8.8	2.1
Cheese & Asparagus, Waitrose*	1 Serving/100g	242	7.2	242	12.6	31.7	7.2	2.4

RAVIOLI

INFO/WEIGHT	Measure	per Measure		Nutrition Values per 100g / 100ml				
		KCAL	FAT	KCAL	PROT	CARB	FAT	FIBRE
Cheese & Sundried Tomato, Co-Op*	½ Pack/150g	395	10.0	263	12.7	38.7	6.7	2.7
Cheese & Tomato, Fresh, Organic, Tesco*	1 Serving/125g	343	14.0	274	12.5	30.8	11.2	1.1
Cheese & Tomato, Heinz*	1 Can/410g	295	3.7	72	2.6	13.3	0.9	0.8
Cherry Tomato & Mushroom, Somerfield*	1 Pack/400g	436	24.8	109	3.5	9.8	6.2	1.2
Chicken, Tomato & Basil, Finest, Tesco*	1 Serving/200g	358	12.0	179	9.6	21.7	6.0	1.0
Chicken & Mushroom, Finest, Tesco*	½ Pack/125g	268	8.9	214	11.6	25.8	7.1	1.1
Chicken & Rosemary, PB, Waitrose*	½ Pack/125g	266	4.4	213	14.9	30.4	3.5	2.1
Chicken & Tomato, PB, Waitrose*	1 Serving/125g	265	3.4	212	13.5	33.4	2.7	2.8
Feta Cheese, M & S*	1 Serving/100g	195	8.5	195	9.1	20.5	8.5	1.3
Five Cheese, Weight Watchers*	1 Pack/330g	271	9.2	82	3.2	11.1	2.8	0.8
Florentine, Weight Watchers*	1 Serving/241g	220	5.0	91	3.7	14.1	2.1	1.2
Four Cheese, Good Intentions, Somerfield*	1 Pack/353g	367	12.4	104	4.1	14.0	3.5	1.7
Four Cheese, Italian Choice, Asda*	1 Pack/449g	467	26.9	104	3.4	9.0	6.0	2.1
Free Range Duck, TTD, Sainsbury's*	½ Pack/161g	314	11.8	195	11.5	21.0	7.3	2.3
Fresh, Bolognese, Safeway*	1 Serving/120g	200	5.5	167	8.8	22.6	4.6	2.0
Fresh, Pasta Reale*	1 Serving/150g	459	8.9	306	13.1	53.3	5.9	0.0
Garlic & Herb, Italiano, Tesco*	1 Serving/100g	318	13.0	318	11.1	39.1	13.0	2.6
Garlic Mushroom, Finest, Tesco*	1 Serving/250g	553	18.3	221	8.9	30.0	7.3	2.0
Goat's Cheese & Pesto, Asda*	½ Pack/150g	204	5.4	136	6.0	20.0	3.6	0.0
Goats Cheese & Roasted Red Pepper, Finest, Tesco*	½ Pack/125g	308	9.6	246	11.4	32.8	7.7	1.8
in Tomato Sauce, Bettabuy, Morrisons*	1oz/28g	21	0.3	75	2.7	14.0	0.9	1.3
in Tomato Sauce, Canned, Carlini*	1 Can/400g	324	4.0	81	3.1	15.0	1.0	0.5
in Tomato Sauce, Canned, Sainsbury's*	½ Can/200g	166	2.0	83	3.1	15.5	1.0	0.5
in Tomato Sauce, Heinz*	1 Can/410g	299	3.3	73	3.1	13.2	0.8	0.3
in Tomato Sauce, Meat Free, Heinz*	1 Can/410g	308	3.3	75	2.4	14.4	0.8	0.5
Meat, Italian, Fresh, Asda*	½ Pack/150g	261	6.3	174	8.0	26.0	4.2	0.0
Meditteranean Vegetable, HE, Tesco*	1 Serving/125g	199	3.3	159	6.7	27.2	2.6	0.9
Mozzarella Tomato & Basil, Tesco*	1 Serving/125g	304	12.8	243	13.6	24.1	10.2	0.5
Mushroom, Fresh, Budgens*	1 Pack/250g	485	15.0	194	7.7	28.8	6.0	1.7
Mushroom, Fresh, Sainsbury's*	½ Pack/125g	196	5.1	157	7.4	22.6	4.1	1.9
Mushroom, Italian, Fresh, Somerfield*	½ Pack/125g	336	12.3	269	10.8	34.4	9.8	1.8
Mushroom, Italiano, Tesco*	1 Serving/125g	333	16.1	266	10.4	27.0	12.9	3.0
Mushroom, Ready Meals, M & S*	1oz/28g	38	0.5	135	8.1	22.0	1.9	2.2
Mushroom, Safeway*	½ Pack/125g	243	8.6	194	7.5	25.5	6.9	1.8
Mushroom, Wild, Finest, Tesco*	1 Serving/200g	472	12.2	236	10.8	34.4	6.1	1.9
Mushroom & Mascarpone, The Best, Safeway*	1 Pack/175g	466	19.3	266	9.9	31.8	11.0	1.0
Mushroomi, Tesco*	½ Pack/125g	333	16.1	266	10.4	27.0	12.9	3.0
Open, Salmon, Asparagus & Cherry Tomato, Finest, Tesco*	1 Pack/400g	680	39.0	170	9.6	10.8	9.8	1.2
Pancetta & Mozzarella, Finest, Tesco*	1 Serving/125g	344	13.3	275	12.2	32.8	10.6	1.8
Prosciuttoi, Ready Meal, M & S*	1 Pack/100g	195	8.1	195	13.3	17.0	8.1	1.0
Red Onion & Brunello Wine, TTD, Sainsbury's*	1 Serving/125g	235	9.1	188	7.5	23.0	7.3	2.5
Red Pepper, Basil & Chilli, Waitrose*	½ Pack/125g	313	10.5	250	11.6	32.0	8.4	1.7
Rich Beef & Red Wine, Morrisons*	1 Pack/300g	813	20.7	271	12.0	42.8	6.9	2.6
Roast Garlic & Herb, Tesco*	½ Pack/125g	343	13.6	274	12.8	31.1	10.9	1.1
Roasted Pepper, M & S*	1 Pack/400g	540	30.8	135	5.4	11.0	7.7	1.1
Roasted Vegetable, Asda*	½ Pack/150g	218	0.8	145	6.0	29.0	0.5	0.0
SmartPrice, Asda*	1 Can/400g	272	0.4	68	2.7	14.0	0.1	1.3
Smoked Ham, Bacon & Tomato, Italiano, Tesco*	1 Can/125g	303	9.6	242	10.8	32.3	7.7	2.9
Smoked Salmon & Dill, Sainsbury's*	1 Serving/125g	256	8.9	205	8.7	26.5	7.1	0.7
Spinach & Ricotta, Waitrose*	1 Serving/125g	309	9.0	247	10.5	35.0	7.2	1.9
Sweet Pepper & Chilli, Tesco*	½ Pack/125g	324	14.0	259	12.5	27.1	11.2	2.7
Tomato, Cheese & Meat, Sainsbury's*	1 Serving/125g	314	16.1	251	12.4	21.4	12.9	2.2
Tomato, Cheese & Mortadella, Sainsbury's*	1 Serving/125g	273	13.3	218	10.3	20.3	10.6	2.4

	Measure INFO/WEIGHT	per Measure KCAL	FAT	Nutrition Values per 100g / 100ml KCAL	PROT	CARB	FAT	FIBRE
RAVIOLI								
Vegetable, Canned, Sainsbury's*	1 Can/400g	328	2.8	82	2.6	16.3	0.7	0.7
Vegetable, Morrisons*	1 Can/400g	276	1.6	69	2.4	13.9	0.4	0.0
Vegetable, Tesco*	½ Can/200g	164	1.4	82	2.6	16.3	0.7	0.7
Vegetable in Tomato Sauce, Italiana, Weight Watchers*	1 Can/385g	266	8.1	69	1.7	11.0	2.1	0.5
Vegetable in Tomato Sauce, Weight Watchers*	1 Can/385g	266	8.1	69	1.7	11.0	2.1	0.5
Wild Mushroom, Al Forno, TTD, Sainsbury's*	1 Pack/300g	459	23.1	153	7.0	14.0	7.7	1.2
RED BULL*								
Regular, Red Bull*	1 Can/250ml	113	0.0	45	0.0	11.3	0.0	0.0
REDCURRANTS								
Raw, Average	1oz/28g	6	0.0	21	1.1	4.4	0.0	3.4
REEF*								
Orange & Passionfruit, Reef*	1 Bottle/275ml	179	0.0	65	0.0	9.5	0.0	0.0
REFRESHERS								
Barratt*	1 Roll/35.6g	130	0.1	365	0.1	88.0	0.3	0.0
Bassett's*	1oz/28g	106	0.0	377	4.3	78.1	0.0	0.0
RELISH								
Barbeque, Sainsbury's*	1 Serving/50g	50	1.1	100	1.0	19.3	2.1	1.1
Caramelised Onion & Chilli, M & S*	1 Serving/20g	47	0.2	235	1.4	55.1	1.1	1.0
Caramelised Red Onion, Tesco*	1 Serving/10g	28	0.0	280	0.6	69.1	0.1	0.7
Hamburger, Bick's*	1oz/28g	27	0.1	96	1.3	22.3	0.2	0.0
Hot Chilli & Jalapeno, Branston*	1 Squidge/25g	31	0.2	124	2.0	27.6	0.6	1.1
Onion, Sainsbury's*	1 Serving/15g	23	0.1	151	0.9	36.0	0.4	0.7
Onion & Garlic, Spicy, Waitrose*	1 Tbsp/15g	35	0.2	232	0.8	54.2	1.1	1.7
Sweet Onion, Branston*	1 Serving/10g	15	0.0	145	1.0	34.2	0.4	0.6
Sweetcorn, American Style, Maryland, Tesco*	1 Serving/15g	15	0.0	101	1.1	23.9	0.1	0.9
Sweetcorn, Bick's*	1 Tbsp/22g	23	0.0	103	1.3	24.3	0.2	0.0
Tomato & Chilli Texan Style, Tesco*	1 Tbsp/14g	20	0.0	140	1.7	32.0	0.1	1.1
Tomato & Red Pepper, Branston*	1 Serving/15g	24	0.1	158	1.3	37.3	0.4	0.6
Tomato Spicy, Bick's*	1 Serving/28g	28	0.1	99	1.3	23.2	0.2	0.0
REVELS								
Cadbury*	1 Pack/35g	168	7.3	480	5.1	68.0	20.9	0.0
RHUBARB								
Raw, Average	1 Stalk/51g	11	0.1	21	0.9	4.5	0.2	1.8
Stewed with Sugar, Average	1oz/28g	32	0.0	116	0.4	31.2	0.1	2.0
RIBENA*								
Apple Juice Drink, Ribena*	1 Carton/287ml	132	0.0	46	0.0	11.1	0.0	0.0
Blackcurrant, Diluted with Water, Ribena*	1 Serving/180ml	81	0.0	45	0.0	11.0	0.0	0.0
Blackcurrant, Really Light, Ribena*	1 Carton/250ml	8	0.0	3	0.0	0.8	0.0	0.0
Blackcurrant & Cranberry, Ribena*	1 Bottle/500ml	205	0.0	41	0.0	9.9	0.0	0.0
Blackcurrant Juice Drink, Ribena*	1 Carton/288ml	147	0.0	51	0.0	12.6	0.0	0.0
Light, Ribena*	1 Carton/288ml	26	0.0	9	0.1	2.1	0.0	0.0
Orange, Juice Drink, Ribena*	1 Serving/288ml	98	0.0	34	0.1	8.1	0.0	0.0
Really Light, Undiluted, Ribena*	1 Serving/25ml	4	0.0	15	0.0	2.5	0.0	0.0
Strawberry Juice Drink, Ribena*	1 Carton/288ml	138	0.0	48	0.0	11.8	0.0	0.0
RIBS								
Barbeque, Tesco*	1 Serving/250g	425	25.5	170	10.2	6.0	11.5	1.6
in a Chinese Style Coating, Tesco*	1 Serving/250g	420	21.8	168	19.5	5.3	8.7	2.5
Loin, Chinese, Taste Summer, Sainsbury's*	1 Serving/29.7g	38	2.3	128	11.7	2.8	7.8	0.1
Pork, Barbecue, Average	1 Serving/100g	275	17.9	275	21.4	7.2	17.9	0.3
Pork, Chinese Style, Average	1 Serving/300g	736	44.7	245	17.9	10.0	14.9	0.7
Pork, Raw, Average	1oz/28g	47	2.8	169	18.6	1.8	9.9	0.2
Spare, Cantonese, Mini, Sainsbury's*	1 Rib/38g	97	5.0	259	17.2	17.3	13.4	1.0

R

INFO/WEIGHT	Measure	per Measure		Nutrition Values per 100g / 100ml				
		KCAL	FAT	KCAL	PROT	CARB	FAT	FIBRE

RIBSTEAKS

Chinese Marinade Style, Dalepak*	1 Steak/100g	191	11.9	191	13.7	7.3	11.9	0.4
Smokey Barbecue Style, Dalepak*	1 Serving/75g	164	9.8	219	16.1	8.8	13.1	0.8

RICCOLI

Egg, Fresh, Waitrose*	1oz/28g	81	1.0	289	11.4	53.1	3.4	2.1

RICE

& Vegetable Mix, Broccoli, Sweetcorn & Peas, Birds Eye*	1 Bag/160g	181	5.3	113	3.5	17.3	3.3	2.1
Arborio, Dry, Average	1 Serving/80g	279	0.6	348	7.1	78.3	0.8	0.8
Balti Style, Quick, Sainsbury's*	1 Serving/228g	192	1.1	84	4.3	15.7	0.5	2.0
Basmati, & Wild, Cooked, Sainsbury's*	½ Pack/125g	150	0.8	120	3.1	25.7	0.6	1.3
Basmati, & Wild, Dry Weight, Tilda*	1 Serving/70g	244	0.3	349	9.4	77.0	0.5	1.0
Basmati, Boil in the Bag, Dry, Average	1 Serving/50g	176	0.4	352	8.4	77.9	0.8	0.5
Basmati, Brown, Dry, Average	1 Serving/50g	177	1.5	353	9.5	71.8	3.0	2.2
Basmati, Cooked, Average	1 Serving/140g	189	2.5	135	3.6	26.0	1.8	0.7
Basmati, Dry Weight, Average	1 Serving/60g	212	0.6	353	8.1	77.9	1.0	0.6
Basmati, Easy Cook, Dry, Average*	1 Serving/40g	135	0.2	338	8.0	75.5	0.5	0.8
Basmati, Indian, Dry, Average	1 Serving/75g	260	0.7	347	8.4	76.1	0.9	0.1
Basmati, Microwave, Cooked, Average	1 Serving/125g	182	2.3	146	2.7	30.1	1.9	0.0
Basmati, White, Dry, Average	1 Serving/75g	262	0.5	349	8.1	77.1	0.6	2.2
Basmati, White, Egg Fried, Pouch, Tilda*	½ Pack/125g	144	3.6	115	2.7	19.4	2.9	3.0
Basmati, White, Mushroom, Pouch, Tilda*	½ Pack/125g	149	3.5	119	2.6	20.9	2.8	2.9
Basmati, White, Pilau Pouch, Tilda*	½ Pack/125g	150	2.9	120	2.6	22.1	2.3	2.2
BBQ & Spicy, M & S*	1 Pack/250g	463	18.0	185	6.1	23.7	7.2	1.2
Beef, Savoury, Batchelors*	1 Pack/120g	431	2.8	359	8.9	75.7	2.3	2.5
Black, Artemide, Eat Well, M & S*	1 Serving/75g	251	2.0	335	8.5	73.3	2.6	4.0
Brown, American, Easy Cook, Average	1 Serving/75g	262	1.6	350	7.4	75.3	2.2	1.5
Brown, Basmati, Wholegrain, Dry, Sainsbury's*	1 Serving/40g	134	0.5	335	9.7	71.1	1.3	1.4
Brown, Cooked, Average	1 Serving/140g	173	1.5	123	2.6	26.6	1.1	0.9
Brown, Dry, Average	1 Serving/75g	266	2.3	355	7.5	76.2	3.0	1.4
Brown, Long Grain, Dry, Average	1 Serving/50g	182	1.4	364	7.6	76.8	2.9	2.1
Brown, Whole Grain, Cooked, Average	1 Serving/170g	223	1.9	132	2.7	27.8	1.1	1.3
Brown, Whole Grain, Dry, Average	1 Serving/40g	138	1.2	344	7.4	71.6	2.9	3.0
Chicken, Savoury, Batchelors*	1 Pack/124g	455	1.9	367	8.9	79.4	1.5	2.6
Chicken, Savoury, Cooked, Safeway*	1 Serving/151g	213	2.3	141	3.6	28.3	1.5	2.2
Chicken, Savoury, SmartPrice, Asda*	½ Pack/168g	210	1.5	125	3.2	26.0	0.9	2.4
Chicken, Savoury, Tesco*	1 Serving/87g	177	1.9	204	6.4	39.4	2.2	6.7
Chicken & Sweetcorn, Savoury, Asda*	½ Pack/60g	195	1.7	325	10.0	65.0	2.8	10.0
Chinese Savoury, Batchelors*	1 Serving/50g	177	1.2	354	9.9	73.1	2.4	2.8
Chinese Style, Express, Uncle Ben's*	1 Pack/250g	393	5.5	157	3.4	30.9	2.2	0.4
Chinese Style Savoury Five Spice, Made Up, Tesco*	1 Serving/141g	217	4.4	154	3.2	28.2	3.1	2.2
Coconut, M & S*	½ Pack/124g	217	5.0	175	3.1	31.8	4.0	0.3
Coconut, Thai, Sainsbury's*	½ Pack/100g	178	9.1	178	2.6	21.3	9.1	1.9
Coconut & Lime, Asda*	1 Pack/360g	695	17.6	193	4.5	32.7	4.9	0.9
Coriander & Herb, Packet, Cooked, Sainsbury's*	¼ Pack/150g	204	0.8	136	2.5	30.4	0.5	1.5
Coriander & Herbs, Batchelors*	1/3 Pack/76g	280	2.7	369	7.9	79.6	3.5	5.0
Curry, Savoury, Somerfield*	½ Pack/160g	194	1.4	121	2.2	26.0	0.9	1.3
Egg, Chinese Style, Morrisons*	1 Serving/250g	285	11.9	114	2.1	16.8	4.8	0.7
Egg Fried, Asda*	1 Pack/228.8g	286	5.7	125	3.6	22.0	2.5	2.3
Egg Fried, Average	1 Serving/300g	624	31.8	208	4.2	25.7	10.6	0.4
Egg Fried, Chinese Style, Tesco*	1 Portion/250g	418	10.5	167	4.4	27.9	4.2	0.7
Egg Fried, Chinese Takeaway, Iceland*	1 Pack/340g	374	7.8	110	4.2	18.1	2.3	1.1
Egg Fried, Chinese Takeaway, Tesco*	1 Serving/200g	250	3.0	125	4.7	23.3	1.5	1.8
Egg Fried, Express, Uncle Ben's*	½ Pack/124.9g	216	5.2	173	4.0	29.9	4.2	0.3
Egg Fried, HE, Tesco*	1 Serving/250g	285	3.3	114	3.5	22.2	1.3	1.8

R

RICE

INFO/WEIGHT	Measure	per Measure		Nutrition Values per 100g / 100ml				
		KCAL	FAT	KCAL	PROT	CARB	FAT	FIBRE
Egg Fried, M & S*	½ Pack/150g	315	10.5	210	4.2	32.4	7.0	0.3
Egg Fried, Micro, Tesco*	1 Pack/250g	313	9.3	125	4.6	18.3	3.7	6.4
Egg Fried, Safeway*	1 Serving/180g	351	7.2	195	4.9	34.8	4.0	0.7
Egg Fried, Sainsbury's*	1 Pack/250g	433	9.5	173	4.5	30.3	3.8	0.8
Express Microwave, Uncle Ben's*	1 Serving/250g	370	4.3	148	3.2	30.0	1.7	0.0
for Pudding, Dry Weight, Spar*	1 Serving/50g	181	0.5	361	6.5	86.8	1.0	0.5
for Pudding, Dry Weight, Tesco*	1 Serving/50g	175	0.6	350	7.3	77.3	1.2	0.2
Fried, Chicken, Chinese Takeaway, Iceland*	1 Pack/340g	510	15.6	150	6.5	20.7	4.6	0.6
Fried, Duck, Chicken & Pork Celebration, Sainsbury's*	1 Pack/450g	545	16.2	121	7.9	14.2	3.6	1.5
Garlic & Butter Flavoured, Batchelors*	1 Serving/50g	175	1.4	350	8.0	79.8	2.8	5.0
Garlic & Coriander Flavoured, Patak's*	1 Serving/125g	186	2.8	149	2.6	28.9	2.2	0.0
Garlic & Herb, Sainsbury's*	¼ Pack/50g	66	0.4	132	2.3	28.8	0.8	1.1
Golden Savoury, Dry Weight, Batchelors*	½ Pack/62g	226	1.7	364	10.1	74.7	2.8	2.4
Golden Savoury, Nirvana*	1 Pack/120g	142	0.8	118	2.5	25.4	0.7	2.9
Golden Savoury, Safeway*	1 Serving/205g	221	1.6	108	2.6	22.6	0.8	1.2
Golden Vegetable, Express, Uncle Ben's*	1 Pack/250g	373	4.8	149	3.4	29.7	1.9	0.6
Golden Vegetable, Savoury, Asda*	1 Portion/75g	111	0.8	148	2.8	32.0	1.0	0.7
Golden Vegetable, Savoury, Morrisons*	1 Serving/50g	71	0.4	141	3.4	30.1	0.8	1.1
Golden Vegetable, Savoury, Sainsbury's*	¼ Pack/100g	122	1.0	122	2.9	25.4	1.0	0.3
Golden Vegetable Savoury, Made Up, Tesco*	½ Pack/184g	220	1.7	120	2.7	24.5	0.9	1.8
House Special & Egg Fried, Somerfield*	1 Pack/448.5g	592	23.3	132	5.5	15.7	5.2	1.0
Imperial Red, Merchant Gourmet*	1oz/28g	85	0.7	305	8.6	61.2	2.5	8.6
Lemon Pepper, in 5, Crosse & Blackwell*	½ Pack/163.4g	200	2.1	123	2.7	25.2	1.3	4.0
Lemon Pepper Speciality, Asda*	1 Serving/52g	67	0.7	129	2.0	27.0	1.4	0.1
Long Grain, & Wild, Dry, Average	1 Serving/75g	254	1.5	338	7.6	72.6	2.0	1.7
Long Grain, American, Cooked, Average	1 Serving/160g	229	2.8	143	3.1	28.8	1.8	0.3
Long Grain, American, Dry, Average	1 Serving/50g	175	0.5	350	7.2	77.9	1.1	0.6
Long Grain, Boil in the Bag, Uncle Ben's*	1 Serving/62.5g	215	0.8	344	7.3	76.0	1.3	1.0
Long Grain, Dry, Average	1 Serving/50g	169	0.5	337	7.4	75.5	1.0	1.7
Long Grain, Microwavable, Cooked, Average	1 Serving/150g	180	0.9	120	2.7	25.8	0.6	0.7
Long Grain, Thai Fragrant, Tesco*	1 Serving/50g	175	0.2	349	7.3	79.1	0.4	0.8
Mexican, Ready Meals, Waitrose*	1 Pack/300g	432	7.5	144	2.6	27.8	2.5	0.5
Mexican Style, Old El Paso*	1 Serving/75g	268	0.8	357	9.0	78.0	1.0	0.0
Mild Curry, Cooked, Tesco*	1 Serving/154g	217	1.7	141	3.1	29.7	1.1	2.1
Mild Curry, Savoury, Batchelors*	1 Pack/120g	426	2.5	355	8.0	76.1	2.1	1.6
Mixed Vegetable, Savoury, Dry Weight, Tesco*	1 Serving/163g	611	4.4	375	7.8	79.1	2.7	2.9
Mushroom, Express, Uncle Ben's*	1 Pack/250g	393	4.8	157	3.3	31.8	1.9	0.5
Mushroom, Savoury, Asda*	½ Pack/60g	222	1.5	370	8.3	78.3	2.5	2.2
Mushroom, Savoury, Somerfield*	½ Pack/160g	144	1.1	90	2.1	18.8	0.7	1.5
Mushroom & Coconut, Organic, Waitrose*	1 Pack/300g	474	15.0	158	3.7	24.5	5.0	1.4
Mushroom & Pepper, Savoury, Cooked, Morrisons*	1 Serving/200g	204	1.6	102	2.3	21.5	0.8	0.0
Mushroom & Pepper, Savoury, Safeway*	½ Pack/194g	227	1.0	117	2.7	25.4	0.5	0.7
Mushroom Pilau, Bombay Brasserie, Sainsbury's*	1 Pack/400g	672	17.2	168	3.7	28.6	4.3	0.7
Mushroom Savoury, Batchelors*	½ Pack/61g	217	1.3	356	10.7	73.6	2.1	2.8
Mushroom Savoury, Bettabuy, Morrisons*	1 Serving/128.4g	131	1.0	102	2.3	21.5	0.8	0.0
Paella, Savoury, Tesco*	1 Serving/60g	220	2.8	367	8.4	72.7	4.7	4.5
Peri Peri Spicy, Nando's*	1 Pot/100g	204	1.5	204	3.6	42.8	1.5	0.0
Pilau, Cooked, Average	1 Serving/140g	244	6.2	174	3.5	30.3	4.4	0.8
Pilau, Dry, Average	1oz/28g	101	0.7	362	8.5	78.2	2.4	3.4
Pilau, Indian Mushroom, Sainsbury's*	1 Serving/100g	119	2.4	119	3.0	21.3	2.4	1.9
Pilau, Indian Take Away, Tesco*	1 Box/100g	135	3.3	135	2.7	23.7	3.3	2.2
Pilau, Mushroom, Sainsbury's*	1 Pack/250g	400	13.8	160	3.4	24.1	5.5	2.4
Pilau, Spinach, Bombay Brasserie, Sainsbury's*	1 Pack/401g	642	17.3	160	3.5	26.9	4.3	0.8

R

RICE

INFO/WEIGHT	Measure	per Measure		Nutrition Values per 100g / 100ml				
		KCAL	FAT	KCAL	PROT	CARB	FAT	FIBRE
Pudding, Short Grain, Morrisons*	1oz/28g	36	1.2	129	3.9	19.9	4.3	0.0
Risotto, Dry, Average	1 Serving/50g	174	0.7	348	7.8	76.2	1.3	2.4
Saffron, Cooked, Average	1 Serving/150g	209	4.7	139	2.6	25.3	3.2	0.5
Spanish Style Savoury, Safeway*	1 Pack/394g	449	3.5	114	2.7	23.7	0.9	1.4
Special Fried, Asda*	1oz/28g	42	1.4	149	5.4	21.0	4.9	1.5
Special Fried, Cantonese, Sainsbury's*	½ Pack/250g	443	10.0	177	4.9	30.4	4.0	1.2
Special Fried, Chinese, Tesco*	1 Serving/300g	618	33.3	206	6.5	19.9	11.1	0.8
Special Fried, Chinese Takeaway, Iceland*	1 Pack/350g	630	17.5	180	5.5	28.2	5.0	1.2
Special Fried, M & S*	1 Pack/450g	923	35.1	205	6.2	27.2	7.8	0.5
Special Fried, Sainsbury's*	1 Serving/166g	272	7.6	164	5.1	25.5	4.6	0.7
Special Fried, Somerfield*	1 Pack/200g	316	8.0	158	5.0	25.0	4.0	0.0
Special Fried, Tesco*	1 Pack/300g	681	27.6	227	6.8	29.1	9.2	1.3
Special Fried, Waitrose*	1 Serving/350g	532	22.4	152	6.1	17.6	6.4	3.2
Spicy Mexican Style, Savoury, Made Up, Tesco*	1 Serving/164g	213	2.5	130	2.9	26.3	1.5	2.4
Spicy Mexican Style, Savoury, Tesco*	1 Serving/164g	584	7.4	356	9.0	69.9	4.5	6.0
Steamed, Asda*	1 Serving/200g	252	2.6	126	2.6	26.0	1.3	2.0
Sticky Thai, Safeway*	1 Pack/200g	260	3.6	130	2.5	25.6	1.8	1.4
Stir Fry, Oriental Style, Oriental Express*	1 Serving/150g	216	5.1	144	4.2	24.1	3.4	1.9
Sweet & Sour, Rice Bowl, Uncle Ben's*	1 Pack/350g	364	2.1	104	5.2	19.5	0.6	0.0
Sweet & Sour, Savoury, Batchelors*	1 Serving/135g	419	2.8	310	9.4	75.6	2.1	3.1
Sweet & Sour, Savoury, Cooked, Tesco*	½ Pack/153g	214	2.1	140	2.7	29.1	1.4	2.3
Sweet & Sour, Savoury, Sainsbury's*	1 Serving/145g	198	0.7	137	2.4	30.8	0.5	1.0
Sweet & Sour, Savoury, Somerfield*	1 Pack/120g	127	1.2	106	2.0	23.0	1.0	0.0
Sweet & Sour Savoury, Cooked, Asda*	½ Pack/126g	154	1.1	122	2.5	26.0	0.9	3.0
Sweet & Spicy, Express, Uncle Ben's*	1 Pack/250g	418	10.0	167	2.7	30.1	4.0	0.0
Tandoori, Savoury, Batchelors*	1 Serving/120g	430	3.0	358	10.3	73.5	2.5	3.0
Thai, Cooked, Average	1 Serving/100g	136	1.8	136	2.5	27.4	1.8	0.3
Thai, Dry, Average	1 Serving/50g	174	0.2	348	7.1	78.9	0.5	0.9
Thai, Fragrant, Dry, Average	1 Serving/75g	272	0.5	363	7.2	82.0	0.7	0.3
Thai Sticky, Tesco*	1 Serving/250g	358	6.3	143	2.5	27.6	2.5	0.4
Thai Style, Lemon Chicken, Savoury, Tesco*	1 Pack/105g	382	5.1	364	9.3	70.6	4.9	5.0
Thai Style Lemon Chicken, Made Up, Tesco*	½ Pack/138g	192	2.3	139	3.4	27.5	1.7	2.1
Tomato & Basil, Express, Uncle Ben's*	1 Pack/250g	455	10.8	182	3.4	32.3	4.3	0.6
Valencia for Paella, Asda*	1 Serving/125g	435	1.0	348	6.0	79.0	0.8	0.0
Vegetable, Golden, Safeway*	1 Serving/125g	111	0.6	89	2.9	18.2	0.5	1.9
Vegetable, Original, Birds Eye*	1oz/28g	29	0.2	105	4.0	20.8	0.6	1.1
Vegetable, Savoury, Co-Op*	½ Pack/60g	210	0.6	350	9.0	76.0	1.0	3.0
Vegetable, Savoury, M & S*	1 Pack/500g	700	11.0	140	3.0	27.3	2.2	1.6
Vegetable Pilau, Express, Uncle Ben's*	½ Pack/125g	195	3.9	156	3.0	29.0	3.1	0.6
White, Cooked, Average	1 Serving/140g	182	1.1	130	2.6	28.7	0.8	0.2
White, Cooked, Frozen, Average	1 Serving/150g	168	0.8	112	2.9	23.9	0.6	1.2
White, Flaked, Dry Weight, Average	1oz/28g	97	0.3	346	6.6	77.5	1.2	0.0
White, Fried	1oz/28g	37	0.9	131	2.2	25.0	3.2	0.6
White, Long Grain, Dry Weight, Average	1 Serving/50g	181	1.0	362	7.1	79.1	1.9	0.4
White, Microwave, Cooked, Average	1 Serving/150g	158	0.8	105	2.7	22.4	0.5	1.1
Whole Grain, Boil in Bag, Uncle Ben's*	1 Pack/125g	420	2.8	336	8.0	71.0	2.2	4.7
Whole Grain, Dry, Average	1 Serving/50g	171	1.2	342	8.2	72.0	2.3	4.1
Whole Grain, Express, Uncle Ben's*	1 Bag/250g	400	6.3	160	3.7	30.7	2.5	2.0
Wild, Giant Canadian, Dry Weight, Tilda*	1 Serving/75g	263	0.6	350	11.5	74.2	0.8	1.9
with Brocolli, Sweetcorn & Peas, SteamFresh, Birds Eye*	1 Bag/170g	192	5.6	113	3.5	17.3	3.3	2.1
with Mixed Vegetables, White & Wild, Steam Rice, Tesco*	1 Pack/150g	158	1.4	105	3.1	21.1	0.9	1.7
Yellow, Ready Cooked, Tesco*	1oz/28g	32	0.4	113	2.7	27.1	1.3	0.1

R

	Measure INFO/WEIGHT	per Measure KCAL	FAT	Nutrition Values per 100g / 100ml KCAL	PROT	CARB	FAT	FIBRE
RICE &								
Red Kidney Beans, Average	1oz/28g	49	1.0	175	5.6	32.4	3.5	2.5
Vegetables, M & S*	1 Serving/250g	250	4.5	100	3.2	17.7	1.8	2.0
RICE BOWL								
Beef with Black Bean Sauce, Uncle Ben's*	1 Pack/350g	368	4.9	105	5.6	17.4	1.4	0.0
Chicken Tikka Masala, Uncle Ben's*	1 Pack/350g	382	8.4	109	5.9	15.9	2.4	0.0
Free From, Sainsbury's*	1 Serving/182g	146	1.1	80	1.6	17.1	0.6	1.4
Honey BBQ Chicken, Uncle Ben's*	1 Pack/350g	420	2.1	120	5.4	23.1	0.6	0.0
Sweet 'n' Sour, Sharwood's*	1 Serving/350g	438	12.3	125	4.8	18.6	3.5	0.8
Thai Green, Sharwood's*	1 Bowl/350g	550	26.6	157	4.8	17.3	7.6	0.9
Thai Red, Sharwood's*	1 Bowl/350g	487	18.6	139	4.7	18.1	5.3	1.0
RICE CAKES								
Barbeque, Tesco*	1 Cake/9g	28	0.2	328	9.6	66.8	2.5	6.2
BGTY, Sainsbury's*	1 Cake/5.9g	22	0.2	372	8.0	78.7	2.8	5.1
Black & White Sesame, Clearspring*	1 Cake/8g	31	0.2	385	7.4	82.2	2.9	0.0
Brink*	1 Cake/15g	56	0.3	370	8.8	78.8	2.2	0.0
Caramel, Jumbo, Tesco*	1 Cake/10g	34	0.3	340	7.0	74.0	3.0	5.0
Caramel, Large, Tesco*	1 Cake/10g	34	0.3	344	6.5	73.9	2.5	5.1
Caramel, Less Than 3% Fat, Sainsbury's*	1 Pack/35g	134	0.6	382	5.6	86.4	1.6	1.8
Caramel, Snack Size, Tesco*	1 Bag/35g	133	1.0	379	5.5	82.7	2.9	0.9
Caramel Flavour, Kallo*	1 Cake/9.9g	38	0.5	383	6.2	78.9	4.8	3.9
Cheese, Jumbo, Free From, Tesco*	1 Serving/10g	44	1.8	439	8.1	62.1	17.6	3.8
Cheese & Onion, Namchow*	1 Serving/38g	141	1.2	377	7.2	79.5	3.3	0.0
Co-Op*	1 Cake/20g	80	0.6	402	8.0	84.0	3.1	0.0
Crispy, Somerfield*	1oz/28g	134	4.8	479	5.0	77.0	17.0	0.0
Dark Chocolate, Organic, Kallo*	1 Cake/12g	57	2.9	471	6.8	57.2	24.1	7.4
Honey, Kallo*	2 Cakes/20.6g	80	0.5	388	5.4	86.6	2.2	1.6
Lightly Salted, PB, Waitrose*	1 Cake/8g	31	0.2	387	8.3	82.4	2.7	2.1
Lightly Salted, Thick Slice, Low Fat, Kallo*	1 Slice/7.5g	28	0.2	372	8.0	78.7	2.8	5.1
Low Fat, Kallo*	1 Cake/10g	38	0.2	375	6.2	83.1	2.2	3.9
Milk Chocolate, Organic, Kallo*	1 Rice Cake/11g	57	3.2	509	6.5	56.2	28.7	3.5
Multigrain, Ryvita*	3 Cakes/11.2g	42	0.5	384	9.1	76.2	4.7	5.3
Plain, Finger Foods, Organic, Organix*	3 Cakes/6g	22	0.1	370	6.5	83.0	1.4	3.2
Salt & Vinegar, Jumbo, Tesco*	1 Cake/8.9g	31	0.2	347	8.4	72.7	2.5	6.0
Salt & Vinegar, Sainsbury's*	1 Cake/30g	121	2.5	403	8.3	73.3	8.3	2.7
Salt & Vinegar, Snack, Tesco*	1 Pack/35g	116	0.6	332	7.5	71.5	1.8	1.1
Savoury, Jumbo, HL, Tesco*	1 Cake/8.4g	31	0.2	369	11.9	75.0	2.4	3.6
Sesame Teriyaki, Clearspring*	1 Cake/7.4g	28	0.2	377	6.5	82.8	2.2	0.0
Slightly Salted, Organic, Thin Slice, Kallo*	1 Slice/4.6g	17	0.1	372	8.0	78.7	2.8	5.1
Slightly Salted, Thick Slice, Organic, Kallo*	1 Slice/7.5g	28	0.2	372	8.0	78.7	2.8	5.1
Thin Slice, No Added Salt, Organic, Kallo*	1 Cake/5g	19	0.1	372	8.0	78.7	2.8	5.1
Thin Slice, Organic, Hawkwood*	2 Slices/11g	40	0.4	378	7.6	79.1	3.5	3.4
RICE CRACKERS								
Barbecue, Sakata*	½ Pack/50g	204	1.3	407	7.3	85.2	2.6	1.6
Barbecue Flavour, Tesco*	1 Bag/25g	102	1.9	409	6.7	78.8	7.4	1.7
Chilli, Temptations, Tesco*	1 Serving/25g	128	7.2	512	4.4	58.0	28.8	0.0
Cracked Pepper, Sakata*	½ Pack/50g	200	1.5	400	7.3	84.4	3.0	2.0
Japanese, Holland and Barratt*	1 Serving/50g	201	4.4	403	11.3	69.8	8.7	1.7
Japanese, Julian Graves*	1 Serving/25g	92	0.4	369	8.8	79.5	1.7	3.8
Mix, M & S*	½ Pack/62.5g	227	0.1	360	6.5	82.9	0.1	1.6
Sainsbury's*	1 Serving/20g	87	1.9	433	11.2	74.3	9.4	1.0
Sea Salt & Vinegar, Go Ahead, McVitie's*	1 Serving/25g	102	1.4	408	6.6	80.6	5.4	1.8
Sour Cream & Herbs, Go Ahead, McVitie's*	1 Serving/25g	106	2.0	422	7.1	78.2	8.0	1.8
Thai, M & S*	1 Serving/55g	209	1.8	380	7.0	80.2	3.3	1.2

R

	INFO/WEIGHT	KCAL	FAT	KCAL	PROT	CARB	FAT	FIBRE
RICE CRACKERS								
Thai, Sesame & Soy Sauce, M & S*	1 Pack/54.5g	212	2.6	385	7.6	77.8	4.8	1.4
Thai, Wakama*	1 Cracker/2g	8	0.1	400	6.9	86.9	2.7	0.5
Thai Chilli, Nature's Harvest*	1 Pack/75g	401	22.3	535	4.6	61.5	29.7	4.2
with Tamari, Clearspring*	1 Bag/50g	190	0.8	380	8.2	83.4	1.5	0.3
RICE MILK								
Organic, Provamel*	1 Serving/250ml	123	3.8	49	0.1	9.5	1.5	0.0
Original, Rice Dream*	1 Serving/150ml	71	1.5	47	0.1	9.4	1.0	0.1
RICE PUDDING								
50% Less Fat, Asda*	½ Can/212g	170	1.6	85	3.3	16.2	0.8	0.2
Apple, Mullerrice, Muller*	1 Pot/200g	224	4.4	112	3.2	19.8	2.2	0.4
Canned, Average	1oz/28g	25	0.7	89	3.4	14.0	2.5	0.2
Canned, Basics, Sainsbury's*	½ Can/212.5g	176	1.9	83	3.1	15.5	0.9	0.1
Canned, BGTY, Sainsbury's*	1 Can/425g	349	3.4	82	3.1	15.7	0.8	0.1
Clotted Cream, M & S*	1 Pudding/185g	431	30.7	233	3.0	19.2	16.6	0.2
Clotted Cream, Tesco*	1 Pudding/190g	400	25.3	211	2.7	19.9	13.3	0.1
COU, M & S*	1 Pot/170.6g	145	2.9	85	2.4	15.5	1.7	0.5
Creamed, Asda*	1 Serving/215.4g	196	3.4	91	3.2	16.0	1.6	0.0
Creamed, Canned, Ambrosia*	1 Can/425g	383	8.1	90	3.1	15.2	1.9	0.0
Creamed, HL, Tesco*	1 Can/425g	340	2.6	80	3.0	15.1	0.6	0.2
Creamed, Low Fat, Ambrosia*	1 Serving/150g	129	1.4	86	3.3	16.1	0.9	0.0
Creamed, Pot, Ambrosia*	1 Pot/150g	156	3.8	104	3.3	17.0	2.5	0.1
Creamed, Value, Tesco*	1 Can/425g	361	3.4	85	3.1	16.0	0.8	0.1
Creamed, Weight Watchers*	1 Pot/130.1g	108	0.9	83	3.2	16.0	0.7	0.3
Creamed with Sultanas & Nutmeg, Ambrosia*	½ Can/200g	210	5.8	105	3.2	16.6	2.9	0.1
Creamy, Ambrosia*	½ Tin/212g	197	4.0	93	3.2	15.7	1.9	0.0
Low Fat, Ambrosia*	½ Tin/212g	176	1.7	83	3.2	15.7	0.8	0.1
Low Fat, No Added Sugar, Weight Watchers*	½ Can/212g	155	3.2	73	3.7	11.4	1.5	0.0
Organic, Ambrosia*	1 Can/425g	455	15.7	107	3.4	15.1	3.7	0.0
Original, Mullerrice, Muller*	1 Pot/200g	212	5.2	106	3.7	16.9	2.6	0.3
Raspberry, Mullerrice, Muller*	1 Std Pot/200g	218	4.4	109	3.2	19.1	2.2	0.6
Strawberry, Mullerrice, Muller*	1 Pot/200g	220	4.4	110	3.2	19.3	2.2	0.4
Vanilla Custard, Mullerrice, Muller*	1 Pot/200g	230	5.0	115	3.4	19.8	2.5	0.3
with Strawberry Sauce, Ambrosia*	1 Pot/160g	174	3.2	109	2.7	19.8	2.0	0.1
with Summer Fruit Compote, Onken*	1 Pot/160g	195	5.4	122	2.5	20.3	3.4	0.5
RICE SALAD								
Chicken Tikka, COU, M & S*	1 Pack/390g	410	3.9	105	5.1	18.7	1.0	0.6
Hot Smoked Salmon, Deli Meal, M & S*	1 Pack/380g	570	26.2	150	6.5	15.1	6.9	0.2
Indian Style, with Chickpeas & Yoghurt Dressing, M & S*	1 Pack/220g	264	7.0	120	3.7	19.3	3.2	3.4
Mexican, with Beans, COU, M & S*	1 Serving/250g	250	3.5	100	6.0	15.6	1.4	1.2
Rainbow, M & S*	1 Serving/261.5g	341	8.4	130	2.5	23.3	3.2	1.5
Red, with Feta, M & S*	1 Pack/244.4g	439	20.7	180	4.8	21.0	8.5	1.3
Spanish Style, with Chicken, M & S*	1 Serving/220g	319	12.8	145	5.8	17.4	5.8	0.5
RICE STICKS								
Chakri, Cofresh*	1 Pack/100g	480	20.5	480	7.8	66.1	20.5	0.0
Mature Cheese & Red Onion Flavour, Weight Watchers*	1 Pack/20g	82.6	1.1	413	5.4	77.3	9.1	0.2
Salt & Vinegar, Weight Watchers*	1 Serving/20g	73	1.5	365	7.7	79.7	1.7	2.4
Thai Sweet Chilli Flavour, Weight Watchers*	1 Serving/20g	72.6	1.5	363	7.6	79.5	1.6	2.2
RIGATONI								
Carbonara, Tesco*	1 Serving/205g	236	11.9	115	5.2	10.6	5.8	1.2
Dry, Average	1 Serving/80g	272	1.2	340	11.4	68.5	1.5	2.7
Tomato & Cheese, PB, Waitrose*	1 Pack/400g	664	9.2	166	7.6	28.6	2.3	2.3
RISOTTO								
Balls, Mushroom, Occasions, Sainsbury's*	1 Ball/25g	76	3.5	304	3.8	41.2	13.8	1.7

R

	Measure INFO/WEIGHT	per Measure		Nutrition Values per 100g / 100ml				
		KCAL	FAT	KCAL	PROT	CARB	FAT	FIBRE
RISOTTO								
Balls, Sun Dried Tomato, Occasions, Sainsbury's*	1 Ball/25g	71	3.8	285	6.8	30.8	15.0	2.9
Beef, Vesta*	1 Serving/100g	346	5.9	346	15.3	57.8	5.9	5.6
Butternut Squash, TTD, Sainsbury's*	1 Pack/450g	630	28.8	140	3.5	17.2	6.4	0.3
Caramelised Onion & Gruyere Cheese, M & S*	1 Pack/200g	350	20.6	175	3.0	17.8	10.3	1.7
Chargrilled Chicken, Ready Meal, M & S*	1 Pack/365g	493	25.2	135	6.4	11.6	6.9	0.7
Cheese Flavour, Made Up, Ainsley Harriott*	1 Sachet/140g	565	14.6	404	7.8	69.6	10.4	9.1
Chicken, BGTY, Sainsbury's*	1 Pack/327g	356	6.2	109	7.5	15.5	1.9	1.0
Chicken, Co-Op*	1 Pack/340g	442	17.0	130	6.0	16.0	5.0	2.0
Chicken, Enjoy, Birds Eye*	1 Pack/500g	735	31.5	147	8.5	14.0	6.3	0.5
Chicken, Lemon & Wild Rocket, Sainsbury's*	1 Pack/360g	683	41.0	190	16.2	5.6	11.4	0.1
Chicken, Ready Meal, M & S*	1 Pack/360g	450	15.8	125	6.7	14.4	4.4	0.9
Chicken & Asparagus, Eat Smart, Safeway*	1 Pack/380g	418	5.7	110	6.2	16.8	1.5	0.6
Chicken & Bacon, Italiano, Tesco*	1 Pack/450g	653	20.3	145	5.9	20.2	4.5	1.5
Chicken & Lemon, Weight Watchers*	1 Pack/330g	313	8.9	95	5.7	11.9	2.7	0.4
Chicken & Mushroom, Finest, Tesco*	1 Pack/400g	496	11.2	124	7.4	17.2	2.8	0.5
Chicken & Mushroom, Good Intentions, Somerfield*	1 Pack/300g	345	5.4	115	5.7	19.0	1.8	0.3
Chicken & Sun Dried Tomato, Waitrose*	1 Pack/350g	385	22.1	110	6.0	7.2	6.3	0.3
Haddock & Mushroom, COU, M & S*	1 Pack/400g	320	3.2	80	6.4	12.1	0.8	2.0
Hot Smoked Salmon & Spinach, M & S*	½ Pack/300g	420	24.0	140	6.4	11.0	8.0	0.6
Italian Red Wine with Creamed Spinach, Sainsbury's*	1 Pack/400g	596	27.6	149	2.4	19.3	6.9	0.4
King Prawn, Pea & Mint, M & S*	½ Pack/300g	405	18.6	135	3.8	15.9	6.2	0.9
King Prawn & Snow Crab, M & S*	1 Pack/365g	402	16.4	110	4.1	12.7	4.5	0.5
Lemon & Mint, PB, Waitrose*	1 Pack/350g	462	13.0	132	3.9	20.7	3.7	1.0
Mushroom, Asda*	1 Pack/340g	340	11.6	100	2.3	15.0	3.4	0.6
Mushroom, BGTY, Sainsbury's*	1 Pack/400g	320	3.2	80	2.6	15.6	0.8	0.6
Mushroom, COU, M & S*	1 Pack/373g	392	10.1	105	3.9	16.7	2.7	1.1
Mushroom, Finest, Tesco*	1 Pack/400g	556	28.0	139	3.9	15.1	7.0	1.2
Mushroom, HL, Tesco*	1 Pack/400g	320	3.2	80	2.6	15.6	0.8	0.6
Mushroom, Italiano, Tesco*	1 Pack/340g	367	6.8	108	2.4	20.0	2.0	4.6
Mushroom, PB, Waitrose*	1 Pack/400g	384	6.4	96	4.3	16.1	1.6	2.1
Mushroom, Ready Meals, M & S*	1 Pack/360g	450	17.6	125	2.8	16.9	4.9	1.0
Mushroom, Safeway*	1 Pack/350g	406	11.2	116	2.7	19.0	3.2	2.9
Mushroom, Somerfield*	1 Pack/300g	333	12.0	111	2.0	16.0	4.0	0.0
Roasted Red Pepper & Italian Cheese, M & S*	1 Pack/400g	500	13.2	125	2.9	20.4	3.3	1.0
Roasted Vegetable, Made Up, Ainsley Harriott*	1 Sachet/140g	766	18.2	547	11.0	96.5	13.0	15.5
Roasted Vegetable & Sunblush Tomato, Finest, Tesco*	½ Pack/200g	306	18.0	153	3.7	14.5	9.0	1.4
Roasted Vegetables, Stir-In, Uncle Ben's*	½ Pack/75g	86	7.3	115	1.7	5.0	9.7	0.0
Salmon & Prawn, Eat Smart, Morrisons*	1 Pack/380.9g	339	5.3	89	4.9	14.1	1.4	0.8
Seafood, Youngs*	1 Pack/350g	424	13.0	121	4.5	17.4	3.7	0.1
Spring Vegetable, M & S*	1 Serving/330g	330	13.2	100	2.0	14.2	4.0	0.9
Tomato & Cheese, GFY, Asda*	1 Pack/400g	428	12.0	107	3.1	17.0	3.0	0.7
Tomato & Mascarpone, M & S*	1 Pack/360g	468	19.1	130	2.7	17.5	5.3	0.9
Vegetable, Average	1oz/28g	41	1.8	147	4.2	19.2	6.5	2.2
Vegetable, Brown Rice, Average	1oz/28g	40	1.8	143	4.1	18.6	6.4	2.4
Vegetable, Great Stuff, Asda*	1 Pack/300g	315	5.7	105	4.3	17.6	1.9	1.3
Wild Mushroom, Made Up, Ainsley Harriott*	1 Sachet/140g	785	21.7	561	12.0	93.3	15.5	14.7
Wild Mushroom & Garlic, Tesco*	1 Pack/320g	522	14.1	163	3.6	27.2	4.4	1.6
RISSOLES								
Lentil, Fried in Vegetable Oil, Average	1oz/28g	59	2.9	211	8.9	22.0	10.5	3.6
RIVELLA*								
Blue, Rivella*	1 Can/330ml	17	0.0	5	0.0	1.3	0.0	0.0
ROCK SALMON								
Raw, Flesh Only, Average	1oz/28g	43	2.7	154	16.6	0.0	9.7	0.0

R

	Measure INFO/WEIGHT	per Measure KCAL	FAT	Nutrition Values per 100g / 100ml KCAL	PROT	CARB	FAT	FIBRE
ROE								
Cod, Average	1 Can/100g	96	2.8	96	17.1	0.5	2.8	0.0
Cod, Hard, Coated in Batter, Fried	1oz/28g	53	3.3	189	12.4	8.9	11.8	0.2
Cod, Hard, Fried in Blended Oil	1oz/28g	57	3.3	202	20.9	3.0	11.9	0.1
Cod, Pressed, John West*	1 Can/200g	220	8.0	110	14.0	5.0	4.0	0.1
Herring, Soft, Fried in Blended Oil	1oz/28g	74	4.4	265	26.3	4.7	15.8	0.2
Herring, Soft, Raw	1oz/28g	25	0.7	91	16.8	0.0	2.6	0.0
Soft Herring, in Brine, Sainsbury's*	1 Can/86g	105	3.2	122	22.2	0.1	3.7	0.0
ROGAN JOSH								
Chicken, with Basmati Rice, Frozen, Patak's*	1 Pack/400g	432	8.4	108	5.7	16.4	2.1	0.7
Chicken, with Pilau Rice, Farmfoods*	1 Pack/325g	354	6.8	109	5.3	17.1	2.1	0.4
Chicken & Rice, Sainsbury's*	1 Pack/500g	675	27.0	135	6.7	14.1	5.4	2.4
King Prawn, with Rice, HL, Tesco*	1 Pack/400g	365	6.0	91	4.8	14.6	1.5	1.6
Lamb, Indian Takeaway, Tesco*	1 Pack/350g	368	12.6	105	9.2	8.2	3.6	1.8
Lamb, M & S*	½ Pack/116.7g	140	7.8	120	9.5	5.4	6.7	4.8
Lamb, Safeway*	1 Pack/350g	515	32.7	147	13.0	2.5	9.3	3.0
Lamb, Sainsbury's*	1 Pack/400g	660	44.4	165	11.3	4.9	11.1	1.9
Lamb, Tesco*	1 Pack/350g	403	20.3	115	10.2	5.0	5.8	1.3
Lamb, Waitrose*	1 Serving/60g	79	4.7	131	12.3	3.0	7.8	1.3
Lamb, with Pilau Rice, Eastern Classics*	1 Pack/400g	604	21.6	151	5.6	19.9	5.4	1.0
Lamb with Basmati Rice, Eat Smart, Safeway*	1 Pack/380g	380	5.7	100	6.9	14.0	1.5	1.9
Prawn, COU, M & S*	1 Pack/400g	360	2.4	90	4.9	16.2	0.6	0.8
Prawn & Pilau Rice, BGTY, Sainsbury's*	1 Pack/401g	353	3.2	88	4.8	15.3	0.8	1.9
ROLL								
All Day Breakfast, Asda*	1 Roll/220g	581	26.4	264	10.0	29.0	12.0	0.0
Bacon, M & S*	2 Rolls/18g	40	3.3	220	14.2	0.4	18.3	0.0
Beef, Weight Watchers*	1 Roll/174g	276	4.4	159	10.8	23.1	2.5	1.0
Brie & Grapes, M & S*	1 Roll/57g	174	10.4	306	11.1	24.5	18.2	1.4
Cheese & Chutney, M & S*	1 Roll/165g	256	1.2	155	13.9	23.1	0.7	1.2
Cheese & Onion, Asda*	1 Serving/66.8g	200	12.1	298	7.0	27.0	18.0	2.0
Cheese & Onion, King Size, Pork Farms*	1 Serving/130g	443	28.6	341	7.4	28.4	22.0	0.0
Cheese & Onion, M & S*	1 Roll/25g	80	5.1	320	9.6	24.7	20.5	1.3
Cheese & Onion, Sainsbury's*	1 Roll/67g	205	13.6	306	8.0	22.9	20.3	1.9
Cheese & Onion, Tesco*	1 Roll/66.6g	204	12.1	305	7.3	28.0	18.1	1.9
Cheese & Pickle, Sainsbury's*	1 Roll/136g	359	13.6	264	10.6	35.1	10.0	0.0
Chicken & Beef Duo, M & S*	1 Serving/146.9g	235	3.8	160	12.0	22.1	2.6	2.7
Chicken Salad, HE, Tesco*	1 Serving/224g	289	5.8	129	10.3	16.0	2.6	1.1
Chunky Cheese & Mustard, Finest, Tesco*	1 Roll/88g	260	9.0	295	10.9	40.0	10.2	2.4
Cornish, in Pastry, Pork Farms*	1 Roll/75.1g	226	15.1	301	6.6	24.5	20.1	0.0
Egg & Bacon, Sub, Shapers, Boots*	1 Serving/169.3g	319	7.3	189	11.0	27.0	4.3	1.3
Egg & Cress, HL, Tesco*	1 Pack/175g	322	6.8	184	9.6	27.7	3.9	1.2
Egg Mayo & Cress, Fullfillers*	1 Roll/125g	266	11.8	213	10.0	25.7	9.4	0.0
Egg Mayonnaise, & Cress, White, Soft, Somerfield*	1 Serving/211g	475	17.3	225	9.4	28.2	8.2	2.1
Ham, Darwins Deli*	1 Serving/125g	298	7.5	238	11.0	37.4	6.0	0.0
Ham & Cheese, in Pastry, Pork Farms*	1 Roll/70.1g	216	12.5	308	8.0	28.8	17.9	0.0
Ham & Tomato, Taste!*	1 Serving/112.2g	211	4.8	188	10.4	27.0	4.3	0.0
Ham Salad, BGTY, Sainsbury's*	1 Roll/178g	292	3.4	164	10.8	25.9	1.9	0.0
Ham Salad, Good Intentions, Somerfield*	1 Pack/213.8g	325	4.7	152	8.7	24.3	2.2	1.6
Ham Salad, HL, Tesco*	1 Roll/203g	284	5.3	140	9.8	19.3	2.6	0.0
Leicester Ham & Cheese, Sub, Waitrose*	1 Pack/206.4ml	581	31.1	282	12.6	24.0	15.1	13.0
Lincolnshire Sausage, COU, M & S*	1 Roll/175g	280	4.7	160	10.0	23.2	2.7	2.6
Mushroom & Bacon, Crusty, M & S*	1 Roll/160g	424	20.2	265	8.7	29.0	12.6	2.3
Roast Chicken & Mayonnaise, Big, Sainsbury's*	1 Pack/185g	479	27.4	259	9.6	21.8	14.8	0.0
Roast Chicken Salad, Improved, Shapers, Boots*	1 Pack/187.6g	303	3.6	161	11.0	25.0	1.9	1.6

	Measure INFO/WEIGHT	per Measure KCAL	FAT	Nutrition Values per 100g / 100ml KCAL	PROT	CARB	FAT	FIBRE
ROLL								
Roast Pork, Stuffing & Apple Sauce, Boots*	1 Roll/218.1g	602	26.2	276	10.0	32.0	12.0	1.8
Steak & Onion, M & S*	1 Serving/150g	308	10.5	205	11.0	24.5	7.0	3.8
Tuna & Sweetcorn with Mayonnaise, Shell*	1 Pack/180g	536	26.3	298	13.1	28.6	14.6	0.0
Tuna Cheese Melt, Boots*	1 Roll/198.7g	613	35.8	308	13.0	23.0	18.0	1.2
Tuna Mayo & Cucumber, Taste!*	1 Serving/110.9g	274	12.5	247	9.0	27.3	11.3	0.0
Tuna Mayonnaise, with Cucumber, Yummies*	1 Serving/132.3g	339	18.5	257	10.4	22.5	14.0	0.0
Turkey, Stuffed, GFY, Asda*	½ Pack/225g	320	9.5	142	14.0	12.0	4.2	0.8
Turkey Salad, Northern Bites*	1 Roll/230.7g	323	8.3	140	8.6	19.6	3.6	3.0
ROLO								
Little, Nestle*	1 Pack/26g	129	6.2	491	4.0	65.5	23.5	0.5
Nestle*	1 Pack/57g	268	11.7	471	3.2	68.5	20.5	0.3
ROLY POLY								
Jam, Aunt Bessie's*	1 Serving/100g	384	16.3	384	5.4	53.9	16.3	1.7
Jam and Custard, Safeway*	1 Serving/112g	299	10.0	267	3.8	43.0	8.9	0.8
Jam, Frozen, Asda*	¼ Pack/104g	380.6	5.2	366	5.0	54.0	15.0	1.8
ROOT BEER								
Average	1 Can/330ml	135	0.0	41	0.0	10.6	0.0	0.0
ROSEMARY								
Dried	1 Tsp/1g	3	0.2	331	4.9	46.4	15.2	0.0
Fresh	1oz/28g	28	1.2	99	1.4	13.5	4.4	0.0
ROSTI								
Oven Baked, McCain*	1 Rosti/100g	194	9.3	194	2.6	25.0	9.3	2.3
Peppered Steak, British Classics, Tesco*	1 Pack/450g	599	27.9	133	9.0	10.7	6.2	1.7
Potato, Cakes, with Onion, M & S*	1 Rosti/76g	95	4.4	125	1.3	16.7	5.8	2.5
Potato, Chicken & Sweetcorn Bake, Asda*	1 Serving/400g	440	18.8	110	7.0	10.0	4.7	0.6
Potato, Fresh, Safeway*	1 Rost/100g	138	5.5	138	2.8	19.2	5.5	2.8
Potato, McCain*	1 Rosti/95g	161	8.6	169	2.2	19.6	9.1	0.0
Potato, Mini, Party Bites, Sainsbury's*	1 Serving/100g	218	11.5	218	2.5	26.2	11.5	3.0
Potato, Mini, Party Range, Tesco*	1 Rosti/16.7g	33	1.9	193	2.1	20.6	11.4	3.3
Potato, Onion & Gruyere, Finest, Tesco*	½ Pack/200g	206	10.6	103	3.2	10.5	5.3	2.0
Potato, Spinach & Mozzarella, Tesco*	1 Serving/140g	228	7.7	163	3.8	24.5	5.5	2.0
Potato & Leek, Sainsbury's*	½ Pack/190g	296	20.9	156	4.5	9.8	11.0	0.3
Potato & Root Vegetable, COU, M & S*	1 Cake/100g	85	2.7	85	1.6	13.3	2.7	1.5
Potato Cakes, Baby, M & S*	1 Rosti/22.9g	40	1.5	175	3.5	25.1	6.7	1.6
Spinach & Mozzarella, Vegetarian, Tesco*	1 Rosti/140g	245	13.6	175	4.8	17.0	9.7	2.3
Vegetable, Waitrose*	1 Pack/400g	248	9.2	62	1.4	8.8	2.3	1.3
ROUGHY								
Orange, Raw	1oz/28g	35	2.0	126	14.7	0.0	7.0	0.0
ROULADE								
Chocolate, Finest, Tesco*	1 Serving/80g	222	4.5	277	3.4	53.2	5.6	2.3
Chocolate, Sainsbury's*	1 Serving/72g	264	15.7	367	5.7	36.9	21.8	1.8
Lemon Meringue, M & S*	1/6 Roulade/71g	250	7.6	350	3.2	60.2	10.7	3.6
Lemon Meringue, TTD, Sainsbury's*	1 Serving/100g	277	9.8	277	2.4	44.7	9.8	0.5
Orange & Lemon Meringue, Co-Op*	1 Serving/82g	287	9.8	350	3.0	57.0	12.0	0.3
Raspberry, Finest, Tesco*	1 Slice/67g	203	11.7	303	3.3	33.2	17.4	1.7
Smoked Salmon & Asparagus, Sainsbury's*	1 Serving/60g	122	9.6	204	13.0	2.2	16.0	0.3
Smoked Salmon & Spinach, Finest, Tesco*	1 Serving/60g	91	6.1	152	11.5	3.6	10.2	0.6
Toffee Pecan, Finest, Tesco*	1 Serving/60g	218	8.9	363	3.6	53.8	14.8	0.5
RUM								
37.5% Volume	1 Pub Shot/35ml	72	0.0	207	0.0	0.0	0.0	0.0
40% Volume	1 Pub Shot/35ml	78	0.0	222	0.0	0.0	0.0	0.0
White	1 Pub Shot/35ml	72	0.0	207	0.0	0.0	0.0	0.0

R

	Measure INFO/WEIGHT	per Measure KCAL	FAT	Nutrition Values per 100g / 100ml KCAL	PROT	CARB	FAT	FIBRE
RUSKS								
Banana, Farleys*	1 Serving/17.1g	70	1.5	409	7.3	75.1	8.8	2.9
Original, Farleys*	1 Rusk/17g	69	1.2	406	7.1	77.7	7.1	2.4

R

	INFO/WEIGHT	KCAL	FAT	KCAL	PROT	CARB	FAT	FIBRE
SAAG								
Aloo, Canned, Tesco*	½ Can/200g	124	3.8	62	1.8	9.3	1.9	2.0
Aloo, Fresh, Sainsbury's*	1 Pack/400g	388	13.2	97	2.0	14.7	3.3	4.8
Aloo, Jar, Sainsbury's*	½ Jar/135g	122	5.8	90	1.6	11.0	4.3	1.7
Aloo, North Indian, Sainsbury's*	1 Pack/300g	354	24.0	118	2.4	9.0	8.0	1.6
Aloo, Packet, Sainsbury's*	½ Pack/150g	185	12.5	123	2.1	9.9	8.3	2.7
Aloo, Safeway*	1 Pack/300g	390	24.0	130	2.2	12.3	8.0	2.8
Aloo, Sainsbury's*	1 Pack/300g	441	31.8	147	2.1	10.7	10.6	3.5
Aloo, Tesco*	1 Serving/200g	144	7.0	72	2.1	8.0	3.5	2.0
Aloo Gobi, Waitrose*	1 Pack/300g	240	13.8	80	2.6	7.1	4.6	2.9
Chicken, M & S*	1 Pack/400g	420	12.0	105	7.5	12.2	3.0	2.8
Chicken, Masala, Sainsbury's*	1oz/28g	36	2.0	127	13.2	2.4	7.2	2.3
Chicken, Masala, Waitrose*	1 Pack/400g	520	30.0	130	13.8	1.8	7.5	2.5
Chicken, Safeway*	1 Pack/350g	504	29.4	144	11.6	5.4	8.4	1.4
Gobi Aloo, Indian, Tesco*	1 Pack/225g	225	16.4	100	2.1	6.5	7.3	1.8
Gobi Aloo, Indian Takeaway, Sainsbury's*	1 Pack/334g	164	3.7	49	1.7	8.0	1.1	1.5
Gobi Aloo, M & S*	1 Pack/225g	270	19.1	120	1.9	9.3	8.5	2.4
Gobi Aloo, Morrisons*	½ Pack/175g	275	17.9	157	2.5	13.8	10.2	2.2
Gobi Aloo, Tesco*	1 Serving/175g	166	8.9	95	2.1	9.5	5.1	1.9
Paneer, Sainsbury's*	1 Pack/300g	387	29.1	129	6.0	4.3	9.7	2.3
SAFFRON								
Average	1 Tsp/0.7g	3	0.1	310	11.4	61.5	5.9	0.0
SAGE								
Dried, Ground	1 Tsp/1g	3	0.1	315	10.6	42.7	12.7	0.0
Fresh	1oz/28g	33	1.3	119	3.9	15.6	4.6	0.0
SAGO								
Raw	1oz/28g	99	0.1	355	0.2	94.0	0.2	0.5
SALAD								
3 Bean, with Fresh Mint Vinaigrette, M & S*	1 Pack/350g	95	2.4	27	1.7	3.5	0.7	2.3
3 Bean & Mixed Leaf, with Mint Dresssing, M & S*	1 Pack/315g	284	16.1	90	2.8	8.0	5.1	5.8
Alfresco Style, Tesco*	1 Serving/200g	40	0.6	20	0.9	3.3	0.3	2.1
All Seasons, Sainsbury's*	1oz/28g	3	0.1	12	1.0	1.5	0.2	1.2
American Ranch, Asda*	1 Serving/220g	253	19.8	115	2.5	6.0	9.0	2.0
American Style, Morrisons*	1 Serving/25g	5	0.1	22	1.1	3.9	0.3	2.3
Aromatic Herb, Waitrose*	¼ Pack/27g	4	0.1	15	0.9	1.7	0.5	1.0
Assorted, Asda*	1 Serving/100g	22	0.6	22	2.4	1.7	0.6	0.0
Baby Leaf, Asda*	1 Serving/80g	10	0.2	12	2.1	0.2	0.3	1.7
Baby Leaf, Florette*	1 Serving/40g	5	0.1	12	2.0	0.4	0.3	1.0
Baby Leaf, Fully Prepared, Sainsbury's*	½ Bag/63g	10	0.3	16	1.3	1.9	0.4	1.5
Baby Leaf, Italian Style, M & S*	1 Serving/55g	74	7.2	135	1.6	2.7	13.1	1.4
Baby Leaf, M & S*	1 Pack/100g	20	0.2	20	3.0	1.7	0.2	0.5
Baby Leaf, Organic, Sainsbury's*	1 Serving/20g	3	0.1	14	1.5	1.4	0.3	1.1
Baby Leaf, Sainsbury's*	1 Serving/60g	12	1.1	20	2.8	1.1	1.9	1.9
Baby Leaf, Seasonal, Organic, Sainsbury's*	1 Serving/30g	3	0.1	10	1.6	0.4	0.3	1.2
Baby Leaf, Seasonal, Tesco*	½ Pack/45g	9	0.3	20	1.8	1.6	0.7	2.1
Baby Leaf, Sweet, Seasonal, M & S*	½ Bag/60g	9	0.2	15	2.4	0.6	0.4	1.8
Baby Leaf, with Purple Basil, Finest, Tesco*	½ Pack/42.5g	7	0.1	17	2.9	0.9	0.2	1.8
Baby Leaf, with Watercress, Tesco*	1 Serving/30g	6	0.2	19	1.8	1.3	0.7	1.8
Baby Leaf & Herb, Asda*	1 Serving/50g	7	0.1	14	2.3	0.7	0.2	2.4
Baby Plum & Sundried Tomato Salad, Waitrose*	1 Serving/200g	226	17.8	113	1.3	6.8	8.9	0.8
Baby Spinach & Red Mustard, M & S*	1 Pack/170g	264	26.7	155	1.7	1.1	15.7	0.1
Baby Tomato, Tesco*	1 Pack/205g	35	0.6	17	0.8	2.8	0.3	0.9
Bacon Caesar, M & S*	1oz/28g	48	3.9	170	5.5	5.7	14.0	1.2
Bacon Caesar, Sainsbury's*	1 Pack/256g	415	32.5	162	4.7	12.0	12.7	1.4

SALAD

INFO/WEIGHT	Measure per Measure KCAL	FAT	Nutrition Values per 100g / 100ml KCAL	PROT	CARB	FAT	FIBRE
Bag, Tesco*	1 Serving/200g	38	0.8	19	0.9	3.0	0.4	1.4
Bagel Egg, Tesco*	1 Pack/185g	474	20.0	256	10.2	29.5	10.8	1.7
Basil, Pesto & Pine Nuts, Italian Style, Finest, Tesco*	½ Pack/90g	144	12.5	160	5.1	3.6	13.9	1.2
Bean, M & S*	1 Serving/80g	72	0.7	90	6.4	14.3	0.9	3.9
Bean, Mint & Coriander, Somerfield*	1 Pack/250g	288	2.8	115	7.0	19.4	1.1	4.7
Bean, Mixed, Vinaigrette, Tesco*	1 Can/400g	280	2.0	70	3.2	13.1	0.5	1.9
Bean, Retail	1oz/28g	41	2.6	147	4.2	12.8	9.3	3.0
Bean, Three, M & S*	1 Pack/225g	225	2.9	100	5.8	16.7	1.3	3.9
Bean & Chorizo, Tapas Selection, Sainsbury's*	1 Serving/22g	29	1.4	132	8.1	10.7	6.3	1.9
Bean & Sweetcorn, Side, M & S*	1 Serving/125g	131	9.0	105	2.5	7.0	7.2	1.3
Beetroot	1oz/28g	28	1.9	100	2.0	8.4	6.8	1.7
Beetroot, 1% Fat, M & S*	1 Serving/225g	131	6.1	58	1.1	7.7	2.7	1.7
Beetroot, Co-Op*	1 Pack/250g	100	0.8	40	0.9	8.0	0.3	2.0
Beetroot, Cous Cous & Quinoa, Tesco*	1 Serving/100g	70	0.6	70	2.3	12.9	0.6	2.3
Beetroot, GFY, Asda*	1 Pack/250g	130	1.0	52	1.1	11.0	0.4	2.3
Beetroot, HL, Tesco*	1 Pot/200g	110	0.4	55	1.7	11.5	0.2	1.3
Beetroot, M & S*	1 Serving/225g	124	0.7	55	1.0	12.0	0.3	3.0
Beetroot, Morrisons*	1 Pot/250g	138	1.0	55	1.2	11.6	0.4	1.6
Beetroot, Organic, M & S*	1oz/28g	20	1.0	73	1.5	9.1	3.4	1.9
Beetroot, Sainsbury's*	1 Tub/200g	148	2.4	74	1.7	14.1	1.2	1.7
Beetroot & Carrot, Continental, Iceland*	1 Serving/100g	24	0.2	24	1.2	4.3	0.2	2.1
Beetroot & Cherry Tomato, & Lemon Dressing, M & S*	1 Pack/215g	86	4.1	40	1.3	5.2	1.9	1.5
Beetroot & Lettuce, Asda*	1 Serving/30g	5	0.0	16	1.4	2.7	0.0	2.5
Birchall*	1 Serving/300g	48	0.6	16	0.8	2.8	0.2	0.9
Bistro, Asda*	1 Serving/180g	29	0.0	16	1.4	2.7	0.0	2.5
Bistro, Morrisons*	1 Serving/20g	5	0.0	23	1.2	4.2	0.2	2.0
Bistro, Sainsbury's*	1 Pack/150g	26	0.3	17	1.9	2.0	0.2	2.0
Bistro, Washed Ready to Eat, Tesco*	1 Pack/140g	22	0.7	16	1.1	1.7	0.5	1.0
Bocconcini Mozzarella, with Sun Ripened Tomato, M & S*	½ Pack/100g	250	21.4	250	9.8	4.9	21.4	2.0
Cabbage & Leek, Crunchy Mix, Sainsbury's*	½ Pack/126.3g	24	0.8	19	1.2	2.1	0.6	1.9
Caesar, & New Potatoes with Asparagus, M & S*	1 Pack/200g	270	15.2	135	3.1	13.8	7.6	1.7
Caesar, Bacon, M & S*	1 Serving/250g	400	31.3	160	7.1	4.1	12.5	1.3
Caesar, Chicken & Bacon, Gourmet, M & S*	1 Salad/250g	550	43.5	220	9.0	7.3	17.4	0.7
Caesar, Chicken & Bacon, Tesco*	1 Pack/200g	506	40.2	253	6.6	11.4	20.1	1.0
Caesar, Co-Op*	¼ Pack/50g	88	7.5	175	3.0	6.0	15.0	2.0
Caesar, Finest, Tesco*	1 Bowl/220g	374	30.6	170	4.9	5.1	13.9	1.6
Caesar, Florette*	1 Serving/100g	163	12.4	163	2.7	10.2	12.4	1.8
Caesar, GFY, Asda*	½ Pack/87.4g	76	2.6	87	8.0	7.0	3.0	1.5
Caesar, HE, Tesco*	1 Serving/100g	101	6.2	101	3.2	8.0	6.2	0.7
Caesar, M & S*	1 Pack/268.4g	510	40.5	190	5.7	8.3	15.1	1.3
Caesar, Morrisons*	1 Serving/115g	194	18.1	169	3.6	5.9	15.7	0.3
Caesar, Pizza Express*	1 Serving/125.5g	199	18.7	159	3.7	2.8	15.0	0.0
Caesar, Sainsbury's*	½ Bag/128g	227	19.3	177	3.6	6.7	15.1	1.0
Caesar, Somerfield*	1 Bag/300g	432	33.3	144	4.4	6.6	11.1	2.6
Caesar, Washed & Ready to Eat, Somerfield*	½ Bag/125g	155	10.9	124	5.0	6.5	8.7	0.8*
Caesar, with Romaine Lettuce, Kit, BGTY, Sainsbury's*	½ Pack/130g	135	7.3	104	3.6	9.8	5.6	1.7
Cajun Chicken, David lloyd leisure*	1 Pack/300g	429	10.0	143	11.7	17.7	3.3	1.0
Cannelini Bean & Chorizo, Sainsbury's*	1 Pack/250g	228	8.0	91	5.3	10.2	3.2	1.6
Cannellini Bean & Chicken, M & S*	1 Serving/225g	250	14.7	111	5.9	7.4	6.5	3.1
Cannellini Bean & Tuna, M & S*	1 Serving/255g	215	11.6	84	5.3	5.4	4.5	2.1
Caribbean Chicken, Shapers, Boots*	1 Pack/220g	222	5.1	101	5.8	14.0	2.3	1.2
Carrot, M & S*	1 Pack/215.4g	280	7.3	130	3.1	22.4	3.4	2.7
Carrot, with Fresh Coriander Vinaigrette, M & S*	½ Pack/105g	137	3.6	130	2.8	21.9	3.4	3.5

SALAD

INFO/WEIGHT	per Measure KCAL	FAT	Nutrition Values per 100g / 100ml KCAL	PROT	CARB	FAT	FIBRE
Carrot & Beetroot, with Balsamic Dressing, Eat Well, M & S* ½ Pack/200g	80	3.5	40	1.0	6.3	1.8	1.7
Carrot & Nut, with French Dressing, Average 1oz/28g	61	4.9	218	2.1	13.7	17.6	2.4
Carrot & Sultana, BGTY, Sainsbury's* ½ Pack/100g	55	0.3	55	0.6	12.4	0.3	0.0
Carrot & Sultana, HL, Tesco* 1 Tub/225g	142	1.4	63	1.2	13.2	0.6	2.5
Celery, Nut & Sultana, Waitrose* 1oz/28g	54	4.6	192	2.8	8.4	16.4	1.0
Chargrilled Chicken, Safeway* 1 Serving/200g	280	7.2	140	8.9	17.9	3.6	1.4
Chargrilled Chicken, Tesco* 1 Serving/300g	384	14.4	128	6.1	15.0	4.8	2.4
Chargrilled Chicken, Weight Watchers* 1 Pack/181.5g	265	3.8	146	11.7	20.0	2.1	2.2
Chargrilled Chicken & Bacon, Tesco* 1 Pack/300g	657	37.8	219	7.8	18.7	12.6	0.9
Chargrilled Chicken & Pesto, Sainsbury's* 1 Pack/250g	375	15.3	150	7.9	15.8	6.1	1.3
Chargrilled Chicken Wholefood, M & S* 1 Pot/219g	230	4.2	105	10.1	11.6	1.9	4.8
Chargrilled Pepper with Cous Cous, Asda* 1 Pack/325.2g	426	10.7	131	4.3	21.0	3.3	0.0
Chargrilled Vegetable, M & S* 1 Tub/165g	91	5.4	55	1.4	5.3	3.3	2.6
Charlotte New Potato, with Mint Vinaigrette, M & S* 1 Serving/110g	99	3.0	90	1.5	14.4	2.7	1.1
Cheese, Layered, Sainsbury's* 1 Pack/235g	367	25.6	156	4.3	10.1	10.9	2.0
Cheese, Layered, Tesco* 1 Serving/225g	437	32.0	194	5.8	10.8	14.2	0.8
Cheese & Coleslaw, Tesco* 1 Serving/125g	135	10.9	108	3.4	3.4	8.7	1.1
Cherry Tomato, All Good Things* 1 Pack/185g	31	0.6	17	0.8	2.8	0.3	1.4
Cherry Tomato, Fresh, Safeway* 1 Pack/170g	31	0.5	18	0.8	2.9	0.3	0.9
Cherry Tomato, Large, Fresh, Safeway* 1 Serving/245g	49	1.0	20	1.0	3.1	0.4	1.9
Chick Pea & Cous Cous, Tesco* 1 Serving/250g	245	6.5	98	3.2	15.5	2.6	0.0
Chick Pea & Spinach, M & S* 1 Serving/260g	299	10.7	115	7.3	12.5	4.1	2.7
Chicken, Avacado & Bacon, M & S* 1 Serving/235g	235	13.6	100	8.5	2.8	5.8	2.8
Chicken, Caesar, Tesco* 1 Pack/300g	330	13.5	110	6.8	10.6	4.5	0.8
Chicken, Chef's, Italian, Pret a Manger* 1 Pack/309g	322	24.1	104	6.9	3.2	7.8	1.8
Chicken, HE, Tesco* 1 Salad/216g	296	3.0	137	8.4	22.6	1.4	1.2
Chicken, Italian Style, Snack Pot, Carb Check, Heinz* 1 Pot/218g	131	4.4	60	5.9	4.3	2.0	1.0
Chicken, Layer, HE, Tesco* 1 Pack/400g	268	4.4	67	5.8	8.4	1.1	2.1
Chicken, Roast, & Coleslaw, Boots* 1 Serving/245g	392	34.3	160	4.5	3.9	14.0	1.3
Chicken, Roast, 93 Cals, Shapers, Boots* 1 Pack/232.5g	93	0.9	40	8.6	0.6	0.4	1.8
Chicken, Safeway* 1 Serving/200g	279	7.2	140	8.9	17.9	3.6	1.4
Chicken, Sweet Chilli, BGTY, Sainsbury's* 1 Serving/200g	206	0.8	103	6.0	18.7	0.4	0.0
Chicken, Sweetcorn & Pasta, Safeway* 1 Serving/200g	230	3.6	115	7.5	16.3	1.8	1.0
Chicken, Tesco* 1 Serving/300g	348	22.2	116	5.3	7.0	7.4	1.0
Chicken, Tomato, & Basil, Safeway* 1 Serving/200g	330	17.8	165	6.9	14.2	8.9	0.6
Chicken, Tomato Chilli, & Rice, COU, M & S* 1 Pack/340g	357	5.1	105	6.8	16.0	1.5	0.9
Chicken & Bacon, Asda* 1 Pack/381.0g	480	22.9	126	7.0	11.0	6.0	0.0
Chicken & Bacon, Carb Control, Tesco* 1 Serving/188g	244	14.7	130	13.2	1.7	7.8	0.5
Chicken & Bacon, Layered, Asda* 1 Serving/375g	473	22.5	126	7.0	11.0	6.0	1.6
Chicken & Bacon Ranch, Sainsbury's* 1 Pack/210g	315	15.8	150	8.4	12.1	7.5	0.9
Chicken & Rice, Safeway* 1 Serving/200g	220	2.6	110	6.4	17.6	1.3	1.4
Chicken Caesar, Asda* 1 Pack/273g	535	43.7	196	10.0	3.0	16.0	1.9
Chicken Caesar, Eat Well, M & S* 1 Pack/395g	595	24.6	150	9.9	18.7	6.2	2.1
Chicken Caesar, Fresh, Sainsbury's* 1 Serving/200g	278	20.0	139	6.0	6.2	10.0	1.2
Chicken Caesar, M & S* ½ Pack/140g	266	20.0	190	6.7	8.7	14.3	0.8
Chicken Caesar, TTD, Sainsbury's* 1 Serving/190g	308	23.4	162	11.1	1.6	12.3	1.5
Chicken Caesar Bistro, M & S* ½ Pack/135g	189	14.3	140	5.0	6.5	10.6	0.6
Chicken Fajita, Shapers, Boots* 1 Pack/258g	181	3.4	70	7.0	7.4	1.3	2.7
Chicken Noodle, Thai Style, Sainsbury's* 1 Pack/260g	283	7.5	109	6.6	14.2	2.9	1.3
Chicken Noodle & Sweet Chilli, Shapers, Boots* 1 Pack/197g	266	5.1	135	12.0	16.0	2.6	0.9
Chicken Pesto Pasta, Royal London Hospital* 1oz/28g	37	1.0	132	10.4	15.3	3.5	0.0
Chicken with Mayonnaise, Waitrose* 1 Pack/208g	406	19.8	195	10.3	17.1	9.5	2.5
Chilli, Tomato, Chick Pea & Butterbean, Tesco* 1 Pack/130g	146	6.0	112	3.4	14.3	4.6	0.5

SALAD

	Measure INFO/WEIGHT	per Measure KCAL	FAT	Nutrition Values per 100g / 100ml KCAL	PROT	CARB	FAT	FIBRE
Chilli Chicken & Spicy Cous Cous, HE, Tesco*	1 Serving/190g	251	4.6	132	6.5	21.1	2.4	1.5
Citrus, Tesco*	1 Tin/400g	160	0.0	40	0.3	9.6	0.0	0.5
Classic, with Chive Dressing, M & S*	½ Pack/137.5g	76	5.8	55	0.9	3.3	4.2	1.6
Classic Caesar, M & S*	½ Pack/112g	174	14.2	155	2.9	6.8	12.7	0.5
Classic Caesar, Reduced Fat, M & S*	1 Serving/115g	132	5.6	115	4.8	12.7	4.9	0.5
Classic with Green Herb Dressing, Co-Op*	1 Serving/90g	86	8.1	95	1.0	2.0	9.0	1.0
Classics, M & S*	1 Pack/255g	140	12.0	55	1.1	2.4	4.7	1.3
Coleslaw, Classics, M & S*	1 Pot/190g	124	4.4	65	1.9	8.8	2.3	1.3
Coleslaw & Potato, 3% Fat, M & S*	1oz/28g	20	1.0	72	2.7	7.7	3.4	1.5
Coleslaw Layered, Fresh, Asda*	1 Tub/197g	209	17.7	106	1.2	5.0	9.0	1.5
Continental, Budgens*	1 Serving/55g	8	0.2	14	1.2	1.4	0.4	2.1
Continental, Co-Op*	1 Serving/80g	12	0.3	15	1.0	2.0	0.4	1.0
Continental Four Leaf, Sainsbury's*	½ Pack/100g	13	0.2	13	1.2	1.7	0.2	1.9
Continental Leaf, Asda*	1oz/28g	4	0.1	16	1.4	1.4	0.5	1.4
Continental Style, Co-Op*	1 Bag/100g	15	0.3	15	1.0	2.0	0.3	0.5
Coronation Chicken, Sainsbury's*	1 Pack/200g	334	17.0	167	8.5	14.0	8.5	1.1
Coronation Chicken, Salad Bar, Asda*	1oz/28g	82	6.4	293	5.7	16.4	22.7	0.7
Coronation Chicken & Rice, Asda*	1oz/28g	67	4.8	241	6.7	15.2	17.0	0.4
Coronation Rice, Tesco*	1 Serving/50g	104	7.6	207	2.0	15.9	15.1	0.8
Cosmopolitan, Fresh, Sainsbury's*	1 Serving/10g	2	0.1	15	1.2	1.6	0.4	1.9
Cous Cous, & Roasted Vegetable, Waitrose*	1 Pack/220g	396	13.4	180	5.1	26.1	6.1	1.2
Cous Cous, BFY, Morrisons*	½ Pot/113g	164	4.0	145	4.6	23.8	3.5	0.5
Cous Cous, BGTY, Sainsbury's*	1 Pot/200g	236	4.4	118	4.7	19.7	2.2	2.8
Cous Cous, Tesco*	1 Serving/25g	35	0.4	141	4.8	26.9	1.6	0.6
Cous Cous, Waitrose*	1 Pot/200g	344	10.0	172	4.9	26.9	5.0	1.4
Cous Cous, with Mixed Peppers & Cucumber, GFY, Asda*	¼ Pot/56g	66	0.1	117	3.9	25.0	0.2	1.5
Cous Cous & Roast Vegetable, GFY, Asda*	1 Serving/100g	120	1.6	120	3.5	23.0	1.6	2.7
Cous Cous with Chargrilled Chicken, Sainsbury's*	1 Pack/240g	446	20.9	186	7.4	19.6	8.7	0.0
Crisp, Mix, Somerfield*	1 Pack/215g	34	0.6	16	0.9	2.4	0.3	1.6
Crisp, Mixed, Morrisons*	1 Pack/230g	39	0.7	17	1.0	2.8	0.3	0.0
Crisp & Crunchy, Asda*	1 Pack/250g	55	1.5	22	0.8	3.3	0.6	1.4
Crisp & Crunchy with French Dressing, GFY, Asda*	1/3 Pack/116g	26	0.7	22	0.8	3.3	0.6	1.4
Crisp & Light, M & S*	1 Serving/170g	51	1.4	30	0.5	5.4	0.8	1.0
Crisp & Sweet, Asda*	½ Pack/85g	14	0.3	17	0.8	2.7	0.3	1.4
Crisp & Sweet Lettuce Leaves, Florette*	¼ Pack/70g	10	0.4	14	0.8	1.7	0.5	0.9
Crisp Leaf, Somerfield*	1 Serving/80g	14	0.1	17	1.1	2.8	0.1	1.3
Crisp Mixed, Safeway*	1 Serving/60g	12	0.2	20	1.2	3.0	0.3	2.0
Crisp Mixed, Tesco*	1 Pack/200g	40	0.6	20	1.1	3.2	0.3	2.0
Crispy, Co-Op*	1 Serving/80g	13	0.2	16	0.8	3.0	0.3	1.0
Crispy, Florette*	1 Portion/100g	22	0.3	22	1.5	3.4	0.3	3.0
Crispy, Somerfield*	1 Pack/140g	17	0.0	12	1.0	2.0	0.0	0.0
Crispy, Tesco*	1oz/28g	6	0.1	20	1.2	3.0	0.3	1.6
Crispy Duck & Herb, M & S*	½ Pack/140g	378	25.6	270	20.7	3.7	18.3	1.4
Crispy Green, Safeway*	1 Bag/165g	21	0.5	13	1.0	1.6	0.3	1.1
Crispy Green, Sainsbury's*	1 Serving/70g	8	0.1	12	0.9	1.6	0.2	0.8
Crispy Leaf, Asda*	1oz/28g	4	0.1	14	0.8	1.6	0.5	0.9
Crispy Leaf, Sainsbury's*	½ Pack/75g	9	0.3	12	1.0	1.2	0.4	1.5
Crispy Medley, Waitrose*	1 Serving/50g	8	0.3	15	0.8	1.7	0.5	0.9
Crunchy, Basics, Sainsbury's*	1 Pack/200g	40	0.4	20	1.3	3.4	0.2	2.2
Crunchy, Fully Prepared, Sainsbury's*	½ Pack/150g	24	0.2	16	1.1	3.0	0.1	1.7
Crunchy, Simple, M & S*	1 Serving/50g	8	0.3	15	1.0	1.6	0.5	1.8
Crunchy, Tesco*	1 Serving/56g	11	0.2	19	1.2	2.8	0.3	2.1
Crunchy, Waitrose*	½ Pack100g	18	0.4	18	1.0	2.6	0.4	1.5

	Measure INFO/WEIGHT	per Measure KCAL	FAT	Nutrition Values per 100g / 100ml KCAL	PROT	CARB	FAT	FIBRE
SALAD								
Crunchy Layered, Tesco*	1 Serving/54g	15	0.2	27	1.1	4.9	0.3	1.7
Crunchy Shredded, Safeway*	1 Serving/50g	10	0.2	19	1.2	2.9	0.3	1.5
Crunchy Spring, Side, M & S*	1 Serving/160g	32	0.3	20	0.9	4.1	0.2	1.3
Eat Me Keep Me, Tesco*	1 Serving/80g	14	0.2	18	0.8	3.0	0.3	1.7
Egg, Fresh4you*	1 Pack/55g	139	12.2	252	8.3	4.6	22.2	0.0
Egg & Baby Spinach, Waitrose*	1 Pack/215g	167	13.5	78	3.5	1.8	6.3	1.0
Egg & Coleslaw, Boots*	1 Pot/233g	405	37.3	174	3.0	4.6	16.0	1.0
Egg & New Potato, GFY, Asda*	1 Pack/230g	123	5.0	53	3.4	5.0	2.2	1.3
Egg & Potato, Fresh, M & S*	1 Serving/250g	150	7.3	60	3.0	4.6	2.9	0.9
Endive & Radicchio, Somerfield*	1 Pack/150g	20	0.0	13	2.0	1.0	0.0	0.0
English Garden, Tesco*	1 Serving/180g	22	0.4	12	0.7	1.8	0.2	0.7
Exotic, with Mango & Chilli Dressing, Co-Op*	½ Pack/65g	25	0.4	38	0.6	7.7	0.6	0.8
Family, Florette*	1 Serving/50g	15	0.1	29	1.1	5.5	0.2	3.0
Family, Somerfield*	1 Serving/67g	12	0.3	18	0.8	2.9	0.4	1.3
Feta Cheese & Sunblushed Tomato, M & S*	1 Serving/190g	361	21.1	190	5.5	17.2	11.1	2.1
Fine Cut, Asda*	½ Bag/87.5g	21	0.3	24	1.2	4.3	0.3	2.1
Fine Noodle with Duck Breast, COU, M & S*	1 Pack/280g	294	3.1	105	5.5	18.9	1.1	1.1
Florida, Retail, Average	1oz/28g	63	5.7	224	0.9	9.7	20.5	1.0
Four Leaf, M & S*	1 Serving/130g	20	0.4	15	0.9	2.0	0.3	1.4
Four Leaf, Tesco*	1oz/28g	4	0.1	15	0.8	1.8	0.5	0.9
French Goat's Cheese, Extra Fine, Asda*	1 Pack/185g	463	35.2	250	8.4	11.4	19.0	0.8
French Style, M & S*	1 Pack/140g	140	13.6	100	1.0	2.5	9.7	0.9
French Style, Morrisons*	1 Pack/200g	28	1.0	14	0.8	1.7	0.5	0.0
Fresh & Crispy, Tesco*	1 Serving/230g	30	0.7	13	0.7	1.9	0.3	1.3
Funky Leaf, Spinach, Rocket etc, Jamie Oliver*	1 Pack/150g	177	9.9	118	0.7	14.2	6.6	1.2
Fusion, Fully Prepared, Sainsbury's*	½ Pack/62.5g	15	0.5	24	3.7	0.3	0.8	3.4
Garden, Asda*	1 Pack/175g	32	0.5	18	0.7	3.1	0.3	1.6
Garden, Fresh, Safeway*	½ Pack/105g	27	0.3	26	1.1	4.8	0.3	1.1
Garden, Safeway*	1oz/28g	6	0.1	23	1.1	4.0	0.3	2.0
Garden, Shapers, Boots*	1 Box/225g	86	1.1	38	1.3	7.1	0.5	1.3
Garden, Sweet & Crispy, Tesco*	1 Bag/225g	54	0.9	24	1.0	4.2	0.4	1.4
Garden, Sweet & Crunchy, Tesco*	1 Pack/225g	54	0.9	24	1.0	4.2	0.4	1.4
Garden, Tesco*	1 Serving/225g	34	0.7	15	1.0	2.0	0.3	0.9
Garden, Tray, Asda*	½ Pack/87.5g	16	0.3	18	0.7	3.1	0.3	1.6
Garden, with Watercress, M & S*	1 Salad/80g	10	0.1	12	1.5	1.4	0.1	1.4
Garden, with Yoghurt & Mint Dressing, GFY, Asda*	1 Serving/195g	51	2.0	26	1.1	3.2	1.0	0.0
Gourmet Chargrilled Chicken & Bacon, Atkins*	1 Pack/245g	311	20.1	127	12.0	2.5	8.2	1.0
Gourmet Continental, Waitrose*	1 Serving/150g	23	0.8	15	0.8	1.7	0.5	0.9
Greek	1oz/28g	36	3.5	130	2.7	1.9	12.5	0.8
Greek, BGTY, Sainsbury's*	1 Serving/198.5g	133	5.0	67	2.0	9.0	2.5	0.8
Greek, Classic, Tesco*	1 Pack/255g	293	23.7	115	2.6	5.2	9.3	1.2
Greek, Gourmet, M & S*	1 Pack/315g	425	39.1	135	3.6	2.5	12.4	1.4
Greek, Side, Waitrose*	1 Pack/150g	156	12.2	104	3.2	4.6	8.1	0.9
Greek, Tesco*	1 Serving/200g	188	14.2	94	3.2	4.3	7.1	0.9
Greek Style, Deli, M & S*	1 Pack/200g	230	19.6	115	3.6	3.3	9.8	1.2
Greek Style, Delphi*	1 Serving/220g	306	27.1	139	3.7	3.5	12.3	0.9
Greek Style, Fresh, Food Counter, Sainsbury's*	1 Serving/166g	247	23.2	149	1.9	2.7	14.0	0.0
Greek Style, Waitrose*	½ Pack/125g	54	2.8	43	1.9	4.0	2.2	1.2
Greek Style, with Herb Dressing, Tesco*	1 Pack/240g	305	28.3	127	3.2	2.0	11.8	1.0
Greek Style, with Houmous Dip, & Pitta, Sainsbury's*	1 Bowl/195g	296	17.4	152	5.4	12.5	8.9	2.6
Greek Style, with White Wine Vinaigrette, Tesco*	1 Pack/235g	256	22.3	109	3.5	2.3	9.5	1.5
Greek Style Feta, Tip & Mix, M & S*	1 Pack/195g	215	18.3	110	4.0	2.5	9.4	1.6
Greek Style Layered, PB, Waitrose*	1 Pack/280g	134	7.8	48	2.4	3.2	2.8	0.7

S

	Measure INFO/WEIGHT	per Measure KCAL	FAT	Nutrition Values per 100g / 100ml KCAL	PROT	CARB	FAT	FIBRE
SALAD								
Green, Complete, Sainsbury's*	1/3 Pack/54.8g	92	6.7	168	4.2	10.3	12.2	1.4
Green, Crispy, Fresh, Sainsbury's*	1 Serving/40g	5	0.1	12	0.9	1.6	0.2	0.8
Green, Fresh, Safeway*	½ Pack/98g	14	0.3	14	0.9	1.9	0.3	0.8
Green, M & S*	1oz/28g	4	0.1	13	0.8	1.7	0.3	0.9
Green, Mixed, Average	1oz/28g	3	0.1	12	0.7	1.8	0.3	1.0
Green Lentil, Red Pepper & Spinach, Waitrose*	1 Container/250g	485	20.0	194	8.6	22.0	8.0	2.9
Green Side, M & S*	1 Serving/200g	30	0.4	15	0.9	2.5	0.2	0.0
Green Side, Sainsbury's*	1 Pack/200g	28	0.2	14	1.2	2.1	0.1	1.4
Green Side, Tesco*	1 Serving/100g	12	0.3	12	0.7	1.6	0.3	1.3
Green with Chives, Tesco*	½ Pack/90g	13	0.4	14	1.0	1.6	0.4	1.7
Green with Honey & Mustard Dressing, M & S*	1 Pack/200g	120	9.6	60	0.9	2.7	4.8	0.8
Green with Sweetcorn & Radish, Fresh, Safeway*	1 Pack/210g	55	0.6	26	1.1	4.8	0.3	1.1
Ham, Antony Worrall Thompson's*	1 Pack/202.4g	257	2.6	127	9.8	19.1	1.3	2.7
Herb, Asda*	1 Serving/20g	2	0.1	12	1.8	0.6	0.3	2.0
Herb, M & S*	1 Pack/100g	20	0.4	20	2.9	1.4	0.4	1.9
Herb, Organic, Sainsbury's*	1 Serving/100g	17	0.5	17	1.8	1.3	0.5	1.8
Herb, Sainsbury's*	1 Pack/120g	22	0.6	18	2.7	0.8	0.5	2.2
Herb, Somerfield*	½ Pack/50g	13	0.6	26	1.9	2.0	1.1	1.7
Herb, Tesco*	1oz/28g	4	0.1	16	1.1	1.8	0.5	0.9
Herb Garden, Morrisons*	1 Serving/28g	4	0.1	14	0.9	1.7	0.5	0.0
Honey Smoked Salmon & New Potato, M & S*	1 Pack/270g	270	14.3	100	5.5	7.5	5.3	1.5
Houmous, Delicious, Boots*	1 Pack/230g	154	4.4	67	5.3	7.4	1.9	3.1
Iceberg & Cabbage, Asda*	½ Pack/125g	24	0.4	19	1.0	3.1	0.3	1.5
Italian, Complete, Sainsbury's*	1 Pack/160g	237	14.4	148	5.4	11.4	9.0	1.6
Italian Style, Asda*	1 Serving/20g	3	0.1	15	1.1	1.6	0.5	1.2
Italian Style, Organic, Waitrose*	½ Pack/45g	7	0.2	15	0.8	1.7	0.5	0.9
Italian Style, Side, Crispy, with Tomato Dressing, Waitrose*	1 Pack/170g	83	5.1	49	1.3	4.3	3.0	1.2
Italian Style, Tesco*	1/3 Pack/40g	6	0.2	16	1.0	1.9	0.5	1.2
Italian Wild Rocket & Parmesan, Sainsbury's*	1 Serving/50g	89	7.4	177	7.5	3.4	14.8	0.5
Jardin, Tesco*	1 Serving/50g	7	0.3	14	0.8	1.8	0.6	1.4
King Prawn, GFY, Asda*	1 Serving/175g	112	2.6	64	4.7	8.0	1.5	1.3
King Prawn, Thai Style, M & S*	1 Pack/295g	266	7.4	90	4.4	12.6	2.5	1.3
King Prawn & New Potato, COU, M & S*	1 Pack/300g	180	6.9	60	3.0	6.9	2.3	0.8
King Prawn & Pasta, COU, M & S*	1 Pack/270g	284	6.5	105	5.9	15.1	2.4	2.7
Layered with Egg, Somerfield*	1 Pot/300g	543	54.0	181	3.0	3.0	18.0	0.0
Layered with Tuna, Somerfield*	1 Pot/255g	599	56.1	235	5.0	5.0	22.0	0.0
Leafy, Tesco*	1oz/28g	4	0.1	14	1.2	1.5	0.4	1.9
Leafy, with Tatsoi, Sainsbury's*	1 Bag/ 115g	17	0.4	15	1.0	1.6	0.3	1.7
Leafy, with Tatsoi, Somerfield*	1 Pack/25g	4	0.2	17	1.3	1.6	0.6	1.7
Leafy, with Tatsoi, Tesco*	1 Serving/42g	6	0.2	14	1.2	1.5	0.4	1.9
Leafy Mixed, Co-Op*	1 Bag/200g	40	0.6	20	1.0	4.0	0.3	1.0
Leafy Mixed, Safeway*	1oz/28g	4	0.1	14	0.9	1.5	0.5	1.0
Leaves, Oriental Mix, Waitrose*	1 Bag/100g	18	0.6	18	1.5	1.7	0.6	1.9
Leek & Pork Deli, Continental, Aldi*	¼ Tub/63g	68	3.2	108	1.9	13.9	5.0	2.3
Lemon Cous Cous & Roasted Pepper, COU, M & S*	1 Pack/340g	306	7.8	90	3.2	14.6	2.3	1.8
Lentil & Wild Rice, TTD, Sainsbury's*	1 Serving/100g	181	7.6	181	4.7	23.6	7.6	2.5
Mediterranean, Asda*	1 Pack/135g	27	0.4	20	0.9	3.3	0.3	1.5
Mediterranean, Side, Sainsbury's*	1 Pack/170g	44	2.2	26	0.9	2.7	1.3	1.3
Mediterranean Style, Asda*	½ Pack/135g	22	0.0	16	1.0	3.0	0.0	0.0
Mediterranean Style, Morrisons*	1 Serving/90g	13	0.2	14	1.5	1.9	0.2	0.0
Mediterranean Style, Safeway*	1 Serving/25g	5	0.2	20	1.7	1.9	0.6	2.0
Mexican Style Bean & Cheese, M & S*	½ Pot/150g	150	5.3	100	6.1	11.2	3.5	4.8
Mixed, Crisp, Mild, Tesco*	½ Pack/145g	29	0.4	20	1.2	3.0	0.3	2.1

S

SALAD

	Measure INFO/WEIGHT	KCAL	FAT	KCAL	PROT	CARB	FAT	FIBRE
Mixed, Florette*	1 Serving/100g	20	0.2	20	1.3	3.4	0.2	3.0
Mixed, Iceland*	1 Serving/50g	12	0.1	24	1.2	4.3	0.2	2.1
Mixed, Sainsbury's*	1 Serving/100g	21	0.2	21	1.4	3.4	0.2	2.1
Mixed, Sweet & Crispy, Tesco*	1 Serving/200g	48	0.6	24	1.0	4.2	0.3	2.0
Mixed, Tesco*	1 Serving/100g	24	0.3	24	1.0	4.2	0.3	2.0
Mixed Bean, Asda*	½ Can/145g	126	3.6	87	5.0	11.0	2.5	6.0
Mixed Bean, Canned, Waitrose*	1 Can/270g	251	1.6	93	6.4	15.5	0.6	5.5
Mixed Bean, Morrisons*	1 Serving/145g	129	1.7	89	5.8	13.7	1.2	0.0
Mixed Bean, Sainsbury's*	1 Can/270g	227	2.4	84	5.4	13.5	0.9	3.8
Mixed Bean, Tesco*	1 Serving/70g	49	0.4	70	3.2	13.1	0.5	1.9
Mixed Bean with Onions & Peppers, Safeway*	½ Can/210g	141	1.3	67	4.0	11.4	0.6	2.7
Mixed Leaf, Asda*	1 Serving/100g	21	0.2	21	1.5	3.2	0.2	2.1
Mixed Leaf, Tomato, Feta, Boots*	1 Pack/179g	218	17.0	122	3.7	5.4	9.5	1.0
Mixed Leaf, Tomato & Olive, Tesco*	1 Serving/170g	150	13.3	88	1.0	3.4	7.8	0.0
Mixed Leaf & Baby Basil, A Taste of Italy, Florette*	1 Pack/155g	143	8.2	92	2.7	8.5	5.3	1.0
Mixed Leaf Medley, Waitrose*	1 Serving/25g	4	0.1	15	0.8	1.7	0.5	1.4
Mixed Leaf Tomato & Olive, Tesco*	1 Serving/170g	150	13.3	88	1.0	3.4	7.8	2.0
Mixed Leaf with Olive Oil Dressing, Pizza Express*	1 Pack/240g	326	33.8	136	0.9	2.1	14.1	0.7
Mixed Leaves, Bondelle*	1 Serving/50g	11	0.1	21	1.4	3.3	0.2	0.0
Mixed Leaves, Somerfield*	1 Pack/140g	17	0.0	12	1.0	2.0	0.0	0.0
Mixed Leaves, Tesco*	1 Serving/20g	3	0.1	14	0.9	1.6	0.4	0.9
Mixed Pepper, Asda*	½ Pack/100g	24	0.3	24	1.0	4.3	0.3	1.7
Mixed Vegetable, Aldi*	1 Serving/200g	120	4.0	60	0.6	10.0	2.0	0.0
Mixed with Peppers & Iceberg Lettuce, Somerfield*	1 Pack/200g	50	0.0	25	1.0	5.0	0.0	0.0
Moroccan Styles, COU, M & S*	½ Pack/100g	160	1.2	160	5.0	32.8	1.2	4.8
Mozarella & Cherry Tomato, Shapers, Boots*	1 Bowl/194g	184	14.2	95	4.1	3.3	7.3	0.9
Mozerella & Tomato, M & S*	1 Serving/310g	400	14.8	129	5.5	15.5	4.8	0.9
Mozzarella & Rocket, Asda*	1 Serving/265g	435	31.8	164	7.0	7.0	12.0	1.5
Mozzarella & Sunkissed Tomato, Tesco*	1 Bag/160g	270	22.9	169	4.6	4.3	14.3	2.1
Mozzarella & Tomato, Pizza Express*	1 Serving/100g	288	22.3	288	15.2	5.9	22.3	0.1
Nantaise, Waitrose*	1 Pack/160g	34	0.6	21	1.5	2.9	0.4	2.0
New Potato, Co-Op*	1 Serving/50g	98	8.0	195	1.0	10.0	16.0	2.0
New Potato, Less Than 5% Fat, M & S*	1 Serving/110g	88	3.4	80	1.3	12.1	3.1	1.5
New Potato, Luxury, Morrisons*	½ Tub/125g	341	30.8	273	1.7	11.2	24.6	0.0
New Potato, M & S*	1 Serving/60g	114	9.8	190	0.9	9.9	16.3	1.3
New Potato, Santini Tomatoes, Egg & Salad Cream, M & S*	1 Pack/305g	153	6.7	50	2.9	7.1	2.2	1.9
New Potato, Tuna & Egg, M & S*	1 Pack/340g	255	12.9	75	3.8	6.7	3.8	0.7
New Potato & Free Range Egg, M & S*	1 Pack/305g	214	11.6	70	2.5	7.0	3.8	0.8
New Potato & Free Range Egg, Side, Sainsbury's*	1 Pack/290g	174	12.2	60	2.5	3.1	4.2	1.4
New Potato & King Prawn, M & S*	1 Pack/210g	221	9.5	105	5.6	10.2	4.5	1.7
New Potato & Sweet Chilli Prawn, M & S*	1 Pack/210g	147	1.1	70	2.8	14.0	0.5	0.7
New Potato & Tuna Sweetcorn, Eat Well, M & S*	1 Pack/190g	133	3.4	70	5.4	8.4	1.8	1.9
Nicoise, Tesco*	1 Pack/260g	286	21.8	110	3.2	5.3	8.4	1.4
Noodle, Sweet Chilli Chicken, Shapers, Boots*	1 Serving/197g	256	4.1	130	11.0	17.0	2.1	1.1
Noodle, Thai Style, BGTY, Sainsbury's*	1 Pack/185g	150	3.5	81	2.7	13.5	1.9	0.0
Noodle & King Prawn, PB, Waitrose*	1 Pack/225g	223	2.3	99	5.0	17.4	1.0	1.0
Noodle with Thai Style Chicken, M & S*	½ Pot/145g	160	7.1	110	5.2	11.6	4.9	1.4
Orchard, Panera*	1 Serving/132g	210	12.0	159	3.8	11.4	9.1	1.5
Orzo & Sunbaked Tomato, BGTY, Sainsbury's*	1 Tub/275.5g	292	6.1	106	3.1	18.5	2.2	2.5
Pancetta, Express, Pizza Express*	1 Salad/90g	200	17.9	223	7.4	3.3	20.0	0.0
Pasta, Chicken & Sweetcorn, Morrisons*	1 Serving/220g	255	3.5	116	6.7	18.7	1.6	1.0
Pasta, Spinach & Pinenut, Safeway*	1 Serving/200g	295	14.4	148	5.3	15.2	7.2	1.7
Pasta, Tomato, Morrisons*	1 Serving/50g	46	0.6	92	3.0	17.3	1.2	2.4

SALAD

	Measure INFO/WEIGHT	per Measure KCAL	FAT	Nutrition Values per 100g / 100ml KCAL	PROT	CARB	FAT	FIBRE
Pasta, Tuna & Sweetcorn, Morrisons*	1 Serving/100g	227	15.1	227	5.0	16.1	15.1	2.2
Pasta & Cheese, Asda*	1 Serving/125g	319	23.8	255	6.0	15.0	19.0	1.2
Pasta & Cheese, Somerfield*	½ Pack/225g	342	23.4	152	3.6	11.8	10.4	1.5
Pasta & Chesse, Safeway*	1 Serving/225g	554	41.4	246	4.8	15.2	18.4	0.0
Pasta & Garlic, Iceland*	1 Serving/75g	149	10.7	199	2.2	15.4	14.3	1.6
Pasta & Ham, Safeway*	1 Pot/225g	284	10.1	126	4.5	16.9	4.5	0.3
Pasta & Mushroom, Waitrose*	1 Pack/200g	320	19.4	160	4.1	14.0	9.7	0.6
Pasta & Pepper Side, Tesco*	1 Pack/230g	278	15.2	121	2.4	13.0	6.6	1.3
Pasta & Sweetcorn, Less Than 3% Fat, M & S*	½ Pack/100g	85	1.4	85	2.8	14.7	1.4	1.5
Pasta & Tomato, GFY, Asda*	1 Pack/300g	348	9.3	116	3.0	19.0	3.1	1.6
Potato, 30% Less Fat, BGTY, Sainsbury's*	1 Serving/60g	64	3.7	106	1.7	11.1	6.1	1.1
Potato, 60% Less Fat, Asda*	1/3 Pack/83g	81	4.2	97	2.0	11.0	5.0	1.6
Potato, Asda*	¼ Pot/57g	67	4.0	117	0.9	12.5	7.0	1.1
Potato, Baby, TTD, Sainsbury's*	1 Tub/300g	528	45.9	176	1.9	7.6	15.3	0.0
Potato, Chunky, Somerfield*	1oz/28g	59	6.2	212	1.0	3.0	22.0	0.0
Potato, Creamy, Asda*	1oz/28g	61	5.2	219	1.0	11.9	18.6	0.7
Potato, Creamy, Waitrose*	1 Serving/100g	163	11.9	163	1.3	12.7	11.9	1.1
Potato, Eat Smart, Safeway*	½ Pack/121g	85	2.4	70	1.7	10.2	2.0	1.9
Potato, Finest, Tesco*	1 Serving/25g	59	5.2	235	2.4	9.7	20.6	1.2
Potato, From Salad Selection, Sainsbury's*	1 Serving/50g	102	8.8	204	1.0	10.5	17.5	1.3
Potato, GFY, Asda*	½ Pack/125g	145	8.8	116	1.3	12.0	7.0	0.0
Potato, Half Fat, Safeway*	1 Serving/125g	175	11.9	140	0.9	11.6	9.5	1.1
Potato, Healthy Choice, Somerfield*	1 Tub/300g	312	16.5	104	1.4	12.2	5.5	1.5
Potato, Heinz*	½ Can/97g	137	8.2	141	1.4	14.8	8.5	0.8
Potato, HL, Tesco*	1 Sm Serving/25g	29	1.2	115	1.7	15.4	4.8	1.2
Potato, Iceland*	1 Serving/75g	162	14.7	216	1.1	8.9	19.6	0.6
Potato, Light, 70% Less Fat, Morrisons*	1/3 Pack/100g	95	3.9	95	1.9	11.9	3.9	2.2
Potato, Luxury, Asda*	1 Serving/50g	119	10.5	237	1.0	11.0	21.0	0.0
Potato, M & S*	1oz/28g	55	4.8	195	1.2	8.5	17.3	1.3
Potato, PB, Waitrose*	½ Pot/125g	99	3.8	79	2.4	10.5	3.0	1.0
Potato, Salad Bar, Asda*	1oz/28g	52	4.3	187	0.6	11.6	15.4	1.1
Potato, Side, Waitrose*	1 Pack/250g	181	11.0	72	3.0	5.2	4.4	1.0
Potato, Spar*	1 Serving/50g	180	18.2	360	1.8	10.2	36.3	1.2
Potato, Tesco*	1 Pot/125g	206	16.9	165	1.3	9.5	13.5	1.3
Potato, Value, Tesco*	½ Pack/125g	138	8.1	110	1.0	12.0	6.5	0.4
Potato, with Onions & Chives, Co-Op*	1 Serving/50g	80	6.0	160	1.0	12.0	12.0	1.0
Potato & Cheese, Pasta & Mixed Leaf, Waitrose*	1 Serving/205g	267	17.4	130	3.2	10.1	8.5	1.1
Potato & Cheese, Sainsbury's*	1 Serving/125g	200	16.4	160	2.7	7.9	13.1	3.4
Potato & Egg, Fresh, Safeway*	1 Serving/105g	84	3.8	80	8.4	3.0	3.6	1.6
Potato & Egg, Somerfield*	½ Pack/157.9g	90	4.7	57	2.5	5.1	3.0	1.2
Potato & Egg, with Mayonnaise, Tesco*	½ Tub/150g	115	8.5	77	2.9	3.1	5.7	1.2
Potato Baby, with Mint, TTD, Sainsbury's*	1 Serving/100g	204	17.0	204	2.0	10.8	17.0	0.7
Potato Layered, Tesco*	1 Pack/350g	284	17.2	81	1.3	7.8	4.9	1.3
Potato with Mayonnaise	1oz/28g	67	5.8	239	1.6	12.2	20.8	0.9
Potato with Mayonnaise, Retail	1oz/28g	80	7.4	287	1.5	11.4	26.5	0.8
Potato with Reduced Calorie Dressing, Retail	1oz/28g	27	1.1	97	1.3	14.8	4.1	0.8
Prawn, King, with Noodles, Delicious, Boots*	1 Pack/228g	251	3.7	110	6.3	18.0	1.6	1.8
Prawn, King & Rice Noodle, M & S*	1 Pack/320g	208	2.6	65	2.9	11.6	0.8	0.9
Prawn, Layered, Asda*	1 Pack/197g	217	9.9	110	4.3	12.0	5.0	1.0
Prawn, Layered, Large Pack, Eat Well, M & S*	1 Pack/447.1g	380	18.8	85	4.1	8.8	4.2	1.2
Prawn, Layered, Sainsbury's*	1 Pack/275g	355	21.2	129	3.6	11.2	7.7	1.1
Prawn, Layered, Single Size, Asda*	1 Serving/197g	217	9.9	110	4.3	12.0	5.0	1.0
Prawn, Layered, Small Pack, Eat Well, M & S*	1 Pack/220g	198	8.4	90	4.4	9.9	3.8	1.0

SALAD

Measure INFO/WEIGHT		per Measure		Nutrition Values per 100g / 100ml				
		KCAL	FAT	KCAL	PROT	CARB	FAT	FIBRE
Prawn, Somerfield*	1 Serving/343g	490	25.0	143	5.6	13.8	7.3	0.5
Prawn, Tesco*	1 Pack/280g	314	14.0	112	4.7	12.0	5.0	0.9
Prawn & Avacado, M & S*	1 Serving/220g	176	15.0	80	3.0	2.0	6.8	3.1
Prawn & Egg, Leaf, Shapers, Boots*	1 Pack/182g	193	14.4	106	6.7	2.1	7.9	1.0
Prawn Cocktail, HL, Tesco*	1 Serving/300g	279	3.0	93	5.7	15.3	1.0	2.0
Prawn Cocktail, Shapers, Boots*	1 Pack/245g	120	5.9	49	4.7	2.2	2.4	0.7
Prawn Cocktail, Tesco*	1 Pack/300g	360	18.0	120	5.7	10.9	6.0	0.8
Prawn Satay & Noodle, Tesco*	1 Serving/250g	320	17.0	128	7.1	9.5	6.8	1.2
Red Thai Chicken with Noodles, Tesco*	1 Pack/300g	342	1.5	114	7.2	20.2	0.5	1.4
Ribbon, M & S*	1oz/28g	5	0.1	17	0.8	3.2	0.2	1.7
Rice, Courgette & Pine Nut, BGTY, Sainsbury's*	1/3 Pot/65g	68	1.0	105	2.7	20.0	1.6	1.5
Roast Chicken, Layered, HL, Tesco*	1 Salad/400g	268	4.4	67	5.8	8.4	1.1	2.1
Roast Chicken, Tesco*	1 Salad/300g	348	22.2	116	5.3	7.0	7.4	1.0
Roasted Artichoke & Pepper, M & S*	1 Serving/220g	638	53.9	290	4.1	12.8	24.5	5.1
Roasted Mediterranean Vegetable, Tesco*	½ Pack/125g	150	7.9	120	3.3	14.4	6.3	1.4
Roasted Vegetable, Feta & Cous Cous, Somerfield*	1 Pack/299.4g	490	17.3	164	5.0	22.9	5.8	1.6
Roasted Vegetables & Cous Cous, Sainsbury's*	1 Pot/225g	378	24.1	168	5.3	12.6	10.7	1.9
Rocket, Leafy, Asda*	1 Serving/75g	10	0.1	13	1.5	1.4	0.1	1.8
Rocket, Morrisons*	1 Serving/100g	14	0.5	14	0.8	1.7	0.5	0.0
Rocket, Tesco*	1oz/28g	4	0.1	14	0.8	1.7	0.5	0.9
Rocket, Wild, Safeway*	1 Serving/25g	6	0.1	25	3.3	2.3	0.3	1.7
Ruby, Tesco*	1 Serving/48g	12	0.2	25	1.4	4.1	0.4	2.2
Salad, Bistro, Somerfield*	½ Pack/50g	7	0.3	14	0.8	1.6	0.5	1.4
Salade Nicoise, M & S*	1 Pack/300g	270	20.2	90	5.8	1.7	6.7	2.1
Salmon & Roquette, M & S*	1 Serving/255g	306	20.4	120	3.9	8.5	8.0	1.0
Santa Plum Tomato & Avocado, M & S*	1 Pack/240g	348	32.2	145	1.7	4.1	13.4	0.2
Santa Plum Tomato with Dressing, M & S*	1 Pack/225g	135	10.8	60	0.9	3.1	4.8	0.9
Santa Tomato, Side, M & S*	1 Pack/225g	146	12.4	65	0.8	3.3	5.5	0.9
Sea Food, Family Mart*	1 Serving/100g	29	0.6	29	1.6	4.1	0.6	0.0
Seafood, Marinated, M & S*	1 Serving/90g	108	5.8	120	13.4	2.3	6.4	0.8
Seafood, Marinated, Waitrose*	1 Tub/160g	235	10.6	147	16.3	5.5	6.6	0.0
Seafood, Sunkis*	1 Tub/100g	83	3.9	83	4.6	7.4	3.9	0.0
Seasonal, Organic, Waitrose*	¼ Pack/25g	4	0.1	15	0.8	1.7	0.5	0.9
Selection, Fresh, M & S*	1 Pack/230g	32	0.7	14	0.7	2.1	0.3	0.9
Selection, Side, M & S*	1 Serving/255g	153	12.8	60	1.1	2.5	5.0	1.3
Shredded Beetroot, Asda*	1 Serving/140g	29	0.4	21	1.1	3.5	0.3	1.5
Side, Fresh & Crispy, Tesco*	1 Salad/230g	30	0.7	13	0.7	1.9	0.3	1.3
Side, Garden, with Cherry Tomatoes, Waitrose*	1 Pack/170g	25	0.7	15	0.8	2.0	0.4	1.3
Simply Chicken, Ginsters*	1 Pack/186.5g	316	6.9	170	11.4	22.7	3.7	0.0
Skipjack Tuna, John West*	1 Can/192g	190	11.7	99	7.3	3.7	6.1	0.0
Smoked Ham, Weight Watchers*	1 Pack/181g	233	3.6	129	11.0	16.6	2.0	3.0
Spicy Rice, Waitrose*	1 Serving/200g	318	13.2	159	3.2	21.7	6.6	0.9
Spinach, Rocket, & Watercress, Asda*	1 Serving/100g	21	0.6	21	2.8	1.2	0.6	1.9
Spinach, Waitrose*	1 Pack/100g	25	0.8	25	2.8	1.6	0.8	2.1
Spinach, Watercress & Rocket, Safeway*	1 Serving/60g	14	0.4	24	3.0	1.5	0.7	1.8
Sugar Plum Tomato, Fresh, Safeway*	1 Serving/160g	46	2.1	29	1.1	3.2	1.3	1.2
Summer, M & S*	1oz/28g	6	0.1	20	0.8	3.6	0.4	1.2
Sweet, Baby Leaf Mix, Co-Op*	1 Serving/50g	8	0.3	15	0.8	2.0	0.5	2.0
Sweet, Crunchy, Mixed, Co-Op*	1 Serving/100g	30	0.2	30	1.0	6.0	0.2	2.0
Sweet, Shredded, Tesco*	1 Serving/100g	20	0.4	20	1.1	2.9	0.4	1.9
Sweet, Waitrose*	1 Serving/50g	7	0.2	14	0.8	1.9	0.4	1.4
Sweet & Crispy, Fresh, Safeway*	1 Serving/90g	19	0.3	21	0.9	3.7	0.3	1.5
Sweet & Crispy, M & S*	1 Serving/140g	49	1.4	35	1.7	4.7	1.0	1.6

SALAD

	Measure INFO/WEIGHT	per Measure KCAL	FAT	Nutrition Values per 100g / 100ml KCAL	PROT	CARB	FAT	FIBRE
Sweet & Crispy, Side, Sainsbury's*	¼ Bag/93g	23	0.2	25	1.3	4.4	0.2	2.2
Sweet & Crispy, Somerfield*	1 Pack/100g	25	0.0	25	1.0	5.0	0.0	0.0
Sweet & Crunchy, Co-Op*	1 Serving/100g	20	0.5	20	1.0	3.0	0.5	1.0
Sweet & Crunchy, Morrisons*	1 Serving/100g	20	0.3	20	0.8	4.0	0.3	1.3
Sweet & Crunchy, Sainsbury's*	1 Pack/150g	23	0.2	15	0.9	2.6	0.1	1.8
Sweet & Crunchy, Somerfield*	1 Bag/250g	48	0.8	19	0.9	3.2	0.3	1.7
Sweet & Crunchy, Tesco*	1 Pack/285g	54	1.0	19	0.8	3.3	0.4	1.9
Sweet & Sour Prawn Noodle, HE, Tesco*	1 Pack/190g	122	1.3	64	5.0	9.4	0.7	0.4
Sweet Carrot, 3% Fat, M & S*	1oz/28g	21	0.3	75	1.3	16.7	1.2	1.4
Sweet Carrot & Sultana, M & S*	1 Serving/100g	55	0.7	55	0.8	11.4	0.7	2.6
Sweet Chilli Chicken Noodle, COU, M & S*	1 Pack/340g	408	7.8	120	6.8	17.4	2.3	1.2
Sweet Green, M & S*	1 Serving/150g	23	0.5	15	1.5	1.3	0.3	2.0
Sweet Leaf, Fully Prepared, Fresh, Sainsbury's*	¼ Pack/75g	12	0.1	16	0.8	3.0	0.1	2.1
Sweet Leaf, M & S*	1 Pack/110g	39	0.9	35	1.5	5.3	0.8	2.1
Sweet Leaf, Sainsbury's*	1 Serving/100g	21	0.5	21	0.8	3.2	0.5	1.5
Sweet Leaf & Carrot, Asda*	½ Pack/164g	34	0.5	21	0.9	3.6	0.3	1.4
Sweet Leafy, Organic, Tesco*	1 Serving/250g	45	1.0	18	0.8	2.7	0.4	1.9
Sweet Pepper, Medley, Waitrose*	½ Pack/100g	22	0.4	22	0.9	3.8	0.4	1.5
Sweet Pepper Side, Tesco*	1 Serving/54g	22	0.2	41	1.3	8.0	0.4	2.1
Sweet Pepper with Corn, Tesco*	1 Pack/270g	103	1.4	38	1.3	7.2	0.5	1.5
Tabbouleh, HL, Tesco*	1 Serving/200g	194	3.6	97	3.5	16.8	1.8	1.3
Tabbouleh & Feta, Tesco*	1 Pack/225g	302	11.3	134	5.4	16.7	5.0	0.6
Tabbouleh Feta, Finest, Tesco*	1 Pack/225g	266	11.7	118	4.2	13.7	5.2	0.6
Tabbouleh Style, PB, Waitrose*	1 Pack/225g	234	8.8	104	2.8	14.3	3.9	2.6
Tender Leaf, with Mizuna, Tesco*	1 Serving/30g	5	0.1	15	1.6	1.4	0.3	1.7
Tenderleaf, Waitrose*	1 Serving/200g	30	1.0	15	0.9	1.6	0.5	1.1
Tenderleaf, with Mizuna, Sainsbury's*	1 Serving/50g	10	0.3	20	3.6	0.2	0.6	2.2
Thai Style Chicken, M & S*	1 Serving/195g	205	3.7	105	6.7	15.1	1.9	1.9
Thai Style Noodle, King Prawns, Gourmet Salad, M & S*	1 Pack/425g	489	2.1	115	5.2	24.4	0.5	1.9
Three Bean, in Water, Wholefoods, Tesco*	½ Can/123g	135	1.2	110	7.7	17.6	1.0	5.3
Three Bean, Pot, Tesco*	1 Pot/210g	204	9.2	97	4.1	10.2	4.4	2.3
Three Bean, Sainsbury's*	1 Serving/125g	108	6.3	86	4.2	6.0	5.0	0.0
Three Bean, Tinned, Tesco*	1 Tin/160g	176	1.6	110	7.7	17.6	1.0	5.3
Three Bean, with Mint Vinaigrette, COU, M & S*	1 Pack/250g	213	4.3	85	5.9	12.1	1.7	8.2
Three Bean & Pesto, Italian Style, Boots*	1 Serving/290g	374	12.5	129	8.3	14.0	4.3	1.8
Tiger Prawn & Pasta, GFY, Asda*	1 Serving/200g	250	5.8	125	4.6	20.0	2.9	2.0
Tomato, Avocado & Rocket, M & S*	1 Pack/350g	508	46.9	145	1.7	4.1	13.4	0.2
Tomato, Lettuce & Cucumber, Classics, M & S*	1 Serving/275g	151	11.6	55	0.9	3.3	4.2	1.6
Tomato & Mozzarella, M & S*	1 Pack/220g	264	16.5	120	9.8	2.8	7.5	1.1
Tomato & Onion	1oz/28g	20	1.7	72	0.8	4.0	6.1	1.0
Tortellini & Chargrilled Vegetable, Tesco*	1 Serving/300g	492	23.1	164	5.1	18.7	7.7	1.7
Tuna, American, Lidl*	1oz/28g	25	0.8	91	7.4	8.5	3.0	0.0
Tuna, Breton Style, Snack Pot, Carb Check, Heinz*	1 Pot/219g	239	13.8	109	8.4	4.6	6.3	1.5
Tuna, HE, Tesco*	1 Serving/300g	399	21.9	133	6.2	10.5	7.3	0.9
Tuna, Layered, Tesco*	1 Serving/370g	466	29.2	126	4.4	9.4	7.9	1.0
Tuna, Mexican, Lidl*	1oz/28g	30	0.9	108	9.3	10.5	3.2	0.0
Tuna, with Lemon Dressing, Tesco*	1 Serving/300g	282	24.0	94	4.2	1.4	8.0	1.0
Tuna & Three Bean, Healthily Balanced, M & S*	1 Serving/350g	333	10.2	95	8.7	8.8	2.9	4.6
Tuna & Tomato, Boots*	1 Pack/171g	150	10.3	88	6.5	2.0	6.0	1.0
Tuna Layer, COU, M & S*	1 Pack/340g	255	8.2	75	5.1	8.7	2.4	1.3
Tuna Layered, M & S*	1 Pack/450g	428	21.2	95	5.6	8.5	4.7	1.0
Tuna Layered, Waitrose*	1 Bowl/300g	636	58.8	212	4.0	4.8	19.6	1.0
Tuna Nicoise, BGTY, Sainsbury's*	1 Pack/300g	315	6.0	105	6.3	15.5	2.0	2.5

	Measure INFO/WEIGHT	per Measure KCAL	FAT	Nutrition Values per 100g / 100ml KCAL	PROT	CARB	FAT	FIBRE
SALAD								
Tuna Nicoise, Finest, Tesco*	1 Serving/250g	430	23.5	172	8.5	13.3	9.4	0.8
Tuna Nicoise, M & S*	½ Pack/255g	306	22.4	120	6.0	3.7	8.8	0.2
Tuna Nicoise, New Potato & Free Range Egg, M & S*	1 Pack/500g	525	39.5	105	5.4	4.8	7.9	1.8
Tuna Nicoise, No Mayonnaise, Shapers, Boots*	1 Pack/276.4g	132	3.6	48	4.0	5.0	1.3	0.8
Tuna Nicoise, Potatoes & Free Range Egg, Sainsbury's*	1 Pack/270g	200	11.1	74	4.9	4.4	4.1	1.1
Tuna Nicoise, Shapers, Boots*	1 Pack/262g	152	5.0	58	5.9	4.5	1.9	0.5
Tuscan Style Bean & Sunblush Tomato, Waitrose*	1 Pot/225g	308	10.8	137	5.6	17.9	4.8	1.0
Vegetable, Canned	1oz/28g	40	2.7	143	1.6	13.0	9.8	1.2
Vegetable, Heinz*	1 Can/195g	259	16.6	133	1.5	12.6	8.5	1.3
Waldorf, Average	1 Serving/100g	193	17.7	193	1.4	7.5	17.7	1.3
Watercress, Baby Spinach & Rocket, Somerfield*	1 Serving/100g	25	0.9	25	3.0	1.2	0.9	1.7
Watercress, Morrisons*	1 Bag/100g	17	0.7	17	1.7	1.2	0.7	0.0
Watercress, Mustard Leaf & Mizuna, M & S*	½ Pack/60g	9	0.2	15	2.4	0.4	0.3	3.0
Watercress, Safeway*	1 Serving/50g	9	0.4	17	1.7	1.2	0.7	0.0
Watercress, Spinach & Rocket, Tesco*	1 Serving/30g	7	0.2	22	3.0	0.8	0.8	1.9
Watercress, Spinach & Rocket, Waitrose*	1 Bag/135g	28	1.1	21	2.2	1.2	0.8	1.5
Watercress & Spinach, Asda*	1 Serving/50g	11	0.3	21	2.8	1.2	0.6	1.9
Wheat with Roasted Vegetables, Sainsbury's*	1 Pack/220g	339	18.3	154	3.3	17.0	8.3	4.5
Wild Rocket, Safeway*	1 Serving/75g	14	0.4	18	1.3	2.1	0.5	1.1
Wild Rocket, Spinach & Watercress, Asda*	1 Serving/100g	21	0.6	21	2.8	1.2	0.6	1.9
Wild Rocket & Chard, Waitrose*	½ Bag/53.3g	8	0.3	15	0.8	1.7	0.5	1.4
with Sweetcorn, Side, Tesco*	1 Serving/135g	51	0.7	38	1.3	7.2	0.5	1.5
World Fusion, Somerfield*	1 Serving/100g	17	0.6	17	1.3	1.6	0.6	1.7
Young, Whole Leaf, Tesco*	1 Pack/200g	28	1.0	14	0.8	1.6	0.5	1.4
SALAD BOWL								
Avocado & Tomato, Sainsbury's*	1 Pack/180g	97	4.7	54	1.0	6.7	2.6	1.3
Chicken & Bacon, Layered, Tesco*	1 Serving/200g	328	23.4	164	3.5	11.3	11.7	2.2
Coleslaw, Tesco*	1 Bowl/300g	327	30.3	109	1.0	3.4	10.1	1.3
Crispy, M & S*	1 Serving/250g	88	1.3	35	1.3	6.6	0.5	1.2
Egg Layered, Tesco*	1 Pack/410g	726	57.8	177	4.2	8.4	14.1	1.3
French Style, Sainsbury's*	1oz/28g	15	1.0	55	1.0	4.8	3.5	1.5
French Style, Way to Five, Sainsbury's*	1 Pack/264g	103	5.8	39	0.7	4.2	2.2	2.2
Goats Cheese, Sainsbury's*	1 Serving/100g	161	11.9	161	5.8	7.6	11.9	1.3
Greek Style, M & S*	1 Bowl/255g	242	20.9	95	2.5	2.4	8.2	0.7
Greek Style, Somerfield*	1 Bowl/225g	178	14.0	79	2.2	3.5	6.2	1.1
Honey & Mustard Chicken, Fresh, Sainsbury's*	1 Serving/300g	408	23.7	136	5.9	10.3	7.9	1.7
Large, Sainsbury's*	1/6 Pack/52g	12	0.2	23	0.9	4.3	0.3	1.1
Mixed, Medley, Waitrose*	¼ Pack/60g	9	0.3	15	0.9	1.7	0.5	1.0
Mixed, Waitrose*	¼ Pack/64.3g	9	0.3	14	0.8	1.6	0.5	1.4
Pasta, Somerfield*	1 Pack/320g	541	25.9	169	3.3	20.8	8.1	1.5
Pasta with Sun Dried Tomato Dressing, WTF, Sainsbury's*	1 Bowl/320g	470	19.2	147	3.2	20.0	6.0	1.5
Prawn, Sainsbury's*	1 Bowl/400g	632	46.8	158	3.7	9.4	11.7	1.2
Red Cheddar & Edam, WTF, Sainsbury's*	½ Pack/224g	240	9.4	107	4.4	12.8	4.2	1.1
Roast Chicken, Layered, HL, Tesco*	1 Pack/400g	280	4.4	70	5.8	8.4	1.1	2.1
Tomato, Sainsbury's*	½ Bowl/150g	93	6.8	62	0.9	4.4	4.5	1.6
Tomato, Wtf, Sainsbury's*	1 Bowl/300g	174	12.3	58	0.8	4.5	4.1	2.8
Tomato & Basil, M & S*	1 Serving/225g	225	22.7	100	0.8	3.7	10.1	1.1
Tuna, BGTY, Sainsbury's*	½ Pack/175g	180	2.6	103	7.0	15.4	1.5	1.7
Tuna, Fresh, Asda*	1 Serving/160g	184	11.2	115	8.0	5.0	7.0	0.0
Tuna, Layered, Tesco*	1 Pack/200g	280	14.2	140	6.8	11.0	7.1	1.3
Tuna, Sainsbury's*	1 Serving/200g	336	21.4	168	6.1	11.7	10.7	1.5
with Crunchy Coleslaw, M & S*	1 Pack/325g	455	44.9	140	1.0	2.5	13.8	2.0

S

	Measure INFO/WEIGHT	per Measure KCAL	FAT	Nutrition Values per 100g / 100ml KCAL	PROT	CARB	FAT	FIBRE
SALAD CREAM								
Average	1 Tsp/5g	17	1.4	335	1.7	18.6	27.9	0.1
Extra Light, Heinz*	1 Serving/20g	28	1.4	138	1.9	15.1	7.2	0.0
Light, Morrisons*	1 Tbsp/15g	32	2.3	214	0.4	18.2	15.6	0.0
Light Choices, Tesco*	1 Tbsp/15g	21	1.5	140	1.4	11.4	9.8	0.5
Reduced Calorie, Average	1 Tsp/5g	6	0.4	130	1.0	12.9	7.9	0.2
Waistline, Crosse & Blackwell*	1 Tbsp/15g	21	1.3	139	0.8	15.1	8.4	0.2
SALAD KIT								
Caesar, Asda*	½ Pack/113g	154	9.0	136	5.0	11.0	8.0	1.4
Caesar, HL, Tesco*	½ Pack/132.5g	149	11.0	112	3.3	5.9	8.3	1.4
Caesar, New Improved, Tesco*	½ Pack/138g	279	25.3	202	4.7	4.5	18.3	1.3
Caesar, Tesco*	½ Pack/150g	237	19.8	158	3.2	6.7	13.2	0.7
Ranch, HL, Tesco*	1 Serving/115g	69	2.9	60	4.4	5.0	2.5	1.8
SALAD SNACK								
Chargrilled Chicken, Tesco*	1 Pot/300g	384	14.4	128	6.1	15.0	4.8	2.4
Cheese & Tomato, Tesco*	1 Pot/300g	519	20.4	173	6.3	21.7	6.8	2.2
Cheese Layered, Sainsbury's*	1 Pack/190g	397	29.1	209	5.4	12.4	15.3	0.0
Chicken & Bacon, Tesco*	1 Pack/300g	501	31.5	167	7.2	10.9	10.5	3.2
Chicken Caesar, Sainsbury's*	1 Pack/182.2g	164	9.1	90	5.9	5.3	5.0	1.0
Chicken Caesar, Tesco*	1 Serving/300g	420	20.4	140	8.2	11.4	6.8	1.7
Chicken Noodle, Sainsbury's*	1 Snack/240g	278	12.2	116	5.2	12.4	5.1	1.4
Greek Style, BGTY, Sainsbury's*	1 Pack/198.5g	133	5.0	67	2.0	9.0	2.5	0.8
Ham & Mushroom, Tesco*	1 Pot/300g	600	32.1	200	4.7	21.2	10.7	1.4
Hoi Sin Chicken & Noodle, TTD, Sainsbury's*	1 Pack/230g	214	3.5	93	4.7	15.2	1.5	1.8
Pasta, Cheese, Somerfield*	1 Salad/200g	422	28.0	211	8.0	14.0	14.0	0.0
Pasta, Egg Mayo, Asda*	1 Serving/180g	364	27.0	202	4.0	12.8	15.0	0.3
Pasta, Tuna, Asda*	1 Serving/180g	196	6.8	109	5.5	13.2	3.8	0.9
Pasta, Tuna, Sainsbury's*	1 Pot/260g	218	4.2	84	6.0	11.5	1.6	2.3
Pasta, with Honey & Mustard Chicken, Tesco*	1 Pack/300g	609	33.6	203	7.0	18.5	11.2	1.2
Pasta & Tuna, BGTY, Sainsbury's*	1 Pack/260g	218	4.2	84	6.0	11.5	1.6	2.3
Pasta & Tuna, Healthy Selection, Somerfield*	1 Pot/190g	194	5.1	102	6.5	13.0	2.7	1.1
Roast Chicken, Tesco*	1 Pack/300g	324	21.6	108	6.0	4.8	7.2	1.9
Salmon & Dill, Tesco*	1 Pack/300g	600	38.4	200	7.7	13.4	12.8	0.8
Sausage & Tomato, Tesco*	1 Serving/300g	529	27.3	176	4.5	19.1	9.1	4.0
Thai Prawn, Good Intentions, Somerfield*	1 Serving/215g	230	3.7	107	5.0	17.9	1.7	1.1
Tuna, HL, Tesco*	1 Serving/300g	237	3.3	79	7.2	10.1	1.1	1.7
Tuna & Pasta, BGTY, Sainsbury's*	1 Pack/260g	255	5.7	98	5.7	13.9	2.2	1.3
Tuna & Sweetcorn, Good Intentions, Somerfield*	1 Pot/215g	219	6.0	102	6.6	12.7	2.8	0.9
Tuna & Sweetcorn, Tesco*	1 Pack/300g	540	18.3	180	7.3	23.9	6.1	0.7
SALAMI								
Ardennes Pepper, Waitrose*	2 Slices/14g	60	5.4	429	18.6	1.9	38.5	1.1
Average	1 Slice/5g	18	1.3	360	28.4	1.9	26.2	0.0
Danish, Average	1 Serving/17g	89	8.8	524	13.2	1.3	51.7	0.0
Emiliano, Sainsbury's*	1 Serving/70g	209	14.2	298	28.8	0.1	20.3	0.0
German, Average	1 Serving/60g	200	16.4	333	20.3	1.6	27.3	0.1
German, Peppered, Average	3 Slices/25g	86	6.8	342	22.2	2.5	27.1	0.2
Healthy Range, Average	4 Slices/25g	55	3.6	221	22.4	0.7	14.3	0.0
Milano, Average	1 Serving/70g	278	22.6	397	25.9	0.9	32.2	0.0
Napoli, Average	1 Slice/5g	17	1.3	342	27.1	0.8	25.5	0.0
Pepperoni, Italian, Morrisons*	1 Slice/5.7g	23	1.9	406	24.0	0.9	34.0	0.0
Spanish, Wafer Thin, Tesco*	1 Pack/80g	273	18.8	341	25.5	6.8	23.5	0.0
Ungherese, Tesco*	1 Serving/35g	136	11.2	388	24.5	0.5	32.0	0.0
SALBA								
Grain, Salba*	1 Tbsp/12g	46	4.0	383	25.0	33.3	33.3	33.3

S

SALMON

	Measure INFO/WEIGHT	per Measure KCAL	FAT	Nutrition Values per 100g / 100ml KCAL	PROT	CARB	FAT	FIBRE
& Pasta, Frozen, Youngs*	½ Bag/175g	235	7.7	134	7.4	16.3	4.4	1.2
& Prawns, with Fusilli Pasta, Frozen, Youngs*	1 Pack/375g	439	27.8	117	5.6	7.0	7.4	1.1
Crunchies, Tesco*	1 Serving/112g	211	11.0	188	9.0	15.9	9.8	1.3
Crusted, Mediterranean Style, Sainsbury's*	1 Serving/166g	322	19.1	194	18.0	5.3	11.5	0.8
Fillets, & Butter, M & S*	1oz/28g	64	5.0	230	16.7	0.0	18.0	0.0
Fillets, Cajun, Waitrose*	1 Serving/150g	215	9.8	143	20.6	0.4	6.5	0.0
Fillets, Chargrilled, Sainsbury's*	1 Serving/270 g	270	19.5	243	20.9	0.2	17.6	0.0
Fillets, in White Wine & Parsley Dressing, Tesco*	1 Fillet/150g	291	20.4	194	17.5	0.3	13.6	0.6
Fillets, Lime & Coriander, Tesco*	1 Pack/250g	283	5.3	113	18.2	5.4	2.1	0.0
Fillets, Lime & Coriander Marinade, Sainsbury's*	1 Serving/100g	139	4.1	139	24.4	1.3	4.1	0.9
Fillets, Malted Wholegrain Crumb, Birds Eye*	1 Fillet/130g	195	8.2	150	16.8	6.4	6.3	0.5
Fillets, Raw, Average	1 Fillet/79g	149	9.2	189	20.9	0.1	11.7	0.1
Fillets, with Lemon & Herb Butter, Asda*	1 Fillet/125g	305	22.5	244	20.0	0.4	18.0	0.0
Fillets, with Orange & Dill Dressing, Tesco*	1 Serving/300g	540	30.9	180	17.7	4.1	10.3	0.7
Fillets, with Sicilian Citrus Glaze, Sainsbury's*	1 Fillet/144.9g	371	25.8	256	21.9	2.3	17.8	0.0
Flakes, Honey Roast, Average	1oz/28g	56	3.0	198	24.0	1.9	10.7	0.2
Flakes, Scottish Lochmuir, Honey Roast, M & S*	1 Pack/120g	234	11.8	195	25.4	1.7	9.8	0.4
Goan, Limited Edition, Sainsbury's*	1 Pack/351g	358	19.0	102	11.1	2.3	5.4	2.4
Goujons, Average	1 Pack/150g	321	16.4	214	16.4	12.4	11.0	1.1
Gravadlax, Finest, Tesco*	1 Serving/70g	125	6.9	178	22.1	0.2	9.9	0.0
Gravadlax, M & S*	1 Serving/140g	294	16.0	210	18.4	5.3	11.4	0.5
Gravadlax, Scottish, M & S*	1 Serving/70g	147	8.0	210	18.4	5.3	11.4	0.5
Gravadlax, TTD, Sainsbury's*	¼ Pack/35g	64	3.3	182	22.9	1.1	9.5	0.1
Gravadlax, with Mustard Sauce, Waitrose*	1 Serving/100g	191	11.1	191	21.8	1.0	11.1	0.4
Honey Roast, with New Potatoes, Tesco*	1 Pack/390g	351	13.7	90	6.8	7.6	3.5	1.9
Hot Smoked, Average	1 Serving/62g	103	4.4	166	24.0	0.9	7.2	0.1
Lime & Coriander, Tesco*	1 Serving/120g	176	4.4	147	21.4	7.0	3.7	0.7
Mild Oak Smoked, Average	1 Slice/25g	46	2.5	182	22.6	0.1	10.2	0.0
Mousse, Tesco*	1 Mousse/57g	100	7.0	177	13.5	2.9	12.4	0.2
Pink, Average	1 Serving/125g	162	7.2	130	19.5	0.1	5.8	0.1
Pink, in Brine, Average	1oz/28g	43	1.8	153	23.5	0.0	6.6	0.0
Poached, Average	1 Serving/90g	176	10.5	195	22.5	0.2	11.7	0.3
Potted, M & S*	1 Serving/75g	184	14.6	245	17.1	0.5	19.4	1.2
Red, Average	½ Can/90g	141	7.4	156	20.5	0.1	8.2	0.1
Red, in Brine, Average	1oz/28g	47	2.5	169	22.4	0.0	8.9	0.0
Rillettes, John West*	½ Can/62g	169	14.6	272	14.9	0.1	23.5	0.0
Scottish, Poached, Waitrose*	1 Fillet/100g	194	11.9	194	21.8	0.0	11.9	0.0
Smoked, Average	1 Serving/70g	126	7.0	179	21.9	0.5	10.0	0.1
Smoked, Birch & Juniper, Sainsbury's*	½ Pack/30g	47	1.9	156	24.7	0.3	6.4	0.0
Smoked, Scottish, Responsibly Sourced, Sainsbury's*	1 Slice/16.7g	37	2.3	221	23.6	0.1	14.0	0.1
Smoked, Trimmings, Average	1 Serving/55g	101	5.7	184	22.9	0.2	10.3	0.0
Smoked, Wild, Pacific, Alaskan, Silver Oak, M & S*	1 Slice/15g	17	0.2	110	24.7	0.5	1.3	0.4
Tail Joint, Lemon & Herb Butter, M & S*	1 Pack/480g	864	54.7	180	18.8	0.8	11.4	0.2
with Penne Pasta & Dill Sauce, SteamFresh, Birds Eye*	1 Meal/424.1g	335	6.4	79	6.4	9.9	1.5	1.1
Zesty, BFY, Asda*	1 Pack/400g	264	6.8	66	6.8	5.9	1.7	2.0

SALMON &

Spinach, Roulade, Tesco*	1 Serving/60g	155	14.2	258	9.5	1.7	23.7	0.2
Thai Noodles, HE, Tesco*	1 Pack/350g	231	4.2	66	6.7	7.1	1.2	1.5
Vegetables, M & S*	1 Serving/200g	220	13.8	110	6.0	5.2	6.9	0.8

SALMON EN CROUTE

Chilled, Youngs*	1 Pastry/200g	531	37.3	266	9.7	14.8	18.7	2.3
Frozen, Tesco*	1 Serving/166g	365	18.4	220	10.1	19.1	11.1	1.1
Frozen, Youngs*	1 Pastry/185g	542	38.3	293	10.2	16.5	20.7	1.0

S

	Measure INFO/WEIGHT	per Measure KCAL	FAT	Nutrition Values per 100g / 100ml KCAL	PROT	CARB	FAT	FIBRE
SALMON EN CROUTE								
Iceland*	1 Serving/170g	476	31.3	280	8.5	20.1	18.4	1.0
Just Cook, Sainsbury's*	1 Pastry/178.7g	512	35.4	286	10.6	16.3	19.8	2.8
Luxury, M & S*	1oz/28g	59	3.8	210	11.9	9.4	13.7	2.2
M & S*	½ Pack/185g	574	40.5	310	10.4	17.3	21.9	0.6
Retail, Average	1oz/28g	81	5.3	288	11.8	18.0	19.1	0.0
Tesco*	1 Serving/190g	523	37.1	275	8.2	16.1	19.5	3.3
SALMON FLORENTINE								
in a Creamy Cheddar & Spinach Sauce, Go Cook!, Asda*	½ Pack/168.4g	197	7.9	117	17.4	1.3	4.7	0.5
SALMON IN								
Dill Sauce, Youngs*	1 Pack/435g	265	10.0	61	6.1	4.2	2.3	0.1
Lemon Mayonnaise, Weight Watchers*	1 Can/80g	130	8.5	163	10.2	6.4	10.6	0.1
Lime & Coriander, Fillets, Good Choice, Iceland*	½ Pack/150g	189	4.4	126	19.8	5.1	2.9	0.8
Pancetta, Wrapped, Finest, Tesco*	1 Serving/150g	328	25.8	219	14.9	1.0	17.2	0.1
Tomato & Mascarpone Sauce, Fillets, Asda*	½ Pack/181g	279	19.9	154	13.0	0.8	11.0	0.6
Watercress Sauce, Somerfield*	1 Pack/210g	386	29.8	184	12.9	1.2	14.2	1.1
Watercress Sauce, Waitrose*	½ Pack/150g	264	19.4	176	13.7	1.2	12.9	0.1
White Wine & Cream Sauce, Tesco*	1 Serving/170g	279	19.2	164	13.5	2.0	11.3	1.2
SALMON LUNCHBOX								
COU, M & S*	1 Pack/235g	200	3.3	85	5.1	13.1	1.4	0.9
SALMON MOROCCAN								
Style, Fillets, Asda*	1 Serving/240g	454	28.8	189	19.0	1.3	12.0	0.0
SALMON PARCELS								
& Garlic Butter, Finest, Tesco*	1 Serving/164g	321	23.1	196	16.8	0.6	14.1	0.5
Smoked, Tesco*	1 Serving/50g	147	12.7	293	16.4	0.0	25.3	0.2
SALMON PLATTER								
GFY, Asda*	1 Pack/400g	376	15.2	94	7.0	8.0	3.8	1.4
SALMON WITH								
a Cream Sauce, Scottish Fillets, M & S*	1 Serving/200g	360	26.0	180	13.8	1.0	13.0	0.1
Coriander & Lime, Pacific, Asda*	1 Serving/113g	154	3.4	137	27.0	0.5	3.0	0.0
Herb Vegetables, HE, Tesco*	1 Pack/350g	228	9.1	65	6.6	3.8	2.6	0.9
Sweet Potato, Edamama Beans & Quinoa, Waitrose*	1 Pack/349.3g	482	22.7	138	8.8	11.0	6.5	2.7
SALSA								
Bottled, M & S*	½ Jar/136g	95	3.3	70	1.2	12.0	2.4	1.5
Chunky, Sainsbury's*	½ Pot/84.3g	43	1.4	51	1.1	7.8	1.7	1.2
Cool, Tesco*	1 Jar/300g	72	0.3	24	1.2	4.6	0.1	1.1
Fire Roasted Pepper, Somerfield*	1 Pot/120g	50	0.6	42	1.2	8.1	0.5	1.3
Fresh, Asda*	1oz/28g	10	0.2	35	1.2	6.2	0.6	2.0
Fresh, Sainsbury's*	1oz/28g	15	0.6	54	1.7	7.0	2.1	0.9
GFY, Asda*	½ Pot/236g	85	0.9	36	1.1	7.0	0.4	0.7
Hot, Fresh, Chilled, Tesco*	1 Pot/150g	90	3.6	60	1.4	7.5	2.4	1.2
Medium Hot, Discovery*	1 Serving/30g	17	0.1	56	1.4	11.7	0.4	0.8
Original, From Dinner Kit, Old El Paso*	1 Jar/226g	71	0.7	32	1.2	6.0	0.3	0.0
Red Onion & Tomato, Tapas Selection, Sainsbury's*	1 Serving/22g	17	1.0	77	3.0	6.0	4.5	0.9
Red Pepper, Sainsbury's*	1 Serving/85g	31	1.4	37	1.7	3.8	1.7	1.5
Spicy Mango & Lime, Morrisons*	½ Pot/85g	62	0.3	73	1.0	15.9	0.4	1.3
Spicy Red Pepper, Fresh, Waitrose*	½ Pot/85g	27	0.8	32	1.9	4.1	0.9	1.6
Spicy Red Pepper, Sainsbury's*	1 Pot/170g	54	2.4	32	1.4	3.2	1.4	1.3
Taco, Old El Paso*	¼ Jar/58g	23	0.1	40	1.0	8.6	0.1	0.0
Tomato, Chunky, Tesco*	1 Pot/170g	68	2.2	40	1.1	5.9	1.3	1.1
Tomato, Chunky, Tex Mex, Tesco*	1 Serving/50g	26	1.3	52	1.0	6.4	2.5	1.0
Tomato, Mexican Style, Dip, Morrisons*	½ Pack/50g	26	0.9	51	1.2	7.6	1.8	0.8
Tomato, Onion, Coriander & Chilli, Fresh, Waitrose*	1 Serving/50g	33	1.6	65	1.3	8.0	3.1	1.2
Tomato, Spicy, Worldwide Sauces*	1 Serving/25g	8	0.1	30	1.2	5.9	0.2	1.2

S

INFO/WEIGHT	Measure	per Measure		Nutrition Values per 100g / 100ml				
		KCAL	FAT	KCAL	PROT	CARB	FAT	FIBRE

SALSA

Tomato, Vine Ripened, Chunky, M & S*	1 Pot/170g	94	3.7	55	0.9	7.6	2.2	1.5
Tomato, Vine Ripened, Tesco*	½ Tub/100g	47	1.8	47	1.0	6.7	1.8	1.1
Tomato & Avocado, Chunky, COU, M & S*	½ Pack/85.7g	30	1.2	35	0.8	5.4	1.4	1.4

SALT

Alternative, Reduced Sodium, Losalt*	1 Serving/10g	0	0.0	0	0.0	0.0	0.0	0.0
Sea, Organic, M & S*	1oz/28g	132	6.7	472	5.3	54.2	24.0	7.0
Table, Average	1 Tsp/5g	0	0.0	0	0.0	0.0	0.0	0.0

SAMOSAS

Chicken, Mumtaz*	1 Serving/105g	177	8.3	169	19.6	4.9	7.9	0.0
Chicken Tikka, Sainsbury's*	2 Samosas/100g	239	12.9	239	8.3	22.5	12.9	3.1
Co-Op*	1oz/28g	70	2.8	250	6.0	34.0	10.0	2.0
Dim Sum Selection, Sainsbury's*	1 Samosa/12g	24	0.9	196	3.4	28.6	7.6	2.8
Indian Style Selection, Co-Op*	1 Samosa/20.8g	50	2.7	240	5.0	27.0	13.0	3.0
Lamb, Morrisons*	1 Samosa/50g	144	7.9	288	9.8	27.0	15.7	1.5
Lamb, Waitrose*	1oz/28g	87	6.3	310	8.5	18.1	22.6	0.8
Vegetable, Indian Starter Selection, M & S*	1 Samosa/20.7g	61	3.5	290	5.0	29.0	16.9	3.3
Vegetable, Large, Individual, Sainsbury's*	1 Samosa/110g	254	16.5	231	3.3	20.7	15.0	2.1
Vegetable, Large, Tesco*	1 Samosa/64g	148	7.9	231	4.8	25.2	12.4	3.4
Vegetable, M & S*	1 Samosa/45g	115	6.9	255	5.1	24.8	15.3	2.8
Vegetable, Mini, Asda*	1 Samosa/23g	52	2.0	233	6.0	32.0	9.0	2.6
Vegetable, Mini, Indian, Party Selection, Tesco*	1 Samosa/30g	59	1.5	195	3.6	33.9	5.0	2.2
Vegetable, Mini, Indian, Somerfield*	1 Samosa/25.3g	64	3.3	253	5.7	28.1	13.1	3.4
Vegetable, Mini, Indian Snack Selection, Sainsbury's*	1 Samosa/25g	70	4.0	280	4.7	29.8	15.8	3.2
Vegetable, Mini, Indian Snack Selection, Tesco*	1 Samosa/32g	76	4.2	238	4.7	25.5	13.0	3.3
Vegetable, Mini, Waitrose*	1 Samosa/29g	70	3.8	242	3.6	27.1	13.2	3.1
Vegetable, Morrisons*	1 Samosa/60g	101	3.5	169	4.9	24.1	5.8	2.0
Vegetable, Northern Indian, Sainsbury's*	1 Samosa/50g	126	5.9	252	5.8	30.6	11.8	2.6
Vegetable, Retail, Average	1 Samosa/110g	239	10.2	217	5.1	30.0	9.3	2.5
Vegetable, Somerfield*	1 Serving/50g	127	6.6	253	5.7	28.1	13.1	3.4
Vegetable, Waitrose*	1 Samosa/50g	118	7.2	236	3.7	23.1	14.3	2.7
Vegetable Lightly Spiced, Sainsbury's*	1 Samosa/50.2g	112	6.3	223	4.0	23.5	12.5	1.2

SANDWICH

All Day Breakfast, BGTY, Sainsbury's*	1 Pack/188g	294	4.5	156	9.6	22.7	2.4	0.0
All Day Breakfast, Finest, Tesco*	1 Pack/275g	660	41.5	240	9.7	16.4	15.1	1.6
All Day Breakfast, Ginsters*	1 Pack/241.3g	537	26.5	223	10.8	20.3	11.0	0.0
All Day Breakfast, HL, Tesco*	1 Pack/223.1g	328	8.0	147	11.9	16.8	3.6	2.7
Avocado, & Spinach, M & S*	1 Pack/241.7g	581	27.3	240	4.0	21.0	11.3	4.8
Bacon, & Brie, Asda*	1 Pack/181g	603	38.2	333	13.3	22.9	21.1	1.3
Bacon, & Brie, Finest, Tesco*	1 Pack/201.1g	571	33.6	284	14.1	19.4	16.7	2.1
Bacon, & Brown Sauce, Ashberry*	1 Pack/419.1g	1207	53.6	288	12.0	31.0	12.8	0.0
Bacon, & Egg, Boots*	1 Pack/179g	480	28.6	268	12.0	19.0	16.0	1.4
Bacon, & Egg, Deep Fill, Ginsters*	1 Pack/210g	590	38.2	281	11.5	18.8	18.2	0.0
Bacon, & Egg, Deep Fill, Spar*	1 Pack/191g	579	38.0	303	12.2	18.7	19.9	0.0
Bacon, & Egg, Free Range, Daily Bread*	1 Serving/175g	425	22.9	243	10.1	21.5	13.1	0.0
Bacon, & Egg, Free Range, M & S*	1 Pack/214g	503	22.7	235	14.1	20.0	10.6	1.7
Bacon, & Egg, Ginsters*	1 Pack/210g	523	24.4	249	13.2	22.0	11.6	0.0
Bacon, & Egg, HL, Tesco*	1 Serving/178.3g	328	9.3	184	11.5	22.7	5.2	1.7
Bacon, & Egg, Sainsbury's*	1 Pack/215g	535	25.6	249	12.3	23.2	11.9	0.0
Bacon, & Egg, Taste!*	1 Pack/186.8g	496	28.6	265	12.8	19.1	15.3	0.0
Bacon, & Egg, Tesco*	1 Pack/188g	481	24.2	256	14.1	21.0	12.9	1.9
Bacon, & Tomato, COU, M & S*	1 Pack/168.8g	270	4.6	160	9.5	25.6	2.7	2.5
Bacon, Brie, & Mango Chutney, Daily Bread*	1 Serving/212.6g	556	22.8	261	12.7	28.6	10.7	0.0
Bacon, Lettuce & Tomato, Shapers, Boots*	1 Pack/175.2g	272	7.5	155	11.0	18.0	4.3	5.9

S

SANDWICH

INFO/WEIGHT	Measure	per Measure		Nutrition Values per 100g / 100ml				
		KCAL	FAT	KCAL	PROT	CARB	FAT	FIBRE
Bacon, Lettuce & Tomato, Weight Watchers*	1 Pack/152.9g	237	2.4	155	9.4	25.8	1.6	2.4
Bap, Chicken, & Sweetcorn, Sainsbury's*	1 Serving/169.9g	462	23.6	272	12.5	24.2	13.9	0.0
Bap, Chicken, Chargrilled, Malted, Co-Op*	1 Bap/201g	492	26.1	245	9.0	23.0	13.0	2.0
Bap, Ham, & Salad, Co-Op*	1 Bap/163.9g	295	4.9	180	8.0	30.0	3.0	2.0
Bap, Tuna, & Sweetcorn, Malted, Co-Op*	1 Bap/212g	530	27.6	250	9.0	24.0	13.0	2.0
Beef, & Horseradish, Roast, So Good, Somerfield*	1 Pack/188g	404	11.5	215	12.4	27.6	6.1	1.8
Beef, & Horseradish, Sainsbury's*	1 Pack/187g	389	13.3	208	12.0	24.1	7.1	0.0
Beef, & Horseradish, Shapers, Boots*	1 Pack/156g	276	2.7	177	12.0	28.0	1.7	1.8
Beef, & Onion, Co-Op*	1 Pack/221g	530	24.3	240	11.0	24.0	11.0	1.0
Beef, & Onion, Roast, HL, Tesco*	1 Pack/185.3g	278	3.5	150	13.3	20.0	1.9	2.7
Beef, & Pate, M & S*	1 Pack/187.9g	310	7.3	165	11.2	21.6	3.9	2.4
Beef, & Salad, Roast, Daily Bread*	1 Pack/202g	319	8.3	158	9.0	21.4	4.1	0.0
Beef, Roast, Daily Bread*	1 Pack/199.3g	281	5.4	141	8.7	20.0	2.7	0.0
Beef, Roast, Handmade, Tesco*	1 Pack/223g	439	15.8	197	12.5	20.7	7.1	1.6
Beef, Roast, Healthy, Woolworths*	1 Pack/191g	283	7.4	148	10.5	17.9	3.9	0.0
Beef, Roast, Sainsbury's*	1 Pack/173.9g	426	17.4	245	9.4	29.3	10.0	0.0
Beef, Tomato & Horseradish, Asda*	1 Pack/168.9g	255	4.4	151	10.0	22.0	2.6	2.7
Beef, Topside, Deli*	1 Serving/191g	447	21.1	234	15.4	18.3	11.0	0.0
BLT, & Chicken Salad, Co-Op*	1 Pack/230g	472	20.7	205	10.0	21.0	9.0	2.0
BLT, Asda*	1 Sandwich/172g	325	11.9	189	9.9	21.8	6.9	4.6
BLT, Beech-Smoked, Pret a Manger*	1 Sandwich/248g	493	28.8	199	8.5	15.4	11.6	1.6
BLT, BGTY, Sainsbury's*	1 Pack/196g	331	4.4	169	10.4	27.0	2.2	0.0
BLT, COU, M & S*	1 Pack/174g	278	4.7	160	9.5	25.6	2.7	2.5
BLT, Deep Fill, Safeway*	1 Pack/202g	565	24.2	280	14.0	29.2	12.0	2.2
BLT, Deep Fill, Spar*	1 Pack/165.9g	408	11.6	246	10.7	35.1	7.0	0.0
BLT, Deep Fill, Tesco*	1 Pack/231g	635	38.1	275	11.8	19.8	16.5	1.2
BLT, Deep Filled, Asda*	1 Pack/206g	606	35.0	294	13.3	21.8	17.0	3.0
BLT, GFY, Asda*	1 Pack/171g	294	6.0	172	9.0	26.0	3.5	1.6
BLT, Ginsters*	1 Pack/192g	516	30.0	269	15.6	21.2	15.6	0.0
BLT, Healthy Selection, Budgens*	1 Pack/183g	361	13.4	197	10.0	22.9	7.3	2.5
BLT, Healthy Selection, Somerfield*	1 Pack/149.7g	217	3.1	145	9.4	22.2	2.1	2.5
BLT, HL, Tesco*	1 Pack/190g	287	2.7	151	10.1	24.5	1.4	1.6
BLT, Impress*	1 Pack/188.6g	382	13.4	202	11.5	22.8	7.1	0.0
BLT, M & S*	1 Serving/181g	381	14.7	210	10.7	23.8	8.1	1.8
BLT, Safeway*	1 Pack/230g	529	5.3	230	15.9	35.4	2.3	3.9
BLT, Shapers, Boots*	1 Pack/169g	254	6.3	150	10.7	18.9	3.7	5.9
BLT, Somerfield*	1 Pack/157g	425	23.1	270	10.3	23.8	14.7	2.3
BLT, Sutherland*	1 Pack/216g	624	37.9	289	9.1	23.8	17.5	0.0
BLT, Tesco*	1 Pack/203g	520	29.2	256	11.9	19.5	14.4	1.5
BLT, Waitrose*	1 Pack/210g	578	31.5	275	9.3	25.6	15.0	2.3
BLT, with Mayo, Safeway*	1 Pack/168g	462	28.1	275	10.4	20.7	16.7	2.3
Brie, & Grape, Finest, Tesco*	1 Pack/209g	527	31.6	252	8.5	20.6	15.1	1.5
Brie, with Apple & Grapes, Sainsbury's*	1 Pack/220g	473	24.2	215	8.2	20.8	11.0	0.0
Brunch, Triple, Sainsbury's*	1 Pack/263.8g	575	25.6	218	12.4	20.4	9.7	4.2
Cajun Chicken, in a Soft Wrap, Sainsbury's*	1 Pack/230.5g	378	13.6	164	10.7	17.1	5.9	4.4
Chargrilled Vegetable & Houmous, HL, Tesco*	1 Pack/167g	250	4.0	150	5.9	25.3	2.4	2.0
Cheddar, & Celery, M & S*	1 Pack/200g	540	31.8	270	9.7	22.4	15.9	1.5
Cheddar, & Coleslaw, Simply, Boots*	1 Pack/185g	538	33.3	291	9.2	23.0	18.0	1.8
Cheddar, & Ham, British, M & S*	1 Serving/164.6g	396	18.6	240	15.1	20.0	11.3	1.7
Cheddar, & Ham, M & S*	1 Pack/165g	396	18.6	240	15.1	20.0	11.3	1.7
Cheddar, & Ham, Oldfields*	1 Pack/246.0g	674	39.6	274	11.7	20.5	16.1	2.0
Cheddar, & Ham, Smoked, Deep Filled, Tesco*	1 Serving/203.2g	572	33.1	282	14.3	19.5	16.3	1.2
Cheddar, & Pickle, Mature, Sainsbury's*	1 Pack/171g	588	27.0	344	14.3	38.7	15.8	7.0

S

SANDWICH

INFO/WEIGHT	Measure	per Measure		Nutrition Values per 100g / 100ml				
		KCAL	FAT	KCAL	PROT	CARB	FAT	FIBRE
Cheddar, & Salad, Mature, Upper Crust*	1 Pack/225.1g	466	22.1	207	9.5	20.3	9.8	0.0
Cheddar, & Tomato, Mature, Big, Sainsbury's*	1 Pack/233g	596	25.6	256	12.9	26.3	11.0	0.0
Cheddar, Oldfields*	1 Pack/121.1g	384	17.3	317	12.8	33.2	14.3	1.5
Cheddar, Red Leicester, & Onion, Tesco*	1 Pack/182g	604	38.9	332	11.0	23.8	21.4	2.5
Cheddar Cheese Ploughmans, M & S*	1 Pack/226g	565	36.4	250	10.5	19.4	16.1	1.5
Cheese, & Celery, M & S*	1 Pack/200g	480	27.0	240	10.9	18.5	13.5	2.7
Cheese, & Coleslaw, Asda*	1 Pack/262g	799	51.4	305	10.1	22.1	19.6	3.3
Cheese, & Coleslaw, M & S*	1 Pack/186g	498	32.4	268	10.2	17.6	17.4	3.2
Cheese, & Coleslaw, Shapers, Boots*	1 Pack/224g	338	4.7	151	11.0	22.0	2.1	3.2
Cheese, & Ham, & Pickle, Co-Op*	1 Serving/185g	370	7.4	200	13.0	27.0	4.0	3.0
Cheese, & Ham, & Pickle, HL, Tesco*	1 Pack/201.3g	312	4.2	155	13.1	21.0	2.1	1.7
Cheese, & Ham, & Pickle, Simply, Boots*	1 Pack/225g	551	29.3	245	11.0	21.0	13.0	2.4
Cheese, & Ham, & Pickle, Tesco*	1 Serving/215g	497	24.7	231	11.7	20.3	11.5	1.8
Cheese, & Ham, Baxter & Platts*	1 Pack/168g	408	21.8	243	11.3	20.5	13.0	1.7
Cheese, & Ham, Eat Smart, Safeway*	1 Pack/170g	254	4.3	149	12.5	19.2	2.5	4.1
Cheese, & Ham, Smoked, Co-Op*	1 Pack/167g	334	8.4	200	15.0	24.0	5.0	2.0
Cheese, & Ham, Smoked, Tesco*	1 Pack/178.2g	490	24.2	275	12.8	25.1	13.6	2.6
Cheese, & Marmite, No Mayonnaise, Boots*	1 Pack/156g	420	20.0	269	12.2	26.3	12.8	1.7
Cheese, & Onion, Deep Fill, Tesco*	1 Pack/212g	742	51.9	350	12.3	20.2	24.5	1.3
Cheese, & Onion, GFY, Asda*	1 Pack/156g	317	4.1	203	14.0	31.0	2.6	2.7
Cheese, & Onion, M & S*	1 Serving/187.8g	461	24.3	245	11.2	21.3	12.9	2.9
Cheese, & Onion, Tesco*	1 Pack/178g	573	37.9	322	11.6	21.0	21.3	3.5
Cheese, & Onion, Waitrose*	1 Pack/176g	579	38.7	329	12.5	20.2	22.0	2.8
Cheese, & Pickle, & Tomato, Somerfield*	1 Pack/166.5g	317	7.1	191	12.5	25.6	4.3	3.5
Cheese, & Pickle, BHS*	1 Pack/177.7g	504	22.6	283	12.5	29.6	12.7	1.8
Cheese, & Pickle, Shapers, Boots*	1 Pack/165g	342	8.1	207	9.8	31.0	4.9	2.3
Cheese, & Pickle, Tesco*	1 Pack/140g	400	19.3	286	12.7	27.8	13.8	1.4
Cheese, & Pickle, Virgin Trains*	1 Pack/158g	444	19.6	281	11.5	31.1	12.4	0.0
Cheese, & Salad, Budgens*	1 Pack/168.9g	250	3.0	148	10.9	21.9	1.8	1.6
Cheese, & Salad, COU, M & S*	1 Pack/188g	244	3.0	130	12.1	17.0	1.6	2.4
Cheese, & Salad, Shapers, Boots*	1 Pack/205g	308	5.1	150	9.7	22.0	2.5	2.2
Cheese, & Salad, Tesco*	1 Serving/188g	429	22.4	228	10.1	20.2	11.9	2.1
Cheese, & Spring Onion, Asda*	1 Pack/159.6g	578	40.0	361	13.0	21.0	25.0	1.9
Cheese, & Spring Onion, Co-Op*	1 Pack/164g	607	42.6	370	12.0	21.0	26.0	3.0
Cheese, & Spring Onion, Sainsbury's*	1 Serving/177g	605	39.5	342	11.4	24.0	22.3	1.1
Cheese, & Tomato, Asda*	1 Pack/154g	388	19.7	252	11.0	23.2	12.8	3.7
Cheese, & Tomato, Co-Op*	1 Pack/155.3g	365	18.5	235	10.6	21.8	11.9	1.9
Cheese, & Tomato, Organic, M & S*	1 Pack/165g	559	35.3	339	11.8	24.8	21.4	1.9
Cheese, & Tomato, Sainsbury's*	1 Pack/215.9g	542	26.4	251	12.9	22.8	12.2	0.0
Cheese, & Tomato, Spar*	1 Pack/124g	294	13.0	237	11.1	24.4	10.5	0.0
Cheese, & Tomato, Tesco*	1 Pack/182g	582	38.9	320	9.2	22.6	21.4	1.1
Cheese, Asda*	1 Pack/262g	618	31.4	236	12.2	20.3	12.0	3.0
Cheese, Ham, BLT, Triple Pack, Asda*	1 Pack/260g	614	31.2	236	12.2	20.3	12.0	3.0
Cheese, Savoury, Northern Bites*	1 Serving/210g	212	4.0	101	3.6	18.5	1.9	0.0
Cheese, Savoury, Sandwich King*	1 Pack/135.2g	328	11.2	243	11.6	30.2	8.3	0.0
Cheese, Three, & Onion, Boots*	1 Pack/169g	566	33.8	335	11.0	28.0	20.0	1.9
Cheese & Onion, Eat Smart, Morrisons*	1 Pack/142.1g	260	2.4	183	14.1	27.8	1.7	2.9
Cheese & Tomato, Simply, Ginsters*	1 Pack/175g	438	25.6	250	8.0	21.5	14.6	3.0
Chicken, & Avocado, Tesco*	1 Serving/219.2g	558	31.5	255	11.9	19.5	14.4	2.4
Chicken, & Bacon, & Lettuce, Tesco*	1 Pack/208.3g	500	22.1	240	13.9	21.9	10.6	1.7
Chicken, & Bacon, & Salad, Dash*	1 Serving/217g	449	15.8	207	9.9	25.3	7.3	0.0
Chicken, & Bacon, Antony Worrall Thompson's*	1 Pack/191.1g	577	27.3	302	16.0	25.9	14.3	2.1
Chicken, & Bacon, Baton, Tesco*	1 Pack/201g	511	26.3	254	9.4	24.7	13.1	1.7

S

SANDWICH

	Measure INFO/WEIGHT	per Measure KCAL	FAT	Nutrition Values per 100g / 100ml KCAL	PROT	CARB	FAT	FIBRE
Chicken, & Bacon, Big Fill, Somerfield*	1 Pack/209.6g	567	28.4	270	12.0	25.0	13.5	2.3
Chicken, & Bacon, COU, M & S*	1 Pack/178.6g	250	3.6	140	13.5	15.8	2.0	3.8
Chicken, & Bacon, Deep Filled, Ginsters*	1 Pack/200g	540	32.2	270	13.1	18.3	16.1	0.0
Chicken, & Bacon, Good Intentions, Somerfield*	1 Pack/209g	335	7.1	160	11.9	19.9	3.4	2.7
Chicken, & Bacon, HL, Co-Op*	1 Pack/179g	277	3.4	155	12.3	21.8	1.9	3.4
Chicken, & Bacon, HL, Tesco*	1 Pack/193g	318	6.2	165	13.5	19.5	3.2	2.7
Chicken, & Bacon, M & S*	1 Pack/185g	509	27.2	275	15.9	20.2	14.7	2.1
Chicken, & Bacon, Roast, Boots*	1 Pack/175g	413	14.0	236	15.4	26.3	8.0	2.2
Chicken, & Bacon, Shapers, Boots*	1 Pack/179g	317	9.0	177	14.0	19.0	5.0	3.1
Chicken, & Bacon, Tesco*	1 Pack/195g	486	24.2	249	14.3	20.0	12.4	2.7
Chicken, & Bacon, Waitrose*	1 Serving/191.1g	495	23.5	259	11.8	25.3	12.3	2.2
Chicken, & Chorizo, Sainsbury's*	1 Pack/215g	436	20.0	203	12.2	17.8	9.3	3.0
Chicken, & Coleslaw, Tesco*	1 Pack/160g	305	7.1	191	12.0	25.7	4.4	2.4
Chicken, & Ham, Oak Smoked, Big, Sainsbury's*	1 Pack/244g	461	17.6	189	12.3	18.8	7.2	0.0
Chicken, & Ham, Roast, Tesco*	1 Pack/228g	561	31.9	246	13.3	16.6	14.0	1.2
Chicken, & Mayo, The Sandwich Company*	1 Pack/72g	251	10.7	348	17.8	35.9	14.8	0.0
Chicken, & Mayo, Wholemeal, Sodhexo*	1 Pack/128g	346	17.4	270	13.1	24.0	13.6	3.6
Chicken, & Pesto, with Rocket, Woolworths*	1 Pack/195g	326	17.2	167	5.0	16.9	8.8	0.0
Chicken, & Ranch Coleslaw, Sainsbury's*	1 Pack/238.8g	425	11.0	178	12.2	21.7	4.6	1.8
Chicken, & Salad, Co-Op*	1 Pack/195g	449	21.5	230	10.0	24.0	11.0	2.0
Chicken, & Salad, COU, M & S*	1 Pack/194g	262	3.7	135	9.8	19.0	1.9	1.6
Chicken, & Salad, Daily Bread*	1 Serving/187g	270	15.4	144	9.6	13.4	8.2	0.0
Chicken, & Salad, Deep Filled, Asda*	1 Pack/247g	551	18.3	223	18.1	22.2	7.4	1.3
Chicken, & Salad, Deep Filled, Co-Op*	1 Pack/213g	437	19.2	205	10.0	20.0	9.0	1.0
Chicken, & Salad, Deep Filled, Tesco*	1 Pack/237.8g	440	19.5	185	13.1	14.6	8.2	2.8
Chicken, & Salad, Eat Smart, Safeway*	1 Pack/183g	265	4.2	145	13.7	17.1	2.3	0.8
Chicken, & Salad, GFY, Asda*	1 Pack/194g	252	2.9	130	12.0	17.0	1.5	2.6
Chicken, & Salad, Ham & Cheese, Twin, Tesco*	1 Pack/189g	434	21.5	230	10.8	21.1	11.4	2.3
Chicken, & Salad, Healthy Choice, Somerfield*	1 Pack/185.6g	284	4.5	153	10.7	22.1	2.4	2.8
Chicken, & Salad, HL, Co-Op*	1 Pack/196g	265	3.5	135	10.4	19.1	1.8	3.9
Chicken, & Salad, HL, Tesco*	1 Pack/207g	290	3.9	140	13.9	16.8	1.9	2.7
Chicken, & Salad, Low Fat, Waitrose*	1 Pack/188g	291	8.1	155	10.4	18.6	4.3	2.1
Chicken, & Salad, Roast, BGTY, Sainsbury's*	1 Pack/204g	298	4.7	146	10.4	21.0	2.3	2.0
Chicken, & Salad, Roast, COU, M & S*	1 Pack/196g	265	4.7	135	8.9	19.6	2.3	2.2
Chicken, & Salad, Roast, Feel Good, Shell*	1 Pack/190.6g	327	9.0	171	9.8	22.4	4.7	0.0
Chicken, & Salad, Roast, Finest, Tesco*	1 Pack/224g	475	21.5	212	16.2	15.1	9.6	3.1
Chicken, & Salad, Roast, Shapers, Boots*	1 Pack/230g	308	5.8	134	11.0	17.0	2.5	3.7
Chicken, & Salad, Roast, Waitrose*	1 Pack/217g	482	24.1	222	9.4	21.1	11.1	2.0
Chicken, & Salad, Roast, Weight Watchers*	1 Pack/186g	266	8.0	143	10.3	15.8	4.3	2.8
Chicken, & Salad, Sainsbury's*	1 Pack/240.1g	425	14.2	177	12.1	18.8	5.9	0.0
Chicken, & Salad, Shell*	1 Pack/201.0g	404	19.7	201	8.7	19.4	9.8	0.0
Chicken, & Salad, Tesco*	1 Pack/193g	386	17.6	200	11.9	17.6	9.1	1.5
Chicken, & Salad, Waitrose*	1 Pack/208g	406	19.8	195	10.3	17.1	9.5	2.5
Chicken, & Salad, Wild Bean Cafe*	1 Pack/210g	273	1.1	130	12.4	18.9	0.5	2.8
Chicken, & Salad, with Mayo, BGTY, Sainsbury's*	1 Serving/200g	314	4.8	157	12.0	21.9	2.4	0.0
Chicken, & Stuffing, Big Fill, Somerfield*	1 Pack/200g	510	22.0	255	12.9	25.7	11.0	1.3
Chicken, & Stuffing, M & S*	1 Pack/166g	398	17.1	240	13.9	23.1	10.3	5.6
Chicken, & Stuffing, Roast, Deep Fill, Tesco*	1 Serving/220g	532	26.8	242	14.0	19.0	12.2	1.3
Chicken, & Stuffing, Roast, M & S*	1 Pack/204g	490	20.8	240	13.4	23.0	10.2	3.0
Chicken, & Stuffing, Roast, Tesco*	1 Sandwich/200g	450	14.4	225	15.0	24.8	7.2	1.9
Chicken, & Stuffing, Shapers, Boots*	1 Serving/184.7g	327	5.2	177	13.0	25.0	2.8	2.2
Chicken, & Stuffing, Tesco*	1 Pack/323g	1043	58.8	323	10.4	29.4	18.2	1.0
Chicken, & Stuffing, Waitrose*	1 Pack/183g	450	18.8	246	12.8	25.6	10.3	1.5

SANDWICH

	Measure INFO/WEIGHT	per Measure KCAL	FAT	Nutrition Values per 100g / 100ml KCAL	PROT	CARB	FAT	FIBRE
Chicken, & Sweet Chilli, Flora Light, Flora*	1 Pack/154g	296	5.7	192	13.1	27.0	3.7	1.9
Chicken, & Sweetcorn, M & S*	1 Pack/208.1g	385	14.2	185	12.3	19.3	6.8	2.7
Chicken, & Sweetcorn, Shapers, Boots*	1 Pack/180g	324	6.3	180	12.0	25.0	3.5	2.0
Chicken, & Sweetcorn, with Mayo, Benedicts*	1 Pack/185g	437	19.8	236	12.2	20.6	10.7	0.0
Chicken, & Watercress, Chargrilled, M & S*	1 Pack/173g	285	2.9	165	12.8	23.9	1.7	2.1
Chicken, Bacon, & Avocado, M & S*	1 Pack/242g	508	28.3	210	10.7	15.8	11.7	3.2
Chicken, Bacon, & Cheese, Club, M & S*	1 Pack/383.3g	804	37.2	210	11.9	18.5	9.7	1.9
Chicken, Bacon & Avocado, Finest, Tesco*	1 Pack/208.7g	480	24.6	230	13.9	16.8	11.8	3.8
Chicken, Bacon & Sweet Chilli, Feel Good, Shell*	1 Pack/173.5g	365	8.7	211	14.1	29.2	5.0	0.0
Chicken, Bacon & Tomato, BGTY, Sainsbury's*	1 Pack/190g	270	4.4	142	11.4	19.0	2.3	0.0
Chicken, BBQ, on Malted Bread, Fresh Bite*	1 Pack/225.8g	341	5.4	151	9.0	23.4	2.4	0.0
Chicken, BLT, Taste!*	1 Pack/238.5g	459	19.8	192	10.3	19.0	8.3	0.0
Chicken, Breast, BGTY, Sainsbury's*	1 Pack/165g	251	0.8	152	12.2	24.7	0.5	0.0
Chicken, Caesar, & Salad, Sainsbury's*	1 Pack/186g	299	7.1	161	11.2	20.4	3.8	0.0
Chicken, Caesar, Finest, Tesco*	1 Pack/199g	454	19.9	228	15.4	19.2	10.0	1.4
Chicken, Chargrill, Choice*	1 Serving/161g	320	8.1	199	15.2	23.3	5.0	1.9
Chicken, Chargrilled, Ginsters*	1 Pack/209g	431	17.3	206	11.3	21.6	8.3	0.0
Chicken, Chargrilled, No Mayo, Rustlers*	1 Pack/150g	228	1.2	152	16.0	20.1	0.8	0.0
Chicken, Chargrilled, Pitta Pocket, M & S*	1 Pack/208g	279	7.3	134	11.2	14.5	3.5	1.6
Chicken, Cheese, Bacon, Big, Sainsbury's*	1 Pack/254g	734	45.5	289	11.7	18.0	17.9	0.0
Chicken, Chinese, Low Calorie, Tesco*	1 Pack/169g	270	4.2	160	11.8	22.6	2.5	2.0
Chicken, Coronation, Indulgence, Taste!*	1 Pack/159.0g	396	18.8	249	9.1	26.5	11.8	0.0
Chicken, Coronation, M & S*	1 Pack/210g	420	20.4	200	11.2	20.2	9.7	3.1
Chicken, Coronation, Taste!*	1 Pack/178.2g	367	13.4	206	10.6	24.0	7.5	0.0
Chicken, Coronation, Woolworths*	1 Serving/159g	396	18.8	249	9.1	26.5	11.8	0.0
Chicken, Flame Grilled, Rustlers*	1 Pack/150g	347	14.3	231	16.3	20.1	9.5	0.0
Chicken, Ham, Prawn, Triple Pack, HL, Tesco*	1 Pack/246.5g	349	5.2	142	10.7	20.2	2.1	2.2
Chicken, Lemon, &with Mint, Brambles*	1 Pack/161.0g	338	8.7	210	13.4	24.6	5.4	3.2
Chicken, Mexican, Healthy Choices, Shell*	1 Serving/167.9g	376	11.8	224	12.2	28.1	7.0	0.0
Chicken, No Mayo, Daily Bread*	1 Pack/160.3g	278	7.0	174	8.6	23.8	4.4	0.0
Chicken, No Mayo, M & S*	1 Pack/142g	220	4.3	155	15.0	17.5	3.0	3.1
Chicken, No Mayo, Roast, COU, M & S*	1 Pack/160g	240	3.5	150	15.8	16.8	2.2	3.1
Chicken, No Mayonnaise, Waitrose*	1 Pack/173g	332	9.5	192	11.6	24.0	5.5	2.1
Chicken, Red Thai, Foo-Go*	1 Pack/188.4g	358	14.9	190	10.2	19.4	7.9	4.4
Chicken, Red Thai, Taste!*	1 Pack/164g	335	9.8	204	11.5	26.1	6.0	0.0
Chicken, Roast, Breast, BGTY, Sainsbury's*	1 Pack/174g	275	4.4	158	14.8	20.9	2.5	1.8
Chicken, Roast, Shapers, Boots*	1 Pack/163g	259	2.1	159	16.0	21.0	1.3	2.5
Chicken, Roast, Tesco*	1 Pack/158g	412	19.8	261	13.1	23.9	12.5	1.5
Chicken, Rustlers*	1 Pack/150g	347	14.3	231	16.3	20.1	9.5	0.0
Chicken, Salad, Aldi*	1 Pack/195.4g	338	4.5	173	11.5	23.8	2.3	2.0
Chicken, Salad, M & S*	1 Pack/225.8g	350	9.3	155	10.6	18.8	4.1	3.0
Chicken, Shell*	1 Pack/121g	334	15.7	276	13.9	25.9	13.0	0.0
Chicken, Simply, Brambles*	1 Pack/136.2g	283	4.2	208	14.0	31.0	3.1	1.3
Chicken, Simply, Eat Smart, Safeway*	1 Pack/147g	250	3.2	170	14.5	23.0	2.2	1.4
Chicken, Spicy, Deep Filled, Co-Op*	1 Pack/216g	421	15.1	195	10.0	24.0	7.0	3.0
Chicken, Sundried Tomato & Herb, Bells*	1 Pack/198g	400	18.8	202	10.2	18.9	9.5	0.0
Chicken, Tandoori, Finest, Tesco*	1 Pack/224g	421	16.8	188	10.8	19.2	7.5	1.4
Chicken, Tandoori, Waitrose*	1 Pack/181g	302	5.6	167	11.6	23.0	3.1	4.1
Chicken, Thai, Deep Fill, Spar*	1 Pack/142.6g	292	6.6	204	13.9	26.8	4.6	0.0
Chicken, Tikka, & Yoghurt, Taste!*	1 Pack/215.3g	436	21.1	203	8.2	20.4	9.8	0.0
Chicken, Tikka, Asda*	1 Pack/186g	316	8.7	170	11.0	21.0	4.7	1.5
Chicken, Tikka, COU, M & S*	1 Pack/185g	268	3.3	145	12.1	20.5	1.8	3.2
Chicken, Tikka, HE, Tesco*	1 Pack/159g	270	4.3	170	14.5	21.9	2.7	1.8

S

SANDWICH

INFO/WEIGHT	Measure	per Measure		Nutrition Values per 100g / 100ml				
		KCAL	FAT	KCAL	PROT	CARB	FAT	FIBRE
Chicken, Tikka, M & S*	1 Pack/180g	391	19.6	217	10.4	19.5	10.9	2.0
Chicken, Tikka, Naan, Ready to Go, M & S*	1 Pack/298g	641	23.2	215	9.9	26.5	7.8	4.0
Chicken, Tikka, Weight Watchers*	1 Pack/158g	250	2.2	158	13.1	23.2	1.4	2.9
Chicken, with Mayo, on Thick Softgrain, Tasties*	1 Pack/192g	338	15.2	176	9.5	16.1	7.9	0.0
Chicken & Stuffing, Roast, Shapers, Boots*	1 Pack/186.2g	324	3.9	174	14.0	25.0	2.1	3.1
Chicken Salad, HL, Tesco*	1 Serving/190g	247	3.4	130	12.3	15.8	1.8	4.5
Chicken Tikka, Bellini & Blake*	1 Pack/179g	354	10.4	198	11.5	24.6	5.8	1.3
Classic, Triple Pack, Somerfield*	1 Serving/250g	653	36.5	261	10.2	22.1	14.6	2.5
Club, New York Style, Sainsbury's*	1 Serving/212g	608	33.5	287	13.3	22.8	15.8	2.7
Corned Beef, & Tomato, & Onion, Salad Garden*	1 Pack/137g	338	14.8	247	14.2	23.0	10.8	0.0
Corned Beef, on White, Simply, Brambles*	1 Pack/126g	325	10.8	258	14.2	30.8	8.6	1.4
Coronation Chicken, in Pitta Bread, COU, M & S*	1 Serving/207g	269	2.5	130	9.2	20.4	1.2	2.0
Cracking Eggs, Pret a Manger*	1 Sandwich/294g	494	27.9	168	6.8	14.0	9.5	1.6
Crayfish, & Rocket, Foo-Go*	1 Pack/198.5g	425	15.1	214	9.6	26.8	7.6	3.0
Crayfish, & Rocket, Go Eat*	1 Pack/163g	289	7.0	177	10.6	24.6	4.3	1.9
Crayfish, & Rocket, Shapers, Boots*	1 Pack/172.2g	291	3.8	169	11.0	26.0	2.2	2.5
Crayfish & Avocado, Pret a Manger*	1 Sandwich/279g	436	23.5	156	5.7	14.3	8.4	2.5
Cream Cheese, & Salad, Choice*	1 Serving/156.4g	293	7.3	188	7.8	28.1	4.7	0.0
Duck, Peking, No Mayo, Boots*	1 Pack/221.7g	400	10.2	180	7.7	27.0	4.6	1.7
Edam, & Tomato, & Spring Onion, BHS*	1 Serving/184.1g	313	9.4	170	8.6	22.5	5.1	3.2
Egg, & Bacon, & Lincolnshire Sausage, Waitrose*	1 Pack/249g	655	32.9	263	11.3	24.7	13.2	0.9
Egg, & Cress, BGTY, Sainsbury's*	1 Pack/166g	281	7.0	169	9.7	23.1	4.2	3.8
Egg, & Cress, Co-Op*	1 Pack/159g	398	23.9	250	9.0	21.0	15.0	0.0
Egg, & Cress, COU, M & S*	1 Pack/192g	240	5.2	125	9.8	15.5	2.7	2.8
Egg, & Cress, Free Range, Co-Op*	1 Pack/154.2g	370	18.5	240	8.0	25.0	12.0	3.0
Egg, & Cress, Free Range, M & S*	1 Pack/192g	307	9.0	160	10.7	17.8	4.7	3.0
Egg, & Cress, Free Range, Sainsbury's*	1 Pack/204g	404	16.9	198	10.5	20.3	8.3	3.3
Egg, & Cress, M & S*	1 Pack/182g	331	17.7	182	10.1	13.6	9.7	3.2
Egg, & Cress, Organic, M & S*	1 Pack/185g	444	26.3	240	9.6	18.0	14.2	3.6
Egg, & Cress, Sainsbury's*	1 Pack/170g	384	19.7	226	10.6	19.8	11.6	0.0
Egg, & Ham, Asda*	1 Pack/262g	590	33.5	225	10.4	16.8	12.8	2.1
Egg, & Salad, Co-Op*	1 Pack/190g	285	7.6	150	7.0	22.0	4.0	4.0
Egg, & Salad, Free Range, Sainsbury's*	1 Pack/224.5g	450	16.9	200	8.5	24.5	7.5	0.0
Egg, & Salad, Free Range, Waitrose*	1 Pack/180g	281	11.5	156	7.6	16.9	6.4	3.3
Egg, & Salad, HE, Tesco*	1 Pack/169g	279	8.3	165	7.6	22.5	4.9	2.0
Egg, & Salad, HL, Tesco*	1 Pack/182g	264	7.6	145	7.2	18.6	4.2	1.8
Egg, & Tomato, Deep Fill, Spar*	1 Serving/183.2g	348	13.5	190	8.2	22.8	7.4	0.0
Egg, & Tomato, on Softgrain Bread, Daily Bread*	1 Pack/160.3g	278	7.0	174	8.6	23.8	4.4	0.0
Egg, & Tomato, Organic, Waitrose*	1 Pack/192g	359	18.6	187	9.7	15.3	9.7	4.0
Egg, & Tomato, Tesco*	1 Pack/172g	311	10.8	181	8.5	22.6	6.3	2.3
Egg, Co-Op*	1 Pack/190g	285	7.0	150	6.8	22.1	3.7	3.7
Egg, Mayo, Free Range, Pret a Manger*	1 Sandwich/185g	426	23.4	231	9.1	19.9	12.7	1.6
Egg & Cress, Healthy Choice, Somerfield*	1 Pack/150g	234	5.4	156	8.9	22.0	3.6	3.3
Egg & Cress, on Wheat Germ Bread, Tesco*	1 Pack/173.8g	365	15.8	210	11.0	20.5	9.1	2.1
Egg Mayo, Free Range, Asda*	1 Serving/178g	311	10.1	175	9.3	21.5	5.7	2.1
Egg Mayonnaise, & Bacon, Boots*	1 Serving/200g	426	14.0	213	13.5	23.5	7.0	2.8
Egg Mayonnaise, & Cress, BHS*	1 Serving/187.8g	462	23.9	246	10.0	24.7	12.7	1.9
Egg Mayonnaise, & Cress, Co-Op*	1 Pack/159g	405	24.0	255	8.8	20.8	15.1	1.9
Egg Mayonnaise, & Cress, Go Simple, Asda*	1 Pack/169g	370	18.6	219	10.0	20.0	11.0	1.7
Egg Mayonnaise, & Cress, Shapers, Boots*	1 Pack/156g	292	7.6	187	11.0	25.0	4.9	2.6
Egg Mayonnaise, & Gammon Ham, Strollers*	1 Pack/169.5g	399	19.3	236	13.0	20.5	11.4	0.0
Egg Mayonnaise, & Salad, Superdrug*	1 Pack/169g	286	12.3	169	7.6	18.3	7.3	2.4
Egg Mayonnaise, Boots*	1 Pack/183.6g	449	23.9	244	9.7	22.0	13.0	2.3

SANDWICH

INFO/WEIGHT	Measure	per Measure		Nutrition Values per 100g / 100ml				
		KCAL	FAT	KCAL	PROT	CARB	FAT	FIBRE
Egg Mayonnaise, Deep Fill, Benedicts*	1 Pack/195g	560	21.6	287	9.6	36.3	11.1	0.0
Egg Mayonnaise, Free Range, Finest, Tesco*	1 Pack/217g	412	19.1	190	10.9	16.8	8.8	2.3
Egg Mayonnaise, Good Intentions, Somerfield*	1 Pack/150.3g	263	6.2	175	10.8	23.7	4.1	3.0
Egg Mayonnaise, HE, Tesco*	1 Pack/162g	253	6.0	156	9.3	21.4	3.7	2.8
Egg Mayonnaise, HL, Tesco*	1 Pack/162.2g	253	6.0	156	9.3	21.4	3.7	2.8
Egg Mayonnaise, on Malted Wheatgrain, Taste!*	1 Serving/169g	394	20.8	233	10.6	20.0	12.3	0.0
Egg Mayonnaise, Shell*	1 Pack/189g	522	29.1	276	9.8	24.7	15.4	0.0
Egg Mayonnaise, Simply, Boots*	1 Pack/181g	449	27.2	248	9.2	19.0	15.0	2.9
Egg Mayonnaise, Simply, Ginsters*	1 Serving/163g	365	15.9	224	10.1	24.1	9.8	3.1
Egg Mayonnaise, Waitrose*	1 Pack/180g	396	20.5	220	10.1	19.1	11.4	3.4
Fat B*d, Fresh! Gourmet Organics*	1 Pack/164.6g	428	20.4	260	12.2	26.2	12.4	2.0
Fish, Triple, Co-Op*	1 Serving/233.3g	419	9.3	180	10.0	26.0	4.0	3.0
Gammon, & Salad, Tasties*	1 Pack/172g	261	6.0	152	9.6	20.6	3.5	0.0
Ham, & Mustard, Eat Smart, Safeway*	1 Pack/139g	250	3.1	180	13.7	26.3	2.2	2.0
Ham, & Mustard, Salad, BGTY, Sainsbury's*	1 Pack/182.5g	261	3.8	143	8.7	22.4	2.1	2.6
Ham, & Mustard, Simply, Ginsters*	1 Pack/157.1g	399	19.8	254	11.7	23.5	12.6	0.0
Ham, & Mustard, Smoked, M & S*	1 Pack/163.8g	385	17.2	235	10.8	24.4	10.5	2.2
Ham, & Mustard, Smoked, Tesco*	1 Pack/156g	385	19.5	247	11.1	22.4	12.5	1.0
Ham, & Mustard, Somerfield*	1 Pack/144g	301	11.7	209	10.9	24.8	8.1	1.9
Ham, & Mustard, Tesco*	1 Pack/147g	437	27.9	297	10.6	20.8	19.0	1.2
Ham, & Philadelphia Light, Dry Cured, Boots*	1 Pack/172g	339	9.3	197	12.8	24.4	5.4	2.5
Ham, & Salad, & Mustard, Darwins Deli*	1 Serving/180g	574	13.7	319	14.0	48.5	7.6	0.0
Ham, & Salad, Big Fill, Somerfield*	1 Pack/222g	515	25.3	232	9.4	22.9	11.4	2.3
Ham, & Salad, Co-Op*	1 Pack/193g	299	9.7	155	9.0	19.0	5.0	1.0
Ham, & Salad, Fulfilled*	1 Serving/183g	288	6.4	157	11.8	19.9	3.5	0.0
Ham, & Salad, Ginsters*	1 Pack/179g	287	6.2	161	8.9	23.6	3.5	0.0
Ham, & Salad, Healthy, Spar*	1 Serving/181g	286	6.7	158	8.4	22.7	3.7	0.0
Ham, & Salad, Healthy Options, Oldfields*	1 Pack/156g	229	3.0	147	8.7	24.0	1.9	0.0
Ham, & Salad, Safeway*	1 Pack/272g	403	4.9	148	8.3	24.5	1.8	1.9
Ham, & Salad, Select*	1 Serving/180g	266	4.7	148	8.0	23.2	2.6	0.0
Ham, & Salad, Shapers, Boots*	1 Pack/195g	269	2.7	138	9.4	22.0	1.4	1.8
Ham, & Salad, Tesco*	1 Pack/163g	215	3.3	132	10.0	17.0	2.0	2.0
Ham, & Salad, Wild Bean Cafe*	1 Pack/212.0g	301	5.5	142	10.7	18.8	2.6	2.0
Ham, & Salad, with Mustard, Finest, Tesco*	1 Pack/200g	466	21.0	233	15.3	19.3	10.5	1.3
Ham, & Soft Cheese, Tesco*	1 Serving/164g	333	12.1	203	11.6	22.5	7.4	2.2
Ham, & Swiss Cheese, Big, Sainsbury's*	1 Pack/218g	652	36.4	299	11.6	25.4	16.7	0.5
Ham, & Swiss Cheese, M & S*	1 Pack/159g	393	20.0	247	14.7	18.9	12.6	3.3
Ham, & Tomato, Brambles*	1 Pack/159.1g	288	7.3	181	11.1	24.1	4.6	3.3
Ham, & Tomato, GFY, Asda*	1 Pack/173g	254	2.9	147	10.0	23.0	1.7	1.4
Ham, & Tomato, Honey Roast, Feel Good, Shell*	1 Pack/170.9g	388	18.8	227	9.8	22.1	11.0	0.0
Ham, & Turkey, & Salad, Sutherland*	1 Pack/185g	303	4.8	164	9.8	25.2	2.6	0.0
Ham, & Turkey, Asda*	1 Pack/190g	393	19.4	207	12.9	15.8	10.2	2.3
Ham, & Turkey, with Salad, Co-Op*	1 Pack/188g	263	5.6	140	9.0	21.0	3.0	2.0
Ham, & Turkey, with Salad, HL, Co-Op*	1 Serving/181.3g	290	5.4	160	10.0	24.0	3.0	3.0
Ham, Asda*	1 Pack/262g	618	31.4	236	12.2	20.3	12.0	3.0
Ham, Cheese, & Pickle, Leicester, Waitrose*	1 Pack/205g	513	24.4	250	11.9	23.7	11.9	2.1
Ham, Cheese, & Pickle, M & S*	1 Pack/197g	459	25.8	233	13.0	15.9	13.1	2.4
Ham, Cheese, & Pickle, Taste!*	1 Pack/173.9g	414	21.8	238	11.1	20.3	12.5	0.0
Ham, Cheese & Pickle, in a Soft Wrap, Sainsbury's*	1 Pack/195g	503	23.2	258	10.9	26.8	11.9	0.9
Ham, Just Ham, Shoprite*	1 Pack/148g	286	7.1	193	12.4	25.0	4.8	0.0
Ham, M & S*	1 Pack/200g	220	5.2	110	17.2	3.2	2.6	0.0
Ham, Tomato, & Lettuce, Oldfields*	1 Pack/215.9g	393	17.5	182	12.3	19.0	8.1	3.5
Ham & Cheese, Eat Smart, Morrisons*	1 Serving/183g	273	4.6	149	12.5	19.2	2.5	4.1

S

SANDWICH	Measure INFO/WEIGHT	per Measure KCAL	FAT	Nutrition Values per 100g / 100ml KCAL	PROT	CARB	FAT	FIBRE
Ham & Salad, British, COU, M & S*	1 Pack/204g	255	4.3	125	6.7	19.9	2.1	2.9
Ham Salad, Light Choices, HL, Tesco*	1 Pack/190g	266	5.3	140	11.0	19.8	2.8	2.1
Ham Smoked, on a Roll, Cafe Life, Brambles*	1 Pack/210.9g	485	12.4	230	9.0	35.2	5.9	2.2
Houmous, & Crunchy Salad, Oldfields*	1 Pack/180g	256	7.6	142	6.3	20.0	4.2	0.0
Houmous, Tomato, & Red Onion, Daily Bread*	1 Serving/184g	367	17.7	199	6.9	22.7	9.6	0.0
Huomous & Carrot, Shapers, Boots*	1 Pack/204.4g	323	10.2	158	7.5	21.0	5.0	5.2
King Prawn, & Wild Rocket, Honduran, M & S*	1 Serving/195.7g	451	23.9	230	9.4	20.3	12.2	1.4
King Prawn, Sainsbury's*	1 Pack/203.8g	424	16.3	208	11.6	22.3	8.0	0.0
King Prawn & Harissa, Foo-Go*	1 Pack/180g	282	6.8	157	9.1	21.6	3.8	3.4
Lemon Chicken & Mangetout Salad, COU, M & S*	1 Pack/185.7g	260	5.0	140	10.6	19.0	2.7	3.7
Mozzarella, & Pepperoni, Sainsbury's*	1 Pack/171.2g	380	12.1	222	10.5	29.0	7.1	0.0
Mozzarella, & Roast Vegetables, Felix Van Den Berghe*	1 Pack/157.9g	330	13.3	209	9.5	23.8	8.4	0.0
Mozzarella, & Tomato, Waitrose*	1 Pack/193.0g	359	18.1	186	9.7	15.7	9.4	2.3
Mozzarella, Pesto & Pine Nuts, Sainsbury's*	1 Pack/180g	423	17.5	235	10.2	26.8	9.7	2.8
New York Deli, Boots*	1 Pack/245g	397	12.5	162	10.0	19.0	5.1	1.7
New York Deli, Extra Special, Asda*	1 Pack/200.5g	403	15.4	201	12.4	20.6	7.7	3.8
Pastrami, & Gherkin, BGTY, Sainsbury's*	1 Pack/230g	357	6.0	155	9.8	23.1	2.6	3.0
Pitta, Falafel, Houmous & Salad, Benedicts*	1 Pack/220.1g	405	13.0	184	6.8	26.1	5.9	0.0
Ploughman's, Cheddar, Heinz*	1 Pack/208.3g	551	27.7	265	9.3	27.1	13.3	2.4
Ploughman's, Cheddar Cheese, Deep Fill, Asda*	1 Pack/228.6g	472	22.9	206	9.0	20.0	10.0	4.3
Ploughman's, Cheese, BGTY, Sainsbury's*	1 Pack/193g	326	8.1	169	9.8	22.8	4.2	3.6
Ploughman's, Deep Fill, Ginsters*	1 Pack/232g	636	40.8	274	9.6	20.8	17.6	0.0
Ploughman's, Deep Fill, Tesco*	1 Pack/245g	551	27.4	225	10.9	20.2	11.2	1.4
Ploughman's, Taste!*	1 Pack/205g	492	27.3	240	9.5	20.6	13.3	0.0
Ploughman's Wedge, with Branston, Tesco*	1 Pack/246.9g	605	31.9	245	9.2	22.6	12.9	2.2
Ploughmans, Cheese, Delicious, Boots*	1 Pack/197.1g	404	17.7	205	9.7	21.0	9.0	2.6
Ploughmans, Cheese, HL, Tesco*	1 Pack/197.6g	328	5.5	166	10.9	24.4	2.8	2.3
Pork, & Apple Sauce, Bells*	1 Pack/179.5g	340	8.1	190	11.5	26.1	4.5	0.0
Prawn, & Egg, Deep Filled, Asda*	1 Pack/250g	570	30.0	228	12.0	17.0	12.0	2.3
Prawn, & Egg, Safeway*	1 Pack/216g	400	17.3	185	9.4	18.8	8.0	1.0
Prawn, Marie Rose, Waitrose*	1 Pack/164g	226	5.6	138	8.8	18.0	3.4	1.9
Prawn, Salad, COU, M & S*	1 Pack/200g	230	3.6	115	8.0	16.6	1.8	3.8
Prawn, Thai Style, Ginsters*	1 Pack/183.0g	313	9.0	171	9.2	22.5	4.9	0.0
Prawn Cocktail, Delicious, Boots*	1 Pack/206g	344	13.0	167	7.7	20.0	6.3	2.9
Prawn Cocktail, HE, Tesco*	1 Pack/154g	245	4.2	159	11.0	22.0	2.7	1.8
Prawn Mayonnaise, Co-Op*	1 Pack/154g	285	6.0	185	9.7	27.3	3.9	3.2
Prawn Mayonnaise, COU, M & S*	1 Pack/155g	240	3.6	155	10.2	22.9	2.3	2.8
Prawn Mayonnaise, Daily Bread*	1 Pack/156.5g	373	17.2	239	11.9	23.0	11.0	0.0
Prawn Mayonnaise, Delicatessen, Waitrose*	1 Pack/168.5g	283	10.3	168	10.3	17.9	6.1	3.1
Prawn Mayonnaise, Eat Smart, Morrisons*	1 Pack/165.5g	245	3.8	148	9.5	22.2	2.3	3.5
Prawn Mayonnaise, GFY, Asda*	1 Pack/160g	251	4.5	157	10.0	23.0	2.8	2.8
Prawn Mayonnaise, Ginsters*	1 Pack/152g	415	27.1	273	12.4	17.8	17.8	0.0
Prawn Mayonnaise, HL, Co-Op*	1 Pack/154g	246	3.6	160	10.0	24.0	2.3	3.0
Prawn Mayonnaise, Light Choices, HL, Tesco*	1 Pack/157g	243	5.5	155	10.7	20.1	3.5	2.1
Prawn Mayonnaise, M & S*	1 Pack/156g	328	12.0	210	10.0	24.7	7.7	2.2
Prawn Mayonnaise, Oatmeal Bread, Co-Op*	1 Pack/159g	445	22.3	280	11.0	28.0	14.0	2.0
Prawn Mayonnaise, Oatmeal Bread, Waitrose*	1 Pack/180g	463	27.0	257	10.2	20.4	15.0	3.2
Prawn Mayonnaise, on Oatmeal Bread, Taste!*	1 Pack/144.1g	320	12.0	222	12.6	24.3	8.3	1.5
Prawn Mayonnaise, Safeway*	1 Pack/168g	402	22.2	239	9.0	21.1	13.2	3.1
Prawn Mayonnaise, Sainsbury's*	1 Pack/150.9g	323	14.0	214	11.6	20.9	9.3	0.0
Prawn Mayonnaise, Sayers Bakery*	1 Pack/154.8g	449	27.7	290	9.7	22.5	17.9	2.1
Prawn Mayonnaise, Shapers, Boots*	1 Pack/161g	254	4.0	158	9.0	25.0	2.5	1.8
Prawn Mayonnaise, Simply, Boots*	1 Pack/261g	736	47.0	282	11.0	19.0	18.0	2.2

SANDWICH

	Measure INFO/WEIGHT	KCAL	FAT	KCAL	PROT	CARB	FAT	FIBRE
Prawn Mayonnaise, Tesco*	1 Pack/152.2g	350	16.3	230	10.2	22.2	10.7	2.6
Prawn Mayonnaise, Triple, Asda*	1 Pack/248.0g	635	39.7	256	9.0	19.0	16.0	3.4
Prawn Mayonnaise, Triple, Tesco*	1 Pack/231g	603	33.0	261	9.5	23.5	14.3	1.6
Prawn Mayonnaise, Upper Crust*	1 Pack/207.9g	343	10.4	165	9.2	20.9	5.0	0.0
Prawn Mayonnaise, Waitrose*	1 Pack/172.9g	389	18.5	225	10.6	21.6	10.7	2.4
Rib, BBQ, Rustlers*	1 Pack/170g	444	20.2	261	14.6	23.8	11.9	0.0
Roast Chicken Salad, Eat Well, M & S*	1 Pack/213.9g	385	15.8	180	11.1	17.1	7.4	1.9
Salmon, & Black Pepper, Smoked, Fulfilled*	1 Pack/120g	293	10.3	244	13.8	29.0	8.6	0.0
Salmon, & Cucumber, Brown Bread, Waitrose*	1 Pack/150g	296	10.7	197	10.5	22.7	7.1	1.4
Salmon, & Cucumber, HL, Co-Op*	1 Pack/193g	290	5.0	150	10.0	22.0	2.6	2.0
Salmon, & Cucumber, HL, Tesco*	1 Serving/155g	256	3.6	165	11.3	24.8	2.3	1.6
Salmon, & Cucumber, M & S*	1 Pack/168g	329	13.9	196	11.0	19.5	8.3	2.6
Salmon, & Cucumber, Red, BGTY, Sainsbury's*	1 Pack/192g	278	4.4	145	9.4	21.7	2.3	2.4
Salmon, & Cucumber, Red, M & S*	1 Pack/183g	375	17.0	205	11.1	18.5	9.3	1.4
Salmon, & Cucumber, Red, Tesco*	1 Pack/144g	284	9.2	197	11.1	23.8	6.4	1.9
Salmon, & Cucumber, Safeway*	1 Serving/173g	346	14.4	200	11.1	19.8	8.3	1.9
Salmon, & Cucumber, Shapers, Boots*	1 Pack/181.3g	272	6.9	150	10.0	19.0	3.8	2.9
Salmon, & Cucumber, Tesco*	1 Pack/156.1g	320	10.1	205	11.8	24.8	6.5	1.8
Salmon, & Cucumber, White Bread, Waitrose*	1 Pack/161.4g	304	8.5	189	9.8	25.5	5.3	1.7
Salmon, & Rocket, Poached, M & S*	1 Pack/180g	495	26.8	275	13.5	21.2	14.9	2.1
Salmon, & Soft Cheese, Smoked, Waitrose*	1 Pack/154g	300	10.0	195	14.8	19.2	6.5	4.2
Salmon, Poached, M & S*	1 Pack/179.1g	385	15.0	215	10.2	24.1	8.4	1.9
Salmon, Smoked, Daily Bread*	1 Pack/121.8g	296	10.6	243	13.5	28.0	8.7	0.0
Salmon, Smoked & Cream Cheese, M & S*	1 Pack/183.7g	450	22.4	245	12.7	20.8	12.2	1.8
Sausage, Egg & Bacon, Boots*	1 Pack/325g	887	52.0	273	9.3	23.0	16.0	2.2
Sausage, Speedy Snacks*	1 Serving/92.5g	259	9.5	279	11.6	35.2	10.2	0.0
Sausage, Triple Pack, GFY, Asda*	1 Pack/215g	424	9.7	197	9.0	30.0	4.5	2.3
Seafood, Mixed, Tesco*	1 Pack/184g	502	30.9	273	7.3	23.2	16.8	0.8
Seafood Cocktail, Asda*	1 Pack/190g	486	30.0	256	6.7	21.3	15.8	1.6
Seafood Cocktail, Waitrose*	1 Pack/210.2g	267	6.3	127	7.3	17.6	3.0	8.1
Seafood Medley, M & S*	1 Pack/227g	468	28.1	206	7.2	16.3	12.4	3.5
Spicy Falafel & Houmous Salad, Delifresh*	1 Pack/209.3g	429	19.7	205	6.1	24.0	9.4	2.6
Spinach, Feta & Rocket, Amy's Kitchen*	1 Serving/128g	260	9.0	203	8.6	26.6	7.0	2.3
Spinach Feta, Amy's Kitchen*	1 Roll/128g	262	9.0	205	8.6	27.0	7.0	2.3
Steak, Hot, M & S*	1 Roll/190g	513	15.2	270	11.9	37.0	8.0	3.2
Sub, Beef, & Onion, M & S*	1 Pack/207g	611	31.7	295	13.3	25.6	15.3	1.5
Sub, Beef, & Onion, Roast, Sainsbury's*	1 Serving/174g	426	17.4	245	9.4	29.3	10.0	0.0
Sub, Chicken, Caesar, Chargrilled, Sainsbury's*	1 Pack/216g	611	30.5	283	13.4	25.6	14.1	0.0
Sub, Chicken & Bacon, Sainsbury's*	1 Pack/190g	554	27.0	291	13.4	27.4	14.2	0.8
Sub, Chicken Caesar, Sainsbury's*	1 Roll/210.0g	590	34.4	281	11.3	22.1	16.4	1.9
Sub, Egg Mayonnaise, Daily Bread*	1 Pack/165.2g	441	22.3	267	9.6	29.6	13.5	0.0
Three Cheese Salad, Shapers, Boots*	1 Pack/168.7g	248	2.2	147	11.0	23.0	1.3	2.7
Tuna, & Cucumber, BGTY, Sainsbury's*	1 Pack/178g	268	3.2	151	11.3	22.3	1.8	3.1
Tuna, & Cucumber, Co-Op*	1 Serving/268.4g	509	13.4	190	12.0	25.0	5.0	2.0
Tuna, & Cucumber, GFY, Asda*	1 Pack/175.7g	253	2.8	144	11.9	20.5	1.6	2.9
Tuna, & Cucumber, Good Sense, Spar*	1 Pack/196.5g	277	3.9	141	14.6	16.0	2.0	2.7
Tuna, & Cucumber, Healthy Choice, Sutherland*	1 Pack/179g	249	4.1	139	9.7	19.7	2.3	2.4
Tuna, & Cucumber, HL, Co-Op*	1 Pack/192g	250	3.5	130	10.9	17.9	1.8	3.0
Tuna, & Cucumber, Less Than 350 Cals, Ginsters*	1 Serving/193g	298	7.5	154	10.8	19.0	3.9	3.1
Tuna, & Cucumber, Low Fat, Heinz*	1 Serving/183.4g	276	2.9	151	12.3	21.6	1.6	6.8
Tuna, & Cucumber, M & S*	1 Pack/187.2g	365	13.7	195	13.4	18.4	7.3	1.5
Tuna, & Cucumber, on a Roll, M & S*	1 Roll/160g	320	12.0	200	11.8	21.6	7.5	3.2
Tuna, & Cucumber, PB, Waitrose*	1 Pack/177.8g	240	3.6	135	11.0	18.3	2.0	3.6

S

SANDWICH

Measure INFO/WEIGHT	per Measure KCAL	per Measure FAT	Nutrition Values per 100g / 100ml KCAL	PROT	CARB	FAT	FIBRE

	Measure INFO/WEIGHT	KCAL	FAT	KCAL	PROT	CARB	FAT	FIBRE
Tuna, & Cucumber, Shapers, Boots*	1 Pack/186.3g	285	4.7	153	11.0	22.0	2.5	2.2
Tuna, & Cucumber, Weight Watchers*	1 Pack/173.3g	279	2.9	161	11.4	25.1	1.7	1.4
Tuna, & Salad, Bloomer, M & S*	1 Pack/230.8g	601	37.0	260	11.8	17.8	16.0	2.6
Tuna, & Salad, Classic*	1 Pack/230.3g	449	15.9	195	8.7	27.3	6.9	2.1
Tuna, & Salad, M & S*	1 Pack/250g	575	31.5	230	12.5	16.8	12.6	2.1
Tuna, & Salad, Maxi, Greenhalgh's*	1 Serving/215.5g	389	18.9	181	8.3	17.4	8.8	1.0
Tuna, & Salad, on White, Tesco*	1 Pack/190g	352	13.3	185	9.8	20.8	7.0	1.1
Tuna, & Salad, Tesco*	1 Pack/197g	339	14.6	172	9.9	16.5	7.4	2.8
Tuna, & Sweetcorn, Ginsters*	1 Pack/163.3g	306	8.2	188	10.5	25.5	5.0	0.0
Tuna, & Sweetcorn, in a Baguette, Asda*	1 Pack/209g	487	16.3	233	9.8	30.9	7.8	2.9
Tuna, & Sweetcorn, Light Choices, HL, Tesco*	1 Pack/167.6g	285	3.2	170	11.2	25.9	1.9	2.8
Tuna, & Sweetcorn, M & S*	1 Pack/195g	390	14.8	200	12.2	20.5	7.6	2.8
Tuna, & Sweetcorn, on Malt Bread, Tesco*	1 Pack/175g	350	8.2	200	11.6	27.5	4.7	2.2
Tuna, & Sweetcorn, Sainsbury's*	1 Pack/183g	392	15.6	214	12.1	22.3	8.5	0.0
Tuna, & Sweetcorn, Shapers, Boots*	1 Pack/170g	295	4.4	174	12.4	25.3	2.6	2.0
Tuna, Healthy Options, Spar*	1 Pack/150g	269	3.6	179	14.3	24.9	2.4	0.0
Tuna, Mayo, Wheat Free, Pret a Manger*	1 Sandwich/295g	540	26.0	183	7.4	17.9	8.8	4.5
Tuna, Mayonnaise & Cucumber, Finest, Tesco*	1 Pack/225g	484	19.1	215	11.6	23.1	8.5	1.7
Tuna, Mediterranean, COU, M & S*	1 Pack/260g	364	5.7	140	10.3	19.6	2.2	1.6
Tuna, Melt, Swedish Bread, Shapers, Boots*	1 Pack/163g	254	3.6	156	14.0	20.0	2.2	2.1
Tuna Mayonnaise, & Cucumber, Classic*	1 Serving/185g	429	22.8	232	10.6	19.8	12.3	0.0
Tuna Mayonnaise, & Cucumber, Daily Bread*	1 Pack/190.3g	391	16.5	206	12.1	19.8	8.7	0.0
Tuna Mayonnaise, & Cucumber, Darwins Deli*	1 Pack/155g	370	14.6	239	9.6	21.9	9.4	0.0
Tuna Mayonnaise, & Cucumber, Simply, Boots*	1 Pack/200g	498	26.0	249	12.0	21.0	13.0	2.4
Tuna Mayonnaise, & Sweetcorn, Asda*	1 Pack/178g	438	24.0	246	13.3	17.7	13.5	2.1
Tuna Mayonnaise, & Sweetcorn, Whistlestop*	1 Pack/139.5g	377	17.7	271	13.6	25.5	12.7	0.0
Tuna Mayonnaise, on White Bread, Oldfields*	1 Pack/141.7g	395	18.2	278	15.2	27.4	12.8	2.0
Tuna Nicoise, on Gluten Free Bread, Starbucks*	1 Sandwich/207g	408	17.2	197	9.2	21.4	8.3	2.9
Tuna Salad, Mediterranean Style, Waitrose*	1 Pack/210g	274	4.0	130	8.6	19.6	1.9	2.1
Tuna Savoury, Bells*	1 Pack/149g	295	10.0	198	11.8	22.5	6.7	1.0
Turkey, & Bacon, COU, M & S*	1 Pack/165g	256	4.0	155	12.0	21.0	2.4	1.7
Turkey, & Cheese, & Bacon, Bernard Matthews*	1 Serving/192.0g	482	21.5	251	9.2	28.3	11.2	0.0
Turkey, & Cranberry, COU, M & S*	1 Pack/180g	279	3.1	155	12.1	22.8	1.7	2.9
Turkey, & Cranberry Salad, Fullfillers*	1 Serving/180g	319	5.8	177	13.0	23.3	3.2	0.0
Turkey, & Salad, Brambles*	1 Pack/169.9g	248	2.0	146	9.3	24.5	1.2	2.0
Turkey, & Salad, HE, Wild Bean Cafe*	1 Serving/230g	315	2.5	137	10.0	21.5	1.1	1.8
Turkey, & Stuffing, M & S*	1 Pack/190g	352	9.3	185	12.3	23.1	4.9	1.9
Turkey, & Stuffing, Shapers, Boots*	1 Pack/196.9g	321	3.2	163	13.0	24.0	1.6	2.7
Turkey, & Suffing, & Bacon, Bernard Matthews*	1 Pack/127.3g	250	8.7	196	12.0	21.6	6.8	2.0
Turkey, Gibsons*	1 Pack/138g	260	5.3	188	12.5	26.0	3.8	0.0
Turkey, Pork Sausage, & Stuffing, Somerfield*	1 Pack/209.3g	475	19.5	227	11.6	24.3	9.3	2.1
Vegetable, & Chilli Bean, Roasted, M & S*	1 Pack/200g	340	11.4	170	5.2	24.5	5.7	2.1
Vegetable, Chargrilled, Eat Smart, Safeway*	1 Pack/183g	265	4.2	145	7.4	23.4	2.3	2.8
Vegetable, Grilled, Safeway*	1 Pack/150g	236	5.9	157	5.6	24.9	3.9	2.4
Vegetable, M & S*	1 Serving/180g	252	4.1	140	6.1	23.5	2.3	2.1
Vegetable, Roasted, Open, COU, M & S*	1 Pack/150g	260	2.2	173	8.4	31.3	1.5	4.4
Wedge, Ham, & Salad, HE, Tesco*	1 Pack/198g	269	3.4	136	7.1	23.0	1.7	1.0
Wensleydale, & Carrot, M & S*	1 Pack/183g	430	22.5	235	9.9	21.4	12.3	2.8
Wild Red Salmon & Cucumber, Eat Well, M & S*	1 Pack/180.6g	352	15.4	195	11.0	19.0	8.5	2.6
Zip, Zap, Zing, Fresh! Gourmet Organics*	1 Pack/164g	267	8.0	163	5.9	24.2	4.9	3.1

SANDWICH FILLER

	Measure INFO/WEIGHT	KCAL	FAT	KCAL	PROT	CARB	FAT	FIBRE
Beef & Onion, Deli, Asda*	1 Serving/50g	79	6.5	157	10.0	0.1	13.0	1.1
Cajun Chicken, Sainsbury's*	1 Serving/60g	109	8.1	182	13.4	1.8	13.5	1.8

SANDWICH FILLER

	Measure INFO/WEIGHT	per Measure KCAL	per Measure FAT	Nutrition Values per 100g / 100ml KCAL	PROT	CARB	FAT	FIBRE
Cheese & Bacon, Tesco*	1 Serving/50g	199	18.8	398	12.2	2.6	37.6	1.2
Cheese & Ham, Sainsbury's*	1 Serving/25g	124	12.3	497	12.4	0.8	49.3	0.3
Cheese & Onion, Deli, Asda*	1 Serving/57g	217	21.1	381	10.0	2.0	37.0	2.0
Cheese & Onion, Reduced Fat, Morrisons*	1 Serving/50g	119	9.4	237	11.7	5.2	18.8	2.3
Cheese & Onion, Sainsbury's*	1 Serving/56g	188	17.4	336	10.8	3.4	31.0	0.7
Cheese & Onion, Tesco*	1 Pack/170g	687	66.6	404	11.2	1.6	39.2	1.6
Cheese & Spring Onion, HE, Tesco*	1 Serving/85g	185	13.1	218	13.2	6.8	15.4	0.6
Cheese & Spring Onion, M & S*	1 Serving/56g	199	18.8	355	8.5	5.0	33.6	0.2
Cheese & Spring Onion, Morrisons*	1 Portion/50g	236	22.3	472	12.9	4.6	44.6	1.1
Chicken, Bacon & Sweetcorn, Sainsbury's*	1 Serving/60g	123	9.4	205	12.0	4.0	15.7	0.9
Chicken, Sweetcorn & Bacon, Tesco*	1 Serving/50g	167	14.9	334	12.3	4.3	29.7	1.6
Chicken, Sweetcorn & Sage, HE, Tesco*	1 Serving/125g	105	1.6	84	9.4	8.8	1.3	1.3
Chicken & Stuffing, Sainsbury's*	½ Tub/120g	397	37.8	331	6.5	5.3	31.5	1.7
Chicken & Sweetcorn, Deli, M & S*	1 Serving/85g	238	20.3	280	13.2	3.9	23.9	1.4
Chicken & Sweetcorn, Eat Smart, Morrisons*	½ Pot/85g	157	11.6	185	13.0	2.5	13.6	3.3
Chicken & Sweetcorn, Sainsbury's*	1 Serving/75g	175	14.9	233	11.0	2.7	19.8	1.9
Chicken & Sweetcorn, Tesco*	1/3 Pot/100g	183	14.2	183	11.2	2.6	14.2	3.3
Chicken Caesar, BGTY, Sainsbury's*	½ Jar/85.4g	116	6.1	137	15.6	2.5	7.2	2.2
Chicken Tikka, BGTY, Sainsbury's*	½ Pot/85g	99	2.6	117	16.5	6.0	3.0	1.0
Chicken Tikka, Deli, Asda*	1 Serving/50g	151	12.5	301	13.0	6.0	25.0	0.8
Chickpea, Moroccan Style, Sainsbury's*	½ Tub/120g	160	9.4	133	4.1	11.7	7.8	4.2
Corned Beef & Onion, Deli, Asda*	1 Serving/50g	170	15.5	340	12.0	3.3	31.0	0.7
Coronation Chicken, Asda*	½ Pack/125g	288	19.0	230	13.3	10.1	15.2	2.6
Coronation Chicken, BGTY, Sainsbury's*	1 Portion/50g	73	3.5	146	11.9	8.9	7.0	1.4
Coronation Chicken, Sainsbury's*	1 Serving/48g	146	11.8	305	12.1	8.9	24.6	1.2
Coronation Chicken, Tesco*	1 Tbsp/30g	84	6.5	279	14.7	6.1	21.8	0.7
Coronation Chicken, Waitrose*	1 Pack/170g	554	43.2	326	11.1	13.2	25.4	2.0
Coronation Tuna, BGTY, Sainsbury's*	1 Tin/80g	90	2.1	112	16.5	5.7	2.6	1.0
Creamy Chicken Tikka, Sainsbury's*	1 Pack/382.3g	432	11.1	113	17.0	4.9	2.9	1.0
Egg & Smoked Bacon, BGTY, Sainsbury's*	1 Pot/240g	374	27.1	156	9.7	3.8	11.3	0.5
Egg Mayonaise, BFY, Morrisons*	1 Serving/50g	71	5.3	142	10.0	1.7	10.6	0.0
Egg Mayonnaise, BGTY, Sainsbury's*	1 Serving/75g	84	4.9	112	9.7	3.6	6.5	0.5
Egg Mayonnaise, Deli, Asda*	1 Serving/50g	114	10.0	227	11.0	0.8	20.0	0.3
Egg Mayonnaise, Deli, Somerfield*	1 Serving/40g	120	11.7	301	9.7	0.2	29.2	0.0
Egg Mayonnaise, Free Range, Tesco*	1 Serving/50g	105	8.9	209	11.3	0.9	17.8	1.6
Egg Mayonnaise, Sainsbury's*	1 Serving/60g	129	11.0	215	10.4	2.0	18.4	0.5
Egg Mayonnaise, Tesco*	1 Serving/50g	114	10.0	228	10.2	1.9	20.0	0.5
Poached Salmon & Cucumber, Deli, M & S*	1 Pot/170g	349	27.7	205	14.0	1.0	16.3	0.5
Prawn Marie Rose, Sainsbury's*	1 Serving/60g	121	10.6	201	8.1	2.5	17.6	0.9
Prawn Mayonaise, Deli, Asda*	1 Serving/50g	170	16.5	339	9.0	1.6	33.0	0.4
Prawn Mayonnaise, GFY, Asda*	1 Serving/57g	101	7.4	177	12.0	3.0	13.0	0.1
Prawn Mayonnaise, Waitrose*	1 Pot/170g	537	52.9	316	8.9	0.2	31.1	0.0
Seafood, BGTY, Sainsbury's*	1oz/28g	36	2.0	128	8.7	7.6	7.0	0.5
Seafood Cocktail, Sainsbury's*	½ Tub/120g	314	27.6	262	5.7	8.1	23.0	1.0
Smoked Salmon & Soft Cheese, M & S*	1 Pack/170g	451	40.6	265	11.1	4.9	23.9	0.0
Tuna, Carb Check, Heinz*	1 Serving/52g	84	6.2	161	6.6	6.3	12.0	0.7
Tuna & Sweetcorn, BGTY, Sainsbury's*	1 Portion/50g	57	2.5	113	10.5	6.5	5.0	1.4
Tuna & Sweetcorn, COU, M & S*	½ Pot/85g	77	1.7	90	11.6	5.7	2.0	1.3
Tuna & Sweetcorn, Deli, Asda*	1 Serving/50g	148	13.0	296	12.0	3.4	26.0	1.4
Tuna & Sweetcorn, GFY, Asda*	1/3 Pot/57g	71	2.3	125	12.0	10.0	4.1	0.8
Tuna & Sweetcorn, HL, Tesco*	1 Serving/60g	69	3.2	115	11.2	5.0	5.3	1.4
Tuna Mayonnaise, BGTY, Sainsbury's*	1 Serving/100g	114	3.4	114	17.6	3.5	3.4	0.1

S

	Measure INFO/WEIGHT	per Measure KCAL	FAT	Nutrition Values per 100g / 100ml KCAL	PROT	CARB	FAT	FIBRE
SANDWICH FILLING								
Cheese & Onion, Asda*	1 Serving/56g	288	28.5	515	9.8	4.4	50.9	0.3
Cheese & Onion, Co-Op*	1 Serving/56g	269	26.3	480	10.0	4.0	47.0	0.5
Cheese & Onion, GFY, Asda*	1 Serving/80g	206	16.8	257	11.0	6.0	21.0	0.8
Chicken Tikka, Asda*	1 Serving/28g	80	5.6	284	13.0	13.0	20.0	0.7
Crab, BGTY, Sainsbury's*	1oz/28g	36	2.0	128	8.7	7.6	7.0	0.5
Egg Mayonnaise, Asda*	1oz/28g	72	6.5	258	10.3	1.9	23.3	0.7
Egg Mayonnaise, Co-Op*	1oz/28g	66	5.9	235	10.0	1.0	21.0	1.0
Houmous & Vegetable, Asda*	1/3 Tub/57g	133	9.7	233	8.0	12.0	17.0	3.5
Tuna & Sweetcorn, Reduced Fat, Co-Op*	1 Serving/50g	103	7.0	205	13.0	7.0	14.0	0.9
Tuna & Sweetcorn with Mayo, Morrisons*	1 Serving/50g	153	13.0	305	11.4	5.4	25.9	1.9
SANDWICH SPREAD								
Beef, Classic, Shippam*	1 Pot/75g	133	8.9	177	15.5	2.2	11.8	0.0
Chicken, Classic, Shippam*	1 Serving/35g	64	4.4	182	15.5	1.8	12.5	0.0
Chicken Tikka, Asda*	1 Serving/50g	77	5.0	154	7.0	9.0	10.0	0.2
Crab, Classic, Shippam*	1 Jar/35g	60	3.8	170	13.1	4.6	10.9	0.0
Cucumber, Heinz*	1oz/28g	46	3.2	164	1.7	12.7	11.6	0.6
Original, Heinz*	1oz/28g	63	3.7	225	1.0	24.9	13.1	0.8
Salmon, Classic, Shippam*	1 Serving/35g	70	4.9	200	14.7	4.2	14.1	0.0
Tuna & Mayonnaise, Shippam*	1 Pot/75g	189	13.9	252	18.3	3.1	18.5	0.0
SARDINES								
Boneless, in Tomato Sauce, John West*	1 Serving/95g	156	9.5	164	17.0	1.5	10.0	0.0
COOK!, M & S*	1 Serving/128g	262	18.0	205	16.4	1.2	14.1	0.1
Grilled	1oz/28g	55	2.9	195	25.3	0.0	10.4	0.0
in Barbecue Sauce, Princes*	1 Can/120g	182	9.6	152	15.1	5.0	8.0	0.0
in Brine, Canned, Drained	1oz/28g	48	2.7	172	21.5	0.0	9.6	0.0
in Brine, Drained, Tesco*	1 Tin/84g	144	8.1	172	21.5	0.0	9.6	0.0
in Oil, Canned, Drained	1oz/28g	62	3.9	220	23.3	0.0	14.1	0.0
in Smoky Barbecue Sauce, Princes*	1 Can/120g	182	9.6	152	15.1	5.0	8.0	0.0
in Spring Water, Portuguese, Sainsbury's*	1 Can/90g	165	9.3	183	22.4	0.0	10.3	0.0
in Tomato Sauce, Brunswick*	1 Tin/106g	141	7.4	133	15.5	2.1	7.0	0.2
in Tomato Sauce, Canned	1oz/28g	45	2.8	162	17.0	1.4	9.9	0.0
Piccanti, in Olive Oil, Drained, Canned, Waitrose*	1 Can/88g	265	22.4	301	17.9	0.3	25.4	0.0
Raw	1oz/28g	46	2.6	165	20.6	0.0	9.2	0.0
SATAY								
Chicken, Breast, Iceland*	1 Satay/9.7g	15	0.1	155	34.1	2.7	0.9	0.1
Chicken, Breast, Party Bites, Sainsbury's*	1 Stick/10g	16	0.1	157	34.1	2.7	0.9	0.1
Chicken, GFY, Asda*	1 Serving/168.1g	242	6.0	144	22.0	6.0	3.6	0.8
Chicken, Indonesian, Bighams*	1 Serving/240g	314	15.4	131	12.2	6.2	6.4	0.6
Chicken, Indonesian, Mini, Sainsbury's*	1 Stick/10g	17	0.7	171	23.0	4.0	7.0	0.7
Chicken, Kebab, Waitrose*	½ Pack/125g	246	13.5	197	18.9	6.0	10.8	0.5
Chicken, M & S*	1 Satay/43g	90	5.5	210	19.1	4.4	12.7	0.7
Chicken, Mini, Iceland*	1 Satay/8g	19	1.1	236	23.0	4.5	14.0	0.7
Chicken, Morrisons*	1 Satay/10g	17	0.7	171	23.5	3.5	7.0	0.7
Chicken, Occasions, Sainsbury's*	1 Satay/10g	15	0.6	150	22.0	2.0	6.0	0.7
Chicken, Oriental, Tesco*	1 Serving/100g	160	5.0	160	23.6	5.1	5.0	0.4
Chicken, Party, Mini, Tesco*	1 Satay/10g	13	0.3	133	23.7	3.4	2.8	1.0
Chicken, Sticks, Asda*	1 Stick/20g	43	2.8	216	18.0	4.5	14.0	0.0
Chicken, Stuffed, Asda*	½ Pack/168.1g	242	6.0	144	22.0	6.0	3.6	0.8
Chicken, Taste Original*	1 Stick/20g	33	1.3	164	23.0	2.5	6.5	0.7
Chicken, Tesco*	1 Pack/200g	165	6.0	83	12.1	1.9	3.0	0.4
Chicken, Thai, Skewers, Sainsbury's*	½ Pack/125g	219	10.5	175	17.8	7.1	8.4	2.3
Chicken, Thai Cocktail Sel & Peanut Sauce, Somerfield*	1oz/28g	43	1.7	152	23.0	2.0	6.0	0.0
Chicken, with Peanut Sauce, Waitrose*	1 Serving/350g	690	37.8	197	18.9	6.0	10.8	0.5

S

	Measure INFO/WEIGHT	per Measure KCAL	FAT	Nutrition Values per 100g / 100ml KCAL	PROT	CARB	FAT	FIBRE
SATAY								
Chicken & Turkey, Co-Op*	1 Pack/120g	264	16.8	220	20.0	4.0	14.0	0.1
Chicken & Turkey, Morrisons*	1 Stick/20g	39	2.5	197	20.3	1.0	12.4	2.3
Chicken & Turkey, Sainsbury's*	1 Stick/20g	44	2.8	222	20.0	4.0	14.0	1.9
Selection, Safeway*	1 Satay/10g	20	0.8	200	26.0	9.0	8.0	3.0
Szechuan Style, Occasions, Sainsbury's*	1 Satay/10g	20	0.9	196	22.8	6.4	8.8	0.5
SATAY TIKKA								
Chicken, Cocktail Selection, Somerfield*	1oz/28g	48	2.0	171	24.0	4.0	7.0	0.0
Chicken, Mini, Asda*	1 Pack/80g	178	12.4	222	15.5	5.2	15.5	2.4
SATSUMAS								
Weighed with Peel, Average	1 Med/80g	21	0.1	26	0.6	6.0	0.1	0.9
SAUCE								
Apple, Baxters*	1 Tbsp/15g	7	0.1	49	0.1	11.1	0.4	0.7
Apple, Bramley, Asda*	1 Serving/20g	17	0.0	86	0.2	21.0	0.1	1.0
Apple, Bramley, M & S*	1 Tbsp/15g	21	0.0	140	0.2	32.6	0.3	0.4
Apple, Bramley, Morrisons*	1 Tbsp/20g	24	0.0	122	0.2	30.0	0.1	1.1
Apple, Bramley, Safeway*	1 Serving/50g	61	0.1	121	0.2	29.9	0.1	1.0
Apple, Bramley, Sainsbury's*	1 Tbsp/15g	17	0.0	111	0.2	27.2	0.1	1.8
Apple, Bramley, Tesco*	1 Tbsp/15g	19	0.0	130	0.2	31.7	0.1	1.0
Apple, Heinz*	1 Tbsp/15g	8	0.0	56	0.3	13.4	0.2	1.5
Apple, SmartPrice, Asda*	1 Tsp/5g	5	0.0	101	0.3	25.0	0.0	0.9
Apple, Value, Tesco*	1 Serving/50g	29	0.0	58	0.1	14.4	0.0	0.5
Apple & Brandy, Asda*	1 Serving/125g	56	0.0	45	0.2	11.0	0.0	0.0
Apricot & Almond Tagine, Sainsbury's*	1/3 Jar/120g	98	1.9	82	2.0	17.9	1.6	2.5
Aromatic Cantonese, Express, Uncle Ben's*	1 Serving/170g	172	0.2	101	0.6	24.6	0.1	0.0
Arrabbiata, Asda*	½ Pot/150g	84	3.3	56	1.6	7.4	2.2	0.6
Arrabbiata, Don Pomodoro*	½ Pot/185g	231	20.4	125	0.5	6.0	11.0	0.0
Arrabbiata, Italian, Tesco*	½ Pot/175g	72	0.5	41	1.3	8.3	0.3	1.1
Arrabiatta, Fresh, Waitrose*	1 Serving/100g	52	2.5	52	1.4	5.9	2.5	2.0
Balti, Cooking, Sharwood's*	1/3 Jar/140g	105	4.9	75	1.6	9.4	3.5	3.0
Balti, Cooking, Shere Khan*	1 Jar/425g	261	20.0	61	0.9	3.9	4.7	0.0
Balti, Curry, Tesco*	1 Serving/200g	126	9.2	63	1.7	4.3	4.6	1.7
Balti, Indian Style, Iceland*	1 Serving/220g	154	5.7	70	1.6	10.1	2.6	0.5
Balti, Reduced Fat, HL, Cook in, Co-Op*	½ Jar/225g	135	5.4	60	2.0	7.5	2.4	2.3
Balti, Tomato & Coriander, Canned, Patak's*	1 Serving/70g	58	4.2	83	0.8	6.5	6.0	1.2
Barbecue, Asda*	1 Serving/135g	128	0.3	95	1.2	22.0	0.2	0.6
Barbecue, Cooking, BGTY, Sainsbury's*	¼ Jar/124g	46	0.2	37	0.4	8.4	0.2	0.7
Barbecue, Original, Sainsbury's*	1 Tbsp/15g	19	0.0	127	0.9	29.6	0.1	0.3
Barbecue, Smoky, Ainsley Harriott*	1 Serving/10g	15	0.0	153	0.8	36.4	0.1	0.0
Barbeque, Cook in, Homepride*	1 Tin/500g	375	7.5	75	0.7	14.6	1.5	0.6
Basil & Pesto, M & S*	1 Serving/65g	348	30.5	535	7.5	20.7	46.9	1.4
BBQ, Heinz*	1 Serving/20g	29	0.1	143	1.1	32.9	0.3	0.5
BBQ, Hellmann's*	1 Serving/10g	13	0.1	125	0.8	27.7	0.7	0.0
BBQ, HP*	1 Serving/20ml	29	0.0	143	0.8	33.1	0.2	0.0
BBQ, Smokey Tomato, HP*	1oz/28g	40	0.1	143	0.8	33.1	0.2	0.0
BBQ, Spicy Mayhem, HP*	1 Serving/2g	3	0.0	156	0.9	36.7	0.1	0.0
Bearnaise, Sainsbury's*	1 Tbsp/15g	59	6.2	393	0.6	5.0	41.0	0.0
Bhuna, Cooking, Sharwood's*	1/3 Jar/140g	116	7.6	83	1.2	7.6	5.4	1.6
Black Bean, Asda*	1 Serving/55g	55	0.8	100	2.9	19.0	1.4	0.0
Black Bean, Canton, Stir Fry, Blue Dragon*	½ Pack/60g	53	1.2	88	2.8	14.8	2.0	1.5
Black Bean, Crushed, Stir Fry Sensations, Amoy*	1 Pouch/150g	150	4.4	100	2.4	16.9	2.9	1.0
Black Bean, Finest, Tesco*	1 Jar/350g	252	1.8	72	0.8	16.1	0.5	0.8
Black Bean, Fresh, Sainsbury's*	1 Sachet/50ml	78	1.3	156	6.7	27.5	2.6	1.7
Black Bean, Ready to Stir Fry, M & S*	1 Sachet/120g	78	1.1	65	2.5	11.5	0.9	1.4

	Measure INFO/WEIGHT	per Measure		Nutrition Values per 100g / 100ml				
		KCAL	FAT	KCAL	PROT	CARB	FAT	FIBRE
SAUCE								
Black Bean, Sharwood's*	1 Serving/97.5g	96	1.5	98	2.2	18.8	1.5	0.6
Black Bean, Stir Fry, Asda*	1 Pack/125g	113	3.0	113	3.5	18.0	3.0	0.8
Black Bean, Stir Fry, Fresh, M & S*	1 Pot/120g	120	0.7	100	2.6	20.3	0.6	1.4
Black Bean, Stir Fry, Morrisons*	½ Jar/237g	438	25.6	185	4.1	17.3	10.8	1.5
Black Bean, Stir Fry, Sainsbury's*	½ Pack/75ml	91	3.2	121	3.3	17.6	4.3	1.7
Black Bean, Stir Fry, Sharwood's*	1 Jar/195g	191	2.9	98	2.2	18.8	1.5	0.6
Black Bean, Stir Fry, Tesco*	½ Jar/220g	297	10.8	135	3.4	18.1	4.9	2.5
Black Bean, Uncle Ben's*	1 Serving/125g	89	1.6	71	2.0	12.8	1.3	0.0
Black Bean, Wing Yip*	½ Jar/61g	75	3.0	123	3.2	17.3	4.9	0.0
Black Bean & Green Pepper, Stir Fry, Sharwood's*	1 Serving/150g	83	0.5	55	2.0	11.0	0.3	0.5
Black Bean & Red Pepper, Sharwood's*	½ Jar/212.5g	132	3.0	62	1.9	10.5	1.4	1.2
Black Pepper, Lee Kum Kee*	1 Serving/90g	107	3.0	119	3.2	19.0	3.3	1.4
Black Pepper, Stir Fry, Blue Dragon*	½ Sachet/60g	47	2.6	79	1.6	8.4	4.4	0.1
Bolognese, Emilia Romagna, Fresh, Sainsbury's*	½ Pot/150g	99	4.8	66	5.9	3.4	3.2	1.7
Bolognese, for Beef, Tesco*	½ Pack/175g	177	10.2	101	5.4	6.9	5.8	0.8
Bolognese, Fresh, Safeway*	½ Pot/153g	182	11.0	119	7.3	6.3	7.2	1.6
Bolognese, Italiano, Tesco*	1 Serving/175g	194	13.1	111	5.9	4.8	7.5	0.8
Bolognese, Loyd Grossman*	¼ Jar/106g	80	3.1	75	2.0	10.2	2.9	1.4
Bolognese, Original, Dolmio*	¼ Jar/125g	66	1.5	53	1.3	9.2	1.2	0.8
Bourguignon, Beef Tonight, Knorr*	1 Serving/150g	86	3.9	57	0.6	7.6	2.6	0.4
Bramley Apple, Colman's*	1 Tbsp/15ml	16	0.0	107	0.2	26.5	0.0	1.3
Branston Smooth, Crosse & Blackwell*	1 Serving/25g	35	0.0	139	0.6	34.0	0.1	1.4
Bread, Luxury, M & S*	1 Serving/115g	196	16.2	170	3.2	8.1	14.1	2.2
Bread, Made with Semi-Skimmed Milk	1 Serving/45g	42	1.4	93	4.3	12.8	3.1	0.3
Brown, Asda*	1 Serving/10g	10	0.0	97	0.7	23.0	0.2	0.4
Brown, Bottled	1 Tsp/6g	6	0.0	99	1.1	25.2	0.0	0.7
Brown, Iceland*	1 Serving/20g	16	0.0	82	0.7	19.3	0.2	1.1
Brown, Tesco*	1 Tsp/10g	10	0.0	104	0.7	25.1	0.1	0.6
Burger, Hellmann's*	1 Tbsp/15g	36	3.2	240	1.1	12.0	21.0	0.0
Butter & Tarragon, Chicken Tonigh, Knorr*	¼ Jar/125g	133	13.0	106	1.0	2.1	10.4	0.7
Carbonara, Less Than 5% Fat, GFY, Asda*	½ Tub/150g	122	6.8	81	5.0	5.0	4.5	0.5
Chasseur, Cook in, Homepride*	1 Can/390g	160	0.4	41	0.7	9.2	0.1	0.4
Cheddar Cheese, Dry, Knorr*	1 Serving/10g	47	3.2	469	7.8	38.0	31.8	0.3
Cheese, Fresh, Italiano, Tesco*	½ Tub/175g	236	16.1	135	6.8	6.2	9.2	0.0
Cheese, Fresh, Waitrose*	1 Pot/350g	459	34.3	131	5.1	5.7	9.8	0.0
Cheese, Instant, Morrisons*	1 Serving/14g	38	2.8	272	7.9	14.3	20.3	0.0
Cheese, Italian, Tesco*	½ Carton/175g	238	15.6	136	5.8	8.3	8.9	0.0
Cheese, Italian Style, Finest, Tesco*	½ Pot/175g	355	20.8	203	10.1	14.0	11.9	0.0
Cheese, Made with Semi-Skimmed Milk	1 Serving/60g	107	7.6	179	8.1	9.1	12.6	0.2
Cheese, Made with Whole Milk	1 Serving/60g	118	8.8	197	8.0	9.0	14.6	0.2
Cheese, Sainsbury's*	1 Serving/125g	140	9.4	112	5.0	6.1	7.5	1.2
Chilli, Amoy*	1 Tsp/6g	2	0.0	25	1.0	5.2	0.0	1.0
Chilli, Hot, Blue Dragon*	1 Tbsp/15ml	14	0.0	96	0.5	23.0	0.2	0.0
Chilli, Hot, Mexican, Morrisons*	¼ Jar/125g	73	0.6	58	2.2	11.2	0.5	2.0
Chilli, HP*	1 Tsp/6g	8	0.0	134	1.2	32.3	0.1	0.0
Chilli, Iceland*	1 Serving/115g	75	0.8	65	2.7	12.0	0.7	1.6
Chilli, Medium, Deliciously Good, Homepride*	1 Jar/460g	258	2.3	56	2.3	10.4	0.5	1.2
Chilli, Sweet, Thai, Dipping, Blue Dragon*	1 Serving/30g	56	0.2	188	0.5	45.2	0.6	1.3
Chilli, Tesco*	1 Tsp/5ml	5	0.2	90	1.3	14.0	3.2	1.1
Chilli & Garlic, Blue Dragon*	1 Serving/30ml	26	0.1	85	1.1	19.7	0.2	0.0
Chilli & Garlic, Lea & Perrins*	1 Tsp/6g	4	0.0	60	1.0	14.9	0.0	0.0
Chilli & Garlic, Stir Fry, M & S*	1 Serving/82.5g	120	1.0	145	0.7	32.4	1.2	1.1
Chilli Con Carne, Cook in, BGTY, Sainsbury's*	¼ Jar/125g	69	0.6	55	1.7	11.0	0.5	2.5

SAUCE

INFO/WEIGHT	Measure	per Measure		Nutrition Values per 100g / 100ml				
		KCAL	FAT	KCAL	PROT	CARB	FAT	FIBRE
Chilli Con Carne, Cook in, Homepride*	1 Can/390g	234	2.3	60	2.5	11.2	0.6	0.0
Chilli Con Carne, Hot, Uncle Ben's*	1 Jar/500g	295	3.0	59	2.3	10.9	0.6	1.7
Chilli Soy, Amoy*	1 Tbsp/15g	8	0.0	55	4.6	9.1	0.0	0.0
Chinese, Curry, Farmfoods*	1 Sachet/200g	220	17.6	110	0.6	7.1	8.8	0.7
Chinese, Stir Fry, Sachet, Fresh, Sainsbury's*	½ Sachet/51ml	83	5.7	163	1.7	14.1	11.1	1.8
Chinese Stir Fry, Sainsbury's*	½ Sachet/75.3g	61	1.9	81	0.4	14.1	2.5	1.0
Chip Shop Curry, Knorr*	1 Sachet/150ml	146	6.9	97	1.7	12.4	4.6	0.7
Chocolate, Sainsbury's*	1 Serving/25g	81	1.6	323	1.8	64.7	6.3	2.7
Chocolate Flavour, Dry, Lyle's*	1 Serving/10g	31	0.1	305	1.0	74.0	0.5	0.0
Chop Suey, Stir Fry, Sharwood's*	1 Jar/160g	120	2.4	75	0.7	14.6	1.5	0.2
Chow Mein, Stir Fry, Asda*	½ Jar/97.5g	97	1.0	99	1.6	21.0	1.0	0.1
Chow Mein, Stir Fry, Blue Dragon*	1 Sachet/120g	110	3.5	92	1.1	15.4	2.9	0.4
Chow Mein, Stir Fry, Morrisons*	½ Sachet/50g	85	2.6	170	1.3	29.0	5.1	0.7
Cooking, Balti, Asda*	¼ Jar/145g	155	10.2	107	1.9	9.0	7.0	1.1
Coronation Chicken, Cook in, Homepride*	1 Serving/250g	233	10.5	93	0.8	13.2	4.2	0.0
Country French, Chicken Tonigh, Knorr*	¼ Jar/125g	113	10.0	90	0.5	4.1	8.0	0.7
Country French, Low Fat, Chicken Tonight, Knorr*	¼ Jar/125g	56	3.6	45	0.4	4.4	2.9	0.7
Cracked Black Pepper, M & S*	1 Serving/160g	160	13.0	100	1.6	4.7	8.1	0.3
Cranberry, Sainsbury's*	1 Tsp/15g	23	0.0	154	0.8	37.1	0.3	1.3
Cranberry, Tesco*	1 Tsp/15g	23	0.0	156	0.1	38.8	0.0	0.9
Cranberry, Waitrose*	1 Tbsp/20g	31	0.0	156	0.2	38.5	0.2	14.0
Cranberry & Port, M & S*	1 Serving/75g	71	0.3	95	2.3	20.2	0.4	2.1
Cranberry Jelly, Baxters*	1 Tsp/15g	40	0.0	268	0.0	67.0	0.0	0.0
Cranberry Jelly, Morrisons*	1 Tsp/12g	23	0.0	189	0.2	47.0	0.0	0.1
Cream, Graddsås, Ikea*	1 Serving/60ml	72	6.6	120	1.0	4.0	11.0	0.0
Creamy Lemon & Dill, Fresh, Sainsbury's*	1/3 Pot/100g	88	7.2	88	1.9	4.0	7.2	0.9
Creamy Mushroom, Cooking, M & S*	1 Jar/510g	663	57.6	130	1.3	5.4	11.3	0.5
Creamy Mushroom, Knorr*	1 Serving/125g	111	9.6	89	0.4	4.5	7.7	0.4
Creamy Peppercorn & Whisky, Baxters*	1 Pack/320g	422	34.6	132	1.9	6.7	10.8	0.2
Creole Style, Aldi*	1 Serving/160g	158	3.5	99	1.3	18.6	2.2	0.0
Cumberland Sausage, Colman's*	¼ Jar/126g	43	0.3	34	0.7	7.4	0.2	0.8
Curry, Cook in, Homepride*	½ Can/250g	140	4.8	56	1.1	8.6	1.9	0.5
Curry, Creamy, Chicken Tonight, Knorr*	½ Jar/250g	208	18.5	83	0.6	3.6	7.4	0.8
Curry, Green Thai, BGTY, Sainsbury's*	¼ Jar/125g	61	3.3	49	0.6	5.7	2.6	1.4
Curry, Green Thai, Finest, Tesco*	1 Serving/350g	420	37.1	120	1.4	4.8	10.6	0.7
Curry, Green Thai, Sharwood's*	1 Serving/403g	431	30.6	107	1.1	8.4	7.6	0.1
Curry, Mild, Tesco*	1 Jar/500g	420	14.0	84	1.1	13.4	2.8	0.8
Curry, Red Thai, BGTY, Sainsbury's*	1 Serving/124g	77	4.8	62	0.6	6.0	3.9	1.4
Curry, Red Thai, Finest, Tesco*	1 Jar/350g	389	31.5	111	1.3	6.2	9.0	0.9
Curry, Red Thai, Sharwood's*	1 Serving/138g	150	11.0	109	1.2	7.9	8.0	0.2
Curry, Sweet	1 Serving/115g	105	6.4	91	1.2	9.6	5.6	1.4
Curry, Thai Coconut, Uncle Ben's*	1 Serving/125g	128	6.0	102	1.4	13.2	4.8	0.0
Curry, Value, Tesco*	1 Can/390g	355	17.6	91	1.6	11.0	4.5	1.3
Curry, Yellow Thai, Cooking, Sainsbury's*	1 Jar/500g	785	70.0	157	2.3	5.4	14.0	2.3
Dark Soy, Sesame & Ginger, for Fish, Schwartz*	1 Pack/300g	279	4.2	93	1.3	18.8	1.4	0.5
Dhansak, Medium, Sharwood's*	1 Jar/420g	370	13.4	88	3.6	11.1	3.2	1.0
Diane, Safeway*	½ Pot/85g	40	3.0	47	0.8	3.3	3.5	0.3
Dill & Lemon, Delicate, for Fish, Schwartz*	1 Pack/300g	387	34.2	129	1.1	5.6	11.4	0.5
Dill & Mustard, for Gravadlax, Dry, Waitrose*	1 Sachet/35g	123	9.0	352	2.5	27.8	25.7	0.6
Dopiaza, Cooking, Tesco*	1 Serving/166g	176	11.0	106	2.2	9.4	6.6	1.9
Dopiaza, Medium, Cook in, Sharwood's*	½ Bottle/210g	193	10.7	92	1.4	10.2	5.1	0.6
Enchilada, Medium, Old El Paso*	1 Can/270g	92	4.6	34	0.0	5.0	1.7	0.0
Fajita, Asda*	¼ Jar/125g	79	5.4	63	1.0	5.0	4.3	1.0

S

SAUCE

INFO/WEIGHT	Measure KCAL	FAT	KCAL	PROT	CARB	FAT	FIBRE
Fish, Nuoc Mam, Thai, Blue Dragon*	1 Tsp/5ml	7	0.0	145	5.9	30.9	0.1	0.0
Four Cheese, Asda*	½ Jar/155g	242	21.7	156	3.5	3.9	14.0	0.1
Four Cheese, Reduced Fat, Morrisons*	½ Tub/175g	161	9.5	92	6.1	4.8	5.4	0.5
Fruity, HP*	1 Tsp/6g	8	0.0	141	1.2	35.1	0.1	0.0
Garlic, Heinz*	1 Serving/10ml	32	3.0	323	1.0	12.1	29.9	1.2
Garlic, Lea & Perrins*	1 Tsp/6g	20	1.7	337	1.8	17.8	29.0	0.0
Green Peppercorn, Dry, Sainsbury's*	1 Tbsp/15ml	68	7.3	455	0.4	3.8	48.5	0.1
Green Tandoori, M & S*	1 Jar/385g	501	38.1	130	3.6	6.8	9.9	1.5
Green Thai, Loyd Grossman*	½ Jar/175g	182	11.2	104	1.6	10.0	6.4	0.8
Green Thai, Stir Fry, Fresh Ideas, Tesco*	1 Pack/50g	91	8.3	182	2.1	6.2	16.6	0.1
Green Thai, Stir Fry, Sainsbury's*	½ Pack/75g	112	8.0	149	1.2	11.9	10.7	1.0
Hearty Cumberland, Sausages Tonight, Knorr*	¼ Jar/127.3g	42	0.1	33	0.7	7.4	0.1	0.8
Hoi Sin, M & S*	½ Pot/50ml	80	1.0	160	3.2	31.8	2.0	2.2
Hoi Sin, Sharwood's*	1 Tbsp/15g	32	0.0	211	2.7	49.5	0.3	0.1
Hoi Sin, Stir Fry, Asda*	1 Serving/100g	165	0.8	165	2.6	36.9	0.8	1.0
Hoi Sin & Garlic, Blue Dragon*	1 Serving/60g	80	1.6	133	1.2	26.1	2.6	0.0
Hoi Sin & Spring Onion, Stir Fry, Sharwood's*	1 Jar/165g	196	1.5	119	1.3	26.5	0.9	0.8
Hoisin & Plum, Dipping, Finest, Tesco*	1 Serving/50g	78	0.3	156	2.3	35.3	0.6	1.4
Hoisin & Plum, Stir Fry, HL, Tesco*	1 Serving/250g	148	3.3	59	2.1	9.7	1.3	1.3
Hollandaise, Classic, for Fish, Schwartz*	1 Sachet/300g	456	49.2	152	0.7	0.4	16.4	2.0
Hollandaise, Classic, Knorr*	1 Serving/100ml	202	20.5	202	0.6	3.9	20.5	0.4
Hollandaise, Dry, M & S*	1oz/28g	115	12.2	410	0.9	3.6	43.6	0.5
Hollandaise, Dry, Maille*	1 Serving/30g	149	15.2	495	1.0	10.8	50.6	0.0
Hollandaise, Finest, Tesco*	1 Serving/98g	473	44.5	485	1.4	17.2	45.6	0.3
Hollandaise, Homemade, Average	1oz/28g	198	21.3	707	4.8	0.0	76.2	0.0
Hollandaise, M & S*	1 Serving/10g	41	4.4	410	0.9	3.6	43.6	0.5
Hollandaise, Sainsbury's*	1 Tbsp/15g	72	7.6	478	0.2	5.9	50.4	0.4
Honey & Coriander, Stir Fry, Blue Dragon*	1 Pack/120g	115	0.7	96	0.5	22.1	0.6	0.3
Honey & Mustard, Chicken Tonight, Knorr*	1 Serving/175g	186	8.2	106	0.8	15.1	4.7	0.6
Honey & Mustard, for Cooking, Asda*	1 Serving/200g	234	14.0	117	0.6	13.0	7.0	0.0
Honey & Mustard, Low Fat, Chicken Tonight, Knorr*	¼ Jar/125g	100	2.9	80	1.0	13.8	2.3	0.8
Horseradish, Colman's*	1 Tbsp/15ml	17	0.9	112	1.9	9.8	6.2	2.6
Horseradish, Creamed, Colman's*	1 Tsp/16g	37	2.1	229	4.3	21.4	13.3	0.0
Horseradish, Creamed, M & S*	1 Tsp/5g	16	1.5	325	2.4	12.1	29.3	2.5
Horseradish, Creamed, Waitrose*	1 Tbsp/16g	30	1.6	185	2.4	19.6	9.9	2.3
Horseradish, Creamy, Sainsbury's*	1 Tsp/5g	11	0.6	223	2.8	28.9	11.8	1.6
Horseradish, Hot, Tesco*	1 Tsp/5g	9	0.5	185	2.3	19.7	10.6	2.3
Horseradish, Sainsbury's*	1 Dtsp/10g	15	0.7	145	1.5	17.8	6.6	2.4
Horseradish Cream, Tesco*	1 Serving/15g	29	1.8	195	2.3	18.7	11.9	2.1
Hot Bean, Har Har Pickle Food Factory*	1 Tbp/10g	4	0.0	40	0.0	10.0	0.0	10.0
Hot Chilli, Asda*	1 Bottle/150ml	126	0.5	84	0.3	20.0	0.3	0.0
Hot Chilli, Sharwood's*	1 fl oz/30ml	36	0.2	120	0.5	29.4	0.6	1.3
Hot Pepper	1oz/28g	7	0.4	26	1.6	1.7	1.5	0.0
Hot Pepper, Encona*	1 Tsp/5ml	3	0.1	52	0.5	10.5	1.2	0.0
HP*	1 Tbsp/15g	18	0.0	119	1.1	27.1	0.2	0.0
Italian, Tomato & Mascarpone, Tesco*	½ Tub/175g	159	11.0	91	2.7	5.9	6.3	0.7
Italian Tomato & Herb, for Pasta, BGTY, Sainsbury's*	½ Jar/250g	138	0.8	55	2.1	10.9	0.3	0.0
Italian Tomato & Herb, Sainsbury's*	¼ Jar/126g	88	2.5	70	2.0	11.1	2.0	1.4
Italian Tomato & Mascarpone, Sainsbury's*	½ Tub/175g	158	10.2	90	2.6	6.8	5.8	1.2
Jalfrezi, Cooking, Asda*	1 Jar/570g	519	35.9	91	1.2	7.4	6.3	1.7
Jalfrezi, Cooking, Sainsbury's*	1 Serving/250g	160	6.0	64	1.0	9.6	2.4	1.7
Jalfrezi, Spice & Stir, Geeta's*	½ Jar/175g	156	11.2	89	1.4	6.5	6.4	1.4
Jamaican Jerk, Stir It Up, Chicken Tonight, Knorr*	1 Jar/80g	506	43.1	633	3.9	20.9	53.9	5.4

SAUCE

	Measure INFO/WEIGHT	per Measure KCAL	FAT	KCAL	PROT	CARB	FAT	FIBRE
Jambalaya, Cajun, Seasoned Pioneers*	1 Pack/400g	248	20.4	62	0.8	3.2	5.1	1.0
Jeera & Tamarind, Daal, Indian, Seasoned Pioneers*	1 Pouch/400g	228	12.0	57	1.8	7.2	3.0	1.6
Kaffir Lime Chilli & Basil, Stir Fry, Sainsbury's*	1 Serving/150g	158	9.6	105	1.2	10.6	6.4	1.0
Korma, Asda*	1 Serving/225g	434	33.8	193	2.5	12.0	15.0	2.2
Korma, Coconut & Cream, Mild, in Glass Jar, Patak's*	1 Serving/135g	235	19.8	174	1.3	9.1	14.7	0.8
Korma, Cooking, BGTY, Sainsbury's*	¼ Jar/125g	100	3.4	80	1.1	12.9	2.7	1.2
Korma, Cooking, HE, Tesco*	¼ Jar/125g	120	8.0	96	1.9	7.4	6.4	0.6
Korma, Indian Style, Iceland*	¼ Jar/112g	150	10.2	134	1.5	11.4	9.1	1.0
Korma, Sharwood's*	1 Serving/105g	150	10.3	143	1.4	12.2	9.8	1.8
Lemon & Ginger, Stir Fry, Finest, Tesco*	¼ Jar/85g	144	0.2	169	0.2	41.7	0.2	0.2
Lemon & Sesame, Stir Fry, Sharwood's*	1 Serving/100g	125	0.1	125	0.1	30.9	0.1	0.1
Lemon Pepper, Californian Style, Stir It Up, Knorr*	1 Serving/35g	231	20.8	659	5.2	26.1	59.3	2.7
Lime & Coriander, Tangy, for Fish, Schwartz*	1 Pack/300g	381	37.2	127	1.1	2.7	12.4	1.3
Lime Honey & Ginger, Stir Fry, Sharwood's*	1 Serving/50g	35	0.1	69	0.3	16.6	0.1	0.2
Mediterranean Vegetables, Stir in, BGTY, Sainsbury's*	1 Jar/150g	123	6.5	82	1.9	9.0	4.3	1.4
Mint, Baxters*	1oz/28g	17	0.1	62	1.7	13.2	0.3	0.0
Mint, Sainsbury's*	1 Dtsp/10g	13	0.0	126	2.5	28.7	0.1	4.0
Mint, SmartPrice, Asda*	1 Serving/5g	3	0.0	52	0.1	13.0	0.0	1.2
Mint Garden, Fresh, Tesco*	1 Tsp/5g	2	0.0	40	2.6	3.6	0.4	1.5
Moglai, Tomato & Fennel, Cooking, Patak's*	1 Jar/283g	374	25.2	132	3.1	9.7	8.9	1.8
Mornay, Cheese, Asda*	¼ Pot/71g	114	9.0	161	6.8	6.6	12.7	0.4
Mushroom, Creamy, Asda*	1 Serving/125g	76	4.6	61	0.8	6.0	3.7	0.5
Mushroom, Creamy, Chicken Tonight, Knorr*	¼ Jar/125g	101	7.9	81	0.8	5.4	6.3	0.3
Mushroom, Creamy, Tesco*	½ Pot/175g	142	10.2	81	1.5	5.6	5.8	0.4
Mushroom, Schwartz*	1 Pack/170g	207	19.2	122	1.2	3.9	11.3	0.5
Mushroom, TTD, Sainsbury's*	1 Serving/150g	251	23.7	167	2.6	3.5	15.8	1.4
Mushroom & Garlic, 95% Fat Free, Homepride*	1 Serving/220g	154	9.2	70	0.9	7.0	4.2	0.3
Napoletana, Fresh, Sainsbury's*	½ Pot/150g	95	4.5	63	1.7	7.3	3.0	2.3
Napoletana, Italian, Tesco*	1 Pot/350g	179	4.2	51	1.5	8.5	1.2	1.0
Olive & Tomato, Stir Through, Sacla*	Spoonful/30g	54	5.3	181	2.1	3.3	17.7	5.4
Onion, Made with Semi-Skimmed Milk	1 Serving/60g	52	3.0	86	2.9	8.4	5.0	0.4
Onion, Made with Skimmed Milk	1 Serving/60g	46	2.4	77	2.9	8.4	4.0	0.4
Orange & Dill Sauce, for Fish, Zesty, Schwartz*	1 Pack/300g	180	1.5	60	0.4	13.5	0.5	0.5
Oriental Sweet & Sour, Express, Uncle Ben's*	1 Serving/170g	221	3.2	130	0.8	27.5	1.9	0.0
Oyster, Blue Dragon*	1 Tsp/5ml	6	0.0	121	3.4	26.9	0.0	0.0
Oyster, Stir Fry, Sainsbury's*	1 Tbsp/15g	9	0.0	61	1.6	13.3	0.1	0.2
Oyster & Garlic, Stir Fry, Straight to Wok, Amoy*	½ Pack/50g	98	1.5	195	4.9	37.0	3.0	0.0
Oyster & Spring Onion, Stir Fry, Blue Dragon*	1 Serving/80g	74	0.6	92	1.6	19.9	0.7	1.1
Oyster Flavoured, Amoy*	1 Tsp/5ml	5	0.0	108	2.0	25.0	0.0	0.0
Pad Thai, Blue Dragon*	1 Serving/50g	111	3.0	222	2.0	40.0	6.0	0.7
Panang, Thai, Seasoned Pioneers*	1 Pouch/400g	280	18.0	70	1.5	5.6	4.5	0.6
Parsley, Fresh, Sainsbury's*	½ Pot/150g	117	7.7	78	2.0	5.9	5.1	0.5
Parsley, Instant, Dry, Asda*	1 Serving/23g	82	1.6	355	7.0	66.0	7.0	4.4
Pasta Bake, Cheese & Bacon, Homepride*	1 Jar/500g	395	28.0	79	2.2	4.8	5.6	0.5
Pasta Bake, Creamy Tomato & Bacon, Homepride*	1 Serving/110g	99	6.9	90	1.9	6.5	6.3	0.0
Pasta Bake, Creamy Tomato & Herb, Homepride*	1 Serving/125g	128	8.8	102	1.5	8.3	7.0	0.9
Peanut, Sainsbury's*	1 Sachet/70g	185	9.2	264	1.9	34.7	13.1	1.6
Peking, Sizzle & Stir, Chicken Tonight, Knorr*	1 Jar/510g	617	45.4	121	0.8	9.4	8.9	1.6
Peking Lemon, Stir Fry, Blue Dragon*	1 Serving/35g	58	0.7	166	0.3	36.8	1.9	0.1
Pepper, Creamy, Schwartz*	1 Pack/170g	116	9.2	68	1.5	3.4	5.4	1.0
Pepper, Creamy, Tesco*	1 Serving/85ml	128	11.4	151	1.2	6.4	13.4	0.5
Pepper & Brandy, Pour Over, Knorr*	1oz/28g	29	2.5	104	1.0	4.0	9.0	0.0
Pepper & Tomato, Spicy, Stir Through, M & S*	½ Jar/95g	166	14.6	175	1.6	7.5	15.4	0.0

SAUCE

	Measure INFO/WEIGHT	per Measure KCAL	FAT	KCAL	PROT	CARB	FAT	FIBRE
Peppercorn, Creamy, Asda*	¼ Jar/137g	137	11.0	100	1.1	6.0	8.0	0.2
Peppercorn, Creamy, Chicken Tonight, Knorr*	¼ Jar/125g	110	9.8	88	0.3	3.8	7.8	0.4
Peppercorn, with Fresh Cream & Brandy, M & S*	½ Pack/100g	110	8.2	110	3.1	5.6	8.2	0.3
Peri-Peri, Hot, Nando's*	1oz/28g	18	0.7	63	0.1	4.5	2.7	1.4
Pesto, Basil, M & S*	1 Serving/65g	348	30.5	535	7.5	20.7	46.9	1.4
Pesto, Green, Asda*	1 Tsp/5g	21	2.2	429	4.7	3.5	44.0	1.4
Pesto, Green, BGTY, Sainsbury's*	1 Serving/50g	71	5.6	142	5.8	5.0	11.1	1.7
Pesto, Green, Fresh, Sainsbury's*	1 Serving/60g	328	31.7	546	9.4	8.3	52.8	0.1
Pesto, Green, Fresh, Tesco*	1oz/28g	141	13.4	505	6.5	12.2	48.0	0.1
Pesto, Green, Italiano, Tesco*	1 Serving/50g	251	24.5	502	9.6	5.6	49.0	1.2
Pesto, Green, Romano*	½ Jar/50g	234	23.1	467	5.1	7.8	46.2	0.0
Pesto, Green, Sainsbury's*	1oz/28g	126	12.0	451	5.9	10.1	43.0	2.0
Pesto, Green, Tesco*	¼ Jar/47.5g	192	20.0	405	5.6	0.6	42.2	4.4
Pesto, Green Basil, Stir-In, Fresh, Chilled, Waitrose*	½ Pot/72.5g	324	31.5	447	8.8	5.2	43.4	1.2
Pesto, Italian, Co-Op*	1 Tsp/10g	43	4.4	430	5.0	4.0	44.0	2.0
Pesto, Italian, Waitrose*	1 Serving/50g	179	18.9	358	3.7	1.1	37.7	2.8
Pesto, Knorr*	1 Serving/100g	216	21.1	216	2.7	3.8	21.1	0.0
Pesto, Red, Italian, Tesco*	1 Serving/37.5g	128	11.5	340	8.2	8.2	30.6	1.2
Pesto, Red, M & S*	1oz/28g	93	9.3	331	3.6	6.9	33.2	3.5
Pesto, Red, Morrisons*	1 Tbsp/15g	68	6.8	452	5.9	5.2	45.3	1.9
Pesto, Red, Tesco*	¼ Jar/50g	163	15.2	325	5.6	6.3	30.3	6.0
Pesto, Red Pepper, Barilla*	1 Serving/25g	91	7.3	364	2.8	22.9	29.0	0.0
Pimenton Bravas, Spanish, Seasoned Pioneers*	1 Pouch/400g	196	12.4	49	1.0	4.1	3.1	0.8
Plum & Ginger, Stir Fry, Asda*	½ Jar/97g	94	0.7	97	0.7	22.0	0.7	0.3
Prawn Cocktail, Frank Cooper*	1 Tbsp/15g	47	4.0	316	0.8	18.3	26.7	0.1
Puttanesca, Fresh, Waitrose*	½ Pot/176.1g	118	7.7	67	1.8	6.2	4.4	1.2
Red Pepper, Fresh, Asda*	¼ Pot/82g	35	1.0	43	1.4	6.8	1.2	1.1
Red Pepper, GFY, Asda*	1 Serving/100g	43	1.1	43	1.2	7.0	1.1	0.0
Red Thai, Loyd Grossman*	1oz/28g	35	1.8	125	2.8	13.7	6.5	1.5
Red Wine, Cook in, Homepride*	¼ Can/98g	47	0.6	48	0.5	10.1	0.6	0.0
Red Wine & Herb, Safeway*	1 Jar/680g	347	10.2	51	1.1	8.3	1.5	0.5
Red Wine Cooking., Homepride*	1 Serving/250ml	115	1.5	46	0.4	9.8	0.6	0.0
Roasted Peanut Satay, Stir Fry Sensations, Amoy*	1 Pouch/160g	354	19.8	221	4.7	21.9	12.4	1.0
Roasted Vegetable, Stir in, Dolmio*	1oz/28g	38	2.9	135	1.5	9.1	10.3	0.0
Rogan Josh, Medium, Sharwood's*	½ Jar/210g	151	7.6	72	1.4	8.6	3.6	0.5
Rogan Josh, Sharwood's*	½ Jar/210g	149	8.0	71	1.5	7.7	3.8	3.5
Royal Korma, Tilda*	1 Pack/400ml	824	73.2	206	1.9	8.4	18.3	0.7
Satay, Indonesian, Sharwood's*	1oz/28g	45	3.0	159	5.4	10.0	10.8	5.1
Satay, Stir Fry & Dipping, Finest, Tesco*	1 Tsp/5g	22	1.7	432	9.0	20.7	34.8	2.7
Sausage Casserole, Cook in, Homepride*	½ Jar/250g	93	0.5	37	0.7	8.0	0.2	0.6
Seafood, 25% Less Fat, Tesco*	1 Tsp/5g	17	1.4	344	2.7	18.2	28.5	0.3
Seafood, Asda*	1 Serving/10g	45	4.2	448	1.6	16.0	42.0	0.2
Seafood, BGTY, Sainsbury's*	1 Serving/50g	94	5.6	188	1.4	20.3	11.2	0.3
Seafood, Colman's*	1 Serving/14ml	41	3.2	296	0.9	21.5	22.9	0.4
Seafood, GFY, Asda*	1 Dstp/10ml	31	2.7	313	0.6	17.0	27.0	0.0
Seafood, Organic, Simply Delicious*	1 Serving/35g	192	18.9	549	2.3	13.6	53.9	0.3
Seafood, Sainsbury's*	1 Tbsp/15g	50	4.2	330	0.7	17.6	28.2	0.1
Seafood, Tesco*	1 Serving/10g	47	4.4	465	1.8	15.6	43.5	0.3
Smoked Bacon & Tomato, Stir in, Dolmio*	½ Tub/75g	124	9.6	165	5.5	6.9	12.8	0.8
Soy, Average	1 Tsp/5ml	3	0.0	64	8.7	8.3	0.0	0.0
Soy, Dark, Amoy*	1 Tsp/5ml	5	0.0	106	0.9	25.6	0.0	0.0
Soy, Light, Amoy*	1 Tbsp/15g	6	0.0	40	2.5	7.5	0.0	0.0
Soy, Light, Asda*	1 Tbsp/15ml	7	0.0	47	0.8	11.0	0.0	0.0

S

SAUCE

	INFO/WEIGHT	KCAL	FAT	KCAL	PROT	CARB	FAT	FIBRE
Soy, Light, Sharwood's*	1 Tsp/5ml	2	0.0	37	2.7	6.4	0.2	0.0
Soy, Naturally Brewed, Kikkoman*	1 Tbsp/15g	11	0.0	74	10.3	8.1	0.0	0.0
Soy, Reduced Salt, Amoy*	1 Tsp/5ml	3	0.0	56	4.0	10.0	0.0	0.0
Soy, Rich, Sharwood's*	1 Tsp/5ml	4	0.0	79	3.1	16.6	0.4	0.0
Soy Ginger & Garlic, Stir Fry, Asda*	1 Pack/100ml	82	0.3	82	0.8	19.0	0.3	0.0
Soya, Japanese, Waitrose*	1 Tbsp/15g	11	0.1	74	7.7	9.4	0.6	0.8
Spanish Chicken, Chicken Tonight, Knorr*	½ Jar/250g	115	3.5	46	1.5	7.0	1.4	0.6
Spiced Tomato Tagine, Sainsbury's*	1 Jar/355g	227	5.7	64	1.7	10.6	1.6	4.3
Spicy Sweet & Sour, Sharwood's*	1 Serving/138g	142	0.7	103	0.7	23.8	0.5	0.4
Spicy Szechuan, Safe To Eat*	1 Pouch/400g	124	2.4	31	1.0	4.8	0.6	0.3
Spicy Szechuan Tomato, Stir Fry, Sharwood's*	½ Jar/97.5g	77	0.3	79	1.3	17.9	0.3	0.8
Sticky Ribz, Ainsley Harriott*	1 Serving/50g	107	0.1	214	0.4	52.2	0.1	0.0
Stir Fry, Chinese, Tesco*	1 Pack/125g	464	40.7	371	1.9	14.2	32.6	1.3
Stroganoff, Mushroom, Creamy, M & S*	1 Serving/75g	86	6.9	115	3.3	4.8	9.2	0.6
Sun Dried Tomato, Heinz*	1 Serving/10ml	7	0.1	73	1.5	14.9	0.6	0.9
Sun Dried Tomato, Mozzarella & Basil, Safeway*	½ Pot/159.1g	175	10.7	110	3.5	8.7	6.7	1.4
Sun Dried Tomato, Stir-In, Dolmio*	½ Pot/75g	115	8.5	153	1.7	11.1	11.3	1.0
Swedish Mustard & Dill, Safeway*	1 Serving/20g	32	2.0	162	17.1	1.5	9.8	0.2
Sweet & Sour, Aromatic, Stir Fry Sensations, Amoy*	1 Pack/160g	312	0.5	195	0.4	46.8	0.3	0.8
Sweet & Sour, Chinese, Sainsbury's*	½ Jar/150g	222	0.2	148	0.2	36.6	0.1	0.1
Sweet & Sour, Classic, Canned, Homepride*	1 Can/500g	440	0.5	88	0.3	21.5	0.1	0.5
Sweet & Sour, Cook In, Glass Jar, Homepride*	1 Jar/500g	335	0.5	67	0.3	16.2	0.1	0.5
Sweet & Sour, Cooking, Chinese, Sainsbury's*	¼ Jar/125g	155	0.1	124	0.6	30.1	0.1	0.7
Sweet & Sour, Cooking, HL, Tesco*	1/3 Jar/170g	46	0.3	27	1.1	5.1	0.2	3.9
Sweet & Sour, Extra Pineapple, Uncle Ben's*	1 Serving/165g	144	0.0	87	0.3	21.4	0.0	0.0
Sweet & Sour, Fresh, Safeway*	1 Sachet/50g	101	2.6	201	0.9	37.8	5.1	0.3
Sweet & Sour, GFY, Asda*	½ Jar/163.8g	77	0.3	47	0.4	11.0	0.2	0.3
Sweet & Sour, HL, Tesco*	1 Jar/510g	326	0.5	64	0.4	15.4	0.1	0.5
Sweet & Sour, Just Stir Fry, Sainsbury's*	1 Pouch/150ml	257	8.9	171	0.6	29.0	5.9	2.0
Sweet & Sour, Light, Uncle Ben's*	1 Serving/200g	120	0.1	60	0.6	14.2	0.0	0.0
Sweet & Sour, Oriental, Chicken Tonight, Knorr*	½ Jar/262g	217	2.6	83	0.4	20.8	1.0	0.5
Sweet & Sour, Original, Uncle Ben's*	1 Pack/300g	264	0.0	88	0.5	21.7	0.0	0.0
Sweet & Sour, PB, Waitrose*	1 Serving/175g	140	0.4	80	0.6	18.9	0.2	1.1
Sweet & Sour, Peking Style, Finest, Tesco*	1 Serving/175g	147	0.2	84	0.6	20.1	0.1	0.5
Sweet & Sour, Spicy, Uncle Ben's*	1 Jar/400g	364	0.4	91	0.6	22.1	0.1	0.0
Sweet & Sour, Stir Fry, Asda*	1 Serving/63g	146	3.2	232	0.8	46.0	5.0	0.0
Sweet & Sour, Stir Fry, Blue Dragon*	1 Sachet/120g	137	1.3	114	0.6	25.6	1.1	0.6
Sweet & Sour, Stir Fry, M & S*	1 Pack/120g	150	0.5	125	0.7	29.8	0.4	1.3
Sweet & Sour, Stir Fry, Sharwood's*	1 Jar 160g	168	0.8	105	0.6	24.5	0.5	0.8
Sweet & Sour, Stir Fry, Tesco*	½ Jar/222g	164	0.4	74	0.6	17.0	0.2	0.4
Sweet & Sour, Stir Fry, Waitrose*	1 Serving/50ml	94	2.2	187	1.2	35.6	4.4	1.8
Sweet & Sour, Take-Away	1oz/28g	44	1.0	157	0.2	32.8	3.4	0.0
Sweet Barbecue, Deliciously Good, Homepride*	1/3 Jar/149g	110	3.3	74	1.4	12.0	2.2	1.2
Sweet Chilli, Asda*	1 Tbsp/15ml	18	0.2	123	0.4	30.0	0.1	0.8
Sweet Chilli, Dipping, Thai, Amoy*	1 Serving/10g	14	0.3	142	0.5	34.2	2.8	0.3
Sweet Chilli, Sharwood's*	1 Bottle/150ml	326	0.6	217	0.7	52.8	0.4	1.7
Sweet Chilli, Stir Fry, Additions, Tesco*	1 Serving/50g	106	3.8	211	0.3	35.2	7.6	0.6
Sweet Chilli & Coriander, Sizzling, Homepride*	1 Serving/100g	51	0.2	51	0.7	11.5	0.2	0.0
Sweet Chilli & Garlic, Stir Fry & Dipping, Tesco*	½ Jar/95ml	78	0.0	82	0.3	20.1	0.0	0.1
Sweet Chilli & Lemon Grass, Stir Fry, Sharwood's*	1 Serving/155g	127	0.2	82	0.3	19.7	0.1	0.3
Sweet Chilli & Lime, Chinatown, Knorr*	1 Jar/525g	635	17.3	121	0.6	22.0	3.3	0.5
Sweet Chilli & Red Pepper, Sharwood's*	1/3 Jar/141g	99	0.1	70	0.6	16.6	0.1	1.1
Sweet Chilli Dipping, M & S*	1 Tbsp/15g	34	0.1	225	0.9	53.2	0.7	0.6

S

SAUCE

	INFO/WEIGHT	KCAL	FAT	KCAL	PROT	CARB	FAT	FIBRE
Sweet Pepper, Stir in, Dolmio*	½ Pot/75g	103	7.7	137	1.5	9.7	10.3	0.0
Sweet Soy & Sesame, Uncle Ben's*	1 Serving/100g	110	1.7	110	0.7	23.0	1.7	0.0
Szechuan, Cooking, Safeway*	1 Jar/440g	458	22.0	104	1.3	13.0	5.0	1.2
Szechuan, Spicy Tomato, Stir Fry, Blue Dragon*	1 Sachet/120g	151	6.7	126	1.3	17.6	5.6	2.0
Szechuan, Stir Fry, Sharwood's*	1 Jar/150g	126	1.7	84	3.0	15.5	1.1	0.4
Tabasco	1 Tsp/5ml	1	0.0	12	1.3	0.8	0.8	0.6
Tamarind & Lime, Stir Fry, Sainsbury's*	1 Serving/75g	88	5.6	117	1.1	11.4	7.4	0.8
Tartare	1oz/28g	84	6.9	299	1.3	17.9	24.6	0.0
Tartare, Baxters*	1oz/28g	144	14.9	515	1.0	8.0	53.3	0.3
Tartare, Rich, Colman's*	1 Serving/20ml	57	4.6	284	1.2	17.0	23.0	0.6
Tartare, Sainsbury's*	1 Serving/20ml	94	9.8	469	0.4	5.8	49.0	1.0
Tartare, Tesco*	1 Tbsp/15g	43	3.3	287	1.5	19.6	21.8	0.3
Teriyaki, Asda*	1 Serving/98g	99	0.1	101	2.1	23.0	0.1	0.0
Teriyaki, Stir Fry, Blue Dragon*	½ Pack/60g	104	0.0	173	2.0	28.6	0.0	0.0
Teriyaki, Stir Fry, Sharwood's*	1 Jar/150g	144	0.5	96	0.9	22.5	0.3	0.3
Thai, Ginger & Lemon Grass, Stir Fry, Sainsbury's*	½ Jar/160g	144	9.0	90	1.9	8.1	5.6	1.3
Thai Chilli, Dipping, Sainsbury's*	1 Tbsp/15g	30	0.0	201	0.2	49.8	0.0	5.0
Thai Chilli, Sharwood's*	1 Bottle/150ml	264	0.5	176	0.2	43.0	0.3	0.5
Thai Fish, Nuoc Mam, Amoy*	1 Tbsp/15ml	12	0.0	80	13.4	6.7	0.0	0.0
Thai Green, Sainsbury's*	¼ Pack/125g	170	11.9	136	1.8	10.8	9.5	2.1
Thai Satay, Sharwood's*	1oz/28g	160	13.4	573	17.2	18.0	48.0	6.3
Tikka, BFY, Morrisons*	½ Jar/237.5g	259	8.1	109	2.3	17.2	3.4	1.3
Tikka, Cooking, BGTY, Sainsbury's*	1 Jar/500g	370	9.5	74	1.2	12.9	1.9	0.3
Tikka, Indian Style, Iceland*	1 Serving/225g	284	16.9	126	1.7	12.9	7.5	2.2
Tikka Masala, 98% Fat Free, Homepride*	1oz/28g	14	0.5	49	1.4	7.9	1.7	0.8
Tikka Masala, Cooking, Sharwood's*	1 Tsp/2g	2	0.2	122	1.2	11.9	7.8	0.9
Tikka Masala, Fresh, Somerfield*	1 Pack/250g	308	20.0	123	3.0	10.0	8.0	0.0
Tikka Masala, GFY, Asda*	½ Jar/250g	190	8.0	76	2.9	9.0	3.2	0.5
Tikka Masala, Hot & Spicy, in Glass Jar, Patak's*	1 Serving/140g	147	11.1	105	1.9	6.6	7.9	1.1
Tikka Masala, Jar, Sharwood's*	1 Jar/435g	492	33.1	113	1.4	9.6	7.6	1.4
Tikka Masala, Lemon & Coriander, Canned, Patak's*	1 Serving/70g	120	9.1	172	2.5	11.0	13.0	1.1
Tikka Masala, Sizzle & Stir, Chicken Tonight, Knorr*	1/3 Jar/168g	336	29.1	200	2.0	8.4	17.3	2.6
Tikka Masala, Sizzle & Stir, Knorr*	1 Jar/455g	851	75.1	187	1.2	8.3	16.5	3.9
Tikka Masala, Spicy, Sharwood's*	1 Jar/420g	449	29.8	107	1.2	9.6	7.1	0.1
Tikka Masala for One, Express, Uncle Ben's*	1 Sachet/170g	168	10.7	99	1.5	9.0	6.3	0.0
Toffee, GFY, Asda*	1 Serving/5g	15	0.1	306	2.2	68.0	2.8	0.0
Toffee, Luxury, Rowse*	1 Serving/20g	67	0.7	336	1.9	73.9	3.7	0.4
Toffee Fudge, Sainsbury's*	1 Serving/40g	134	1.5	336	1.9	73.9	3.7	0.4
Tomato, Organic, Heinz*	1 Tsp/5g	5	0.0	105	1.3	24.0	0.1	0.9
Tomato, Pizza Topping, Napolina*	1 Serving/70g	34	1.5	49	0.9	6.3	2.2	0.6
Tomato & Basil, Cooking, BGTY, Sainsbury's*	1 Jar/500g	335	6.5	67	2.6	11.3	1.3	0.7
Tomato & Basil, Eat Smart, Safeway*	1 Serving/250g	150	6.3	60	1.7	7.4	2.5	1.4
Tomato & Basil, Fresh, Organic, Waitrose*	¼ Pot/175g	77	3.0	44	1.0	6.2	1.7	0.8
Tomato & Basil, Tesco*	½ Jar/175g	84	5.8	48	0.7	3.8	3.3	0.8
Tomato & Garlic, for Pasta, Asda*	¼ Jar/125g	80	2.9	64	2.7	8.0	2.3	1.1
Tomato & Marscapone, Finest, Tesco*	1 Serving/350g	270	17.5	77	2.7	5.4	5.0	0.8
Tomato & Marscapone, Italiano, Tesco*	1 Serving/175g	194	15.2	111	2.8	5.4	8.7	0.6
Tomato & Mascarpone, BGTY, Sainsbury's*	1 Pot/300g	150	9.0	50	2.0	3.6	3.0	3.6
Tomato & Mascarpone, Fresh, Tesco*	½ Pot/175g	207	15.2	118	2.8	7.1	8.7	0.6
Tomato & Mascarpone, Light Choices, Tesco*	½ Pot/175g	77	3.5	44	1.6	4.9	2.0	0.8
Tomato & Onion, Cook in, Homepride*	1 Can/390g	183	2.0	47	0.9	9.8	0.5	0.0
Tomato & Roasted Garlic, Stir in, Dolmio*	½ Pack/75g	94	7.7	125	1.2	7.7	10.2	0.0
Tomato & Worcester, Table, Lea & Perrins*	1 Serving/10g	10	0.1	102	0.8	23.0	0.5	0.7

	Measure INFO/WEIGHT	per Measure KCAL	FAT	Nutrition Values per 100g / 100ml KCAL	PROT	CARB	FAT	FIBRE
SAUCE								
Tomato Frito, Heinz*	1 Serving/16g	13	0.6	80	1.5	9.7	3.9	0.8
Vine Ripened Tomato & Aromatic Basil, Discovery*	1 Serving/125g	161	9.0	129	1.8	14.3	7.2	0.0
Vongole, Sainsbury's*	½ Pot/150g	107	4.5	71	3.1	7.8	3.0	1.9
Watercress, & Stilton, Creamy, for Fish, Schwartz*	1 Pack/300g	141	12.3	47	0.6	2.0	4.1	0.7
Watercress, for Fish, M & S*	½ Pack/90g	144	13.4	160	4.4	2.4	14.9	0.5
Watercress & Creme Fraiche, COU, M & S*	½ Pack/153.8g	100	2.8	65	3.2	9.2	1.8	0.5
White, for Lasagne, Dolmio*	1 Jar/470g	451	34.3	96	0.6	7.0	7.3	0.0
White, Savoury, Made with Semi-Skimmed Milk	1oz/28g	36	2.2	128	4.2	11.1	7.8	0.2
White, Savoury, Made with Whole Milk	1oz/28g	42	2.9	150	4.1	10.9	10.3	0.2
White Granules, Sauce in Seconds, Dry, Asda*	1 Pack/57g	237	6.8	415	3.7	73.0	12.0	0.9
White Wine, Chardonnay, M & S*	1 Serving/160ml	184	16.0	115	1.4	4.6	10.0	0.9
White Wine, Dry, Alcohol Boiled Off	1 Serving/125ml	4	0.0	3	0.1	0.6	0.0	0.0
White Wine & Cream, Homepride*	1 Serving/150g	122	6.8	81	1.1	9.0	4.5	0.3
White Wine & Mushroom, BGTY, Sainsbury's*	¼ Jar/125g	81	2.5	65	2.8	9.0	2.0	0.3
White Wine & Tarragon, French, for Fish, Schwartz*	½ Pack/150g	186	16.7	124	1.1	5.0	11.1	0.8
Wild Mushroom, Finest, Tesco*	½ Pack/175g	158	11.9	90	1.9	5.2	6.8	0.4
Wild Mushroom & Creme Fraiche, NCGF Co*	½ Carton/150g	69	4.7	46	1.7	2.8	3.1	0.7
Worcestershire, Average	1 Tsp/5g	3	0.0	65	1.4	15.5	0.1	0.0
Worcestershire, Lea & Perrins*	1 Tsp/5ml	4	0.0	88	1.1	22.0	0.0	0.0
Yellow Bean, Stir Fry, Sainsbury's*	½ Jar/100g	126	1.3	126	1.8	26.7	1.3	0.8
Yellow Bean, Stir Fry, Sharwood's*	½ Jar/97.5g	101	0.6	104	1.1	23.5	0.6	0.1
Yellow Bean & Cashew, Tesco*	½ Jar/210g	170	6.1	81	1.6	11.9	2.9	0.3
SAUCE MIX								
Bacon & Mushroom Tagliatelle, Schwartz*	1 Pack/33g	110	1.0	333	7.5	69.2	2.9	8.3
Beef Bourguignon, Colman's*	1/3 Pack/13.3g	40	0.2	308	4.9	68.6	1.6	2.2
Beef Stroganoff, Colman's*	1 Pack/40g	140	3.6	350	11.6	56.1	8.9	2.7
Bombay Potatoes, Schwartz*	1 Pack/33g	84	4.0	254	16.1	20.1	12.1	31.1
Bread, Colman's*	1 Pack/40g	131	0.4	327	11.4	67.9	1.1	3.2
Bread, Knorr*	½ Pint/40g	177	9.3	442	7.9	49.9	23.3	2.1
Cajun Chicken, Schwartz*	1 Pack/38g	108	0.5	285	6.4	61.9	1.3	0.5
Cheddar Cheese, Colman's*	1 Pack/40g	163	6.2	407	18.3	48.8	15.4	1.2
Cheddar Cheese, Schwartz*	1 Pack/40g	144	3.0	361	18.4	55.1	7.4	2.3
Cheese, Knorr*	1 Pack/58g	132	2.8	227	7.8	38.0	4.9	1.8
Cheese, Made Up, Somerfield*	1 Serving/65ml	53	1.8	81	4.7	9.3	2.8	0.4
Chicken Chasseur, Colman's*	1 Pack/45g	128	0.7	284	8.0	59.2	1.6	3.8
Chicken Chasseur, Schwartz*	1 Pack/40g	126	1.8	316	9.6	59.1	4.6	6.8
Chicken Supreme, Colman's*	½ Pack/20g	72	1.8	358	12.1	56.7	9.2	2.4
Chilli Con Carne, Hot, Colman's*	1 Serving/13g	41	0.4	317	10.4	62.4	2.9	7.0
Chilli Con Carne, Schwartz*	1 Serving/10g	29	0.4	293	7.9	57.2	3.6	9.5
Coq Au Vin, Colman's*	1 Pack/50g	151	0.9	301	5.6	65.6	1.8	3.3
Cream, for Meatballs, Ikea*	1 Pack/40g	179	9.4	448	9.6	49.2	23.6	0.0
Creamy Cheese & Bacon, for Pasta, Colman's*	1 Pack/50g	182	4.1	364	16.7	56.1	8.1	1.9
Creamy Pepper & Mushroom, Colman's*	½ Pack/12.5g	43	0.5	332	9.6	64.6	3.8	3.0
for Garlic Mushrooms, Creamy, Schwartz*	1 Pack/35g	109	1.6	311	7.6	59.7	4.7	4.2
Four Cheese, Colman's*	1 Pack/35g	127	3.9	362	17.1	48.4	11.1	1.8
Hollandaise, Colman's*	1 Pack/27g	100	3.0	372	6.4	61.6	11.1	1.8
Hollandaise, Schwartz*	1 Pack/25g	99	3.2	394	10.6	59.2	12.8	3.7
Lamb Hotpot, Colman's*	1 Serving/13.5g	40	0.2	297	6.9	63.3	1.7	2.1
Lasagne, Mediterranean Vegetable, Schwartz*	1 Serving/29.9g	79	1.3	263	9.3	46.0	4.4	15.2
Lemon Butter, for Fish, Schwartz*	1 Serving/9g	32	0.7	357	6.1	65.3	8.0	5.8
Mexican Chilli Chicken, Schwartz*	1 Pack/35g	105	2.0	299	7.0	55.1	5.6	12.0
Onion, Colman's*	½ Pack/17g	55	0.2	325	9.1	69.4	1.3	4.8
Parsley, Colman's*	1 Pack/20g	63	0.3	314	7.2	67.9	1.5	3.7

S

	Measure INFO/WEIGHT	per Measure KCAL	FAT	Nutrition Values per 100g / 100ml KCAL	PROT	CARB	FAT	FIBRE
SAUCE MIX								
Parsley, Creamy, Schwartz*	1 Pack/26g	96	2.8	371	11.5	57.2	10.7	3.8
Parsley & Chive, for Fish, Schwartz*	1 Serving/19g	66	1.6	348	9.0	58.9	8.5	7.7
Pepper, Creamy, Colman's*	1 Pack/25g	88	2.8	352	13.0	50.0	11.0	0.0
Pepper, Creamy, Schwartz*	1 Pack/25g	86	1.7	342	17.9	52.0	6.9	7.0
Peppercorn, Mild, Creamy, Schwartz*	1 Pack/25g	88	2.2	352	13.8	55.0	8.6	5.0
Pork & Mushroom, Creamy, Schwartz*	¼ Pack/10g	29	0.4	289	8.6	54.7	4.0	12.1
Savoury Mince, Schwartz*	1 Pack/35g	109	0.7	310	14.6	58.3	2.0	1.8
Shepherd's Pie, Schwartz*	1 Pack/38g	104	1.0	273	7.9	54.4	2.6	11.1
Spaghetti Bolognese, Colman's*	1 Pack/45g	135	0.4	300	8.9	64.1	0.9	5.2
Spaghetti Bolognese, Schwartz*	1 Pack/40g	114	0.6	285	9.2	59.0	1.6	7.0
Spaghetti Carbonara, Schwartz*	½ Pack/16g	67	3.2	421	10.4	49.4	20.1	7.2
Stroganoff, Mushroom, Schwartz*	1 Pack/35g	113	1.9	324	10.0	59.2	5.3	9.6
Sweet & Sour, Colman's*	1 Pack/40g	133	0.2	333	2.6	79.9	0.4	2.2
Thai Green Curry, Schwartz*	1 Pack/41g	137	3.3	333	7.6	57.6	8.1	13.0
Thai Red Curry, Schwartz*	1 Serving/20g	68	1.4	342	5.9	63.5	7.1	7.6
Three Cheese, for Vegetables, Schwartz*	1 Pack/40g	168	8.2	421	17.4	41.7	20.5	4.8
Tuna & Mushroom Pasta Melt, Schwartz*	1 Pack/40.1g	122	2.8	304	10.2	49.7	7.1	7.7
Tuna & Pasta Bake, Colman's*	1 Pack/45g	144	2.4	319	10.4	57.1	5.4	5.2
Tuna Napolitana, Schwartz*	1 Pack/30g	107	3.9	357	10.3	49.6	13.1	0.5
White, Dry Weight, Bisto*	1 Serving/10g	50	2.8	496	3.2	57.4	28.2	0.4
White, Made Up with Semi-Skimmed Milk	1oz/28g	20	0.7	73	4.0	9.6	2.4	0.0
White, Made Up with Skimmed Milk	1oz/28g	17	0.3	59	4.0	9.6	0.9	0.0
White, Savoury, Colman's*	1 Pack/25g	84	0.7	335	10.7	66.5	2.9	2.6
White, Savoury, Knorr*	½ Pack/16g	46	0.9	290	7.8	52.2	5.6	5.2
White Wine, with Herbs, Creamy, Schwartz*	1 Pack/26g	86	1.7	330	8.0	60.0	6.5	9.1
Wholegrain Mustard, Creamy, Schwartz*	1 Pack/25g	93	2.8	370	12.9	54.4	11.2	7.5
SAUERKRAUT								
Average	1oz/28g	4	0.0	13	1.3	1.9	0.1	1.1
SAUSAGE								
& Bacon, Wrap, Asda*	1 Wrap/25g	63	4.2	252	15.9	9.0	16.9	1.3
Beef, Average	1 Sausage/60g	151	11.1	252	14.5	7.0	18.5	0.6
Beef, with Onion & Red Wine, Finest, Tesco*	1 Sausage/63g	117	6.9	185	13.2	8.5	10.9	1.2
Billy Bear, Kids, Tesco*	1 Slice/20g	37	2.2	185	13.7	7.5	11.2	0.4
Bockwurst, Average	1 Sausage/45g	114	10.4	253	10.8	0.8	23.0	0.0
Bratwurst, Frozen, Lidl*	1 Sausage/80g	235	21.4	294	12.8	0.5	26.8	0.0
Cambridge Gluten Free, Waitrose*	1 Sausage/56.8g	121	9.3	213	14.6	1.9	16.3	1.3
Cheese & Leek, Tesco*	1 Sausage/55g	135	7.5	246	6.9	24.0	13.6	1.7
Chicken, Manor Farm*	1 Sausage/65g	126	8.1	194	13.7	6.6	12.5	1.2
Chicken & Tarragon, Butchers Choice, Sainsbury's*	1 Sausage/47g	106	6.8	225	18.1	5.8	14.4	0.2
Chicken & Turkey, Morrisons*	1 Sausage/56.6g	86	4.1	152	16.0	5.8	7.2	1.1
Chilli Beef, Boston Style, Waitrose*	1 Sausage/66.5g	136	9.8	203	14.7	3.4	14.6	0.9
Chipolata, Average	1 Sausage/28g	81	6.5	291	12.1	8.7	23.1	0.7
Chipolata, Chicken & Sweet Chilli, TTD, Sainsbury's*	1 Chipolata/38g	77	5.0	206	18.4	5.4	13.3	1.2
Chipolata, Lamb & Rosemary, Tesco*	1 Sausage/31.6g	69	4.9	218	11.3	8.3	15.5	0.0
Chipolata, Pork, Extra Lean, BGTY, Sainsbury's*	1 Chipolata	46	2.1	189	16.9	10.9	8.6	0.5
Chipolata, Pork & Tomato, Organic, Tesco*	1 Chipolata/28g	79	6.7	283	12.2	4.3	24.1	0.9
Chipolata, Premium, Average	1 Serving/80g	187	13.8	234	14.9	4.7	17.3	1.2
Chorizo, Average	1 Serving/80g	250	19.4	313	21.1	2.6	24.2	0.2
Chorizo, Lean, Average	1 Sausage/67g	131	9.2	195	15.7	2.3	13.7	0.8
Chorizo, Wafer Thin, Tesco*	¼ Pack/25g	79	5.8	315	23.3	3.5	23.0	0.0
Classic Toulouse, TTD, Sainsbury's*	1 Sausage/45.4g	147	11.6	324	21.4	2.3	25.5	0.8
Cocktail, Average	1oz/28g	90	7.5	323	12.1	8.6	26.7	0.9
Cocktail, with BBQ Dip, Asda*	1 Pack/105g	227	12.6	216	9.0	19.0	12.0	0.7

SAUSAGE

	Measure INFO/WEIGHT	per Measure KCAL	FAT	Nutrition Values per 100g / 100ml KCAL	PROT	CARB	FAT	FIBRE
Cumberland, Average	1 Sausage/57g	167	13.0	293	13.9	8.6	22.8	0.8
Cumberland, Healthy Range, Average	1 Sausage/52.6g	75	2.1	142	17.4	9.0	4.1	0.9
Duck & Orange, TTD, Sainsbury's*	1 Sausage/40.9g	123	10.6	301	13.8	3.2	25.9	0.9
Extrawurst, German, Waitrose*	1 Slice/28.3g	80	7.1	281	13.0	1.0	25.0	0.0
Free From Wheat & Gulten, Sainsbury's*	1 Serving/22.8g	62	4.8	268	15.2	4.5	21.0	1.8
French Saucisson, Tesco*	1 Slice/5g	19	1.4	379	26.7	4.1	28.4	0.0
Garlic, Average	1 Slice/11g	25	2.0	227	15.7	0.8	18.2	0.0
German, Bierwurst, Selection, Sainsbury's*	1 Slice/4g	8	0.6	224	15.0	1.0	17.8	0.1
German, Extrawurst, Selection, Sainsbury's*	1 Slice/3g	9	0.8	279	13.1	0.5	25.0	0.1
German, Schinkenwurst, Selection, Sainsbury's*	1 Slice/3g	8	0.7	251	13.1	0.3	21.9	0.1
Hot Mustard Porker, Tesco*	1 Sausage/52g	143	10.3	275	16.1	8.1	19.8	3.1
Irish, Average	1 Sausage/40g	119	8.3	298	10.7	17.2	20.7	0.7
Lamb & Mint, M & S*	1oz/28g	63	4.6	225	13.3	6.6	16.3	1.7
Lincolnshire, Average	1 Sausage/42g	122	9.1	291	14.6	9.2	21.8	0.6
Lincolnshire, Healthy Range, Average	1 Sausage/50g	89	4.3	177	15.8	9.0	8.6	0.8
Lorne, Average	1 Sausage/25g	78	5.8	312	10.8	16.0	23.1	0.6
Mediterranean Style, 95% Fat Free, Bowyers*	1 Sausage/50g	60	1.6	120	13.9	8.9	3.2	0.0
Mediterranean Style Paprika, Waitrose*	1 Sausage/67g	190	16.1	283	12.1	4.6	24.0	1.9
Mortadella, Sainsbury's*	1 Slice/13g	34	2.8	261	17.3	0.1	21.2	0.1
Pancetta, & Parmesan, TTD, Sainsbury's*	1 Sausage/58g	156	10.8	269	20.8	4.7	18.6	1.2
Polish Kabanos, Sainsbury's*	1 Sausage/25g	92	7.6	366	23.0	0.1	30.4	0.1
Polony, Slicing, Value, Tesco*	1 Serving/40g	92	6.6	229	10.0	10.0	16.5	1.0
Polony Slicing, Asda*	1oz/28g	60	3.9	214	11.0	11.0	14.0	0.0
Pork, & Fresh Bramley Apple, Waitrose*	1 Sausage/67g	137	9.3	206	14.0	5.9	14.0	0.8
Pork, & Sweet Chilli, Waitrose*	1 Sausage/67g	146	10.2	219	15.6	4.6	15.3	0.8
Pork, Apricot & Herb, Waitrose*	1 Sausage/67g	165	11.1	246	11.2	12.9	16.6	1.3
Pork, Average	1 Sausage/50g	152	11.9	305	12.8	9.8	23.8	0.8
Pork, Bacon & Cheese, Asda*	¼ Pack/114g	329	23.9	289	18.0	7.0	21.0	0.4
Pork, Battered, Thick, Average	1oz/28g	126	10.2	448	17.3	21.7	36.3	2.0
Pork, Chilli & Coriander, Grilled, Sainsbury's*	1 Sausage/54g	123	8.3	228	18.9	3.5	15.4	1.8
Pork, Chilli & Coriander, Grilled, TTD, Sainsbury's*	1 Sausage/58.8g	173	13.2	294	19.9	3.3	22.4	1.5
Pork, Cumberland, Light Choices, Tesco*	2 Sausages/114g	143	3.6	125	15.3	8.2	3.2	1.9
Pork, Extra Lean, Average	1 Sausage/54g	84	3.7	155	17.3	6.1	6.9	0.9
Pork, Free From, Tesco*	1 Sausage/57g	124	8.6	218	12.1	8.5	15.0	2.2
Pork, Frozen, Fried	1oz/28g	88	6.9	316	13.8	10.0	24.8	0.0
Pork, Frozen, Grilled	1oz/28g	81	5.9	289	14.8	10.5	21.2	0.0
Pork, Garlic & Herb, Average	1 Sausage/75.6g	204	16.6	269	12.0	6.0	21.9	1.2
Pork, Grilled, Extra Lean, ½ the Fat, Waitrose*	1 Sausage/56.7g	89	4.6	157	13.7	7.2	8.2	0.6
Pork, Grilled, GFY, Asda*	1 Sausage/46.6g	68	1.9	146	16.9	10.5	4.0	1.4
Pork, Ham & Asparagus, Tesco*	1 Sausage/75.7g	173	12.9	228	14.9	3.8	17.0	1.1
Pork, Honey Roast, Westways*	1 Sausage/66g	158	11.6	240	13.9	4.7	17.6	0.0
Pork, Premium, Average	1 Sausage/74g	191	13.6	258	14.9	8.3	18.4	1.0
Pork, Premium, Extra Lean, Waitrose*	1 Sausage/57.1g	89	4.9	156	17.2	2.7	8.5	1.8
Pork, Reduced Fat, Chilled, Grilled	1oz/28g	64	3.9	230	16.2	10.8	13.8	1.5
Pork, Reduced Fat, Healthy Range, Average	1 Sausage/57g	86	3.4	151	15.7	9.1	6.0	0.9
Pork, Roasted Pepper & Chilli, COU, M & S*	1 Sausage/57g	57	1.1	100	15.2	7.1	2.0	2.1
Pork, Skinless, Average	1oz/28g	81	6.6	291	11.7	8.2	23.6	0.6
Pork, Smoked Bacon, & Garlic, Finest, Tesco*	1 Sausage/67g	115	8.4	173	14.7	0.2	12.6	0.4
Pork, Thick, Average	1 Sausage/38.8g	116	8.7	296	13.3	10.0	22.4	1.0
Pork, Thick, Reduced Fat, Healthy Range, Average	1 Sausage/52g	90	3.8	173	14.1	12.3	7.4	0.8
Pork & Apple, Average	1 Sausage/57g	146	10.7	256	14.5	7.5	18.8	1.9
Pork & Beef, Average	1 Sausage/45g	133	10.2	295	8.7	13.7	22.7	0.5
Pork & Chilli, Tesco*	1 Sausage/67g	124	8.0	186	16.4	3.2	12.0	1.1

S

	Measure INFO/WEIGHT	per Measure KCAL	FAT	Nutrition Values per 100g / 100ml KCAL	PROT	CARB	FAT	FIBRE
SAUSAGE								
Pork & Herb, Average	1 Sausage/75g	231	19.5	308	13.2	5.5	26.0	0.4
Pork & Herb, Healthy Range, Average	1 Sausage/59g	75	1.4	127	16.1	10.8	2.4	1.1
Pork & Leek, Average	1oz/28g	73	5.6	262	14.6	6.0	20.0	1.1
Pork & Onion, Gluten Free, Asda*	1 Sausage/40.9g	105	7.0	257	20.0	6.0	17.0	1.8
Pork & Stilton, Average	1 Sausage/57g	180	15.2	317	13.2	5.9	26.7	0.3
Pork & Sundried Tomato, TTD, Sainsbury's*	1 Sausage/67g	161	10.4	240	20.9	4.3	15.5	0.2
Pork & Tomato, Grilled, Average	1 Sausage/46.5g	126	9.6	273	13.9	7.5	20.8	0.4
Pork with Mozzarella, Italian Style, Tesco*	1 Sausage/75.6g	206	15.4	271	12.0	10.1	20.3	1.0
Premium, Chilled, Fried	1oz/28g	77	5.8	275	15.8	6.7	20.7	0.0
Premium, Chilled, Grilled	1oz/28g	82	6.3	292	16.8	6.3	22.4	0.0
Rich Venison & Redcurrant, Grilled, TTD, Sainsbury's*	1 Sausage/46g	138	10.4	299	21.2	3.0	22.5	1.8
Round, Breakfast Pack, Healthy Choice, Asda*	1 Sausage/53g	85	2.6	160	23.0	6.0	4.9	0.0
Saucisson Montagne, Waitrose*	1 Slice/5g	21	1.8	421	20.7	1.9	36.7	0.0
Schinkenwurst, German, Waitrose*	1 Slice/12.5g	29	2.3	224	16.0	0.8	17.6	0.0
Smoked, Average	1 Sausage/174g	588	52.2	338	13.0	4.0	30.0	0.0
Smoky Cajun, TTD, Sainsbury's*	1 Sausage/46.4g	115	7.5	250	24.2	1.6	16.3	0.9
Spanish, Wafer Thin, Asda*	1 Slice/4g	12	0.8	298	25.4	4.1	20.0	0.0
Spicy Pork, Polenta & Sun Dried Tomato, Waitrose*	1 Sausage/67g	165	11.9	247	11.8	9.8	17.8	0.9
Spicy Pork & Pepper, Sainsbury's*	1 Sausage/33g	86	5.7	260	20.1	6.0	17.3	1.6
Toulouse, M & S*	1 Sausage/57g	123	8.9	215	12.4	5.8	15.6	1.3
Toulouse, So Good, Somerfield*	1 Sausage/67g	197	15.3	296	15.2	7.2	22.9	0.8
Toulouse, TTD, Sainsbury's*	1 Sausage/67g	186	14.0	277	22.0	0.3	20.9	1.2
Toulouse Style, Extra Special, Asda*	2 Sausages/117g	302	23.2	258	17.3	2.6	19.8	2.1
Tuna, Mediterranean Style, Sainsbury's*	1 Sausage/50g	102	4.8	204	15.1	14.7	9.5	1.2
Tuna & Herb, Sainsbury's*	1 Sausage/47g	109	5.9	231	19.6	10.0	12.5	1.5
Turkey, Average	1 Sausage/57g	90	4.6	157	15.7	6.3	8.0	0.0
Turkey & Chicken, Average	1 Sausage/56.7g	126	8.3	222	14.5	8.2	14.6	1.8
Turkey & Ham, Tesco*	1 Sausage/57g	101	5.7	178	13.8	8.3	10.0	1.0
Tuscan, M & S*	1 Sausage/66g	145	10.6	220	14.9	4.6	16.0	0.6
Venison, & Red Wine, TTD, Sainsbury's*	1 Sausage/66g	150	8.8	226	19.7	6.8	13.3	1.7
Venison, Oisin, M & S*	1 Serving/25g	41	2.3	165	16.8	3.8	9.3	0.7
with Baked Beans, Heinz*	1 Serving/70g	135	7.3	193	13.3	11.5	10.4	2.5
SAUSAGE & MASH								
BGTY, Sainsbury's*	1 Serving/490g	387	10.8	79	4.7	10.1	2.2	1.8
British Classic, Tesco*	1 Pack/450g	675	42.8	150	5.1	11.1	9.5	0.9
Eat Smart, Morrisons*	1 Pack/400g	312	11.6	78	4.3	10.5	2.9	1.3
GFY, Asda*	1 Pack/400g	330	10.0	83	4.3	10.8	2.5	1.8
Iceland*	1 Pack/440g	484	26.0	110	3.8	10.4	5.9	1.6
Light Choices, HE, Tesco*	1 Pack/450g	405	10.4	90	4.4	12.3	2.3	1.1
Onion, M & S*	1 Pack/300g	315	17.1	105	4.1	9.0	5.7	1.5
Pork & Leek Sausages, Gravy, Mashed Potato, HL, Tesco*	1 Pack/450g	405	10.4	90	4.4	12.3	2.3	1.0
Vegetarian, Safeway*	1 Pack/450g	450	21.2	100	5.5	8.9	4.7	1.8
Vegetarian, Tesco*	1 Pack/410g	398	15.6	97	4.6	11.1	3.8	2.0
with Onion Gravy, Tesco*	1 Pack/500g	525	27.0	105	3.0	11.1	5.4	1.6
with Red Wine & Onion Gravy, BGTY, Sainsbury's*	1 Pack/379.5g	315	7.2	83	5.0	11.4	1.9	2.0
SAUSAGE MEAT								
Pork, Average	1oz/28g	96	8.2	344	9.9	10.2	29.5	0.7
SAUSAGE ROLL								
Asda*	1 Roll/64g	216	16.0	337	7.0	21.0	25.0	0.8
Basics, Party Size, Somerfield*	1 Roll/13g	45	2.9	343	7.0	29.0	22.0	0.0
BGTY, Sainsbury's*	1 Roll/65g	200	11.4	308	9.6	27.9	17.6	1.4
Buffet, HE, Tesco*	1 Roll/30g	83	3.8	278	9.6	31.2	12.8	1.5
Cocktail, M & S*	1 Roll/14.3g	50	3.2	350	10.4	26.4	22.3	2.2

S

	Measure INFO/WEIGHT	per Measure KCAL	per Measure FAT	Nutrition Values per 100g / 100ml KCAL	PROT	CARB	FAT	FIBRE
SAUSAGE ROLL								
Cocktail, Mini, Sainsbury's*	1 Roll/15g	54	3.6	361	9.0	27.6	23.8	2.6
Co-Op*	1 Roll/66g	244	17.8	370	8.0	25.0	27.0	2.0
Farmfoods*	1 Roll/34g	101	6.7	297	6.7	22.9	19.8	0.4
Ginsters*	1 Roll/139.8g	552	42.1	394	9.1	21.7	30.1	1.1
Go Large, Asda*	1 Roll/170g	660	47.6	388	9.0	25.0	28.0	0.9
HE, Tesco*	1 Roll/70g	195	9.0	278	9.6	31.2	12.8	1.5
Jumbo, Sainsbury's*	1 Roll/145g	492	34.4	339	8.2	23.2	23.7	1.5
Kingsize, Pork Farms*	½ Roll/49.9g	242	15.9	483	10.5	39.9	31.8	0.0
Large, Freshbake*	1 Roll/52g	153	9.5	294	6.6	25.9	18.3	4.6
Large, Frozen, Tesco*	1 Roll/50g	183	11.9	365	6.0	31.0	23.8	0.9
Lincolnshire, Geo Adams*	1 Serving/130g	475	31.6	365	8.3	28.2	24.3	1.1
M & S*	1 Roll/32g	122	9.1	380	10.5	21.0	28.4	0.9
Mini, Tesco*	1 Roll/15g	53	3.7	356	9.0	23.9	24.9	1.5
Mini, Waitrose*	1 Roll/35g	124	9.2	353	13.0	16.1	26.3	1.0
Party, Sainsbury's*	1 Roll/12g	54	4.0	422	8.7	26.7	31.1	1.2
Party, Value, Tesco*	1 Roll/12g	33	1.4	274	6.8	35.9	11.5	0.6
Party Size, Tesco*	2 Rolls/28g	105	6.7	375	6.0	33.7	23.8	0.9
Pork, Morrisons*	1 Roll/70g	195	9.0	278	9.6	31.2	12.8	1.5
Pork Farms*	1 Roll/54g	196	12.9	363	7.9	30.0	23.9	0.0
Puff Pastry	1oz/28g	107	7.7	383	9.9	25.4	27.6	1.0
Puff Pastry, Sainsbury's*	1 Roll/65g	250	18.1	384	8.3	25.0	27.9	0.9
Reduced Fat, Sainsbury's*	1 Roll/66g	191	9.4	289	10.5	29.8	14.2	1.8
Sainsbury's*	1 Roll/66.6g	246	16.2	367	9.5	27.8	24.2	2.7
Snack, GFY, Asda*	1 Roll/34g	112	7.0	329	9.4	26.5	20.6	0.9
Snack, Sainsbury's*	1 Roll/34g	130	8.5	383	9.7	29.9	25.0	2.1
Snack Size, Safeway*	1 Roll/28.8g	106	6.8	365	7.7	30.0	23.4	1.6
Snack Size, Tesco*	1 Roll/32g	118	8.8	369	9.1	21.7	27.4	2.3
Somerfield*	1 Roll/35g	149	10.2	426	9.0	32.0	29.0	0.0
Tesco*	1 Roll/67g	241	17.7	360	8.1	21.3	26.4	2.3
Value, Tesco*	1 Roll/64g	211	13.2	330	6.8	29.1	20.7	4.1
Waitrose*	1 Roll/75g	287	19.6	383	10.1	27.0	26.1	1.3
SAUSAGE ROLL VEGETARIAN								
Linda McCartney*	1 Roll/52g	142	7.0	273	9.7	28.2	13.5	2.5
SAUSAGE VEGETARIAN								
Asda*	1 Sausage/43g	81	3.9	189	20.0	7.0	9.0	2.9
Cumberland, Cauldron*	1 Sausage/50g	78	4.3	156	8.8	10.8	8.6	4.6
Cumberland, Waitrose*	1 Sausage/50g	80	3.4	160	12.6	12.3	6.7	2.4
Glamorgan, Organic, Cauldron*	1 Sausage/41.3g	67	3.8	162	12.5	7.3	9.2	1.7
Granose*	1oz/28g	63	3.8	226	8.5	17.5	13.5	0.0
Leek & Cheese, Organic, Cauldron*	1 Sausage/41g	80	4.1	194	14.4	11.3	10.1	1.7
Lincolnshire, Asda*	1 Sausage/57g	98	4.5	172	17.0	8.0	8.0	1.4
Lincolnshire, Chilled, Cauldron*	1 Sausage/50g	91	5.0	181	10.5	12.2	10.0	4.1
Lincolnshire, Frozen, Tesco*	1 Sausage/50g	78	2.5	155	15.5	10.8	5.0	3.0
Linda McCartney*	1 Sausage/50g	101	4.4	202	22.6	8.2	8.8	1.6
Mushroom & Tarragon, Wicken Fen*	1 Sausage/47g	82	3.5	175	10.1	17.0	7.4	2.4
Realeat*	1 Sausage/40g	66	3.9	165	17.2	2.0	9.8	8.1
Safeway*	2 Sausages/89.7g	149	8.8	165	17.2	2.0	9.8	8.1
SAVOURY EGGS								
Mini, Asda*	1 Egg/20g	64	4.4	318	9.8	20.0	22.1	2.3
Mini, Iceland*	1 Egg/20g	66	4.8	327	11.0	17.5	23.7	1.1
Mini, Tesco*	1 Egg/20g	55	3.5	274	9.2	20.2	17.4	2.3
Snack, Tesco*	1 Egg/45g	133	8.9	295	9.0	19.6	19.7	1.8

S

	Measure INFO/WEIGHT	per Measure		Nutrition Values per 100g / 100ml				
		KCAL	FAT	KCAL	PROT	CARB	FAT	FIBRE

SCALLOPS
Asda*	1oz/28g	33	0.4	118	23.2	1.4	1.4	0.0
Breaded, with Plum & Chilli Dipping Sauce, Tesco*	1 Pack/210g	441	15.1	210	10.6	25.6	7.2	0.8
Hotbake Shells, Sainsbury's*	1 Serving/140g	241	15.7	172	9.5	8.4	11.2	0.8
King, Finest, Tesco*	1 Pack/170g	129	1.5	76	16.9	0.1	0.9	0.0
King, Trimmed By Hand, Sainsbury's*	1 Pack/200g	142	0.2	71	16.0	1.4	0.1	0.2
Lemon & Pepper, TTD, Sainsbury's*	1 Serving/100g	213	8.4	213	13.8	20.6	8.4	1.7
Lemon Grass & Ginger, Tesco*	½ Pack/112g	90	1.1	80	15.2	2.5	1.0	0.6
New England, Fresh, M & S*	½ Pack/110g	77	0.1	70	15.5	1.2	0.1	1.2
Queen, Kintyre*	1 Serving/100g	105	1.4	105	23.2	0.1	1.4	0.1
Queen, Scottish, Sainsbury's*	1 Pack/200g	350	11.0	175	30.4	0.8	5.5	0.0
Steamed, Average	1oz/28g	33	0.4	118	23.2	3.4	1.4	0.0
with Roasted Garlic Butter, Finest, Tesco*	1 Serving/100g	201	14.3	201	16.2	1.8	14.3	0.4

SCAMPI
Breaded, Average	½ Pack/255g	565	27.4	222	10.7	20.5	10.7	1.0
Wholetails, in Crunchy Crumb, Morrisons*	1 Pack/250g	508	21.8	203	9.6	19.9	8.7	1.7

SCHNITZEL VEGETARIAN
Breaded, Tivall*	1 Schnitzel/100g	172	8.0	172	16.0	9.0	8.0	5.0

SCONE
3% Fat, M & S*	1 Scone/65g	179	1.6	275	7.2	55.1	2.5	2.3
All Butter, Tesco*	1 Scone/41g	126	3.2	308	7.2	52.3	7.8	1.6
Cheese, Average	1 Scone/40g	145	7.1	363	10.1	43.2	17.8	1.6
Cheese, Finest, Tesco*	1 Scone/70g	255	11.3	364	11.3	42.6	16.1	1.1
Cheese, Mature Cheddar, M & S*	1 Scone/65g	257	14.2	395	10.3	38.9	21.9	1.6
Cheese, Sainsbury's*	1 Scone/70g	250	13.0	357	10.6	36.9	18.6	2.0
Cheese & Black Pepper, Mini, M & S*	1 Scone/18g	67	3.3	370	10.2	41.1	18.3	1.7
Cherry, M & S*	1 Scone/60g	202	7.3	337	6.9	49.7	12.2	1.9
Cream, Sainsbury's*	1 Scone/50g	173	8.7	345	4.6	42.5	17.4	3.1
Derby, Asda*	1 Scone/59g	202	5.9	342	7.0	56.0	10.0	0.0
Derby, Mother's Pride*	1 Scone/60g	208	8.4	347	5.2	49.8	14.0	1.5
Derby, Somerfield*	1 Scone/60g	208	8.4	347	5.3	49.9	14.0	1.9
Derby, Tesco*	1 Scone/60g	201	6.1	335	7.2	53.7	10.2	2.0
Devon, M & S*	1 Scone/59.2g	224	9.6	380	7.1	50.8	16.2	1.5
Devon, Sainsbury's*	1 Scone/54g	201	8.4	372	7.1	51.1	15.5	1.6
Devon, Waitrose*	1 Scone/71.8g	269	9.5	373	7.5	56.0	13.2	2.3
Fresh Cream, Finest, Tesco*	1 Serving/133g	469	23.2	354	4.6	44.5	17.5	1.7
Fresh Cream, Tesco*	1 Scone/79.5g	244	10.0	304	15.8	32.3	12.5	0.9
Fresh Cream, TTD, Sainsbury's*	1 Serving/110g	379	15.9	346	5.8	48.1	14.5	2.6
Fresh Cream with Strawberry Jam, Tesco*	1 Scone/83g	290	15.6	352	4.7	40.7	18.9	1.1
Fruit	1 Scone/40g	126	3.9	316	7.3	52.9	9.8	0.0
Fruit, Economy, Sainsbury's*	1 Scone/34g	111	3.2	326	7.9	52.5	9.4	1.7
Fruit, Ready 2 Bake, Aunt Bessie's*	1 Scone/65.9g	234	8.4	355	8.6	51.6	12.7	3.1
Fruit, Ready to Bake, Aunt Bessie's*	1 Scone/65.9g	234	8.4	355	8.6	51.6	12.7	3.1
Fruit, SmartPrice, Asda*	1 Scone/41g	139	4.1	338	7.0	55.0	10.0	3.0
Fruit, Somerfield*	1 Scone/35g	116	3.5	332	8.0	53.0	10.0	0.0
Fruit, Waitrose*	1 Scone/58g	190	4.8	325	6.3	56.5	8.2	2.2
Luxury, Hovis*	1 Scone/85g	267	7.9	314	5.6	51.8	9.3	2.2
Plain, Average	1 Scone/40g	145	5.8	362	7.2	53.8	14.6	1.9
Potato, Average	1 Scone/40g	118	5.7	296	5.1	39.1	14.3	1.6
Potato, Mother's Pride*	1 Scone/37g	77	0.8	207	4.7	42.0	2.2	4.3
Potato, Warburton's*	1 Scone/58.7g	116	5.8	196	4.7	22.3	9.8	4.1
Strawberry, Fresh Cream, Sainsbury's*	1 Scone/60g	218	11.2	363	6.5	42.5	18.6	1.4
Sultana, BGTY, Sainsbury's*	1 Scone/63g	178	1.8	283	7.7	56.7	2.8	2.4
Sultana, Finest, Tesco*	1 Scone/70g	238	7.6	340	8.9	50.9	10.9	2.1

S

	Measure INFO/WEIGHT	per Measure KCAL	per Measure FAT	per 100g KCAL	PROT	CARB	FAT	FIBRE
SCONE								
Sultana, Less Than 5% Fat, M & S*	1 Scone/66.7g	200	3.0	300	7.6	57.8	4.5	2.1
Sultana, M & S*	1 Scone/64g	200	3.0	313	8.0	60.5	4.7	2.2
Sultana, Sainsbury's*	1 Scone/53.8g	177	5.9	327	6.9	50.2	11.0	6.5
Sultana, Somerfield*	1 Scone/34g	108	2.8	318	5.7	55.4	8.2	0.0
Sultana, Tesco*	1 Scone/60g	189	5.0	315	7.1	52.5	8.4	2.6
Sultana, Value, Tesco*	1 Scone/40g	134	4.0	335	6.5	53.8	10.1	2.7
Wholemeal	1 Scone/40g	130	5.8	326	8.7	43.1	14.4	5.2
Wholemeal, Fruit	1 Scone/40g	130	5.1	324	8.1	47.2	12.8	4.9
SCONE MIX								
Fruit, Asda*	1 Scone/47.5g	144	2.4	301	7.0	57.0	5.0	3.7
SCOTCH EGGS								
Asda*	1 Egg/114g	286	19.2	251	11.2	13.7	16.8	1.4
Budgens*	1 Egg/113g	294	19.9	260	11.4	13.8	17.6	0.0
Finest, Tesco*	1 Egg/114g	280	20.1	247	11.6	10.4	17.7	1.1
Free Range, Sainsbury's*	1 Egg/112.7g	284	19.0	252	12.4	12.5	16.9	2.5
Ginsters*	1 Egg/95g	228	15.1	240	15.3	9.7	15.9	0.6
M & S*	1 Egg/120g	318	22.8	265	10.7	13.0	19.0	2.2
Mini, 40% Less Fat, Sainsbury's*	1 Egg/20g	46	2.6	231	12.8	15.3	13.2	1.4
Mini, Sainsbury's*	1 Egg/12.2g	37	2.7	307	10.8	15.7	22.5	1.0
Morrisons*	1 Egg/113.9g	286	19.2	251	11.2	13.7	16.8	1.4
Retail	1 Egg/120g	301	20.5	251	12.0	13.1	17.1	0.0
Sainsbury's*	1 Egg/116g	319	22.4	275	11.1	14.2	19.3	0.9
Super Mini, Asda*	1 Egg/12.5g	37	2.5	305	10.0	19.0	21.0	2.1
Tesco*	1 Egg/113.5g	270	15.8	238	10.2	16.9	13.9	2.2
SEA BASS								
Raw, Average	1oz/28g	32	1.0	113	20.3	0.0	3.5	0.1
SEA BREAM								
Fillets, Raw, Average	1oz/28g	27	0.8	96	17.5	0.0	2.9	0.0
SEAFOOD COCKTAIL								
Asda*	1oz/28g	26	0.4	92	14.0	5.7	1.5	0.1
Average	1oz/28g	24	0.4	87	15.6	2.9	1.5	0.0
Premium Quality, Lyons Seafoods*	1 Serving/100g	76	0.9	76	13.2	3.7	0.9	1.1
Somerfield*	1oz/28g	23	0.6	81	14.0	2.0	2.0	0.0
SEAFOOD MEDLEY								
Sainsbury's*	½ Pack/175g	158	3.3	90	14.3	4.0	1.9	0.5
Steam Cuisine, M & S*	1 Pack/400g	320	12.4	80	8.5	4.5	3.1	1.3
SEAFOOD MIX								
Asda*	1 Serving/213g	175	2.3	82	12.0	6.0	1.1	0.0
SEAFOOD SELECTION								
Asda*	½ Pack/125g	159	2.1	127	16.6	11.3	1.7	0.3
Fresh, Tesco*	1 Pack/234g	187	2.3	80	17.7	0.1	1.0	0.0
Luxury, Safeway*	1 Pack/250g	215	5.0	86	13.8	3.1	2.0	0.0
M & S*	1 Serving/200g	170	2.0	85	17.4	1.6	1.0	0.5
Mussels, King Prawns & Squid, Tesco*	½ Pack/200g	140	3.0	70	13.7	0.1	1.5	0.0
Sainsbury's*	½ Pack/125g	85	1.3	68	14.6	0.8	1.0	2.5
Somerfield*	1 Serving/200g	170	3.2	85	15.9	1.7	1.6	0.4
SEAFOOD STICKS								
Average	1 Stick/15g	16	0.0	106	8.0	18.4	0.2	0.2
Low Price, Sainsbury's*	1 Stick/16g	16	0.1	101	7.3	16.0	0.9	0.6
with Cocktail Dip, Asda*	1 Pot/95g	126	4.8	133	6.0	16.0	5.0	0.1
with Garlic & Lemon Dip, Asda*	1 Pot/97.9g	184	11.8	188	7.0	13.0	12.0	0.0
SEASONING								
Aromat, Knorr*	1oz/28g	46	1.0	164	12.4	20.5	3.6	1.0

S

	Measure INFO/WEIGHT	per Measure KCAL	per Measure FAT	Nutrition Values per 100g / 100ml KCAL	PROT	CARB	FAT	FIBRE
SEASONING CUBES								
for Potato, Mint, Perfect Potato, Knorr*	1 Cube/10g	56	5.1	560	5.1	21.2	50.5	1.8
for Rice, Pilau, Knorr*	1 Cube/10g	31	2.3	305	11.4	13.9	22.6	1.4
for Rice, Saffron, Knorr*	1 Cube/10g	29	1.8	291	13.8	17.5	18.4	2.2
for Stir Fry, Oriental Spices, Knorr*	1 Cube/10g	41	3.1	414	9.7	25.0	30.6	1.1
Oriental Spice, Knorr*	1 Cube/10g	41	3.1	409	9.5	23.7	30.7	0.0
Perfect Pasta, Knorr*	1 Cube/10g	28	2.4	278	10.3	5.2	24.0	0.0
Wild Mushroom, Knorr*	1 Cube/10g	37	2.7	365	10.3	21.3	26.5	0.2
SEASONING MIX								
Beef Taco, Colman's*	1 Pack/30g	76	3.6	252	9.1	26.9	12.0	14.0
Cajun, Sizzle & Grill, Schwartz*	1 Tsp/4g	7	0.2	182	9.8	23.0	5.6	24.4
Chicken, Chargrilled, Grill & Sizzle, Schwartz*	1 Tsp/5g	12	0.2	232	8.2	40.8	4.0	13.1
Chicken Fajitas, Schwartz*	1 Pack/35g	99	0.9	283	10.9	54.1	2.5	10.8
Chilli, Old El Paso*	1 Pack/39g	117	2.0	301	7.0	57.0	5.0	0.0
Chinese Curry, Youngs*	1 Serving/22g	109	6.8	495	8.3	46.4	30.7	0.0
Fajita, Asda*	1 Serving/8g	20	0.6	251	6.0	41.0	7.0	0.9
Fajita, Chicken, Colman's*	1 Pack/40g	138	2.5	344	9.4	62.5	6.3	4.8
Italian Herb, Schwartz*	1 Tsp/1g	3	0.0	338	11.0	64.5	4.0	0.0
Lamb, Simply Shake, Schwartz*	1oz/28g	54	0.9	193	12.1	53.1	3.1	23.9
Mediterranean Roast Vegetable, Schwartz*	1 Pack/30g	86	1.2	288	6.9	56.1	4.0	10.3
Moroccan Spiced Vegetables, Schwartz*	1 Pack/40g	99	2.0	247	12.2	38.4	4.9	22.0
Potato Wedges, Cajun, Schwartz*	1 Serving/100g	295	7.6	295	9.1	47.6	7.6	14.3
Potato Wedges, Garlic & Herb, Schwartz*	1 Pack/38g	106	1.9	278	11.4	47.1	4.9	11.7
Potato Wedges, Nacho Cheese, Schwartz*	1 Serving/10g	30	1.0	299	13.6	39.3	9.7	7.7
Potato Wedges, Onion & Chive, Schwartz*	1 Pack/38g	113	0.7	297	10.9	59.4	1.8	6.5
Season-All, Schwartz*	1 Tsp/6g	4	0.1	72	2.3	11.6	1.8	0.0
Shepherd's Pie, Colman's*	1 Pack/50g	141	0.7	282	12.5	54.7	1.4	4.3
Shotz, Cajun Chicken, Schwartz*	1 Pack/3g	8	0.2	268	9.9	45.6	5.2	0.0
Shotz, Moroccan Chicken, Schwartz*	1 Pack/3g	9	0.2	312	9.7	56.7	5.2	0.0
Shotz, Seven Pepper Steak, Schwartz*	1 Pack/3g	7	0.1	246	8.2	47.8	2.4	0.0
Spanish Roasted Vegetables, Schwartz*	1 Pack/15g	22	0.9	147	9.1	14.1	6.0	22.6
Taco, Old El Paso*	¼ Pack/9g	30	0.4	334	5.5	69.0	4.0	0.0
Thai Seven Spice, Schwartz*	1 Serving/10g	24	0.4	243	7.5	44.1	4.1	0.0
SEAWEED								
Crispy, Average	1oz/28g	182	17.3	651	7.5	15.6	61.9	7.0
Irish Moss, Raw	1oz/28g	2	0.1	8	1.5	0.0	0.2	12.3
Kombu, Dried, Raw	1oz/28g	12	0.4	43	7.1	0.0	1.6	58.7
Nori, Dried, Raw	1oz/28g	38	0.4	136	30.7	0.0	1.5	44.4
Wakame, Dried, Raw	1oz/28g	20	0.7	71	12.4	0.0	2.4	47.1
SEED MIX								
Chilli & Garlic, The Food Doctor*	1 Serving/30g	161	13.0	536	29.3	3.7	43.2	16.0
Original, The Food Doctor*	1 Serving/30g	157	13.3	522	28.2	3.7	44.4	17.7
Salad Sprinkle, Nature's Harvest*	1 Serving/8g	48	4.1	598	20.0	14.6	51.1	4.9
SEEDS								
Melon, Average	1 Tbsp/15g	87	7.2	583	28.5	9.9	47.7	0.0
Pomegranate, Sainsbury's*	1 Pack/150g	77	0.3	51	1.3	11.8	0.2	0.6
Poppy, Asda*	1 Serving/2g	11	0.9	556	21.0	19.0	44.0	0.0
Pumpkin, Average	1 Tbsp/10g	57	4.6	568	27.9	13.0	45.9	3.9
Pumpkin, Whole, Roasted, Salted, Average	1 Serving/50g	261	21.1	522	33.0	13.4	42.1	3.9
Sesame, Tesco*	1 Tsp/4g	24	2.3	598	18.2	0.9	58.0	7.9
Sunflower, Average	1 Tbsp/10g	59	4.9	585	23.4	15.0	48.7	5.7
SEMOLINA								
Average	1oz/28g	98	0.5	348	11.0	75.2	1.8	2.1
Pudding, Creamed, Ambrosia*	1 Can/425g	344	7.2	81	3.3	13.1	1.7	0.2

S

	Measure INFO/WEIGHT	per Measure KCAL	FAT	Nutrition Values per 100g / 100ml KCAL	PROT	CARB	FAT	FIBRE
SHALLOTS								
Pickled, in Hot & Spicy Vinegar, Tesco*	1 Onion/18g	14	0.0	77	1.0	18.0	0.1	1.9
Raw, Average	1oz/28g	6	0.1	20	1.5	3.3	0.2	1.4
SHANDY								
Bitter, Original, Ben Shaws*	1 Can/330ml	89	0.0	27	0.0	6.0	0.0	0.0
Homemade, Average	1 Pint/568ml	148	0.0	26	0.2	2.9	0.0	0.0
Lemonade, Schweppes*	1 Can/330ml	76	0.0	23	0.0	5.1	0.0	0.0
Lemonade, Traditional Style, Tesco*	1 Can/330ml	63	0.0	19	0.0	4.7	0.0	0.0
SHARK								
Raw	1oz/28g	29	0.3	102	23.0	0.0	1.1	0.0
SHARON FRUIT								
Average	1oz/28g	20	0.0	73	0.8	18.6	0.0	1.6
SHERBET LEMONS								
M & S*	1oz/28g	107	0.0	382	0.0	93.9	0.0	0.0
SHERRY								
Dry, Average	1 Glass/120ml	139	0.0	116	0.2	1.4	0.0	0.0
Medium	1 Serving/50ml	58	0.0	116	0.1	5.9	0.0	0.0
Sweet	1 Serving/50ml	68	0.0	136	0.3	6.9	0.0	0.0
SHORTBREAD								
All Butter, Assorted, Aldi*	1oz/28g	143	7.5	511	6.5	61.0	26.8	2.0
All Butter, Deans*	1 Biscuit/15g	77	3.8	511	4.9	65.7	25.4	1.2
All Butter, Round, Luxury, M & S*	1 Biscuit/20g	105	5.8	525	6.2	60.0	29.0	2.0
All Butter, Royal Edinburgh, Asda*	1 Finger/18g	93	5.1	519	5.8	60.3	28.3	1.8
All Butter, Scottish, M & S*	1 Biscuit/34g	173	9.5	510	5.7	58.9	27.8	2.3
All Butter, Thins, M & S*	1 Biscuit/10.3g	49	2.1	485	5.8	68.4	21.1	3.5
All Butter, Trufree*	1 Biscuit/11g	58	3.1	524	2.0	66.0	28.0	0.9
Average	1oz/28g	139	7.3	498	5.9	63.9	26.1	1.9
Belgian Chocolate Chunk, Asda*	1 Serving/20g	106	6.2	531	7.0	56.0	31.0	1.8
Caramel, Millionaires, Fox's*	1 Serving/16g	75	3.9	483	6.1	57.9	25.3	0.1
Choc Chip, Fair Trade, Co-Op*	1 Biscuit/19g	100	6.0	526	5.3	57.9	31.6	2.6
Chocolate, Waitrose*	1oz/28g	144	7.8	516	5.5	61.2	27.7	1.8
Chocolate & Caramel, TTD, Sainsbury's*	1 Serving/55g	245	15.2	446	4.7	45.0	27.7	1.3
Chocolate Caramel, Co-Op*	1 Cake/50.5g	245	13.1	485	5.0	59.0	26.0	0.5
Chocolate Chip, Jacob's*	1 Biscuit/17g	87	4.7	513	5.2	61.2	27.5	1.8
Chocolate Chip, Tesco*	1 Serving/20g	105	6.1	525	7.5	50.0	30.6	3.0
Chocolate Chunk, Starbucks*	1 Biscuit/90g	484	28.4	538	5.7	57.9	31.5	1.4
Clotted Cream, Cornish Traditional, Furniss*	2 Biscuits/15g	81	4.3	541	6.6	63.6	28.9	1.7
Clotted Cream, Finest, Tesco*	1 Biscuit/20g	109	6.4	543	5.2	58.0	32.2	1.7
Clotted Cream, Fingers, Furniss*	1 Finger/15g	80	4.1	533	6.8	65.3	27.3	1.7
Cookies, Organic, Evernat*	1oz/28g	149	8.8	532	5.9	56.7	31.3	0.0
Crawfords*	1 Biscuit/12.5g	64	3.3	533	6.6	65.0	27.4	2.0
Double Choc Chip, Petit Four, Scottish, Tesco*	1 Serving/50g	266	15.0	531	5.1	60.4	30.0	1.7
Dutch, M & S*	1 Biscuit/17.0g	90	5.2	530	5.7	58.2	30.6	0.9
Fingers, All Butter, Co-Op*	1 Finger/16g	85	4.9	520	6.0	58.0	30.0	2.0
Fingers, All Butter, McVitie's*	1 Finger/20g	106	5.4	530	6.5	64.7	27.2	0.0
Fingers, All Butter, Royal Edinburgh Bakery*	1 Biscuit/17g	88	4.8	519	5.8	60.3	28.3	1.8
Fingers, All Butter, Scottish, M & S*	1 Biscuit/17.6g	90	4.9	510	5.7	58.9	27.8	4.7
Fingers, All Butter, Scottish, Tesco*	1 Finger/17.8g	94	5.2	520	6.0	58.5	29.1	1.8
Fingers, All Butter, Tesco*	1 Finger/13g	67	3.7	519	5.8	60.3	28.3	1.8
Fingers, Asda*	1 Finger/18g	93	5.1	519	5.8	60.3	28.3	18.0
Fingers, Deans*	1 Finger/24g	115	5.9	488	5.1	60.1	24.8	1.4
Fingers, Highland, Organic, Sainsbury's*	1 Serving/16g	84	4.8	527	5.8	58.7	29.9	1.9
Fingers, Highland, Sainsbury's*	1 Biscuit/10g	53	3.0	527	5.8	58.7	29.9	1.9
Fingers, Light & Buttery, TTD, Sainsbury's*	1 Finger/20g	105	5.8	528	5.1	61.6	29.0	0.7

S

	Measure INFO/WEIGHT	per Measure KCAL	FAT	Nutrition Values per 100g / 100ml KCAL	PROT	CARB	FAT	FIBRE
SHORTBREAD								
Fingers, Scottish, Finest, Tesco*	1 Pack/165g	822	39.4	498	5.1	65.5	23.9	2.0
Hearts, with Milk Chocolate, M & S*	1 Biscuit/25g	125	6.5	500	7.2	59.5	25.8	3.0
Highland, Organic, Duchy Originals*	1 Biscuit/16g	80	4.2	515	5.2	61.8	27.4	1.7
Highland Demerara Rounds, Sainsbury's*	1 Biscuit/20g	113	5.8	565	5.5	70.5	29.0	2.0
Millionaire, M & S*	1 Portion/65g	325	17.9	500	4.0	58.9	27.6	1.0
Orange Marmalade & Oatflake, Deans*	1 Biscuit/20g	105	5.9	524	6.7	59.3	29.6	3.2
Organic, Waitrose*	1 Biscuit/12.5g	64	3.2	495	5.8	63.0	24.4	1.8
Pecan & Caramel, TTD, Sainsbury's*	1 Slice/52g	259	15.3	497	5.1	53.1	29.4	1.6
Pure Butter, Jacob's*	1 Biscuit/20g	105	5.9	525	5.7	58.6	29.7	1.8
Rounds, All Butter, Farmhouse, TTD, Sainsbury's*	1 Biscuit/20g	108	6.2	538	5.0	59.5	31.1	1.6
Rounds, Safeway*	1 Biscuit/19.9g	108	6.2	538	5.4	59.2	31.1	1.6
Shrewsbury, M & S*	1oz/28g	128	6.5	458	7.5	63.9	23.3	4.5
Stem Ginger, Waitrose*	1 Biscuit/15g	71	3.3	487	4.7	66.0	22.7	1.6
SHRIMP								
Boiled, Average	1 Serving/60g	70	1.4	117	23.8	0.0	2.4	0.0
Dried, Average	1oz/28g	69	0.7	245	55.8	0.0	2.4	0.0
Frozen, Average	1oz/28g	20	0.2	73	16.5	0.0	0.8	0.0
in Brine, Canned, Drained, Average	1oz/28g	26	0.3	94	20.8	0.0	1.2	0.0
SKATE								
Grilled	1oz/28g	22	0.1	79	18.9	0.0	0.5	0.0
in Batter, Fried in Blended Oil	1oz/28g	47	2.8	168	14.7	4.9	10.1	0.2
Raw	1oz/28g	18	0.1	64	15.1	0.0	0.4	0.0
SKIPS								
Bacon, KP Snacks*	1 Pack/17.1g	81	3.8	474	6.5	62.1	22.2	2.3
Cheesy, KP Snacks*	1 Bag/17g	89	5.0	524	6.2	58.5	29.5	1.0
Pickled Onion, KP Snacks*	1 Pack/13.1g	67	3.9	512	3.4	56.4	30.3	1.4
Prawn Cocktail, KP Snacks*	1 Bag/17g	89	5.1	523	3.1	60.6	29.9	1.4
SKITTLES								
Fruits, Mars*	1 Serving/36g	145	1.5	404	0.0	91.5	4.2	0.0
SLICES								
Beef, Minced, Morrisons*	1 Slice/143g	457	29.6	320	8.8	24.6	20.7	1.0
Beef, Minced Steak & Onion, Tesco*	1 Slice/150g	425	27.2	283	8.7	21.3	18.1	1.6
Beef, Minced with Onion, Sainsbury's*	1 Slice/120g	328	19.7	273	6.8	24.5	16.4	1.1
Belgian Chocolate, Weight Watchers*	1 Slice/30.1g	99	2.0	329	5.9	61.3	6.7	2.3
Cheddar Cheese & Onion, Ginsters*	1 Slice/180g	583	40.9	324	7.1	22.8	22.7	1.0
Chicken, Spicy, Deep Fill, Ginsters*	1 Slice/180g	499	30.6	277	9.2	21.8	17.0	1.4
Chicken & Ham, Taste!*	1 Slice/154.8g	357	15.3	230	10.8	24.2	9.9	0.0
Chicken & Leek, Taste!*	1 Slice/155g	406	19.1	262	10.1	27.6	12.3	0.0
Chicken & Mushroom, Asda*	1 Serving/128g	355	21.8	277	7.0	24.0	17.0	2.1
Chicken & Mushroom, Ginsters*	1 Slice/155g	420	27.1	271	6.6	21.8	17.5	1.7
Chicken & Mushroom, Morrisons*	1 Slice/158g	446	28.1	282	7.3	23.3	17.8	1.0
Chicken & Mushroom, Sainsbury's*	1 Slice/164g	427	26.5	259	7.3	21.3	16.1	1.0
Chicken & Mushroom, Tesco*	1 Slice/165g	457	28.9	277	9.2	20.6	17.5	0.9
Iced Lemon, GFY, Asda*	1 Serving/30g	67	0.8	223	3.0	47.0	2.5	0.7
Minced Steak & Onion, Sainsbury's*	1 Slice/165g	475	29.9	288	15.2	16.0	18.1	2.5
Peppered Steak, Asda*	1 Serving/164g	483	31.1	295	9.0	22.0	19.0	1.2
Pork & Egg, Gala, Tesco*	1 Slice/105g	333	24.2	317	10.3	17.2	23.0	3.4
Prawn & Avocado, Plait, Extra Special, Asda*	1 Serving/198g	331	6.7	167	11.0	23.0	3.4	1.3
Salmon, & Watercress, Honey Roast, Plait, Asda*	1 Plait/166g	421	16.6	254	13.0	28.0	10.0	0.4
Sausage Meat, with Onion Gravy, Lattice, Asda*	1 Serving/278g	595	38.9	214	10.0	12.0	14.0	1.7
Spinach & Ricotta, Safeway*	1 Slice/165g	487	33.7	295	6.0	21.2	20.4	2.9
Spinach & Ricotta, Sainsbury's*	1 Slice/165g	500	35.3	303	6.5	21.1	21.4	2.9
Steak, Peppered, Deep Fill, Ginsters*	1 Slice/180g	513	36.2	285	9.4	16.1	20.1	3.1

	Measure INFO/WEIGHT	per Measure		Nutrition Values per 100g / 100ml				
		KCAL	FAT	KCAL	PROT	CARB	FAT	FIBRE
SLICES								
Steak, Peppered, Ginsters*	1 Slice/155g	415	24.5	268	9.9	21.5	15.8	1.9
Steak & Onion, Aberdeen Angus, Tesco*	1 Slice/165g	444	27.7	269	8.7	20.7	16.8	1.3
SLIMFAST*								
Meal Bar, Chocolate Crunch, Slim Fast*	1 Bar/60g	206	5.9	343	23.9	42.8	9.9	7.7
Meal Bar, Fruits of the Forest, Slim Fast*	1 Bar/60g	211	6.1	351	23.7	42.1	10.1	7.3
Meal Bar, Yoghurt & Muesli, Slim Fast*	1 Bar/60g	208	6.5	347	23.9	42.2	10.8	7.4
Milk Shake, Banana, Canned, Slim Fast*	1 Can/325ml	215	8.5	66	4.2	10.6	2.6	4.9
Milk Shake, Chocolate, Powder, Dry, Slim Fast*	2 Scoops/37.5g	136	2.8	363	13.9	59.0	7.5	10.9
Milk Shake, Chocolate, Ready to Drink	1 Bottle/325ml	211	5.2	65	4.6	8.0	1.6	1.5
Milk Shake, Chocolate, Ready to Drink, Slim Fast*	1 Bottle/325ml	211	5.2	65	4.6	8.0	1.6	1.5
Milk Shake, Vanilla, Powder, Dry, Slim Fast*	1 Serving/35g	126	2.3	360	13.4	60.9	6.5	11.0
Smoothie, Forest Fruits, Slim Fast*	1 Bottle/325ml	205	6.2	63	4.1	7.2	1.9	1.1
Snacks, Chocolate Caramel Bar, Slim Fast*	1 Bar/26g	99	3.2	382	3.4	69.6	12.4	1.2
Snacks, Sour Cream & Chive Pretzels, Slim Fast*	1 Pack/23g	96	2.0	416	9.5	75.2	8.6	3.4
Soup, Chicken & Vegetable Pasta, Hearty's*	1 Pack/295ml	212	5.6	72	6.6	7.0	1.9	0.7
SMARTIES								
Mini Eggs, Nestle*	1 Lge Bag/112g	535	22.4	478	4.8	69.6	20.0	0.7
Nestle*	1 Tube/43g	198	7.1	461	4.0	73.6	16.6	0.6
SMIRNOFF*								
Ice, Smirnoff*	1 Bottle/275ml	188	0.0	68	1.8	12.0	0.0	0.0
SMOOTHIE								
Banana, Dairy, Probiotic, Boots*	1 Bottle/250ml	148	1.3	59	1.6	12.0	0.5	1.0
Banana, Dairy, Tesco*	1 Bottle/250ml	165	1.0	66	1.6	14.0	0.4	0.4
Banana, M & S*	1 Bottle/500ml	400	2.0	80	1.8	16.8	0.4	1.2
Banana, Shapers, Boots*	1 Bottle/251.4ml	176	0.8	70	2.8	14.0	0.3	0.8
Banana Fruit, with Yoghurt, Tesco*	1 Bottle/1000ml	610	7.0	61	2.1	11.3	0.7	0.4
Blackberries & Blueberries, Innocent*	1 Bottle/250ml	120	0.3	48	0.5	12.0	0.1	2.1
Blackberry & Blueberry, Innocent*	1 Bottle/250ml	120	0.3	48	0.6	11.5	0.1	0.0
Blackcurrant & Apple, for Kids, Innocent*	1 Carton/180ml	112	0.4	62	0.4	14.5	0.2	0.8
Blueberry, Blackberry & Strawberry, COU, M & S*	1 Bottle/250ml	150	0.8	60	0.8	13.1	0.3	0.3
Blueberry & Pear, COU, M & S*	1 Bottle/250ml	113	0.8	45	0.3	10.4	0.3	0.3
Boysenberry & Raspberry, Fruit, TTD, Sainsbury's*	1 Bottle/250ml	108	0.3	43	0.7	10.0	0.1	1.6
Cherries & Strawberries, Innocent*	1 Bottle/250ml	123	0.3	49	0.6	12.6	0.1	0.0
Cranberries & Raspberries, Innocent*	1 Bottle/250ml	113	0.0	45	0.5	12.0	0.0	2.3
Cranberries & Strawberries, Innocent*	1 Bottle/250ml	103	0.5	41	0.5	9.5	0.2	0.0
Cranberry & Raspberry, Juice Republic*	1 Bottle/250mls	183	1.0	73	0.5	16.0	0.4	0.0
Guavas, Mangoes & Goji Berries, Innocent*	1 Bottle/250ml	113	0.3	45	0.6	12.0	0.1	2.1
Mango & Orange, Smoothie Smile*	1 Bottle/250ml	130	1.0	52	0.4	11.7	0.4	0.0
Mango & Passion Fruit, Innocent*	1 Sm Bottle/250ml	140	0.8	56	0.5	14.8	0.3	1.7
Mangoes, Coconuts & Lemongrass, Innocent*	1 Bottle/250ml	165	3.0	66	0.6	14.1	1.2	1.0
Mangoes & Passion Fruits, Pure Fruit, Innocent*	1 Glass/200ml	112	0.4	56	0.6	14.7	0.2	2.0
Orange, Banana & Pineapple, Innocent*	1 Bottle/250ml	120	1.0	48	0.6	10.8	0.4	0.0
Orange, Mandarin & Guava, PJ Smoothies*	1 Bottle/250ml	123	0.0	49	0.7	10.9	0.0	1.6
Orange, Mango, Banana & Passion Fruit, Asda*	1 Serving/100ml	55	0.2	55	0.8	12.0	0.2	1.1
Orange, Mango & Apricot, COU, M & S*	1 Bottle/250ml	113	0.5	45	0.6	10.7	0.2	0.5
Orange, Mango & Pineapple, PJ Smoothies*	1 Carton/100ml	54	0.0	54	0.6	12.2	0.0	0.0
Orange, Strawberry & Guava, Sainsbury's*	1 Serving/300ml	159	0.6	53	0.3	12.0	0.2	0.8
Orange & Mango, Fruit, Morrisons*	1 Bottle/250ml	145	0.0	58	0.5	14.0	0.0	0.7
Oranges, Bananas & Pineapples, Innocent*	1 Bottle/250ml	143	0.3	57	0.6	14.1	0.1	0.0
Oranges Mangos & Bananas, PJ Smoothies*	1 Bottle/250ml	115	0.0	46	0.6	10.9	0.0	0.0
Pineapple, Banana & Mango Fruit, Finest, Tesco*	1 Bottle/250ml	150	0.3	60	0.5	14.0	0.1	0.8
Pineapple, Banana & Pear, Princes*	1 Bottle/250ml	153	0.5	61	0.5	13.9	0.2	0.5
Pineapple, Mango & Passionfruit, Sainsbury's*	1 Bottle/250ml	163	0.3	65	0.7	15.2	0.1	1.0

S

	Measure INFO/WEIGHT	per Measure		Nutrition Values per 100g / 100ml				
		KCAL	FAT	KCAL	PROT	CARB	FAT	FIBRE
SMOOTHIE								
Pineapples, Bananas & Coconuts, Innocent*	1 Bottle/250ml	183	3.0	73	0.7	15.3	1.2	1.0
Pomegranates & Raspberries, Innocent*	1 Bottle/250ml	150	0.3	60	0.6	15.4	0.1	2.0
Raspberry, Banana & Peach, Sainsbury's*	1 Bottle/250.9ml	138	0.3	55	0.8	12.8	0.1	1.5
Raspberry & Bio Yoghurt, M & S*	1 Bottle/500ml	275	1.5	55	2.0	10.8	0.3	0.9
Raspberry & Blueberry, Plus, Tesco*	1 Serving/100ml	59	0.3	59	2.6	11.6	0.3	0.5
Strawberries & Bananas, PJ Smoothies*	1 Bottle/330ml	155	0.3	47	0.4	11.0	0.1	0.0
Strawberries & Bananas, Pure Fruit, Innocent*	1 Bottle/250ml	143	0.3	57	0.5	14.4	0.1	1.3
Strawberry, Dairy, Finest, Tesco*	1 Bottle/250ml	163	0.3	65	2.9	13.2	0.1	0.1
Strawberry, Raspberry & Banana, Waitrose*	1 Bottle/250ml	123	0.3	49	0.7	10.8	0.1	0.8
Strawberry & Banana, Fruit, Finest, Tesco*	1 Bottle/250ml	135	0.8	54	0.3	12.5	0.3	0.5
Strawberry & Banana, Morrisons*	1 Bottle/250ml	135	0.0	54	0.5	13.0	0.0	0.6
Strawberry & Banana, Tesco*	1 Sm Bottle/250ml	113	0.5	45	0.6	10.1	0.2	0.8
Strawberry & Raspberry, COU, M & S*	1 Bottle/250ml	125	0.3	50	0.5	11.7	0.1	2.4
Strawberry & Raspberry, Fruity, Sainsbury's*	1 Glass/200ml	106	0.0	53	0.6	11.9	0.0	2.4
Strawberry & Raspberry, Shapers, Boots*	1 Bottle/250ml	123	0.5	49	0.3	12.0	0.2	0.6
Strawberry Dairy, Shapers, Boots*	1 Bottle/250ml	120	0.8	48	1.7	9.7	0.3	0.5
Strawberry with Yoghurt, Finest, Tesco*	1 Serving/100ml	62	1.2	62	2.1	10.5	1.2	0.6
Summer Fruits, Tesco*	1 Bottle/250ml	140	0.0	56	0.2	13.8	0.0	0.5
Vanilla Bean, M & S*	1 Bottle/500ml	450	13.0	90	3.3	13.9	2.6	0.0
Yoghurt, Vanilla Bean & Honey, Innocent*	1 Bottle/250g	235	6.5	94	3.5	14.5	2.6	0.0
SMOOTHIES								
Iced, Blackcurrant, Ribena*	1 Serving/90g	70	0.1	78	0.2	19.1	0.1	11.8
Strawberries & Bananas, Innocent*	1 Serving/250ml	138	0.3	55	0.6	14.6	0.1	1.5
SNACK MIX								
Bowl, Bombay, Tesco*	¼ Bowl/131g	626	34.9	477	19.5	40.0	26.6	3.6
Bowl, Oriental Style, Tesco*	¼ Bowl/80g	298	0.6	373	7.2	84.2	0.8	1.0
Roasted, Organic, Clearspring*	1 Bag/60.1g	271	17.1	451	37.5	11.1	28.5	14.4
SNACK POT								
Potato & Vegetable, Quick Snack, Made Up, Tru Free*	1 Pack/245.8g	236	7.4	96	1.0	15.0	3.0	1.0
Potato & Vegetable, Wheat & Gluten Free, Trufree*	1 Pot/244.6g	225	8.6	92	1.3	13.8	3.5	1.1
Rice & Lentil, Quick Snack, Made Up, Tru Free*	1 Pack/270g	291	5.0	108	3.0	20.4	1.9	0.6
SNACK SALAD								
Prawn, Lime & Chilli, Good Intentions, Somerfield*	1 Pack/226g	276	9.3	122	4.1	17.3	4.1	1.8
SNACK STOP								
Bolognese Style, Big, Made Up, Crosse & Blackwell*	1 Pot/407.1g	403	4.5	99	2.8	19.5	1.1	0.0
Cheese & Pepperoni, Made Up, Crosse & Blackwell*	1 Pack/237g	237	9.7	100	2.9	13.3	4.1	0.0
Chicken & Mushroom Flavour Pasta, Crosse & Blackwell*	1 Pot/60g	251	5.3	418	10.3	74.3	8.8	0.0
Creamy Cheese Pasta, Made Up, Crosse & Blackwell*	1 Pot/218.3g	251	6.3	115	3.0	19.2	2.9	0.0
Creamy Chicken Pasta, Made Up, Crosse & Blackwell*	1 Pot/247g	210	4.0	85	2.7	15.7	1.6	0.0
Macaroni Cheese, Light, Made Up, Crosse & Blackwell*	1 Pack/248g	260	7.4	105	3.2	16.4	3.0	0.9
Mushroom Pasta Twirls, Made Up, Crosse & Blackwell*	1 Pot/248g	248	6.7	100	3.1	15.9	2.7	0.9
Roast Onion & Potato, Made Up, Crosse & Blackwell*	1 Pot/210g	210	7.8	100	1.7	14.4	3.7	0.0
Roast Parsnip & Potato, Made Up, Crosse & Blackwell*	1 Pot/210g	200	7.6	95	1.7	13.6	3.6	0.0
Spicy Tomato Pasta, Crosse & Blackwell*	1 Pot/412g	358	6.2	87	2.4	15.9	1.5	0.0
Sun Ripened Tomato & Herb, Crosse & Blackwell*	1 Pot/ 237g	201	2.6	85	2.6	16.1	1.1	0.0
SNACK-A-JACKS								
Barbecue, Jumbo, Quaker*	1 Cake/10g	38	0.2	380	8.0	83.0	2.0	1.7
Barbecue, Snack, Quaker*	1 Bag/30g	123	1.8	410	7.5	81.0	6.0	1.0
Caramel, Jumbo, Quaker*	1 Cake/10g	39	0.2	390	5.5	87.0	2.1	1.4
Caramel, Snack, Quaker*	1 Bag/30g	122	0.9	405	6.0	88.0	3.0	0.8
Cheese, Jumbo, Quaker*	1 Cake/10g	38	0.3	380	8.5	81.0	2.5	1.7
Cheese, Snack, Quaker*	1 Bag/30g	125	2.4	415	8.5	77.0	8.0	0.9
Cheese & Onion, Snack, Quaker*	1 Bag/30g	120	2.3	400	6.7	77.0	7.5	1.5

	Measure INFO/WEIGHT	per Measure KCAL	per Measure FAT	Nutrition Values per 100g / 100ml KCAL	PROT	CARB	FAT	FIBRE
SNACK-A-JACKS								
Chocolate & Caramel, Delights, Quaker*	1 Cake/15g	62	0.9	415	6.0	83.0	6.0	1.6
Chocolate Chip, Delights, Quaker*	1 Cake/15g	62	1.1	410	6.0	81.0	7.0	1.7
Prawn Cocktail, Snack, Quaker*	1 Pack/30g	123	2.3	410	7.0	78.0	7.5	0.8
Roast Chicken, Snack, Quaker*	1 Pack/30g	125	2.4	415	7.0	77.5	8.0	1.0
Salt & Vinegar, Snack, Quaker*	1 Std Bag/30g	123	2.3	410	7.0	79.0	7.5	0.9
Sour Cream & Chive, Snack, Quaker*	1 Std Bag/30g	125	2.3	415	8.0	79.0	7.5	1.3
SNAPPER								
Red, Fried in Blended Oil	1oz/28g	35	0.9	126	24.5	0.0	3.1	0.0
Red, Weighed with Bone, Raw	1oz/28g	25	0.4	90	19.6	0.0	1.3	0.0
SNICKERS								
Cruncher, Mars*	1 Bar/40g	209	12.0	523	9.0	57.0	30.0	2.3
Mars*	1 Bar/64.5g	323	18.1	501	9.3	52.9	28.1	0.0
SORBET								
Blackcurrant, Del Monte*	1oz/28g	30	0.0	106	0.4	27.1	0.1	0.0
Blackcurrant, Iceland*	¼ Pot/100g	100	0.0	100	0.0	25.0	0.0	0.0
Exotic Fruit, Sainsbury's*	1 Serving/75g	90	1.5	120	1.2	24.1	2.0	0.0
Jamaican Me Crazy, Ben & Jerry's*	1 Tub/391g	411	0.0	105	0.0	27.5	0.0	1.0
Lemon	1 Scoop/60g	79	0.0	131	0.9	34.2	0.0	0.0
Lemon, Asda*	1 Serving/100g	120	0.0	120	0.0	30.0	0.0	0.0
Lemon, Sainsbury's*	¼ Pot/89g	100	0.0	112	0.0	28.1	0.0	0.1
Lemon, Tesco*	1 Serving/75g	80	0.0	106	0.0	26.2	0.0	0.4
Lemon, The Real Ice Company*	1 Serving/100g	117	0.1	117	0.1	29.1	0.1	0.4
Lemon, Zesty, Haagen-Dazs*	1 Serving/125ml	120	0.0	96	0.0	24.8	0.0	1.0
Lemon Harmony, Haagen-Dazs*	1 Serving/90ml	214	10.2	238	1.5	32.5	11.3	0.0
Mango, Del Monte*	1 Sorbet/500g	575	0.5	115	0.2	29.6	0.1	0.0
Mango, Organic, M & S*	1 Serving/100g	99	0.1	99	0.3	24.1	0.1	0.9
Mango, Tesco*	1 Serving/100g	107	0.0	107	0.1	26.5	0.0	0.3
Mango, Waitrose*	1 Pot/100g	90	0.0	90	0.1	22.1	0.0	0.6
Orange, Del Monte*	1 Sorbet/500g	625	0.5	125	0.2	32.1	0.1	0.0
Passion Fruit, Fat Free, M & S*	1 Sorbet/125g	129	0.0	103	0.4	25.0	0.0	0.4
Peach & Strawberry, Haagen-Dazs*	1oz/28g	30	0.0	108	0.0	27.0	0.0	0.0
Peach & Vanilla Fruit Swirl, HL, Tesco*	1 Pot/73g	93	0.6	127	1.1	28.9	0.8	0.5
Pineapple, Del Monte*	1 Sorbet/500g	600	0.5	120	0.3	30.6	0.1	0.0
Raspberry, Haagen-Dazs*	½ Cup/105g	120	0.0	114	0.2	28.6	0.0	1.9
Raspberry, Sticks, Haagen-Dazs*	1oz/28g	28	0.0	99	0.2	24.2	0.1	0.0
Raspberry, Tesco*	1 Serving/70ml	97	0.0	138	0.5	34.0	0.0	0.0
Raspberry, Waitrose*	1 Pot/750ml	690	0.8	92	0.5	22.2	0.1	1.1
Raspberry & Blackberry, Fat Free, M & S*	1 Sorbet/125g	140	0.0	112	0.4	27.5	0.0	0.6
Strawberry, M & S*	1oz/28g	27	0.0	95	0.3	23.4	0.1	0.5
Strawberry & Champagne, Sainsbury's*	¼ Pot/89g	95	0.0	107	0.2	25.5	0.0	0.6
Swirl, Raspberry & Blackcurrant, Safeway*	1 Serving/50g	58	0.0	115	0.6	27.0	0.0	1.6
SOUFFLE								
Cheese	1oz/28g	71	5.4	253	11.4	9.3	19.2	0.3
Cheese, Mini, Waitrose*	1 Souffle/14g	32	2.4	232	16.0	2.9	17.4	2.4
Chocolate, Gu*	1 Pot/70g	307	24.9	439	6.3	24.4	35.6	2.9
Plain	1oz/28g	56	4.1	201	7.6	10.4	14.7	0.3
Ricotta & Spinach, M & S*	1 Serving/120g	186	13.3	155	8.0	6.2	11.1	2.1
Strawberry, M & S*	1 Serving/95g	171	10.1	180	1.6	19.5	10.6	0.9
SOUP								
Asparagus, Batchelors*	1 Serving/223g	143	6.2	64	0.5	9.2	2.8	0.4
Asparagus, Fresh, Finest, Tesco*	½ Pot/300g	153	8.1	51	1.6	5.0	2.7	1.0
Asparagus, Fresh, M & S*	1 Serving/300g	135	10.8	45	1.1	2.5	3.6	0.9
Asparagus, in a Cup, BGTY, Sainsbury's*	1 Sachet/18g	72	1.5	400	1.7	77.8	8.3	2.8

S

SOUP

	Measure INFO/WEIGHT	per Measure KCAL	per Measure FAT	Nutrition Values per 100g / 100ml KCAL	PROT	CARB	FAT	FIBRE
Asparagus, Knorr*	1 Serving/100g	28	1.0	28	0.4	4.5	1.0	0.1
Asparagus, M & S*	1 Serving/300g	180	13.5	60	1.1	3.3	4.5	0.7
Asparagus, NCGF Co*	½ Carton/300g	111	5.1	37	0.9	4.5	1.7	0.9
Asparagus, Simmer & Serve, Dried, Sainsbury's*	1/3 Pack/100ml	35	1.6	35	0.4	4.8	1.6	0.3
Asparagus, Slimline, Cup, Waitrose*	1 Sachet/204ml	51	1.4	25	0.4	4.3	0.7	0.7
Asparagus, Waitrose*	1 Serving/300g	60	3.6	20	0.9	1.5	1.2	0.9
Asparagus & Chicken, Waitrose*	1 Can/415g	166	4.6	40	2.1	5.3	1.1	0.7
Asparagus & Creme Fraiche, Morrisons*	½ Pot/300g	186	11.7	62	1.3	5.4	3.9	0.5
Aubergine & Red Pepper, Flame Grilled, NCGF Co*	1 Carton/600g	144	0.6	24	0.9	4.8	0.1	0.4
Autumn Vegetable, Vie, Knorr*	1 Pack/500ml	190	10.0	38	0.7	4.3	2.0	0.7
Autumn Vegetable & Lentil, Heinz*	1 Can/400g	184	1.2	46	2.3	8.6	0.3	1.0
Bean, Italian Style, Tesco*	1 Can/300g	153	3.6	51	2.8	7.3	1.2	1.1
Beef, Big, Heinz*	1 Can/400g	180	2.8	45	2.4	7.2	0.7	0.9
Beef & Tomato, Cup a Soup, Batchelors*	1 Portion/252g	83	1.6	33	0.6	6.3	0.6	0.4
Beef & Vegetable, Big, Heinz*	½ Can/200g	102	1.8	51	3.2	7.6	0.9	1.0
Beef & Vegetable, Chunky, Canned, Sainsbury's*	1 Can/400g	176	2.4	44	2.7	7.0	0.6	0.0
Beef & Vegetable, Chunky, Meal, Tesco*	1 Can/400g	344	19.2	86	7.0	5.3	4.8	0.6
Beef & Vegetable, for One, Fresh, Tesco*	1 Pot/300g	102	3.0	34	2.9	3.3	1.0	1.1
Beef & Vegetable, Fresh, NCGF Co*	½ Carton/300g	177	6.6	59	4.5	5.4	2.2	0.7
Beef & Vegetable Broth, Chunky, Canned, M & S*	1 Can/415g	166	3.3	40	1.9	6.4	0.8	0.6
Beef & Vegetable Mighty, Asda*	1 Can/400g	192	2.8	48	3.6	6.8	0.7	1.7
Beef & Winter Vegetable, Favourites, Baxters*	1 Can/415g	195	4.6	47	2.3	6.9	1.1	0.4
Beef Broth, Big, Heinz*	1 Serving/200g	86	1.4	43	2.2	6.9	0.7	1.0
Beef Chilli Baked Potato Big, Heinz*	1 Can/400g	232	3.6	58	3.4	9.1	0.9	1.3
Beijing, Vitasia*	1 Can/400ml	168	4.0	42	1.1	7.2	1.0	0.0
Big Red Tomato, Heinz*	½ Can/210g	63	0.8	30	0.5	6.4	0.4	0.0
Blended Autumn Vegetable, Heinz*	½ Can/200g	114	6.0	57	1.2	6.4	3.0	0.7
Blended Carrot & Coriander, Heinz*	½ Can/200g	104	5.4	52	0.7	6.2	2.7	0.6
Blended Leek & Bacon, Heinz*	½ Can/200g	108	5.8	54	1.9	5.0	2.9	0.5
Blended Sweetcorn & Yellow Pepper, Heinz*	½ Can/200g	98	4.2	49	0.9	6.6	2.1	0.6
Boston Bean & Ham, NCGF Co*	½ Carton/300g	171	0.6	57	2.4	7.8	0.2	1.6
Broccoli, Baxters*	1 Can/425g	191	7.7	45	1.3	5.9	1.8	0.4
Broccoli & Cauliflower, Cup, BFY, Morrisons*	1 Sachet/15g	56	2.1	376	4.9	57.2	14.2	4.9
Broccoli & Cheddar, Heinz*	1 Can/430g	340	24.1	79	2.6	4.4	5.6	0.6
Broccoli & Potato, Organic, Baxters*	1 Can/425g	162	3.4	38	1.5	6.2	0.8	0.7
Broccoli & Stilton, Canned, Sainsbury's*	½ Can/200g	108	7.0	54	2.0	3.7	3.5	0.6
Broccoli & Stilton, Canned, Tesco*	1 Can/400g	240	14.0	60	1.7	5.0	3.5	0.4
Broccoli & Stilton, Classics, Fresh, Tesco*	½ Pot/300g	180	8.4	60	2.9	5.8	2.8	1.1
Broccoli & Stilton, Fresh, Sainsbury's*	½ Pot/300ml	156	9.9	52	3.0	2.6	3.3	1.8
Broccoli & Stilton, NCGF Co*	1 Carton/600ml	336	26.4	56	2.3	1.8	4.4	0.7
Broccoli & Stilton, Somerfield*	½ Pack/250g	140	9.8	56	1.6	3.5	3.9	1.5
Broccoli with Mustard, NCGF Co*	1 Carton/568g	204	10.8	36	1.3	3.3	1.9	1.2
Butternut Squash, Fresh, Waitrose*	½ Pot/300g	153	8.7	51	0.5	5.8	2.9	0.8
Butternut Squash & Red Pepper, Baxters*	1 Tin/415g	158	4.2	38	0.7	6.5	1.0	0.6
Cantonese Hot & Sour Noodle, Baxters*	1 Serving/215g	133	2.8	62	1.4	11.1	1.3	0.5
Carrot, Onion & Chick Pea, Healthy Choice, Baxters*	1 Can/415ml	170	0.8	41	1.9	8.0	0.2	1.2
Carrot, Orange & Ginger, Go Organic*	1 Jar/495g	119	4.0	24	0.5	3.6	0.8	1.4
Carrot, Parsnip & Sweet Potato, Classic, Baxters*	1 Carton/600g	348	16.8	58	0.9	7.2	2.8	1.3
Carrot, Potato & Coriander, Weight Watchers*	1 Can/295g	74	0.3	25	0.5	5.5	0.1	0.6
Carrot & Butter Bean, Baxters*	½ Can/207.4g	112	3.9	54	1.6	7.7	1.9	1.7
Carrot & Coriander, Baxters*	1 Can/425g	174	6.4	41	0.8	6.0	1.5	0.8
Carrot & Coriander, Canned, BGTY, Sainsbury's*	½ Can/200g	62	2.0	31	0.8	4.8	1.0	0.9
Carrot & Coriander, Canned, M & S*	½ Can/210g	95	5.0	45	0.4	5.9	2.4	0.9

SOUP

	Measure INFO/WEIGHT	per Measure KCAL	FAT	Nutrition Values per 100g / 100ml KCAL	PROT	CARB	FAT	FIBRE
Carrot & Coriander, Canned, Tesco*	1 Can/400g	220	11.6	55	0.7	5.7	2.9	0.8
Carrot & Coriander, Carton, Campbell's*	1 Serving/250ml	110	5.5	44	0.7	5.4	2.2	0.0
Carrot & Coriander, Classic Homestyle, M & S*	1 Can/425g	170	8.5	40	0.6	5.6	2.0	0.7
Carrot & Coriander, Classics, Fresh, Tesco*	½ Pot/300g	120	6.3	40	0.7	4.6	2.1	1.4
Carrot & Coriander, Fresh, Asda*	1 Pack/315g	98	1.6	31	0.7	5.8	0.5	3.0
Carrot & Coriander, Fresh, Co-Op*	½ Carton/300g	105	6.0	35	0.6	3.0	2.0	2.0
Carrot & Coriander, Fresh, Low Fat, Sainsbury's*	½ Pot/300g	95	4.5	32	0.7	3.8	1.5	1.5
Carrot & Coriander, Fresh, M & S*	½ Pot/300g	90	4.5	30	0.4	4.2	1.5	0.5
Carrot & Coriander, Fresh, Morrisons*	½ Pot/300g	120	7.2	40	1.1	3.2	2.4	0.9
Carrot & Coriander, Fresh, NCGF Co*	½ Carton/300g	129	6.6	43	0.6	5.2	2.2	1.2
Carrot & Coriander, Fresh, Waitrose*	½ Pot/300g	150	10.2	50	0.5	4.4	3.4	0.9
Carrot & Coriander, GFY, Asda*	1 Carton/600g	132	4.2	22	0.5	3.3	0.7	1.2
Carrot & Coriander, PB, Waitrose*	½ Can/207.5g	33	0.4	16	0.5	3.1	0.2	1.0
Carrot & Coriander, Seeds of Change*	1 Pack/500g	185	9.0	37	0.6	4.7	1.8	1.1
Carrot & Coriander, Selection, Campbell's*	1 Carton/500ml	185	5.0	37	0.6	6.4	1.0	0.6
Carrot & Coriander, Somerfield*	½ Pot/300g	108	8.1	36	0.5	2.3	2.7	2.2
Carrot & Coriander, Soup in a Mug, HL, Tesco*	1 Serving/21g	81	2.2	385	4.8	66.4	10.7	5.1
Carrot & Ginger, Fresh, Sainsbury's*	1 Pot/600g	150	5.4	25	0.4	3.9	0.9	1.0
Carrot & Lentil, Microwave, Heinz*	1 Can/303.2g	94	0.3	31	1.5	6.1	0.1	0.8
Carrot & Orange	1oz/28g	6	0.1	20	0.4	3.7	0.5	1.0
Carrot & Orange, Baxters*	1 Can/415g	174	2.1	42	1.0	8.3	0.5	0.4
Carrot & Orange, Fresh, Finest, Tesco*	½ Tub/300g	150	5.7	50	0.7	7.5	1.9	1.1
Carrot & Orange, Fresh, Sainsbury's*	½ Carton/300g	54	0.3	18	0.4	4.2	0.1	0.9
Carrot & Parsnip, M & S*	1 Can/425g	170	7.2	40	0.6	6.0	1.7	1.0
Carrot with Creme Fraiche, Baxters*	1 Can/415g	170	7.1	41	0.5	5.9	1.7	0.7
Cauliflower Cheese, Safeway*	1 Serving/300g	135	6.9	45	2.3	3.7	2.3	0.8
Celeriac & Leek with Horseradish, NCGF Co*	½ Carton/300g	108	8.7	36	0.7	1.8	2.9	1.1
Chicken, Campbell's*	1 Can/295g	142	10.6	48	1.1	3.5	3.6	0.0
Chicken, Coconut & Lemon Grass, Fresh, Waitrose*	½ Pot/300g	303	24.9	101	2.6	4.1	8.3	0.8
Chicken, Condensed, 99% Fat Free, Campbell's*	1 Can/295g	77	2.1	26	1.0	3.8	0.7	0.1
Chicken, Cream Of, Canned	1oz/28g	16	1.1	58	1.7	4.5	3.8	0.0
Chicken, Cream Of, Fresh, Tesco*	½ Tub/300g	129	5.1	43	1.8	5.0	1.7	0.6
Chicken, Cup, Calorie Counter, Dry, Co-Op*	1 Sachet/12.5g	42	1.4	320	6.0	49.0	11.0	7.0
Chicken, Fresh, Sainsbury's*	½ Carton/300g	126	5.7	42	2.2	4.0	1.9	0.3
Chicken, From Heinz, Canned, Weight Watchers*	1 Can/295g	88	2.9	30	1.2	4.0	1.0	0.0
Chicken, Green Thai, Waitrose*	½ Pot/300g	246	16.2	82	3.8	4.6	5.4	0.9
Chicken, in a Cup, Dry, Symingtons*	1 Serving/22g	93	4.0	424	7.0	57.7	18.4	11.7
Chicken, Jamaican Jerk & Pumpkin, Sainsbury's*	½ Pot/300g	141	5.1	47	2.7	5.1	1.7	0.2
Chicken, Mushroom & Potato, Big, Heinz*	½ Can/200g	132	4.6	66	3.4	8.1	2.3	0.4
Chicken, Mushroom & Rice, Chilled, M & S*	½ Pot/300g	225	10.2	75	3.2	7.3	3.4	1.8
Chicken, NCGF Co*	1 Carton/600g	510	32.4	85	3.8	5.4	5.4	0.6
Chicken, Red Thai, Chunky, Fresh, Sainsbury's*	½ Pot/300g	165	9.9	55	0.9	5.4	3.3	0.9
Chicken, Thai, Fresh, Finest, Tesco*	½ Tub/300g	180	11.1	60	3.9	2.9	3.7	0.7
Chicken, Thai, GFY, Asda*	1 Serving/200g	85	3.0	43	1.7	5.5	1.5	0.5
Chicken, Thai, Spicy, Baxters*	1 Can/415g	278	14.5	67	1.8	7.1	3.5	0.3
Chicken, Thai & Coconut, Safeway*	1 Serving/300g	235	15.5	78	3.4	4.6	5.2	0.9
Chicken, Thai Style, Morrisons*	1 Serving/250g	240	15.5	96	4.6	5.5	6.2	1.2
Chicken, Thai Style, Thick & Creamy, in a Mug, Tesco*	1 Sachet/28g	107	4.0	390	3.7	61.3	14.5	5.1
Chicken & Broccoli, Soup a Cups, GFY, Asda*	1 Cup/226.1ml	52	1.4	23	0.5	4.0	0.6	0.4
Chicken & Broccoli Cup a Soup, Asda*	1 Serving/16g	55	1.4	341	7.0	58.0	9.0	6.0
Chicken & Country Vegetable, Soupfulls, Batchelors*	1 Serving/400g	164	3.6	41	5.1	3.0	0.9	1.3
Chicken & Ham, Chunky, Canned, Sainsbury's*	½ Can/200g	80	1.2	40	2.7	6.0	0.6	0.9
Chicken & King Prawn, Noodle, Fresh, Tesco*	1 Pot/400g	180	1.6	45	4.7	5.5	0.4	0.4

S

SOUP

	Measure INFO/WEIGHT	per Measure KCAL	FAT	Nutrition Values per 100g / 100ml KCAL	PROT	CARB	FAT	FIBRE
Chicken & Leek, Big, Heinz*	½ Can/200g	128	4.4	64	2.9	8.1	2.2	0.6
Chicken & Leek, Cup a Soup, Made Up, Batchelors*	1 Serving/259g	96	4.7	37	0.5	4.7	1.8	0.7
Chicken & Leek, Soup in a Cup, Made Up, Sainsbury's*	1 Serving/200ml	82	3.3	41	0.4	6.2	1.7	0.1
Chicken & Mushroom, Extra, Slim a Soup, Batchelors*	1 Serving/257.1g	90	1.5	35	1.4	5.9	0.6	0.3
Chicken & Mushroom in a Cup, Sainsbury's*	1 Sachet/223ml	107	4.2	48	0.7	7.1	1.9	0.1
Chicken & Pasta Big, Heinz*	½ Can/200g	68	0.8	34	1.8	5.9	0.4	0.8
Chicken & Red Pepper Noodle, Fresh, Tesco*	1 Serving/400ml	200	1.2	50	3.6	8.5	0.3	0.4
Chicken & Sweetcorn, Asda*	1 Pot/600g	246	8.4	41	2.2	4.9	1.4	1.6
Chicken & Sweetcorn, Baxters*	1 Can/425g	166	3.8	39	1.6	6.2	0.9	0.6
Chicken & Sweetcorn, Canned, BGTY, Sainsbury's*	½ Can/200g	56	0.8	28	1.5	4.5	0.4	0.2
Chicken & Sweetcorn, Canned, HL, Tesco*	½ Can/200g	70	0.6	35	1.6	6.5	0.3	0.3
Chicken & Sweetcorn, Canned, Tesco*	1 Can/400ml	240	6.0	60	1.6	8.2	1.5	0.7
Chicken & Sweetcorn, Cantonese, Fresh, Sainsbury's*	½ Pot/300ml	135	1.5	45	2.1	7.9	0.5	0.5
Chicken & Sweetcorn, Cup, Morrisons*	1 Serving/14g	53	2.1	375	8.4	51.2	15.2	0.0
Chicken & Sweetcorn, Cup Soup, Asda*	1 Sachet/200ml	109	3.9	55	0.7	8.5	2.0	0.3
Chicken & Sweetcorn, Fresh, Asda*	1 Pack/500g	260	9.5	52	2.6	6.0	1.9	0.0
Chicken & Sweetcorn, Fresh, Sainsbury's*	1 Bottle/600ml	312	12.6	52	2.8	5.4	2.1	1.2
Chicken & Sweetcorn, GFY, Asda*	1 Can/400g	108	2.0	27	1.5	4.2	0.5	0.2
Chicken & Sweetcorn, Light Choice, Tesco*	½ Can 200g	84	0.8	42	1.7	7.9	0.4	0.2
Chicken & Sweetcorn, NCGF Co*	1 Carton/600g	282	5.4	47	1.0	8.7	0.9	0.5
Chicken & Tarragon, Thick & Creamy, Batchelors*	1 Sachet/281g	118	6.5	42	0.8	5.7	2.3	0.3
Chicken & Vegetable, Big, Heinz*	½ Can/200g	94	1.2	47	2.9	7.4	0.6	0.9
Chicken & Vegetable, Chunky, Canned, Sainsbury's*	½ Can/200g	94	1.6	47	4.0	6.0	0.8	1.6
Chicken & Vegetable, Chunky, Meal, Canned, Tesco*	1 Can/410g	176	2.1	43	2.3	7.2	0.5	0.7
Chicken & Vegetable, Chunky, Safeway*	1 Can/400g	156	2.0	39	2.5	6.2	0.5	0.6
Chicken & Vegetable, Fresh, Somerfield*	½ Pot/300g	177	8.4	59	2.9	5.6	2.8	3.0
Chicken & Vegetable, Loyd Grossman*	1 Pouch/420g	286	16.0	68	0.5	8.0	3.8	0.6
Chicken & Vegetable, Mighty, Asda*	1 Can/410g	176	5.3	43	2.5	6.8	1.3	0.7
Chicken & Vegetable, PB, Waitrose*	1 Can/415g	141	2.5	34	1.8	5.4	0.6	1.0
Chicken & Vegetable, Soup in a Mug, Value, Tesco*	1 Serving/19g	75	2.5	395	4.4	64.1	13.4	1.6
Chicken & Vegetable, Soup to Go, Asda*	1 Pot/330g	144	4.9	44	2.4	5.1	1.5	0.7
Chicken & Vegetable Broth, Canned, BFY, Morrisons*	½ Can/205g	50	0.4	24	1.2	4.5	0.2	0.5
Chicken & Vegetable with Pasta, Select, Campbell's*	1 Can/480ml	220	1.0	46	2.9	7.9	0.2	0.8
Chicken Broth, Baxters*	1 Can/425g	132	1.7	31	1.5	5.4	0.4	0.6
Chicken Broth, Somerfield*	1 Pot/600g	240	7.2	40	2.5	4.3	1.2	0.8
Chicken Mulligatawny, Fresh, Finest, Tesco*	½ Pot/300g	237	8.4	79	3.8	9.7	2.8	0.8
Chicken Noodle, Asda*	1 Can/400g	144	3.6	36	1.9	5.0	0.9	0.5
Chicken Noodle, Batchelors*	1 Pack/284g	71	0.6	25	1.6	4.2	0.2	0.3
Chicken Noodle, Canned, Sainsbury's*	½ Can/216.7g	78	0.7	36	1.7	7.4	0.3	0.7
Chicken Noodle, Chunky, Campbell's*	½ Can/200g	86	1.2	43	2.8	6.5	0.6	0.0
Chicken Noodle, Clear, From Heinz, Weight Watchers*	1 Can/295g	50	0.3	17	0.7	3.1	0.1	0.2
Chicken Noodle, Cup, Asda*	1 Sachet/13g	40	0.2	305	9.0	63.0	1.9	3.6
Chicken Noodle, Dry, Morrisons*	1oz/28g	88	1.1	314	13.1	56.0	4.0	5.1
Chicken Noodle, Dry, Symingtons*	½ Pack/15g	48	0.4	318	8.6	65.4	2.4	2.4
Chicken Noodle, Heinz*	½ Can/200g	55	0.5	28	1.2	5.1	0.3	0.2
Chicken Noodle, Simmer & Serve, Dried, Sainsbury's*	1 Pack/600ml	102	1.2	17	0.8	2.9	0.2	0.0
Chicken Noodle, Soup in a Cup, Made Up, Sainsbury's*	1 Serving/200ml	44	0.2	22	0.7	4.7	0.1	0.2
Chicken Noodle, with Sweetcorn, Baxters*	1 Can/415g	141	2.5	34	1.4	5.8	0.6	0.2
Chilli, Meal, Chunky, Canned, Tesco*	½ Can/200g	120	2.4	60	5.0	6.3	1.2	1.6
Chinese Chicken Noodle, Dry, Knorr*	1 Pack/45g	138	2.0	307	15.1	51.8	4.4	2.9
Chowder, Bacon & Corn, M & S*	½ Pot/300g	195	10.8	65	2.5	6.0	3.6	1.8
Chowder, Clam, New England, Select, Campbell's*	1 Cup/240ml	221	14.4	92	2.5	6.0	6.0	0.8
Chowder, Prawn, Manhattan, Fresh, Sainsbury's*	1 Serving/300g	177	6.9	59	1.6	7.9	2.3	0.1

SOUP

	Measure INFO/WEIGHT	per Measure KCAL	FAT	Nutrition Values per 100g / 100ml KCAL	PROT	CARB	FAT	FIBRE
Chowder, Seafood, Baxters*	½ Can/213.3g	160	9.6	75	3.3	5.4	4.5	0.4
Chowder, Smoked Haddock, Canned, Tesco*	½ Can/200g	140	8.2	70	1.8	6.8	4.1	0.2
Cock-A-Leekie, Traditional, Baxters*	1 Can/425g	98	2.1	23	1.0	3.7	0.5	0.3
Country Garden, Vegetarian, Canned, Baxters*	1 Can/415g	137	2.1	33	1.0	6.0	0.5	0.8
Country Mushroom, Baxters*	1 Pot/600g	378	24.6	63	0.9	5.5	4.1	0.1
Country Mushroom, Selection, Campbell's*	1 Serving/250ml	80	4.5	32	0.6	3.4	1.8	0.5
Country Vegetable, Asda*	1 Serving/125g	59	3.6	47	0.6	4.5	2.9	0.8
Country Vegetable, Chilled, M & S*	½ Pot/300g	105	6.3	35	0.5	3.2	2.1	1.0
Country Vegetable, Chunky, Asda*	½ Pot/300g	105	2.7	35	0.7	6.0	0.9	0.6
Country Vegetable, Chunky, Healthy Choice, Baxters*	1 Pot/273.9g	126	0.8	46	2.0	8.8	0.3	1.7
Country Vegetable, Erin*	1 Bowl/250ml	78	2.4	31	0.9	4.8	1.0	0.3
Country Vegetable, Fresh, Asda*	1 Carton/500g	195	2.0	39	1.9	7.0	0.4	0.0
Country Vegetable, Fresh, Chilled, M & S*	1 Pot/600g	210	12.6	35	0.5	3.2	2.1	1.0
Country Vegetable, Fresh, Morrisons*	½ Pot/295.5g	130	5.3	44	1.1	5.9	1.8	1.0
Country Vegetable, Fresh, Sainsbury's*	½ Pot/300g	123	2.7	41	1.6	6.6	0.9	2.5
Country Vegetable, From Heinz, Weight Watchers*	1 Can/295g	91	0.6	31	1.1	6.1	0.2	1.0
Country Vegetable, Heinz*	1oz/28g	14	0.1	51	2.3	9.3	0.5	1.1
Country Vegetable, M & S*	½ Can/207.5g	90	1.9	43	1.7	6.9	0.9	1.3
Country Vegetable, Thick, Asda*	½ Can/200g	109	6.0	55	0.8	5.5	3.0	1.5
Courgette & Parmesan, Fresh, Sainsbury's*	1 Pack/300ml	198	16.8	66	1.5	2.5	5.6	0.4
Cream of Asparagus, Baxters*	1 Can/415g	278	17.8	67	1.1	6.0	4.3	0.2
Cream of Asparagus, Cup a Soup, Batchelors*	1 Sachet/223g	143	6.2	64	0.5	9.2	2.8	0.4
Cream of Celery, Asda*	1 Can/410g	189	11.1	46	0.6	4.8	2.7	0.2
Cream of Celery, Campbell's*	1 Serving/150g	71	5.1	47	0.6	3.2	3.4	0.0
Cream of Chicken, Asda*	1 Can/410g	209	13.9	51	1.2	4.0	3.4	0.1
Cream of Chicken, Batchelors*	1 Pack/289g	165	9.5	57	1.1	5.6	3.3	0.3
Cream of Chicken, Baxters*	½ Can/209g	144	8.8	69	1.8	6.1	4.2	0.1
Cream of Chicken, Campbell's*	1 Can/590g	283	21.2	48	1.1	3.5	3.6	0.0
Cream of Chicken, Canned, Sainsbury's*	½ Can/200g	96	5.4	48	2.3	3.7	2.7	0.2
Cream of Chicken, Condensed, Made Up, Heinz*	½ Can/295g	124	8.3	42	1.1	3.1	2.8	0.0
Cream of Chicken, Co-Op*	½ Can/200g	120	8.0	60	0.8	5.0	4.0	0.1
Cream of Chicken, for One, Heinz*	1 Can/290g	142	7.8	49	1.5	4.5	2.7	0.1
Cream of Chicken & Mushroom, Campbell's*	1 Can/250g	140	11.0	56	0.9	3.5	4.4	0.0
Cream of Chicken & Mushroom, Heinz*	½ Can/200g	98	5.8	49	1.3	4.6	2.9	0.1
Cream of Leek, Baxters*	1 Can/415g	237	17.4	57	1.1	3.8	4.2	0.7
Cream of Leek in Seconds, Dry, Knorr*	1 Pack/64g	326	21.6	509	5.9	45.2	33.8	1.4
Cream of Mushroom, Asda*	1 Can/410g	185	11.1	45	1.1	4.1	2.7	0.1
Cream of Mushroom, Canned, Sainsbury's*	1 Can/400g	220	20.8	55	0.6	1.4	5.2	0.1
Cream of Mushroom, Classics, Canned, Heinz*	1 Can/290g	151	8.1	52	1.5	5.2	2.8	0.1
Cream of Mushroom, Co-Op*	1 Pack/400g	240	16.0	60	1.0	5.0	4.0	0.0
Cream of Mushroom, Cup a Soup, Batchelors*	1 Serving/219g	125	6.1	57	0.6	7.5	2.8	0.4
Cream of Mushroom, Dry, Knorr*	1 Serving/25g	125	8.0	500	5.2	47.8	31.8	1.0
Cream of Mushroom, Fresh, Waitrose*	1 Pot/600g	282	17.4	47	0.9	4.3	2.9	0.5
Cream of Mushroom, Packet, Knorr*	1 Pack/75g	389	26.5	518	5.2	44.8	35.3	0.9
Cream of Mushroom, Soupreme*	1 Serving/200g	100	5.8	50	1.4	4.5	2.9	0.3
Cream of Mushroom Condensed, Made Up, Heinz*	1oz/28g	12	0.8	42	0.9	3.5	2.7	0.1
Cream of Potato & Leek, Canned, Sainsbury's*	½ Can/200g	80	3.0	40	0.6	6.1	1.5	0.0
Cream of Sweetcorn, Campbell's*	1 Serving/80g	41	2.2	51	0.6	6.2	2.7	0.3
Cream of Tomato, Asda*	½ Can/205g	137	7.0	67	1.0	8.0	3.4	0.0
Cream of Tomato, Diluted with Water, Campbell's*	½ Can/295g	195	9.4	66	0.8	8.5	3.2	0.0
Cream of Tomato, Dry, Knorr*	1 Pack/90g	392	21.2	435	4.3	51.3	23.6	3.3
Cream of Tomato, Favourites, Baxters*	1 Can/415g	257	11.2	62	1.0	8.4	2.7	0.3
Cream of Tomato, for One, Heinz*	1 Can/300g	189	10.8	63	0.8	6.9	3.6	0.4

SOUP

	Measure INFO/WEIGHT	per Measure KCAL	FAT	Nutrition Values per 100g / 100ml KCAL	PROT	CARB	FAT	FIBRE
Cream of Tomato, Fresh, Sainsbury's*	½ Pot/300ml	126	3.6	42	0.9	7.0	1.2	0.6
Cream of Tomato, Fresh, Waitrose*	½ Pot/300g	99	2.1	33	1.1	5.6	0.7	1.5
Cream of Tomato, Heinz*	½ Can/200g	114	6.0	57	0.9	6.7	3.0	0.4
Cream of Tomato, Microwaveable Cup, Heinz*	1 Cup/275ml	169	9.4	61	0.8	6.9	3.4	0.4
Cream of Tomato, Morrisons*	1 Serving/205g	141	6.2	69	1.2	9.4	3.0	0.6
Cream of Tomato, Organic, Heinz*	1 Can/400g	220	10.4	55	1.0	7.0	2.6	0.4
Cream of Tomato, SmartPrice, Asda*	1 Can/400g	174	6.8	44	0.4	6.7	1.7	0.7
Cream of Tomato & Basil, Somerfield*	1 Pack/450g	279	18.0	62	1.0	5.0	4.0	0.0
Cream of Vegatable, Cup Soup, Soupreme*	1 Serving/27g	95	2.8	352	4.8	59.6	10.5	6.3
Cream of Vegetable, Cup a Soup, Batchelors*	1 Sachet/33g	134	5.3	406	5.8	59.8	16.0	6.2
Cream of Vegetable, Cup a Soup, Soupreme*	1 Pack/20.5g	73	2.2	356	4.9	59.5	10.7	6.3
Creamy Chicken & Mushroom, Baxters*	1 Tin/415g	216	11.2	52	1.6	5.3	2.7	0.1
Creamy Mushroom, Asda*	1 Pot/500g	228	14.0	46	1.1	4.0	2.8	1.3
Creamy Mushroom, Fresh, Asda*	1 Serving/250g	110	6.8	44	1.1	3.8	2.7	1.3
Creamy Potato & Spring Onion, NCGF Co*	½ Carton/300g	168	8.7	56	1.0	6.4	2.9	1.1
Creamy Tomato, Fresh, Asda*	1 Pot/500g	202	12.0	40	0.7	4.0	2.4	0.5
Creamy Tomato, Seeds of Change*	1 Pack/350g	238	6.0	68	1.2	12.0	1.7	0.4
Crofter's Thick Vegetable, Dry, Knorr*	1 Pack/66g	240	8.1	364	10.8	52.9	12.2	3.3
Cullen Skink, Baxters*	1 Can/415g	357	13.7	86	6.4	7.7	3.3	0.4
English Broccoli & Stilton, Dry, Knorr*	1 Pack/65g	331	24.6	509	11.7	30.3	37.9	1.6
Farmhouse Chicken Leek, Dry, Knorr*	1 Pack/54g	248	15.7	459	10.3	39.3	29.0	1.5
Farmhouse Vegetable, Canned, BGTY, Sainsbury's*	½ Can/200ml	52	1.6	26	0.5	4.4	0.8	0.9
Farmhouse Vegetable, Fresh, Avonmore*	½ Carton/250g	138	5.0	55	1.9	7.4	2.0	0.8
Farmhouse Vegetable, Soup-A-Cup, GFY, Asda*	1 Sachet/218.5ml	59	1.1	27	0.6	4.9	0.5	0.4
Farmhouse Vegetable, Thick, Co-Op*	1 Can/400g	140	1.6	35	1.0	7.0	0.4	0.3
Fire Roasted Tomato & Red Pepper, Asda*	½ Tub/265.1g	114	6.9	43	0.7	4.1	2.6	1.0
Flame Roasted Red Pepper & Tomato, Baxters*	½ Can/207.1g	116	5.8	56	0.9	6.8	2.8	0.6
Florentine Pea, The Best, Safeway*	½ Pot/300g	165	7.5	55	2.5	4.9	2.5	1.4
Florida Spring Vegetable, Dry, Knorr*	1 Pack/36g	104	2.0	290	7.8	52.2	5.6	5.2
French Onion	1oz/28g	11	0.6	40	0.2	5.7	2.1	1.0
French Onion, Favourites, Baxters*	½ Can/207g	56	0.2	27	0.9	5.5	0.1	0.7
French Onion, Fresh, Morrisons*	1 Serving/500g	155	4.5	31	0.8	5.0	0.9	0.5
French Onion, GFY, Asda*	½ Pot/253g	91	1.3	36	1.9	6.0	0.5	0.4
French Onion, Simmer & Serve, Dried, Sainsbury's*	1/3 Sachet/204ml	37	0.2	18	0.3	3.8	0.1	0.2
French Onion & Cider, Waitrose*	1 Can/425g	94	0.4	22	0.5	4.8	0.1	0.4
Garden Vegetable, Baxters*	1 Serving/200g	70	1.2	35	0.9	6.6	0.6	0.8
Garden Vegetable, Heinz*	1 Can/400g	160	3.2	40	0.9	7.2	0.8	0.9
Gazpacho, NCGF Co*	1 Carton/600g	246	16.2	41	0.9	3.3	2.7	0.8
Golden Vegetable, Asda*	1 Pack/300g	150	6.0	50	1.9	6.0	2.0	0.0
Golden Vegetable, Calorie Counter, Cup, Co-Op*	1 Sachet/12g	40	1.2	335	7.0	54.0	10.0	5.0
Golden Vegetable, Cup, Calorie Counter, Co-Op*	1 Sachet/10.9g	35	1.1	320	7.0	50.0	10.0	9.0
Golden Vegetable, Dry, Knorr*	1 Pack/76g	299	14.4	394	10.4	45.4	19.0	3.3
Golden Vegetable, Slim a Soup, Batchelors*	1 Sachet/207g	58	1.7	28	0.5	4.7	0.8	0.7
Golden Vegetable, Soup-A-Slim, Asda*	1 Sachet/15g	50	1.2	336	6.0	60.0	8.0	1.9
Green Vegetables & Lentil, Lima*	1 Serving/300g	96	3.6	32	1.6	3.7	1.2	0.5
Haggis Broth, Baxters*	1 Can/425g	221	8.1	52	1.8	6.8	1.9	0.7
Highlander's Broth, Baxters*	½ Can/206.4g	97	3.1	47	1.8	6.5	1.5	0.6
Italian Bean & Pasta, Baxters*	1 Tin/415g	180	1.2	43	2.0	7.9	0.3	1.1
Italian Bean & Pasta, Healthy Choice, Baxters*	1 Can/415g	170	0.8	41	1.7	8.2	0.2	1.3
Italian Chicken Broth, Healthy Choice, Baxters*	½ Can/210g	84	1.7	40	1.5	6.6	0.8	0.8
Italian Minestrone, Dry, Knorr*	1 Pack/62g	193	2.5	311	11.5	57.1	4.1	7.8
Italian Minestrone, M & S*	1 Can/425g	191	2.1	45	2.2	9.0	0.5	0.8
Italian Style Tomato, Safeway*	½ Pot/248g	134	7.2	54	1.3	5.7	2.9	0.9

S

SOUP

	Measure INFO/WEIGHT	per Measure KCAL	per Measure FAT	Nutrition Values per 100g / 100ml KCAL	PROT	CARB	FAT	FIBRE
Italian Style Tomato & Basil, Co-Op*	1 Pack/500g	200	10.0	40	1.0	4.0	2.0	0.6
Italian Tomato & Basil, Go Organic*	1 Jar/495g	183	10.4	37	1.2	3.3	2.1	0.8
Lamb & Vegetable, Big Soup, Canned, Heinz*	½ Can/200g	116	2.4	58	2.8	9.0	1.2	1.3
Leek & Chicken, Knorr*	1 Serving/300ml	82	5.2	27	0.6	2.4	1.7	0.1
Leek & Maris Piper Potato, Chilled, M & S*	1 Serving/300g	165	11.4	55	0.6	4.5	3.8	0.9
Leek & Potato, Chunky, Meal, Canned, Tesco*	½ Can/200g	60	2.6	30	1.0	3.5	1.3	1.0
Leek & Potato, Creamy, Fresh, Asda*	1 Serving/300g	156	9.6	52	2.1	3.7	3.2	0.9
Leek & Potato, Cup a Soup, Batchelors*	1 Sachet/28g	121	4.9	432	5.2	63.2	17.6	1.8
Leek & Potato, Eat Smart, Safeway*	½ Pot/225g	113	5.4	50	1.1	6.0	2.4	0.6
Leek & Potato, Fresh, Sainsbury's*	½ Pot/300ml	141	7.2	47	1.0	5.3	2.4	0.4
Leek & Potato, Fresh, So Organic, Sainsbury's*	1 Serving/300g	108	4.2	36	0.9	4.9	1.4	0.6
Leek & Potato, Fresh, Somerfield*	½ Carton/300g	123	4.5	41	1.3	5.5	1.5	0.7
Leek & Potato, Fresh, Tesco*	½ Tub/300g	171	10.5	57	1.0	5.3	3.5	0.7
Leek & Potato, in a Cup, BGTY, Sainsbury's*	1 Sachet/196ml	53	1.4	27	0.3	4.9	0.7	0.2
Leek & Potato, Slim a Soup, Batchelors*	1 Serving/204g	57	1.4	28	0.4	5.0	0.7	0.2
Leek & Potato, Soup in a Cup, Made Up, Waitrose*	1 Sachet/204ml	47	1.0	23	0.3	4.3	0.5	0.5
Leek & Potato, Soup in a Mug, HL, Tesco*	1 Serving/16g	54	0.9	336	4.3	67.1	5.6	7.4
Leek & Potato, Weight Watchers*	1 Sachet/214.8ml	58	1.1	27	0.5	5.1	0.5	0.1
Lentil, Asda*	½ Can/202g	89	0.4	44	2.6	8.0	0.2	0.7
Lentil, Average	1 Serving/220g	218	8.4	99	4.4	12.7	3.8	1.1
Lentil, Campbell's*	1 Can/295g	139	1.8	47	2.6	7.7	0.6	0.0
Lentil, Canned	1 Serving/220g	86	0.4	39	3.1	6.5	0.2	1.2
Lentil, Carrot & Cumin, Canned, BGTY, Sainsbury's*	1 Can/400g	204	3.6	51	2.3	8.4	0.9	0.1
Lentil, Low Fat, Amy's Kitchen*	1 Can/411g	242	7.0	59	3.1	7.7	1.7	3.6
Lentil, Tomato & Vegetable, M & S*	1 Can/415g	170	3.4	41	2.0	6.3	0.8	1.4
Lentil, Wholesome, Heinz*	1 Can/300g	120	0.6	40	2.3	7.4	0.2	1.0
Lentil & Bacon, Baxters*	1 Can/415g	228	5.4	55	2.9	7.8	1.3	0.8
Lentil & Bacon, Canned, Tesco*	1 Serving/200g	96	1.4	48	3.2	7.2	0.7	0.5
Lentil & Bacon, Chunky, Fresh, Sainsbury's*	½ Pot/300g	117	2.4	39	2.3	5.7	0.8	2.0
Lentil & Bacon, Safeway*	1 Can/400g	160	1.6	40	2.7	6.3	0.4	2.9
Lentil & Chick Pea, Fresh, Organic, Tesco*	1 Serving/300ml	117	2.4	39	1.9	6.1	0.8	0.5
Lentil & Parsley, Simply Organic*	1 Pot/600g	390	1.8	65	4.4	11.8	0.3	1.4
Lentil & Tomato, NCGF Co*	½ Pack/284g	162	3.1	57	3.6	8.1	1.1	0.7
Lentil & Tomato, Spicy, Chunky, Fresh, Tesco*	½ Pot/300g	195	5.4	65	2.6	9.7	1.8	1.3
Lentil & Vegetable with Bacon, Organic, Baxters*	½ Can/211.4g	93	1.5	44	1.9	7.6	0.7	1.0
Lobster Bisque, Baxters*	1 Can/415g	187	8.7	45	3.0	3.6	2.1	0.2
Lobster Bisque, NCGF Co*	½ Carton/300g	108	1.8	36	3.2	4.4	0.6	0.4
Londoner's Pea Souper, NCGF Co*	½ Carton/300g	153	6.0	51	4.3	4.1	2.0	1.1
Mediterranean Fish, Waitrose*	½ Pot/300g	108	2.7	36	3.4	3.5	0.9	0.7
Mediterranean Tomato, Fresh, Organic, Sainsbury's*	1 Serving/250ml	78	3.5	31	1.3	3.3	1.4	1.0
Mediterranean Tomato, in a Cup, Waitrose*	1 Sachet/18g	52	1.5	289	8.3	45.6	8.3	10.0
Mediterranean Tomato, Instant, Weight Watchers*	1 Serving/200ml	50	0.2	25	0.7	5.2	0.1	0.1
Mediterrenean Tomato, Baxters*	1 Tin/415g	129	0.8	31	0.9	6.3	0.2	0.7
Melon & Carrot, NCGF Co*	1 Serving/300g	60	1.2	20	0.6	3.6	0.4	0.6
Minestrone, Average	1oz/28g	18	0.8	63	1.8	7.6	3.0	0.9
Minestrone, Baxters*	1 Can/425g	145	2.1	34	1.5	5.9	0.5	0.9
Minestrone, Canned	1oz/28g	9	0.2	32	1.4	5.1	0.8	0.6
Minestrone, Canned, M & S*	½ Can/200g	60	1.0	30	1.2	5.7	0.5	1.5
Minestrone, Chilled, M & S*	½ Pot/300g	135	3.9	45	2.0	5.8	1.3	1.9
Minestrone, Chunky, Big Soup, Canned, Heinz*	½ Can/200g	82	1.9	41	1.6	6.7	1.0	1.3
Minestrone, Chunky, Classic, Fresh, Tesco*	½ Pot/300g	126	2.1	42	1.2	7.8	0.7	1.2
Minestrone, Chunky, Classic, Meal, Canned, Tesco*	½ Can/205g	94	1.2	46	2.0	8.3	0.6	1.2
Minestrone, Chunky, COU, M & S*	1 Bowl/400g	300	7.2	75	3.0	11.8	1.8	0.8

S

SOUP

INFO/WEIGHT	Measure		per Measure		Nutrition Values per 100g / 100ml				
			KCAL	FAT	KCAL	PROT	CARB	FAT	FIBRE
Minestrone, Chunky, Fresh, Baxters*	1 Serving/250g		95	1.8	38	1.5	6.5	0.7	1.1
Minestrone, Chunky, Fresh, Sainsbury's*	½ Pot/302.9g		94	0.6	31	1.4	6.1	0.2	2.3
Minestrone, Chunky, Waitrose*	1 Can/415g		195	3.3	47	1.6	8.3	0.8	1.1
Minestrone, Classic, Canned, Heinz*	1 Can/400g		168	6.4	42	1.0	5.8	1.6	0.8
Minestrone, Cup a Soup, Batchelors*	1 Sachet/257.1g		90	1.8	35	0.6	6.6	0.7	0.7
Minestrone, for One, Heinz*	1 Can/300g		96	2.1	32	1.4	5.2	0.7	0.7
Minestrone, Fresh, Asda*	½ Pot/254.3g		89	2.3	35	0.8	6.0	0.9	1.2
Minestrone, Fresh, Baxters*	1 Box/568ml		233	5.7	41	1.8	6.2	1.0	0.6
Minestrone, Fresh, Safeway*	½ Pot/250g		83	1.3	33	1.0	6.2	0.5	0.8
Minestrone, Fresh, Waitrose*	1 Pack/600g		240	8.4	40	1.1	5.8	1.4	0.8
Minestrone, Healthy Choice, Baxters*	½ Can/207.5g		67	0.4	32	0.9	6.6	0.2	0.8
Minestrone, Mighty, Dry, Asda*	1 Serving/38.2g		130	0.5	343	9.0	74.0	1.2	2.4
Minestrone, NCGF Co*	½ Carton/300g		111	4.2	37	1.5	4.7	1.4	0.9
Minestrone, Organic, Seeds of Change*	1 Pack/350g		228	11.6	65	1.4	7.4	3.3	0.9
Minestrone, Packet, Dry, Knorr*	1 Pack/61g		178	2.7	292	9.2	53.9	4.4	6.5
Minestrone, Simmer, Dry, Asda*	1 Pack/50g		131	0.6	262	6.0	57.0	1.1	15.0
Minestrone, Soup a Slim, Asda*	1 Serving/17g		53	0.2	311	6.0	69.0	1.2	4.5
Minestrone, with Croutons, Cup a Soup, Batchelors*	1 Serving		93	1.3	37	0.7	7.3	0.5	0.3
Minestrone, with Croutons, in a Cup, Sainsbury's*	1 Sachet/225ml		72	0.9	32	0.9	6.3	0.4	0.5
Minestrone, with Croutons, in a Mug, Tesco*	1 Sachet/23g		83	1.9	360	9.0	62.6	8.1	2.7
Minestrone, with Croutons, Slim a Soup, Batchelors*	1 Serving/203g		55	1.2	27	0.6	4.8	0.6	0.6
Minestrone, with Pasta, Chunky, Co-Op*	1 Pack/400g		140	2.4	35	1.0	6.0	0.6	0.7
Minestrone with Wholemeal Pasta, Baxters*	1 Tin/400g		136	0.8	34	0.9	7.0	0.2	1.0
Minted Lamb Hot Pot, Big Soup, Canned, Heinz*	1 Can/400g		220	4.8	55	2.6	8.5	1.2	1.0
Miso, Instant, Blue Dragon*	1 Sachet/18g		25	0.7	139	10.0	14.4	3.9	0.0
Miso, Instant, Dry, Sanchi*	1 Sachet/8g		27	0.6	336	18.4	48.6	7.6	0.0
Miso, Organic, Instant, Sanchi*	1 Sachet/10g		27	0.3	270	14.0	47.0	3.0	0.0
Miso, Wakama*	1 Sachet/8g		27	0.6	336	18.7	48.6	7.6	0.0
Miso, with Tofu, Instant, Kikkoman*	1 Sachet/10g		35	1.0	350	30.0	30.0	10.0	0.0
Miso, with Tofu, Instant, Wakama*	1 Serving/8g		27	0.6	338	17.0	51.0	7.3	0.0
Moroccan Chicken, Waitrose*	½ Pot/300g		147	4.2	49	3.8	5.4	1.4	4.5
Moroccan Lentil, Waitrose*	½ Pot/300g		153	1.5	51	3.5	8.2	0.5	3.4
Mulligatawny	1 Serving/220g		213	15.0	97	1.4	8.2	6.8	0.9
Mulligatawny, Asda*	1 Can/400g		172	4.4	43	2.2	6.0	1.1	0.3
Mulligatawny, Canned, Tesco*	1 Can/400g		188	4.0	47	1.3	8.1	1.0	0.3
Mulligatawny Beef Curry, Heinz*	1oz/28g		15	0.5	54	2.0	7.2	1.9	0.6
Mushroom, Chilled, M & S*	½ Pot/300g		165	11.7	55	2.1	2.4	3.9	0.9
Mushroom, Cream Of, Canned	1 Serving/220g		101	6.6	46	1.1	3.9	3.0	0.1
Mushroom, Cream Of, Fresh, Tesco*	½ Tub/300g		129	6.3	43	1.3	4.7	2.1	0.3
Mushroom, Dry, Symingtons*	1 Serving/23g		80	2.1	348	17.8	48.4	9.2	6.7
Mushroom, for One, Heinz*	1 Tin/290g		148	7.8	51	1.4	5.1	2.7	0.1
Mushroom, From Heinz, Canned, Weight Watchers*	1 Tin/300g		81	1.8	27	1.0	4.4	0.6	0.1
Mushroom, Low Fat, Fresh, Sainsbury's*	½ Pot/300g		132	8.7	44	0.7	3.7	2.9	0.6
Mushroom, Morrisons*	1 Serving/500g		250	18.0	50	1.3	3.2	3.6	0.3
Mushroom, Wild, NCGF Co*	1 Carton/600g		228	9.6	38	1.2	4.8	1.6	0.6
Mushroom, Wild, Tesco*	1 Carton/400g		360	30.4	90	0.8	4.3	7.6	0.2
Mushroom, with Croutons, Soup in a Mug, Tesco*	1 Pack/26g		113	4.6	435	6.1	63.3	17.5	2.9
Mushroom & Tarragon, Fresh, TTD, Sainsbury's*	½ Pot/300ml		201	12.6	67	1.4	5.8	4.2	0.7
Mushroom Potage, Baxters*	1 Can/415g		320	21.6	77	1.5	6.1	5.2	0.3
Oxtail, Baxters*	1 Tin/415g		187	5.4	45	1.9	6.4	1.3	0.5
Oxtail, Canned	1 Serving/220g		97	3.7	44	2.4	5.1	1.7	0.1
Oxtail, Canned, Sainsbury's*	1 Can/400g		132	1.6	33	2.3	5.1	0.4	0.2
Oxtail, Canned, Tesco*	1 Can/400g		152	2.8	38	2.0	5.9	0.7	0.3

SOUP

INFO/WEIGHT	Measure KCAL	FAT	KCAL	PROT	CARB	FAT	FIBRE
Oxtail, Cup of Soup, Batchelors*	1 Serving/251.5g	83	3.3	33	0.9	4.4	1.3	0.3
Oxtail, Heinz*	1oz/28g	10	0.1	37	1.6	6.5	0.5	0.3
Parsnip, Fresh, Morrisons*	½ Pot/250g	100	3.8	40	0.9	5.8	1.5	1.4
Parsnip, Spicy, Canned, BGTY, Sainsbury's*	1 Can/400g	196	3.6	49	2.8	7.5	0.9	0.5
Parsnip, Spicy, Fresh, Tesco*	1 Serving/300g	123	6.3	41	0.8	4.6	2.1	1.9
Parsnip & Apple, COU, M & S*	1 Can/415g	187	10.4	45	0.7	5.4	2.5	1.2
Parsnip & Honey, Fresh, Sainsbury's*	½ Container/300g	192	12.6	64	1.1	5.4	4.2	1.5
Pea, Artichoke & Parmesan, The Best, Morrisons*	½ Pot/300g	171	7.8	57	2.8	5.6	2.6	1.0
Pea & Ham	1oz/28g	20	0.6	70	4.0	9.2	2.1	1.4
Pea & Ham, Baxters*	1 Can/425g	213	2.1	50	3.0	8.3	0.5	0.9
Pea & Ham, Canned, Asda*	1 Can/400g	140	4.0	35	2.0	4.5	1.0	1.4
Pea & Ham, Canned, Tesco*	1 Serving/300g	180	3.3	60	2.6	9.0	1.1	0.8
Pea & Ham, Fresh, Sainsbury's*	1 Serving/400ml	160	2.0	40	1.9	7.0	0.5	0.3
Pea & Ham, M & S*	1oz/28g	25	1.8	90	3.9	4.0	6.6	2.7
Pea & Ham, Morrisons*	1 Serving/250g	93	2.8	37	2.0	4.8	1.1	1.2
Pea & Mint, Fresh, M & S*	1 Serving/164g	49	0.2	30	1.8	6.3	0.1	1.5
Pea & Mint, Fresh, Sainsbury's*	½ Pot/300g	141	6.9	47	1.8	4.8	2.3	2.3
Pea & Mint, Fresh, Tesco*	1 Serving/300g	207	13.2	69	2.4	5.1	4.4	0.0
Pea & Mint, Fresh, Waitrose*	1 Serving/300g	126	3.9	42	2.8	4.7	1.3	2.9
Plum Tomato & Basil, NCGF Co*	½ Carton/300g	132	6.0	44	1.3	5.2	2.0	1.3
Pork, Chinese Dumpling, New Cultural Revolution*	1 Serving/250ml	156	4.0	62	6.4	6.0	1.6	0.4
Potato, Leek & Bacon, Fresh, Baxters*	½ Pot/300g	249	16.8	83	2.0	6.1	5.6	0.7
Potato, Leek & Chicken, Canned, BGTY, Sainsbury's*	½ Can/200g	62	0.8	31	1.6	5.3	0.4	0.4
Potato & Leek	1oz/28g	15	0.7	52	1.5	6.2	2.6	0.8
Potato & Leek, Canned, Baxters*	1 Can/415g	183	3.3	44	1.2	8.1	0.8	0.9
Potato & Leek, Classics, Canned, Heinz*	1 Can/400g	184	7.2	46	0.8	6.7	1.8	0.6
Potato & Leek, Fresh, Morrisons*	½ Carton/300g	204	12.0	68	1.8	6.2	4.0	0.7
Potato & Leek with Peppers & Chicken, Stockmeyer*	½ Can/200g	118	4.8	59	2.6	6.7	2.4	0.8
Pumpkin, NCGF Co*	½ Pint/284ml	97	3.1	34	0.4	5.5	1.1	0.6
Pumpkin, Spicy, Fresh, Sainsbury's*	½ Pot/300g	88	3.0	29	0.9	4.2	1.0	1.3
Puy Lentil & Tomato, Healthy Choice, Baxters*	½ Tin/207g	118	0.6	57	3.1	10.5	0.3	2.7
Puy Lentil & Vine Ripened Tomato, Finest, Tesco*	1 Pot/600g	360	7.8	60	2.8	9.2	1.3	1.5
Red Lentil & Ham, Waitrose*	½ Pot/300g	147	3.3	49	3.9	5.8	1.1	2.0
Red Lentil & Tomato, Canned, Tesco*	½ Can/300g	189	3.9	63	4.0	8.9	1.3	1.1
Red Pepper, Tomato & Basil, M & S*	1 Can/415g	83	1.2	20	1.3	2.7	0.3	0.8
Red Pepper & Tomato, Canned, PB, Waitrose*	½ Can/207g	77	3.7	37	0.8	4.5	1.8	0.9
Red Pepper with Tomato, Heinz*	½ Can/200g	102	5.8	51	0.8	5.2	2.9	0.7
Rice & Noodle, Instant, Thai Kitchen*	1 Pack/45g	190	3.0	422	6.7	82.2	6.7	0.0
Roasted Red Pepper, Fresh, Waitrose*	1 Pack/600g	172	9.0	29	0.8	3.0	1.5	1.0
Roasted Red Pepper & Tomato, M & S*	1 Serving/150g	105	7.4	70	1.4	5.0	4.9	0.6
Roasted Vegetable, Chunky, M & S*	1 Can/400g	140	2.4	35	1.3	5.8	0.6	1.1
Roasted Vegetable, Fresh, Sainsbury's*	½ Pot/273ml	71	1.4	26	0.5	4.8	0.5	1.2
Scotch Broth, Baxters*	1 Can/415g	166	3.7	40	1.6	6.4	0.9	0.7
Scotch Broth, Canned, Asda*	1 Can/400g	200	6.4	50	1.9	7.0	1.6	1.4
Scotch Broth, Canned, Heinz*	½ Can/200g	70	1.4	35	1.2	5.8	0.7	0.6
Scotch Broth, Canned, Sainsbury's*	½ Can/200g	100	2.4	50	1.7	8.0	1.2	0.7
Scotch Broth, Canned, Tesco*	½ Can/200g	72	1.8	36	1.4	6.4	0.9	0.8
Scotch Broth, Favourites, Baxters*	1 Serving/415g	166	3.7	40	1.6	6.4	0.9	0.7
Scotch Broth, Fresh, Baxters*	1 Serving/300g	108	2.1	36	1.6	5.9	0.7	0.6
Scotch Broth, M & S*	1 Serving/300g	150	7.2	50	2.1	5.1	2.4	1.1
Scotch Broth, NCGF Co*	1 Carton/600g	240	15.0	40	1.6	2.8	2.5	0.5
Scotch Vegetable, Baxters*	1 Can/425g	183	2.6	43	1.9	7.4	0.6	1.2
Spiced Chickpea & Fresh Red Pepper, M & S*	1 Serving/300g	165	6.9	55	2.2	5.8	2.3	2.5

SOUP

INFO/WEIGHT	Measure	per Measure		Nutrition Values per 100g / 100ml				
		KCAL	FAT	KCAL	PROT	CARB	FAT	FIBRE
Spiced Spinach & Green Lentil, Asda*	½ Pot/250g	123	5.0	49	2.7	5.0	2.0	0.0
Spicy Corn Chowder, NCGF Co*	½ Carton/300g	144	3.9	48	1.4	7.6	1.3	0.6
Spicy Lentil, Organic, Seeds of Change*	1 Pack/350g	249	7.7	71	2.8	9.8	2.2	0.7
Spicy Lentil, Seeds of Change*	1 Pack/422.2g	190	0.8	45	2.5	8.2	0.2	1.9
Spicy Parsnip, PB, Waitrose*	½ Can/216.7g	65	1.5	30	1.0	4.8	0.7	1.1
Spicy Parsnip, Vegetarian, Baxters*	1 Can/425g	217	10.6	51	1.1	6.1	2.5	1.5
Spicy Red Curry, Blue Dragon*	1 Serving/205g	97	5.1	47	0.4	5.8	2.5	0.3
Spicy Red Lentil & Tomato, M & S*	½ Pack/300g	150	2.4	50	2.7	8.0	0.8	1.1
Spicy Tomato & Vegetable, HL, Co-Op*	1 Can/400g	180	3.2	45	2.0	8.0	0.8	2.0
Spinach & Nutmeg, NCGF Co*	½ Carton/300g	114	4.2	38	1.3	5.1	1.4	0.8
Spinach & Watercress, NCGF Co*	½ Carton/298g	60	1.2	20	1.3	2.8	0.4	0.8
Split Pea & Ham, Asda*	1 Serving/300g	129	0.6	43	3.5	6.9	0.2	0.7
Split Peas, Yellow, Simply Organic*	1 Pot/600g	354	3.0	59	4.3	10.4	0.5	2.6
Spring Vegetable, Condensed, Campbell's*	1 Can/295g	62	0.3	21	0.5	4.5	0.1	0.0
Spring Vegetable, Heinz*	1 Can/400g	124	1.6	31	0.8	6.2	0.4	0.7
Stilton, Celery & Watercress, Morrisons*	1 Serving/250g	273	23.0	109	3.9	3.1	9.2	0.3
Sugar Snap Pea & Mint, NCGF Co*	½ Pack/300g	87	3.3	29	1.7	3.0	1.1	1.4
Summer Vegetable, NCGF Co*	½ Carton/300g	148	6.6	49	2.1	5.3	2.2	1.0
Sun Dried Tomato & Basil, Heinz*	1 Serving/275ml	124	5.2	45	0.6	6.5	1.9	0.1
Super Chicken Noodle, Dry, Knorr*	1 Pack/56g	182	2.7	325	14.3	56.0	4.9	1.8
Sweet Cherry Tomato, Fresh, TTD, Sainsbury's*	1 Pack/300g	120	4.5	40	0.7	6.0	1.5	1.0
Sweet Potato, Chilli & Ginger, NCGF Co*	1 Carton/600g	360	14.4	60	1.2	8.3	2.4	1.2
Sweet Potato & Coconut, COU, M & S*	1 Can/415g	166	5.4	40	0.7	6.7	1.3	0.8
Sweetcorn & Chilli, COU, M & S*	½ Can/275g	138	6.6	50	0.9	6.1	2.4	0.4
Sweetcorn & Chilli Chowder, Simply Organic*	½ Pot/300g	126	2.7	42	2.2	6.1	0.9	3.8
Thai Chicken, NCGF Co*	½ Carton/300g	174	10.5	58	2.6	4.1	3.5	0.8
Thai Spiced Mushroom, NCGF Co*	½ Carton/300g	150	6.6	50	1.5	6.0	2.2	0.5
Three Bean, Chunky, M & S*	1 Can/415g	208	5.0	50	2.3	7.5	1.2	1.8
Three Bean, Organic, Seeds of Change*	1 Serving/350g	207	4.6	59	2.1	9.7	1.3	1.6
Tomato, 99% Fat Free, Wattie's*	1 Serving/105g	32	0.4	31	1.0	5.6	0.4	1.1
Tomato, Canned, HL, Tesco*	½ Can/200g	110	4.0	55	0.7	7.5	2.0	0.5
Tomato, Cream Of, Canned	1oz/28g	15	0.8	52	0.8	5.9	3.0	0.7
Tomato, Cream Of, Canned, Tesco*	½ Can/200g	150	7.6	75	0.7	8.5	3.8	0.5
Tomato, Cream Of, Fresh, Tesco*	½ Pot/250g	140	4.8	56	1.4	8.4	1.9	0.4
Tomato, Cup a Soup, Made Up, Batchelors*	1 Sachet/255.6g	92	2.3	36	0.3	6.7	0.9	0.3
Tomato, Fresh, Tesco*	1 Serving/100g	44	2.3	44	0.7	5.2	2.3	0.4
Tomato, From Heinz, Canned, Weight Watchers*	1 Can/295g	74	1.5	25	0.7	4.5	0.5	0.3
Tomato, in a Cup, Symingtons*	1 Sachet/31.5g	99	1.6	308	3.5	62.0	5.0	3.8
Tomato, in a Cup, Tesco*	1 Serving/23g	75	0.7	328	6.4	68.5	3.2	0.1
Tomato, Rice & Sweetcorn, Baxters*	1 Serving/400ml	256	7.2	64	2.0	9.9	1.8	1.1
Tomato, Vegetable Garden, Campbell's*	1 Can/310g	240	2.7	77	1.6	16.1	0.9	0.0
Tomato, Weight Watchers*	1 Can/295g	74	1.4	25	0.7	4.5	0.5	0.5
Tomato & Basil, Campbell's*	1 Pack/500ml	205	6.5	41	0.7	6.7	1.3	1.1
Tomato & Basil, Canned, Eat Well, M & S*	½ Can/207.5g	62	1.5	30	0.6	5.7	0.7	0.6
Tomato & Basil, Cup a Soup, Batchelors*	1 Sachet/255.3g	97	2.6	38	0.5	6.7	1.0	0.5
Tomato & Basil, Cup a Soup, Made Up, GFY, Asda*	1 Serving/250ml	50	0.2	20	0.4	4.4	0.1	0.2
Tomato & Basil, Fresh, Avonmore*	1 Carton/250g	135	7.5	54	1.2	5.5	3.0	0.2
Tomato & Basil, Fresh, Finest, Tesco*	½ Pot/300g	219	14.7	73	1.0	6.3	4.9	0.6
Tomato & Basil, Fresh, Low Fat, Sainsbury's*	½ Carton/300ml	75	1.8	25	1.1	4.1	0.6	0.7
Tomato & Basil, Fresh, M & S*	½ Pot/300g	105	3.6	35	0.8	5.2	1.2	1.5
Tomato & Basil, Fresh, Morrisons*	1 Pot/600g	234	4.2	39	1.5	6.6	0.7	1.0
Tomato & Basil, Fresh, So Organic, Sainsbury's*	½ Carton/200g	100	4.0	50	0.5	7.5	2.0	0.2
Tomato & Basil, Fresh, Somerfield*	1 Serving/294.7g	83	2.4	28	0.7	4.5	0.8	0.8

S

SOUP

	Measure INFO/WEIGHT	per Measure KCAL	FAT	KCAL	PROT	CARB	FAT	FIBRE
Tomato & Basil, Fresh, Tesco*	½ Pack/300g	138	4.8	46	0.9	6.9	1.6	0.6
Tomato & Basil, Fresh, The Fresh Soup Company*	½ Pot/250g	85	2.3	34	1.3	5.1	0.9	0.6
Tomato & Basil, Fresh, Waitrose*	½ Pot/300g	108	3.6	36	0.9	5.3	1.2	1.3
Tomato & Basil, GFY, Asda*	1 Serving/250ml	100	3.5	40	0.9	6.0	1.4	1.6
Tomato & Basil, Italian, 99% Fat Free, Baxters*	½ Can/208g	119	2.1	57	2.6	9.3	1.0	1.1
Tomato & Basil, Loyd Grossman*	½ Pack/210g	97	4.0	46	0.8	6.4	1.9	0.2
Tomato & Brown Lentil, Healthy Choice, Baxters*	1 Tin/415g	199	0.8	48	2.6	9.0	0.2	2.7
Tomato & Butterbean, Baxters*	1 Can/415g	166	5.0	40	1.2	6.1	1.2	1.0
Tomato & Herb, M & S*	1oz/28g	14	0.4	50	1.3	7.9	1.6	1.3
Tomato & Lebtil, Mediteranean, Weight Watchers*	1 Can/400g	184	2.4	46	2.3	7.8	0.6	1.0
Tomato & Lentil, M & S*	½ Can/211.1g	95	0.4	45	2.3	8.4	0.2	1.5
Tomato & Lentil, Spicy, Canned, BGTY, Sainsbury's*	1 Can/400g	204	3.2	51	2.8	8.3	0.8	0.5
Tomato & Orange, Baxters*	1 Can/425g	179	2.1	42	1.0	8.3	0.5	0.4
Tomato & Red Pepper, Canned, Soupreme*	1 Can/400g	192	8.8	48	0.5	6.6	2.2	0.5
Tomato & Red Pepper, to Go, Asda*	1 Pot/330g	102	4.3	31	0.6	4.3	1.3	0.6
Tomato & Roasted Red Pepper, COU, M & S*	1 Serving/415g	145	0.4	35	1.0	7.6	0.1	0.9
Tomato & Three Bean, Canned, BGTY, Sainsbury's*	½ Can/200g	118	1.8	59	3.7	9.1	0.9	1.7
Tomato & Vegetable, Cup a Soup, Batchelors*	1 Serving/218g	107	2.6	49	1.1	8.5	1.2	0.6
Tomato & Vegetable, Mighty, Asda*	1 Sachet/38g	140	2.2	368	10.5	68.4	5.8	3.7
Tomato & Vegetable, Organic, Baxters*	1 Can/400g	200	3.2	50	1.6	9.2	0.8	0.8
Tomato with Basil, Italian, Baxters*	1 Can/415g	199	3.7	48	2.1	7.9	0.9	0.8
Tuscan Bean, Canned, HL, Tesco*	½ Can/200ml	130	3.6	65	3.5	10.3	1.8	1.3
Tuscan Bean, NCGF Co*	½ Carton/300g	84	2.4	28	1.6	3.7	0.8	1.0
Tuscan Bean, Organic, Fresh, Sainsbury's*	1 Pack/400g	171	3.2	43	2.6	6.3	0.8	2.0
Tuscan Bean, PB, Waitrose*	½ Pot/300g	147	5.4	49	2.0	6.1	1.8	1.8
Tuscan Style Bean & Sausage, Chunky, M & S*	1 Can/415g	249	9.1	60	2.4	7.7	2.2	1.0
Vegetable, 99% Fat Free, Wattie's*	1 Serving/105g	30	0.2	29	0.8	5.9	0.2	0.8
Vegetable, Asda*	1 Can/400g	144	1.6	36	1.1	7.0	0.4	0.8
Vegetable, Average	1 Serving/220g	114	8.8	52	0.9	3.2	4.0	0.9
Vegetable, Bean & Pasta, Organic, Baxters*	1 Can/415g	212	3.3	51	2.2	8.7	0.8	1.4
Vegetable, Canned	1oz/28g	13	0.2	48	1.4	9.9	0.6	1.5
Vegetable, Canned, Tesco*	½ Can/200g	84	0.6	42	0.7	9.2	0.3	0.7
Vegetable, Chunky, Big, Heinz*	½ Can/200g	104	1.8	52	1.7	9.2	0.9	1.6
Vegetable, Chunky, Canned, Sainsbury's*	1 Can/400g	184	2.8	46	1.5	8.3	0.7	1.2
Vegetable, Chunky, Fresh, Organic, Simply Organic*	½ Tub/300g	153	4.5	51	1.9	9.0	1.5	1.4
Vegetable, Chunky, Fresh, Tesco*	1 Serving/300g	123	5.7	41	0.6	5.5	1.9	1.0
Vegetable, Chunky, Organic, Tesco*	½ Pot/300g	150	3.6	50	1.7	8.0	1.2	2.1
Vegetable, Chunky, Tesco*	1 Pot/600g	288	17.4	48	0.8	5.0	2.9	1.3
Vegetable, Condensed, Campbell's*	1 Can/295g	103	2.4	35	0.8	6.2	0.8	0.0
Vegetable, Condensed, Classic, Campbell's*	1 Can/295g	221	5.0	75	1.7	13.2	1.7	1.7
Vegetable, Cup, Soupreme*	1 Sachet/26g	111	5.9	444	8.1	49.7	23.6	2.3
Vegetable, Extra Thick, Canned, Sainsbury's*	1 Can/400g	184	2.4	46	1.5	8.6	0.6	1.4
Vegetable, Fresh, Co-Op*	1 Pack/600g	150	6.0	25	0.6	4.0	1.0	1.0
Vegetable, Fresh, Somerfield*	1 Serving/600g	150	4.8	25	0.7	3.7	0.8	1.1
Vegetable, From Heinz, Canned, Weight Watchers*	1 Can/295g	86	0.9	29	0.9	5.6	0.3	0.8
Vegetable, Heinz*	1 Tin/400g	176	3.2	44	1.0	8.2	0.8	0.9
Vegetable, in a Cup, BGTY, Sainsbury's*	1 Sachet/200g	52	1.6	26	0.5	4.4	0.8	0.9
Vegetable, in a Cup, HL, Tesco*	1 Sachet/18g	66	1.4	367	7.2	66.1	7.8	2.8
Vegetable, Soup in a Mug, HL, Tesco*	1 Sachet/18g	66	1.4	365	7.0	66.3	8.0	2.6
Vegetable, Soup-A-Cups, Asda*	1 Sachet/200ml	59	1.1	30	0.7	5.5	0.6	0.5
Vegetable, Thick & Creamy, Soup in a Mug, Tesco*	1 Serving/26g	104	4.3	399	5.2	57.4	16.5	7.5
Vegetable, Vie, Knorr*	1 Pack/500ml	160	3.5	32	0.9	5.5	0.7	1.2
Vegetable, with Croutons, Soup in a Mug, Tesco*	1 Pack/23g	90	3.7	392	6.2	55.2	16.3	8.0

S

	Measure INFO/WEIGHT	per Measure		Nutrition Values per 100g / 100ml				
		KCAL	FAT	KCAL	PROT	CARB	FAT	FIBRE
SOUP								
Vegetable & Beef, Canned, Sainsbury's*	1 Can/400g	196	8.4	49	1.7	5.7	2.1	2.2
Vegetable & Chilli, Chunky, Fresh, Sainsbury's*	½ Pot/300g	117	1.8	39	1.6	6.9	0.6	2.6
Vegetable & Lentil, Fresh, Somerfield*	½ Carton/306.8g	135	2.8	44	2.6	6.4	0.9	3.6
Vegetable & Rosemary, Fresh, Sainsbury's*	½ Pack/300g	96	3.0	32	0.9	4.9	1.0	1.3
Vegetable Broth, Canned, HL, Tesco*	½ Can/200g	74	0.4	37	1.3	7.5	0.2	1.1
Vegetable Chowder, NCGF Co*	½ Carton/300g	159	5.1	53	2.9	6.6	1.7	1.1
Vine Ripened Tomato & Basil, Fresh, Avonmore*	1 Serving/300g	141	8.1	47	1.0	4.7	2.7	0.3
Vine Tomato, Harissa & Mint, The Best, Morrisons*	1 Pot/600g	294	11.4	49	1.5	6.4	1.9	1.1
Watercress, M & S*	½ Pot/300g	75	5.1	25	1.3	1.5	1.7	0.6
Watercress & Cream, Soup Chef*	1 Jar/780g	413	22.6	53	0.8	5.9	2.9	0.3
Wild Mushroom, in a Cup, BGTY, Sainsbury's*	1 Serving/200ml	56	1.8	28	0.4	4.5	0.9	0.2
Wild Mushroom & Maderia, Fresh, Finest, Tesco*	½ Tub/300g	156	8.7	52	1.5	4.9	2.9	0.5
Winter Vegetable, Chunky, M & S*	1 Tin/415g	166	1.2	40	1.5	7.5	0.3	0.4
Winter Vegetable, NCGF Co*	½ Pack/300g	162	3.3	54	2.4	8.7	1.1	1.5
Winter Vegetable, Organic, Sainsbury's*	½ Can/200g	100	2.0	50	2.3	7.9	1.0	1.3
Winter Vegetable, with Yellow Split Peas, Baxters*	½ Can/207.5g	83	0.4	40	1.5	8.1	0.2	1.3
Wonton, Blue Dragon*	1 Can/410g	103	5.3	25	1.2	2.0	1.3	0.2
SOUP MIX								
Minestrone, Made Up, Sainsbury's*	1 Serving/200ml	44	0.0	22	0.3	6.0	0.0	0.3
Scotch Broth, Made Up, Sainsbury's*	1 Serving/175g	32	0.4	18	0.2	3.8	0.2	0.6
Soup & Broth Mix, Wholefoods, Tesco*	¼ Pack/125g	456	2.4	365	14.7	71.4	1.9	7.3
SOUTHERN COMFORT								
37.5% Volume	1 Pub Shot/35ml	72	0.0	207	0.0	0.0	0.0	0.0
SOYA								
Chunks, Dried, Cooked, Sainsbury's*	1oz/28g	27	0.1	98	14.0	9.8	0.3	1.1
Mince, Dry Weight, Sainsbury's*	1 Serving/50g	164	0.4	328	47.2	33.2	0.8	3.6
SOYA MILK								
Banana Flavour, Provamel*	1 Serving/250ml	195	5.5	78	3.8	10.4	2.2	0.6
Choco Flavour, Provamel*	1 Serving/250ml	208	6.0	83	3.8	11.1	2.4	1.1
Chocolate, So Good Beverages*	1 Serving/250ml	160	2.5	64	3.6	10.8	1.0	0.0
Fat Free, Original, So Good Beverages*	1 Serving/250ml	100	0.3	40	3.6	6.4	0.1	0.0
Flavoured, Average	1floz/30mls	12	0.5	40	2.8	3.6	1.7	0.0
No Added Sugar, Unsweetened, Average	1 Serving/250ml	85	4.8	34	3.3	0.9	1.9	0.4
Omega Original, So Good Beverages*	1 Serving/250ml	130	3.0	52	3.6	6.8	1.2	0.0
Omega Vanilla, So Good Beverages*	1 Serving/250ml	130	3.0	52	3.6	7.6	1.2	0.0
Original, No Added Sugar, So Good Beverages*	1 Serving/250ml	80	2.5	32	3.6	2.0	1.0	0.8
Original, So Good Beverages*	1 Serving/250ml	140	5.0	56	3.6	5.6	2.0	0.0
Sweetened, Average	1 Glass/200ml	94	4.2	47	3.4	3.7	2.1	0.4
Uht, Non Dairy, Alternative to Milk, Waitrose*	1 Glass/250ml	103	4.8	41	3.3	2.7	1.9	0.2
Unsweetened, Organic, Waitrose*	1 Serving/60ml	19	1.1	31	3.3	0.2	1.9	0.0
Unsweetened, Uht, Organic, Tesco*	1 Serving/150ml	47	2.9	31	3.4	0.1	1.9	0.6
Vanilla, Fat Free, So Good Beverages*	1 Serving/250ml	140	0.3	56	3.6	10.4	0.1	0.0
Vanilla Flavour, Organic, Provamel*	1 Serving/250ml	150	5.5	60	3.8	6.2	2.2	0.6
SPAGHETTI								
Canned in Tomato Sauce	1oz/28g	18	0.1	64	1.9	14.1	0.4	0.7
Chicken, BGTY, Sainsbury's*	1 Serving/300g	281	2.7	94	9.8	11.6	0.9	2.3
Cooked, Average	1oz/28g	33	0.2	119	4.1	24.8	0.7	1.1
Dry, Average	1oz/28g	98	0.4	350	12.1	72.1	1.5	2.4
Dry, Carb Check, Heinz*	1 Serving/75g	219	1.7	292	52.7	15.2	2.3	20.8
Durum Wheat, Dry, Average	1oz/28g	97	0.1	348	12.4	71.8	0.4	1.5
Fresh, Cooked, Average	1 Serving/125g	182	2.2	146	6.1	26.9	1.7	1.8
Fresh, Dry, Average	1 Serving/100g	278	3.0	278	10.8	53.0	3.0	2.2
in Tomato & Cheese, Sainsbury's*	1 Serving/300g	345	10.2	115	4.4	16.8	3.4	1.4

S

	Measure INFO/WEIGHT	per Measure KCAL	FAT	Nutrition Values per 100g / 100ml KCAL	PROT	CARB	FAT	FIBRE
SPAGHETTI								
in Tomato Sauce, Heinz*	1 Can/400g	244	0.8	61	1.7	13.0	0.2	0.5
in Tomato Sauce, HP*	1 Can/410g	247	0.8	60	1.5	13.1	0.2	0.4
in Tomato Sauce, Organic, Sainsbury's*	½ Can/205g	133	0.4	65	1.8	13.9	0.2	1.0
in Tomato Sauce, Sainsbury's*	Small Tin/212g	123	0.8	58	1.7	11.8	0.4	0.5
in Tomato Sauce, Tesco*	1 Can/410g	246	0.8	60	1.6	12.9	0.2	0.5
in Tomato Sauce, Value, Tesco*	½ Can/205g	131	0.8	64	1.9	13.3	0.4	0.5
in Tomato Sauce, Whole Wheat, Sainsbury's*	1 Serving/205g	125	1.2	61	2.0	11.9	0.6	1.1
in Tomato Sauce, with Parsley, Weight Watchers*	1 Sm Can/200g	98	0.4	49	1.8	10.0	0.2	0.6
Quick Dry, Average, COOK*	1 Serving/50g	176	0.9	351	12.8	70.8	1.9	2.7
Trufree*	1 Serving/75g	263	1.5	350	8.0	75.0	2.0	2.5
Wheat Free, Tesco*	1 Serving/100g	340	2.0	340	8.0	72.5	2.0	2.5
Whole Wheat, Cooked, Average	1oz/28g	32	0.3	113	4.7	23.2	0.9	3.5
Whole Wheat, Dry, Average	1 Serving/100g	326	2.6	326	13.5	62.2	2.6	8.0
with Sausages, Heinz*	1 Can/400g	352	13.6	88	3.5	10.8	3.4	0.5
with Tomato & Cheese, Tesco*	½ Pack/250g	280	6.5	112	4.0	18.1	2.6	1.1
SPAGHETTI & MEATBALLS								
American, Superbowl, Asda*	1 Pack/453.4g	593	17.7	131	11.0	13.0	3.9	1.1
BGTY, Sainsbury's*	1 Pack/300g	249	2.7	83	5.9	12.7	0.9	3.1
Chicken in Tomato Sauce, Heinz*	1 Can/400g	352	12.0	88	4.1	11.0	3.0	0.5
COU, M & S*	1 Pack/400g	360	8.0	90	6.0	12.3	2.0	2.6
GFY, Asda*	1 Pack/400g	344	6.0	86	7.0	11.0	1.5	1.5
Italian, HL, Tesco*	1 Pack/400g	392	10.0	98	5.4	13.5	2.5	0.4
Italian, Sainsbury's*	1 Pack/450g	495	21.2	110	5.0	11.9	4.7	2.7
Italian, Somerfield*	1 Pack/400g	412	15.6	103	5.4	11.5	3.9	1.3
Sainsbury's*	1 Pack/400g	497	18.4	124	6.5	14.2	4.6	2.8
Somerfield*	½ Pack/450g	518	18.0	115	5.0	15.0	4.0	0.0
Tesco*	1 Serving/475g	641	30.9	135	5.1	14.1	6.5	0.9
Vegetarian, Safeway*	1 Pack/350g	382	13.3	109	5.0	13.7	3.8	0.5
SPAGHETTI BOLOGNESE								
Al Forno, Sainsbury's*	1 Pack/400g	460	19.6	115	7.8	10.0	4.9	1.1
Asda*	1 Pack/400g	536	24.0	134	7.0	13.0	6.0	1.5
Average	1 Serving/450g	581	25.2	129	7.8	12.5	5.6	0.9
Basics, Sainsbury's*	1 Pack/300g	219	4.2	73	4.1	11.1	1.4	1.5
BGTY, Sainsbury's*	1 Pack/450g	392	9.0	87	4.7	12.3	2.0	2.3
Canned, Asda*	½ Can/205g	174	5.7	85	4.2	10.7	2.8	0.6
Canned, Heinz*	1 Can/400g	316	6.0	79	3.4	13.2	1.5	0.5
COOK*	1 Portion/430g	636	24.9	148	7.6	16.2	5.8	1.0
Co-Op*	1 Pack/300g	285	12.0	95	4.0	11.0	4.0	1.0
Cost Cutter, Costcutters*	1 Pack/600g	504	11.4	84	5.7	11.2	1.9	0.9
COU, M & S*	1 Pack/400g	380	8.4	95	7.5	11.7	2.1	1.7
Egg Pasta in Rich Beef Sauce, Waitrose*	1 Serving/250g	253	6.5	101	7.6	11.7	2.6	1.0
Favourites, Morrisons*	1 Pack/300g	261	3.3	87	4.6	14.7	1.1	1.6
Frozen, Tesco*	1 Pack/450g	473	9.0	105	5.8	15.0	2.0	1.8
GFY, Asda*	1 Pack/400g	440	8.0	110	7.0	16.0	2.0	1.3
Good Intentions, Somerfield*	1 Serving/400g	380	9.2	95	6.2	12.4	2.3	1.4
Healthy Choice, Iceland*	1 Pack/400g	428	4.0	107	6.8	17.8	1.0	1.1
HL, Tesco*	1 Pack/400g	420	8.8	105	5.4	15.5	2.2	1.4
HP*	1 Pack/410g	312	7.8	76	3.8	11.3	1.9	0.7
in Tomato & Beef Sauce, Canned, Carlini*	1 Can/410g	324	10.7	79	3.7	10.2	2.6	1.2
Italian, Chilled, Tesco*	1 Pack/400g	520	17.2	130	6.5	15.9	4.3	1.5
Italiano, Pro-Cuisine, Pro Cuisine*	1 Pack/600g	522	11.4	87	5.7	11.7	1.9	0.0
Lean Cuisine, Findus*	1 Pack/320g	275	7.4	86	4.5	11.5	2.3	1.1
M & S*	1 Pack/400g	380	8.4	95	7.5	11.7	2.1	1.7

S

	Measure INFO/WEIGHT	per Measure KCAL	per Measure FAT	Nutrition Values per 100g / 100ml KCAL	PROT	CARB	FAT	FIBRE
SPAGHETTI BOLOGNESE								
PB, Waitrose*	1 Pack/400g	380	6.8	95	6.7	13.4	1.7	1.1
PB, Waitrose*	1 Pack/400g	380	6.8	95	6.7	13.4	1.7	1.1
Quick Pasta, Dry, Sainsbury's*	1 Serving/63g	231	2.8	367	10.8	71.0	4.4	3.3
Ross*	1 Serving/320g	288	3.5	90	4.2	15.7	1.1	0.9
Sainsbury's*	1 Pack/400g	525	18.8	131	6.1	16.0	4.7	2.2
Saucy Spag Bol, M & S*	1 Pack/225g	280	9.0	124	7.3	14.9	4.0	1.5
Somerfield*	1 Pack/300g	339	6.6	113	5.3	18.0	2.2	2.0
Spar*	1 Pack/500g	440	17.5	88	5.6	8.6	3.5	1.5
Weight Watchers*	1 Pack/319.1g	300	7.0	94	5.6	13.0	2.2	0.7
with Mini Meatballs, Frozen, Captain Birds Eye, Birds Eye*	1 Pack, Cooked	401	20.5	98	4.6	17.2	5.0	1.0
SPAGHETTI CARBONARA								
Cappelletti, Canned, Balanced Lifestyle, Carlini*	1 Can/400g	328	11.2	82	4.1	10.0	2.8	0.6
Cheese Flavour Sauce with Bacon, GFY, Asda*	1 Pack/380g	445	6.8	117	3.1	22.0	1.8	0.7
Chicken, Mushroom & Ham, Asda*	1 Pack/700g	686	14.0	98	10.0	10.0	2.0	1.5
Chicken & Asparagus, Sainsbury's*	1 Pack/450g	657	27.5	146	6.6	16.2	6.1	1.1
COU, M & S*	1 Pack/330g	347	6.6	105	5.7	15.5	2.0	1.8
GFY, Asda*	1 Pack/380g	445	6.8	117	3.1	22.0	1.8	0.7
Italian, Chilled, Sainsbury's*	1 Pack/400g	492	15.6	123	5.5	16.1	3.9	1.4
Italian, Fresh, Chilled, Tesco*	1 Pack/430g	606	26.2	141	7.6	13.9	6.1	1.3
Italian Express*	1 Pack/320g	310	11.8	97	4.3	11.6	3.7	1.1
M & S*	1 Pack/360g	630	34.2	175	7.6	14.3	9.5	0.1
Safeway*	1 Pack/360g	569	25.6	158	7.9	15.7	7.1	1.2
SPAGHETTI HOOPS								
& Sausages, Tesco*	1 Serving/205g	185	6.8	90	3.1	11.9	3.3	0.2
'N' Hot Dogs, Heinz*	1 Can/400g	304	9.6	76	2.8	11.0	2.4	0.4
Canned, SmartPrice, Asda*	½ Can/204.8g	127	0.6	62	1.7	13.0	0.3	0.4
in Tomato Sauce, Canned, Heinz*	1 Can /400g	208	0.8	52	1.6	10.8	0.2	1.5
Tesco*	½ Can/205g	123	0.4	60	1.6	12.9	0.2	0.5
SPAGHETTI IN								
Tomato Sauce, Canned, Asda*	1 Lge Can/415g	257	1.7	62	1.5	13.0	0.4	0.7
SPAGHETTI MARINARA								
GFY, Asda*	1 Pack/400g	520	16.8	130	8.0	15.0	4.2	0.9
SPAGHETTI RINGS								
in Tomato Sauce, Canned, Sainsbury's*	1 Serving/213g	136	0.9	64	1.9	13.3	0.4	0.5
SPAGHETTI WITH								
Cheese & Broccoli Sauce, GFY, Asda*	1 Pack/382.1g	447	6.9	117	3.2	22.0	1.8	0.8
Tomato & Mozzarella Sauce, GFY, Asda*	1 Pack/120g	446	6.0	372	10.8	70.8	5.0	2.6
SPAM*								
Pork & Ham, Chopped, Spam*	1 Serving/100g	296	24.2	296	14.5	3.2	24.2	0.0
SPICE BLEND								
Tikka, Sharwood's*	1 Pack/260g	263	14.0	101	2.7	10.2	5.4	1.7
SPICE MIX								
for Burritos, Old El Paso*	½ Packet/22.5g	68	0.9	304	13.0	54.0	4.0	0.0
for Fajitas, Old El Paso*	1 Pack/35g	107	2.1	306	9.0	54.0	6.0	0.0
SPICE PASTE								
Five Spice Ginger & Garlic, Stir Fry, Schwartz*	1 Tbsp/25g	42	1.8	168	4.2	22.1	7.0	0.0
Garlic, Ginger & Spring Onion, Stir Fry, Schwartz*	1 Serving/20g	35	2.2	177	2.5	17.8	10.8	0.0
Lemongrass, Ginger & Coconut, Stir Fry, Schwartz*	1 Squeeze/25g	62	4.5	248	1.8	20.2	17.8	0.0
SPINACH								
Baby, Average	1 Serving/90g	23	0.7	25	2.8	1.6	0.8	2.1
Boiled Or Steamed, Average	1 Serving/80g	17	0.6	21	2.6	0.9	0.8	2.1
Canned, Average	1 Serving/80g	18	0.4	23	3.1	1.5	0.5	3.0
Raw, Average	1 Serving/100g	24	0.8	24	2.9	1.3	0.8	2.1

S

	Measure INFO/WEIGHT	per Measure KCAL	FAT	Nutrition Values per 100g / 100ml KCAL	PROT	CARB	FAT	FIBRE
SPIRALI								
Dry, Average	1 Serving/50g	176	0.8	352	12.2	72.6	1.7	2.8
SPIRITS								
37.5% Volume	1 Pub Shot/35ml	72	0.0	207	0.0	0.0	0.0	0.0
40% Volume	1 Shot/35ml	78	0.0	222	0.0	0.0	0.0	0.0
SPLENDIPS								
Cheesecake, Philadelphia, Kraft*	1 Serving/83g	195	6.9	235	6.1	34.0	8.3	2.9
Chives, Philadelphia, Kraft*	1 Pack/85g	159	4.4	187	7.5	27.0	5.2	1.7
Nachos, Philadelphia, Kraft*	1 Pack/85g	150	6.5	177	6.4	20.0	7.6	1.0
SPLIT PEAS								
Dried, Average	1oz/28g	89	0.5	319	22.1	57.4	1.7	3.2
Green, Dried, Boiled, Average	1 Tbsp/35g	40	0.2	115	8.3	19.8	0.6	3.9
SPONGE FINGERS								
Boudoir, Sainsbury's*	1 Biscuit/5g	20	0.2	396	8.1	82.8	3.6	0.4
Tesco*	1 Finger/5g	19	0.2	386	7.6	80.6	3.7	1.0
SPONGE PUDDING								
Average	1 Portion/170g	578	27.7	340	5.8	45.3	16.3	1.1
Blackberry & Apple, HE, Tesco*	1 Pot/102.5g	159	1.4	155	3.1	32.6	1.4	0.7
Cherry & Almond Flavour, Sainsbury's*	¼ Pudding/110g	334	15.7	304	3.5	40.3	14.3	0.7
Chocolate, BGTY, Sainsbury's*	1 Pudding/105g	137	2.5	131	4.4	23.1	2.4	2.7
Chocolate, Free From, Sainsbury's*	1 Pudding/110g	388	10.2	353	5.2	62.0	9.3	0.3
Chocolate, GFY, Asda*	1 Pudding/105g	187	4.4	178	3.0	32.0	4.2	2.6
Chocolate, HL, Tesco*	1 Serving/125g	239	4.8	191	4.4	34.7	3.8	0.9
Chocolate, M & S*	¼ Pudding/131g	524	32.2	400	6.1	38.6	24.6	1.8
Chocolate, Sainsbury's*	¼ Pudding/110g	464	28.3	422	5.4	42.3	25.7	0.8
Chocolate, Tesco Light Choices*	1 Pudding/115g	196	4.7	170	4.7	28.3	4.1	2.8
Chocolate, Tesco*	1 Pudding/110g	337	16.6	306	4.7	37.7	15.1	1.8
Chocolate, TTD, Sainsbury's*	1 Pot/110g	404	21.7	367	4.1	43.3	19.7	2.3
Chocolate & Chocolate Sauce, HE, Tesco*	1 Pudding/90g	186	3.7	207	3.9	38.7	4.1	2.1
Chocolate & Sauce, Co-Op*	1 Pack/225g	608	29.3	270	5.0	34.0	13.0	0.6
Fruit, Co-Op*	1 Can/300g	1110	48.0	370	3.0	53.0	16.0	2.0
Fruits of the Forest, Asda*	1 Pudding/115g	323	4.4	281	2.8	59.0	3.8	1.3
Jam, Tesco*	1 Pudding/110g	367	13.1	334	3.3	53.3	11.9	0.5
Jam & Custard, Co-Op*	1 Pack/244g	598	22.0	245	3.0	37.0	9.0	0.3
Jam & Custard, Somerfield*	¼ Pudding/62g	143	5.0	231	3.0	38.0	8.0	0.0
Lemon, COU, M & S*	1 Pudding/100g	157	2.3	157	2.0	32.1	2.3	1.9
Lemon, M & S*	1 Pudding/105g	326	16.0	310	4.3	39.4	15.2	2.3
Raspberry Jam, Asda*	½ Pudding/147g	481	16.2	327	3.1	54.0	11.0	4.1
Sticky Toffee, Microwavable, Heinz*	1 Serving/75g	233	9.0	311	3.3	47.4	12.0	0.7
Sticky Toffee, Somerfield*	1 Pudding/440g	1456	56.0	364	3.0	56.0	14.0	0.0
Strawberry, Co-Op*	1 Can/300g	960	39.0	320	2.0	48.0	13.0	0.8
Strawberry Jam, Heinz*	¼ Can/82g	230	6.2	281	2.6	50.4	7.6	0.6
Summer Fruits, BGTY, Sainsbury's*	1 Serving/110g	243	4.7	221	2.7	42.9	4.3	1.0
Syrup, GFY, Asda*	1 Sponge/105g	207	4.3	197	2.0	38.0	4.1	2.6
Syrup, Individual, Tesco*	1 Pudding/110g	391	14.5	355	3.1	55.6	13.2	0.5
Treacle, Heinz*	1 Serving/160g	445	13.0	278	2.5	48.9	8.1	0.6
Treacle, Waitrose*	1 Pudding/105g	385	13.8	367	2.8	59.5	13.1	0.5
with Jam Or Treacle	1oz/28g	93	4.0	333	5.1	48.7	14.4	1.0
SPRATS								
Fried	1oz/28g	116	9.8	415	24.9	0.0	35.0	0.0
Raw	1oz/28g	48	3.1	172	18.3	0.0	11.0	0.0
SPREAD								
Butter Me Up, Light, Tesco*	1 Thin Spread/7g	25	2.7	350	0.3	0.5	38.0	0.0
Butter Me Up, Tesco*	1 Thin Spread/7g	38	4.1	540	0.8	1.2	59.0	0.0

S

SPREAD

INFO/WEIGHT	Measure	per Measure		Nutrition Values per 100g / 100ml				
		KCAL	FAT	KCAL	PROT	CARB	FAT	FIBRE
Butterlicious, Vegetable, Sainsbury's*	1 Thin Spread/7g	44	4.8	628	0.6	1.1	69.0	0.0
Buttersoft, Light, Reduced Fat, Sainsbury's*	1 Serving/10g	54	6.0	544	0.4	0.5	60.0	0.0
Buttery Gold, Somerfield*	1 Thin Spread/7g	44	4.8	627	0.5	1.0	69.0	0.0
Buttery Taste, Benecol*	2 Tsp/12g	69	7.6	575	0.0	0.8	63.3	0.0
Dairy Free, Organic, Pure Spreads*	1 Thin Spread/7g	37	4.1	533	0.5	0.0	59.0	0.0
Diet, Delight*	1 Thin Spread/7g	16	1.6	228	3.6	1.6	23.0	0.0
Enriched Olive, Tesco*	1 Serving/10g	54	5.9	540	0.2	1.2	59.0	0.0
From Soya, Kallo*	1 Thin Spread/7g	27	2.6	380	7.0	6.0	37.0	0.0
Gold, Low Fat, Omega 3, St Ivel*	1 Thin Spread/7g	25	2.7	360	0.5	3.1	38.0	0.0
Gold, Lowest Fat, with Omega 3, St Ivel*	1 Serving/7g	13	1.3	192	0.8	4.3	19.0	1.3
Golden, Light, HE, Tesco*	1 Serving/10g	35	3.8	354	1.5	1.5	38.0	0.0
Heart, Cholesterol Reducing, Dairygold	1 Serving/10g	34	3.6	338	0.7	2.8	36.0	0.0
Irish, Dairy, Original, Low Low*	1 Serving/10g	35	3.8	346	0.4	0.5	38.0	0.0
Light, Benecol*	2 Tsp/12g	40	4.2	333	2.5	0.0	35.0	0.0
Low Fat, Better By Far, Morrisons*	1 Serving/10g	63	6.9	627	0.5	1.0	69.0	0.0
Low-Fat, Average	1 Thin Spread/7g	27	2.8	390	5.8	0.5	40.5	0.0
Morning Gold, Low Fat, Morrisons*	1 Thin Spread/7g	26	2.7	372	7.5	0.0	38.0	0.0
Olive, Gold, Reduced Fat, Sainsbury's*	1 Serving/10g	54	5.9	536	0.1	1.2	59.0	0.0
Olive, Light, Low Fat, HL, Tesco*	1 Serving/15g	52	5.7	348	1.5	0.0	38.0	0.0
Olive, Low Fat, Morrisons*	1 Serving/10g	35	3.8	346	0.9	0.0	38.0	0.0
Olive, Reduced Fat, Asda*	1 Thin Spread/7g	38	4.1	536	0.2	1.1	59.0	0.0
Olive, Reduced Fat, M & S*	1 Thin Spread/7g	38	4.1	536	0.2	1.1	59.0	0.0
Olive, Reduced Fat, Morrisons*	1 Thin Spread/7g	38	4.2	537	0.9	0.0	59.3	0.3
Olive, Reduced Fat, So Organic, Sainsbury's*	1 Serving/4g	21	2.4	537	0.1	0.4	59.5	0.0
Olive, Reduced Fat, Somerfield*	1 Thin Spread/7g	38	4.1	536	0.1	1.1	59.0	0.0
Olive, Waitrose*	1 Serving/10g	53	5.9	534	0.2	0.5	59.0	0.0
Olive Gold, Reduced Fat, Co-Op*	1 Thin Spread/7g	37	4.1	535	0.2	1.0	59.0	0.0
Olive Light, Low Fat, BGTY, Sainsbury's*	1 Thin Spread/ 7g	19	2.0	265	0.1	0.8	29.0	0.0
Olive Oil, 55% Reduced Fat, Benecol*	1 Thin Spread/7g	35	3.9	498	0.3	0.5	55.0	0.0
Olive Oil, Bertolli*	1 Serving/10g	54	5.9	536	0.2	1.0	59.0	0.0
Olivite, Low Fat, Weight Watchers*	Thin Spread/7g	25	2.7	351	0.0	0.2	38.9	0.0
Organic, Dairy Free, M & S*	1 Serving/5g	27	3.0	531	0.0	0.0	59.0	0.0
Pure Gold, Light, 65% Less Fat, Asda*	1 Serving/10g	24	2.5	239	2.5	1.0	25.0	0.0
Soft, Economy, Sainsbury's*	1 Thin Spread/7g	32	3.5	450	0.2	1.0	50.0	0.0
Soft, Reduced Fat, Basics, Sainsbury's*	1 Thin Spread/7g	30	3.4	425	0.0	0.0	48.1	0.0
Soft, Reduced Fat, SmartPrice, Asda*	1 Thin Spread/7g	32	3.5	455	0.2	1.0	50.0	0.0
Soft, Sainsbury's*	1 Serving/75g	473	52.5	630	0.1	0.1	70.0	0.0
Soft, Value, Tesco*	1 Serving/10g	44	4.8	435	0.0	0.0	48.0	0.0
Sunflower, Asda*	1 Serving/10g	64	7.0	635	0.2	1.0	70.0	0.0
Sunflower, Co-Op*	1 Thin Spread/7g	44	4.9	635	0.2	1.0	70.0	0.0
Sunflower, Enriched, Light, HL, Tesco*	1 Serving/6g	21	2.3	350	0.3	1.0	38.0	0.0
Sunflower, Enriched, Tesco*	1 Serving/15g	80	8.9	535	0.1	0.2	59.0	0.0
Sunflower, Light, BFY, Morrisons*	1 Tsp/5g	17	1.9	342	0.0	0.0	38.0	0.0
Sunflower, Light, BGTY, Sainsbury's*	1 Serving/10g	27	2.9	265	0.1	0.8	29.0	0.0
Sunflower, Light, Reduced Fat, Asda*	1 Serving/5g	17	1.9	347	0.3	1.0	38.0	0.1
Sunflower, Low Fat, Aldi*	1 Serving/10g	37	3.8	366	0.2	5.7	38.0	0.0
Sunflower, Low Fat, M & S*	1 Serving/14g	48	5.3	342	0.0	0.0	38.0	1.0
Sunflower, Low Fat, Somerfield*	1 Thin Spread/7g	24	2.7	342	0.0	0.0	38.0	0.0
Sunflower, Lowest, HE, Tesco*	1 Thin Spread/7g	8	0.4	109	2.0	14.0	5.0	10.0
Sunflower, M & S*	1 Serving/10g	63	7.0	630	0.0	0.0	70.0	3.0
Sunflower, Morrisons*	1 Serving/10g	63	7.0	631	0.0	0.2	70.0	0.0
Sunflower, Reduced Fat, Suma*	1 Serving/25g	134	14.9	537	0.0	0.4	59.5	0.0
Sunflower, Sainsbury's*	1 Serving/20g	106	11.8	532	0.1	0.2	59.0	0.0

S

	Measure INFO/WEIGHT	per Measure KCAL	FAT	Nutrition Values per 100g / 100ml KCAL	PROT	CARB	FAT	FIBRE
SPREAD								
Sunflower, Value, Tesco*	1 Thin Spread/7g	31	3.4	439	0.1	0.4	48.6	0.0
Sunflower, Waitrose*	1 Serving/5g	32	3.5	631	0.0	0.2	70.0	0.0
Vegetable, Dairy Free, Free From, Sainsbury's*	1 Thin Spread/7g	44	4.9	630	0.0	0.0	70.0	3.0
Vegetable, Soft, Tesco*	1 Tbsp/15g	99	11.0	661	0.1	1.0	73.0	0.0
Vitalite, St Ivel*	1 Thin Spread/7g	35	3.9	503	0.0	0.0	56.0	0.8
with Soya, Dairy Free, Pure Spreads*	1 Serving/10g	60	6.7	603	0.0	0.0	67.0	0.0
with Sunflower, Dairy Free, Organic, Pure Spreads*	1 Serving/10g	60	6.7	603	0.0	0.0	67.0	0.0
SPRING ONIONS								
Bulbs Only, Raw, Average	1oz/28g	10	0.0	35	0.9	8.5	0.0	1.7
Fresh, Raw, Unprepared, Average	1 Onion/10g	2	0.1	24	2.0	3.0	0.5	1.5
SPRING ROLL								
Mini, Veg, Chinese Snack Selection, Morrisons*	1 Roll/25.1g	52	2.2	207	3.5	28.8	8.7	2.7
SPRING ROLLS								
Cantonese Selection, Sainsbury's*	1 Serving/35.2g	68	2.7	193	4.1	26.9	7.7	1.4
Char Sui Pork & Bacon, M & S*	1 Pack/220g	528	20.7	240	4.8	33.9	9.4	0.6
Chicken, & Chilli, Cantonese, Sainsbury's*	1 Roll/51g	85	2.8	166	9.7	19.4	5.5	0.6
Chicken, & Chilli, Sainsbury's*	1 Roll/50g	93	4.7	185	9.6	15.6	9.3	2.8
Chicken, Asda*	1 Roll/58g	115	5.2	199	4.6	25.0	9.0	3.4
Chicken, Finest, Tesco*	1 Roll/60g	118	5.0	196	10.1	20.1	8.3	1.0
Chicken, Oriental, Asda*	1 Roll/59.6g	107	4.2	178	3.7	25.0	7.0	0.4
Chicken, Oriental Snack Selection, Sainsbury's*	1 Roll/15g	38	1.5	256	11.5	30.3	9.9	1.7
Chicken, Safeway*	1 Roll/50g	125	4.6	250	10.0	30.4	9.2	2.0
Chicken, Tesco*	1 Roll/50g	116	5.6	231	8.1	24.5	11.2	1.5
Chinese Takeaway, Tesco*	1 Roll/50g	101	4.3	201	4.4	26.4	8.6	1.5
Co-Op*	1oz/28g	67	3.1	240	6.0	29.0	11.0	0.4
Dim Sum, Sainsbury's*	1 Roll/12g	26	1.2	216	4.1	28.2	9.6	2.9
Duck, M & S*	1 Roll/30g	75	3.4	250	9.8	27.7	11.2	1.5
Duck, Morrisons*	1 Roll/30g	68	3.1	226	6.2	27.2	10.3	1.2
Duck, Party Bites, Sainsbury's*	1 Roll/20g	49	1.8	245	10.1	31.4	8.8	1.0
Duck with Sweet Chilli Sauce, Waitrose*	1 Roll/72g	66	1.4	92	5.1	14.0	1.9	0.9
M & S*	1 Pack/180g	333	15.1	185	3.5	24.2	8.4	2.3
Mini, Asda*	1 Roll/20g	35	0.6	175	3.5	33.6	3.0	1.9
Mini, Safeway*	1 Serving/30g	63	2.4	210	4.0	30.3	8.0	1.9
Mini, Sainsbury's*	1 Roll/12g	27	1.2	221	4.2	28.7	9.9	1.6
Mini, Tesco*	2 Rolls/40g	92	3.3	230	2.2	36.6	8.2	0.8
Prawn, Cantonese, Sainsbury's*	1 Roll/28g	46	1.7	162	6.8	20.3	6.0	2.5
Prawn, Chinese, Sainsbury's*	1 Roll/28.4g	60	2.9	211	6.2	23.8	10.1	1.2
Prawn, Crispy, M & S*	1 Spring Roll/34.1g	75	3.4	220	10.0	22.2	9.9	1.3
Prawn, Tesco*	3 Rolls/100g	211	9.4	211	8.7	22.8	9.4	1.4
Roast Duck, M & S*	1 Roll/30.9g	85	4.9	275	7.8	26.2	15.7	1.4
Thai, Sainsbury's*	1 Roll/30g	69	3.4	229	2.9	28.8	11.3	3.5
Thai Prawn, Waitrose*	1 Roll/50g	110	4.8	219	8.0	25.4	9.5	2.4
Vegetable, Asda*	1 Roll/62g	126	5.6	203	3.5	27.0	9.0	2.7
Vegetable, Cantonese, Large, Sainsbury's*	1 Roll/63.4g	130	6.3	205	3.6	25.3	9.9	1.5
Vegetable, Cantonese, Sainsbury's*	1 Roll/36.1g	84	4.2	233	3.6	28.1	11.7	1.4
Vegetable, Chilled, Tesco*	1 Roll/67.5g	149	7.6	221	4.0	25.9	11.3	1.6
Vegetable, Chinese, Sainsbury's*	1 Roll/26g	69	2.8	193	4.1	26.9	7.7	1.4
Vegetable, Chinese Takeaway, Sainsbury's*	1 Roll/59g	100	3.7	170	4.0	24.4	6.3	2.8
Vegetable, Cocktail, Tiger Tiger*	1 Roll/15g	38	2.0	254	6.4	26.7	13.4	2.0
Vegetable, Frozen, Tesco*	1 Roll/60g	123	6.4	205	3.5	23.0	10.6	1.3
Vegetable, M & S*	1 Roll/29g	62	3.0	215	3.2	27.7	10.3	2.4
Vegetable, Mini, Nirvana*	1 Roll/26g	54	2.7	208	3.5	25.1	10.4	1.7
Vegetable, Mini, Occasions, Sainsbury's*	1 Roll/24g	52	2.3	216	4.1	28.2	9.6	2.9

	Measure INFO/WEIGHT	per Measure KCAL	FAT	Nutrition Values per 100g / 100ml KCAL	PROT	CARB	FAT	FIBRE
SPRING ROLLS								
Vegetable, Mini, Oriental Selection, Waitrose*	1 Roll/18.2g	35	1.2	192	4.2	28.6	6.8	1.7
Vegetable, Mini, Party Food, M & S*	1 Roll/17g	35	1.6	205	3.5	26.3	9.7	2.0
Vegetable, Mini, Tesco*	1 Roll/17.5g	37	1.5	205	4.4	26.4	8.6	1.5
Vegetable, Oriental Selection, Party, Iceland*	1 Roll/14.9g	36	1.4	241	4.3	34.1	9.7	2.1
Vegetable, Oriental Style, Party, Tesco*	1 Roll/20.2g	47	2.4	235	3.0	29.0	12.0	1.5
Vegetable, Party Delights, Farmfoods*	1 Roll/20g	31	0.9	156	4.4	24.8	4.4	1.5
Vegetable, Safeway*	1 Serving/117g	242	11.0	207	3.5	27.1	9.4	2.7
Vegetable, Somerfield*	1 Roll/60g	107	4.0	179	3.8	26.1	6.6	1.6
Vegetable, Tempura, M & S*	1 Pack/140g	280	12.0	200	2.8	27.9	8.6	1.8
Vegetable, Waitrose*	1 Roll/57g	107	5.3	187	3.7	22.1	9.3	3.4
Vegetable & Chicken, Tesco*	1 Roll/60g	110	4.6	183	6.1	22.2	7.7	2.5
Waitrose*	1 Roll/33g	61	2.8	184	3.6	23.1	8.6	2.5
SQUARES								
Rice Krispies, Chewy, Marshmallow, Kellogg's*	1 Med Bar/18g	75	2.0	415	3.0	76.0	11.0	0.9
Rice Krispies, Chocolate & Caramel, Kellogg's*	1 Bar/21g	90	2.9	430	4.5	71.0	14.0	2.0
Rice Krispies, Crazy Choc, Kellogg's*	1 Bar/18g	76	2.2	422	3.0	76.0	12.0	1.5
SQUASH								
Acorn, Baked, Average	1oz/28g	16	0.0	56	1.1	12.6	0.1	3.2
Acorn, Raw, Average	1oz/28g	11	0.0	40	0.8	9.0	0.1	2.3
Apple, Blackcurrant, Low Sugar, Diluted, Sainsbury's*	1 Glass/250ml	5	0.3	2	0.1	0.2	0.1	0.1
Apple, Cherry & Raspberry, High Juice, Robinson's*	1 Serving/25ml	49	0.0	196	0.2	47.6	0.1	0.0
Apple, Hi Juice, Tesco*	1 fl oz/30ml	52	0.0	173	0.1	42.5	0.0	0.0
Apple, No Added Sugar, Morrisons*	1 Serving/40ml	8	0.0	21	0.1	4.1	0.0	0.0
Apple & Blackcurrant, No Added Sugar, Tesco*	1 Serving/30mls	5	0.0	15	0.2	2.0	0.0	0.0
Apple & Blackcurrant, Special R, Robinson's*	1 Serving/30ml	2	0.0	8	0.1	1.1	0.0	0.0
Blackcurrant, High Juice, Tesco*	1 Serving/75ml	215	0.0	287	0.3	70.0	0.0	0.0
Butternut, Baked, Average	1oz/28g	9	0.0	32	0.9	7.4	0.1	1.4
Butternut, Courgette & Mange Tout, M & S*	1 Pack/80g	24	0.2	30	2.0	5.8	0.2	2.3
Butternut, Raw, Unprepared, Average	1oz/28g	11	0.0	38	1.1	8.3	0.1	1.6
Cherries & Berries, Tesco*	1 Serving/25mls	5	0.0	21	0.2	3.2	0.0	0.0
Dandelion & Burdock, Morrisons*	1 Serving/50ml	2	0.0	3	0.0	0.0	0.0	0.0
Forest Fruits, Fruit & Barley, Diluted, Morrisons*	1 fl oz/30ml	4	0.0	12	0.1	1.7	0.0	0.0
Forest Fruits, High Juice, Undiluted, Robinson's*	1 Serving/25ml	52	0.0	206	0.2	50.0	0.1	0.0
Fruit & Barley, No Added Sugar, Robinson's*	1 fl oz/30ml	4	0.0	14	0.3	2.0	0.0	0.0
Fruit & Barley, Tropical, No Added Sugar, Robinson's*	1 fl oz/30ml	4	0.0	14	0.3	2.0	0.0	0.0
Fruit & Barley Orange, Diluted, Robinson's*	1 Serving/50ml	6	0.0	12	0.2	1.7	0.0	0.1
Grapefruit, High Juice, No Added Sugar, Sainsbury's*	1 Serving/25ml	15	0.3	6	0.1	1.1	0.1	0.1
Lemon, High Juice, Diluted, Sainsbury's*	1 Glass /250ml	98	0.3	39	0.1	9.1	0.1	0.1
Lemon, High Juice, Tesco*	1 Serving/80ml	141	0.1	176	0.3	43.6	0.1	0.0
Lemon, No Sugar, Asda*	1 Serving/200ml	5	0.2	3	0.1	0.3	0.1	0.1
Lemon, Whole, Low Sugar, Sainsbury's*	1 Glass/250ml	5	0.3	2	0.1	0.2	0.1	0.1
Mixed Fruit, Low Sugar, Sainsbury's*	1 Glass/250ml	5	0.3	2	0.1	0.2	0.1	0.1
Mixed Fruit, Tesco*	1 Serving/75ml	13	0.0	17	0.0	3.5	0.0	0.0
Orange, Hi Juice, Tesco*	1 Serving/75ml	140	0.1	187	0.3	45.0	0.1	0.0
Orange, High Juice, Undiluted, Robinson's*	1 Serving/200ml	364	0.2	182	0.3	44.0	0.1	0.0
Orange, No Added Sugar, High Juice, Sainsbury's*	1 Serving/100ml	6	0.1	6	0.1	1.1	0.1	0.1
Orange, Sainsbury's*	1 Glass/250ml	8	0.3	3	0.1	0.5	0.1	0.1
Orange, Special R, Diluted, Robinson's*	1 fl oz/30ml	2	0.0	8	0.2	0.7	0.1	0.0
Orange & Mandarin, Fruit Spring, Robinson's*	1 Serving/440ml	26	0.0	6	0.1	0.8	0.0	0.0
Orange & Mango, Low Sugar, Sainsbury's*	1 Serving/250ml	5	0.3	2	0.1	0.2	0.1	0.1
Orange & Mango, No Added Sugar, Robinson's*	1 Serving/25ml	2	0.0	8	0.2	0.9	0.0	0.0
Orange & Mango, Special R, Diluted, Robinson's*	1 Serving/250ml	20	0.0	8	0.2	0.9	0.0	0.0
Orange & Pineapple, Original, Undiluted, Robinson's*	1 Serving/250ml	138	0.0	55	1.0	13.0	0.0	0.0

S

	Measure INFO/WEIGHT	per Measure KCAL	FAT	Nutrition Values per 100g / 100ml KCAL	PROT	CARB	FAT	FIBRE
SQUASH								
Pink Grapefruit, High Juice, Low Sugar, Tesco*	1 Serving/75ml	12	0.1	16	0.2	3.7	0.1	0.0
Pink Grapefruit, High Juice, Sainsbury's*	1 Serving/250ml	103	0.3	41	0.1	9.9	0.1	0.1
Pink Grapefruit, High Juice, Tesco*	1 Serving/75ml	135	0.1	180	0.2	44.6	0.1	0.0
Pink Grapefruit, High Juice, Undiluted, Robinson's*	1 Glass/250ml	455	0.3	182	0.2	43.3	0.1	0.0
Spaghetti, Baked	1oz/28g	6	0.1	23	0.7	4.3	0.3	2.1
Spaghetti, Including Pips & Rind, Raw	1oz/28g	7	0.2	26	0.6	4.6	0.6	2.3
Summer Fruits, High Juice, Undiluted, Robinson's*	1 fl oz/30ml	61	0.0	203	0.1	49.0	0.1	0.0
Summer Fruits, High Juice, Waitrose*	1 Serving/250ml	102	0.0	41	0.0	10.0	0.0	0.0
Summer Fruits, No Added Sugar, Made Up, Morrisons*	1 Glass/200ml	3	0.0	2	0.0	0.3	0.0	0.0
Tropical, High Juice, Tesco*	1 Glass/75ml	141	0.1	188	0.2	46.6	0.1	0.1
Tropical, No Added Sugar, Diluted, Tesco*	1 Glass/200ml	18	0.0	9	0.2	0.9	0.0	0.0
Tropical Fruits, Sainsbury's*	1 Serving/250ml	95	0.3	38	0.1	9.3	0.1	0.1
Whole Orange, Spar*	1 Serving/250ml	10	0.1	4	0.0	0.8	0.0	0.0
Whole Orange, Tesco*	1 Serving/100ml	45	1.0	45	0.2	10.1	1.0	1.0
SQUID								
Calamari, Battered, Frozen, Youngs*	1 Bag/375g	758	37.9	202	8.1	19.7	10.1	0.8
Calamari, Battered, M & S*	1 Pack/160g	424	25.8	265	14.3	15.8	16.1	0.7
Calamari, Battered, with Tartar Sauce Dip, Tesco*	1 Pack/210g	573	41.0	273	8.9	15.4	19.5	0.6
Calamari, M & S*	1oz/28g	65	4.0	231	13.9	11.5	14.4	0.5
Calamari, Rings in Batter, Waitrose*	½ Pack/85g	227	14.6	267	13.9	14.2	17.2	0.6
Dried, Average	1oz/28g	88	1.3	313	63.3	4.8	4.6	0.0
in Batter, Fried in Blended Oil, Average	1oz/28g	55	2.8	195	11.5	15.7	10.0	0.5
Raw, Average	1oz/28g	23	0.5	81	15.4	1.2	1.7	0.0
STAR FRUIT								
Average	1oz/28g	9	0.1	32	0.5	7.3	0.3	1.3
STARBAR								
Cadbury*	1 Bar/53g	260	14.8	491	10.7	49.0	27.9	0.0
STARBURST								
Fruit Chews, Tropical, Mars*	1 Tube/45g	168	3.3	373	0.0	76.9	7.3	0.0
Joosters, Mars*	1 Pack/45g	160	0.0	356	0.0	88.8	0.1	0.0
Mars*	1 Pack/45g	185	3.4	411	0.3	85.3	7.6	0.0
STEAK								
Au Poivre, Finest, Tesco*	½ Pack/225g	383	20.3	170	16.4	5.0	9.0	0.5
Diane, Finest, Tesco*	1 Serving/225g	331	18.7	147	14.2	3.9	8.3	0.7
STEAK &								
Ale, with Vintage Cheddar Mash, Finest, Tesco*	1 Serving/550g	594	25.3	108	8.0	8.6	4.6	0.6
Vegetable Medley, HE, Tesco*	1 Pack/400g	264	6.4	66	7.6	5.3	1.6	0.8
STEAK & KIDNEY PUDDING								
Fray Bentos*	1 Tin/213g	477	26.8	224	7.8	19.8	12.6	0.0
M & S*	1 Pudding/121g	260	13.4	215	9.2	19.4	11.1	3.2
Sainsbury's*	1 Pudding/435g	1135	62.6	261	10.5	22.3	14.4	0.8
Somerfield*	1 Pudding/190g	488	25.7	257	10.2	23.6	13.5	1.0
Tesco*	1 Serving/190g	437	22.6	230	10.0	20.7	11.9	1.2
Waitrose*	1 Pudding/223g	497	26.1	223	8.9	20.4	11.7	1.2
STEAK CHASSEUR								
HE, Tesco*	1 Pack/450g	347	8.1	77	10.0	5.3	1.8	0.5
STEAK IN								
Rich Gravy, Stewed, Extra Lean, Sainsbury's*	1 Sm Can/220g	249	6.2	113	20.3	1.6	2.8	1.6
STEAK PEPPERED								
with Garlic Butter, Somerfield*	1 Serving/170g	265	9.4	156	24.9	1.7	5.5	0.3
STEAK STEWED								
& Onions with Gravy, John West*	½ Can/205g	269	14.4	131	14.0	3.0	7.0	0.0
Tesco*	½ Can/200g	230	6.0	115	17.5	4.5	3.0	0.0

S

	Measure INFO/WEIGHT	per Measure KCAL	FAT	Nutrition Values per 100g / 100ml KCAL	PROT	CARB	FAT	FIBRE
STEAK STEWED								
with Gravy, John West*	1oz/28g	30	0.8	107	18.0	2.0	3.0	0.2
STEAK WITH								
Red Wine & Shallot Sauce, Rump, Waitrose*	1 Serving/205g	242	11.5	118	16.4	0.9	5.6	0.3
STEAMED PUDDING								
Golden Syrup, Aunty's*	1 Pudding/110g	325	4.5	295	2.9	58.6	4.1	0.7
Sticky Toffee, Aunty's*	1 Serving/110g	331	5.3	301	2.6	58.4	4.8	1.2
Toffee & Date, Aunty's*	1 Serving/110g	320	5.1	291	2.6	59.1	4.6	1.1
STEW								
Beef, Asda*	½ Can/196g	178	4.9	91	10.0	7.0	2.5	1.5
Beef, Meal for One, M & S*	1 Pack/440g	350	8.4	80	7.0	8.7	1.9	2.0
Beef, Value, Tesco*	1 Serving/200g	170	9.8	85	4.0	6.2	4.9	1.0
Beef, with Dumplings, Tesco*	1 Serving/400g	424	14.0	106	4.8	13.9	3.5	0.6
Beef & Dumplings, Asda*	1 Pack/400g	392	13.2	98	6.0	11.0	3.3	0.8
Beef & Dumplings, Birds Eye*	1 Pack/320g	246	6.7	77	4.4	10.0	2.1	0.9
Beef & Dumplings, British Classics, Tesco*	1 Pack/450g	563	29.7	125	7.9	8.6	6.6	0.5
Beef & Dumplings, Countryside*	1 Pack/300g	246	6.9	82	8.1	7.3	2.3	0.5
Beef & Dumplings, Eat Smart, Safeway*	1 Pack/394g	335	9.9	85	8.1	6.8	2.5	1.1
Beef & Dumplings, Farmfoods*	1 Pack/300g	312	13.2	104	4.0	12.0	4.4	1.1
Beef & Dumplings, Frozen, Asda*	1 Pack/400g	392	13.2	98	6.0	11.0	3.3	0.8
Beef & Dumplings, Iceland*	1 Serving/400g	468	20.0	117	4.5	13.5	5.0	0.5
Beef & Dumplings, Morrisons*	1 Pack/400g	440	18.4	110	6.0	11.1	4.6	1.5
Beef & Dumplings, Plumrose*	½ Can/196g	143	3.9	73	6.1	9.0	2.0	0.0
Beef & Dumplings, Ready Meals, Waitrose*	1oz/28g	38	1.6	136	8.0	13.3	5.6	0.8
Beef & Dumplings, Weight Watchers*	1 Pack/327g	262	6.9	80	5.2	10.0	2.1	0.8
Beef with Dumplings, Classic British, Sainsbury's*	1 Pack/450g	531	23.4	118	7.7	10.2	5.2	0.5
Beef with Dumplings, COU, M & S*	1 Pack/454g	431	11.8	95	8.9	9.1	2.6	0.8
Beef with Dumplings, GFY, Asda*	1 Pack/400g	429	9.0	107	11.5	10.3	2.3	0.9
Beef with Dumplings, Sainsbury's*	1 Pack/450g	603	27.5	134	9.3	10.5	6.1	0.7
Chicken, Morrisons*	1 Pack/400g	492	7.6	123	17.6	8.9	1.9	0.5
Chicken & Dumplings, Birds Eye*	1 Pack/320g	282	8.6	88	7.0	8.9	2.7	0.5
Chicken & Dumplings, Tesco*	1 Serving/450g	567	29.7	126	7.6	9.1	6.6	0.7
Irish, Asda*	¼ Can/196g	172	7.8	88	6.0	7.0	4.0	1.0
Irish, Morrisons*	1 Can/392g	243	4.7	62	3.8	8.9	1.2	0.0
Irish, Plumrose*	1 Can/392g	318	9.8	81	7.5	7.2	2.5	0.0
Irish, Sainsbury's*	1 Pack/450g	275	9.5	61	5.7	4.8	2.1	0.5
Irish, SmartPrice, Asda*	1 Can/392g	298	14.1	76	3.0	8.0	3.6	0.9
Irish, Tesco*	1 Can/400g	308	11.2	77	7.0	5.9	2.8	0.8
Lentil & Vegetable, Organic, Simply Organic*	1 Pack/400g	284	6.0	71	3.5	11.0	1.5	1.3
Lentil & Winter Vegetable, Organic, Pure & Pronto*	1 Pack/400g	364	9.6	91	3.6	14.0	2.4	4.0
Mixed Vegetable Topped with Herb Dumplings, Tesco*	1 Pack/420g	508	26.0	121	1.9	14.5	6.2	1.3
STIR FRY								
Baby Leaf, Ready Prepared, M & S*	1 Serving/125g	25	0.1	20	1.7	4.9	0.1	2.5
Baby Vegetable & Pak Choi, Two Step, Tesco*	½ Pack/95g	29	0.8	31	2.1	4.0	0.8	2.3
Bean Sprout, Chinese, Sainsbury's*	1 Pack/300g	144	8.4	48	1.9	5.1	2.8	1.5
Bean Sprout, Ready to Eat, Washed, Sainsbury's*	1 Serving/150g	83	5.9	55	1.5	3.3	3.9	1.8
Bean Sprout & Vegetable, with Red Peppers, Asda*	1 Pack/350g	126	3.9	36	1.8	4.7	1.1	2.3
Bean Sprouts, Asda*	½ Pack/175g	56	0.9	32	2.9	4.0	0.5	1.5
Bean Sprouts, Morrisons*	1 Serving/150g	47	0.6	31	2.0	4.8	0.4	1.8
Bean Sprouts & Vegetables, Asda*	½ Pack/173g	107	6.9	62	2.0	4.5	4.0	1.8
Beef, BGTY, Sainsbury's*	½ Pack/125g	156	5.1	125	22.0	0.1	4.1	0.0
Beef, Less Than 10% Fat, Asda*	1 Pack/227g	275	6.4	121	24.0	0.0	2.8	0.8
Beef, Less Than 3% Fat, BGTY, Sainsbury's*	½ Pack/125g	134	2.6	107	22.1	0.1	2.1	0.1
Cherry Tomato & Noodle, Waitrose*	1 Pack/400g	304	15.2	76	2.1	8.5	3.8	1.5

S

STIR FRY

	Measure INFO/WEIGHT	per Measure KCAL	FAT	Nutrition Values per 100g / 100ml KCAL	PROT	CARB	FAT	FIBRE
Chicken, Safeway*	1 Serving/200g	204	3.2	102	22.0	0.0	1.6	0.0
Chicken Chow Mein, Fresh, Heathly Living, Tesco*	1 Pack/400g	312	4.8	78	5.7	11.4	1.2	1.3
Chicken Chow Mein, Orient Express, Oriental Express*	1 Pack/400g	384	10.8	96	7.3	10.7	2.7	2.2
Chicken Noodle, GFY, Asda*	1 Pack/330g	403	10.9	122	7.0	16.0	3.3	2.4
Chinese, Family, Sainsbury's*	1 Serving/150g	60	3.0	40	2.3	3.3	2.0	3.6
Chinese, with Oriental Sauce, Tesco*	1 Pack/530g	180	2.1	34	2.3	5.4	0.4	1.5
Chinese Chicken, Iceland*	1 Pack/298g	262	4.2	88	6.2	12.7	1.4	2.9
Chinese Chicken, Sizzling, Oriental Express*	1 Pack/400g	400	8.0	100	6.6	13.8	2.0	1.7
Chinese Exotic Vegetable, Sainsbury's*	1 Pack/350g	133	7.7	38	1.7	2.8	2.2	1.8
Chinese Mixed Vegetable, Sainsbury's*	1 Serving/150g	75	4.1	50	1.7	4.7	2.7	0.0
Chinese Mushroom, Sainsbury's*	1 Serving/175g	67	4.2	38	1.7	2.4	2.4	1.7
Chinese Noodles, Oriental Express*	1oz/28g	20	0.1	70	2.7	14.7	0.5	1.4
Chinese Prawn, Asda*	1 Serving/375g	345	2.3	92	3.6	18.0	0.6	1.8
Chinese Prawn, Iceland*	1 Pack/340g	235	4.4	69	3.1	11.1	1.3	2.1
Chinese Prawns, Sizzling, Oriental Express*	1 Pack/375g	341	4.1	91	4.0	16.2	1.1	12.0
Chinese Style, Co-Op*	1 Pack/300g	105	1.2	35	3.0	6.0	0.4	2.0
Chinese Style, Somerfield*	½ Pack/175g	95	4.0	54	1.9	6.3	2.3	0.7
Chinese Style, Tesco*	1 Pack/475g	128	1.4	27	2.1	4.1	0.3	2.1
Chinese Style Chicken, GFY, Asda*	1 Pack/338.3g	362	5.7	107	6.0	17.0	1.7	1.5
Chinese Style Prawn, GFY, Asda*	1 Pack/400g	324	6.4	81	3.6	13.0	1.6	1.6
Chinese Style Rice with Vegetables, Tesco*	1 Serving/550g	495	13.8	90	2.2	14.8	2.5	0.3
Chinese Style Turkey, Asda*	½ Pack/210g	321	6.0	153	23.8	8.1	2.9	0.8
Chinese Vegetable & Oyster Sauce, Asda*	1 Serving/150g	93	3.8	62	1.9	8.0	2.5	0.0
Chinese Vegetables, Oriental Express*	½ Pack/200g	44	0.4	22	1.4	3.7	0.2	2.2
Chinese Vegetables, Tesco*	1 Serving/175g	93	0.7	53	1.6	10.8	0.4	1.3
Chinese Vegetables, with Oyster Sauce, Tesco*	1 Pack/350g	98	0.7	28	2.0	4.6	0.2	1.1
Chow Mein, Safeway*	1 Pack/400g	536	25.6	134	3.8	15.2	6.4	1.9
Exotic, Asda*	1 Serving/250g	103	4.3	41	2.3	4.2	1.7	2.7
Family, Safeway*	1 Serving/150g	83	5.0	55	2.1	4.2	3.3	2.1
Family Pack, Vegetables & Beansprouts, Fresh, Tesco*	1 Pack/600g	108	0.6	18	2.0	2.2	0.1	2.1
Green Vegetable, M & S*	1 Pack/220g	165	13.0	75	3.1	2.5	5.9	2.2
Mexican Vegetables, Lidl*	1 Serving/100g	97	5.7	97	3.4	8.1	5.7	0.0
Mixed Pepper, HL, Tesco*	1 Pack/325g	62	0.3	19	1.9	2.6	0.1	1.5
Mixed Pepper, Tesco*	1/3 Pack/100g	23	0.1	23	1.9	3.7	0.1	1.9
Mixed Pepper & Sweet Chilli Sauce, Asda*	1 Pack/300g	180	6.0	60	1.6	9.0	2.0	2.6
Mixed Pepper & Vegetable, Asda*	½ Pack/150g	42	1.5	28	1.6	3.2	1.0	2.6
Mixed Vegetable, Safeway*	1 Serving/150g	105	5.4	70	2.1	6.2	3.6	2.5
Mixed Vegetables, Sainsbury's*	½ Pack/140g	70	3.8	50	1.7	4.7	2.7	3.0
Mushroom, Asda*	½ Pack/175g	86	4.7	49	2.8	3.3	2.7	2.8
Mushroom, Freshly Prepared, Tesco*	1 Pack/350g	67	0.4	19	2.7	1.9	0.1	1.9
Mushroom, Just Stir Fry, Sainsbury's*	1 Pack/350g	172	9.5	49	2.8	3.3	2.7	2.8
Mushroom, Safeway*	1 Pack/350g	210	12.6	60	2.3	4.2	3.6	2.1
Mushroom, Somerfield*	1 Serving/175g	89	6.0	51	2.2	3.0	3.4	1.0
Noodles & Bean Sprouts, Tesco*	½ Pack/125g	131	2.6	105	4.2	16.1	2.1	0.7
Noodles & Veg, with Soy, Ginger & Garlic Sauce, Tesco*	1 Pack/300g	270	5.4	90	2.7	15.5	1.8	2.4
Orient Inspired, M & S*	1 Serving/250g	50	0.8	20	1.6	3.4	0.3	1.6
Oriental Leaf, M & S*	½ Pack/125g	25	0.6	20	1.9	2.5	0.5	2.2
Oriental Style Pak Choi, M & S*	1 Pack/220g	165	12.5	75	2.2	3.5	5.7	2.4
Oriental Vegetable, Frozen, Asda*	1 Serving/150g	116	6.8	77	2.1	7.0	4.5	1.7
Oriental Vegetables, Safeway*	1 Serving/175g	196	7.7	112	2.6	15.5	4.4	0.5
Singaporean Noodle, Sainsbury's*	½ Pack/160g	202	11.7	126	3.2	11.9	7.3	2.4
SmartPrice, Asda*	1 Pack/350g	126	3.9	36	1.8	4.7	1.1	2.3
Spicy Thai Style Noodle, Tesco*	1 Pack/500g	335	13.0	67	2.6	8.4	2.6	1.3

S

	Measure INFO/WEIGHT	per Measure KCAL	FAT	Nutrition Values per 100g / 100ml KCAL	PROT	CARB	FAT	FIBRE
STIR FRY								
Sweet & Sour, Co-Op*	½ Pack/187g	103	1.7	55	2.0	10.0	0.9	3.0
Sweet & Sour Vegetable, Somerfield*	1 Pack/350g	249	3.5	71	2.0	14.0	1.0	0.0
Tatsoi & Sugar Snap Pea, M & S*	½ Pack/125g	25	0.4	20	2.0	3.0	0.3	1.9
Tender Shoot, Sainsbury's*	½ Pack/126g	113	8.3	90	4.4	2.8	6.6	0.8
Thai, Vegetable, Safeway*	1 Serving/300g	220	13.0	73	2.6	5.6	4.3	2.3
Thai Style, Eastern Inspirations*	1 Pack/330g	92	1.7	28	2.9	3.2	0.5	1.3
Thai Style, M & S*	1 Serving/150g	75	4.5	50	2.3	3.0	3.0	1.2
Thai Style, Tesco*	1 Pack/350g	301	17.9	86	3.9	6.2	5.1	1.9
Tomato & Basil, Sundried, Tesco*	1 Pack/325g	205	11.7	63	1.6	6.2	3.6	2.2
Turkey, Fresh, Good Intentions, Somerfield*	½ Pack/150g	246	6.8	164	31.0	0.0	4.5	0.0
Vegetable, Asda*	1 Pack/300g	132	6.9	44	1.6	4.2	2.3	3.1
Vegetable, Chinese Style, Asda*	1 Pack/300g	81	2.1	27	1.6	3.6	0.7	2.8
Vegetable, Crunchy, Waitrose*	1 Pack/300g	81	0.3	27	1.6	4.8	0.1	2.4
Vegetable, Premium, Sainsbury's*	½ Pack/150g	90	5.3	60	2.8	4.2	3.5	2.7
Vegetable, Ready Prepared, M & S*	½ Pack/150g	38	0.5	25	2.2	3.5	0.3	2.2
Vegetable, Safeway*	½ Pack/150g	68	4.7	45	1.1	3.2	3.1	1.6
Vegetable, Sweet & Crunchy, Waitrose*	1 Pack/300g	69	0.3	23	1.8	3.6	0.1	1.4
Vegetable & Beansprout, Waitrose*	1 Pack/300g	78	0.9	26	1.4	4.5	0.3	2.1
Vegetable & Beansprout, with Peanut Sauce, Tesco*	1 Serving/475g	409	23.8	86	3.9	6.2	5.0	1.9
Vegetable & Mushroom, Asda*	½ Pack/160g	59	2.4	37	2.4	3.4	1.5	3.4
Vegetable & Noodle, Asda*	1 Pack/330g	465	14.9	141	4.0	21.0	4.5	3.0
Vegetable Noodles, BGTY, Sainsbury's*	1 Pack/455g	391	9.1	86	3.2	14.0	2.0	1.4
Vegetables, Family Pack, Co-Op*	½ Pack/300g	90	1.2	30	2.0	5.0	0.4	2.0
Vegetables, Fresh, Asda*	½ Pack/150g	107	7.5	71	1.7	4.9	5.0	1.7
Vegetables, Mixed, with Slices of Pepper, Tesco*	1 Pack/300g	57	0.3	19	1.9	2.6	0.1	1.5
Vegetables, Somerfield*	1 Pack/300g	93	0.0	31	2.0	5.0	0.0	0.0
Vegetables & Bean Sprout, M & S*	1 Pack/350g	105	1.4	30	1.8	4.6	0.4	2.0
Vegetables & Beansprouts, Fresh, Tesco*	1 Pack/600g	108	0.6	18	2.0	2.2	0.1	2.1
Vegetables with Oyster Sauce, Asda*	1 Serving/150g	93	3.8	62	1.9	8.0	2.5	0.0
STOCK								
Beef, Fresh, Tesco*	1 Serving/300ml	54	0.9	18	2.1	1.6	0.3	0.5
Chicken, Asda*	½ Pot/150g	26	1.4	17	1.8	0.7	0.9	0.2
Chicken, Concentrated, M & S*	1 Tsp/5g	16	0.9	315	25.6	12.2	18.1	0.8
Chicken, Fresh, Sainsbury's*	½ Pot/142ml	23	0.1	16	3.7	0.1	0.1	0.3
Chicken, Fresh, Tesco*	1 Serving/300ml	27	0.3	9	1.6	0.5	0.1	0.5
Chicken, Home Prepared, Average	1 fl oz/28ml	5	0.0	16	3.7	0.1	0.1	0.3
Chicken, Knorr*	1 Pack/150g	348	5.6	232	13.1	36.5	3.7	0.4
Chicken, Prepared, Tesco*	1 Serving/300ml	54	0.3	18	2.4	1.8	0.1	0.5
Chicken, Simply, Knorr*	1 Pack/450ml	27	0.0	6	1.5	0.1	0.0	0.1
Fish, Home Prepared, Average	1 Serving/250ml	43	2.0	17	2.3	0.0	0.8	0.0
Vegetable, Concentrated, M & S*	1 Tsp/5g	19	1.0	380	3.3	43.0	19.0	1.2
Vegetable, Cooks Ingredients, Waitrose*	1 Pouch/500ml	15	0.5	3	0.2	0.4	0.1	0.5
Vegetable, Knorr*	1 Serving/9g	18	0.1	199	8.5	39.9	0.6	0.9
Vegetable, Tablets, Sainsbury's*	1 Tablet/11g	1	0.1	7	0.4	0.2	0.5	0.1
STOCK CUBES								
Basil, Herb Cubes, Knorr*	1 Cube/10g	47	3.4	472	6.1	35.9	33.8	0.6
Beef, Dry Weight, Bovril*	1 Cube/5.9g	12	0.2	197	10.8	29.3	4.1	0.0
Beef, Dry Weight, Oxo*	1 Cube/5.8	15	0.3	265	17.3	38.4	4.7	1.5
Beef, Knorr*	1 Cube/9.5g	33	2.4	347	9.5	17.9	25.3	0.0
Beef, Organic, Kallo*	1 Cube/12g	25	1.0	208	16.7	16.7	8.3	0.0
Beef, SmartPrice, Asda*	1 Cube/11g	31	2.5	279	10.0	8.0	23.0	0.0
Beef, Tesco*	1 Serving/7g	17	0.2	260	9.7	48.9	2.8	1.3
Beef, Toro*	1 Cube/60g	90	2.4	150	27.0	1.0	4.0	0.0

	Measure INFO/WEIGHT	per Measure KCAL	FAT	Nutrition Values per 100g / 100ml KCAL	PROT	CARB	FAT	FIBRE
STOCK CUBES								
Beef, Value, Tesco*	1 Cube/10g	19	0.9	189	11.2	17.0	8.5	0.1
Chicken	1 Cube/6g	14	0.9	237	15.4	9.9	15.4	0.0
Chicken, Dry, Oxo*	1 Cube/6g	15	0.2	249	11.7	42.9	3.4	1.6
Chicken, Just Bouillon, Kallo*	1 Cube/12g	30	1.3	247	11.8	26.1	10.6	1.0
Chicken, Knorr*	1 Cube/10g	30	1.9	301	10.1	23.6	18.5	0.2
Chicken, Made Up, Sainsbury's*	1 Serving/200ml	16	0.2	8	0.3	1.4	0.1	0.1
Chicken, Tesco*	1 Cube/11g	32	2.5	290	10.5	11.1	22.6	0.7
Chinese, Dry Weight, Oxo*	1 Cube/5.8g	16	0.4	274	9.5	42.9	7.2	3.6
Fish, Knorr*	1 Cube/10g	32	2.0	321	18.9	15.9	20.2	0.7
Fish, Sainsbury's*	1 Cube/11g	31	2.2	282	19.1	7.3	20.0	0.9
Garlic, Dry Weight, Oxo*	1 Cube/6g	18	0.3	298	13.4	48.5	5.5	3.6
Ham, Knorr*	1 Cube/10g	31	1.9	313	11.8	24.4	18.7	0.0
Indian, Dry Weight, Oxo*	1 Cube/6g	17	0.5	291	11.5	43.9	7.7	6.7
Italian, Dry Weight, Oxo*	1 Cube/6g	19	0.4	309	11.9	48.9	7.3	4.6
Lamb, Made Up, Knorr*	1 Cube/10g	30	2.1	301	14.7	12.9	21.2	0.2
Mexican, Dry Weight, Oxo*	1 Cube/6g	15	0.4	248	11.8	36.8	6.0	3.7
Parsley & Garlic, Herb Cubes, Knorr*	1 Cube/10g	42	2.7	422	8.6	35.2	27.4	1.8
Vegetable, Average	1 Cube/7g	18	1.2	253	13.5	11.6	17.3	0.0
Vegetable, Dry, Oxo*	1 Cube/6g	15	0.2	258	9.8	45.3	4.2	1.7
Vegetable, Knorr*	1 Pack/80g	264	19.2	330	10.0	25.0	24.0	1.0
Vegetable, Low Salt, Organic, Made Up, Kallo*	1 Serving/500ml	50	3.5	10	0.3	0.7	0.7	0.2
Vegetable, Made Up, Organic, Kallo*	2 Cubes/100ml	7	0.4	7	0.1	0.5	0.4	0.1
Vegetable, Made Up, Safeway*	1 Serving/500ml	18	0.9	4	0.2	0.3	0.2	0.0
Vegetable, Organic, Evernat*	1oz/28g	2	0.1	6	0.3	0.0	0.5	0.0
Vegetable, Premium, Made Up, Kallo*	1 Serving/125ml	7	0.4	6	0.4	0.4	0.3	0.1
Vegetable, SmartPrice, Asda*	1 Cube/11g	27	2.1	243	6.0	12.0	19.0	0.0
Vegetable, Tesco*	1 Cube/11.2g	29	2.0	259	10.0	13.6	18.3	1.2
Vegetable, Yeast Free, Made Up, Kallo*	1 Cube/500ml	35	3.0	7	0.3	0.2	0.6	0.1
STORTELLI								
Microwaveable, Dolmio*	1 Serving/220g	299	2.2	136	5.3	26.3	1.0	0.0
STRAWBERRIES								
Fresh, Raw, Average	1oz/28g	8	0.0	28	0.8	6.0	0.1	0.9
in Fruit Juice, Canned, Average	1/3 Can/127g	58	0.0	46	0.5	11.0	0.0	1.0
in Light Syrup, Canned, Drained, Tesco*	1 Can/149g	100	0.1	67	0.5	16.0	0.1	0.7
in Raspberry Sauce, WTF, Sainsbury's*	1 Serving/170g	111	0.2	65	0.7	15.3	0.1	2.3
STRAWBERRIES & CREME FRAICHE								
Shapers, Boots*	1 Pack/100g	77	5.7	77	1.4	5.1	5.7	0.8
STROGANOFF								
Beef, BGTY, Sainsbury's*	1 Pack/400g	416	10.4	104	5.6	14.6	2.6	0.6
Beef, Eat Smart, Morrisons*	1 Pack/400g	344	9.2	86	5.0	11.2	2.3	0.9
Beef, Finest, Tesco*	½ Pack/200g	330	13.4	165	9.4	16.2	6.7	0.7
Beef, Nutrionally Balanced, M & S*	1 Pack/400g	460	10.4	115	8.4	14.7	2.6	1.6
Beef, Sainsbury's*	1 Can/200g	232	12.0	116	12.5	3.0	6.0	0.2
Beef, TTD, Sainsbury's*	1 Pack/400g	656	42.0	164	11.9	5.2	10.5	0.4
Beef, Weight Watchers*	1 Pack/330g	297	7.6	90	4.3	13.0	2.3	0.1
Beef, with Long Grain & Wild Rice, Somerfield*	1 Pack/400g	485	16.4	121	7.3	13.8	4.1	1.6
Beef, with Rice, Naturally Good Food, Tesco*	1 Pack/400g	425	9.4	106	7.1	13.9	2.4	1.3
Chicken, with Rice, BGTY, Sainsbury's*	1 Pack/415g	448	5.4	108	7.0	17.1	1.3	1.1
Chicken & Mushroom, COU, M & S*	1 Serving/400g	400	8.0	100	3.2	16.7	2.0	0.1
Mushroom, Eat Smart, Morrisons*	1 Pack/400g	312	4.4	78	2.6	14.3	1.1	1.0
Mushroom, with Rice, BGTY, Sainsbury's*	1 Serving/450g	419	6.8	93	3.3	16.6	1.5	1.0
Mushroom with Rice, Vegetarian, Health Living, Tesco*	1 Pack/450g	527	21.6	117	3.2	15.2	4.8	1.2
Mushroom with Rice, Vegetarian, HL, Tesco*	1 Pack/450g	527	21.6	117	3.2	15.2	4.8	1.2

S

	Measure INFO/WEIGHT	per Measure KCAL	per Measure FAT	Nutrition Values per 100g / 100ml KCAL	PROT	CARB	FAT	FIBRE
STROGANOFF								
Pork with Rice, HE, Tesco*	1 Pack/450g	482	8.1	107	7.0	15.8	1.8	0.5
STRUDEL								
Apple, Co-Op*	1 Slice/100g	225	12.0	225	3.0	28.0	12.0	3.0
Apple, Frozen, Sainsbury's*	1 Serving/100g	283	15.4	283	3.2	32.8	15.4	1.9
Apple, Safeway*	¼ Strudel/150g	414	21.6	276	3.1	35.7	14.4	2.4
Apple, Sainsbury's*	1/6 Portion/90g	255	13.9	283	3.2	32.8	15.4	1.9
Apple, Tesco*	1 Serving/150g	432	21.6	288	3.3	36.4	14.4	2.8
Apple, with Sultanas, Tesco*	1/6 Strudel/100g	245	12.0	245	2.9	30.9	12.0	0.7
Woodland Fruit, Tesco*	1 Serving/100g	257	13.1	257	3.2	31.5	13.1	1.8
STUFFED PEPPERS								
Filled with Rice, Average	1oz/28g	24	0.7	85	1.5	15.4	2.4	1.3
Filled with Vegetables, Cheese Topping, Average	1oz/28g	31	1.9	111	3.4	9.8	6.7	1.5
Fresh, Asda*	1 Pepper/150g	144	7.5	96	3.8	9.0	5.0	1.2
PB, Waitrose*	1 Pack/300g	243	7.2	81	3.0	11.8	2.4	1.3
Sainsbury's*	1 Serving/137g	169	9.5	123	3.3	11.8	6.9	1.0
Yellow, Italian, Ready to Roast, Sainsbury's*	1 Pack/136g	144	6.8	106	5.3	9.9	5.0	1.3
STUFFING								
Apricot & Walnut, Made Up, Celebrations, Paxo*	1 Serving/50g	81	1.8	161	4.3	28.0	3.5	2.8
Chestnut & Pork, M & S*	1oz/28g	67	4.7	240	6.6	16.3	16.7	2.9
Olde English Chestnut, Sainsbury's*	1 Serving/110g	216	12.8	196	9.4	13.5	11.6	2.1
Parsley, Thyme & Lemon Stuffing, Paxo*	1 Serving/45g	68	0.9	150	4.3	28.4	2.1	2.4
Parsley & Thyme, Co-Op*	1 Serving/28g	95	0.8	340	10.0	67.0	3.0	6.0
Pork, Sage & Onion, M & S*	1 Serving/85g	174	12.3	205	10.2	13.2	14.5	2.8
Sage & Onion, for Chicken, Paxo*	1 Serving/50g	62	0.9	123	3.6	23.0	1.8	1.7
Sage & Onion, Made Up, Paxo*	1 Serving/50g	72	0.6	143	3.2	29.9	1.2	1.9
Sage & Onion, Made Up, Safeway*	1 Serving/60g	90	0.4	150	4.5	30.8	0.7	3.2
Sage & Onion, Somerfield*	1oz/28g	100	1.4	358	6.0	74.0	5.0	0.0
Sage & Onion, with Lemon, Paxo*	1 Serving/50g	61	0.6	122	3.4	24.2	1.2	1.9
Sausagemeat, Sainsbury's*	1 Serving/100g	175	4.2	175	7.0	27.0	4.2	2.3
Sausagemeat & Thyme, Made Up, Celebrations, Paxo*	1 Serving/50g	80	1.8	160	6.3	25.8	3.5	4.0
STUFFING BALLS								
Pork, Sausagemeat, Aunt Bessie's*	1 Ball/25.9g	55	2.1	212	7.2	27.3	8.2	3.0
Sage & Onion, Aunt Bessie's*	1 Ball/26g	63	2.3	243	6.4	34.4	8.9	3.1
Sage & Onion, Meat-Free, Aunt Bessie's*	1 Ball/28g	54	1.9	193	5.4	28.0	6.7	1.7
Sage & Onion, Tesco*	1 Serving/20g	64	4.4	322	10.0	21.1	22.0	1.9
Tesco*	1 Ball/20.6g	65	4.1	315	9.6	23.5	20.0	1.4
STUFFING MIX								
Apple & Herb, Special Recipe, Sainsbury's*	1 Serving/41g	68	0.9	165	3.8	32.4	2.2	2.2
Apple Mustard & Herb, Paxo*	1 Serving/50g	83	1.0	166	4.2	32.8	2.0	4.0
Chestnut, Morrisons*	1 Serving/20g	33	0.7	165	4.6	29.1	3.4	3.7
Chestnut & Cranberry, Celebration, Paxo*	1 Serving/25g	35	0.5	141	4.0	26.7	2.0	2.4
Date & Walnut, TTD, Sainsbury's*	1 Serving/50g	66	0.9	131	4.4	24.2	1.8	3.4
Herb & Onion, Gluten Free, Allergycare*	1 Serving/12g	43	0.3	360	7.9	76.8	2.4	0.0
Parsley, Thyme & Lemon, Sainsbury's*	1 Pack/170g	240	2.2	141	4.2	28.2	1.3	1.3
Sage, Red Onion & Lemon, TTD, Sainsbury's*	1 Serving/50g	53	0.7	106	3.8	23.9	1.3	4.2
Sage & Onion, Asda*	1 Serving/27g	29	0.2	107	3.4	22.0	0.6	1.3
Sage & Onion, Co-Op*	1 Serving/28g	94	0.6	335	10.0	68.0	2.0	6.0
Sage & Onion, Dry Weight, Tesco*	1 Std Pack/170g	578	4.1	340	10.3	69.3	2.4	6.3
Sage & Onion, Made Up, Paxo*	1 Serving/60g	74	1.1	123	3.6	23.0	1.8	1.7
Sage & Onion, Prepared, Tesco*	1 Serving/100g	50	0.4	50	1.5	10.1	0.4	0.9
Sage & Onion, SmartPrice, Asda*	¼ Pack/75g	262	2.8	349	11.0	68.0	3.7	4.7
Sausage Meat, Morrisons*	1 Serving/20g	35	0.5	174	6.8	30.8	2.6	2.9

S

	Measure INFO/WEIGHT	per Measure KCAL	FAT	Nutrition Values per 100g / 100ml KCAL	PROT	CARB	FAT	FIBRE
SUET								
Beef, Shredded, Original, Atora*	1 Pack/250g	2075	218.5	830	0.9	10.1	87.4	0.4
Beef, Tesco*	1 Serving/100g	854	91.9	854	0.6	6.2	91.9	0.1
Vegetable, Average	1oz/28g	234	24.6	836	1.2	10.1	87.9	0.0
Vegetable, Shredded, Atora*	1 Pack/250g	1760	159.8	704	3.8	28.5	63.9	1.2
SUET PUDDING								
Average	1oz/28g	94	5.1	335	4.4	40.5	18.3	0.9
SUGAR								
Brown, Soft, Average	1 Tsp/4g	15	0.0	382	0.0	96.5	0.0	0.0
Canem Demerara, Unrefined, Sainsbury's*	1 Tsp/5.1g	20	0.0	396	0.0	99.0	0.0	0.0
Caster, Average	1 Tbsp/12g	48	0.0	399	0.0	99.8	0.0	0.0
Dark Brown, Muscovado, Average	1 Tsp/7g	27	0.0	380	0.3	94.8	0.0	0.0
Dark Brown, Soft, Average	1 Tsp/5g	18	0.0	369	0.1	92.0	0.0	0.0
Demerara, Average	1 Tsp/5g	18	0.0	368	0.3	99.2	0.0	0.0
for Making Jam, Silver Spoon*	1oz/28g	111	0.0	398	0.0	99.5	0.0	0.0
Fructose, Fruit Sugar, Tate & Lyle*	1 Tsp/4g	16	0.0	400	0.0	100.0	0.0	0.0
Golden, Unrefined, Average	1 Tsp/4g	16	0.0	399	0.0	99.8	0.0	0.0
Granulated, Organic, Average	1 Tsp/4g	16	0.0	398	0.2	99.7	0.0	0.0
Icing, Average	1 Tsp/4g	16	0.0	395	0.0	102.2	0.0	0.0
Light, Silver Spoon*	1 Tsp/5g	12	0.0	240	0.0	60.0	0.0	0.0
White, Granulated, Average	1 Tsp/5g	20	0.0	397	0.0	100.7	0.0	0.0
SULTANAS								
Average	1oz/28g	82	0.1	292	2.5	69.7	0.4	2.0
SUMMER FRUITS								
Asda*	1 Serving/30g	8	0.0	28	0.9	6.0	0.0	2.5
Frozen, Asda*	1 Serving/100g	28	0.0	28	0.9	6.0	0.0	2.5
Frozen, Sainsbury's*	1 Serving/80g	43	0.1	54	0.9	6.9	0.1	2.0
in Syrup, Sainsbury's*	1 Pudding/289g	188	0.3	65	0.5	15.6	0.1	1.2
Mix, Sainsbury's*	1 Serving/80g	26	0.0	32	0.9	7.4	0.0	2.4
SUNDAE								
Banoffee, PB, Waitrose*	1 Pot/115g	143	2.2	124	3.1	23.6	1.9	0.8
Blackcurrant, M & S*	1 Sundae/53g	212	10.2	400	3.0	54.2	19.2	1.9
Chocolate, M & S*	1oz/28g	80	5.1	285	3.1	27.2	18.2	0.0
Chocolate, Sainsbury's*	1 Pot/140g	393	29.8	281	2.5	19.3	21.3	0.6
Chocolate Brownie, Finest, Tesco*	1 Serving/215g	778	56.5	362	2.7	28.7	26.3	2.3
Chocolate Nut	1 Portion/70g	195	10.7	278	3.0	34.2	15.3	0.1
Hot Fudge, Two Scoop, Baskin Robbins*	1 Serving/203g	530	29.0	261	3.9	30.5	14.3	0.0
Strawberry, M & S*	1 Sundae/45g	173	8.0	385	3.4	53.3	17.8	1.0
SUNNY DELIGHT*								
Californian Style, No Added Sugar	1 Serving/200ml	20	0.4	10	0.1	1.4	0.2	0.1
SUSHI								
Aya Set, Waitrose*	1 Pack/110g	200	4.3	182	5.4	31.7	3.9	1.5
California Roll Box, M & S*	1 Box/230g	391	12.0	170	7.0	22.0	5.2	1.1
California Roll Selection, Classics, M & S*	1 Pack/225g	326	6.1	145	7.0	23.2	2.7	1.1
California Set, Taiko Foods*	1 Pack/120g	223	9.1	186	3.8	25.2	7.6	1.7
Californian, Yakatori, M & S*	1 Serving/200g	340	9.4	170	6.4	25.0	4.7	1.0
Californian Roll, Nigiri & Maki Selection, M & S*	1 Serving/145g	203	3.0	140	4.4	25.9	2.1	2.2
Californian Roll & Nigiri, Selection, M & S*	1 Pack/215g	355	5.8	165	7.1	28.0	2.7	1.1
Californian Rolls, Variety, Six Rolls, Sainsbury's*	1 Pack/218g	327	5.9	150	5.2	26.2	2.7	2.0
Californian Rolls Pack, Tesco*	1 Pack/190.2g	310	8.4	163	4.3	24.0	4.4	1.0
Classic, Finest, Tesco*	1 Pack/232g	330	0.9	142	6.6	27.6	0.4	0.6
Deluxe, Shapers, Boots*	1 Serving/235g	355	3.5	151	5.3	29.0	1.5	2.7
Fish Nigiri, Adventurous, Tesco*	1 Pack/200g	270	4.4	135	7.1	21.7	2.2	0.5
Fish Roll, Nigiri & Maki Selection, M & S*	1 Pack/210g	315	4.8	150	6.5	25.8	2.3	1.0

S

SUSHI

INFO/WEIGHT	Measure	per Measure		Nutrition Values per 100g / 100ml				
		KCAL	FAT	KCAL	PROT	CARB	FAT	FIBRE
Fish Selection, M & S*	1 Pack/210g	347	6.5	165	7.4	26.3	3.1	1.4
Fish Selection, Medium, M & S*	1 Pack/189g	302	5.5	160	7.0	27.4	2.9	0.6
GFY, Asda*	1 Pack/220g	352	3.1	160	4.9	32.0	1.4	0.0
Hagi Set, Taiko Foods*	1 Box/370g	688	9.6	186	7.1	33.6	2.6	1.1
Hana Set, Waitrose*	1 Serving/175g	324	4.0	185	5.4	35.7	2.3	1.4
Large, Boots*	1 Pack/324g	480	5.8	148	5.0	28.0	1.8	0.7
Large Pack, Tesco*	1 Pack/250g	358	5.5	143	6.1	24.8	2.2	2.7
Maki Rolls Box, Sainsbury's*	1 Box/127g	197	2.2	155	4.5	30.5	1.7	0.8
Maki Selection, Shapers, Boots*	1 Pack/158g	225	2.1	142	3.5	29.0	1.3	1.1
Medium Pack, Tesco*	1 Pack/139g	211	3.2	152	6.3	26.6	2.3	2.3
Mini, Boots*	1 Pack/99g	153	1.9	155	5.5	29.0	1.9	0.8
Mixed Box, Somerfield*	1 Pack/220g	339	2.4	154	4.6	31.4	1.1	0.0
Nigiri, M & S*	1 Serving/190g	303	5.9	159	7.3	25.3	3.1	0.6
Nigiri Set, Taiko Foods*	1 Serving/165g	252	4.3	153	6.3	26.0	2.6	0.6
Nigri, Californian Roll, Maki Roll, Sainsbury's*	1 Pack/195g	283	2.9	145	5.3	27.4	1.5	1.9
Oriental Fish Box, M & S*	1 Box/205g	318	8.4	155	6.1	23.3	4.1	0.9
Prawn & Salmon Selection, M & S*	1 Serving/175g	255	2.9	146	5.5	27.4	1.7	0.6
Prawn Feast, M & S*	1 Box/219g	350	8.1	160	5.7	25.8	3.7	1.1
Roll Selection, Tesco*	1 Pack/214g	327	5.4	153	5.0	27.6	2.5	1.2
Rolls, Shapers, Boots*	1 Pack/168g	259	4.0	154	4.7	28.0	2.4	0.5
Salmon, Nigri Crayfish, Red Pepper, Sainsbury's*	1 Serving/150g	233	4.5	155	5.5	26.4	3.0	1.0
Salmon & Roll Set, Sainsbury's*	1 Serving/101g	167	2.6	165	4.9	30.4	2.6	0.8
Salmon Feast Box, M & S*	1 Pack/200g	330	5.8	165	5.6	27.0	2.9	1.0
Selection, Boots*	1 Pack/268g	434	9.6	162	5.5	27.0	3.6	1.6
Selection, Shapers, Boots*	1 Pack/189g	301	5.7	159	5.2	28.0	3.0	0.7
Snack Pack, to Go, Eat Well, M & S*	1 Pack/96g	139	0.5	145	3.9	30.7	0.5	0.7
Snack Selection, Tesco*	1 Pack/85g	118	0.3	139	4.2	29.6	0.4	0.5
Tokyo Set, M & S*	1 Pack/150g	240	4.7	160	7.3	25.3	3.1	0.6
Trial Pack, Asda*	1 Pack/115g	186	2.8	162	4.1	31.0	2.4	0.0
Tuna, to Snack Selection, Food to Go, M & S*	1 Serving/150g	225	3.9	150	5.2	26.4	2.6	2.3
Vegetarian, M & S*	1 Pack/196.7g	295	6.3	150	2.5	28.2	3.2	0.9
Vegetarian, Snack Selection, Tesco*	1 Pack/85g	128	0.9	151	3.5	31.7	1.1	1.2
Vegetarian, with Pickled Vegetables, Taiko Foods*	1 Pack/135g	244	4.9	181	5.0	27.8	3.6	1.7
Yo!, Bento Box, Sainsbury's*	1 Pack/208g	530	6.2	255	8.4	48.7	3.0	0.9
Yo!, Salmon Lunch Set, Sainsbury's*	1 Pack/150g	242	4.2	161	5.9	28.1	2.8	0.8

SWEDE

INFO/WEIGHT	Measure	per Measure						
Boiled, Average	1oz/28g	3	0.0	11	0.3	2.3	0.1	0.7
Mash, COU, M & S*	1oz/28g	15	0.3	55	1.1	9.5	1.2	2.1
Raw, Unprepared, Average	1oz/28g	6	0.1	21	0.8	4.4	0.3	1.9

SWEET & SOUR

INFO/WEIGHT	Measure	per Measure						
Beef, Feeling Great, New, Findus*	1 Pack/350g	420	8.8	120	4.5	20.0	2.5	1.3
Chicken, & Noodles, BGTY, Sainsbury's*	1 Pack/400g	356	2.4	89	7.5	13.3	0.6	0.7
Chicken, & Noodles, Chinese Takeaway, Tesco*	1 Pack/350g	350	0.7	100	5.7	18.8	0.2	0.2
Chicken, & Noodles, Takeaway, Tesco*	1 Pack/350g	350	0.7	100	5.7	18.8	0.2	0.2
Chicken, & Rice, Chilled, Tesco*	1 Pack/450g	540	5.9	120	4.9	21.9	1.3	0.9
Chicken, & Rice, Mega, Value, Tesco*	1 Pack/500g	675	9.5	135	4.4	25.0	1.9	1.9
Chicken, & Rice, Morrisons*	1 Pack/400g	452	10.4	113	3.6	18.8	2.6	0.8
Chicken, Breast, Good Choice, Iceland*	1 Breast/170.5g	150	1.7	88	10.9	9.0	1.0	2.0
Chicken, Breasts, Tesco*	1 Serving/185g	172	1.9	93	14.6	6.5	1.0	0.1
Chicken, Canned, Tesco*	1 Can/400g	408	6.4	102	9.6	12.4	1.6	1.1
Chicken, Chinese Takeaway, Sainsbury's*	1 Pack/264g	515	16.9	195	13.1	21.3	6.4	1.0
Chicken, Crispy, Fillets, Tesco*	1 Pack/350g	508	19.6	145	7.2	15.3	5.6	0.9
Chicken, Crispy, Iceland*	1 Serving/125g	221	6.5	177	18.3	14.2	5.2	1.2

INFO/WEIGHT	Measure	per Measure		Nutrition Values per 100g / 100ml				
		KCAL	FAT	KCAL	PROT	CARB	FAT	FIBRE

SWEET & SOUR
Chicken, GFY, Asda*	1 Pack/400g	416	4.0	104	7.0	16.7	1.0	1.1
Chicken, Good Choice, Iceland*	1 Pack/400g	488	0.8	122	4.5	25.6	0.2	0.5
Chicken, in Batter, Cantonese, Chilled, Sainsbury's*	1 Pack/300g	480	18.0	160	8.9	22.4	6.0	0.9
Chicken, in Batter, Cantonese, Sainsbury's*	1 Pack/300g	480	18.0	160	8.9	22.4	6.0	0.9
Chicken, in Crispy Batter, Morrisons*	1 Pack/350g	511	13.7	146	10.1	17.6	3.9	1.2
Chicken, Low Fat, Iceland*	1 Pack/400g	444	6.8	111	8.1	15.7	1.7	1.1
Chicken, M & S*	1 Pack/300g	465	10.8	155	6.6	24.4	3.6	0.8
Chicken, Somerfield*	1 Serving/175g	156	0.2	89	9.5	12.6	0.1	0.6
Chicken, Take It Away, M & S*	1 Pack/200g	200	1.6	100	9.4	13.2	0.8	1.2
Chicken, Tinned, M & S*	1 Serving/481g	553	20.2	115	11.4	7.8	4.2	1.9
Chicken, Waitrose*	1 Serving/400g	372	3.2	93	9.8	11.7	0.8	1.4
Chicken, with Egg Fried Rice, Somerfield*	1 Pack/400g	428	2.8	107	8.5	16.7	0.7	2.0
Chicken, with Egg Rice, Chilled, HL, Tesco*	1 Pack/450g	500	3.2	111	6.8	19.2	0.7	0.6
Chicken, with Mixed Veg & Pineapple, without Rice, Tesco*	1 Pack/350g	301	2.5	86	8.1	11.9	0.7	0.7
Chicken, with Noodles, Feeling Great, Findus*	1 Pack/350g	385	8.8	110	5.0	17.0	2.5	1.5
Chicken, with Noodles, Steamed, HE, Tesco*	1 Pack/370g	289	0.7	78	8.3	10.8	0.2	0.6
Chicken, with Rice, Chilled, BGTY, Sainsbury's*	1 Pack/400g	344	3.6	86	6.0	13.5	0.9	1.0
Chicken, with Rice, Eat Smart, Safeway*	1 Pack/390g	312	3.5	80	5.4	12.2	0.9	1.2
Chicken, with Rice, Farmfoods*	1 Pack/300g	324	2.7	108	5.9	19.2	0.9	0.7
Chicken, with Rice, Good Intentions, Somerfield*	1 Serving/400g	448	2.4	112	6.6	20.1	0.6	0.3
Chicken, with Rice, Kwik Save*	1 Pack/500g	520	1.5	104	4.0	21.9	0.3	0.7
Chicken, with Rice, Nisa, Heritage, Nisa Heritage*	1 Pack/600g	606	4.8	101	6.0	17.4	0.8	0.4
Chicken, with Rice, Oriental Express*	1 Pack/340g	350	2.0	103	4.4	21.3	0.6	0.7
Chicken, with Rice, Value, Tesco*	1 Pack/300g	348	0.9	116	5.9	22.3	0.3	0.7
Chicken, with Vegetable Rice, COU, M & S*	1 Pack/400g	400	5.6	100	6.9	14.9	1.4	1.1
Chicken, without Batter, Cantonese, Chilled, Sainsbury's*	1 Pack/350g	410	4.9	117	8.5	17.6	1.4	1.0
Chicken with Rice, Iceland*	1 Pack/498g	548	4.5	110	4.3	21.1	0.9	0.8
Pork	1oz/28g	48	2.5	172	12.7	11.3	8.8	0.6
Pork, Battered, Sainsbury's*	½ Pack/175g	306	8.8	175	7.3	25.1	5.0	0.6
Pork, Cantonese, & Egg Fried Rice, Farmfoods*	1 Pack/327g	520	19.0	159	4.8	22.0	5.8	0.1
Roasted Vegetables, Cantonese, Sainsbury's*	1 Pack/348g	327	4.2	94	1.1	19.6	1.2	0.9
Vegetables, with Rice, Waitrose*	1 Pack/400g	384	4.4	96	1.9	19.5	1.1	1.1

SWEET POTATO
Baked, Average	1 Potato/130g	150	0.5	115	1.6	27.9	0.4	3.3
Boiled in Salted Water, Average	1 Potato/130g	109	0.4	84	1.1	20.5	0.3	2.3
Raw, Unprepared, Average	1 Med/130g	113	0.4	87	1.2	21.3	0.3	2.4
Steamed, Average	1 Med/130g	109	0.4	84	1.1	20.4	0.3	2.3

SWEET POTATOES
Roast, Oven Baked, McCain*	1 Serving/85g	130	3.5	153	1.2	18.8	4.1	3.5

SWEETBREAD
Lamb, Fried	1oz/28g	61	3.2	217	28.7	0.0	11.4	0.0
Lamb, Raw	1oz/28g	37	2.2	131	15.3	0.0	7.8	0.0

SWEETCORN
& Petit Pois, M & S*	1oz/28g	20	0.4	73	4.6	10.8	1.3	3.6
Baby, & Mangetout, Somerfield*	1 Pack/150g	42	0.5	28	3.2	3.0	0.3	1.9
Baby, Canned, Drained, Average	1oz/28g	6	0.1	23	2.9	2.0	0.4	1.5
Baby, Frozen, Average	1oz/28g	7	0.1	24	2.5	2.7	0.4	1.7
Boiled, Average	1oz/28g	31	0.6	111	4.2	19.6	2.3	2.2
Canned, in Water, No Sugar & Salt, Average	½ Can/125g	99	1.3	79	2.7	15.0	1.1	1.6
Canned, with Sugar & Salt, Average	½ Can/71g	79	0.8	111	3.2	21.9	1.2	1.9
with Peppers, Canned, Average	1 Serving/50g	40	0.2	79	2.7	16.5	0.3	0.6

SWEETENER
Aspartamo, Artificial Sugar, Zen*	1 Tbsp/2g	8	0.0	383	1.8	94.0	0.0	0.0

S

	Measure INFO/WEIGHT	per Measure		Nutrition Values per 100g / 100ml				
		KCAL	FAT	KCAL	PROT	CARB	FAT	FIBRE
SWEETENER								
Canderel, Spoonful, Canderel*	2 Tsp/1g	4	0.0	384	2.9	93.0	0.0	0.0
Granulated, Asda*	1 Tsp/1g	4	0.0	400	0.0	100.0	0.0	0.0
Granulated, Aspartame, Safeway*	1 Tsp/0.5g	4	0.0	392	3.0	95.0	0.0	0.0
Granulated, Low Calorie, Splenda*	1 Tsp/0.5g	2	0.0	391	0.0	97.7	0.0	0.0
Granulated, Safeway*	1 Tsp/1g	4	0.0	392	3.0	95.0	0.0	0.0
Granulated, Silver Spoon*	1 Tsp/0.5g	2	0.0	387	1.0	96.8	0.0	0.0
Granulated, Tesco*	1 Tsp/1g	4	0.0	383	1.8	94.0	0.0	0.0
Low Calorie, Somerfield*	1 Tsp/0.5g	4	0.0	380	3.0	92.0	0.0	0.0
Silver Spoon*	1 Tablet/0.05g	0	0.0	325	10.0	71.0	0.0	0.0
Slendasweet, Sainsbury's*	1 Tsp/1g	4	0.0	395	1.8	97.0	0.0	0.1
Spoonfull, Low Calorie, SupaSweet*	1 Tsp/1g	4	0.0	392	3.0	95.0	0.0	0.0
Sweet' N Low*	1 Sachet/1g	3	0.0	368	0.0	92.0	0.0	0.0
Tablets, Low Calorie, Canderel*	1 Tablet/0.1g	0	0.0	342	13.0	72.4	0.0	0.0
Tablets, Splenda*	1 Tablet/0.1g	0	0.0	345	10.0	76.2	0.0	1.6
Tablets, Tesco*	5 Tablets/5g	1	0.0	20	2.0	2.0	0.5	0.0
Xylosweet, Xylitol*	1 Serving/4g	10	0.0	240	0.0	100.0	0.0	0.0
SWEETS								
Alphabet Candies, Asda*	1 Pack/80g	306	0.0	382	0.5	95.0	0.0	0.0
Aquadrops, Citrus & Apple, Mars*	1 Serving/2.5g	10	0.0	400	0.0	80.0	0.0	0.0
Banana, Baby Foam, M & S*	1/3 Pack/34g	131	0.0	385	4.1	92.7	0.0	0.0
Black Jacks & Fruit Salad, Bassett's*	1 Serving/190g	760	11.8	400	0.7	84.9	6.2	0.0
Blackcurrant & Liquorice, M & S*	1 Sweet/8g	32	0.3	400	0.6	89.0	4.3	0.0
Butter Candies, Original, Werther's*	1 Sweet/5g	21	0.4	424	0.1	85.7	8.9	0.1
Campino, Strawberries & Cream, Bendicks*	1oz/28g	117	2.3	418	0.1	86.2	8.1	0.0
Candy Cane, Average	1oz/28g	100	0.0	357	3.6	85.7	0.0	0.0
Candy Foam Shapes, Fun Fruits, Value, Tesco*	1 Serving/25g	96	0.1	384	3.6	94.0	0.3	0.1
Chew	1oz/28g	107	1.6	381	1.0	87.0	5.6	1.0
Chews, Fruity, Starburst*	1 Sweet/8.3g	34	0.6	404	0.0	83.4	7.4	0.0
Chews, Just Fruit, Fruit-Tella*	1 Serving/42.5g	172	2.8	400	0.9	79.5	6.5	0.0
Chews, Strawberry Mix, Starburst*	1 Chew/3.8g	15	0.3	401	0.0	83.9	7.3	0.0
Chocolate Caramels, Milk, Tesco*	1 Sweet/3.3g	15	0.5	444	2.7	72.1	16.1	0.1
Chocolate Eclairs, Cadbury*	1 Sweet/8g	36	1.4	455	4.5	68.9	17.9	0.0
Chocolate Eclairs, Co-Op*	1 Sweet/8g	38	1.6	480	3.0	71.0	20.0	0.6
Chocolate Eclairs, M & S*	1 Sweet/6.7g	30	1.2	445	3.1	65.8	18.6	0.4
Chocolate Limes, Pascall*	1 Sweet/8g	27	0.2	333	0.3	77.2	2.5	0.0
Cola Bottles, Asda*	1 Serving/100g	329	0.2	329	9.0	73.0	0.2	0.0
Cola Bottles, Fizzy Wizzy, Woolworths*	1 Bag/100g	336	0.0	336	3.5	77.2	0.0	0.0
Cream Caramel, Sula*	1 Sweet/3.37g	10	0.0	297	0.4	86.1	0.0	0.0
Drumstick, Matlow's*	1 Pack/40g	164	2.2	409	0.4	88.3	5.5	0.0
Fizzy Lemon Fish, Asda*	1 Sweet/4.3g	13	0.0	325	5.0	76.0	0.1	0.0
Fizzy Mix, Tesco*	½ Bag/50g	166	0.0	332	5.2	75.2	0.0	0.0
Flipsters, Starburst*	1 Pack/37g	145	0.0	392	0.0	98.1	0.0	0.0
Flumps, Bassett's*	1 Serving/5g	16	0.0	325	4.0	77.0	0.0	0.0
Flying Saucers, Morrisons*	1 Pack/21.9g	73	0.0	333	0.0	84.0	0.0	0.0
Fruit Gums & Jellies	1 Tube/33g	107	0.0	324	6.5	79.5	0.0	0.0
Gummy Mix, Tesco*	1 Pack/100g	327	0.1	327	5.9	75.7	0.1	0.0
Hazardously Sour, Toxic Waste*	5 Sweets/15g	60	0.0	400	0.0	100.0	0.0	0.0
Jelly Babies, Morrisons*	1 Serving/227g	781	0.0	344	5.3	80.7	0.0	0.0
Kisses, Hershey*	1 Kiss/5g	28	1.6	561	7.0	59.0	32.0	0.0
Lances, Fizzy, Strawberry, Somerfield*	1 Lance/3.7g	14	0.1	362	2.8	79.8	2.7	1.5
Lances, Strawberry Flavour, Fizzy, Tesco*	½ Pack/50g	177	1.3	354	2.8	79.8	2.6	1.8
Lovehearts, Giant, Swizzels*	1 Pack/42g	165	0.0	393	0.0	100.0	0.0	0.0
Lovehearts, Swizzels*	1oz/28g	100	0.0	359	0.7	88.2	0.0	0.0

S

	Measure	per Measure		Nutrition Values per 100g / 100ml				
	INFO/WEIGHT	KCAL	FAT	KCAL	PROT	CARB	FAT	FIBRE

SWEETS

Maynards Sours, Bassett's*	1 Pack/52g	166	0.1	320	3.9	74.9	0.1	0.0
Milk Chocolate Eclairs, Sainsbury's*	1 Sweet/8g	33	1.1	442	2.1	75.7	14.5	0.5
Mint Creams, Bassett's*	10 Mints/100g	365	0.0	365	0.0	91.8	0.0	0.0
Percy Pig & Pals, Soft, M & S*	1 Sweet/7.6g	28	0.0	344	5.8	80.0	0.1	0.0
Pic 'n' Mix, Woolworths*	1 Serving/180g	750	6.0	417	0.0	96.7	3.3	0.0
Red & Blacks, M & S*	1 Pack/113g	367	0.2	325	5.7	74.1	0.2	0.0
Rhubarb & Custard, Sainsbury's*	1 Sweet/8g	28	0.0	351	0.1	87.7	0.0	0.0
Scary Mix, Tesco*	1 Bag/100g	327	0.5	327	9.5	71.1	0.5	0.3
Sherbert Cocktails, Sainsbury's*	1 Sweet/9g	36	0.7	400	0.0	83.1	7.5	0.0
Sherbert Lemons, M & S*	1 Serving/20g	76	0.0	380	0.0	93.9	0.0	0.0
Sherbet Lemons, Bassett's*	1 Sweet/6.7g	25	0.0	375	0.0	93.9	0.0	0.0
Shrimps & Bananas, Sainsbury's*	½ Pack/50g	188	0.1	376	2.5	91.3	0.1	0.5
Snakes, Bassett's*	1 Sweet/9.4g	30	0.0	320	3.5	76.8	0.1	0.0
Sour Apple Sticks, Fizzy Wizzy, Woolworths*	1 Stick/5g	18	0.1	358	2.8	79.8	2.7	0.0
Sour Squirms, Bassett's*	1 Serving/6.5g	23	0.0	325	3.1	78.1	0.0	0.0
Strawberry & Cream, Sugar Free, Sula*	1 Serving/10g	27	0.5	267	0.2	90.5	5.4	0.0
Sugar Free, Sula*	1 Sweet/3g	7	0.0	231	0.0	96.1	0.0	0.0
Sweetshop Favourites, Bassett's*	1 Sweet/5g	17	0.0	340	0.0	84.3	0.0	0.0
Toffo*	1 Tube/43g	194	9.5	451	2.2	69.8	22.0	0.0
Wazzly Wobble Drops, Wonka*	1 Bag/42g	186	6.8	443	3.0	71.6	16.1	0.2
Wiggly Worms, Sainsbury's*	1 Serving/10g	32	0.0	317	5.6	72.7	0.4	0.2

SWORDFISH

Grilled, Average	1oz/28g	39	1.5	139	22.9	0.0	5.2	0.0
Raw, Average	1oz/28g	42	2.0	149	21.1	0.0	7.2	0.0

SYRUP

Caramel, for Coffee, Lyle's*	2 Tsps/10ml	33	0.0	329	0.0	83.0	0.0	0.0
Corn, Dark, Average	1 Tbsp/20g	56	0.0	282	0.0	76.6	0.0	0.0
Golden, Average	1 Tbsp/20g	61	0.0	304	0.4	78.3	0.0	0.0
Maple, Amber, No 2, Waitrose*	1 Serving/10g	25	0.0	253	0.0	63.0	0.1	0.2
Maple, Average	1 Tbsp/20g	52	0.0	262	0.0	67.2	0.2	0.0
Maple, Original, Aunt Jemima*	1 Serving/30ml	105	0.0	350	0.0	87.0	0.0	0.0
Strawberry, Milk Shake Mix, Crusha*	1 Serving/20ml	25	0.1	125	0.5	30.0	0.5	0.0

S

	Measure INFO/WEIGHT	per Measure KCAL	FAT	Nutrition Values per 100g / 100ml KCAL	PROT	CARB	FAT	FIBRE
TABOO*								
Average, Taboo*	1 Serving/30ml	69	0.0	230	0.0	33.0	0.0	0.0
TABOULEH								
Average	1oz/28g	33	1.3	119	2.6	17.2	4.6	0.0
TACO SHELLS								
Corn, Crunchy, Old El Paso*	1 Taco/10g	51	2.6	506	7.0	61.0	26.0	0.0
Old El Paso*	1 Taco/12g	57	2.7	478	7.4	60.8	22.8	0.0
Traditional, Discovery*	1 Shell/11g	55	3.2	489	5.7	53.4	28.1	6.0
TADKA DAAL								
Sainsbury's*	½ Pack/150g	138	3.2	92	5.5	12.7	2.1	3.0
TAGINE								
Vegetable, Filo Topped, M & S*	1 Serving/281.8g	310	6.5	110	3.3	18.7	2.3	3.9
TAGLIATELLE								
Basil, M & S*	1 Serving/100g	365	2.8	365	15.1	69.0	2.8	4.0
Bicolore, Asda*	¼ Pack/125g	203	3.0	162	7.0	28.0	2.4	1.4
Ham & Mushroom, Safeway*	1 Serving/400g	480	20.4	120	5.2	12.9	5.1	1.0
Meditarranean Style Chicken, Eat Smart, Safeway*	1 Pack/400g	320	10.0	80	5.6	8.7	2.5	1.4
Multigrain, BGTY, Cooked, Sainsbury's*	1 Serving/190g	295	4.8	155	7.0	26.0	2.5	3.0
Mushroom & Bacon, BGTY, Sainsbury's*	1 Pack/400g	368	9.6	92	4.0	13.5	2.4	1.0
Mushroom & Bacon, Sainsbury's*	1 Pack/450g	585	23.4	130	7.1	13.8	5.2	0.5
Mushroom & Tomato, Asda*	1 Pack/340g	211	4.4	62	2.5	10.0	1.3	1.2
Nests, Dry Weight, Napolina*	1oz/28g	93	0.4	332	11.5	68.0	1.5	3.7
Prawn, Eat Smart, Morrisons*	1 Pack/380g	296	6.8	78	6.1	9.4	1.8	0.9
Prawn, Eat Smart, Safeway*	1 Pack/380g	304	8.0	80	5.1	10.1	2.1	0.8
Red Pepper, Organic, Sainsbury's*	½ Bag/125g	183	1.9	146	5.4	27.8	1.5	1.4
Salmon, PB, Waitrose*	1 Pack/400g	376	10.8	94	5.4	11.7	2.7	0.8
Salmon, PB, Waitrose*	1 Pack/400g	376	10.8	94	5.4	11.7	2.7	0.8
Salmon & King Prawn, HL, Tesco*	1 Pack/400g	480	9.6	120	6.5	17.2	2.4	1.7
Salmon & Prawn, PB, Waitrose*	1 Pack/401.2g	341	13.2	85	6.8	7.1	3.3	1.1
Salmon & Prawn, PB, Waitrose*	1 Pack/401.2g	341	13.2	85	6.8	7.1	3.3	1.1
Smoked Ham, COU, M & S*	1 Pack/400g	360	10.4	90	5.6	10.9	2.6	1.1
Smoked Salmon, Ready Meals, M & S*	1 Pack/360g	612	40.3	170	6.2	10.6	11.2	0.9
Sundried Tomato, Fresh, Morrisons*	1 Pack/250g	748	8.3	299	11.1	56.4	3.3	3.5
Tomato & Basil Chicken, Weight Watchers*	1 Pack/330g	322	4.0	98	7.5	14.1	1.2	0.3
Tricolore, Waitrose*	½ Pack/125g	351	3.6	281	12.0	51.6	2.9	1.6
Vegetables, Retail	1oz/28g	21	0.8	74	1.6	11.0	3.0	0.7
Verdi, Dry, Barilla*	1 Serving/150g	555	5.3	370	14.0	70.5	3.5	0.0
Verdi, Fresh, Average	1 Serving/125g	171	1.8	137	5.5	25.5	1.5	1.8
with Chicken, Garlic & Lemon, BGTY, Sainsbury's*	1 Pack/450g	410	1.4	91	7.8	14.2	0.3	1.7
with Chicken, Garlic & Lemon, New, BGTY, Sainsbury's*	1 Pack/300g	324	3.6	108	9.2	15.1	1.2	1.7
with Chicken & Pancetta, Sainsbury's*	½ Pack/351g	453	19.3	129	9.5	10.4	5.5	0.7
with Ham & Mushroom, New, BGTY, Sainsbury's*	1 Pack/450g	401	10.4	89	5.3	11.8	2.3	1.4
with Roasted Vegetables, Good Intentions, Somerfield*	1 Pack/340g	349	8.2	103	3.7	16.6	2.4	1.7
TAHINI PASTE								
Average	1 Heaped Tsp/19g	115	11.2	607	18.5	0.9	58.9	8.0
TAMARILLOS								
Fresh, Raw, Average	1oz/28g	8	0.1	28	2.0	4.7	0.3	0.0
TAMARIND								
Paste, Barts*	1 Tbsp/15g	20	0.0	133	0.9	32.1	0.1	0.0
Whole, Raw, Weighed with Pod, Average	1oz/28g	67	0.2	239	2.8	62.5	0.6	5.1
TANGERINES								
Weighed with Peel & Pips	1 Med/70g	18	0.1	25	0.7	5.8	0.1	0.9
TANGO*								
Apple, Britvic*	1 Can/330ml	33	0.0	10	0.0	2.1	0.0	0.0

T

	INFO/WEIGHT	KCAL	FAT	KCAL	PROT	CARB	FAT	FIBRE
TANGO*								
Orange, Britvic*	1 Can/330ml	63	0.0	19	0.1	4.4	0.0	0.0
TAPENADE								
Green Olive, The Best, Safeway*	1 Tsp/15g	71	7.1	470	1.6	10.2	47.0	1.7
Olive with Capers & Anchovy, Safeway*	1 Tbsp/20g	103	11.1	513	2.1	1.0	55.6	2.2
TAPIOCA								
Creamed, Ambrosia*	½ Can/212.5g	160	3.4	75	2.6	12.6	1.6	0.2
Raw	1oz/28g	101	0.0	359	0.4	95.0	0.1	0.4
TARAMASALATA								
Average	1oz/28g	141	14.8	504	3.2	4.1	52.9	0.0
BGTY, Sainsbury's*	1oz/28g	71	5.7	253	4.3	13.5	20.2	0.7
HE, Tesco*	1 Pot/170g	430	34.3	253	4.3	13.5	20.2	0.7
M & S*	1 Serving/100g	480	48.9	480	4.9	6.4	48.9	0.7
Reduced Fat, Tesco*	½ Pot/85g	256	23.0	301	3.8	10.5	27.1	1.5
Reduced Fat, Waitrose*	1 Pack/170g	522	48.3	307	4.0	8.9	28.4	1.5
Sainsbury's*	¼ Tub/50g	236	24.1	472	4.0	7.5	48.1	0.0
Smoked Salmon, Tesco*	1 Serving/95g	474	48.2	499	3.1	7.7	50.7	0.3
Somerfield*	½ Pot/85g	434	43.2	510	3.4	9.8	50.8	0.7
Supreme, Waitrose*	1 Serving/20g	84	8.1	421	7.4	6.3	40.7	2.9
Tesco*	1/8 Tub/25g	115	11.2	460	2.9	10.5	44.8	1.0
TARRAGON								
Dried, Ground	1 Tsp/1.6g	6	0.1	295	22.8	42.8	7.2	0.0
Fresh, Average	1 Tbsp/3.8g	2	0.0	49	3.4	6.3	1.1	0.0
TART								
Apple & Fresh Cream, Asda*	½ Tart/50g	134	8.0	267	3.4	33.0	16.0	0.8
Apricot Lattice, Sainsbury's*	1 Slice/125g	321	14.2	257	3.4	35.3	11.4	2.6
Aubergine & Feta, Roast Marinated, Sainsbury's*	1 Serving/105g	227	15.2	216	4.8	16.6	14.5	1.7
Bakewell, Average	1oz/28g	128	8.3	456	6.3	43.5	29.7	1.9
Bakewell, Free From, Tesco*	1 Cake/50g	170	4.6	340	1.6	63.0	9.2	4.8
Bakewell, Large, Tesco*	1 Serving/57g	247	11.2	433	4.3	59.5	19.7	1.7
Bakewell, Lyons*	1/6 Tart/51.6g	206	8.9	397	3.8	56.7	17.2	0.9
Bakewell, M & S*	¼ Tart/75g	345	20.0	460	7.5	48.1	26.7	2.1
Bakewell, Weight Watchers*	1 Cake/43.0g	156	5.0	363	3.6	65.2	11.7	3.2
Caramelised Onion & Goats Cheese, M & S*	1 Tartlet/160g	400	26.4	250	6.0	19.5	16.5	2.7
Cherry Bakewell, Morrisons*	1 Tart/46g	198	9.8	430	4.6	54.9	21.4	1.3
Cherry Tomato & Mascarpone, Asda*	1 Tart/160g	290	18.0	181	4.4	15.6	11.3	1.1
Cherry Tomato & Mascarpone, Extra Special, Asda*	1 Tart/153g	290	18.3	190	4.6	16.0	12.0	1.1
Chocolate, TTD, Sainsbury's*	1 Tart/93.1g	389	25.7	418	4.8	37.6	27.6	3.0
Coconut, M & S*	1 Tart/53g	220	9.6	415	5.8	57.8	18.1	3.6
Coconut & Cherry, Asda*	1 Serving/50g	215	10.0	430	4.4	58.0	20.0	4.0
Coconut & Raspberry, Waitrose*	1 Tart/48g	204	11.5	426	5.0	45.0	24.0	3.9
Congress, Morrisons*	1 Tart/38g	149	5.5	393	6.0	59.7	14.4	2.4
Custard, Individual, Average	1 Tart/94g	260	13.6	277	6.3	32.4	14.5	1.2
Date Pecan & Almond, Sticky, Sainsbury's*	1/8 Pie/75g	298	10.3	397	5.0	63.5	13.7	1.7
Egg Custard, Asda*	1 Tart/80g	215	10.4	269	9.0	29.0	13.0	1.2
Egg Custard, Baked, M & S*	1 Tart/85.5g	235	11.2	275	6.1	32.7	13.1	1.0
Egg Custard, Sainsbury's*	1 Tart/90g	235	11.2	261	6.0	31.4	12.4	1.8
Egg Custard, Somerfield*	1 Tart/85g	206	9.6	242	5.1	29.9	11.3	0.7
Egg Custard, Tesco*	1 Cake/82g	214	10.0	261	6.2	31.5	12.2	1.1
Feta Cheese & Spinach, Puff Pastry, Tesco*	1 Tart/108g	306	19.2	283	7.1	23.5	17.8	0.9
Filo Asparagus Tartlette, M & S*	1 Serving/15g	45	3.1	300	4.4	25.2	20.4	2.1
Frangipane, Lutowska Cherry Amaretto, Sainsbury's*	1 Serving/66g	264	12.9	400	6.0	50.0	19.5	1.3
Fruit, Safeway*	1 Tart/180g	425	20.5	236	2.7	30.6	11.4	0.0
Italian Lemon & Almond, Sainsbury's*	1 Slice/49g	182	11.6	371	7.4	31.9	23.7	4.1

T

	Measure INFO/WEIGHT	per Measure KCAL	FAT	Nutrition Values per 100g / 100ml KCAL	PROT	CARB	FAT	FIBRE
TART								
Jam, Assorted, Asda*	1 Tart/30g	122	4.8	407	2.7	63.0	16.0	2.4
Jam, Assorted, Tesco*	1 Tart/35g	123	5.0	351	3.4	51.9	14.4	1.2
Jam, Average	1 Slice/90g	342	13.4	380	3.3	62.0	14.9	1.6
Jam, Real Fruit, Mr Kipling*	1 Tart/35g	136	5.2	388	3.8	67.9	14.9	1.7
Jam, Real Fruit, Sainsbury's*	1 Tart/37g	142	5.2	383	3.4	60.9	14.0	1.4
Leek & Stilton, Morrisons*	1 Serving/125g	393	26.9	314	6.9	23.1	21.5	0.3
Lemon, M & S*	1/6 Tart/50g	208	14.7	415	5.0	32.7	29.3	0.9
Lemon, Sainsbury's*	1/8 Tart/75g	257	12.9	343	4.9	42.2	17.2	1.1
Lemon & Raspberry, Finest, Tesco*	1 Tart/120g	360	16.8	300	5.2	38.4	14.0	2.9
Lemon Curd, Asda*	1 Tart/30.1g	121	4.5	402	2.8	64.0	15.0	2.2
Lemon Curd, Lyons*	1 Tart/30g	122	5.1	406	3.7	59.3	17.0	0.0
Manchester, M & S*	1oz/28g	104	6.6	370	4.1	36.0	23.5	1.1
Mixed Fruit, Fresh, M & S*	1 Tart/100g	265	15.4	265	3.2	27.8	15.4	2.1
Mixed Fruit, Waitrose*	1 Tart/146g	318	16.4	218	2.3	27.3	11.2	1.0
Normandy Apple & Calvados, Finest, Tesco*	1/6 Tart/100g	256	7.6	256	3.2	41.4	7.6	1.9
Raspberry, Reduced Sugar, Asda*	1 Tart/34g	129	3.4	380	4.6	67.5	10.1	1.2
Red Pepper, Serrano Ham & Goats Cheese, Waitrose*	1 Serving/100g	293	19.2	293	8.7	21.3	19.2	3.2
Roasted Vegetable, Finest, Tesco*	¼ Tart/112.5g	231	13.2	205	3.1	20.6	11.7	2.3
Strawberry, M & S*	1 Tart/120g	294	17.9	245	2.5	25.6	14.9	0.7
Strawberry, Reduced Sugar, Asda*	1 Tart/37g	141	3.7	380	4.6	67.5	10.1	1.2
Strawberry, Sainsbury's*	1 Serving/206g	521	26.2	253	2.6	32.0	12.7	0.7
Strawberry, Waitrose*	1 Serving/101g	241	12.0	239	3.8	29.2	11.9	1.2
Strawberry & Fresh Cream, Finest, Tesco*	1 Tart/129g	350	19.1	271	3.3	31.1	14.8	1.2
Strawberry Custard, Asda*	1 Tart/100g	335	15.0	335	3.1	47.0	15.0	0.0
Strawberry Sundae, Asda*	1 Tart/46g	187	8.3	407	3.3	58.0	18.0	1.3
Toffee Apple, Co-Op*	1 Tart/20g	69	3.2	345	3.0	47.0	16.0	0.7
Toffee Bakewell, Morrisons*	1 Tart/47g	212	8.5	451	3.4	69.5	18.2	1.4
Toffee Pecan, M & S*	1 Tart/91g	414	24.1	455	6.0	48.5	26.5	2.0
Tomato, Mozzarella & Basil Puff, Sainsbury's*	1/3 Tart/120g	318	25.0	265	9.2	10.2	20.8	0.9
Treacle, Average	1oz/28g	103	3.9	368	3.7	60.4	14.1	1.1
Treacle, Large, Tesco*	1/6 Tart/59g	237	6.1	402	3.3	74.1	10.3	1.7
Treacle, Lattice, Lyons*	1/6 Tart/70g	255	8.4	364	4.4	59.3	12.0	1.1
Treacle, Sainsbury's*	1 Serving/100g	369	12.1	369	4.3	60.6	12.1	1.2
Treacle & Pecan, Mini, TTD, Sainsbury's*	1 Tart/27.1g	107	4.2	395	4.4	59.3	15.6	1.7
Treacle Lattice, Mr Kipling*	1/6 Tart/70g	256	8.5	365	4.4	59.8	12.1	1.1
TARTE								
Au Citron, TTD, Sainsbury's*	1/6 Tart/83.8g	259	10.4	309	4.7	44.7	12.4	1.3
Au Citron, Waitrose*	1 Tart/100g	325	18.1	325	4.9	35.7	18.1	1.0
Aux Citron, M & S*	1/8 Tarte/69g	235	10.7	340	4.8	45.2	15.5	1.5
Aux Fruits, Finest, Tesco*	1 Tarte/130g	332	14.8	255	3.4	33.7	11.4	1.5
Aux Pommes, TTD, Sainsbury's*	1 Portion/77.2g	210	7.7	272	2.9	42.5	10.0	2.3
Bacon, Leek & Roquefort, Bistro, Waitrose*	1/6 Tarte/100g	277	18.2	277	8.4	19.8	18.2	0.6
Flamme, Bacon & Creme Fraiche, TTD, Sainsbury's*	½ Flamme/115g	335	24.5	291	6.8	17.9	21.3	1.2
Goats Cheese & Spinach Flambe, Sainsbury's*	1/3 Tart/76.8g	223	16.8	289	7.4	15.9	21.8	0.9
Tatin, Sainsbury's*	1 Serving/120g	244	8.0	203	2.9	32.8	6.7	1.9
TARTLETS								
Caramelised Onion & Gruyere, Sainsbury's*	1 Tart/145g	381	27.6	263	5.8	17.3	19.0	1.3
Cheese & Roast Onion, Asda*	1 Tartlet/50g	135	7.5	270	6.0	28.0	15.0	1.9
Cherry Tomato & Aubergine, M & S*	1 Tartlet/160g	320	20.2	200	3.1	17.8	12.6	1.7
Mushroom, Bacon & Spinach, Safeway*	1 Tartlet/120g	312	24.0	260	7.0	13.0	20.0	1.0
Mushroom & Watercress, Waitrose*	1 Tartlet/120g	308	24.6	257	8.4	19.1	20.5	2.6
Mushroom Medley, BGTY, Sainsbury's*	1 Serving/80g	134	8.0	167	4.7	14.5	10.0	3.4
Onion, Caramelised, Creamy, Somerfield*	1 Tartlet/105g	310	23.1	295	4.0	21.0	22.0	0.0

T

	Measure INFO/WEIGHT	per Measure KCAL	FAT	Nutrition Values per 100g / 100ml KCAL	PROT	CARB	FAT	FIBRE
TARTLETS								
Red Onion & Goats Cheese, Sainsbury's*	1 Tart/112.8g	336	21.8	297	7.0	23.7	19.3	1.5
Roast Pepper & Mascarpone, Sainsbury's*	1 Tart/100g	232	16.4	232	3.5	17.7	16.4	1.5
Roast Vegetable, Filo, Mini, Somerfield*	1oz/28g	71	2.8	255	8.0	34.0	10.0	0.0
Roasted Red Pepper, BGTY, Sainsbury's*	1 Tartlet/80g	143	7.4	179	3.1	21.0	9.2	3.4
Salmon & Watercress, Hot Smoked, Waitrose*	1 Serving/130g	315	19.9	242	8.1	18.0	15.3	3.0
Sausage & Tomato, Sainsbury's*	1 Tartlet/135g	323	21.3	239	4.8	19.5	15.8	1.6
Tomato & Goats Cheese, Waitrose*	1 Tartlet/130g	295	19.0	227	6.6	17.4	14.6	2.0
TEA								
Camomile, Smile, Tetley*	1oz/28g	1	0.0	2	0.0	0.5	0.0	0.0
Decaf, Tetley*	1 Mug/100ml	1	0.0	1	0.0	0.3	0.0	0.0
Earl Grey, Infusion with Water, Average	1 Mug/250ml	3	0.0	1	0.0	0.2	0.0	0.0
Fruit Or Herbal, Made with Water, Twinings*	1 Mug/200ml	8	0.0	4	0.0	1.0	0.0	0.0
Green, with Jasmine, Wellbeing Selection, Flavia*	1 Cup/200ml	14	0.2	7	0.5	1.2	0.1	0.0
Green & Lemon, Twinings*	1 Serving/250ml	65	0.0	26	0.0	7.3	0.0	0.0
Iced, Green, Orange, Lipton*	1 Bottle/500ml	100	0.0	20	0.0	5.0	0.0	0.0
Iced, Lemon, San Benedetto*	1 Bottle/500ml	170	0.1	34	0.1	8.3	0.0	0.0
Iced, Mango, Lipton*	1 fl oz/30ml	10	0.0	33	0.0	8.1	0.0	0.0
Iced, Peach, Twinings*	1 Serving/200ml	60	0.2	30	0.1	7.3	0.1	0.0
Iced, with Lemon, Lipton*	1 Bottle/325ml	98	0.3	30	0.1	7.2	0.1	0.0
Lemon, Instant, Original, Lift*	1 Serving/15g	53	0.0	352	0.0	87.0	0.0	0.0
Lemon, Instant, Reduced Sweetness, Lift*	2 Tsps/7.1g	23	0.0	325	0.0	81.3	0.0	0.0
Lemon, Instant, Tesco*	1 Serving/7g	23	0.0	326	1.0	80.5	0.0	0.0
Made with Water	1 Mug/227ml	0	0.0	0	0.1	0.0	0.0	0.0
Made with Water with Semi-Skimmed Milk	1 Cup/200ml	14	0.4	7	0.5	0.7	0.2	0.0
Made with Water with Skimmed Milk	1 Mug/227ml	14	0.5	6	0.5	0.7	0.2	0.0
Made with Water with Whole Milk	1 Cup/200ml	16	0.8	8	0.4	0.5	0.4	0.0
Peach Flavour, Lift*	1 Cup/15g	58	0.0	384	0.3	95.6	0.0	0.0
Raspberry & Cranberry, T of Life, Tetley*	1 Serving/100ml	36	0.0	36	0.0	9.0	0.0	0.0
with Lemon, Lipton*	1 Bottle/591ml	150	0.0	25	0.0	6.8	0.0	0.0
TEACAKES								
Average	1 Teacake/60g	178	4.5	296	8.0	52.5	7.5	0.0
Chocolate, Tunnock's*	1 Cake/22g	91	4.0	413	5.3	61.0	18.1	0.0
Chocolate Marshmallow, Tunnock's*	1 Teacake/22g	91	4.0	413	5.3	61.0	18.1	0.1
Coconut Snowballs, Tunnock's*	1 Cake/30g	116	6.5	388	3.9	47.0	21.8	0.0
Currant, Sainsbury's*	1 Serving/100g	283	5.4	283	7.7	50.9	5.4	3.8
Fruited, Co-Op*	1 Cake/62g	160	2.0	258	9.7	46.8	3.2	3.2
Fruited, M & S*	1 Cake/60g	156	0.6	260	8.9	53.4	1.0	2.0
Fruity, Warburton's*	1 Teacake/62.5g	160	2.2	256	8.7	48.0	3.5	2.7
Jam, Castello*	1 Teacake/12.8g	60	2.4	470	5.3	70.1	18.4	1.3
Lees'*	1 Cake/19g	81	2.9	426	4.2	67.7	15.4	0.0
Lge, Sainsbury's*	1 Cake/100g	291	6.8	291	8.3	49.1	6.8	3.4
Mallow, Tesco*	1 Cake/14g	63	2.7	450	4.1	65.4	19.1	1.0
Mallow, Value, Tesco*	1 Teacake/14g	63	2.7	450	4.1	65.4	19.1	1.0
Milk Chocolate, Tunnock's*	1 Serving/22g	91	4.0	413	5.3	61.0	18.1	0.0
Morrisons*	1 Cake/64g	172	1.9	268	9.9	50.7	2.9	2.8
Richly Fruited, Waitrose*	1 Cake/72g	205	2.7	285	7.8	55.0	3.7	2.2
Sainsbury's*	1 Cake/70g	171	2.5	244	8.0	45.0	3.6	2.6
Somerfield*	1 Teacake/62g	165	2.7	267	10.6	46.3	4.4	2.2
Tesco*	1 Cake/61g	163	2.1	267	7.8	51.1	3.5	2.4
Toasted, Average	1 Teacake/60g	197	5.0	329	8.9	58.3	8.3	0.0
Value, Tesco*	1 Teacake/68g	180	2.4	265	9.6	47.8	3.6	4.9
with Fruit, Morning Fresh, Aldi*	1 Cake/65g	155	2.2	239	7.4	44.6	3.4	2.3
with Sultanas, Raisins & Currants, Sainsbury's*	1 Teacake/73g	207	2.9	284	8.2	53.7	4.0	2.5

	Measure INFO/WEIGHT	per Measure KCAL	FAT	Nutrition Values per 100g / 100ml KCAL	PROT	CARB	FAT	FIBRE
TEMPEH								
Average	1oz/28g	46	1.8	166	20.7	6.4	6.4	4.3
TEQUILA								
Average	1 Pub Shot/35ml	78	0.0	224	0.0	0.0	0.0	0.0
TERRINE								
Lobster & Prawn, Slices, M & S*	1 Serving/55g	107	7.4	195	18.2	0.7	13.4	0.7
Prawn, TTD, Sainsbury's*	1 Serving/60g	115	9.4	192	9.0	3.7	15.7	0.4
Salmon, Poached, Tesco*	1 Pack/113g	349	30.6	309	15.5	0.8	27.1	0.0
Salmon, Reduced Fat, Tesco*	1 Serving/56g	100	7.0	179	15.5	1.1	12.5	3.5
Salmon, Smoked, Finest, Tesco*	1 Serving/25g	71	5.8	285	13.2	5.1	23.3	0.0
Salmon, Three, M & S*	1 Serving/80g	168	12.2	210	17.6	0.8	15.3	0.9
Salmon, with Prawn & Lobster, M & S*	1 Serving/55g	107	7.4	195	18.2	0.7	13.4	0.7
Salmon & Crayfish, Slice, Finest, Tesco*	1 Slice/110g	149	5.7	135	21.9	0.1	5.2	0.1
Salmon & King Prawn, Waitrose*	1 Serving/75g	98	4.0	130	19.3	1.3	5.3	0.0
Salmon & Lemon, Luxury, Tesco*	1 Segment/50g	98	7.9	196	10.6	3.2	15.7	0.8
Trout, TTD, Sainsbury's*	1 Serving/60g	138	10.7	230	14.7	2.6	17.9	0.2
TEX MEX PLATTER								
M & S*	1 Pack/415g	934	60.6	225	12.6	10.5	14.6	0.9
THAI BITES								
Lightly Salted, Jacob's*	1 Pack/25g	94	0.8	375	6.9	79.7	3.2	0.1
Mild Thai Flavour, Jacob's*	1 Bag/25g	93	0.8	373	6.9	79.0	3.3	1.0
Oriental Spice, Jacob's*	1 Bag/25g	99	1.1	397	7.3	82.5	4.2	0.2
Roasted Chilli Flavour, Fusions, Jacob's*	1 Bag/30g	109	1.7	363	5.5	72.3	5.8	1.2
Seaweed Flavour, Jacob's*	1 Pack/25g	94	0.8	377	7.1	80.0	3.2	0.5
THYME								
Dried, Ground	1 Tsp/1.2g	3	0.1	276	9.1	45.3	7.4	0.0
Fresh, Average	1 Tsp/0.8g	1	0.0	95	3.0	15.1	2.5	0.0
TIA MARIA								
Original	1 Pub Shot/35ml	105	0.0	300	0.0	0.0	0.0	0.0
TIC TAC								
Fresh Mint, Ferrero*	2 Tic Tacs/1g	4	0.0	390	0.0	97.5	0.0	0.0
Lime & Orange, Ferrero*	2 Tic Tacs/1g	4	0.0	386	0.0	95.5	0.0	0.0
Orange, Ferrero*	2 Tic Tacs/1g	4	0.0	385	0.0	95.5	0.0	0.0
Spearmint, Ferrero*	1 Box/16g	62	0.0	390	0.0	97.5	0.0	0.0
TIDGY PUDS								
Aunt Bessie's*	4 Puds/16.9g	55	2.5	326	9.6	38.4	14.8	2.1
Tryton Foods*	1oz/28g	97	3.9	346	11.3	43.5	14.1	2.1
TIDGY TOADS								
Aunt Bessie's*	1 Serving/45g	125	5.9	278	14.7	25.3	13.2	1.1
TIKKA MASALA								
Cauliflower & Potato, with Pilau Rice, Safeway*	1 Serving/414.3g	435	17.0	105	2.4	13.9	4.1	2.2
Chicken, & Pilau Basmati Rice, Frozen, Patak's*	1 Pack/400g	580	20.0	145	9.9	15.1	5.0	0.2
Chicken, & Pilau Rice, Asda*	1 Pack/400g	608	19.6	152	7.0	20.0	4.9	1.5
Chicken, & Pilau Rice, BGTY, Sainsbury's*	1 Pack/400g	380	4.8	95	8.1	13.0	1.2	1.1
Chicken, & Pilau Rice, GFY, Asda*	1 Pack/400g	440	8.0	110	6.0	17.0	2.0	0.8
Chicken, & Pilau Rice, Safeway*	1 Pack/399g	654	29.9	164	7.5	16.5	7.5	1.4
Chicken, & Pilau Rice, Waitrose*	1 Pack/500g	797	34.5	159	8.2	16.1	6.9	0.8
Chicken, & Rice, HL, Co-Op*	1 Pack/395g	395	8.3	100	7.1	13.0	2.1	1.0
Chicken, & Rice, HL, Tesco*	1 Pack/450g	480	8.6	107	6.1	16.3	1.9	0.8
Chicken, & Rice, M & S*	1 Pack/400g	700	35.2	175	7.4	17.0	8.8	1.0
Chicken, & Rice, Morrisons*	1 Pack/400g	544	10.0	136	6.0	22.3	2.5	0.9
Chicken, & Vegetable, HL, Tesco*	1 Pack/450g	360	12.2	80	6.8	6.9	2.7	1.8
Chicken, Asda*	1 Pack/340g	388	20.4	114	9.0	6.0	6.0	1.5
Chicken, Birds Eye*	1 Serving/400g	420	7.2	105	5.6	16.6	1.8	0.3

	Measure INFO/WEIGHT	per Measure KCAL	FAT	Nutrition Values per 100g / 100ml KCAL	PROT	CARB	FAT	FIBRE
TIKKA MASALA								
Chicken, Boiled Rice & Nan, Meal for One, GFY, Asda*	1 Pack/605g	823	18.8	136	6.0	21.0	3.1	0.0
Chicken, Breast, GFY, Asda*	1 Pack/380g	486	14.4	128	19.0	4.5	3.8	0.2
Chicken, Feeling Great, Findus*	1 Pack/350g	420	12.3	120	5.5	17.0	3.5	2.0
Chicken, Good Choice, Iceland*	1 Pack/398g	486	6.0	122	6.6	20.4	1.5	0.6
Chicken, Good Intentions, Somerfield*	1 Pack/400g	612	8.4	153	7.6	26.0	2.1	1.7
Chicken, Healthy Choice, Iceland*	1 Pack/399g	431	4.4	108	6.5	18.0	1.1	0.9
Chicken, Hot, Sainsbury's*	1 Pack/400g	604	37.2	151	13.2	3.6	9.3	1.5
Chicken, Hot, Tesco*	1 Pack/400g	588	34.4	147	8.7	8.6	8.6	1.0
Chicken, Indian, Medium, Sainsbury's*	1 Pack/400g	848	61.2	212	13.2	5.3	15.3	0.1
Chicken, Indian Meal for One, BGTY, Sainsbury's*	1 Serving/241.0g	200	1.9	83	13.9	5.1	0.8	1.0
Chicken, Indian Takeaway, Iceland*	1 Pack/400g	484	28.4	121	8.9	6.0	7.1	1.9
Chicken, Indian Takeaway, Tesco*	1 Serving/125g	100	3.3	80	8.9	4.9	2.6	2.1
Chicken, Large, Sainsbury's*	1 Pack/650g	1105	68.9	170	11.7	7.0	10.6	0.3
Chicken, Low Fat, Iceland*	1 Pack/400g	360	4.0	90	7.8	12.5	1.0	0.5
Chicken, Medium Spiced, Tesco*	½ Pack/175g	231	13.1	132	10.2	5.9	7.5	0.9
Chicken, Medium Spiced, without Rice, Tesco*	½ Pack/175g	231	13.1	132	10.2	5.9	7.5	0.9
Chicken, Microwave Meal, Good Choice, Iceland*	1 Pack/400g	488	6.0	122	6.6	20.4	1.5	0.6
Chicken, Morrisons*	1 Pack/340g	561	34.7	165	12.4	5.9	10.2	1.7
Chicken, Safeway*	1 Pack/350g	525	27.3	150	12.5	6.3	7.8	2.4
Chicken, Sharwood's*	1 Pack/375g	563	25.1	150	7.2	15.1	6.7	0.8
Chicken, SmartPrice, Asda*	1 Pack/300g	414	18.0	138	13.0	8.0	6.0	1.6
Chicken, Somerfield*	1 Pack/350g	553	37.8	158	11.7	3.6	10.8	1.5
Chicken, The Authentic Food Company*	1 Serving/375g	510	31.5	136	10.6	5.5	8.4	0.9
Chicken, Tinned, Asda*	½ Can/200g	238	14.0	119	8.0	6.0	7.0	0.9
Chicken, Tinned, M & S*	½ Can/213g	309	18.1	145	14.5	2.9	8.5	2.2
Chicken, Waitrose*	½ Pack/200g	298	19.4	149	12.8	2.6	9.7	1.6
Chicken, with Basmati Rice, Eat Smart, Safeway*	1 Pack/363g	290	5.1	80	6.4	9.6	1.4	0.7
Chicken, with Fruit & Nut Pilau Rice, Sainsbury's*	1 Pack/500g	885	45.5	177	7.6	16.1	9.1	2.8
Chicken, with Golden Rice, Iceland*	1 Pack/500g	885	41.5	177	6.2	19.4	8.3	1.1
Chicken, with Pilau Rice, Eat Smart, Safeway*	1 Pack/400g	396	8.4	99	5.7	14.3	2.1	1.6
Chicken, with Pilau Rice, Frozen, Waitrose*	1 Pack/399g	674	32.3	169	9.3	14.6	8.1	2.1
Chicken, with Pilau Rice, Indian, Budgens*	1 Serving/400g	416	3.6	104	8.0	16.0	0.9	1.8
Chicken, with Pilau Rice, PB, Waitrose*	1 Pack/400g	476	10.0	119	8.2	15.8	2.5	1.8
Chicken, with Pilau Rice, PB, Waitrose*	1 Pack/400g	476	10.0	119	8.2	15.8	2.5	1.8
Chicken, with Rice, Sainsbury's*	1 Pack/500g	960	41.0	192	8.3	21.2	8.2	0.1
Chicken, with Rice, Tesco*	1 Serving/475g	713	34.2	150	7.7	13.6	7.2	1.1
Chicken, with Rice & Naan Bread, JD Wetherspoon*	1 Serving/708g	1069	36.1	151	7.0	19.9	5.1	1.2
Chicken, with White Rice, Good Choice, Iceland*	1 Serving/400g	356	4.0	89	5.4	14.7	1.0	0.6
Green, Asda*	1 Jar/340g	401	30.6	118	1.2	8.0	9.0	0.4
HE, Tesco*	1 Serving/220g	191	10.3	87	1.0	10.2	4.7	0.5
Prawn, COU, M & S*	1 Pack/400g	400	6.4	100	6.9	14.7	1.6	1.9
Prawn, King, PB, Waitrose*	1 Pack/400g	372	3.6	93	5.2	16.0	0.9	1.7
Prawn, King, PB, Waitrose*	1 Pack/400g	372	3.6	93	5.2	16.0	0.9	1.7
Vegetable, Aldi*	1 Can/400g	496	33.6	124	1.9	10.3	8.4	1.4
Vegetable, Asda*	1 Pack/340g	316	20.7	93	2.0	7.4	6.1	1.1
Vegetable, Canned, Waitrose*	1 Can/200g	152	4.4	76	3.6	10.5	2.2	0.0
Vegetable, Indian, Tesco*	1 Pack/225g	234	13.5	104	2.4	10.4	6.0	2.4
Vegetable, Waitrose*	1 Serving/196g	149	4.3	76	3.6	10.5	2.2	3.8
Vegetable, with Rice, Patak's*	1 Pack/298g	247	7.2	83	2.9	12.3	2.4	1.4
Vegetable, with Rice, Tesco*	1 Pack/450g	500	19.4	111	2.6	15.5	4.3	0.9
Vegetarian, with Pilau Rice, Tesco*	1 Serving/440g	519	17.2	118	5.0	15.6	3.9	1.5
TIME OUT								
Break Pack, Cadbury*	1 Serving/20.4g	106	6.1	530	6.2	58.3	30.7	0.0

T

	Measure INFO/WEIGHT	per Measure KCAL	FAT	Nutrition Values per 100g / 100ml KCAL	PROT	CARB	FAT	FIBRE
TIME OUT								
Chocolate Fingers, Cadbury*	2 Fingers/35g	186	10.7	530	6.2	58.3	30.7	0.0
Orange, Snack Size, Cadbury*	1 Finger/11g	61	3.6	555	5.0	59.4	32.9	0.0
TIRAMISU								
Asda*	1 Pot/100g	252	11.0	252	4.3	34.0	11.0	0.5
BGTY, Sainsbury's*	1 Pot/90g	140	2.4	156	4.5	28.3	2.7	0.3
Family Size, Tesco*	1 Serving/125g	356	18.1	285	4.3	34.5	14.5	4.3
HL, Tesco*	1 Pot/90g	172	3.9	191	7.8	27.4	4.3	2.0
Italian, Co-Op*	1 Pack/90g	230	9.0	255	5.0	37.0	10.0	0.4
Italian, Safeway*	1 Serving/125g	353	17.5	282	4.4	34.4	14.0	1.6
Sainsbury's*	1 Serving/100g	263	10.0	263	4.4	40.2	10.0	0.1
Single Size, Tesco*	1 Pot/100g	290	12.9	290	3.8	35.1	12.9	4.5
Trifle, Sainsbury's*	1 Serving/100g	243	15.7	243	2.3	23.2	15.7	0.6
Waitrose*	1 Pot/90g	221	11.2	246	6.4	27.2	12.4	0.0
TOAD IN THE HOLE								
& Potatoes, M & S*	1 Serving/100g	200	12.9	200	6.4	14.6	12.9	0.9
Average	1oz/28g	78	4.9	277	11.9	19.5	17.4	1.1
Co-Op*	1 Pack/170g	366	25.3	215	7.8	12.3	14.9	2.6
Large, Great Value, Asda*	¼ Pack/81.2g	237	13.8	293	10.0	25.0	17.0	2.3
Tesco*	1 Serving/188g	461	28.4	245	8.5	18.7	15.1	2.6
Vegetarian, Aunt Bessie's*	1 Pack/190.2g	502	19.4	264	15.6	27.5	10.2	2.7
with Three Sausages, Asda*	1 Pack/150g	435	27.0	290	10.0	22.0	18.0	1.0
TOAST TOPPERS								
Chicken & Mushroom, Heinz*	1 Serving/56g	31	0.8	56	5.1	5.7	1.4	0.2
Ham & Cheese, Heinz*	1oz/28g	27	1.1	96	7.4	7.3	4.1	0.1
Mushroom & Bacon, Heinz*	1 Serving/56g	53	2.5	94	6.9	6.6	4.4	0.2
TOASTIE								
Cheese & Pickle, M & S*	1 Toastie/136g	320	9.1	235	10.4	33.5	6.7	2.6
Ham & Cheddar, British, M & S*	1 Pack/128g	269	8.6	210	15.5	22.3	6.7	1.3
Ham & Cheese, Tesco*	1 Serving/138g	388	18.2	281	11.5	29.1	13.2	1.0
TOFFEE CRISP								
Biscuit, Nestle*	1 Biscuit/22.5g	116	6.3	516	3.9	62.6	27.8	1.1
Mini, Nestle*	1 Bar/18g	94	5.0	516	3.7	63.1	27.6	1.1
Snack Size, Nestle*	1 Bar/30g	155	8.3	516	3.7	63.1	27.6	1.1
TOFFEES								
Assorted, Bassett's*	1 Toffee/8g	35	1.1	434	3.8	73.1	14.0	0.0
Assorted, Sainsbury's*	1 Sweet/8g	37	1.3	457	2.2	76.5	15.8	0.2
Brazil Nut, Diabetic, Thorntons*	1 Serving/20g	93	7.0	467	3.2	49.0	35.1	0.5
Butter, Double Devon, M & S*	1 Toffee/7.3g	35	1.5	480	1.8	73.2	19.9	0.0
Butter, SmartPrice, Asda*	1 Toffee/8.4g	35	1.2	440	1.3	75.0	15.0	0.0
Chewy, Werther's*	1 Toffee/5g	22	0.8	436	3.5	71.3	15.2	0.1
Chocolate Coated, Thorntons*	1 Bag/100g	521	30.7	521	3.5	57.9	30.7	0.3
Dairy, Tesco*	1 Toffee/8g	37	1.3	464	1.8	77.0	16.6	0.3
Dairy, Waitrose*	1 Toffee/14g	64	2.0	458	2.0	80.2	14.3	0.5
Devon Butter, Thorntons*	1 Sweet/9g	40	1.5	444	1.7	72.2	16.7	0.0
Liquorice, Thorntons*	1 Bag/100g	506	29.4	506	1.9	58.8	29.4	0.0
Milk Chocolate Smothered, Thorntons*	1 Pack/125g	655	38.5	524	4.3	57.5	30.8	1.1
Mixed, Average	1oz/28g	119	5.2	426	2.2	66.7	18.6	0.0
TOFU								
Average	1 Pack/250g	297	16.5	119	13.4	1.4	6.6	0.1
Beech Smoked, Organic, Cauldron*	½ Pack/110g	124	7.8	113	10.9	1.0	7.1	0.5
Firm Silken Style, Blue Dragon*	1 Pack/216g	134	5.8	62	6.9	2.4	2.7	0.0
Fresh, Kong Nam*	1 Pack/800g	552	29.6	69	7.7	1.3	3.7	0.1
Fried, Average	1oz/28g	75	4.0	268	28.6	9.3	14.1	0.0

	Measure INFO/WEIGHT	per Measure KCAL	per Measure FAT	Nutrition Values per 100g / 100ml KCAL	PROT	CARB	FAT	FIBRE
TOFU								
Original, Organic, Cauldron*	½ Pack/125g	131	7.5	105	12.1	0.6	6.0	0.5
Pieces, Golden Marinated, Organic, Cauldron*	½ Pack/75g	173	11.9	230	19.3	2.4	15.9	0.7
Sheets, Dried, H.k. Huizenhou Foods*	10g	5	0.4	50	4.0	5.0	4.0	0.0
Smoked, Organic, Evernat*	1oz/28g	36	1.8	127	16.3	0.8	6.6	0.0
TOMATO PASTE								
Average	1 Tbsp/20g	19	0.0	96	5.0	19.2	0.2	1.5
Sun Dried, Average	1 Serving/10g	39	3.5	385	3.2	13.9	35.2	0.0
TOMATO PUREE								
Average	1oz/28g	21	0.1	76	4.5	14.1	0.2	2.3
Sun Dried, & Olive Oil & Herbs, GIA*	1 Serving/20g	41	4.3	204	2.6	0.5	21.6	0.0
TOMATOES								
Cherry, Average	1 Serving/73g	14	0.2	19	0.9	3.3	0.3	1.0
Cherry, on the Vine, Average	1 Serving/50g	9	0.2	18	0.7	3.1	0.3	1.0
Cherry, Tinned, Napolina*	1 Tin/400g	92	2.4	23	1.2	3.3	0.6	0.0
Chopped, Canned, Average	1 Serving/130g	27	0.2	21	1.1	3.9	0.1	0.8
Chopped, Italian, Average	½ Can/200g	47	0.2	23	1.3	4.4	0.1	0.9
Chopped, Italian, with Olives, Waitrose*	1 Can/400g	184	7.2	46	1.4	6.0	1.8	0.8
Chopped, with Chilli, Sainsbury's*	½ Can/200g	44	1.0	22	1.0	3.5	0.5	0.9
Chopped, with Chilli & Peppers, Asda*	1 Pack/400g	92	1.2	23	1.0	4.0	0.3	0.0
Chopped, with Garlic, Average	½ Can/200g	43	0.3	21	1.2	3.8	0.1	0.8
Chopped, with Herbs, Average	½ Can/200g	42	0.3	21	1.1	3.8	0.1	0.8
Chopped, with Onion & Herbs, Napolina*	1 Can/400g	84	0.4	21	1.0	4.0	0.1	0.4
Chopped, with Onions, Italian, Tesco*	½ Can/200g	46	0.4	23	1.4	4.0	0.2	0.9
Chopped, with Peppers & Onions, Sainsbury's*	½ Can/200g	40	0.2	20	1.2	3.5	0.1	0.9
Creamed, Sainsbury's*	¼ Carton/127.3g	28	0.1	22	1.2	4.0	0.1	1.2
Fresh, Raw, Average	1 Med/85g	15	0.2	18	0.8	3.2	0.3	1.1
Fried in Blended Oil	1 Tomato/85g	77	6.5	91	0.7	5.0	7.7	1.3
Green Tiger, Raw, M & S*	1 Serving/80g	12	0.2	15	0.7	3.1	0.3	1.0
Grilled, Average	1oz/28g	14	0.3	49	2.0	8.9	0.9	2.9
Plum, Baby, Average	1 Serving/50g	9	0.2	18	1.5	2.3	0.3	1.0
Plum, in Tomato Juice, Average	1 Can/400g	71	0.4	18	1.0	3.3	0.1	0.7
Plum, in Tomato Juice, Premium, Average	1 Can/400g	93	1.2	23	1.3	3.8	0.3	0.7
Pomodorino, TTD, Sainsbury's*	1 Portion/80g	14	0.3	18	0.8	3.0	0.4	1.0
Ripened on the Vine, Average	1 Serving/100g	18	0.3	18	0.7	3.0	0.3	0.7
Semi Dried, in Olive Oil, TTD, Sainsbury's*	1 Serving/20g	33	1.6	167	4.2	19.5	8.0	0.0
Stuffed with Rice, Average	1oz/28g	59	3.8	212	2.1	22.2	13.4	1.1
Sun Dried, Average	3 Pieces/20g	43	3.2	214	4.7	13.0	15.9	3.3
Sun Dried, in Oil, GIA*	1 Serving/10g	15	1.4	153	1.9	7.5	13.9	0.0
Sun Dried, in Olive Oil, M & S*	1 Jar/280g	644	57.1	230	3.9	7.9	20.4	6.7
Sun Dried, in Seasoned Oil, Asda*	1 Serving/50g	113	9.5	225	4.6	9.0	19.0	9.0
Sun Dried, Italian, Merchant Gourmet*	1 Serving/50g	56	0.4	111	5.7	20.4	0.7	1.3
Sun Dried, Marinated, Waitrose*	1 Tomato/10g	32	2.4	315	5.9	20.0	23.5	3.1
Sun Dried, Moist, Waitrose*	1 Serving/25g	44	0.5	175	11.8	27.4	2.0	7.2
Sun Dried, with Chianti, TTD, Sainsbury's*	½ Pot/150g	108	5.3	72	1.8	8.2	3.5	1.0
Sun Dried, with Herbs & Olive Oil, Waitrose*	1 Serving/50g	73	5.3	145	3.4	9.1	10.5	7.1
TONGUE								
Lunch, Average	1oz/28g	51	3.0	181	20.1	1.8	10.7	0.0
Slices, Average	1oz/28g	56	3.9	201	18.7	0.0	14.0	0.0
TONIC WATER								
Average	1 Glass/250ml	83	0.0	33	0.0	8.8	0.0	0.0
Diet, Asda*	1 Glass/200ml	2	0.0	1	0.0	0.0	0.0	0.0
Indian, Diet, Schweppes*	1 Glass/100ml	1	0.0	1	0.0	0.0	0.0	0.0
Indian, Schweppes*	1 Serving/500ml	110	0.0	22	0.0	5.1	0.0	0.0

T

INFO/WEIGHT	Measure		per Measure		Nutrition Values per 100g / 100ml				
			KCAL	FAT	KCAL	PROT	CARB	FAT	FIBRE
TONIC WATER									
Indian, Slimline, Schweppes*	1 Serving/188ml		3	0.0	2	0.4	0.1	0.0	0.0
Low Calorie, Tesco*	1 Serving/200ml		4	0.0	2	0.0	0.5	0.0	0.0
M & S*	1 Bottle/500ml		100	0.0	20	0.0	4.8	0.0	0.0
Quinine, Schweppes*	1 Glass/125ml		46	0.0	37	0.0	9.0	0.0	0.0
Soda Stream*	1 Glass/100ml		15	0.0	15	0.0	3.2	0.0	0.0
TOOTY FROOTIES									
Rowntree's*	1 Bag/45.1g		179	1.6	397	0.1	91.5	3.5	0.0
TOPIC									
Mars*	1 Bar/47g		234	12.3	498	6.2	59.6	26.2	1.7
TOPPING									
Bruschetta, Sainsbury's*	1 Sm Tin/230g		60	1.8	26	1.2	3.6	0.8	1.1
Cake Covering, Milk Chocolate Flavoured, Tesco*	1 Pack/300g		1761	116.4	587	2.1	57.3	38.8	2.6
Creamy, Tip Top, Nestle*	1 Serving/50g		54	3.2	107	3.5	8.6	6.4	0.1
for Cappuccino, Creamy, Flavia*	1 Serving/15g		38	1.0	253	14.7	33.3	6.7	0.0
Pizza, Italian Tomato & Herb, Sainsbury's*	1/5 Jar/50g		19	0.2	38	1.6	7.1	0.4	1.1
Pizza, Traditional Tomato with Basil, Napolina*	1 Jar/250g		153	6.5	61	1.2	7.8	2.6	0.7
Pizza, with Herbs, Napolina*	1 Serving/100g		49	2.2	49	0.9	6.3	2.2	0.6
TORCHIETTI									
Egg, with Parmesan & Rocket, TTD, Sainsbury's*	¼ Pot/62.5g		123	5.7	195	7.1	21.4	9.0	1.6
TORTE									
Chocolate, Safeway*	1/6 Torte/55g		122	5.8	221	4.1	27.6	10.5	1.5
Chocolate, Tesco*	1 Serving/50g		126	6.0	251	3.6	32.3	11.9	1.0
Chocolate Orange & Almond, Gu*	1 Serving/65g		273	19.8	420	5.0	28.2	30.5	2.7
Chocolate Truffle, Waitrose*	1 Serving/116g		359	20.1	309	4.6	30.1	17.3	1.4
Lemon, Farmfoods*	1/6 Cake/70g		137	7.0	195	4.3	21.9	10.0	0.5
Lemon, Somerfield*	1 Serving/45g		71	1.2	157	0.8	32.6	2.6	0.8
Lemon, Tesco*	1 Serving/62g		142	6.1	230	2.3	32.9	9.9	0.5
Raspberry, Safeway*	1/6 Serving/54g		93	4.0	172	1.2	25.1	7.4	1.5
TORTELLI									
Gorgonzola & Walnut, Specially Selected, Aldi*	1 Pack/200g		536	20.8	268	11.4	32.1	10.4	1.3
TORTELLINI									
3 Cheese, Sainsbury's*	1 Serving/50g		196	4.4	391	14.4	63.8	8.7	3.0
Aubergine & Pecorino, Sainsbury's*	½ Pack/150g		354	6.5	236	8.9	40.3	4.3	3.2
Basil, Mozerella & Tomato, Weight Watchers*	½ Pack/125g		278	3.4	222	9.0	40.5	2.7	4.8
Beef & Red Wine, Italian, Asda*	½ Pack/150.3g		242	4.2	161	9.0	25.0	2.8	0.0
Beef & Red Wine, Italiano, Tesco*	1 Serving/150g		324	4.8	216	11.7	35.3	3.2	3.3
Cheese, Canned, Italiana, Weight Watchers*	1 Can/395g		245	6.3	62	2.3	9.7	1.6	0.4
Cheese, Fresh, Sainsbury's*	½ Pack/180g		329	9.0	183	7.6	26.8	5.0	1.7
Cheese, HL, Tesco*	1 Serving/400g		368	11.2	92	3.2	13.4	2.8	0.6
Cheese, Tomato & Basil, Tesco*	1 Serving/150g		387	8.1	258	13.0	39.5	5.4	3.3
Cheese & Ham, Italiano, Tesco*	½ Pack/150g		396	12.3	264	12.8	34.8	8.2	3.0
Four Cheese, Italian, Asda*	1 Serving/150g		296	7.5	197	8.0	30.0	5.0	3.4
Four Cheese, Tesco*	½ Pack/150g		405	11.9	270	12.3	37.3	7.9	3.4
Four Cheese & Tomato, Italian, Asda*	1 Serving/150g		249	5.7	166	8.0	25.0	3.8	0.0
Four Cheese with Tomato & Basil Sauce, Tesco*	1 Pack/400g		500	14.8	125	6.1	16.9	3.7	0.6
Garlic, Basil & Ricotta, Asda*	½ Pack/175g		319	10.5	182	6.0	26.0	6.0	2.6
Garlic & Herb, Fresh, Sainsbury's*	½ Pack/150g		365	11.7	243	11.1	32.2	7.8	1.8
Ham & Cheese, Fresh, Asda*	½ Pack/150g		255	9.0	170	6.0	23.0	6.0	1.7
Ham & Cheese, Tesco*	1 Serving/225g		578	12.6	257	13.5	38.1	5.6	1.8
Meat, Italian, Tesco*	1 Serving/125g		333	9.5	266	10.6	38.9	7.6	2.3
Mozzarella & Tomato, Fresh, Asda*	1oz/28g		46	1.1	166	8.0	25.0	3.8	0.0
Mushroom, Asda*	1 Serving/125g		218	5.3	174	6.0	28.0	4.2	2.3
Mushroom, BGTY, Sainsbury's*	½ Can/200g		180	6.2	90	2.2	13.2	3.1	0.7

	Measure INFO/WEIGHT	per Measure KCAL	per Measure FAT	Nutrition Values per 100g / 100ml KCAL	PROT	CARB	FAT	FIBRE
TORTELLINI								
Mushroom, PB, Waitrose*	1 Pack/250g	573	9.0	229	9.4	39.8	3.6	2.4
Pepperoni, Italian, Asda*	½ Pack/150g	250	6.0	167	6.7	26.0	4.0	0.0
Pesto & Goats Cheese, Sainsbury's*	½ Pack/125g	259	10.1	207	8.9	24.6	8.1	2.6
Pork & Beef, BGTY, Sainsbury's*	½ Can/200g	148	3.0	74	3.7	11.2	1.5	0.6
Sausage & Ham, Italiano, Tesco*	1 Pack/300g	816	27.9	272	13.1	34.0	9.3	3.7
Smoked Bacon & Tomato, Asda*	1 Pack/300g	591	15.0	197	9.0	29.0	5.0	0.0
Smoked Ham & Cheese, Ready Meals, Waitrose*	1oz/28g	73	1.7	261	12.9	38.7	6.1	1.3
Spicy Pepperoni, Fresh, Asda*	½ Pack/150g	249	6.0	166	7.0	26.0	4.0	0.0
Spinach & Ricotta, Canned, Somerfield*	1 Can/250g	283	15.0	113	12.0	4.0	6.0	0.0
Spinach & Ricotta, Italian, Asda*	½ Pack/150g	189	3.6	126	5.0	21.0	2.4	0.6
Spinach & Ricotta, Pasta Reale*	½ Pack/125g	314	6.4	251	10.4	44.5	5.1	3.7
Spinach & Ricotta, Sainsbury's*	1oz/28g	109	2.4	388	15.0	62.5	8.7	2.2
Spinach & Ricotta, Verdi, Asda*	1 Serving/125g	186	5.6	149	6.0	21.0	4.5	2.4
TORTELLONI								
Arrabbiata, Sainsbury's*	½ Pack/210g	407	11.8	194	7.1	28.8	5.6	2.6
Beef & Pancetta, Aberdeen Angus, Grandi, Budgens*	½ Pack/125g	314	5.4	251	12.4	40.5	4.3	2.9
Bell Pepper & Sundried Tomato, Morrisons*	½ Pack/150g	375	6.5	250	12.1	40.7	4.3	2.9
Carbonara, Italian, Fresh, Sainsbury's*	½ Pack/210g	405	12.6	193	8.4	26.3	6.0	2.2
Cheese, Garlic & Herb, Co-Op*	1 Serving/125g	331	7.5	265	10.0	43.0	6.0	0.0
Cheese, Heinz*	1 Can/395g	233	7.1	59	2.1	8.6	1.8	0.5
Cheese, Tomato, & Basil, Sainsbury's*	½ Pack/150g	272	9.8	181	8.0	22.7	6.5	1.7
Cheese & Ham, Co-Op*	½ Pack/150g	405	10.7	270	12.0	39.3	7.1	1.9
Cheese & Ham, Fresh, Budgens*	1 Serving/100g	268	6.5	268	12.6	42.0	6.5	2.2
Cheese & Pesto, Somerfield*	1 Pack/250g	788	30.0	315	12.0	40.0	12.0	0.0
Cheese & Smoked Ham, Waitrose*	1 Serving/250g	625	17.0	250	11.5	35.8	6.8	1.8
Cheese & Sun Dried Tomato, Fresh, Safeway*	½ Pack/199g	364	12.3	183	7.7	24.2	6.2	2.7
Cheese Garlic & Herb, Fresh, Budgens*	½ Pack/125g	334	7.5	267	10.3	46.1	6.0	3.3
Chicken & Ham, Morrisons*	1 Serving/150g	366	5.9	244	12.3	38.6	3.9	2.4
Chicken & Ham, Safeway*	1 Serving/125g	203	4.8	162	8.8	23.1	3.8	3.8
Chorizo & Tomato, Morrisons*	1 Serving/150g	447	12.9	298	12.8	45.1	8.6	2.6
Five Cheese, Safeway*	1 Serving/150g	275	9.3	183	7.8	24.2	6.2	2.7
Five Cheese, Sainsbury's*	1 Serving/125g	285	11.6	228	10.8	25.2	9.3	2.9
Four Cheese, Express, Dolmio*	1 Pack/220g	411	16.7	187	7.6	22.1	7.6	0.0
Four Cheese, Waitrose*	½ Pack/125g	298	8.4	238	10.3	34.2	6.7	1.6
Fresh, Morrisons*	1 Serving/150g	431	14.6	287	11.2	41.0	9.7	2.4
Garlic & Herb, Cooked, Pasta Reale*	1 Pack/300g	546	11.7	182	6.7	30.1	3.9	0.9
Garlic Mushroom & Onion, Eat Smart, Safeway*	1 Serving/125g	231	2.5	185	9.3	31.4	2.0	1.4
Goats Cheese & Basil, Somerfield*	1 Serving/250g	650	17.0	260	11.1	38.7	6.8	1.8
Goats Cheese & Pesto, Sainsbury's*	½ Pack/150g	311	12.2	207	8.9	24.6	8.1	2.6
Goats Cheese & Red Pepper, Morrisons*	1 Pack/150g	450	16.7	300	11.5	38.4	11.1	3.8
Italian Style Sausage & Red Wine, Morrisons*	½ Pack/150g	420	10.8	280	11.1	45.5	7.2	2.7
Meat, Italian, Asda*	½ Pack/150g	266	6.8	177	7.0	27.0	4.5	2.4
Meat & Cheese, Fresh, Sainsbury's*	½ Pack/125g	304	10.5	243	13.5	28.3	8.4	2.5
Mediterranean Vegetable, PB, Waitrose*	½ Pack/125g	286	4.5	229	9.1	40.1	3.6	2.5
Mozzarella, Tomato & Basil, Italian, Somerfield*	½ Pack/125g	314	5.1	251	10.5	43.1	4.1	1.9
Mushroom, PB, Waitrose*	½ Pack/125g	300	4.0	240	10.9	41.8	3.2	2.2
Olive & Ricotta, Sainsbury's*	½ Pack/175.2g	403	18.4	230	8.8	25.1	10.5	2.3
Parma Ham & Parmesan, Safeway*	1 Serving/125g	269	8.4	215	9.9	27.8	6.7	1.5
Pasta, Fresh, Cream Cheese, Garlic & Herb, Morrisons*	1 Serving/150g	401	9.0	267	10.3	46.1	6.0	3.2
Porcini & Pancetta, TTD, Sainsbury's*	1 Serving/175g	294	11.0	168	7.1	20.8	6.3	3.4
Potato & Rosemary, Fresh, Sainsbury's*	½ Pack/175g	364	15.4	208	5.7	26.6	8.8	2.3
Red Pepper & Mozzarella, Cooked, Somerfield*	½ Pack/124g	325	8.2	263	10.8	40.1	6.6	1.8
Roasted Vegetable, TTD, Sainsbury's*	½ Pack/125g	259	11.1	207	8.4	23.3	8.9	4.0

	Measure INFO/WEIGHT	per Measure KCAL	per Measure FAT	Nutrition Values per 100g / 100ml KCAL	PROT	CARB	FAT	FIBRE
TORTELLONI								
Sicilian Style & Tuna, Morrisons*	½ Pack/150g	398	8.9	265	12.1	43.0	5.9	2.3
Smoked Ham, Bacon & Tomato, Italiano, Tesco*	½ Pack/148.3g	445	17.4	300	12.0	35.7	11.7	2.5
Spicy Red Pepper & Tomato, Pasta Reale*	½ Pack/125g	310	5.5	248	10.0	42.0	4.4	3.3
Spinach & Ricotta, Chilled, Italiano, Tesco*	½ Pack/150g	413	12.8	275	10.4	38.1	8.5	3.3
Spinach & Ricotta, Fresh, Morrisons*	½ Pack/125g	248	8.1	198	7.8	27.0	6.5	3.1
Spinach & Ricotta, Fresh, Safeway*	½ Pack/202g	341	9.7	169	7.4	24.0	4.8	2.4
Spinach & Ricotta, Fresh, Waitrose*	½ Pack/125g	328	8.8	262	11.3	38.4	7.0	2.4
Spinach & Ricotta, Italian, Somerfield*	1 Serving/125g	320	7.9	256	10.9	38.8	6.3	2.2
Spinach & Ricotta, Sainsbury's*	½ Pack/150g	456	15.1	217	7.8	30.2	7.2	2.4
Spinach & Ricotta, Waistline, Crosse & Blackwell*	1 Serving/300g	219	7.2	73	2.9	10.1	2.4	1.3
Spinach & Ricotta Cheese, Co-Op*	½ Pack/126g	315	6.3	250	10.0	41.0	5.0	4.0
Sundried Tomato & Mozzarella, M & S*	1 Pack/280g	448	15.1	160	6.6	21.1	5.4	1.6
Taleggio & Leek, Fresh, Sainsbury's*	½ Pack/175g	450	12.4	257	9.7	38.8	7.1	2.6
Tomato & Mozzarella, Fresh, Asda*	½ Pack/150g	236	4.2	157	8.0	25.0	2.8	0.0
Tomato & Mozzarella, Fresh, Sainsbury's*	½ Pack/150g	291	12.0	194	7.5	23.0	8.0	3.4
Tomato & Mozzarella, Sainsbury's*	1 Serving/175g	340	14.0	194	7.5	23.0	8.0	3.4
Trio, Fresh, Tesco*	½ Pack/125g	323	8.9	258	12.8	35.8	7.1	2.0
Walnut & Gorgonzola, Fresh, Sainsbury's*	½ Pack/210g	414	12.2	197	8.4	27.8	5.8	2.4
with Tomato, Basil, & Paprika, Easy Cook, Napolina*	1 Pack/120g	481	14.5	401	12.4	60.7	12.1	0.0
TORTIGLIONI								
Dry, Average	1 Serving/75g	266	1.4	355	12.5	72.2	1.9	2.1
TORTILLA CHIPS								
Blazing BBQ, Sainsbury's*	1 Serving/50g	237	11.8	474	6.8	58.9	23.5	4.6
Blue, Organic, Sainsbury's*	1 Serving/50g	252	11.7	504	7.7	65.8	23.4	5.6
Chilli, Organic, Evernat*	1oz/28g	137	6.2	490	8.0	65.0	22.0	0.0
Chilli Flavour, Somerfield*	1 Serving/50g	242	12.1	484	6.8	60.1	24.1	5.3
Classic Mexican, Phileas Fogg*	1 Serving/35g	162	6.7	464	5.9	67.2	19.1	3.8
Cool, Asda*	1 Pack/100g	475	23.0	475	8.0	59.0	23.0	4.9
Cool, Salted, Sainsbury's*	1 Serving/50g	253	13.7	506	6.5	58.6	27.3	4.3
Cool, Tesco*	1 Serving/40g	190	9.9	474	6.3	56.7	24.7	7.8
Cool Flavour, Safeway*	1 Serving/50g	227	10.8	454	6.6	58.3	21.6	7.2
Cool Flavour, Sainsbury's*	1 Serving/50g	232	9.4	463	5.7	68.1	18.7	3.7
Co-Op*	1 Serving/25g	123	6.3	490	7.0	59.0	25.0	5.0
Easy Cheesy!, Sainsbury's*	1 Serving/50g	249	13.1	498	7.1	58.7	26.1	4.5
Lightly Salted, M & S*	1 Serving/20g	98	4.8	490	7.2	61.5	24.1	4.5
Lightly Salted, SmartPrice, Asda*	¼ Bag/50g	251	13.0	502	7.0	60.0	26.0	5.0
Lightly Salted, Tesco*	1 Serving/50g	248	13.8	495	4.8	56.8	27.6	7.5
Lightly Salted, Waitrose*	1 Serving/40g	187	8.6	468	7.1	61.2	21.6	6.5
Nacho Cheese Flavour, M & S*	1 Serving/30g	144	6.7	480	7.5	62.0	22.4	4.2
Nacho Cheese Flavour, Morrisons*	1 Serving/25g	126	6.6	504	7.2	59.4	26.4	3.6
Nachos Kit, Asda*	1 Serving/100g	448	24.0	448	7.0	51.0	24.0	0.7
Salsa, Asda*	1 Serving/25g	122	6.0	488	6.0	62.0	24.0	6.0
Salsa, M & S*	½ Bag/75g	364	18.8	485	5.7	59.1	25.1	6.1
Taco, Tesco*	1 Serving/50g	248	12.7	495	7.4	59.3	25.4	4.4
TORTILLAS								
Asda*	1 Tortilla/34g	97	2.0	286	8.0	50.0	6.0	1.9
Corn, Gluten Free, Discovery*	1 Tortilla/16g	39	0.4	243	5.4	53.8	2.3	3.8
Corn, Soft, Old El Paso*	1 Tortlla/37.5g	118	4.1	315	10.0	44.0	11.0	0.0
Flour, 10 Pack, Asda*	1 Tortilla/30g	95	2.1	315	9.0	54.0	7.0	2.5
Flour, American Style, Sainsbury's*	1 Tortilla/34.5g	110	2.5	313	8.6	53.9	7.0	2.5
Flour, Bakery, Asda*	1 Tortilla/42.6g	130	3.0	303	9.1	50.9	7.1	2.6
Flour, From Dinner Kit, Old El Paso*	1 Tortilla/42g	144	4.9	344	8.7	51.1	11.7	0.0
Flour, Mexican Style, Morrisons*	1 Tortilla/33g	103	2.3	313	8.6	53.9	7.0	2.5

T

	Measure INFO/WEIGHT	per Measure KCAL	FAT	Nutrition Values per 100g / 100ml KCAL	PROT	CARB	FAT	FIBRE
TORTILLAS								
Flour, Salsa, Old El Paso*	1 Tortilla/41g	132	3.7	323	9.0	52.0	9.0	0.0
Flour, Soft, Discovery*	1 Tortilla/40g	119	2.8	298	8.0	49.6	7.1	2.4
Flour, Soft, Garlic & Coriander, Discovery*	1 Wrap/40g	116	2.4	289	8.1	50.6	6.0	1.7
Flour, Soft, Old El Paso*	1 Tortilla/41g	141	2.9	343	10.7	60.0	7.0	0.0
Flour, Wheat, Waitrose*	1 Wrap/62g	203	6.1	327	8.5	51.5	9.8	0.5
Made with Wheat Flour	1oz/28g	73	0.3	262	7.2	59.7	1.0	2.4
Plain, Morrisons*	1 Serving/35g	92	0.9	263	8.5	51.2	2.7	2.5
Plain, Wrap, HL, Tesco*	1 Wrap/50g	140	1.4	280	8.5	54.2	2.8	3.3
Plain, Wrap, Morrisons*	1 Wrap/63.3g	190	3.7	300	8.4	52.2	5.9	2.7
Plain, Wraps, Tesco*	1 Tortilla/64g	192	3.8	300	8.4	52.2	5.9	2.7
White, Wraps, M & S*	1 Wrap/64.2g	170	2.4	265	7.9	49.0	3.8	1.6
Wholewheat, Magnifico*	1 Wrap/34.1g	86	2.7	252	9.8	35.7	7.8	7.1
Wrap, 8 Pack, Asda*	1 Serving/34g	97	2.0	286	8.0	50.0	6.0	1.9
Wrap, BGTY, Sainsbury's*	1 Wrap/50g	125	1.1	250	7.8	50.1	2.2	2.9
Wrap, Low Carb, Tesco*	1 Tortilla/17g	77	1.5	453	39.4	53.5	8.8	23.5
Wrap, Low Fat, M & S*	1 Serving/180g	225	4.0	125	6.3	20.6	2.2	1.9
Wrap, Morrisons*	1 Serving/60g	132	2.1	220	6.2	42.0	3.5	1.7
Wrap, Organic, Sainsbury's*	1 Wrap/56g	167	4.3	298	8.6	48.8	7.7	2.1
Wrap, Organic, Tesco*	1 Tortilla/56.6g	173	4.4	306	8.1	51.0	7.7	2.0
Wrap, Spicy Tomato, Morrisons*	1 Wrap/55g	158	3.1	288	8.6	50.5	5.7	0.7
Wrap, Tomato & Herb, Tesco*	1 Serving/63g	165	3.5	262	7.9	45.1	5.5	2.1
Wrap, Tomato & Herbs, Sainsbury's*	1 Tortilla/52g	157	3.1	302	7.8	54.1	6.0	2.4
Wrap, Wholemeal, Morrisons*	1 Wrap/50g	177	4.0	354	10.0	60.4	8.0	6.6
Wraps, Deli, Multigrain, Mission*	1 Wrap/61.3g	185	4.0	302	8.3	52.6	6.5	3.6
Wraps, Plain, Sainsbury's*	1 Tortilla/56g	175	3.9	313	8.6	53.9	7.0	2.5
TRAIL MIX								
Average	1oz/28g	121	8.0	432	9.1	37.2	28.5	4.3
TREACLE								
Black, Average	1 Tbsp/20g	51	0.0	257	1.2	67.2	0.0	0.0
TRIFLE								
Average	1oz/28g	45	1.8	160	3.6	22.3	6.3	0.5
Banana & Mandarin, Co-Op*	¼ Trifle/125g	238	13.8	190	2.0	21.0	11.0	0.1
Blackforest, BGTY, Sainsbury's*	1 Pot/125g	171	5.6	137	2.1	21.9	4.5	1.6
Chocolate, HL, Tesco*	1 Serving/150g	189	4.1	126	4.0	21.4	2.7	4.6
Chocolate, Light, Cadbury*	1 Pot/88.2g	163	6.6	185	5.5	23.4	7.5	0.0
Chocolate, Tesco*	1 Serving/125g	313	19.0	250	4.3	24.0	15.2	0.7
Cream Mandarin, GFY, Asda*	1 Serving/113g	151	5.0	134	1.6	27.0	4.4	0.2
Fruit, Sainsbury's*	1 Serving/125g	233	12.5	186	2.3	21.7	10.0	0.3
Fruit Cocktail, Co-Op*	1 Trifle/125g	213	10.0	170	2.0	23.0	8.0	0.2
Fruit Cocktail, COU, M & S*	1 Trifle/140g	175	3.2	125	2.8	23.1	2.3	0.5
Fruit Cocktail, Individual, Tesco*	1 Pot/113g	175	8.8	155	1.7	19.6	7.8	0.6
Fruit Cocktail, Luxury Devonshire, St Ivel*	1 Trifle/125g	211	9.9	169	1.9	22.6	7.9	0.2
Fruit Cocktail, M & S*	1 Serving/165g	272	13.7	165	2.4	19.6	8.3	0.9
Fruit Cocktail, Somerfield*	1 Trifle/125g	211	10.0	169	2.0	23.0	8.0	0.0
Raspberry, Co-Op*	1 Trifle/125g	206	10.0	165	2.0	22.0	8.0	0.3
Raspberry, Individual, Safeway*	1 Pot/125g	259	12.8	207	2.7	26.2	10.2	0.0
Raspberry, Sainsbury's*	1 Pot/125g	204	9.8	163	1.7	21.5	7.8	0.6
Raspberry, Tesco*	1 Pot/150g	210	9.8	140	1.7	18.5	6.5	1.0
Strawberry, BGTY, Sainsbury's*	1 Pot/125g	135	2.6	108	2.4	19.9	2.1	0.5
Strawberry, Co-Op*	1 Serving/123g	234	13.5	190	2.0	21.0	11.0	0.2
Strawberry, COU, M & S*	1 Pot/140g	154	2.8	110	2.8	20.6	2.0	1.2
Strawberry, HL, Tesco*	1 Trifle/150g	173	2.7	115	2.3	22.2	1.8	1.5
Strawberry, Individual, Safeway*	1 Pot/125g	215	10.0	172	2.3	22.0	8.0	0.5

T

	Measure INFO/WEIGHT	per Measure KCAL	FAT	Nutrition Values per 100g / 100ml KCAL	PROT	CARB	FAT	FIBRE
TRIFLE								
Strawberry, Individual, Waitrose*	1 Pot/150g	206	8.6	137	1.8	19.7	5.7	1.0
Strawberry, Low Fat Goodies, Danone*	1 Pot/115g	148	2.1	129	2.2	26.0	1.8	0.3
Strawberry, Luxury Devonshire, St Ivel*	1 Trifle/125g	208	9.9	166	2.0	21.7	7.9	0.2
Strawberry, Sainsbury's*	¼ Tub/150g	261	15.5	174	2.2	18.1	10.3	1.0
Strawberry, Tesco*	1 Serving/83g	137	7.6	165	1.5	19.1	9.2	0.8
Summerfruit, BGTY, Sainsbury's*	1 Trifle/125g	151	5.5	121	1.2	19.2	4.4	0.5
TRIFLE MIX								
Strawberry Flavour, Bird's*	1oz/28g	119	2.9	425	2.7	78.0	10.5	1.2
TRIPE &								
Onions, Stewed	1oz/28g	26	0.8	93	8.3	9.5	2.7	0.7
TROFIE								
Waitrose*	1 Serving/75g	256	1.0	341	12.5	68.8	1.3	3.7
TROMPRETTI								
Fresh, Waitrose*	1 Serving/125g	339	3.0	271	11.7	50.6	2.4	2.0
Tricolour, Fresh, Tesco*	1 Pack/250g	675	8.5	270	11.2	48.6	3.4	4.0
TROTTOLE								
Dry, Sainsbury's*	1 Serving/90g	338	1.5	375	12.3	73.1	1.7	2.5
Tricolore, Sainsbury's*	1 Serving/90g	321	1.5	357	12.3	73.1	1.7	2.5
TROUT								
Fillets, Arbroath, Hot, Smoked, Rainbow, M & S*	½ Pack/63g	85	3.4	135	20.8	1.0	5.4	0.5
Raw, Average	1 Serving/120g	159	6.5	132	20.6	0.0	5.4	0.0
Roasting, Lemon & Rosemary, TTD, Sainsbury's*	1 Fish/269.9g	475	28.6	176	20.2	0.0	10.6	0.5
Rosemary Crusted, Finest, Tesco*	1 Fillet/150g	353	26.3	235	16.1	3.1	17.5	1.0
Smoked, Average	1oz/28g	39	1.5	139	22.7	0.3	5.2	0.1
TUACA*								
Alcoholic Beverage, Average, Tuaca*	1 Serving/25ml	67	0.0	267	0.0	0.0	0.0	0.0
TUNA								
Chunks, in Brine, Average, Drained	1 Can /130g	141	0.7	108	25.9	0.0	0.5	0.0
Chunks, in Brine, Yellowfin, Drained, Princes*	1 Can/130g	137	0.7	105	25.0	0.0	0.5	0.0
Chunks, in Spring Water, Average, Drained	1 Can /130g	140	0.8	108	25.4	0.0	0.6	0.1
Chunks, in Sunflower Oil, Average, Drained	1 Can/138g	260	12.6	189	26.5	0.0	9.2	0.0
Chunks, Skipjack, in Brine, Average	1 Can/138g	141	0.8	102	24.3	0.0	0.6	0.0
Coronation, BGTY, Sainsbury's*	1 Can/80g	90	2.1	112	16.5	5.7	2.6	1.0
Coronation Style, By John West, Weight Watchers*	1 Can/80g	75	2.0	94	9.3	8.7	2.5	0.4
Coronation Style, Canned, Average	1 Can/80g	122	7.6	152	10.2	6.5	9.5	0.6
Fillets, in Tomato Sauce, Princes*	1 Can/120g	131	3.0	109	19.0	2.5	2.5	0.0
Flakes, in Brine, Average	1oz/28g	29	0.2	104	24.8	0.0	0.6	0.0
Flakes, in Brine, Makes Sense!, Somerfield*	1 Tin/130g	130	0.8	100	23.5	0.0	0.6	0.0
French Style, Light Lunch, John West*	1 Pack/240g	221	6.2	92	7.9	9.4	2.6	0.9
in a Light Lemon Mayo, Slimming World, Princes*	1 Can/80g	99	3.8	124	16.8	3.5	4.8	0.0
in a Light Mayonnaise. Slimming World, Princes*	1 Can/80g	96	3.3	120	17.3	3.6	4.1	0.0
in a Red Chilli & Lime Dressing, Princes*	1 Sachet/85g	102	2.8	120	21.5	1.0	3.3	0.0
in a Tikka Dressing, Slimming World, Princes*	1 Can/80g	108	4.6	135	16.8	4.0	5.7	0.0
in a Tikka Dressing, Slimming World*	1 Serving/85g	116	3.8	137	18.6	5.5	4.5	0.0
in Chilli Sauce, Safeway*	1 Serving/100g	158	7.9	158	16.8	4.8	7.9	0.5
in Olive Oil, Yellowfin, John West*	1 Sm Can/56g	106	5.0	189	27.0	0.0	9.0	0.0
in Sweet & Sour Sauce, Safeway*	1 Can/185g	148	3.0	80	10.9	5.6	1.6	1.0
in Thousand Island Dressing, John West*	1 Can/185g	287	13.0	155	18.0	5.1	7.0	0.2
in Water, Average	1 Serving/120g	126	1.0	105	24.0	0.1	0.8	0.0
Light Lunch, French Style, John West*	1 Tub/240.2g	221	6.2	92	7.9	9.4	2.6	0.9
Light Lunch, Indian Style, John West*	1 Pack/240g	401	23.0	167	7.7	12.3	9.6	0.6
Light Lunch, Mediterranean Style, John West*	1 Pack/240g	218	6.0	91	7.9	9.3	2.5	1.7
Light Lunch, Nicoise Style, John West*	1 Pack/250g	245	5.8	98	10.3	9.0	2.3	2.7

T

	Measure INFO/WEIGHT	per Measure KCAL	FAT	Nutrition Values per 100g / 100ml KCAL	PROT	CARB	FAT	FIBRE

TUNA

	Measure INFO/WEIGHT	KCAL	FAT	KCAL	PROT	CARB	FAT	FIBRE
Light Lunch, Tomato Salsa Style, John West*	1 Pack/250g	180	2.8	72	8.0	7.5	1.1	1.1
Lime & Black Pepper, John West*	1 Serving/85g	133	7.8	156	15.6	2.8	9.2	0.0
Puertorican Style, Tinned, Natura*	1 Tin/185g	157	8.3	85	9.0	1.0	4.5	0.0
Steaks, Chargrilled, Italian, Sainsbury's*	1 Serving/125g	199	8.0	159	25.1	0.2	6.4	0.5
Steaks, Fishermans Choice*	2 Steaks/300g	390	11.7	130	23.1	0.0	3.9	0.0
Steaks, Fresh, Morrisons*	1 Serving/180g	245	2.3	136	31.5	0.2	1.3	0.0
Steaks, in Brine, Average	1 Sm Can/99g	106	0.5	107	25.6	0.0	0.6	0.0
Steaks, in Cajun Marinade, Sainsbury's*	1 Steak/100g	141	2.4	141	29.8	0.0	2.4	0.0
Steaks, in Olive Oil, Average	1 Serving/111g	211	10.7	190	25.8	0.0	9.6	0.0
Steaks, in Oriental Sauce, Good Choice, Iceland*	1 Pack/260g	333	1.8	128	22.3	8.1	0.7	0.4
Steaks, in Sunflower Oil, Average	1 Can/150g	276	12.9	184	26.7	0.0	8.6	0.0
Steaks, in Water, Average	1 Serving/200g	215	0.8	107	25.6	0.0	0.4	0.0
Steaks, Lemon & Herb Marinade, Seared, Sainsbury's*	½ Pack/118.6g	192	8.8	161	23.4	0.1	7.4	0.0
Steaks, Marinated, Sainsbury's*	1 Serving/100g	153	5.3	153	25.1	1.3	5.3	0.5
Steaks, Raw, Average	1 Serving/140g	185	2.8	132	28.5	0.1	2.0	0.2
Steaks, Skipjack, in Brine, Average	½ Can/75g	73	0.4	98	23.2	0.0	0.6	0.0
Steaks, Thai Style Butter, Tesco*	1 Serving/110g	191	9.1	174	24.7	0.0	8.3	0.0
Steaks, TTD, Sainsbury's*	100g/100g	136	1.1	136	31.5	0.0	1.1	0.0
Steaks, with Lime & Coriander Dressing, Tesco*	1 Serving/150g	156	0.6	104	21.6	3.6	0.4	0.6
Steaks, with Sweet Red Pepper Glaze, Sainsbury's*	1 Steak/100g	135	0.1	135	28.5	5.0	0.1	0.1
Steaks, Yellowfin, Fisherman's Choice*	1 Steak/150g	195	5.9	130	23.1	0.0	3.9	0.0
with a Twist, French Dressing, John West*	1 Pack/85g	135	8.2	159	15.2	2.8	9.7	0.1
with a Twist, Oven Dried Tomato & Herb, John West*	1 Pack/85g	129	6.8	152	16.1	3.9	8.0	0.1
with Basil Butter, Microwave Easy Steam, Sainsbury's*	1 Pack/170g	292	14.5	172	23.3	0.5	8.5	0.1
with Onion, John West*	1oz/28g	33	0.6	118	19.0	6.0	2.0	0.0
with Salsa Verde, Sainsbury's*	1 Serving/125g	310	20.0	248	25.5	0.6	16.0	0.0

TUNA IN

	Measure INFO/WEIGHT	KCAL	FAT	KCAL	PROT	CARB	FAT	FIBRE
a Tomato & Herb Dressing, Weight Watchers*	1 Can/80g	79	2.9	99	11.6	5.1	3.6	0.5

TUNA MAYONNAISE

	Measure INFO/WEIGHT	KCAL	FAT	KCAL	PROT	CARB	FAT	FIBRE
& Sweetcorn, Canned, BGTY, Sainsbury's*	1 Can/80g	78	1.8	97	15.2	4.0	2.3	0.7
Garlic & Herb, John West*	½ Can/92g	243	20.4	264	12.0	4.0	22.2	0.2
Light, Slimming World*	1 Serving/80g	96	3.3	120	17.3	3.6	4.1	0.0
with Sweetcorn, John West*	½ Can/92g	231	19.0	251	12.0	4.5	20.6	0.2
with Sweetcorn, Weight Watchers*	1 Can/80g	114	6.3	142	11.5	6.2	7.9	0.1

TUNA MEAL

	Measure INFO/WEIGHT	KCAL	FAT	KCAL	PROT	CARB	FAT	FIBRE
Italian, Light, All Day, John West*	1 Serving/100g	141	5.0	141	11.0	13.0	5.0	0.0

TUNA SNACK POT

	Measure INFO/WEIGHT	KCAL	FAT	KCAL	PROT	CARB	FAT	FIBRE
Italian, Weight Watchers*	1 Pot/240g	245	8.6	102	9.1	8.5	3.6	0.5
Oriental, Weight Watchers*	1 Pot/240g	269	7.0	112	9.0	12.6	2.9	0.3
Provencale, Weight Watchers*	1 Pot/240g	266	8.2	111	9.8	10.2	3.4	0.5

TURBOT

	Measure INFO/WEIGHT	KCAL	FAT	KCAL	PROT	CARB	FAT	FIBRE
Grilled	1oz/28g	34	1.0	122	22.7	0.0	3.5	0.0
Raw	1oz/28g	27	0.8	95	17.7	0.0	2.7	0.0

TURKEY

	Measure INFO/WEIGHT	KCAL	FAT	KCAL	PROT	CARB	FAT	FIBRE
Breast, Butter Basted, Average	1 Serving/75g	110	3.6	146	23.7	1.9	4.9	0.4
Breast, Canned, Average	1 Can/200g	194	4.7	97	18.3	0.7	2.4	0.1
Breast, Diced, Healthy Range, Average	1oz/28g	30	0.4	108	23.9	0.1	1.3	0.1
Breast, Fillets, Flamegrilled, Bernard Matthews*	1 Pack/200g	252	7.2	126	22.5	0.9	3.6	0.2
Breast, Fillets, Marinated, Lidl*	1 Serving/250g	238	2.5	95	19.0	2.5	1.0	0.0
Breast, Honey Roast, Sliced, Average	1 Serving/50g	57	0.7	115	24.0	1.6	1.4	0.3
Breast, Joint, Lemon & Pepper Basted, Tesco*	¼ Pack/132g	238	14.8	180	19.7	0.0	11.2	0.0
Breast, Joint, Raw, Average	1 Serving/125g	134	2.6	108	21.3	0.7	2.1	0.6
Breast, Joint, with Sage & Onion Stuffing, Waitrose*	1 Serving/325g	377	13.3	116	19.2	1.4	4.1	0.1

TURKEY

INFO/WEIGHT	Measure	per Measure KCAL	FAT	Nutrition Values per 100g / 100ml KCAL	PROT	CARB	FAT	FIBRE
Breast, Raw, Average	1oz/28g	33	0.6	117	24.1	0.5	2.0	0.1
Breast, Roasted, Average	1oz/28g	37	0.9	131	24.6	0.7	3.3	0.1
Breast, Roll, Cooked, Average	1 Slice/10g	9	0.1	92	17.6	3.5	0.8	0.0
Breast, Slices, Cooked, Average	1 Slice/20g	23	0.3	114	24.1	1.2	1.4	0.3
Breast, Smoked, Sliced, Average	1 Slice/20g	23	0.4	113	23.4	0.7	2.0	0.0
Breast, Steaks, in Crumbs, Average	1 Steak/76g	217	14.1	286	13.7	16.4	18.5	0.2
Breast, Steaks, Raw, Average	1oz/28g	30	0.3	107	24.3	0.0	1.1	0.0
Breast, Steaks, Thai, Bernard Matthews*	1 Serving/175g	280	4.7	160	29.4	4.6	2.7	0.0
Breast, Strips, Chinese Style, Sainsbury's*	¼ Pack/163g	319	7.3	196	26.4	12.5	4.5	0.5
Breast, Strips, for Stir Fry, Average	1 Serving/175g	205	2.7	117	25.6	0.1	1.6	0.0
Breast, Stuffed, Just Roast, Sainsbury's*	1 Serving/100g	155	6.6	155	21.1	2.9	6.6	0.6
Dark Meat, Raw, Average	1oz/28g	29	0.7	104	20.4	0.0	2.5	0.0
Dark Meat, Roasted, Average	1oz/28g	50	1.8	177	29.4	0.0	6.6	0.0
Drummers, Golden, Bernard Matthews*	1 Drummer/57g	147	10.3	258	13.1	11.0	18.0	1.1
Drummers, Golden, Grilled, Bernard Matthews*	1 Drummer/50g	147	10.6	294	15.6	10.0	21.2	1.0
Drumsticks, Tesco*	1 Serving/200g	272	12.6	136	19.9	0.0	6.3	0.0
Escalope, Average	1 Escalope/138g	341	19.3	247	13.5	16.7	14.0	0.6
Escalope, Cheese & Leek Sauce, Bernard Matthews*	1 Escalope/141g	357	23.1	254	8.8	17.7	16.4	1.5
Escalope, Creamy Pepper Topped, Tesco*	1 Escalope/165g	337	17.7	204	11.5	15.3	10.7	1.7
Escalope, in Pepper Sauce, Bernard Matthews*	1 Escalope/143g	350	21.5	245	9.4	18.2	15.0	1.5
Escalope, Lemon & Pepper, Average	1 Escalope/143g	371	22.6	260	12.6	16.7	15.8	0.5
Escalope, Spicy Mango, Bernard Matthews*	1 Escalope/136g	354	17.4	260	11.6	24.6	12.8	0.0
Escalope, Tomato & Herb, Bernard Matthews*	1 Escalope/143g	336	19.2	236	10.5	18.0	13.5	0.0
Fillets, Chinese Marinated, Bernard Matthews*	1 Pack/200g	304	6.6	152	23.4	7.2	3.3	0.0
Goujons, Cooked, Bernard Matthews*	4 Goujons/128g	355	23.3	277	11.8	16.6	18.2	1.1
Joint, Butter Basted, Asda*	1 Serving/100g	193	8.0	193	30.0	0.2	8.0	0.2
Leg, Roast, Bernard Matthews*	1 Leg/567g	777	30.6	137	15.4	0.5	5.4	1.2
Light Meat, Raw, Average	1oz/28g	29	0.2	105	24.4	0.0	0.8	0.0
Medallions, Tomato Salsa, Morrisons*	½ Pack/125.2g	184	3.1	147	30.4	0.8	2.5	0.9
Mince, Average	1oz/28g	45	2.0	161	23.9	0.0	7.2	0.0
Mince, Free From, Sainsbury's*	1 Serving/100g	148	6.2	148	23.0	0.1	6.2	0.0
Mince, Lean, Healthy Range, Average	1oz/28g	33	1.1	118	20.3	0.0	4.1	0.0
Rashers, Average	1 Rasher/26g	26	0.4	101	19.1	2.3	1.6	0.0
Rashers, Smoked, Average	1 Serving/75g	76	1.4	101	19.8	1.5	1.8	0.0
Rashers, Unsmoked, Mattessons*	1 Rasher/25.3g	25	0.4	99	19.7	1.6	1.6	0.9
Ready to Roast, with Stuffing & Bacon, M & S*	1 Third/169g	245	10.5	145	20.2	2.1	6.2	1.1
Roast, Meat & Skin, Average	1oz/28g	48	1.8	171	28.0	0.0	6.5	0.0
Roast, Meat Only, Average	1 Serving/100g	157	3.2	157	29.9	0.0	3.2	0.0
Roast, Sugar Marinade, Slices, M & S*	½ Pack/120g	156	1.9	130	29.0	0.2	1.6	0.5
Roll, Dinosaur, Cooked, Bernard Matthews*	1 Slice/10g	17	1.0	170	13.6	6.0	10.2	1.1
Schnitzel, Lidl*	1 Schnitzel/115g	210	8.1	183	19.0	11.0	7.0	0.0
Steaks, Breaded, Bernard Matthews*	1 Steak/110g	319	20.0	290	11.0	20.5	18.2	1.5
Sticks, Honey Roast, Mini, Tesco*	1 Serving/90g	101	1.7	112	20.0	3.6	1.9	0.0
Sticks, with Nacho Cheese Dip, Tesco*	1 Serving/35g	161	16.8	459	5.5	1.5	47.9	0.0
Strips, Stir-Fried, Average	1oz/28g	46	1.3	164	31.0	0.0	4.5	0.0
Thigh, Diced, Average	1oz/28g	33	1.2	117	19.7	0.0	4.3	0.0
Thigh, Diced, Lean, BGTY, Sainsbury's*	1 Serving/200g	242	8.8	121	20.3	0.1	4.4	0.1
Thigh, Joint, Cooked, Sainsbury's*	1 Serving/150g	366	20.9	244	27.7	2.1	13.9	0.1
Tikka, Deli Fillets, Bernard Matthews*	1 Pack/130g	148	2.0	114	21.3	4.9	1.5	1.3
Wafer Thin, Cooked, Average	1 Slice/10g	12	0.4	122	19.0	3.2	3.7	0.0
Wafer Thin, Honey Roast, Average	1 Slice/10g	11	0.2	109	19.2	4.2	1.7	0.2
Wafer Thin, Smoked, Average	1 Slice/10g	12	0.4	119	18.1	3.6	3.7	0.0
Whole, Raw, Average	½ Joint/254g	389	16.8	153	22.6	0.9	6.6	0.1

T

	Measure INFO/WEIGHT	per Measure KCAL	FAT	Nutrition Values per 100g / 100ml KCAL	PROT	CARB	FAT	FIBRE
TURKEY DINNER								
Roast, Asda*	1 Pack/400g	344	6.4	86	7.0	11.0	1.6	2.0
Roast, Iceland*	1 Meal/400g	374	7.2	94	8.4	10.9	1.8	1.3
Roast, Meal for One, M & S*	1 Pack/370g	460	16.2	125	9.1	12.4	4.4	2.7
Roast, Sainsbury's*	1 Pack/450g	354	9.0	79	6.8	8.4	2.0	1.9
TURKEY HAM								
Average	1 Serving/75g	81	2.9	108	15.6	2.8	3.9	0.0
TURKEY IN								
BBQ Marinade, Steaks, Asda*	1 Serving/225g	356	5.2	158	30.0	4.4	2.3	0.9
TURKEY WITH								
Cranberry & Orange Glaze, Breast Joint, Sainsbury's*	1 Serving/180g	281	5.2	156	29.6	3.0	2.9	1.0
Sage & Onion, Breast Joint, Glazed, GFY, Asda*	1 Serving/100g	101	1.7	101	19.0	2.5	1.7	1.0
Sausagemeat, Sage & Onion Stuffing, Breast, Tesco*	1 Serving/300g	417	18.6	139	17.9	2.8	6.2	0.8
Stuffing, Breast, Cooked, Somerfield*	1oz/28g	29	0.6	104	17.0	6.0	2.0	0.0
TURKISH DELIGHT								
Assorted Flavours, Julian Graves*	1 Square/30g	110	0.0	366	0.5	91.1	0.1	0.0
Dark Chocolate Covered, Thorntons*	1 Chocolate/10g	39	1.1	390	2.7	69.0	11.0	2.0
Fry's*	1 Bar/51g	186	3.7	365	2.0	73.3	7.2	0.0
Milk Chocolate, M & S*	1 Pack/55g	220	4.7	400	1.6	79.0	8.5	0.0
Sultans*	1 Serving/16g	58	0.0	360	0.0	90.0	0.0	0.0
with Mixed Nuts, Hazer Baba*	1 Piece/12g	47	0.2	389	1.6	88.5	1.7	0.0
with Rose, Hazer Baba*	1 Square/18g	70	0.3	389	1.6	88.6	1.7	0.0
TURMERIC								
Powder	1 Tsp/3g	11	0.3	354	7.8	58.2	9.9	0.0
TURNIP								
Boiled, Average	1oz/28g	3	0.1	12	0.6	2.0	0.2	1.9
Raw, Unprepared, Average	1oz/28g	6	0.1	23	0.9	4.7	0.3	2.4
TURNOVER								
Apple, Bramley, Tesco*	1 Turnover/88g	304	22.8	346	2.7	25.4	25.9	0.9
Apple, Dutch, Sainsbury's*	1 Serving/33g	130	5.5	393	3.6	56.9	16.8	1.4
Apple, Fresh Cream, Sainsbury's*	1 Turnover/84g	292	20.9	347	4.1	26.9	24.8	2.5
Apple, Tesco*	1 Turnover/88g	294	19.7	334	3.2	29.8	22.4	0.9
Rasperry, Fresh Cream, Asda*	1 Cake/100g	411	23.0	411	6.0	45.0	23.0	2.1
TWIGLETS								
Curry, Jacob's*	1 Bag/30g	134	6.5	448	8.0	55.7	21.5	6.0
Original, Jacob's*	1 Bag/30g	117	3.2	390	12.0	61.3	10.8	11.8
TWIRL								
Cadbury*	1 Finger/22g	116	6.6	525	8.1	55.9	30.1	0.0
TWIRLS								
Salt & Vinegar, Tesco*	1 Bag/80g	349	14.0	436	3.9	65.8	17.5	2.4
TWISTS								
Black Olive & Basil, Finest, Tesco*	¼ Pack/31g	151	7.9	483	11.3	53.1	25.1	3.9
Tomato & Herb, Shapers, Boots*	1 Pack/20g	94	4.2	468	3.7	66.0	21.0	3.9
TWIX								
Fun Size, Mars*	1 Bar/21g	103	5.0	492	4.7	65.1	23.7	1.5
King Size, Master Foods*	1 Finger/42.5g	208	10.1	490	4.7	65.5	23.7	0.0
Mars*	1 Biscuit/25g	123	5.9	492	4.8	65.6	23.6	1.6
Top, Mars*	1 Bar/28g	143	7.8	511	5.2	60.2	27.7	0.0
TZATZIKI								
Average	1oz/28g	18	1.4	66	3.7	2.0	4.9	0.2
Fresh, Sainsbury's*	1oz/28g	35	3.0	126	4.0	3.7	10.6	0.3
Greek, Authentic, Total, Fage*	1 Serving/50g	50	3.5	99	4.9	4.1	7.0	1.0
Morrisons*	½ Pot/85g	82	5.4	97	3.6	6.4	6.3	0.5
Somerfield*	½ Pot/85g	108	8.0	127	5.8	4.8	9.4	1.5

T

	Measure INFO/WEIGHT	per Measure KCAL	FAT	Nutrition Values per 100g / 100ml KCAL	PROT	CARB	FAT	FIBRE
TZATZIKI								
Tesco*	½ Pack/100g	132	10.2	132	5.1	4.9	10.2	2.2
Waitrose*	1 Serving/50g	54	2.7	108	6.7	8.4	5.3	0.8

T

	Measure INFO/WEIGHT	per Measure		Nutrition Values per 100g / 100ml				
		KCAL	FAT	KCAL	PROT	CARB	FAT	FIBRE
VANILLA								
Bean, Average	1oz/28g	81	0.0	288	0.0	13.0	0.0	0.0
Flavouring, Supercook*	1 Tsp/4g	2	0.0	50	6.3	0.0	0.0	0.0
Madagascan, Extra Special, Asda*	1 Pot/150g	233	10.8	155	3.5	19.0	7.2	0.0
VANILLA EXTRACT								
Average	1 Tbsp/13g	37	0.0	288	0.1	12.7	0.1	0.0
Pure, Nielsen Massey Vanillas*	1 Tsp/5mls	8	0.0	160	0.1	39.5	0.2	0.1
VEAL								
Escalope, Fried, Average	1oz/28g	55	1.9	196	33.7	0.0	6.8	0.0
Escalopes, Breaded, M & S*	1 Escalope/130g	293	13.9	225	13.6	18.7	10.7	0.4
Mince, Raw, Average	1oz/28g	40	2.0	144	20.3	0.0	7.0	0.0
VEGEMITE								
Australian, Kraft*	1 Tsp/5g	9	0.0	173	23.5	19.7	0.0	0.0
Kraft*	1 Serving/4g	8	0.0	189	25.4	19.4	0.7	0.0
VEGETABLE ARRABIATA								
Roast, HE, Tesco*	1 Pack/450g	437	5.0	97	3.3	18.4	1.1	1.1
VEGETABLE CHIPS								
Cassava, Average	1oz/28g	99	0.1	353	1.8	91.4	0.4	4.0
Mixed Root, Tyrells*	1oz/28g	133	8.3	476	5.7	35.4	29.8	12.8
Parsnip, Golden, Kettle Chips*	½ Pack/50g	258	18.8	515	4.6	39.5	37.6	8.4
Sweet Potato, Kettle Chips*	½ Pack/50g	242	16.4	483	2.4	44.4	32.8	9.3
VEGETABLE FAT								
Pure, Trex*	1 Tbsp/12g	108	12.0	900	0.0	0.0	100.0	0.0
VEGETABLE FINGERS								
Crispy, Captain Birds Eye, Birds Eye*	1 Finger/29g	55	2.5	191	4.8	23.8	8.5	1.8
Crispy Crunchy, Dalepak*	1 Finger/28g	62	3.1	223	4.2	26.7	11.0	15.0
VEGETABLE GREEN								
M & S*	1 Serving/250g	63	1.3	25	3.0	1.8	0.5	1.8
VEGETABLE MEDLEY								
& New Potato, Asda*	½ Pack/175g	102	3.9	58	2.5	7.0	2.2	5.0
Asda*	1 Pack/300g	84	0.6	28	2.8	3.9	0.2	2.9
Classic, Waitrose*	½ Pack/125g	39	0.6	31	2.3	4.1	0.5	2.8
Crunchy, M & S*	1 Pack/250g	75	2.0	30	3.1	2.8	0.8	2.5
Frozen, M & S*	1 Pack/500g	175	4.0	35	3.4	3.9	0.8	3.1
Green, Sainsbury's*	1 Pack/220g	178	14.3	81	3.0	2.5	6.5	2.9
HL, Tesco*	1 Serving/125g	59	2.3	47	3.7	4.1	1.8	4.1
Mediterranean Style, Asda*	1 Pack/410g	226	7.4	55	1.7	8.0	1.8	1.3
Roast, Four Seasons*	1 Pack/375g	203	12.0	54	2.8	3.5	3.2	2.7
with Herby Butter, M & S*	1 Pack/300g	180	10.8	60	1.4	5.2	3.6	1.5
VEGETABLE SELECTION								
Baby, Tesco*	½ Pack/100g	25	0.4	25	1.6	3.7	0.4	1.0
Chefs, M & S*	1 Pack/250g	88	1.3	35	2.6	4.5	0.5	2.9
Fresh, Finest, Tesco*	1 Pack/250g	183	14.5	73	1.9	3.2	5.8	2.2
Garden, Tesco*	1 Pack/275g	124	9.1	45	1.2	2.7	3.3	1.2
Lightly Buttered & Seasoned, M & S*	1 Pack/300g	195	10.8	65	1.6	6.3	3.6	2.8
M & S*	1 Pack/300g	180	7.5	60	1.5	7.5	2.5	2.7
Ready to Cook, Morrisons*	1 Serving/150g	51	0.9	34	2.4	4.8	0.6	2.3
Roast, COU, M & S*	1 Serving/250g	95	2.0	38	1.2	6.1	0.8	0.6
Winter, M & S*	1 Bag/400g	80	0.0	20	2.2	3.2	0.0	3.1
Winter, Ready to Roast, Safeway*	½ Pack/175g	140	4.7	80	0.8	12.4	2.7	3.5
with Herb Butter, Waitrose*	1 Pack/300g	270	16.8	90	1.9	8.1	5.6	2.1
VEGETABLES								
& Feta Cheese, Roasted, BGTY, Sainsbury's*	1 Pack/200g	264	4.4	132	6.4	21.7	2.2	0.0
Baby, Frozen, Asda*	1 Serving/100g	25	0.3	25	1.9	3.7	0.3	1.9

V

VEGETABLES

INFO/WEIGHT	Measure	per Measure KCAL	FAT	Nutrition Values per 100g / 100ml KCAL	PROT	CARB	FAT	FIBRE
Baby Mix, Freshly Frozen, Iceland*	1 Serving/100g	26	0.3	26	1.8	3.9	0.3	1.9
Broccoli & Cauliflower, Layered, M & S*	½ Pack/135g	95	4.6	70	1.5	7.6	3.4	1.2
Chinese, Stir Fry, Tesco*	1 Pack/350g	98	0.8	28	2.3	4.3	0.2	2.1
Chinese Glazed, Tesco*	1 Pack/200g	110	4.4	55	1.3	7.7	2.2	1.2
Chinese Inspired, Crisp, M & S*	1 Pack/250g	63	0.8	25	1.7	4.6	0.3	1.9
Crispy, Ready to Cook, Sainsbury's*	1 Serving/100g	24	0.3	24	1.8	3.6	0.3	2.2
Farmhouse Mix, Frozen, Asda*	1 Serving/100g	25	0.8	25	2.5	2.2	0.8	0.0
Favourite Five Selection, M & S*	½ Pack/125g	25	0.8	20	1.8	2.4	0.6	2.9
for Roasting, M & S*	½ Pack/223.5g	190	12.5	85	1.2	7.7	5.6	2.4
Italiano Marinated, Roasted, Tesco*	½ Tub/100g	121	8.6	121	1.7	9.2	8.6	0.8
Julienne, Tesco*	1 Serving/100g	30	0.3	30	1.1	5.7	0.3	1.9
Layered, with Butter, Waitrose*	1 Pack/280g	207	16.2	74	1.7	3.6	5.8	2.4
Mediterranean, in Tomato Sauce, COU, M & S*	1 Pack/300g	105	2.1	35	2.5	4.3	0.7	2.2
Mediterranean, Ready to Roast, Waitrose*	1 Serving/200g	128	8.0	64	1.3	5.6	4.0	1.6
Mediterranean Roasted, Sainsbury's*	1 Serving/150g	119	5.4	79	2.2	9.5	3.6	3.4
Mediterranean Style, Asda*	½ Pack/205g	113	3.7	55	1.7	7.9	1.8	1.3
Mediterranean Style, COOK!, M & S*	½ Pack/200g	60	1.8	30	1.2	5.5	0.9	1.0
Mediterranean Style, Finest, Tesco*	½ Pack/150g	155	12.2	103	1.5	5.5	8.1	3.0
Mediterranean Style, Roasting, Tesco*	1 Serving/200g	72	2.0	36	1.1	5.7	1.0	1.3
Oriental Inspired, M & S*	1 Pack/260g	78	1.3	30	1.9	4.6	0.5	2.7
Oriental Stir Fry, Frozen, Sainsbury's*	½ Pack/225g	142	8.8	63	1.5	5.4	3.9	1.5
Oven Roasted, Somerfield*	1oz/28g	36	1.4	129	1.0	19.0	5.0	0.0
Ready to Roast Mediterranean, Woolworths*	1 Punnet/660g	378	31.7	57	1.9	1.6	4.8	3.2
Roast, M & S*	1 Pack/420g	273	17.6	65	1.4	4.9	4.2	0.4
Roasted, & Olive Sauce, TTD, Sainsbury's*	1 Serving/75g	42	1.8	56	1.7	6.9	2.4	2.0
Roasted, Italian, M & S*	1 Serving/95g	219	20.0	230	1.8	7.1	21.0	1.7
Roasted, Mediterranean, Tesco*	½ Pack/172.7g	95	3.1	55	1.3	7.6	1.8	2.0
Roasted, Selection, COU, M & S*	1 Pack/250g	88	2.0	35	1.2	6.1	0.8	0.6
Roasted Mediterranean, The Best*	1 Serving/125g	100	5.8	80	2.3	7.0	4.6	3.6
Roasted Root, Extra Special, Asda*	½ Pack/205g	160	3.1	78	1.1	15.0	1.5	6.0
Roasted Winter, HL, Tesco*	½ Pack/200g	160	5.0	80	1.9	12.7	2.5	3.6
Roasting, Tesco*	1 Serving/350g	152	1.9	43	1.2	8.0	0.5	3.0
Root, Honey Roast, Sainsbury's*	1 Pack/400g	748	34.8	187	0.0	25.8	8.7	5.2
Root, Ready to Roast, Sainsbury's*	½ Pack/200g	188	8.6	94	1.3	13.0	4.3	2.2
Seasonal, Pack, Sainsbury's*	1 Serving/261g	60	0.8	23	0.7	4.6	0.3	2.0
Special Mix, Sainsbury's*	1 Serving/80g	54	1.4	68	3.4	9.7	1.7	3.2
Steam & Serve, Morrisons*	1 Serving/120g	66	1.3	55	2.4	8.8	1.1	2.6
Stew Pack, Budgens*	1 Serving/80g	32	0.2	40	0.9	8.4	0.3	1.2
Stir Fry, Tesco*	1 Serving/150g	38	0.2	25	0.9	5.0	0.1	1.4
Sun Dried Tomato, Selection, Finest, Tesco*	1 Pack/340g	303	17.3	89	1.8	8.9	5.1	1.1
Sweet & Crunchy, Safeway*	1 Bag/200g	86	1.2	43	2.3	7.0	0.6	2.4
Sweet & Crunchy, Tesco*	1 Serving/50g	22	0.3	43	2.3	7.0	0.6	2.4
Sweet Summer, Safeway*	1 Serving/115g	60	0.8	52	3.7	7.8	0.7	3.5
Szechuan Style, Ready Prepared, Waitrose*	1 Pack/300g	132	3.9	44	2.3	5.7	1.3	1.9
Vietnamese, Wok, Findus*	1 Serving/100g	25	0.5	25	1.5	4.5	0.5	0.0
Winter, Fresh, Asda*	1 Bag/250g	75	2.5	30	3.0	2.2	1.0	2.3
Winter, Ready to Roast, Fresh, Sainsbury's*	1 Pack/272g	226	7.6	83	1.2	13.2	2.8	0.0
Winter, Sainsbury's*	1 Serving/125g	38	1.0	30	2.0	3.6	0.8	2.2
Winter Crunchy, M & S*	½ Pack/125g	31	1.0	25	2.0	3.1	0.8	2.7
Winter Selection, Somerfield*	1 Pack/250g	90	2.0	36	2.6	4.7	0.8	3.0
with Sun Dried Tomato, Roasted, Finest, Tesco*	½ Pack/150g	153	10.8	102	1.9	7.3	7.2	1.2
Wok, Chinese, Stir Fry, Classic, Findus*	1 Pack/500g	150	2.5	30	1.0	5.0	0.5	3.5
Wok, Sambal Oelek, Findus*	1 Serving/200g	170	0.8	85	3.0	17.0	0.4	0.0

	Measure INFO/WEIGHT	per Measure KCAL	per Measure FAT	Nutrition Values per 100g / 100ml KCAL	PROT	CARB	FAT	FIBRE
VEGETARIAN								
Chicken Style Pieces, Sainsbury's*	1 Pack/375g	754	26.3	201	25.5	9.0	7.0	0.6
VEGETARIAN MINCE								
Meat Free, Asda*	1oz/28g	49	1.2	176	27.0	7.0	4.4	4.1
Vegemince, Realeat*	1 Serving/125g	218	12.5	174	18.0	3.0	10.0	3.0
VENISON								
Grill Steak, Average	1 Grillsteak/150g	179	3.8	119	19.0	5.0	2.5	1.0
Roasted, Average	1oz/28g	46	0.7	165	35.6	0.0	2.5	0.0
Steak, Raw, Average	1oz/28g	30	0.5	108	22.8	0.0	1.9	0.0
VENISON IN								
Red Wine & Port, Average	1oz/28g	21	0.7	76	9.8	3.5	2.6	0.4
VERMICELLI								
Dry	1oz/28g	99	0.1	355	8.7	78.3	0.4	0.0
Egg, Cooked, Average	1 Serving/185g	239	2.6	129	5.0	24.0	1.4	1.0
VERMOUTH								
Dry	1 Shot/50ml	55	0.0	109	0.1	3.0	0.0	0.0
Sweet	1 Shot/50ml	76	0.0	151	0.0	15.9	0.0	0.0
VIMTO*								
Cordial, No Added Sugar, Diluted	1 Glass/250ml	6	0.3	2	0.1	0.4	0.1	0.0
Cordial, Original, Diluted	1 Serving/200ml	60	0.0	30	0.0	7.4	0.0	0.0
Grape, Blackcurrant & Raspberry Juice Drink, Fizzy	1 Can/330ml	147	0.0	45	0.0	11.0	0.0	0.0
VINAIGRETTE								
Balsamic, Newman's Own*	1 Serving/20g	67	7.0	333	0.5	3.9	35.0	0.0
Balsamic Vinegar & Pistachio, Finest, Tesco*	1 Tbsp/15ml	56	5.9	370	0.2	2.8	39.2	0.0
French, Real, Briannas*	2 Tbsp/30ml	150	17.0	500	0.0	0.0	56.7	0.0
French Style, Finest, Tesco*	1 Tbsp/15ml	93	9.8	620	0.6	6.3	65.3	0.2
Light, Hellmann's*	1 Serving/15ml	7	0.0	49	0.1	10.9	0.0	0.3
Luxury French, Hellmann's*	1 Tsp/5ml	15	1.3	305	0.8	16.0	26.1	0.4
Olive Oil & Lemon, Amoy*	½ Sachet/15ml	38	3.6	250	0.3	3.0	24.0	0.0
Paul Newman, Newman's Own*	1 Tbsp/20ml	68	7.3	340	0.5	4.0	36.5	0.0
Waistline, 99% Fat Free, Crosse & Blackwell*	1 Tbsp/15ml	1	0.0	9	1.0	0.7	0.2	0.2
with Mustard, Delhaize*	1 Serving/20g	93	10.2	464	0.8	0.7	50.9	0.0
VINE LEAVES								
Preserved in Brine	1oz/28g	4	0.0	15	3.6	0.2	0.0	0.0
Stuffed, Mediterranean Deli, M & S*	1 Leaf/37g	39	1.5	105	2.6	14.2	4.1	1.2
Stuffed, Sainsbury's*	1 Parcel/37.5g	47	2.1	124	2.9	15.3	5.7	3.1
Stuffed with Rice	1oz/28g	73	5.0	262	2.8	23.8	18.0	0.0
Stuffed with Rice, Dolmades, M & S*	1 Leaf/38.1g	40	1.6	105	2.6	14.2	4.1	1.2
Stuffed with Rice & Mixed Herbs, Sainsbury's*	1 Leaf/36.7g	44	1.8	120	2.6	16.3	4.9	1.2
VINEGAR								
Balsamic	1 Tsp/5ml	0	0.0	3	0.3	0.6	0.0	0.0
Balsamic, M & S*	1 Tbsp/20g	24	0.0	120	0.9	29.1	0.0	0.3
Balsamic, of Modena, Asda*	1 Tbsp/15ml	16	0.0	109	0.4	27.0	0.1	0.0
Balsamic, of Modena, Monari Federzoni*	1 Tsp/5ml	3	0.0	69	0.6	16.0	0.0	0.0
Balsamic, of Modena, TTD, Sainsbury's*	1 Tbsp/15ml	18	0.3	120	2.0	25.0	2.0	2.0
Malt	1 Tbsp/15g	1	0.0	4	0.4	0.6	0.0	0.0
Rice, White, Amoy*	1 Tsp/5ml	0	0.0	4	0.0	1.0	0.0	0.0
VODKA								
37.5% Volume	1 Pub Shot/35ml	72	0.0	207	0.0	0.0	0.0	0.0
40% Volume	1 Shot/35ml	78	0.0	222	0.0	0.0	0.0	0.0
VOL AU VENTS								
Broccoli, M & S*	1oz/28g	105	7.4	375	6.8	28.5	26.4	1.0
Chicken & Mushroom, M & S*	1oz/28g	98	6.8	350	7.7	25.2	24.3	2.1
Garlic Mushroom, Mini, Asda*	1 Serving/17g	59	4.6	347	5.0	21.0	27.0	0.0

V

VOL AU VENTS	Measure INFO/WEIGHT	per Measure KCAL	per Measure FAT	Nutrition Values per 100g / 100ml KCAL	PROT	CARB	FAT	FIBRE
Ham & Cheese, M & S*	1oz/28g	106	7.5	380	8.8	25.7	26.7	1.8
Mushroom, Sainsbury's*	1 Serving/14g	49	3.1	350	6.9	30.8	22.1	1.4
Mushroom & Roast Garlic, M & S*	1 Serving/19g	65	4.6	345	6.2	25.2	24.3	1.9
Prawn, M & S*	1oz/28g	101	6.9	360	8.0	26.2	24.7	1.9
Seafood, Party, Youngs*	1 Serving/17g	60	4.2	354	8.3	26.0	24.8	1.0
Tomato, M & S*	1oz/28g	87	5.7	310	4.5	26.7	20.4	1.7

	Measure INFO/WEIGHT	per Measure		Nutrition Values per 100g / 100ml				
		KCAL	FAT	KCAL	PROT	CARB	FAT	FIBRE
WAFERS								
Cafe Curls, Rolled, Askeys*	1 Curl/5g	21	0.4	422	5.8	80.3	8.6	0.0
Caramel, Dark Chocolate, Tunnock's*	1 Wafer/26g	128	6.6	492	5.2	60.7	25.4	0.0
Caramel, M & S*	1oz/28g	136	6.6	486	5.4	63.1	23.5	0.5
Caramel, Milk Chocolate, M & S*	1oz/28g	133	6.4	475	5.9	61.9	22.8	3.1
Caramel, Milk Chocolate Coated, Value, Tesco*	1 Bar/23.1g	109	4.6	475	5.6	67.6	20.2	0.6
Caramel, Tunnock's*	1 Biscuit/26g	118	5.2	454	4.6	68.0	20.1	0.0
Caramel Log, Tunnock's*	1 Biscuit/32g	152	7.7	474	4.2	64.3	24.0	0.0
Chocolate, Cadbury*	1oz/28g	147	8.3	526	7.0	61.2	29.8	0.0
Chocolate Curl, Mini, M & S*	1 Biscuit/4.7g	25	1.4	530	6.5	57.0	30.6	3.2
Cream, Tunnock's*	1 Biscuit/20g	103	5.6	513	6.6	63.2	28.0	0.0
for Ice Cream, Askeys*	2 Wafers/3g	12	0.1	388	11.4	79.0	2.9	0.0
Hazelnut, Elledi*	2 Biscuits/15.6g	77	3.8	493	6.3	62.4	24.3	0.0
Orange, Highlights, Cadbury*	1 Wafer/19g	80	2.7	430	5.2	70.6	14.3	1.4
WAFFLES								
Belgian, TTD, Sainsbury's*	1 Waffle/25.1g	123	7.4	490	6.0	50.6	29.3	1.2
Sweet, American Style, Sainsbury's*	1 Waffle/35.0g	160	8.9	457	7.2	50.6	25.3	1.1
Toasting, McVitie's*	1 Waffle/24.9g	118	6.3	474	6.0	52.6	25.5	0.6
WAGON WHEEL								
Chocolate, Burton's*	1 Wheel/39g	165	5.7	424	5.3	67.4	14.6	1.9
Jammie, Burton's*	1 Biscuit/40g	168	5.6	420	5.1	67.7	14.1	1.9
WALNUT WHIP								
Nestle*	1 Whip/35g	173	8.8	494	5.3	61.3	25.2	0.7
Vanilla, Nestle*	1 Whip/34g	160	8.1	486	5.7	60.5	24.6	0.0
WALNUTS								
Average	6 Halves/20g	138	13.7	691	15.6	3.2	68.5	3.5
WASABI								
Paste, Ready Mixed, Japanese, Yutaka*	1 Tsp/5g	14	0.4	286	2.7	53.0	7.0	0.0
WATER								
Berry Blast, Revive, Volvic*	1 Bottle/500ml	10	0.0	2	0.3	0.4	0.0	0.0
Blackcurrants, Juicy, Innocent*	1 Bottle/420ml	155	0.4	37	0.1	8.7	0.1	0.0
Cranberries & Raspberries, Juicy, Innocent*	1 Bottle/380ml	118	1.1	31	0.1	6.7	0.3	0.0
Cranberry & Blueberry, Lightly Sparkling, Waitrose*	1 Glass/250mls	10	0.0	4	0.0	0.7	0.0	0.0
Elderflower Presse, Bottle Green*	1 Serving/250ml	88	0.0	35	0.0	8.9	0.0	0.0
Grapefruit, Slightly Sparkling, Tesco*	1 Serving/200ml	4	0.0	2	0.0	0.2	0.0	0.0
Lemon, Vittel*	1 Bottle/500ml	6	0.0	1	0.0	0.0	0.0	0.0
Lemon & Lime, Sugar Free, Touch of Fruit, Volvic*	1 Bottle/150ml	2	0.0	1	0.0	0.0	0.0	0.0
Mineral Or Tap	1 Glass/200ml	0	0.0	0	0.0	0.0	0.0	0.0
Peach & Raspberry, Still, M & S*	1 Bottle/500ml	10	0.0	2	0.0	0.0	0.0	0.0
Raspberry & Apple, Still, Shapers, Boots*	1 Serving/250ml	10	0.0	4	0.0	0.8	0.0	0.0
Skinny, Bo-Synergy*	1 Bottle/500ml	9	0.0	2	0.0	0.3	0.0	0.0
Spring, Apple & Blackcurrant, Hadrian*	1 Bottle/365ml	3	0.0	1	0.1	0.1	0.0	0.0
Spring, Apple & Mango, Sparkling, Asda*	1 Glass/200ml	2	0.0	1	0.0	0.2	0.0	0.0
Spring, Apple & Raspberry, Shapers, Boots*	1 Bottle/500ml	10	0.0	2	0.0	0.2	0.0	0.0
Spring, Apple & Raspberry, Sparkling, Tesco*	1 Glass/330ml	7	0.0	2	0.0	0.5	0.0	0.0
Spring, Apple & Raspberry Flavoured, Sainsbury's*	1 fl oz/30ml	1	0.0	2	0.1	0.1	0.1	0.1
Spring, Elderflower & Pear, Sainsbury's*	1 Glass/250g	5	0.3	2	0.1	0.2	0.1	0.1
Spring, Lemon & Lime, Slightly Sparkling, Tesco*	1 Serving/200ml	4	0.2	2	0.1	0.2	0.1	0.1
Spring, Peach Flavour, Sparkling, Co-Op*	1 Glass/250ml	2	0.0	1	0.0	0.0	0.0	0.0
Spring, Peach Flavoured, No Added Sugar, Asda*	1 Glass/200ml	4	0.0	2	0.0	0.2	0.0	0.0
Spring, Strawberry & Aloe Vera, Botanical, M & S*	1 Bottle/500ml	5	0.0	1	0.0	0.2	0.0	0.0
Spring, Strawberry & Kiwi, Still, Shapers, Boots*	1 Glass/250ml	3	0.0	1	0.0	0.1	0.0	0.9
Spring, White Grape & Blackberry, Tesco*	1 Glass/200ml	4	0.0	2	0.0	0.5	0.0	0.0
Spring, with Grapefruit, Tesco*	1 Serving/200ml	4	0.0	2	0.0	0.2	0.0	0.0

W

	Measure	per Measure		Nutrition Values per 100g / 100ml				
	INFO/WEIGHT	KCAL	FAT	KCAL	PROT	CARB	FAT	FIBRE
WATER								
Strawberry & Guava, Still, M & S*	1 Glass/250ml	5	0.0	2	0.0	0.1	0.0	0.0
WATER CHESTNUTS								
Raw, Average	1oz/28g	10	0.0	34	1.0	7.8	0.1	0.1
with Bamboo Shoots, Sainsbury's*	1 Serving/50g	29	0.1	58	2.0	12.0	0.2	1.1
WATER ICE								
Raspberry, Iceland*	1 Ice/75ml	67	0.0	89	0.0	22.2	0.0	0.2
WATERMELON								
Flesh Only, Average	1 Serving/250g	75	0.8	30	0.4	7.0	0.3	0.4
WHEAT BRAN								
Average	1 Tbsp/7g	14	0.4	206	14.1	26.8	5.5	36.4
Coarse, Holland & Barrett*	1 Tbsp/4g	8	0.2	206	14.1	26.8	5.5	36.4
Natural, Jordans*	2 Tbsp/20g	38	1.2	188	16.3	17.4	5.9	44.5
WHEAT CRUNCHIES								
Crispy Bacon, KP Snacks*	1 Pack/30g	151	8.1	502	9.2	55.4	27.0	2.4
Golden Wonder*	1 Pack/35g	172	8.7	491	11.1	55.9	24.8	0.0
Salt & Vinegar, Golden Wonder*	1 Bag/34g	165	8.5	484	10.5	54.5	24.9	2.8
Spicy Tomato, KP Snacks*	1 Bag/30g	151	8.1	502	9.0	55.8	26.9	2.5
Worcester Sauce, Golden Wonder*	1 Bag/35g	172	8.9	492	9.3	56.4	25.5	3.9
WHEAT GERM								
Average	1oz/28g	100	2.6	357	26.7	44.7	9.2	15.6
Natural, Jordans*	2 Tbsp/16g	54	1.5	340	28.0	36.0	9.3	13.1
WHELKS								
Boiled	1oz/28g	25	0.3	89	19.5	0.0	1.2	0.0
WHISKEY								
37.5% Volume	1 Pub Shot/35ml	72	0.0	207	0.0	0.0	0.0	0.0
40% Volume	1 Pub Shot/35ml	78	0.0	222	0.0	0.0	0.0	0.0
Jack Daniel's*	1 Pub Shot/35ml	78	0.0	222	0.0	0.0	0.0	0.0
Teacher's*	1 Pub Shot/35ml	78	0.0	222	0.0	0.0	0.0	0.0
WHISKY								
Scotch, 37.5% Volume	1 Pub Shot/35ml	72	0.0	207	0.0	0.0	0.0	0.0
Scotch, 40% Volume	1 Pub Shot/35ml	78	0.0	222	0.0	0.0	0.0	0.0
WHITE PUDDING								
Average	1oz/28g	126	8.9	450	7.0	36.3	31.8	0.0
WHITEBAIT								
in Flour, Fried	1oz/28g	147	13.3	525	19.5	5.3	47.5	0.2
WHITECURRANTS								
Raw, Average	1oz/28g	7	0.0	26	1.3	5.6	0.0	3.4
WHITING								
in Crumbs, Fried in Blended Oil	1 Serving/180g	344	18.5	191	18.1	7.0	10.3	0.2
Raw	1oz/28g	23	0.2	81	18.7	0.0	0.7	0.0
Steamed	1 Serving/85g	78	0.8	92	20.9	0.0	0.9	0.0
WIENER SCHNITZEL								
Average	1oz/28g	62	2.8	223	20.9	13.1	10.0	0.4
WINE								
Cherry, Lambrini*	100ml	64	0.0	64	0.0	0.0	0.0	0.0
Diet, Lambrini*	100ml	35	0.0	35	0.0	0.0	0.0	0.0
Elderberry & Lemon, Ame*	1 Glass/350mls	130	0.0	37	0.0	6.4	0.0	0.0
Fruit, Average	100ml	92	0.0	92	0.0	5.5	0.0	0.0
Grape & Apricot, Ame*	1 Serving/100ml	39	1.0	39	1.3	6.7	1.0	0.0
Mulled, Homemade, Average	1 Glass/120ml	227	0.0	196	0.1	25.2	0.0	0.0
Mulled, Sainsbury's*	1 Serving/125ml	113	0.0	90	0.0	8.6	0.0	0.0
Original, Lambrini*	1 Glass/100ml	70	0.0	70	0.0	0.0	0.0	0.0
Red, Average	1 Glass/120ml	80	0.0	68	0.1	0.2	0.0	0.0

W

INFO/WEIGHT	Measure	per Measure		Nutrition Values per 100g / 100ml				
		KCAL	FAT	KCAL	PROT	CARB	FAT	FIBRE

WINE
Red, Non Alcoholic, Ame*	1 Glass/100ml	34	0.0	34	0.0	5.7	0.0	0.0
Rose, Medium, Average	1 Glass/120ml	83	0.0	71	0.1	2.5	0.0	0.0
Rose, White Zinfandel, Ernest & Julio Gallo*	1 Glass/125ml	89	0.0	71	0.0	0.0	0.0	0.0
Sparkling, Alcohol Free, Sainsbury's*	1 Glass/175ml	35	0.0	20	0.0	4.9	0.0	0.0
White, Dry, Average	1 Glass/120ml	77	0.0	66	0.1	0.6	0.0	0.0
White, Medium, Average	1 Glass/120ml	87	0.0	74	0.1	3.0	0.0	0.0
White, Non Alcoholic, Ame*	1 Glass/120ml	46	0.0	38	0.0	9.5	0.0	0.0
White, Sparkling, Average	1 Glass/120ml	87	0.0	74	0.3	5.1	0.0	0.0
White, Sweet, Average	1 Glass/120ml	110	0.0	94	0.2	5.9	0.0	0.0

WINE GUMS
Co-Op*	1 Sweet/6g	20	0.0	337	3.5	80.8	0.0	0.0
Haribo*	1 Pack/175g	609	0.4	348	0.1	86.4	0.2	0.4
Maynards*	1 Gum/6.2g	20	0.0	325	5.8	74.2	0.6	0.0
Mini, Rowntree's*	1 Sm Bag/36g	125	0.0	348	6.7	80.5	0.0	0.0
Sainsbury's*	1 Sweet/6.1g	19	0.0	314	7.7	70.3	0.2	0.0
SmartPrice, Asda*	1 Sweet/6.0g	20	0.0	332	4.0	79.0	0.0	0.0
Sour, Bassett's*	¼ Bag/50g	160	0.0	319	3.7	78.0	0.0	0.0

WINKLES
Boiled	1oz/28g	20	0.3	72	15.4	0.0	1.2	0.0

WISPA
Cadbury*	1 Bar/40g	210	12.9	525	6.8	53.0	32.3	0.8

WONTON
Prawn, Dim Sum Selection, Sainsbury's*	1 Wonton/10g	26	1.2	259	11.3	26.8	11.8	1.3
Prawn, Oriental Selection, Waitrose*	1 Wonton/17.9g	45	2.0	252	9.1	29.2	11.0	1.1
Prawn, Oriental Snack Selection, Sainsbury's*	1 Wonton/20g	53	2.7	265	10.6	25.6	13.4	2.0

WOTSITS
BBQ, Walkers*	1 Bag/21g	108	6.3	515	4.5	57.0	30.0	1.3
Flamin' Hot, Walkers*	1 Bag/19g	99	5.7	520	5.0	57.0	30.0	1.2
Prawn Cocktail, Walkers*	1 Pack/21g	111	6.5	530	5.5	57.0	31.0	1.1
Really Cheesy, Walkers*	1 Bag/18g	95	5.8	545	5.5	56.0	33.0	1.1

WRAP
All Day Breakfast, M & S*	1 Pack/196g	529	31.4	270	10.8	21.2	16.0	1.4
American Deli, Shapers, Boots*	1 Pack/171.7g	249	4.5	145	9.5	21.0	2.6	2.0
Aromatic Duck, Safeway*	1 Pack/180g	376	17.5	209	9.1	21.3	9.7	1.6
BBQ Steak, M & S*	1 Pack/261g	535	20.9	205	10.5	22.6	8.0	1.8
Beef Fajita, Boots*	1 Pack/200g	352	8.4	176	9.5	25.5	4.2	3.2
Bombay Potato, Whistlestop*	1 Wrap/180g	343	15.0	191	4.2	24.7	8.3	0.3
Brie & Cranberry, M & S*	1 Pack/224.5g	549	27.8	245	6.1	27.3	12.4	1.7
Cajun, GFY, Asda*	1 Pack/176.3g	231	2.1	131	9.0	21.0	1.2	0.9
Cajun Chicken, Sandwich King*	1 Pack/138.2g	386	19.8	279	12.3	25.1	14.4	0.0
Cajun Chicken Pizzatilla, M & S*	1 Pack/228.6g	560	28.3	245	12.1	21.0	12.4	1.9
Chargrilled Chicken, PB, Waitrose*	1 Pack/230g	361	6.7	157	10.3	22.7	2.9	2.9
Cheese & Bean, Tesco*	1 Pack/105g	235	9.5	224	7.0	28.6	9.0	1.0
Chicken, Barbecue, Shapers, Boots*	1 Pack/196.4g	271	3.5	138	15.0	16.0	1.8	3.5
Chicken, Cheddar & Peppers, Cajun, Sainsbury's*	1 Pack/242g	535	26.6	221	10.4	19.8	11.0	2.1
Chicken, Eat Smart, Safeway*	1 Pack/153g	230	2.9	150	12.5	19.7	1.9	2.0
Chicken, M & S*	1 Pack/246.5g	531	24.9	215	8.2	23.4	10.1	1.6
Chicken, Mediterranean Style, Waitrose*	1 Pack/182.7g	296	11.0	162	8.3	18.6	6.0	2.3
Chicken, Mexican Style, Co-Op*	1 Pack/163g	367	14.7	225	11.0	26.0	9.0	3.0
Chicken, Moroccan, BGTY, Sainsbury's*	1 Pack/207.2g	315	3.1	152	9.4	25.3	1.5	0.0
Chicken, Morrocan, Shapers, Boots*	1 Serving/154g	251	2.3	163	10.0	27.0	1.5	1.9
Chicken, Salsa, Light Choices, Tesco*	1 Pack/219.4g	340	5.9	155	9.7	22.6	2.7	1.9
Chicken, Southern Fried, Fresh for You, Tesco*	1 Pack/206.4g	485	24.4	235	8.6	22.7	11.8	2.0

W

WRAP

	Measure INFO/WEIGHT	per Measure KCAL	per Measure FAT	Nutrition Values per 100g / 100ml KCAL	PROT	CARB	FAT	FIBRE
Chicken, Thai, Spiced, Salad, Eat Well, M & S*	1 Pack/122g	92	1.5	75	5.2	9.5	1.2	1.5
Chicken & Bacon, Simple Solutions, Tesco*	1 Pack/300g	474	23.4	158	20.7	1.2	7.8	0.5
Chicken & Bacon Caesar, COU, M & S*	1 Pack/170g	260	4.2	153	10.7	22.0	2.5	2.1
Chicken & Bacon Caesar Salad, Asda*	1 Pack/160g	565	35.2	353	18.0	20.8	22.0	0.9
Chicken Caesar, COU, M & S*	1 Pack/168.8g	270	3.5	160	9.3	26.0	2.1	1.2
Chicken Caesar, Delicious, Boots*	1 Pack/217.3g	402	14.6	185	14.0	17.0	6.7	3.8
Chicken Caesar, Good Intentions, Somerfield*	1 Pack/184g	357	7.9	194	13.0	25.7	4.3	1.1
Chicken Caesar, HE, Tesco*	1 Pack/170g	296	4.0	174	12.0	26.2	2.4	2.6
Chicken Caesar, HL, Tesco*	1 Pack/200g	296	4.0	148	10.2	22.3	2.0	2.2
Chicken Caesar, M & S*	1 Pack/221g	519	21.4	235	12.0	24.9	9.7	1.6
Chicken Caesar, Tesco*	1 Pack/214g	503	25.7	235	10.6	21.3	12.0	1.3
Chicken Fajita, Asda*	1 Pack/180g	369	16.9	205	9.4	20.6	9.4	0.4
Chicken Fajita, Daily Bread*	1 Pack/191g	392	10.5	205	9.4	29.4	5.5	0.0
Chicken Fajita, Eat Smart, Morrisons*	1 Pack/176g	264	4.2	150	9.7	22.4	2.4	1.6
Chicken Fajita, Finest, Tesco*	1 Pack/213g	422	15.6	198	9.0	24.0	7.3	1.9
Chicken Fajita, PB, Waitrose*	1 Serving/218g	368	5.7	169	10.5	26.0	2.6	1.9
Chicken Fajita, Shapers, Boots*	1 Pack/215.6g	291	5.2	135	14.0	15.0	2.4	3.1
Chicken Fajita, Tesco*	1 Pack/220g	407	11.7	185	10.6	23.2	5.3	1.8
Chicken Fillet with Cheese & Bacon, Asda*	1 Pack/164.1g	366	21.3	223	25.0	1.4	13.0	0.0
Chicken Nacho, HL, Tesco*	1 Pack/222.9g	390	10.0	175	12.3	21.2	4.5	2.6
Chicken Salad, Roast, Sainsbury's*	1 Pack/214g	443	19.9	207	10.0	20.9	9.3	2.5
Chicken Southern Style, Ginsters*	1 Pack/150g	290	9.6	193	9.5	25.1	6.4	0.8
Chicken Thai Style, Boots*	1 Pack/156g	290	10.0	186	11.0	21.0	6.4	2.2
Chicken Tikka, Finest, Tesco*	1 Pack/227g	402	14.3	177	5.1	24.9	6.3	2.0
Chicken Tikka, Ginsters*	1 Pack/150g	278	8.0	185	8.9	25.5	5.3	1.6
Chicken Tikka, HL, Tesco*	1 Pack/206g	317	4.7	154	11.3	22.1	2.3	1.3
Chicken Tikka, Shaw & Lisle*	1 Pack/195g	311	6.1	159	9.4	18.2	3.1	0.0
Chicken Tikka Masala, Patak's*	1 Pack/150g	252	9.9	168	7.8	19.3	6.6	0.0
Chinese Chicken, Asda*	1 Pack/200g	404	12.0	202	9.0	28.0	6.0	0.0
Coronation Chicken, Waitrose*	1 Pack/163.6g	284	8.4	173	10.1	21.3	5.1	2.2
Cous Cous, Moroccan Style, Tesco*	1 Serving/240g	370	6.5	154	5.3	27.3	2.7	1.3
Crayfish & Rocket, HL, Tesco*	1 Pack/163.6g	270	5.1	165	7.5	25.9	3.1	1.9
Dhansak Prawn, M & S*	1 Pack/208.1g	385	15.0	185	7.1	23.3	7.2	2.4
Duck, Food to Go, M & S*	1 Pack/257g	474	13.8	185	8.5	25.5	5.4	1.0
Duck, Hoi Sin, Delicious, Boots*	1 Pack/214g	393	10.9	184	10.0	25.0	5.1	1.8
Duck, Hoisin, COU, M & S*	1 Pack/180g	270	3.8	150	10.8	22.0	2.1	2.4
Duck, Hoisin, Nutritionally Balanced, M & S*	1 Pack/220g	385	8.1	175	10.3	25.3	3.7	1.8
Egg Mayonnaise, Tomato & Cress, Sainsbury's*	1 Pack/255g	592	38.3	232	7.3	17.7	15.0	0.0
Feta Cheese Flat Bread, COU, M & S*	1 Pack/180g	225	4.0	125	6.3	20.6	2.2	1.9
Goats Cheese & Tomato, TTD, Sainsbury's*	1 Pack/204g	420	17.1	206	7.0	25.6	8.4	0.0
Greek Feta Salad, Shapers, Boots*	1 Pack/157.5g	242	5.7	153	6.4	24.0	3.6	1.2
Greek Salad, Sainsbury's*	1 Pack/167g	242	6.2	145	6.7	21.2	3.7	1.8
Ham, Cheese & Pickle Tortilla, Weight Watchers*	1 Pack/170.1g	296	4.8	174	10.9	26.4	2.8	1.2
Hoisin Duck, Tesco*	1 Pack/218.9g	405	12.9	185	9.1	22.9	5.9	2.4
Houmous & Chargrilled Vegetables, Shapers, Boots*	1 Pack/192.3g	250	4.6	130	7.6	20.0	2.4	3.3
King Prawn, Shapers, Boots*	1 Pack/154.4g	226	2.2	147	9.2	24.0	1.4	2.1
Mexican Bean, BGTY, Sainsbury's*	1 Pack/216g	341	5.3	158	9.2	24.9	2.5	1.5
Mexican Chicken, M & S*	1 Serving/218g	447	22.5	205	8.6	19.7	10.3	1.3
Mexican Sweet Potato & Three Bean, M & S*	1 Pack/250g	550	26.8	220	6.2	24.8	10.7	2.1
Mexican Three Bean, M & S*	1 Pack/246.8g	580	27.2	235	7.6	26.4	11.0	1.4
Monterey Jack & Ham, Tesco*	1 Pack/200g	522	28.2	261	7.9	25.9	14.1	0.2
Nacho Chicken, COU, M & S*	1 Wrap/183.9g	285	4.8	155	11.2	21.2	2.6	3.1
Peking Duck, Asda*	1 Pack/172g	427	18.4	248	9.4	28.5	10.7	1.1

WRAP

Measure INFO/WEIGHT	per Measure KCAL	per Measure FAT	Nutrition Values per 100g / 100ml KCAL	PROT	CARB	FAT	FIBRE
WRAP							
Peking Duck, Finest, Tesco* — 1 Pack/200g	378	8.4	189	8.4	29.5	4.2	0.3
Peking Duck, Waitrose* — 1 Pack/182g	319	6.4	175	10.0	25.9	3.5	1.6
Piri Piri Chicken, Burger King* — 1 Wrap/225g	348	4.0	155	11.6	23.1	1.8	1.3
Red Thai Chicken, BGTY, Sainsbury's* — 1 Pack/194g	384	7.6	198	11.3	29.3	3.9	1.0
Roasted Vegetable & Feta, BGTY, Sainsbury's* — 1 Serving/200g	318	8.0	159	5.8	25.0	4.0	0.0
Sausage & Bacon, Asda* — 1 Wrap/25g	63	4.2	252	15.9	9.0	16.9	1.3
Sicilian Lemon & Roasted Vegetable, COU, M & S* — 1 Pack/177.8g	240	3.7	135	4.9	23.8	2.1	1.9
Smoked Salmon, Finest, Tesco* — 1 Pack/58g	113	8.4	194	15.5	0.6	14.4	0.3
Smoked Salmon & Prawn, Finest, Tesco* — 1 Serving/58.5g	84	5.4	143	14.3	1.0	9.1	0.0
Sushi Salmon & Cucumber, Waitrose* — 1 Pack/180g	299	6.5	166	6.3	27.2	3.6	1.6
Sweet & Sour Prawn, Eat Smart, Safeway* — 1 Pack/204g	275	2.4	135	6.4	24.0	1.2	1.4
Sweet Chili Chicken, Waitrose* — 1 Pack/200g	390	14.7	195	10.3	22.0	7.4	2.4
Sweet Chilli Chicken, Shapers, Boots* — 1 Pack/194.6g	290	3.5	149	13.0	20.0	1.8	3.7
Tandoori Chicken, GFY, Asda* — 1 Pack/167g	281	4.5	168	10.0	26.0	2.7	1.7
Thai Prawn, COU, M & S* — 1 Pack/181g	235	2.9	130	8.3	20.4	1.6	1.9
Tortilla, Chicken, Asda* — 1 Pack/125g	253	2.3	202	9.6	36.9	1.8	3.3
Tortilla, Chicken Fajita, Sutherland* — 1 Pack/158g	379	14.2	240	13.0	27.0	9.0	0.0
Tortilla, Vegetable, Asda* — 1 Pack/125g	245	2.8	196	6.8	37.2	2.2	0.8
Tuna, Sweetcorn & Red Pepper, BGTY, Sainsbury's* — 1 Pack/178g	306	8.2	172	11.5	21.2	4.6	2.1
Tuna Crunch, BGTY, Sainsbury's* — 1 Wrap/260g	364	9.6	140	8.8	17.8	3.7	2.4
Tuna Nicoise, BGTY, Sainsbury's* — 1 Pack/181g	273	7.1	151	11.0	18.0	3.9	0.0
Tuna Nicoise, HE, Tesco* — 1 Pack/117g	160	2.7	137	8.3	20.6	2.3	0.5
Turkey, Bacon & Cranberry, COU, M & S* — 1 Pack/143.8g	230	2.2	160	9.6	27.1	1.5	2.3
Yellow Thai Prawn, COU, M & S* — 1 Pack/171.4g	266	5.0	155	7.6	23.4	2.9	1.7
WRAP KIT							
Moroccan Style, Sainsbury's* — 1 Wrap/62g	205	9.3	332	8.0	41.1	15.1	3.6

	Measure INFO/WEIGHT	per Measure KCAL	FAT	Nutrition Values per 100g / 100ml KCAL	PROT	CARB	FAT	FIBRE
YAM								
Baked	1oz/28g	43	0.1	153	2.1	37.5	0.4	1.7
Boiled, Average	1oz/28g	37	0.1	133	1.7	33.0	0.3	1.4
Raw	1oz/28g	32	0.1	114	1.5	28.2	0.3	1.3
YEAST								
Bakers, Compressed	1oz/28g	15	0.1	53	11.4	1.1	0.4	0.0
Dried, Average	1 Tbsp/6g	10	0.1	169	35.6	3.5	1.5	0.0
Extract	1 Tsp/9g	16	0.0	180	40.7	3.5	0.4	0.0
YOGHURT								
0.1% Fat, Lidl*	1 Pot/150g	119	0.2	79	4.0	15.6	0.1	0.0
Activia, Danone*	1 Pot/132g	125	4.2	94	3.5	12.8	3.2	2.0
Adore Vanilla with Choc Flakes, Ehrmann*	1 Pot/150g	215	10.5	143	3.1	17.0	7.0	0.0
Apple, Light, Muller*	1 Pot/200g	108	0.2	54	4.4	9.0	0.1	0.0
Apple & Blackberry, Bio, Sainsbury's*	1 Pot/125g	134	3.4	107	4.1	16.6	2.7	0.2
Apple & Blackberry, Custard Style, Co-Op*	1 Pot/150g	195	8.0	130	3.7	15.9	5.3	0.1
Apple & Blackberry, Fruity, Low Fat, Sainsbury's*	1 Pot/125g	125	1.3	100	4.3	18.5	1.0	0.4
Apple & Blackberry, Organic, Yeo Valley*	1 Pot/125g	121	4.1	97	4.3	12.5	3.3	0.1
Apple & Cinnamon, COU, M & S*	1 Pot/150g	68	0.2	45	4.2	6.1	0.1	0.2
Apple & Cinnamon, Dessert, Low Fat, Sainsbury's*	1 Pot/125g	115	2.1	92	4.5	14.7	1.7	0.1
Apple & Cinnamon, Jubileum, Tine*	1 Pot/125g	166	6.5	133	3.2	18.5	5.2	0.0
Apple & Cranberry, Smooth, Bio, Fat Free, Shape*	1 Pot/120g	86	0.1	72	4.2	13.5	0.1	0.0
Apple & Custard, Low Fat, Sainsbury's*	1 Pot/125g	116	1.9	93	4.3	15.5	1.5	0.2
Apple & Pear, Low Fat, Sainsbury's*	1 Pot/125g	115	1.9	92	4.3	15.2	1.5	0.2
Apple & Prune, Fat Free, Yeo Valley*	1 Pot/125g	98	0.1	78	5.1	14.1	0.1	0.2
Apple & Spice Bio, Virtually Fat Free, Shape*	1 Pot/120g	67	0.1	56	5.6	7.3	0.1	0.2
Apple Danish Fruit Pudding Style, HE, Tesco*	1 Pot/125g	99	0.9	79	4.1	14.1	0.7	0.2
Apple Pie, Simply Desserts, Muller*	1 Pot/175g	278	8.1	159	4.6	24.7	4.6	0.7
Apricot, Bio, Low Fat, Benecol*	1 Pot/125g	98	0.8	78	3.9	14.3	0.6	0.0
Apricot, Custard Style, Shapers, Boots*	1 Pot/146g	82	1.2	56	3.9	8.3	0.8	0.2
Apricot, Fat Free, Bio Live, Rachel's Organic*	1 Pot/142g	81	0.1	57	3.5	10.5	0.1	0.0
Apricot, French Style Smooth, Tesco*	1 Pot/125g	123	3.8	98	3.6	14.1	3.0	0.0
Apricot, Fruity, Mullerlight, Muller*	1 Pot/200g	100	0.2	50	4.1	7.5	0.1	0.1
Apricot, HL, Tesco*	1 Pot/125g	68	0.4	54	5.1	7.9	0.3	1.1
Apricot, Jubileum, Tine*	1 Pot/135g	146	6.5	108	3.1	13.3	4.8	0.0
Apricot, Layered Fruit, Thick & Creamy, Sainsbury's*	1 Pot/125g	141	3.4	113	4.1	18.0	2.7	0.2
Apricot, Light, HL, Tesco*	1 Pot/125g	54	0.3	43	4.1	6.3	0.2	0.9
Apricot, Low Fat, Organic, Sainsbury's*	1 Pot/125g	103	1.3	82	5.3	13.0	1.0	0.1
Apricot, Low Fat, Organic, Somerfield*	1 Pot/150g	153	3.0	102	6.0	17.0	2.0	0.0
Apricot, Low Fat, Sainsbury's*	1 Pot/125g	93	1.4	74	3.5	12.5	1.1	0.4
Apricot, Low Fat, Tesco*	1 Pot/125g	113	2.3	90	4.3	14.1	1.8	0.0
Apricot, Organic, Bio Live, Yeo Valley*	1 Pot/125g	125	5.0	100	4.4	11.6	4.0	0.1
Apricot, Organic, Low Fat, Tesco*	1 Pot/125g	111	1.3	89	5.3	14.6	1.0	0.2
Apricot, Pro Activ, Flora*	1 Pot/125ml	70	0.6	56	4.0	7.9	0.5	1.8
Apricot, Smooth Set French, Sainsbury's*	1 Pot/125g	100	1.5	80	3.5	13.6	1.2	0.0
Apricot & Mango, 25% Extra Fruit, Low Fat, Asda*	1 Pot/125g	120	1.4	96	4.6	17.0	1.1	0.0
Apricot & Mango, Best There Is, Yoplait*	1 Pot/125g	130	2.0	104	4.7	17.4	1.6	0.0
Apricot & Mango, Low Fat, Tesco*	1 Pot/125g	126	2.3	101	4.9	16.3	1.8	0.0
Apricot & Mango, Thick & Creamy, Sainsbury's*	1 Pot/150g	179	5.4	119	4.3	17.3	3.6	0.2
Apricot & Nectarine, HE, Tesco*	1 Pot/175g	79	0.2	45	2.1	8.9	0.1	0.3
Apricot & Passion Fruit, Fat Free, Yeo Valley*	1 Pot/125g	94	0.1	75	5.3	13.2	0.1	0.1
Apricot Bio, HE, Tesco*	1 Pot/125g	58	0.1	46	4.2	7.1	0.1	0.1
Apricot Tart Style, Sveltesse, Nestle*	1 Pot/125g	98	0.3	78	4.8	14.2	0.2	0.1
Banana, Childrens, Co-Op*	1 Pot/125g	124	3.3	99	3.7	15.1	2.6	0.2
Banana, Custard Style, Asda*	1 Pot/150g	224	9.0	149	3.7	20.0	6.0	0.2

YOGHURT

INFO/WEIGHT	Measure	per Measure KCAL	FAT	Nutrition Values per 100g / 100ml KCAL	PROT	CARB	FAT	FIBRE
Banana, Low Fat, Asda*	1 Pot/150g	149	1.5	99	4.6	18.0	1.0	0.1
Banana, Low Fat, Sainsbury's*	1 Pot/125g	116	1.9	93	4.4	15.4	1.5	0.1
Banana, Low Fat, Tesco*	1 Pot/125g	128	2.1	102	4.9	16.8	1.7	0.1
Banana & Custard, Smooth, Mullerlight, Muller*	1 Pot/200g	102	0.2	51	4.1	8.6	0.1	0.6
Banana & Orange, Low Fat, 25% Extra Fruit, Asda*	1 Pot/125g	125	1.4	100	4.6	18.0	1.1	0.0
Banana Choco Flakes, Crunch Corner, Muller*	1 Pot/150g	215	7.7	143	4.1	22.5	5.1	0.3
Banana Smooth, M & S*	1 Pot/150g	165	2.6	110	4.8	19.3	1.7	0.2
Banana Toffee, Low Fat, Somerfield*	1 Pot/125g	123	1.4	98	4.1	18.0	1.1	0.0
Banoffee, Dessert, Low Fat, Sainsbury's*	1 Pot/125g	123	2.1	98	4.5	16.1	1.7	0.2
Banoffee, Eat Smart, Safeway*	1 Pot/125g	68	0.1	54	4.7	8.5	0.1	0.0
Banoffee, Fat Free, Bio, Eat Smart, Safeway*	1 Pot/125g	69	0.1	55	4.7	8.5	0.1	0.0
Banoffee, Low Fat, Asda*	1 Pot/125g	126	1.5	101	4.6	18.2	1.2	1.0
Banoffee, Thick & Creamy, Safeway*	1 Pot/150g	189	6.0	126	4.3	18.2	4.0	0.1
Bio, Low Fat, Spelga*	1 Pot/125g	125	2.1	100	3.9	17.0	1.7	0.0
Bio Activia, with Raspberry, Danone*	1 Pot/125g	113	3.5	90	3.5	12.8	2.8	2.0
Bio Fruits with Cherries, 0% Fat, Danone*	1 Pot/125g	65	0.1	52	3.6	9.1	0.1	0.0
Black Cherry, Bodyline*	1 Pot/113g	50	0.1	44	3.0	7.7	0.1	0.3
Black Cherry, Extra Fruity, Low Fat, Safeway*	1 Pot/150g	143	1.4	95	3.9	17.7	0.9	0.5
Black Cherry, Extremely Fruity, Bio, M & S*	1 Pot/150g	165	2.3	110	4.9	18.4	1.5	0.2
Black Cherry, Extremely Fruity, M & S*	1 Pot/200g	220	3.0	110	4.9	18.4	1.5	0.2
Black Cherry, Fat Free, BGTY, Sainsbury's*	1 Pot/125g	103	0.1	82	4.2	16.0	0.1	0.1
Black Cherry, Fayrefield Foods*	1 Pot/140g	185	7.1	132	4.0	17.4	5.1	0.0
Black Cherry, Juicy, Shapers, Boots*	1 Pot/152g	91	1.7	60	4.0	8.4	1.1	0.5
Black Cherry, Live, Turners Dairies*	1 Pot/125g	86	0.4	69	4.9	11.9	0.3	0.0
Black Cherry, Low Fat, Asda*	1 Pot/150g	143	1.5	95	4.6	17.4	1.0	0.2
Black Cherry, Low Fat, Sainsbury's*	1 Pot/125g	116	1.8	93	4.2	15.9	1.4	0.2
Black Cherry, Low Fat, Somerfield*	1 Pot/150g	116	1.5	77	3.0	14.0	1.0	0.0
Black Cherry, Low Fat, Value, Tesco*	1 Pot/125g	100	0.9	80	2.3	16.0	0.7	0.1
Black Cherry, PB, Waitrose*	1 Pot/150g	120	0.2	80	4.2	15.6	0.1	0.3
Black Cherry, Seriously Fruity, Low Fat, Waitrose*	1 Pot/170g	155	1.5	91	4.1	16.5	0.9	0.5
Black Cherry, So Good Beverages*	1 Pot/120g	92	1.6	77	2.1	16.6	1.3	0.0
Black Cherry, Swiss, Finest, Tesco*	1 Pot/150g	195	8.9	130	3.5	15.7	5.9	0.5
Black Cherry, Thick & Creamy, Waitrose*	1 Pot/125g	139	3.1	111	3.7	18.3	2.5	0.4
Black Cherry, Thick & Fruity, Weight Watchers*	1 Pot/120g	58	0.1	48	4.2	7.5	0.1	0.1
Black Cherry, Very Cherry, Activ8, Ski, Nestle*	1 Pot/120g	116	2.0	97	4.3	16.1	1.7	0.2
Black Cherry, Virtually Fat Free, Shapers, Boots*	1 Pot/125g	71	0.1	57	5.3	8.8	0.1	0.1
Blackberry, BGTY, Sainsbury's*	1 Pot/150g	107	0.6	71	3.4	13.5	0.4	1.6
Blackberry, Boysenberry & William Pear, M & S*	1 Pot/150g	188	9.8	125	4.0	13.6	6.5	2.4
Blackberry, Farmhouse, BGTY, Sainsbury's*	1 Pot/150g	107	0.6	71	3.4	13.5	0.4	1.6
Blackberry, Fat Free, BGTY, Sainsbury's*	1 Pot/150g	101	0.2	67	3.4	13.6	0.1	1.6
Blackberry, Sveltesse, Nestle*	1 Pot/125g	68	0.1	54	4.9	8.2	0.1	0.4
Blackberry & Apple, BGTY, Sainsbury's*	1 Pot/122g	61	0.2	50	4.7	7.2	0.2	0.3
Blackberry & Apple, HL, Tesco*	1 Pot/176g	86	0.2	49	2.1	10.0	0.1	1.5
Blackberry & Raspberry, Fruit Corner, Muller*	1 Pot/175g	186	6.8	106	3.8	14.0	3.9	1.0
Blackberry & Raspberry Flip, Morrisons*	1 Pot/175g	207	8.1	118	3.4	15.8	4.6	0.5
Blackcherry, Everyday, Low Fat, Co-Op*	1 Pot/125g	88	0.9	70	3.0	13.0	0.7	0.0
Blackcurrant, BGTY, Sainsbury's*	1 Pot/200g	100	0.4	50	4.8	7.3	0.2	0.1
Blackcurrant, Bio Live, Organic, Yeo Valley*	1 Pot/150g	152	5.9	101	4.1	12.4	3.9	0.2
Blackcurrant, Childrens, Co-Op*	1 Pot/125g	120	3.4	96	3.7	14.2	2.7	0.2
Blackcurrant, Extra Special, Asda*	1 Pot/100g	163	9.0	163	2.6	18.0	9.0	0.0
Blackcurrant, Fat Free, BGTY, Sainsbury's*	1 Pot/125g	64	0.1	51	4.6	8.0	0.1	1.6
Blackcurrant, Fruity, Mullerlight, Muller*	1 Pot/200g	102	0.2	51	4.1	7.9	0.1	0.8
Blackcurrant, Low Fat, Sainsbury's*	1 Pot/125g	116	1.8	93	4.2	15.9	1.4	0.6

Y

YOGHURT

INFO/WEIGHT	Measure	per Measure		Nutrition Values per 100g / 100ml				
		KCAL	FAT	KCAL	PROT	CARB	FAT	FIBRE
Blackcurrant, Low Fat, Tesco*	1 Pot/125g	113	2.3	90	4.3	14.1	1.8	0.0
Blackcurrant, Munch Bunch, Nestle*	1 Pot/100g	107	3.1	107	4.4	15.3	3.1	0.5
Blackcurrant, Thick & Creamy, Sainsbury's*	1 Pot/150g	171	5.4	114	4.3	15.9	3.6	0.4
Blackcurrant, Vitually Fat Free, Morrisons*	1 Pot/200g	114	0.4	57	5.4	8.4	0.2	0.2
Blackcurrant & Raspberry, Mullerlight, Muller*	1 Pot/175g	95	0.2	54	3.1	9.7	0.1	0.7
Blackcurrant & Vanilla, TTD, Sainsbury's*	1 Pot/143g	136	4.1	95	3.6	13.6	2.9	1.0
Blackcurrant with Liquorice, Tesco*	1 Pot/150g	138	1.7	92	4.6	15.8	1.1	0.4
Blueberry, Fruit Bottom, Stonyfield*	1 Pot/170g	120	2.0	71	3.5	12.4	1.2	0.6
Blueberry, Fruit Corner, Muller*	1 Pot/175g	184	6.8	105	3.8	13.7	3.9	0.4
Blueberry, Low Fat, Somerfield*	1 Pot/150g	131	1.5	87	4.0	16.0	1.0	0.0
Blueberry, Wholemilk, Organic, Sainsbury's*	1 Pot/150g	123	5.3	82	3.5	9.2	3.5	0.1
Blueberry Bio, Co-Op*	1 Pot/125g	141	3.5	113	4.5	16.5	2.8	0.4
Blueberry Flip, Morrisons*	1 Pot/175g	201	8.1	115	3.1	15.1	4.6	0.5
Blueberry Loganberry, Layered, Bio, Sainsbury's*	1 Pot/125g	134	3.4	107	4.0	16.6	2.7	0.2
Blueberry Muffin, Fat Free, Eat Smart, Safeway*	1 Pot/125g	66	0.1	53	4.7	8.2	0.1	0.3
Boysenberry, Low Fat, Yoplait*	1 Pot/100g	49	0.1	49	5.3	6.7	0.1	0.0
Cappuccino, Thick & Creamy, Safeway*	1 Pot/150g	228	8.4	152	4.5	20.8	5.6	0.0
Caramelised Orange, COU, M & S*	1 Pot/145g	65	0.1	45	4.2	6.1	0.1	0.2
Cereals, Fibre, Bio Activia, Danone*	1 Pot/125g	124	4.3	99	3.7	13.5	3.4	3.0
Champagne Rhubarb, Finest, Tesco*	1 Pot/150g	203	10.8	135	3.4	13.7	7.2	1.4
Champagne Rhubarb & Vanilla, M & S*	1 Pot/150g	195	8.7	130	3.8	15.7	5.8	0.8
Cherry, 0% Fat, Yoplait*	1 Pot/125g	70	0.1	56	3.8	9.8	0.1	0.0
Cherry, 0.1% Fat, Shape, Danone*	1 Pot/120g	56	0.1	47	4.6	6.8	0.1	2.1
Cherry, Bio, Low Fat, Benecol*	1 Pot/150g	122	0.9	81	3.8	15.2	0.6	0.0
Cherry, Fat Free, Activia, Danone*	1 Pot/125g	70	0.1	56	4.5	9.3	0.1	0.9
Cherry, Fruit Corner, Muller*	1 Pot/175g	187	6.8	107	3.9	14.0	3.9	0.4
Cherry, Fruity, Mullerlight, Muller*	1 Pot/150g	72	0.2	48	4.2	6.9	0.1	0.2
Cherry, Greek Style, Shape, Danone*	1 Pot/125g	143	3.4	114	6.0	16.4	2.7	0.0
Cherry, HE, Tesco*	1 Pot/200g	96	0.2	48	4.2	7.5	0.1	0.0
Cherry, Low Fat, Asda*	1 Pot/125g	120	1.4	96	4.6	17.0	1.1	0.0
Cherry, Somerfield*	1 Pot/125g	61	0.0	49	5.0	7.0	0.0	0.0
Cherry & Vanilla Flavour, Light, Brooklea*	1 Pot/200g	138	0.2	69	5.5	11.4	0.1	0.6
Cherry Bakewell Tart Flavour, Muller*	1 Pot/175g	119	0.4	68	4.8	11.8	0.2	0.2
Cherry Bio, Co-Op*	1 Pot/125g	144	3.5	115	4.5	17.0	2.8	0.1
Cherry Flip, BFY, Morrisons*	1 Pot/175g	93	0.5	53	3.9	8.7	0.3	0.4
Cherry Morello Bio, Tesco*	1 Pot/124g	51	0.2	41	4.4	5.4	0.2	0.9
Cherry Pie Layered, Custard Style, HE, Tesco*	1 Pot/125g	99	1.0	79	4.1	13.9	0.8	0.2
Chocolate, GFY, Asda*	1 Pot/200g	110	1.0	55	4.7	8.0	0.5	0.1
Chocolate, Seriously Smooth, Waitrose*	1 Pot/125g	158	3.0	126	6.0	20.1	2.4	0.1
Chocolate, Village Dairy*	1 Pot/125g	181	3.8	145	6.3	23.5	3.0	0.0
Chocolate, Vitaline*	1 Pot/125g	103	0.6	82	3.5	15.8	0.5	0.0
Citrus Fruit, Tesco*	1 Pot/117g	53	0.1	45	4.2	6.5	0.1	0.1
Cranberry, Fruit Yoghurt, Bio Activia, Danone*	1 Pot/125g	115	4.0	92	3.6	12.3	3.2	1.7
Creamy Cranberry & Raspberry, Shapers, Boots*	1 Pot/150g	86	1.7	57	4.0	7.0	1.1	1.1
Dessert with Honey, PB, Waitrose*	1 Pot/125ml	128	1.5	102	3.5	19.4	1.2	0.1
Devon Toffee, Low Fat, Sainsbury's*	1 Pot/126g	137	1.9	109	4.3	19.6	1.5	0.0
English Plum, The Best, Safeway*	1 Pot/175g	245	11.2	140	3.2	17.4	6.4	0.3
Exotic Fruits French Set Wholemilk, Asda*	1 Pot/125g	125	4.0	100	3.6	14.1	3.2	0.0
Fig, Fruit Yoghurt, Bio Activia, Danone*	1 Pot/125g	121	4.0	97	3.7	13.3	3.2	1.6
Forest Fruits, 0.1% Fat, Shape, Danone*	1 Pot/120g	55	0.1	46	4.6	6.7	0.1	2.1
Forest Fruits, Fat Free, Bio Activia, Danone*	1 Pot/125g	66	0.1	53	4.5	8.5	0.1	1.1
Forest Fruits, French Set Wholemilk, Asda*	1 Pot/125g	125	4.0	100	3.6	14.1	3.2	0.0
Forest Fruits, M & S*	1 Pot/150g	149	2.4	99	4.7	16.8	1.6	0.5

Y

YOGHURT

INFO/WEIGHT	Measure		per Measure		Nutrition Values per 100g / 100ml				
			KCAL	FAT	KCAL	PROT	CARB	FAT	FIBRE
Forest Fruits, Yoplait*	1 Pot/125g		120	3.2	96	3.8	14.4	2.6	0.3
French Set, Low Fat, Iceland*	1 Pot/125g		100	1.5	80	3.6	13.6	1.2	0.0
French Set, Waitrose*	1 Pot/125g		120	3.9	96	3.5	13.4	3.1	0.0
French Style, Whole Milk, Smooth Set, Tesco*	1 Pot/125g		123	3.8	98	3.6	14.1	3.0	0.0
Fruit, Brooklea*	1 Pot/120g		97	0.2	81	2.7	17.0	0.2	0.0
Fruit, Low Fat	1 Pot/120g		108	0.8	90	4.1	17.9	0.7	0.0
Fruit, Low Fat, Safeway*	1 Pot/125ml		88	1.0	70	2.1	13.7	0.8	0.0
Fruit Bio, Low Fat, Sainsbury's*	1 Pot/150g		156	1.7	104	4.6	18.9	1.1	0.3
Fruit Whole Milk	1 Pot/150g		158	4.2	105	5.1	15.7	2.8	0.0
Fruits of the Forest, Nestle*	1 Pot/125g		123	2.0	98	3.4	16.7	1.6	0.0
Fruits of the Forest, Smooth Set, Co-Op*	1 Pot/125g		95	1.1	76	3.7	12.5	0.9	0.0
Fruity Favourites, Organic, Yeo Valley*	1 Pot/125g		126	4.9	101	4.1	12.4	3.9	0.2
Fudge, Devonshire Style, Finest, Tesco*	1 Pot/150g		281	13.8	187	3.7	22.4	9.2	0.0
Fudge, Thick & Creamy, Co-Op*	1 Pot/150g		197	7.5	131	3.8	17.6	5.0	0.0
Fudge, Thick & Creamy, M & S*	1 Pot/150g		195	7.5	130	4.4	17.3	5.0	0.7
Fudge, Thick & Creamy, Waitrose*	1 Pot/150g		197	4.5	131	4.4	21.5	3.0	0.0
Fudge Layer, Indulgent Greek Style, Somerfield*	1 Pot/125g		226	8.8	181	3.0	26.0	7.0	0.0
Get Up & Go, Get Fresh At Home*	1 Pack/100g		113	0.5	113	8.0	19.0	0.5	1.9
Goats Whole Milk	1 Carton/150g		95	5.7	63	3.5	3.9	3.8	0.0
Gooseberry, Custard Style, Co-Op*	1 Pot/150g		216	8.0	144	3.7	19.3	5.3	0.3
Gooseberry, Custard Style, Shapers, Boots*	1 Pot/151g		106	1.1	70	3.9	12.0	0.7	0.2
Gooseberry, Custard Style, Somerfield*	1 Pot/125g		151	6.3	121	3.0	17.0	5.0	0.0
Gooseberry, Low Fat, Live, Bio, Waitrose*	¼ Pot/125g		106	1.1	85	4.8	14.3	0.9	0.5
Gooseberry, Low Fat, Sainsbury's*	1 Pot/125g		113	1.9	90	4.4	14.6	1.5	0.2
Gooseberry, Low Fat, Tesco*	1 Pot/125g		119	2.3	95	4.3	14.5	1.8	0.0
Gooseberry & Vanilla, TTD, Sainsbury's*	1 Pot/150g		143	4.4	95	3.7	13.6	2.9	0.4
Greek, 0% Fat, Strained, Authentic, Total, Fage*	¼ Pot/125g		65	0.0	52	9.0	4.0	0.0	0.0
Greek, 2% Fat, Strained, Authentic, Total, Fage*	1 Pot/150g		101	3.0	67	8.4	3.8	2.0	0.0
Greek, Original, Strained, Total, Fage*	1 Pot/200g		260	20.0	130	6.8	3.2	10.0	0.0
Greek, with Honey, Strained, Total, Fage*	1 Pot/150g		255	12.0	170	5.4	19.0	8.0	0.0
Greek, with Strawberry, 2% Fat, Total, Fage*	1 Pot/150g		140	2.4	93	6.7	12.9	1.6	0.0
Greek Style, Honey Topped, Tesco*	1 Pot/140g		203	12.0	145	3.6	13.4	8.6	0.0
Greek Style, Layered, Honey, Shapers, Boots*	1 Pot/150g		137	3.0	91	4.2	14.0	2.0	0.0
Greek Style, Luxury, Loseley*	1 Pot/175g		226	17.9	129	4.8	4.5	10.2	0.0
Greek Style, Natural, Sainsbury's*	1 Pot/125g		180	13.8	144	4.5	6.6	11.0	0.0
Greek Style, Natural, Tesco*	1 Pot/125g		179	13.8	143	4.5	6.6	11.0	0.0
Greek Style with Honey, Asda*	1 Pot/150g		225	13.1	150	4.0	13.9	8.7	0.0
Greek Style with Strawberries, Asda*	1 Pot/125g		159	8.3	127	3.2	13.6	6.6	0.2
Greek Style with Strawberry, Morrisons*	1 Pot/125g		163	8.3	130	3.3	14.4	6.6	0.0
Greek Style with Toffee & Hazelnuts, Asda*	1 Pot/125g		230	10.8	184	3.7	23.1	8.6	0.1
Greek Style with Tropical Fruits, Asda*	1 Pot/125g		164	8.3	131	3.3	14.5	6.6	0.3
Guava & Orange, Fat Free, Organic, Yeo Valley*	1 Pot/125g		93	0.1	74	5.3	13.0	0.1	0.2
Guava & Passion Fruit, Virtualy Fat Free, Tesco*	1 Pot/125g		56	0.3	45	4.2	6.7	0.2	1.2
Hazelnut, Low Fat, Sainsbury's*	1 Pot/125g		135	3.4	108	4.5	16.4	2.7	0.2
Hazelnut, Low Fat, Spelga*	1 Pot/125g		135	3.1	108	4.4	17.0	2.5	0.0
Hazelnut, Low Fat, Tesco*	1 Pot/150g		159	4.1	106	4.5	16.0	2.7	0.0
Hazelnut, Morrisons*	1 Pot/150g		159	3.9	106	3.9	16.9	2.6	0.0
Hazelnut, Sainsbury's*	1 Pot/150g		183	3.5	122	5.0	20.3	2.3	0.2
Hazelnut, Yoplait*	1 Pot/125g		166	5.0	133	4.6	19.6	4.0	0.0
Hazelnut, Longley Farm*	1 Pot/150g		206	8.5	137	5.5	16.0	5.7	0.0
Hazelnut, Low Fat, Pro-Biotic, Asda*	1 Pot/150g		111	2.4	74	3.5	11.5	1.6	0.0
Hazelnut, Low Fat, Safeway*	1 Pot/150g		179	3.8	119	4.9	19.3	2.5	0.2
Hazelnut, Low Fat, Somerfield*	1 Pot/150g		126	1.5	84	4.0	15.0	1.0	0.0

YOGHURT

	Measure INFO/WEIGHT	per Measure KCAL	FAT	KCAL	PROT	CARB	FAT	FIBRE
Honey, Greek Style, Co-Op*	1 Pot/150g	228	12.8	152	4.0	13.8	8.5	0.0
Honey, Greek Style, Organic, Sainsbury's*	1 Pot/100g	156	8.7	156	4.1	15.3	8.7	0.1
Honey, Low Fat, Asda*	1 Pot/125g	130	1.4	104	4.6	19.0	1.1	0.0
Honey & Ginger, Enhanced, Low Fat, Asda*	1 Pot/150g	150	1.7	100	4.6	18.0	1.1	0.0
Honey & Ginger, Tesco*	1 Pot/150g	150	1.7	100	4.6	18.0	1.1	0.0
Honey & Ginger, Waitrose*	1 Pot/150g	227	11.4	151	3.7	17.0	7.6	0.1
Honey & Muesli, Breakfast Break, Tesco*	1 Pot/170g	207	4.6	122	3.9	20.5	2.7	0.6
Italian Lemon, Amore Luxury, Muller*	1 Pot/150g	219	11.7	146	2.8	16.2	7.8	0.1
Jaffa Orange, Low Fat, Co-Op*	1 Pot/150g	126	1.4	84	3.9	15.0	0.9	0.4
Jaffa Orange, Morrisons*	1 Pot/150g	134	1.7	89	3.6	16.2	1.1	0.0
Jubileum Kiwi, Tine*	1 Pot/135g	149	6.6	110	3.2	13.5	4.9	0.0
Jubileum Raspberry, Tine*	1 Pot/135g	163	6.5	121	3.2	16.1	4.8	0.0
Kiwi, BGTY, Sainsbury's*	1 Pot/125g	61	0.1	49	4.6	7.5	0.1	0.2
Kiwi, Fruit Yoghurt, Bio Activia, Danone*	1 Pot/120g	109	4.0	91	3.7	11.5	3.3	2.0
Kiwi Cereal, Fibre, Bio Activia, Danone*	1 Pot/120g	124	4.0	103	3.8	14.5	3.3	3.0
Layered, Eat Smart, Safeway*	1 Pot/125g	81	0.1	65	4.1	11.3	0.1	0.4
Lemon, COU, M & S*	1 Pot/200g	90	0.2	45	4.2	6.6	0.1	0.4
Lemon, Greek Style, GFY, Asda*	1 Pot/150g	125	4.4	83	4.1	10.0	2.9	0.1
Lemon, Greek Style, Shape, Danone*	1 Pot/125g	140	3.4	112	5.9	15.9	2.7	0.0
Lemon, Low Fat, Asda*	1 Pot/125g	130	1.4	104	4.6	19.0	1.1	0.0
Lemon, Low Fat, Organic, Sainsbury's*	1 Pot/125g	121	1.3	97	5.1	17.0	1.0	0.1
Lemon, Low Fat, Safeway*	1 Pot/150g	155	1.7	103	4.6	18.7	1.1	0.1
Lemon, Smooth Set French, Low Fat, Sainsbury's*	1 Pot/125g	100	1.5	80	3.5	13.6	1.2	0.0
Lemon, Summer, Biopot, Onken*	1 Pot/150g	155	3.9	103	3.9	15.9	2.6	0.1
Lemon, Thick & Fruity, Weight Watchers*	1 Pot/120g	49	0.1	41	4.0	5.8	0.1	0.1
Lemon & Lime, BGTY, Sainsbury's*	1 Pot/125g	66	0.1	53	4.6	8.3	0.1	1.1
Lemon & Lime, Fat Free, Shape, Danone*	1 Pot/120g	61	0.1	51	4.5	7.3	0.1	0.1
Lemon Cheesecake, HL, Light, Tesco*	1 Pot/200g	88	0.2	44	4.2	6.6	0.1	0.1
Lemon Cheesecake, Probiotic, GFY, Asda*	1 Pot/125g	66	0.1	53	4.7	8.4	0.1	0.2
Lemon Cheesecake, Sveltesse, Nestle*	1 Pot/125g	96	0.3	77	4.9	14.0	0.2	0.3
Lemon Curd, Farmhouse, TTD, Sainsbury's*	1 Pot/150g	182	5.6	121	4.1	17.7	3.7	0.2
Lemon Curd, Indulgent, Dessert, Waitrose*	1 Pot/150g	278	13.8	185	4.1	21.5	9.2	0.0
Lemon Lime Mousse, Shapers, Boots*	1 Pot/90g	89	3.8	99	4.2	11.0	4.2	0.1
Lemon Meringue, Eat Smart, Safeway*	1 Pot/125g	68	0.1	54	4.7	8.6	0.1	0.0
Lemon Meringue, Sveltesse, Nestle*	1 Pot/125g	60	0.1	48	4.1	7.7	0.1	0.0
Lemon Smooth Set, Co-Op*	1 Pot/125g	95	1.1	76	3.7	12.5	0.9	0.0
Loganberry, Low Fat, Sainsbury's*	1 Pot/125g	111	1.9	89	4.2	14.5	1.5	0.2
Loganberry, Sainsbury's*	1 Pot/150g	194	9.3	129	3.9	14.2	6.2	0.6
Low Calorie	1 Pot/120g	49	0.2	41	4.3	6.0	0.2	0.0
Mandarin, Fruity, Mullerlight, Muller*	1 Pot/200g	106	0.2	53	4.1	8.4	0.1	0.0
Mandarin, Longley Farm*	1 Pot/150g	161	5.7	107	4.9	13.3	3.8	0.0
Mandarin, Low Fat, Asda*	1 Pot/125g	101	1.5	81	4.6	13.0	1.2	0.0
Mango, 0.1% Fat, Shape, Danone*	1 Pot/120g	55	0.1	46	4.6	6.7	0.1	2.1
Mango, Fruit Yoghurt, Bio Activia, Danone*	1 Pot/125g	121	4.0	97	3.7	13.4	3.2	1.6
Mango, Light, HL, Tesco*	1 Pot/125g	56	0.3	45	4.1	6.6	0.2	0.9
Mango, Light, Muller*	1 Pot/200g	110	0.2	55	4.3	9.2	0.1	0.0
Mango, Virtually Fat Free, Tesco*	1 Pot/125g	56	0.3	45	4.1	6.6	0.2	0.9
Mango & Guava, Sunshine Selection, Sainsbury's*	1 Pot/125g	145	2.4	116	5.4	19.3	1.9	0.3
Mango & Pineapple, BGTY, Sainsbury's*	1 Pot/124g	63	0.2	51	4.6	7.6	0.2	0.2
Mango Bio, HE, Tesco*	1 Pot/125g	59	0.1	47	4.7	6.8	0.1	0.2
Mississippi Mud Pie, Crunchable, Brooklea*	1 Pot/140g	237	6.3	169	4.0	28.0	4.5	0.3
Mixed Berries, Jogood, Imlek*	1 Pot/200g	172	4.4	86	2.9	13.4	2.2	0.0
Mixed Seeds, Probiotic, Yoplait*	1 Pot/125g	139	5.6	111	4.5	13.2	4.5	3.1

Y

YOGHURT

INFO/WEIGHT	Measure	per Measure		Nutrition Values per 100g / 100ml				
		KCAL	FAT	KCAL	PROT	CARB	FAT	FIBRE
Morello Cherry, Amore Luxury, Muller*	1 Pot/150g	216	11.7	144	2.8	16.3	7.8	0.1
Morello Cherry, HE, Tesco*	1 Pot/125g	58	0.1	46	4.2	7.1	0.1	0.1
Morello Cherry, HL, Tesco*	1 Pot/125g	56	0.3	45	4.1	6.6	0.2	0.9
Muesli Nut, Low Fat	1 Pot/120g	134	2.6	112	5.0	19.2	2.2	0.0
Multifruits, Yop Petit Déjeuner, Yoplait*	1 Bottle/180g	155	2.2	86	2.7	16.0	1.2	0.0
Natural, 0.1% Fat, Stirred, Biopot, Onken*	1 Serving/100g	48	0.1	48	5.4	6.4	0.1	0.0
Natural, Bio, BFY, Morrisons*	1 Serving/100g	65	0.2	65	6.5	9.4	0.2	0.0
Natural, Bio, Co-Op*	1 Pot/150g	117	5.4	78	4.8	5.5	3.6	0.0
Natural, Bio, Fat Free, Waitrose*	1 Pot/150g	90	0.2	60	6.1	8.6	0.1	0.0
Natural, Bio, HL, Tesco*	1 Serving/100g	55	0.1	55	5.4	7.6	0.1	0.0
Natural, Bio, Low Fat, Sainsbury's*	1 Serving/100g	48	1.5	48	4.0	4.6	1.5	0.0
Natural, Bio, Very Low Fat, Somerfield*	1 Pot/150g	98	0.0	65	7.0	9.0	0.0	0.0
Natural, Bio, Virtually Fat Free, HL, Tesco*	1 Serving/100g	47	0.2	47	5.5	5.8	0.2	0.1
Natural, Bio Activia, Individual Pots, Danone*	1 Pot/125g	86	4.3	69	4.2	5.5	3.4	0.0
Natural, Bio Life, Easiyo*	1 Pot/150g	95	2.7	63	5.0	6.7	1.8	0.0
Natural, Bio Live, Fat Free, Organic, Waitrose*	½ Pot/250g	145	0.3	58	6.0	8.4	0.1	0.0
Natural, Bio Live, Fat Free, Organic, Yeo Valley*	1 SmPot/150g	87	0.2	58	5.9	8.4	0.1	0.0
Natural, Bio Live, Low Fat, Organic, Waitrose*	¼ Pot/125g	81	1.3	65	5.8	8.3	1.0	0.0
Natural, Bio Live, Organic, Yeo Valley*	1 Pot/100g	82	4.2	82	4.5	6.6	4.2	0.0
Natural, Bio Live, Very Low Fat, Ann Forshaw's*	1 Pot/125g	53	0.1	42	5.0	5.5	0.1	0.0
Natural, Bio Set, Low Fat, Sainsbury's*	1 Pot/150g	78	2.3	52	3.9	5.7	1.5	0.0
Natural, Danone*	1 Pot/125g	71	3.6	57	3.2	3.8	2.9	0.0
Natural, Fat Free, Rachel's Organic*	1 Pot/500g	180	0.5	36	3.9	4.8	0.1	0.0
Natural, Greek, Half Fat, Safeway*	1 Serving/100g	101	5.1	101	5.7	8.1	5.1	0.0
Natural, Greek Style, Asda*	1oz/28g	36	3.0	129	4.6	4.8	10.8	0.0
Natural, Greek Style, BGTY, Sainsbury's*	1 Serving/50g	39	1.4	78	5.5	7.9	2.7	0.0
Natural, Greek Style, Bio Live, Rachel's Organic*	1 Pot/450g	513	40.5	114	3.7	4.6	9.0	0.0
Natural, Greek Style, GFY, Asda*	¼ Pot/125g	100	3.4	80	5.8	8.2	2.7	0.0
Natural, Greek Style, HE, Tesco*	1oz/28g	22	1.1	79	6.5	4.0	4.1	0.0
Natural, Greek Style, HL, Tesco*	1 Serving/100g	80	2.7	80	5.7	8.2	2.7	0.0
Natural, Greek Style, Organic, Tesco*	1oz/28g	37	2.8	133	4.5	6.2	10.0	0.0
Natural, Greek Style, Waitrose*	1 Pot/150g	210	15.5	140	4.8	6.9	10.3	0.0
Natural, Greek Style, with Cow's Milk, Tesco*	1 Pot/150g	215	16.4	143	4.5	6.6	10.9	0.0
Natural, Longley Farm*	1 Pot/150g	119	5.3	79	4.8	7.0	3.5	0.0
Natural, Low Fat, Asda*	1oz/28g	17	0.3	62	6.1	7.1	1.0	0.0
Natural, Low Fat, Bio, Co-Op*	1 Pot/150g	98	1.5	65	6.0	8.0	1.0	0.0
Natural, Low Fat, Bio, Safeway*	1 Serving/100g	72	1.1	72	6.6	8.8	1.1	0.0
Natural, Low Fat, Bio, Sainsbury's*	1 Pot/125g	85	1.9	68	5.6	7.9	1.5	0.0
Natural, Low Fat, Budgens*	1 Serving/112g	65	0.9	58	5.1	7.5	0.8	0.0
Natural, Low Fat, Live, Waitrose*	1 Pot/175g	114	1.8	65	5.8	8.2	1.0	0.0
Natural, Low Fat, Morrisons*	1 Pot/150g	93	1.5	62	6.1	7.1	1.0	0.0
Natural, Low Fat, Organic, Yeo Valley*	1 Serving/100g	68	1.2	68	5.9	8.5	1.2	0.0
Natural, Low Fat, Safeway*	1 Serving/100g	52	1.1	52	4.6	5.9	1.1	0.0
Natural, Low Fat, So Organic, Sainsbury's*	1 Pot/150g	107	1.8	71	6.2	8.8	1.2	0.0
Natural, Low Fat, Somerfield*	1 Pot/150g	78	1.7	52	4.5	5.9	1.1	0.0
Natural, Low Fat, Stirred, Sainsbury's*	1 Serving/124g	83	1.9	67	5.5	7.8	1.5	0.0
Natural, Low Fat, Tesco*	¼ Pot/125g	88	1.9	70	5.5	7.8	1.5	0.0
Natural, Low Fat, TTD, Sainsbury's*	1 Pot/125g	80	2.3	64	6.7	4.6	1.8	0.0
Natural, Low Fat, Ubley*	1 Serving/100g	67	1.5	67	5.5	7.8	1.5	0.0
Natural, Netto*	1 Serving/50g	40	1.9	80	4.8	6.9	3.7	0.0
Natural, Organic, Yeo Valley*	1 Pot/150g	120	5.6	80	4.7	6.9	3.7	0.0
Natural, Probiotic, Eat Smart, Morrisons*	¼ Pot/125g	76	0.4	61	6.3	8.3	0.3	0.0
Natural, Set, Low Fat, Waitrose*	1 Pot/150g	99	1.8	66	5.7	8.1	1.2	0.0

Y

YOGHURT

INFO/WEIGHT	per Measure KCAL	per Measure FAT	KCAL	PROT	CARB	FAT	FIBRE
Natural, Virtually Fat Free, Bio, Safeway*	1 Pot/100g	65	0.2	65	6.4	9.4	0.2	0.0
Natural, Whole Milk, Set, Biopot, Onken*	1 Pot/150g	105	5.6	70	3.8	5.3	3.7	0.0
Natural, Wholemilk, Live Bio, Organic, Waitrose*	1 Pot/100g	88	4.4	88	5.1	7.1	4.4	0.0
Natural, Wholemilk, Organic, Sainsbury's*	1 Pot/125g	86	4.8	69	3.7	5.0	3.8	0.1
Natural with Honey, Greek Style, Sainsbury's*	1 Sm Pot/150g	243	14.1	162	4.0	15.4	9.4	0.0
Nectarine & Orange, Best There Is, Yoplait*	1 Pot/122g	131	2.0	107	4.7	18.0	1.6	0.0
Nectarine & Orange, Channel Island, M & S*	1 Pot/150g	158	5.0	105	4.5	14.7	3.3	0.3
Nectarine & Orange, Fat Free, BFY, Morrisons*	1 Pot/200g	128	0.6	64	5.9	9.5	0.3	0.1
Nectarine & Orange, M & S*	1 Pot/150g	147	2.4	98	4.9	16.0	1.6	0.3
Nectarine & Orange, Virtually Fat Free, Tesco*	1 Pot/125g	58	0.1	46	4.1	7.2	0.1	0.0
Nectarine & Passion Fruit, 0.1% Fat, Shape*	1 Pot/120g	55	0.1	46	4.6	6.7	0.1	2.1
Nectarine & Passion Fruit, BGTY, Sainsbury's*	1 Pot/151g	122	0.6	81	3.2	16.3	0.4	0.6
Nectarine & Raspberry, Low Fat, Somerfield*	1 Pot/150g	134	1.5	89	4.0	17.0	1.0	0.0
Nectarine & Raspberry, Very Low Fat, Somerfield*	1 Pot/125g	60	0.0	48	5.0	7.0	0.0	0.0
Orange, BGTY, Sainsbury's*	1 Pot/125g	63	0.1	50	4.5	7.7	0.1	1.1
Orange, Greek Style, Boots*	1 Pot/140g	207	12.0	148	3.7	14.0	8.6	0.2
Orange, Greek Style, Shape, Danone*	1 Pot/100g	112	2.7	112	6.0	16.0	2.7	0.1
Orange, Low Fat, Tesco*	1 Pot/125g	114	2.3	91	4.3	14.5	1.8	0.0
Orange & Lemon, BGTY, Sainsbury's*	1 Pot/125g	63	0.3	50	4.7	7.3	0.2	0.2
Orange & Nectarine, Light, Spelga*	1 Pot/175g	79	0.4	45	4.4	7.1	0.2	0.0
Orange Blossom Honey, Finest, Tesco*	1 Pot/150g	237	10.7	158	3.5	20.1	7.1	0.0
Orange with Grains, Good Intentions, Somerfield*	1 Pot/125g	91	0.4	73	5.9	11.6	0.3	0.1
Passion Fruit with Elderflower Extract, Tesco*	1 Pot/150g	147	1.7	98	4.7	17.3	1.1	0.2
Peach, BGTY, Sainsbury's*	1 Pot/125g	61	0.3	49	4.7	7.2	0.2	0.2
Peach, Custard Style, Low Fat, Sainsbury's*	1 Pot/125g	110	1.9	88	4.4	14.2	1.5	0.1
Peach, Economy, Sainsbury's*	1 Pot/125g	93	0.5	74	2.8	14.7	0.4	0.0
Peach, Fat Free, Activ8, Ski, Nestle*	1 Pot/120g	89	0.1	74	4.5	13.7	0.1	0.7
Peach, Fat Free, Bio Activia, Danone*	1 Pot/125g	70	0.1	56	4.5	9.3	0.1	1.0
Peach, Forbidden Fruits, Rachel's Organic*	1 Pot/125g	156	7.6	125	3.4	14.0	6.1	0.0
Peach, Honey & Grain, Eat Smart, Safeway*	1 Pot/200g	120	0.4	60	4.7	9.4	0.2	0.3
Peach, Low Fat, Asda*	1 Pot/125g	118	1.3	95	4.7	16.7	1.1	0.2
Peach, Low Fat, Basics, Sainsbury's*	1 Pot/125g	84	1.3	67	4.0	10.4	1.0	0.1
Peach, Low Fat, Probiotic, Tesco*	1 Pot/125g	106	1.8	85	3.9	14.3	1.4	0.3
Peach, Low Fat, Safeway*	1 Pot/150g	141	1.7	94	4.7	16.2	1.1	0.2
Peach, Low Fat, Yeo Valley*	1 Pot/125g	113	1.4	90	4.6	15.3	1.1	0.1
Peach, Smooth Style, Mullerlight, Muller*	1 Pot/125g	61	0.1	49	4.1	7.2	0.1	0.2
Peach, Thick & Fruity, Fat Free, Weight Watchers*	1 Pot/120g	55	0.1	46	4.2	7.1	0.1	0.2
Peach & Apricot, 0.1% Fat, Shape, Danone*	1 Pot/120g	55	0.1	46	4.6	6.7	0.1	2.1
Peach & Apricot, Extremely Fruity, Low Fat, M & S*	1 Pot/170g	170	1.5	100	4.5	18.2	0.9	0.7
Peach & Apricot, Fruit Corner, Muller*	1 Pot/175g	191	6.8	109	3.9	14.5	3.9	0.3
Peach & Apricot, Light, HL, Tesco*	1 Pot/200g	82	0.2	41	3.9	6.2	0.1	1.0
Peach & Lemon Balm, Biowild, Onken*	1 Pot/175g	158	2.6	90	4.3	14.9	1.5	0.1
Peach & Mango, Juicy, Shapers, Boots*	1 Pot/150g	89	1.7	59	4.0	8.3	1.1	0.5
Peach & Mango, Thick & Creamy, Waitrose*	1 Pot/125g	136	3.1	109	3.7	17.8	2.5	0.3
Peach & Mango, Truly Fruity, Brooklea, Aldi*	1 Pot/200g	162	2.8	81	4.6	12.4	1.4	0.0
Peach & Maracuya, Mullerlight, Muller*	1 Pot/200g	102	0.2	51	4.5	8.1	0.1	0.0
Peach & Papaya, Fat Free, Yeo Valley*	1 Pot/125g	94	0.1	75	5.3	13.1	0.1	0.1
Peach & Papaya, Waitrose*	1 Pot/150g	129	0.2	86	4.2	17.1	0.1	0.2
Peach & Passion Fruit, 0.1% Fat, Shape, Danone*	1 Pot/120g	55	0.1	46	4.6	6.7	0.1	2.1
Peach & Passion Fruit, Eat Smart, Safeway*	1 Pot/125g	69	0.1	55	5.2	8.5	0.1	0.3
Peach & Passion Fruit, Layers, Mullerlight, Muller*	1 Pot/175g	95	0.2	54	3.1	9.7	0.1	0.2
Peach & Passion Fruit, Lite Biopot, Onken*	1/5 Pot/100g	45	0.2	45	4.6	6.0	0.2	0.2
Peach & Passion Fruit, Low Fat, Somerfield*	1 Pot/150g	132	1.5	88	4.0	16.0	1.0	0.0

Y

YOGHURT

	Measure INFO/WEIGHT	per Measure KCAL	FAT	Nutrition Values per 100g / 100ml KCAL	PROT	CARB	FAT	FIBRE
Peach & Passion Fruit, Very Low Fat, Somerfield*	1 Pot/125g	61	0.0	49	5.0	7.0	0.0	0.0
Peach & Passion Fruit Flip, Morrisons*	1 Pot/175g	89	0.5	51	3.9	8.2	0.3	0.6
Peach & Passionfruit, BGTY, Sainsbury's*	1 Pot/125g	69	0.1	55	4.9	8.6	0.1	0.1
Peach & Pear, Low Fat, Somerfield*	1 Pot/125g	118	1.3	94	4.5	16.5	1.0	0.2
Peach & Pear, Seriously Fruity, Low Fat, Waitrose*	1 Pot/125g	110	1.3	88	4.5	15.3	1.0	0.3
Peach & Vanilla, HE, Tesco*	1 Pot/125g	55	0.1	44	4.8	6.0	0.1	0.1
Peach & Vanilla, HL, Tesco*	1 Pot/125g	54	0.3	43	4.1	6.3	0.2	1.0
Peach & Vanilla, Thick & Creamy, Co-Op*	1 Pot/150g	180	6.9	120	3.6	16.0	4.6	0.1
Peach & Vanilla Flip, Morrisons*	1 Pot/175g	212	8.1	121	3.4	16.5	4.6	0.6
Peach Melba, Everyday Low Fat, Co-Op*	1 Pot/125g	88	0.9	70	3.0	13.0	0.7	0.0
Peach Melba, Low Fat, Tesco*	1 Pot/125g	100	0.9	80	2.3	16.0	0.7	0.1
Peach Melba, Sveltesse, Nestle*	1 Pot/125g	70	0.1	56	4.7	9.1	0.1	0.2
Peach Melba, Value, Tesco*	1 Pot/125g	100	0.9	80	2.3	16.0	0.7	0.1
Peaches, Farmhouse, BGTY, Sainsbury's*	1 Pot/150g	134	0.6	89	3.2	17.8	0.4	0.3
Peanut Toffee, Low Fat, Somerfield*	1 Pot/150g	131	1.5	87	4.0	15.0	1.0	0.0
Pear, Jubileum, Tine*	1 Pot/125g	168	6.5	134	3.2	18.6	5.2	0.0
Pear, Lidl*	1 Pot/125g	108	0.1	86	4.3	16.1	0.1	0.0
Pear, Rosehip & Marigold, Biowild, Onken*	1 Pot/175g	161	2.6	92	4.4	15.1	1.5	0.3
Pear & Butterscotch, Finest, Tesco*	1 Pot/150g	413	21.0	275	5.0	32.3	14.0	0.5
Pear & Vanilla, Thick & Creamy, Weight Watchers*	1 Pot/120g	54	0.6	45	4.2	5.8	0.5	0.2
Pineapple, Channel Island, M & S*	1 Pot/150g	165	5.0	110	4.3	15.9	3.3	0.3
Pineapple, Eat Smart, Safeway*	1 Pot/125g	66	0.1	53	4.5	8.4	0.1	0.1
Pineapple, Extremely Fruity, M & S*	1 Pot/200g	200	2.8	100	4.3	17.6	1.4	0.1
Pineapple, Finest, Tesco*	1 Pot/200g	220	5.8	110	3.5	17.5	2.9	0.2
Pineapple, HL, Tesco*	1 Pot/125g	69	0.4	55	5.1	8.1	0.3	1.1
Pineapple, Low Fat, Bio, Asda*	1 Pot/150g	144	1.7	96	4.6	17.0	1.1	0.1
Pineapple, Low Fat, Sainsbury's*	1 Pot/125g	110	1.6	88	4.1	15.0	1.3	0.2
Pineapple, Low Fat, Somerfield*	1 Pot/150g	134	1.5	89	4.0	17.0	1.0	0.0
Pineapple, Low Fat, Tesco*	1 Pot/125g	111	2.1	89	4.6	13.4	1.7	0.0
Pineapple, Thick & Creamy, Waitrose*	1 Pot/125g	136	3.1	109	3.6	17.9	2.5	0.2
Pineapple, Thick & Fruity, Weight Watchers*	1 Pot/120g	56	0.1	47	3.9	7.7	0.1	0.9
Pineapple, Virtually Fat Free, Tesco*	1 Pot/125g	55	0.3	44	4.1	6.5	0.2	0.9
Pineapple & Grapefruit, BGTY, Sainsbury's*	1 Pot/125g	68	0.1	54	4.4	8.8	0.1	0.1
Pineapple & Papaya, Tropical Fruit, Ski, Nestle*	1 Pot/120g	114	2.0	95	4.5	15.4	1.7	0.1
Pineapple & Passion Fruit, Soya, Light, Alpro*	1 Pot/120g	62	1.3	52	2.1	7.3	1.1	0.8
Pineapple & Peach, Fruity, Mullerlight, Muller*	1 Pot/200g	100	0.2	50	4.1	7.6	0.1	0.2
Pineapple Or Peach, Low Fat, Organic, Tesco*	1 Pot/125g	108	1.3	86	5.1	14.1	1.0	0.1
Pink Grapefruit, Breakfast Selection, Sainsbury's*	1 Pot/117g	109	1.6	93	4.2	15.9	1.4	0.1
Pink Grapefruit, Low Fat, Sainsbury's*	1 Pot/125g	116	1.8	93	4.2	15.9	1.4	0.1
Pink Grapefruit, Thick & Fruity, Weight Watchers*	1 Pot/120g	49	0.1	41	3.9	6.2	0.1	1.0
Pink Grapefruit Thick & Fruity, Weight Watchers*	1 Pot/120g	49	0.1	41	3.9	6.2	0.1	0.6
Plain, Low Fat	1 Pot/120g	67	1.0	56	5.1	7.5	0.8	0.0
Plain, Whole Milk, Average	1oz/28g	22	0.8	79	5.7	7.8	3.0	0.0
Plum, BGTY, Sainsbury's*	1 Pot/125g	69	0.1	55	4.8	8.8	0.1	0.1
Plum, Bio Live, Summer Selection, Yeo Valley*	1 Pot/125g	126	4.9	101	4.1	12.4	3.9	0.1
Plum, Low Fat, Sainsbury's*	1 Pot/125g	118	2.1	94	4.5	15.2	1.7	0.1
Plum & Hop, Biowild, Onken*	1 Pot/175g	158	2.6	90	4.3	14.9	1.5	0.3
Probiotic, Aldi*	1 Pot/200g	178	2.8	89	4.1	14.2	1.4	0.0
Probiotic, Low Fat, Organic, Glenisk*	1 Pot/150g	92	2.9	61	4.5	6.4	1.9	0.0
Prune, Breakfast Selection, Sainsbury's*	1 Pot/125g	119	1.8	95	4.2	16.3	1.4	0.2
Prune, Fruit Yoghurt, Bio Activia, Danone*	1 Pot/125g	110	3.5	88	3.5	12.2	2.8	0.2
Prune, Probiotic, Tesco*	1 Pot/170g	145	2.4	85	3.9	14.3	1.4	1.0
Prune, Vitality, Low Fat, with Omega 3, Muller*	1 Pot/150g	144	2.9	96	4.7	15.0	1.9	1.1

YOGHURT

	Measure INFO/WEIGHT	per Measure KCAL	FAT	KCAL	PROT	CARB	FAT	FIBRE
Prune, with Fruit Layer, Bio Activia, Danone*	1 Pot/125g	110	3.5	88	3.5	12.2	2.8	0.2
Rasberry, Orange & Grain, Eat Smart, Safeway*	1 Pot/200g	120	0.4	60	4.7	9.1	0.2	0.6
Raspberry, 0.1% Fat, Shape, Danone*	1 Pot/120g	55	0.1	46	4.6	6.7	0.1	2.6
Raspberry, Bio, Low Fat, Benecol*	1 Pot/125g	99	0.8	79	3.8	14.5	0.6	0.0
Raspberry, Eat Smart, Safeway*	1 Pot/127g	70	0.1	55	5.2	8.5	0.1	0.7
Raspberry, Economy, Sainsbury's*	1 Pot/125g	85	1.3	68	3.0	11.9	1.0	0.0
Raspberry, Everyday, Low Fat, Co-Op*	1 Pot/125g	88	0.9	70	3.0	13.0	0.7	0.0
Raspberry, Extremely Fruity, M & S*	1 Pot/200g	190	3.0	95	5.0	15.6	1.5	0.5
Raspberry, Farmhouse, TTD, Sainsbury's*	1 Pot/150g	149	4.2	99	3.6	15.0	2.8	1.6
Raspberry, Fat Free, Activ8, Ski, Nestle*	1 Pot/120g	91	0.1	76	4.6	14.1	0.1	0.7
Raspberry, Fat Free, BGTY, Sainsbury's*	1 Pot/125g	64	0.1	51	4.8	7.7	0.1	1.7
Raspberry, Fat Free, Bio Live, Organic, Yeo Valley*	1 Pot/125g	98	0.1	78	5.2	14.0	0.1	0.4
Raspberry, Fat Free, Farmhouse, BGTY, Sainsbury's*	1 Pot/150g	101	0.2	67	3.4	13.7	0.1	2.0
Raspberry, French Set, Waitrose*	1 Pot/125g	120	3.9	96	3.5	13.4	3.1	2.0
Raspberry, French Set Wholemilk, Asda*	1 Pot/125g	125	4.0	100	3.6	14.1	3.2	0.0
Raspberry, Light, HL, Tesco*	1 Pot/200g	88	0.2	44	3.9	7.0	0.1	1.7
Raspberry, Low Fat, Asda*	1 Pot/150g	126	1.7	84	4.5	14.0	1.1	0.4
Raspberry, Low Fat, Bio, Sainsbury's*	1 Pot/150g	146	1.7	97	4.7	17.0	1.1	0.7
Raspberry, Low Fat, Budgens*	1 Pot/125g	121	1.4	97	4.7	17.0	1.1	0.2
Raspberry, Low Fat, Organic, Sainsbury's*	1 Pot/125g	106	1.2	85	5.1	14.0	1.0	0.2
Raspberry, Low Fat, Probiotic, M & S*	1 Pot/170g	179	2.7	105	4.8	17.6	1.6	0.5
Raspberry, Low Fat, Probiotic, Tesco*	1 Pot/170g	145	2.4	85	3.9	14.3	1.4	0.3
Raspberry, Low Fat, Safeway*	1 Pot/150g	143	1.7	95	4.7	16.5	1.1	0.3
Raspberry, Low Fat, Sainsbury's*	1 Pot/150g	108	1.7	72	3.5	11.0	1.1	0.1
Raspberry, Low Fat, Somerfield*	1 Pot/150g	128	1.5	85	4.0	16.0	1.0	0.0
Raspberry, Low Fat, Tesco*	1 Pot/125g	116	2.3	93	4.3	14.9	1.8	0.0
Raspberry, Meadow Fresh*	1 Pot/125g	130	1.3	104	4.5	18.9	1.0	0.0
Raspberry, Organic, Fat Free, Rachel's Organic*	1 Pot/142g	78	0.1	55	3.6	10.0	0.1	0.0
Raspberry, Organic, Yeo Valley*	1 Pot/150g	152	5.9	101	4.2	12.3	3.9	0.4
Raspberry, Probiotic, Live, Yeo Valley*	1 Pot/125g	106	1.3	85	5.1	14.0	1.0	0.4
Raspberry, Probiotic, Low Fat, Organic, M & S*	1 Pot/170g	128	2.4	75	4.4	11.5	1.4	0.4
Raspberry, Scottish, Finest, Tesco*	1 Pot/150g	195	10.2	130	3.4	12.8	6.8	1.2
Raspberry, Scottish, Seriously Fruity, Waitrose*	1 Pot/170g	139	1.5	82	4.2	14.2	0.9	1.5
Raspberry, Scottish, The Best, Morrisons*	1 Pot/150g	209	10.4	139	3.6	15.6	6.9	1.3
Raspberry, Smooth, Activ8, Ski, Nestle*	1 Pot/120g	113	2.0	94	4.6	14.8	1.7	0.7
Raspberry, Smooth, Mullerlight, Muller*	1 Pot/125g	64	0.1	51	4.2	7.8	0.1	0.6
Raspberry, Smooth Set, Co-Op*	1 Pot/125g	95	1.1	76	3.7	12.5	0.9	0.0
Raspberry, Summer, Biopot, Onken*	1/5 Pot/100g	101	2.6	101	3.9	15.5	2.6	0.6
Raspberry, Sveltesse, Nestle*	1 Pot/125g	61	0.1	49	4.9	7.2	0.1	0.6
Raspberry, Thick & Creamy, Sainsbury's*	1 Pot/150g	179	5.6	119	4.4	17.2	3.7	0.2
Raspberry, Thick & Fruity, Fat Free, Weight Watchers*	1 Pot/120g	49	0.1	41	4.2	5.7	0.1	0.3
Raspberry, Thick & Fruity, Probiotic, COU, M & S*	1 Pot/150g	68	0.2	45	4.2	6.9	0.1	0.6
Raspberry, Value, Tesco*	1 Pot/125g	100	0.9	80	2.3	16.0	0.7	0.1
Raspberry, Virtually Fat Free, Tesco*	1 Pot/125g	51	0.3	41	4.1	5.8	0.2	1.1
Raspberry, Way to Five, Sainsbury's*	1 Pot/151g	104	0.2	69	3.3	13.6	0.1	2.1
Raspberry, with Fruit Layer, Bio Activia, Danone*	1 Pot/125g	108	3.5	86	3.5	11.6	2.8	2.0
Raspberry, with Real Fruit, Low Fat, Morrisons*	1 Pot/150g	134	1.8	89	3.6	16.0	1.2	0.3
Raspberry & Blackberry, Rich & Creamy, Spelga*	1 Pot/150g	188	7.1	125	3.7	17.2	4.7	0.1
Raspberry & Blackberry, Thick & Creamy, Co-Op*	1 Pot/150g	188	6.9	125	3.6	17.3	4.6	0.1
Raspberry & Cranberry, BGTY, Sainsbury's*	1 Pot/125g	65	0.1	52	4.4	8.4	0.1	0.5
Raspberry & Cranberry, Light, HL, Tesco*	1 Pot/125g	55	0.3	44	4.2	6.3	0.2	1.1
Raspberry & Cranberry, Smooth, Mullerlight, Muller*	1 Pot/200g	104	0.2	52	4.2	7.9	0.1	0.5
Raspberry & Redcurrant, Low Fat, Morrisons*	1 Pot/125g	117	2.0	94	4.4	15.4	1.6	0.7

Y

YOGHURT

Measure INFO/WEIGHT		per Measure		Nutrition Values per 100g / 100ml				
		KCAL	FAT	KCAL	PROT	CARB	FAT	FIBRE
Raspberry & Redcurrant, Low Fat, Sainsbury's*	1 Pot/125g	109	1.8	87	4.2	14.5	1.4	0.5
Raspberry Tart, Sveltesse, Nestle*	1 Pot/125g	64	0.1	51	4.5	7.1	0.1	0.1
Red Berry, Healthy Balance, Corner, Muller*	1 Pot/150g	179	4.1	119	5.0	18.0	2.7	0.5
Red Berry, Vitality, Low Fat, Muller*	1 Pot/150g	138	2.9	92	4.3	13.8	1.9	0.7
Red Cherry, Fat Free, Ski, Nestle*	1 Pot 120g	97	0.1	81	4.5	15.6	0.1	0.1
Red Cherry, Fruit Layered, GFY, Asda*	1 Pot/125g	75	0.1	60	3.7	11.0	0.1	0.0
Red Cherry, Very Cherry, Activ8, Ski, Nestle*	1 Pot/120g	115	2.0	96	4.5	15.7	1.7	0.1
Red Fruits, Crumble Style, Sveltesse, Nestle*	1 Pot/125g	100	0.3	80	4.9	14.6	0.2	0.4
Rhubarb, Custard Style, Co-Op*	1 Pot/150g	203	8.0	135	3.7	17.2	5.3	0.3
Rhubarb, Custard Style, Somerfield*	1 Pot/125g	149	6.3	119	3.0	16.0	5.0	0.0
Rhubarb, Eat Smart, Morrisons*	1 Pot/200g	112	0.6	56	5.7	7.9	0.3	0.2
Rhubarb, Eat Smart, Safeway*	1 Pot/125g	69	0.1	55	5.1	7.8	0.1	0.2
Rhubarb, Farmhouse, TTD, Sainsbury's*	1 Pot/150g	149	4.7	99	4.3	13.4	3.1	0.3
Rhubarb, Fruit Yoghurt, Bio Activia, Danone*	1 Pot/125g	113	4.0	90	3.5	11.8	3.2	2.2
Rhubarb, Longley Farm*	1 Pot/150g	165	5.6	110	4.9	14.3	3.7	0.0
Rhubarb, Low Fat, Asda*	1 Pot/150g	122	1.5	81	4.3	13.8	1.0	0.3
Rhubarb, Low Fat, Bio Live, Rachel's Organic*	1 Pot/100g	73	1.7	73	3.5	11.0	1.7	0.0
Rhubarb, Low Fat, Organic, M & S*	1 Pot/170g	119	2.0	70	4.1	10.6	1.2	0.2
Rhubarb, Low Fat, Organic, Sainsbury's*	1 Pot/125g	99	1.3	79	5.1	12.3	1.0	0.2
Rhubarb, Low Fat, Safeway*	1 Pot/150g	137	1.7	91	4.6	15.7	1.1	0.1
Rhubarb, Low Fat, Sainsbury's*	1 Pot/125g	114	2.1	91	4.5	14.5	1.7	0.2
Rhubarb, Low Fat, Tesco*	1 Pot/150g	135	2.7	90	4.3	14.0	1.8	0.0
Rhubarb, M & S*	1 Pot/150g	149	2.1	99	4.4	17.4	1.4	0.3
Rhubarb, Spiced, Thick & Creamy, COU, M & S*	1 Pot/170g	68	0.2	40	4.3	5.8	0.1	0.5
Rhubarb, Very Low Fat, Somerfield*	1 Pot/125g	58	0.0	46	5.0	6.0	0.0	0.0
Rhubarb & Orange, Tesco*	1 Pot/150g	146	1.7	97	4.6	17.1	1.1	0.5
Rhubarb & Vanilla, Summer, Biopot, Onken*	1/5 Pot/100g	106	2.6	106	3.8	16.9	2.6	0.3
Rhubarb Crumble, Crunch Corner, Muller*	1 Pot/150g	239	8.4	159	3.6	23.5	5.6	0.5
Rhubarb Crumble, Layered Style, HE, Tesco*	1 Pot/125g	93	0.9	74	4.1	12.9	0.7	0.2
Rich & Creamy, Spelga*	1 Pot/150g	188	7.1	125	3.7	17.2	4.7	0.1
Simpley Strawberry, Low Fat, Ubley*	1 Pot/125g	115	1.4	92	4.8	15.6	1.1	0.3
Smooth Toffee, Eat Smart, Safeway*	1 Pot/125g	69	0.1	55	5.1	8.7	0.1	0.0
Smooth Toffee & Apple, Low Fat, Co-Op*	1 Pot/125g	150	1.3	120	6.0	22.0	1.0	0.1
Smooth Toffee & Orange, Co-Op*	1 Pot/125g	181	1.3	145	6.0	27.0	1.0	0.0
Smooth Vanilla, Eat Smart, Safeway*	1 Pot/125g	69	0.1	55	5.0	8.3	0.1	0.0
Somerset with Vanilla, TTD, Sainsbury's*	1 Pot/150g	222	9.9	148	4.0	18.1	6.6	0.0
Soya, Plain, Average	1oz/28g	20	1.2	72	5.0	3.9	4.2	0.0
Spanish Orange, Amore Luxury, Muller*	1 Pot/175g	264	13.7	151	2.9	17.2	7.8	0.1
Spiced Orange, Dessert, Low Fat, Sainsbury's*	1 Pot/125g	121	2.1	97	4.5	16.0	1.7	0.1
Sticky Toffee Pudding, Mullerlight, Muller*	1 Pot/175g	109	0.4	62	4.4	9.9	0.2	0.2
Strawberries & Cream, Finest, Tesco*	1 Pot/150g	206	10.4	137	3.4	15.4	6.9	0.5
Strawberries & Cream, TTD, Sainsbury's*	1 Pot/150g	194	8.6	129	3.6	15.8	5.7	0.5
Strawberry, & Muesli, Breakfast, Tesco*	1 Pot/170g	192	4.8	113	4.1	17.9	2.8	0.5
Strawberry, & Whole Grain, Bio Break, Tesco*	1 Pot/175g	175	1.9	100	4.7	17.8	1.1	0.2
Strawberry, 0.1% Fat, Shape, Danone*	1 Pot/120g	55	0.1	46	4.6	6.7	0.1	2.1
Strawberry, Balanced Lifestyle, Aldi*	1 Pot/150g	72	0.5	48	4.1	7.1	0.3	0.5
Strawberry, Bettabuy, Morrisons*	1 Pot/115g	91	1.5	79	4.4	12.8	1.3	0.3
Strawberry, BGTY, Sainsbury's*	1 Pot/125g	64	0.1	51	4.8	7.7	0.1	1.2
Strawberry, Bio, Co-Op*	1 Pot/125g	143	3.5	114	4.5	16.7	2.8	0.1
Strawberry, Bio, HE, Tesco*	1 Pot/125g	61	0.3	49	4.7	7.0	0.2	0.2
Strawberry, Bio Live, Fat Free, Rachel's Organic*	1 Pot/142g	124	4.8	87	3.5	10.5	3.4	0.0
Strawberry, Bio Live, Organic, Yeo Valley*	1 Pot/125g	125	5.0	100	4.4	11.7	4.0	0.1
Strawberry, Bio Virtually Fat Free, Tesco*	1 Pot/125g	50	0.3	40	4.4	5.3	0.2	0.9

YOGHURT

INFO/WEIGHT	Measure	per Measure		Nutrition Values per 100g / 100ml				
		KCAL	FAT	KCAL	PROT	CARB	FAT	FIBRE
Strawberry, Biopot, Lite, Onken*	1 Pot/150g	72	0.3	48	4.7	6.9	0.2	0.2
Strawberry, Carb Control, Tesco*	1 Pot/125g	61	1.3	49	3.7	6.3	1.0	0.2
Strawberry, Childrens, Co-Op*	1 Pot/125g	121	3.4	97	3.5	14.9	2.7	0.2
Strawberry, Custard Style, Shapers, Boots*	1 Pot/150g	117	1.1	78	3.9	14.0	0.7	0.5
Strawberry, Custard Style, Somerfield*	1 Pot/125g	153	6.3	122	3.0	17.0	5.0	0.0
Strawberry, Duo, Co-Op*	1 Pot/175g	219	8.8	125	3.0	17.0	5.0	0.7
Strawberry, Eat Smart, Morrisons*	1 Pot/200g	116	0.6	58	5.7	8.5	0.3	0.3
Strawberry, Eat Smart, Safeway*	1 Pot/125g	69	0.1	55	5.1	8.3	0.1	0.3
Strawberry, Everyday Low Fat, Co-Op*	1 Pot/125g	88	0.9	70	3.0	13.0	0.7	0.0
Strawberry, Farmhouse, BGTY, Sainsbury's*	1 Pot/150g	107	0.6	71	3.2	13.7	0.4	0.5
Strawberry, Fat Free, Activ8, Ski, Nestle*	1 Pot/120g	89	0.2	74	4.5	13.7	0.2	0.3
Strawberry, Fat Free, Bio Activia, Danone*	1 Pot/125g	68	0.1	54	4.7	8.6	0.1	0.8
Strawberry, Fat Free, Bio Live, Organic, Yeo Valley*	1 Pot/125g	108	1.3	86	5.1	14.1	1.0	0.1
Strawberry, Fat Free, Rachel's Organic*	1 Pot/125g	121	2.3	97	4.7	15.4	1.8	0.0
Strawberry, Fat Free, Waitrose*	1 Pot/150g	135	0.2	90	4.6	17.8	0.1	0.1
Strawberry, Fruit Corner, Snack Size, Muller*	1 Pot/95g	108	3.8	114	3.9	15.6	4.0	0.4
Strawberry, Fruit Yoghurt, Bio Activia, Danone*	1 Pot/125g	118	4.0	94	3.5	12.8	3.2	2.0
Strawberry, Fruit'n'creamy, Ubley*	1 Pot/150g	167	4.4	111	4.3	16.9	2.9	0.3
Strawberry, Fruity, Mullerlight, Muller*	1 Pot/200g	102	0.2	51	4.1	7.9	0.1	0.0
Strawberry, Great Stuff, Asda*	1 Pot/60g	58	1.5	97	4.7	14.0	2.5	0.5
Strawberry, Greek Style, Shape, Danone*	1 Pot/120g	136	3.2	113	6.0	16.1	2.7	0.0
Strawberry, Happy Shopper*	1 Pot/150g	131	0.5	87	3.0	18.5	0.3	0.0
Strawberry, Healthy Balance, Corner, Muller*	1 Pot/150g	176	3.2	117	4.2	19.8	2.1	0.5
Strawberry, Light, Brooklea*	1 Pot/200g	154	0.2	77	6.1	12.9	0.1	0.4
Strawberry, Light, Fat Free, Muller*	1 Pot/200g	102	0.2	51	4.1	7.7	0.1	0.2
Strawberry, Light, HL, Tesco*	1 Pot/200g	80	0.2	40	3.5	6.4	0.1	0.8
Strawberry, Light & Refreshing, Campina*	1 Pot/125g	110	1.4	88	2.5	16.9	1.1	0.0
Strawberry, Little Town Dairy*	1 Pot/125g	82	2.0	66	2.9	9.9	1.6	0.0
Strawberry, Live, Turners Dairies*	1 Pot/125g	86	0.4	69	4.9	11.9	0.3	0.0
Strawberry, Low Fat, Asda*	1 Pot/125g	114	1.3	91	4.4	16.0	1.0	0.0
Strawberry, Low Fat, Basics, Sainsbury's*	1 Pot/125g	84	1.6	67	4.3	9.6	1.3	0.1
Strawberry, Low Fat, Benecol*	1 Pot/125g	98	0.8	78	3.7	14.5	0.6	0.0
Strawberry, Low Fat, Budgens*	1 Pot/125g	113	1.4	90	4.6	15.5	1.1	0.1
Strawberry, Low Fat, Co-Op*	1 Pot/125g	113	1.3	90	5.0	16.0	1.0	0.3
Strawberry, Low Fat, Lakeland*	1 Pot/125g	98	1.0	78	4.3	13.4	0.8	0.1
Strawberry, Low Fat, Loseley*	1 Pot/140g	143	2.5	102	5.4	16.0	1.8	0.0
Strawberry, Low Fat, Organic, Sainsbury's*	1 Pot/125g	100	1.3	80	5.3	12.6	1.0	0.1
Strawberry, Low Fat, Organic, Somerfield*	1 Pot/150g	153	3.0	102	6.0	17.0	2.0	0.0
Strawberry, Low Fat, Safeway*	1 Pot/150g	138	1.7	92	4.6	16.0	1.1	0.1
Strawberry, Low Fat, Sainsbury's*	1 Pot/150g	107	1.7	71	3.5	11.7	1.1	0.5
Strawberry, Low Fat, SmartPrice, Asda*	1 Pot/125g	96	0.8	77	2.5	15.2	0.6	0.0
Strawberry, Low Fat, Spelga*	1 Pot/125g	129	2.3	103	4.5	18.0	1.8	0.0
Strawberry, Low Fat, Tesco*	1 Pot/125g	113	2.1	90	4.2	14.4	1.7	0.0
Strawberry, Low Fat, Value, Tesco*	1 Pot/125g	81	0.9	65	2.7	11.8	0.7	0.1
Strawberry, Luscious, Shapers, Boots*	1 Pot/150g	83	1.7	55	4.0	7.3	1.1	0.6
Strawberry, Organic, Low Fat, Morrisons*	1 Pot/150g	158	2.3	105	5.2	17.6	1.5	0.1
Strawberry, Organic, Low Fat, Tesco*	1 Pot/150g	135	1.5	90	6.3	13.7	1.0	0.9
Strawberry, Organic, Yeo Valley*	1 Pot/150g	144	5.0	96	4.3	12.4	3.3	0.1
Strawberry, PB, Waitrose*	1 Pot/150g	136	0.2	91	4.6	17.8	0.1	0.1
Strawberry, Petit Filou, Yoplait*	1 Pot/60g	62	1.7	104	6.6	12.6	2.9	0.2
Strawberry, Probiotic, Tesco*	1 Pot/125g	95	2.8	76	4.4	8.9	2.2	0.1
Strawberry, Redcurrant, Bio Layered, Sainsbury's*	1 Pot/125g	134	3.4	107	4.1	16.5	2.7	0.2
Strawberry, Seriously Fruity, Low Fat, Waitrose*	1 Pot/150g	131	1.5	87	4.5	15.0	1.0	0.3

Y

YOGHURT

INFO/WEIGHT	Measure	per Measure KCAL	FAT	Nutrition Values per 100g / 100ml KCAL	PROT	CARB	FAT	FIBRE
Strawberry, Smooth, Activ8, Ski, Nestle*	1 Pot/120g	113	2.0	94	4.6	14.8	1.7	0.7
Strawberry, Smooth Set, Co-Op*	1 Pot/125g	95	1.1	76	3.7	12.5	0.9	0.0
Strawberry, Soyage, GranoVita*	1 Pot/145g	112	0.6	77	1.8	16.5	0.4	0.0
Strawberry, Sveltesse, Nestle*	1 Pot/125g	61	0.1	49	4.8	7.1	0.1	0.2
Strawberry, Thick & Creamy, Co-Op*	1 Pot/150g	182	6.9	121	3.6	16.4	4.6	0.1
Strawberry, Thick & Creamy, Waitrose*	1 Pot/125g	135	3.1	108	3.7	17.6	2.5	0.4
Strawberry, Thick & Fruity, Probiotic, COU, M & S*	1 Pot/167g	75	0.2	45	4.1	7.3	0.1	0.4
Strawberry, Very Berry, Activ8, Ski, Nestle*	1 Pot/120g	110	2.0	92	4.3	15.0	1.7	0.3
Strawberry, Very Low Fat, Bio, Somerfield*	1 Pot/200g	100	0.0	50	5.0	7.0	0.0	0.0
Strawberry, Virtually Fat Free, Morrisons*	1 Pot/200g	114	0.4	57	5.4	8.4	0.2	0.0
Strawberry, Virtually Fat Free, Organic, Yeo Valley*	1 Pot/125g	98	0.1	78	5.1	14.3	0.1	0.1
Strawberry, Virtually Fat Free, Shapers, Boots*	1 Pot/125g	67	0.1	54	5.2	8.1	0.1	0.1
Strawberry, Virtually Fat Free, Tesco*	1 Pot/125g	53	0.3	42	4.1	6.0	0.2	1.0
Strawberry, Vitality, Low Fat, Muller*	1 Pot/175g	163	3.3	93	4.3	14.0	1.9	0.8
Strawberry, Wholemilk, Organic, Sainsbury's*	1 Pot/150g	123	5.3	82	3.5	9.2	3.5	0.1
Strawberry, Yoplait*	1 Pot/125g	61	0.3	49	4.2	7.6	0.2	0.9
Strawberry & Cornish Clotted Cream, M & S*	1 Pot/150g	218	11.6	145	3.2	15.4	7.7	0.5
Strawberry & French Vanilla, Amore, Muller*	1 Pot/150g	225	11.7	150	2.9	17.0	7.8	0.1
Strawberry & Raspberry, HL, Tesco*	1 Pot/125g	58	0.1	46	4.2	7.0	0.1	0.2
Strawberry & Raspberry, Low Fat, Asda*	1 Pot/150g	143	1.5	95	4.6	17.4	1.0	0.2
Strawberry & Raspberry, Low Fat, Sainsbury's*	1 Pot/125g	109	1.8	87	4.2	14.3	1.4	0.2
Strawberry & Rhubarb, Channel Island, M & S*	1 Pot/150g	158	4.5	105	3.9	15.4	3.0	0.0
Strawberry & Rhubarb, Low Fat, Sainsbury's*	1 Pot/125g	108	1.8	86	4.2	14.1	1.4	0.2
Strawberry & Rhubarb, Low Fat, Somerfield*	1 Pot/125g	108	1.0	86	4.1	15.6	0.8	0.1
Strawberry & Vanilla, Low Fat, Somerfield*	1 Pot/125g	109	1.0	87	4.0	15.9	0.8	0.1
Strawberry Cheesecake, Eat Smart, Safeway*	1 Pot/125g	64	0.1	51	4.7	7.7	0.1	0.3
Strawberry Crumble, Crunch Corner, Muller*	1 Pot/150g	234	8.4	156	3.6	22.9	5.6	0.5
Strawberry Mousse, Shapers, Boots*	1 Pot/90g	88	3.7	97	4.1	11.0	4.1	0.1
Strawberry Orange Balls. Crunch Corner, Muller*	1 Pot/150g	222	8.1	148	4.0	20.8	5.4	0.2
Strawberry Shortcake, Crunch Corner, Muller*	1 Pot/150g	231	8.6	154	3.9	21.0	5.7	0.1
Summer Fruits, Cool Country*	1 Pot/150g	137	2.3	91	3.0	16.3	1.5	0.0
Summer Fruits, Light, Spelga*	1 Pot/175g	79	0.4	45	4.4	7.1	0.2	0.0
Summer Selection, Fat Free, Organic, Yeo Valley*	1 Pot/125g	89	0.1	71	5.2	12.3	0.1	0.2
Summer Selection, Thick & Fruity, COU, M & S*	1 Pot/145g	75	0.2	52	4.2	7.8	0.1	0.5
Summerfruits Bio, Boots*	1 Pot/150g	140	4.1	93	4.1	13.0	2.7	0.4
Timperley Rhubarb, Seriously Fruity, Waitrose*	1 Pot/125g	106	1.3	85	4.6	14.4	1.0	0.0
Toffee, Benecol*	1 Pot/125g	124	0.9	99	3.8	19.3	0.7	0.0
Toffee, Childrens, Co-Op*	1 Pot/125g	143	3.5	114	3.6	18.6	2.8	0.0
Toffee, COU, M & S*	1 Pot/145g	65	0.3	45	4.2	7.7	0.2	0.0
Toffee, Economy, Sainsbury's*	1 Pot/126g	91	1.3	72	3.0	12.8	1.0	0.0
Toffee, Fat Free, Eat Smart, Safeway*	1 Pot/200g	100	0.2	50	4.6	7.7	0.1	0.0
Toffee, Light, HL, Tesco*	1 Pot/200g	80	0.2	40	3.9	5.9	0.1	1.0
Toffee, Live Bio, PB, Waitrose*	1 Pot/150g	156	0.5	104	4.2	21.1	0.3	0.0
Toffee, Low Fat, Asda*	1 Pot/125g	104	0.8	83	2.5	17.0	0.6	0.0
Toffee, Low Fat, Budgens*	1 Pot/125g	145	1.5	116	4.7	21.6	1.2	0.0
Toffee, Low Fat, Co-Op*	1 Pot/150g	125	1.4	83	3.8	15.0	0.9	0.2
Toffee, Low Fat, M & S*	1 Pot/150g	180	2.6	120	4.9	21.6	1.7	0.0
Toffee, Low Fat, Safeway*	1 Pot/150g	174	1.8	116	4.7	21.6	1.2	0.0
Toffee, Low Fat, Somerfield*	1 Pot/150g	149	1.5	99	3.0	19.0	1.0	0.0
Toffee, Low Fat, Tesco*	1 Pot/150g	150	2.7	100	4.9	15.8	1.8	0.8
Toffee, Seriously Smooth, Low Fat, Waitrose*	1 Pot/150g	156	3.2	104	4.7	16.5	2.1	0.1
Toffee, Smooth, Mullerlight, Muller*	1 Pot/200g	102	0.2	51	4.0	7.9	0.1	0.0
Toffee, Very Low Fat Bio, Somerfield*	1 Pot/200g	100	0.0	50	5.0	7.0	0.0	0.0

YOGHURT

Measure INFO/WEIGHT	per Measure KCAL	FAT	Nutrition Values per 100g / 100ml KCAL	PROT	CARB	FAT	FIBRE
YOGHURT							
Toffee, Virtually Fat Free, Boots* — 1 Pot/125g	69	0.1	55	5.1	8.3	0.1	0.0
Toffee Apple, COU, M & S* — 1 Pot/200g	90	0.4	45	4.2	6.3	0.2	0.2
Toffee Apple, Indulgent Greek Style, Somerfield* — 1 Pot/125g	225	8.8	180	3.0	27.0	7.0	0.0
Toffee Flavour, Bio, Virtually Fat Free, Morrisons* — 1 Pot/125g	69	0.3	55	5.3	8.1	0.2	0.0
Toffee Fudge, Low Fat, Sainsbury's* — 1 Pot/125g	146	2.5	117	4.3	20.4	2.0	0.0
Toffee Hoops, Crunch Corner, Muller* — 1 Pot/150g	233	8.3	155	4.0	22.6	5.5	0.2
Treacle Toffee, Dessert, Low Fat, Sainsbury's* — 1 Pot/125g	149	2.4	119	4.3	21.2	1.9	0.0
Tropical, Luscious, Low Fat, Rachel's Organic* — 1 Pot/125g	115	2.0	92	4.0	15.3	1.6	0.0
Tropical Fruit, Greek Style, Asda* — 1 Pot/125g	170	8.8	136	3.3	15.0	7.0	0.0
Tropical Fruit, Greek Style, Shapers, Boots* — 1 Pot/150g	101	2.3	67	3.6	9.8	1.5	0.8
Tropical Fruit, HL, Tesco* — 1 Pot/125g	56	0.3	45	4.1	6.6	0.2	0.9
Valencia Orange, Layered, Bio, GFY, Asda* — 1 Pot/125g	80	0.1	64	3.7	12.0	0.1	0.0
Vanilla, Average — 1 Pot/120g	100	5.4	83	4.5	12.4	4.5	0.8
Vanilla, Benecol* — 1 Pot/125g	99	0.8	79	3.7	14.6	0.6	0.0
Vanilla, BGTY, Sainsbury's* — 1 Pot/200g	98	0.2	49	4.5	7.5	0.1	0.0
Vanilla, Bio, BFY, Morrisons* — 1 Pot/150g	83	0.5	55	5.7	8.4	0.3	0.0
Vanilla, Bio Live, Low Fat, Rachel's Organic* — 1 Pot/142g	104	2.6	73	3.7	10.5	1.8	0.0
Vanilla, Breakfast, Tesco* — 1 Pot/150g	108	0.8	72	2.9	13.9	0.5	0.0
Vanilla, Creamy, Smarties, Nestle* — 1 Pot/120g	200	7.4	167	4.1	23.7	6.2	0.0
Vanilla, Eat Smart, Morrisons* — 1 Pot/200g	116	0.6	58	5.6	8.4	0.3	0.1
Vanilla, French Set Wholemilk, Asda* — 1 Pot/125g	125	4.0	100	3.6	14.1	3.2	0.0
Vanilla, Lifestyle, Co-Op* — 1 Pot/180g	81	0.2	45	5.0	6.0	0.1	0.0
Vanilla, Live, Bio, Bio Green Dairy* — 1 Bottle/250ml	263	7.3	105	2.5	17.7	2.9	0.0
Vanilla, Low Fat, Bio, Sainsbury's* — 1 Pot/150g	147	1.7	98	4.8	17.2	1.1	0.0
Vanilla, Low Fat, Safeway* — 1 Pot/150g	155	1.7	103	4.6	18.7	1.1	0.0
Vanilla, Low Fat, Tesco* — 1 Pot/125g	125	2.1	100	4.9	16.3	1.7	0.0
Vanilla, Organic, Low Fat, Sainsbury's* — 1 Pot/125g	114	1.3	91	5.3	15.3	1.0	0.0
Vanilla, Smooth, Mullerlight, Muller* — 1 Pot/200g	102	0.2	51	4.3	7.5	0.1	0.0
Vanilla, Smooth Set, Co-Op* — 1 Pot/125g	95	1.1	76	3.7	12.5	0.9	0.0
Vanilla, Thick & Creamy, Channel Island, M & S* — 1 Pot/150g	188	6.6	125	4.5	17.5	4.4	1.0
Vanilla, Thick & Creamy, Probiotic, COU, M & S* — 1 Pot/170g	77	0.2	45	4.5	6.3	0.1	0.5
Vanilla, Very Low Fat Bio, Somerfield* — 1 Pot/200g	98	0.0	49	5.0	7.0	0.0	0.0
Vanilla, Virtually Fat Free, Shapers, Boots* — 1 Pot/125g	66	0.1	53	5.0	7.9	0.1	0.0
Vanilla, Virtually Fat Free, Yeo Valley* — 1 Pot/150g	122	0.2	81	5.1	15.0	0.1	0.0
Vanilla & Pineapple, Nestle* — 1 Pot/125g	120	1.9	96	4.2	16.7	1.5	0.0
Vanilla Choco Balls, Crunch Corner, Muller* — 1 Pot/150g	228	7.5	152	4.0	22.0	5.0	0.2
Vanilla Flavour, HL, Light, Tesco* — 1 Pot/200g	90	0.2	45	4.1	7.0	0.1	0.0
Vanilla Flavour, Organic, Low Fat, Tesco* — 1 Pot/125g	114	1.3	91	5.3	15.3	1.0	0.0
Vanilla Toffee, Low Fat, Sainsbury's* — 1 Pot/125g	145	2.3	116	4.3	20.6	1.8	0.0
Very....lemon Curd, Morrisons* — 1 Pot/150g	263	13.7	175	4.1	19.2	9.1	0.0
Walnut & Greek Honey, Amore Luxury, Muller* — 1 Pot/150g	242	13.1	161	3.0	17.6	8.7	0.1
White Peach, Seriously Fruity, Waitrose* — 1 Pot/150g	152	2.6	101	4.8	16.5	1.7	0.2
Wild Blackberry, Seriously Fruity, Waitrose* — 1 Pot/125g	120	1.3	96	4.4	17.2	1.0	0.4
Wild Blackberry, The Best, Safeway* — 1 Pot/175g	254	11.2	145	3.3	17.9	6.4	1.2
Wild Blueberry, Finest, Tesco* — 1 Pot/150g	212	10.2	141	3.4	16.6	6.8	0.5
Winter Medley, COU, M & S* — 1 Pot/150g	68	0.2	45	4.2	6.2	0.1	0.1
with Hazelnut, Low Fat, Safeway* — 1 Pot/150g	182	3.5	121	4.9	20.1	2.3	0.2
with Large Fruit Chunks, Bio, Waitrose* — 1 Pot/170g	170	4.1	100	3.7	15.8	2.4	0.4
Yellow Fruit, Yoplait* — 1 Pot/125g	139	3.6	111	3.3	18.0	2.9	0.0
YOGHURT BREAK							
Forest Fruit, Go Ahead, McVitie's* — 1 Slice/18.1g	68	2.0	375	5.0	64.0	11.0	1.7
Plain, Go Ahead, McVitie's* — 1 Bar/18.3g	72	2.1	394	6.5	66.0	11.5	3.3
Strawberry, Go Ahead, McVitie's* — 1 Slice/18.1g	72	2.0	397	5.9	68.0	11.1	2.1

	Measure INFO/WEIGHT	per Measure		Nutrition Values per 100g / 100ml				
		KCAL	FAT	KCAL	PROT	CARB	FAT	FIBRE

YOGHURT BREAK

Tropical, Go Ahead, McVitie's*	2 Slices/36g	155	4.0	430	5.9	76.3	11.0	2.3

YOGHURT DRINK

Actimel, Mixed Fruit, Danone*	1 Serving/100ml	88	1.5	88	2.7	16.0	1.5	0.0
Actimel, Orange, Danone*	1 fl oz/30ml	26	0.5	88	2.7	16.0	1.5	0.0
Actimel, Original, 0.1% Fat, Danone*	1 Bottle/100g	28	0.1	28	2.8	3.3	0.1	1.9
Actimel, Original, Danone*	1 fl oz/30ml	24	0.5	80	2.8	12.8	1.6	0.0
Actimel, Pineapple, 0.1% Fat, Danone*	1 Bottle/100g	33	0.0	33	2.7	5.5	0.0	1.8
Actimel, Strawberry, Danone*	1 Bottle/100g	74	1.5	74	2.9	11.5	1.5	0.0
Average	1floz/30ml	19	0.0	62	3.1	13.1	0.0	0.0
Ayran, Gazi*	1 Can/330ml	34	1.9	10	0.5	0.8	0.6	0.0
Banana & Honey, Ski Up & Go, Nestle*	1 Bottle/250g	215	2.2	86	0.0	16.0	0.9	0.0
Bioactive, Yagua*	1 Bottle/200ml	84	0.0	42	0.4	9.9	0.0	0.0
Blueberry & Blackcurrant, Orchard Maid*	1 Carton/250ml	148	0.1	59	1.6	13.6	0.0	0.0
Cholesterol Lowering, Asda*	1 Bottle/100g	76	1.4	76	2.9	13.0	1.4	1.0
Danacol, Original, Danone*	1 Bottle/100ml	64	1.0	64	3.2	10.0	1.0	0.0
Danacol, Strawberry, Danone*	1 Bottle/100g	68	1.2	68	3.2	11.2	1.2	0.0
Fristi*	1 Carton/330g	191	0.3	58	2.6	13.6	0.1	0.0
Light, Benecol*	1 Bottle/67.5g	41	1.4	60	2.8	7.3	2.1	0.1
Light, Yakult*	1 Serving/65ml	27	0.1	42	1.4	10.2	0.1	1.8
Mixed Berry, Up & Go, Ski, Nestle*	1 Bottle/250g	218	2.3	87	3.1	16.0	0.9	0.2
Nectarine, Pfirsich, Light, Bifidus, Emmi*	1 Serving/500ml	245	4.0	49	3.0	7.5	0.8	0.0
Omega 3 Plus, Raspberry, Pro Biotic, Flora*	1 Bottle/100g	58	1.6	58	2.6	8.5	1.6	0.0
Orchard Maid*	1 Serving/250g	148	0.1	59	1.6	13.0	0.0	0.0
Original, Benecol*	1 Serving/70g	62	1.6	88	2.6	14.2	2.3	0.0
Peach & Apricot, Benecol*	1 Bottle/67.5g	38	1.5	56	2.8	6.2	2.2	0.0
Peach & Mango, Fristi*	1 Carton/330g	191	0.3	58	2.6	13.6	0.1	0.0
Pro Activ, Orange, Cholesterol, Flora*	1 Bottle/100g	87	2.9	87	2.6	12.5	2.9	0.0
Pro Activ, Original, Blood Pressure, Flora*	1 Bottle/100g	80	1.5	80	3.9	12.7	1.5	0.3
Pro Activ, Original, Cholesterol, Flora*	1 Bottle/100g	87	2.9	87	2.6	12.5	2.9	0.0
Pro Activ, Strawberry, Blood Pressure, Flora*	1 Bottle/100g	80	1.5	80	3.9	12.7	1.5	0.3
Pro Activ, Strawberry, Cholesterol, Flora*	1 Bottle/100g	87	2.9	87	2.6	12.5	2.9	0.0
Probiotic, Orange, Lidl*	1 Serving/125ml	105	2.0	84	2.5	14.7	1.6	0.0
Strawberry, Benecol*	1 Bottle/67.5g	38	1.5	56	2.9	6.2	2.2	0.0
Strawberry, Bio, The Best, Safeway*	1 Bottle/250ml	215	4.8	86	2.7	13.6	1.9	0.6
Strawberry, Fristi*	1 Carton/250g	165	0.3	66	2.6	13.6	0.1	0.0
Strawberry, Yop, Yoplait*	1 Bottle/330g	261	4.3	79	2.8	14.0	1.3	0.0
Sveltesse, 0%, Nestle*	1 Pot/125g	61	0.1	49	4.8	7.3	0.1	0.1
Yakult*	1 Pot/65ml	51	0.1	78	1.4	17.8	0.1	0.0

YORK FRUITS

Terry's*	1 Sweet/9g	30	0.0	328	0.0	81.4	0.0	1.0

YORKIE

King Size, Nestle*	1 Bar/82.9g	446	26.1	537	6.1	57.3	31.5	0.0
Original, Nestle*	1 Bar/68g	365	21.4	537	6.1	57.3	31.5	0.7
Raisin & Biscuit, Nestle*	1 Bar/61g	303	16.0	497	5.5	59.7	26.2	0.9

YORKSHIRE PUDDING

& Beef Dripping, M & S*	4 Puddings/100g	410	30.4	410	9.4	25.2	30.4	3.2
3", Baked, Aunt Bessie's*	1 Pudding/36g	91	2.8	252	9.0	36.4	7.9	1.7
4 Minute, Aunt Bessie's*	1 Pudding/18g	52	2.0	291	10.5	36.6	11.3	2.2
7", Baked, Aunt Bessie's*	1 Pudding/110g	290	9.9	264	8.5	37.4	9.0	2.0
Average	1 Pudding/30g	62	3.0	208	6.6	24.7	9.9	0.9
Baked Sage & Onion, Morrisons*	1 Pudding/19.2g	50	2.2	261	8.6	30.4	11.7	1.2
Batters, in Foils, Frozen, Aunt Bessie's*	1 Pudding/17g	47	1.8	276	9.1	32.6	10.8	1.4
Chicken & Vegetable, COU, M & S*	1 Pudding/150g	195	3.3	130	12.2	14.3	2.2	1.3

	Measure INFO/WEIGHT	per Measure KCAL	per Measure FAT	Nutrition Values per 100g / 100ml KCAL	PROT	CARB	FAT	FIBRE
YORKSHIRE PUDDING								
Filled, Chicken Casserole, Farmfoods*	1 Pack/280g	347	6.4	124	6.5	19.3	2.3	1.3
Filled, with Beef, Morrisons*	1 Serving/350g	515	21.0	147	7.4	15.7	6.0	0.5
Filled, with Sausage, Sainsbury's*	1 Pack/300g	576	31.2	192	6.9	17.5	10.4	0.9
Filled with Beef, Tesco*	1 Pudding/300g	408	15.6	136	6.1	16.2	5.2	1.1
Filled with Beef & Vegetable, Safeway*	1 Pack/300g	396	12.3	132	8.6	15.2	4.1	1.3
Filled with Chicken, GFY, Asda*	1 Pack/380.9g	438	9.9	115	9.0	14.0	2.6	1.5
Filled with Chicken, Tesco*	1 Pack/300g	366	8.7	122	6.5	17.4	2.9	1.3
Filled with Chicken & Vegetable, GFY, Asda*	1 Pack/380g	376	9.9	99	6.0	13.0	2.6	1.1
Frozen, Ovenbaked, Iceland*	1 Pudding/12.4g	35	0.9	290	9.7	45.1	7.9	4.1
Fully Prepared, M & S*	1 Pudding/22g	63	2.9	285	9.4	31.6	13.2	1.2
Giant, Aunt Bessie's*	1 Pudding/110g	290	9.9	264	8.5	37.4	9.0	2.0
Large, Aunt Bessie's*	1 Pudding/39g	108	4.4	277	8.5	35.3	11.4	1.5
Large, Co-Op*	1 Serving/110g	319	18.7	290	8.0	27.0	17.0	4.0
Large, Frozen, Co-Op*	1 Pudding/33.8g	85	2.4	250	10.0	36.0	7.0	2.0
Large, Iceland*	1 Pudding/30g	96	4.1	321	10.5	38.8	13.8	1.7
Large, Safeway*	1 Pudding/45g	123	3.7	273	8.5	41.1	8.3	2.5
Large, The Real Yorkshire Pudding Co*	1 Pudding/34g	103	4.1	304	11.5	37.3	12.1	2.5
Made From Batter Mix, Sainsbury's*	1 Pudding/100g	248	5.3	248	9.9	40.1	5.3	4.0
Minced Beef Filled, Waitrose*	1 Serving/350g	525	24.9	150	7.5	14.1	7.1	1.0
Mini, Asda*	1 Serving/17.4g	48	1.5	281	9.0	41.0	9.0	2.3
Mini, Co-Op*	1 Serving/16g	50	2.0	313	6.3	43.8	12.5	2.5
Mini, Farmfoods*	1 Pudding/3g	8	0.2	281	9.6	43.2	7.7	1.9
Premium, Bisto*	1 Pudding/30g	74	3.3	248	7.3	30.3	10.9	2.1
Ready Baked, SmartPrice, Asda*	1 Pudding/12g	36	1.1	297	10.0	44.0	9.0	2.8
Ready to Bake, Aunt Bessie's*	1 Pudding/17g	42	1.4	246	8.5	35.1	8.0	1.7
Ready to Bake, Sainsbury's*	1 Pudding/18g	48	1.6	263	9.9	35.9	8.9	1.3
Riding Lodge*	1 Pudding/16g	44	1.2	276	10.0	41.5	7.8	0.0
Roast Chicken Filled, COU, M & S*	1 Pudding/150g	210	4.1	140	12.6	15.7	2.7	0.9
Roberts Bakery*	1 Pudding/18.3g	47	1.6	263	9.9	35.9	8.9	1.3
Safeway*	1 Serving/22g	58	1.8	265	8.4	38.9	8.4	2.5
Sage & Onion, Tesco*	1 Pudding/19g	53	2.3	280	8.0	35.0	12.0	2.6
Sainsbury's*	1 Pudding/14g	43	2.0	309	7.9	37.5	14.1	2.9
Sausage & Onion Gravy Filled, Safeway*	1 Pudding/300g	540	27.6	180	6.2	18.0	9.2	1.2
Sausage Filled, Frozen, Tesco*	1 Pack/340g	510	19.7	150	6.6	17.8	5.8	1.8
Steak Filled, COU, M & S*	1 Serving/150g	188	3.8	125	11.0	14.7	2.5	0.8
The Best, Morrisons*	1 Pudding/22g	60	1.8	271	8.3	43.0	8.0	1.6
Traditional, Giant, Asda*	1 Yorkshire/110g	310	11.0	282	10.0	38.0	10.0	2.3
Traditional Style, Medium, Asda*	1 Pudding/35.7g	87	3.2	241	9.0	31.0	9.0	2.4
Traditional Style, Small, Asda*	1 Pudding/20g	52	2.0	262	8.0	35.0	10.0	2.9
Unbaked, Iceland*	1 Serving/30.8g	81	2.7	263	9.9	35.9	8.9	1.3
Value, Tesco*	1 Pudding/16g	45	1.9	282	9.7	34.3	11.8	1.6
with Beef in Gravy, Asda*	1 Serving/290g	406	10.2	140	7.0	20.0	3.5	0.7
YULE LOG								
Christmas Range, Tesco*	1 Serving/30g	131	6.4	442	4.9	56.8	21.7	1.1

	Measure INFO/WEIGHT	per Measure KCAL FAT		Nutrition Values per 100g / 100ml KCAL PROT CARB FAT FIBRE				

BAGEL FACTORY
BAGEL

	Measure INFO/WEIGHT	per Measure KCAL	FAT	KCAL	PROT	CARB	FAT	FIBRE
Bacon, Bagel Factory*	1 Bagel/100g	614	25.9	614	32.2	62.1	25.9	3.8
Salmon & Cream Cheese, Bagel Factory*	1 Serving/300g	515	18.3	172	10.0	19.1	6.1	0.7
Chicken, Tomato & Spinach, Wholemeal, Bagel Factory*	1 Bagel/100g	306	1.9	306	23.0	49.2	1.9	9.1
with Marmite, Wholemeal, Bagel Factory*	1 Bagel/85g	312	1.6	368	24.4	63.4	1.9	11.6

BURGER KING
BAGUETTE

	Measure INFO/WEIGHT	per Measure KCAL	FAT	KCAL	PROT	CARB	FAT	FIBRE
Chicken, BLT, Burger King*	1 Baguette/228g	578	26.0	254	10.1	27.2	11.4	1.8
Chicken, Piri Piri, Burger King*	1 Baguette/225g	348	4.0	155	11.6	23.1	1.8	1.3
Sweet Chilli Chicken, Burger King*	1 Baguette/198g	512	18.0	259	10.6	33.8	9.1	2.0

BURGERS

	Measure INFO/WEIGHT	per Measure KCAL	FAT	KCAL	PROT	CARB	FAT	FIBRE
Angus, 3 Pepper, Burger King*	1 Burger/246g	684	41.0	278	15.0	17.9	16.7	1.2
Angus, 6 Pack, Burger King*	1 Pack/318g	917	42.0	288	16.4	25.2	13.2	1.6
Angus, Burger King*	1 Burger/239g	561	31.0	235	12.6	17.6	13.0	0.8
Angus, Double, Burger King*	1 Burger/323g	814	31.0	252	9.3	13.0	9.6	0.6
Angus, Smoked Bacon & Cheddar, Burger King*	1 Burger/270g	696	41.0	258	14.4	15.6	15.2	0.7
Angus, Smoked Bacon & Cheddar, Double, Burger King*	1 Burger/354g	949	60.0	268	17.5	11.6	17.0	0.6
Angus, Smoky Blue, Burger King*	1 Burger/256g	650	39.0	254	13.3	16.8	15.2	0.8
Cheeseburger, Bacon Double, Burger King*	1 Burger/160g	478	27.0	299	20.0	17.5	16.9	0.6
Cheeseburger, Bacon Double, Extra Large, Burger King*	1 Burger/302g	863	51.0	286	21.2	13.6	16.9	1.3
Cheeseburger, Burger King*	1 Burger/123g	311	13.0	253	13.8	23.6	10.6	0.8
Cheeseburger, Double, Burger King*	1 Burger/173g	463	25.0	268	17.3	16.8	14.5	0.6
Cheeseburger, Supreme, Burger King*	1 Burger/147g	385	20.0	262	12.9	20.4	13.6	1.4
Chicken Flamer, Burger King*	1 Sandwich/162g	308	11.8	190	12.6	18.6	7.3	1.9
Chicken Royale, Burger King*	1 Burger/210g	574	32.0	273	12.4	21.4	15.2	2.4
Hamburger, Burger King*	1 Burger/110g	270	10.0	245	13.6	26.4	9.1	0.9
Ocean Catch, Burger King*	1 Burger/175g	399	18.0	228	9.7	25.1	10.3	1.1
Spicy Bean, Burger King*	1 Burger/247g	506	20.0	205	7.7	25.1	8.1	3.6
Spicy Royale, Burger King*	1 Burger/210g	545	30.0	260	12.4	21.0	14.3	2.4
Whopper, Angry, Burger King*	1 Burger/310g	784	47.1	253	11.6	17.4	15.2	1.3
Whopper, Burger King*	1 Burger/274g	614	34.0	224	10.6	17.2	12.4	1.5
Whopper, Dark, Burger King*	1 Burger/296g	771	34.0	260	11.5	16.6	11.5	1.4
Whopper, Double, Burger King*	1 Burger/355g	841	50.0	237	14.1	13.2	14.1	1.1
Whopper, Double, with Cheese, Burger King*	1 Burger/380g	923	57.0	243	14.5	12.4	15.0	1.1

BURGERS VEGETARIAN

	Measure INFO/WEIGHT	per Measure KCAL	FAT	KCAL	PROT	CARB	FAT	FIBRE
Burger King*	1 Burger/222g	409	15.0	184	5.9	24.3	6.8	2.7

BUTTY

	Measure INFO/WEIGHT	per Measure KCAL	FAT	KCAL	PROT	CARB	FAT	FIBRE
Bacon & Egg, Burger King*	1 Butty/165g	456	23.0	276	13.9	23.6	13.9	1.2
Bacon & Egg, with Brown Sauce, Burger King*	1 Butty/176g	469	23.0	266	13.1	23.3	13.1	1.1
Bacon & Egg, with Ketchup, Burger King*	1 Butty/176g	467	23.0	265	13.1	23.9	13.1	1.1
Bacon, Burger King*	1 Butty/115g	376	17.0	327	15.7	33.0	14.8	1.7
Bacon, with Brown Sauce, Burger King*	1 Butty/126g	389	17.0	309	14.3	31.8	13.5	1.6
Bacon, with Ketchup, Burger King*	1 Butty/126g	387	17.0	307	14.3	32.5	13.5	1.6
Big Breakfast, Burger King*	1 Butty/301g	832	49.0	276	15.6	16.3	16.3	0.7
Big Breakfast, with Brown Sauce, Burger King*	1 Butty/312g	845	49.0	271	15.1	16.0	15.7	0.6
Big Breakfast, with Ketchup, Burger King*	1 Butty/312g	843	49.0	270	15.1	16.4	15.7	0.6
Egg & Cheese, Burger King*	1 Butty/153g	445	25.0	291	11.1	24.2	16.3	1.3
Egg & Cheese, with Brown Sauce, Burger King*	1 Butty/164g	458	25.0	279	10.4	24.4	15.2	1.2
Egg & Cheese, with Ketchup, Burger King*	1 Butty/164g	456	25.0	278	10.4	24.4	15.2	1.2
Sausage, Cumberland & Egg, Burger King*	1 Butty/247g	641	37.0	260	12.6	18.6	15.0	0.8
Sausage, Cumberland & Egg, Brown Sauce, Burger King*	1 Butty/258g	654	37.0	253	12.0	18.6	14.3	0.8
Sausage, Cumberland & Egg, with Ketchup, Burger King*	1 Butty/258g	652	37.0	253	12.0	19.0	14.3	0.8
Sausage, Cumberland, Burger King*	1 Butty/197g	561	31.0	285	13.2	22.8	15.7	1.0

BURGER KING

	Measure INFO/WEIGHT	per Measure KCAL	FAT	Nutrition Values per 100g / 100ml KCAL	PROT	CARB	FAT	FIBRE
BUTTY								
Sausage, Cumberland, with Brown Sauce, Burger King*	1 Butty/208g	574	31.0	276	12.5	22.6	14.9	1.0
Sausage, Cumberland, with Ketchup, Burger King*	1 Butty/208g	572	31.0	275	12.5	23.1	14.9	1.0
CAKE								
Chocolate Fudge, Double, Fusions, Burger King*	1 Serving/155g	244	7.0	157	3.9	25.2	4.5	0.7
CHEESECAKE								
Strawberry, Fusions, Burger King*	1 Serving/170g	342	8.0	201	3.5	34.7	4.7	0.0
CHICKEN								
Bites, Burger King*	1 Portion/78g	176	11.0	226	16.7	12.8	14.1	0.0
Strips, Breaded, Burger King*	1 Portion/132g	342	16.0	259	21.2	18.2	12.1	0.0
Wings, Burger King*	1 Portion/85g	222	15.0	261	20.0	7.1	17.7	1.2
COFFEE								
Black, Large, Burger King*	1 Serving/284ml	3	0.0	1	0.0	0.0	0.0	0.0
Black, Regular, Burger King*	1 Serving/200ml	2	0.0	1	0.0	0.0	0.0	0.0
Cappuccino, Large, Burger King*	1 Serving/284ml	52	0.0	18	1.1	3.5	0.0	0.0
Cappuccino, Regular, Burger King*	1 Serving/200ml	36	0.0	18	1.0	3.0	0.0	0.0
Latte, Large, Burger King*	1 Serving/284ml	95	0.0	33	2.1	6.3	0.0	0.0
Latte, Regular, Burger King*	1 Serving/200ml	67	0.0	34	2.0	6.0	0.0	0.0
COLA								
Coca-Cola, Regular, Burger King*	1 Drink/400g	164	0.0	41	0.0	10.0	0.0	0.0
DIP								
Barbeque Sauce, Pot, Burger King*	1 Serving/25g	31	0.1	125	0.6	28.7	0.3	0.4
Soured Cream & Chive, Burger King*	1 Pot/40g	208	23.0	520	2.5	0.0	57.5	0.0
Sweet Chilli, Burger King*	1 Pot/40g	100	0.0	250	0.0	60.0	0.0	0.0
Tangy Tomato, Burger King*	1 Pot/40g	56	0.0	140	0.0	32.5	0.0	0.0
DIP POT								
Caramel, Burger King*	1 Pot/20g	61	1.0	305	0.0	65.0	5.0	0.0
Chocolate, Burger King*	1 Pot/20g	57	2.0	285	5.0	50.0	10.0	0.0
Raspberry, Burger King*	1 Pot/20g	58	0.0	290	0.0	70.0	0.0	0.0
Sweet Chilli, Burger King*	1 Pot/40g	100	0.0	250	0.0	60.0	0.0	0.0
DOUGHNUTS								
Diddy, Burger King*	1 Serving/84g	256	8.0	305	6.0	48.8	9.5	1.2
DRESSING								
French, Burger King*	1 Sachet/40g	8	0.0	20	90.0	2.5	0.0	0.0
Honey & Mustard, Burger King*	1oz/28g	22	0.7	80	2.5	15.0	2.5	0.0
Thousand Island, Burger King*	1 Sachet/40g	65	6.0	163	0.0	7.5	15.0	0.0
Tomato & Basil, Burger King*	1 Sachet/40g	19	1.0	48	2.5	7.5	2.5	0.0
FRIES								
Large, Burger King*	1 Lge Serving/137g	363	16.7	265	2.7	35.1	12.2	2.7
Regular, Burger King*	1 Portion/111g	294	14.0	265	2.7	35.1	12.6	2.7
Small, Burger King*	1 Serving/74g	196	9.0	265	2.7	35.1	12.2	2.7
Super, Burger King*	1 Portion/174g	461	21.2	265	2.7	35.1	12.2	2.7
HASH BROWNS								
Burger King*	1 Serving/102g	333	22.0	326	2.9	30.4	21.6	2.9
HOT CHOCOLATE								
Burger King*	1 Serving/200ml	78	2.0	39	0.5	7.5	1.0	0.5
ICE CREAM								
Apple Crumble, Bramley, Burger King*	1 Serving/190g	313	11.0	165	3.2	24.2	5.8	0.0
Cookies & Cream, Burger King*	1 Serving/170g	315	11.0	185	3.5	27.7	6.5	0.0
Strawberry Cheesecake, Burger King*	1 Serving/190g	421	12.0	222	4.2	35.3	6.3	0.0
Summer Berry Burst, Fusions, Burger King*	1 Serving/148g	180	3.0	122	2.7	23.0	2.0	0.0
Vanilla & Chocolate, Burger King*	1 Cone/102g	287	14.0	281	2.9	36.3	13.7	2.9
Vanilla & Strawberry, Burger King*	1 Cone/102g	269	12.0	264	2.9	39.2	11.8	1.0

	Measure INFO/WEIGHT	per Measure KCAL	FAT	Nutrition Values per 100g / 100ml KCAL	PROT	CARB	FAT	FIBRE
BURGER KING								
ICE CREAM CONE								
Vanilla & Chocolate, Burger King*	1 Serving/102g	287	14.0	281	2.9	36.3	13.7	2.9
Vanilla & Strawberry, Burger King*	1 Cone/102g	269	12.0	264	2.9	39.2	11.8	1.0
KETCHUP								
Dip Pot, Burger King*	1 Pot/25g	27	0.0	107	1.0	24.7	0.1	0.6
Sachet, Burger King*	1 Sachet/15g	16	0.0	107	0.0	26.7	0.0	0.0
MAYONNAISE								
Burger King*	1 Sachet/12g	81	9.0	675	0.0	0.0	75.0	0.0
Sachet, Burger King*	1 Sachet/12g	81	9.0	675	0.0	0.0	75.0	0.0
MILK SHAKE								
Banana, Regular, Burger King*	1 Serving/145g	170	3.0	117	2.8	22.8	2.1	0.0
Chocolate, Regular, Burger King*	1 Serving/145g	176	3.0	121	2.8	22.8	2.1	0.0
Strawberry, Regular, Burger King*	1 Serving/145g	167	3.0	115	2.8	21.4	2.1	0.0
Vanilla, Regular, Burger King*	1 Serving/124g	124	3.0	100	3.2	16.1	2.4	0.0
ONION RINGS								
Large, Burger King*	1 Serving/120g	348	17.3	290	4.4	36.4	14.4	3.3
Regular, Burger King*	1oz/28g	81	4.0	290	4.4	36.7	14.4	3.3
Super, Burger King*	1 Serving/180g	522	26.0	290	4.4	36.7	14.4	3.3
PIE								
Apple, Burger King*	1 Pie/150g	446	19.0	297	2.7	42.7	12.7	1.3
Apple, with Ice Cream, Burger King*	1 Pie/220g	548	23.0	249	2.7	35.9	10.5	1.4
Dutch Apple, Burger King*	1 Pie/113g	339	13.9	300	1.7	46.0	12.3	0.8
POTATO WEDGES								
Burger King*	1 Portion/100g	147	3.0	147	2.0	21.0	3.0	3.0
SALAD								
Chicken, Flame Grilled, Ia, Burger King*	1 Salad/215g	99	1.0	46	6.5	2.8	0.5	1.9
Chicken, Warm & Crispy, Burger King*	1 Salad/206g	184	7.1	89	6.9	7.8	3.5	2.2
Garden, Ia, Burger King*	1 Salad/165g	35	0.0	21	1.2	3.6	0.0	2.4
TEA								
Regular, White, No Sugar, Burger King*	1 Serving/200ml	22	4.0	11	0.5	1.0	2.0	0.0
CAFFE NERO								
BARS								
Chocolate & Hazelnut, Caffe Nero*	1 Bar/40g	229	15.2	572	8.0	49.5	38.0	1.8
Chocolate, Milk, Caffe Nero*	1 Bar/40g	223	13.6	558	8.0	55.0	34.0	1.0
Exotic Fruit, Organic, Caffe Nero*	1 Bar/64g	239	10.8	374	5.6	50.3	16.8	10.0
Fruit & Seed, Caffe Nero*	1 Bar/64g	196	5.8	303	7.5	48.2	8.9	8.7
Granola, Caffe Nero*	1 Bar/64g	259	13.9	404	5.9	55.3	21.7	0.0
Granola, Organic, Caffe Nero*	1 Bar/64g	269	13.2	420	7.4	51.0	20.7	6.0
Shortbread, Caffe Nero*	1 Pack/50g	243	13.8	485	4.8	54.6	27.6	0.0
BISCOTTI								
Almond, Caffe Nero*	1 Pack/52g	202	8.0	388	9.2	53.1	15.3	2.8
Doppio, Almond & Chocolate, Caffe Nero*	1 Pack/29g	228	9.3	786	15.0	110.0	32.0	0.0
BROWNIE								
Chocolate, Double, Organic, Gluten Free, Caffe Nero*	1 Brownie/77g	331	16.1	425	4.3	55.4	20.7	2.0
BRUSCHETTA								
Parmesan & Roast Onion, Caffe Nero*	1 Pack/50g	239	11.1	479	16.0	53.7	22.2	1.5
Sun Dried Tomato & Basil, Caffe Nero*	1 Pack/50g	224	9.2	448	12.1	58.4	18.3	1.7
CAKE								
Banana & Caramel, Slice, Caffe Nero*	1 Serving/82g	342	19.8	417	4.6	45.5	24.1	0.0
Banana & Sultana, Slice, Caffe Nero*	1 Serving/81g	221	3.8	276	4.7	53.6	4.8	0.0
Carrot & Raisin, Slice, Organic, Caffe Nero*	1 Slice/70g	283	17.3	404	4.1	41.5	24.7	4.4
Chocolate & Orange, Slice, Caffe Nero*	1 Serving/69g	233	9.9	333	4.7	46.7	14.2	1.4
Chocolate & Pecan Fudge Brownie, Caffe Nero*	1 Serving/113g	426	21.6	377	3.6	47.7	19.1	0.0

CAFFE NERO

	Measure INFO/WEIGHT	per Measure KCAL	FAT	Nutrition Values per 100g / 100ml KCAL	PROT	CARB	FAT	FIBRE
CAKE								
Chocolate Fudge, Caffe Nero*	1 Serving/143g	615	32.0	430	5.3	51.8	22.4	1.3
Chocolate Zabaglione, Caffe Nero*	1 Serving/112g	420	28.0	375	5.1	32.5	25.0	3.9
Coffee & Pecan, Slice, Caffe Nero*	1 Serving/87g	389	23.4	447	5.1	46.2	26.9	0.0
Cranberry & Orange, Slice, Caffe Nero*	1 Serving/60g	196	7.2	326	5.1	49.8	11.9	0.0
Fruit, Slice, Organic, Caffe Nero*	1 Slice/69g	223	8.4	319	4.7	48.0	12.0	0.0
Ginger, Spicy, Organic, Caffe Nero*	1 Serving/70g	236	10.6	338	3.9	46.4	15.2	4.1
Lemon Drizzle, Slice, Organic, Caffe Nero*	1 Slice/76g	252	9.9	331	4.3	49.2	13.0	0.7
Mocha, Slice, Caffe Nero*	1 Serving/89g	333	17.9	375	4.8	43.4	20.2	0.0
Panettone, Chocolate, Mini, Caffe Nero*	1 Serving/100g	420	22.3	420	9.0	46.0	22.3	1.0
Panettone, Classic, Mini, Caffe Nero*	1 Serving/100g	385	13.6	385	9.0	51.0	13.6	2.0
Passion, Caffe Nero*	1 Serving/125g	518	39.5	414	5.5	52.8	31.6	0.9
Sponge, Victoria, Caffe Nero*	1 Serving/144g	474	21.7	329	4.5	43.5	15.1	0.4
Toffee & Banana, Organic, Caffe Nero*	1 Serving/70g	188	9.2	268	3.8	33.8	13.1	0.7
White Chocolate & Orange Ganache, Caffe Nero*	1 Serving/135g	558	42.3	413	4.0	29.0	31.3	0.0
CALZONE								
Mozzarella & Tomato, Caffe Nero*	1 Serving/155g	320	11.2	206	9.3	25.5	7.2	1.2
Pepperoni, Spicy, Caffe Nero*	1 Pack/154g	298	10.0	194	8.2	25.9	6.5	1.3
CHEESE TWISTS								
Caffe Nero*	1 Serving/90g	387	22.7	431	14.3	36.4	25.3	1.5
CHEESECAKE								
Apple & Blackberry, Reduced Fat, Caffe Nero*	1 Serving/165g	277	11.7	168	4.2	23.3	7.1	1.3
Apple & Cinnamon, Baked, Caffe Nero*	1 Serving/138g	406	24.7	294	4.1	30.6	17.9	0.0
Blackcurrant, Reduced Fat, Caffe Nero*	1 Serving/119g	248	11.2	209	5.4	25.7	9.4	0.5
Chocolate, Simply, Caffe Nero*	1 Serving/125g	475	25.0	380	4.4	45.6	20.0	0.0
Chocolate, White & Dark, Caffe Nero*	1 Serving/170g	711	52.6	416	5.7	30.8	30.8	0.0
Chocolate, Zucotto, Caffe Nero*	1 Serving/137g	512	36.0	374	4.8	29.6	26.3	0.5
Lemon & Mascarpone, Caffe Nero*	1 Serving/135g	466	30.4	345	5.2	30.2	22.5	1.0
Lemon, Dessert Pot, Caffe Nero*	1 Pot/105g	390	27.2	370	2.6	32.0	25.8	0.9
Rhubarb & Vanilla, Caffe Nero*	1 Serving/135g	424	29.7	314	5.4	26.9	22.0	0.0
Summer Fruit, Caffe Nero*	1 Serving/157g	388	20.7	247	3.4	29.5	13.2	0.0
Toffee Crunch, Caffe Nero*	1 Serving/155g	577	34.9	372	5.8	36.8	22.5	1.0
Toffee Swirl, Caffe Nero*	1 Serving/133g	410	24.1	308	6.3	30.0	18.1	0.0
White Chocolate & Orange, Reduced Fat, Caffe Nero*	1 Serving/120g	310	18.7	258	6.5	23.0	15.6	0.7
CHOCOLATE								
Coin, Caffe Nero*	1 Serving/25g	129	7.0	516	6.3	59.7	27.8	2.1
COFFEE								
Cappuccino, Semi Skimmed Milk, Regular, Caffe Nero*	1 Cup/80.4g	37	1.4	46	3.5	4.7	1.7	0.0
Cappuccino, Skimmed Milk, Regular, Caffe Nero*	1 Regular/80g	27	0.2	34	3.5	4.8	0.3	0.0
Cappuccino, Soya Milk, Regular, Caffe Nero*	1 Serving/80g	36	1.8	45	3.7	2.5	2.2	0.6
Latte, Caramel, Semi Skimmed Milk, Caffe Nero*	1 Latte/421ml	484	25.3	115	2.3	12.3	6.0	0.0
Latte, Chai, Semi Skimmed Milk, Caffe Nero*	1 Serving/405ml	284	10.5	70	3.8	8.3	2.6	0.0
Latte, Chai, Skimmed Milk, Caffe Nero*	1 Serving/405ml	239	5.3	59	3.8	8.4	1.3	0.0
Latte, Frappe, Semi Skimmed, Caffe Nero*	1 Serving/538ml	307	4.3	57	2.6	10.2	0.8	0.0
Latte, Frappe, Skimmed Milk, Caffe Nero*	1 Serving/532g	277	1.1	52	2.6	10.3	0.2	0.0
Latte, Iced, Caffe Nero*	1 Latte/487ml	117	4.4	24	1.8	2.5	0.9	0.0
Latte, Semi Skimmed Milk, Caffe Nero*	1 Regular/150g	69	2.6	46	3.5	4.7	1.7	0.0
Latte, Skimmed Milk, Regular, Caffe Nero*	1 Regular/150g	51	0.5	34	3.5	4.8	0.3	0.0
Latte, Soya Milk, Regular, Caffe Nero*	1 Cup/152g	68	3.3	45	3.7	2.5	2.2	0.6
Mocha Latte, Semi Skimmed Milk, Regular, Caffe Nero*	1 Serving/581g	483	5.8	83	2.8	16.3	1.0	0.4
Mocha Latte, Skimmed Milk, Caffe Nero*	1 Serving/587ml	511	4.1	87	3.8	16.6	0.7	0.8
Mocha, Whipped Cream, Semi Skimmed Milk, Caffe Nero*	1 Cup/180ml	326	19.5	181	4.3	17.2	10.8	0.8
Mocha, White Chocolate, Semi Skimmed Milk, Caffe Nero*	1 Serving/400ml	413	25.3	103	2.4	6.1	6.3	0.0

	Measure INFO/WEIGHT	per Measure KCAL	FAT	Nutrition Values per 100g / 100ml KCAL	PROT	CARB	FAT	FIBRE

CAFFE NERO

COFFEE BEANS

	Measure INFO/WEIGHT	KCAL	FAT	KCAL	PROT	CARB	FAT	FIBRE
Chocolate Coated, Caffe Nero*	1 Serving/25g	117	6.5	469	8.5	50.0	26.2	11.9
Cioccafe, Caffe Nero*	1 Serving/25g	117	6.5	468	8.5	50.0	26.0	0.0
COOKIES								
Belgian Chocolate, Organic, Caffe Nero*	1 Cookie/50g	244	11.3	488	6.4	64.8	22.6	0.0
Chocolate Chip, Organic, Caffe Nero*	1 Cookie/60g	263	12.1	438	4.5	56.6	20.1	1.5
Milk Chocolate Chunk, Caffe Nero*	1 Cookie/71g	338	17.9	470	5.8	55.8	24.9	1.7
Raisin & Oat, Organic, Caffe Nero*	1 Cookie/60g	253	11.6	422	5.1	56.8	19.3	2.4
Triple Chocolate, Caffe Nero*	1 Cookie/71g	333	17.5	463	5.6	55.6	24.3	3.3
White Chocolate & Cranberry, Caffe Nero*	1 Serving/71g	301	10.9	419	4.4	66.3	15.2	1.5
COUS COUS								
Mediterranean, Caffe Nero*	1 Serving/315g	403	21.4	128	2.8	14.0	6.8	2.1
CRISPS								
Mature Cheddar & Spring Onion, Handcooked, Caffe Nero*	1 Pack/50g	241	14.3	481	6.1	54.0	28.6	4.4
Sea Salt & Balsamic Vinegar, Caffe Nero*	1 Pack/50g	241	13.2	482	7.0	54.1	26.4	4.0
Sea Salt, Caffe Nero*	1 Pack/50g	247	13.6	493	8.0	54.0	27.1	4.5
CROISSANT								
Almond, Caffe Nero*	1 Croissant/89g	365	19.0	406	7.5	46.4	21.1	1.7
Apricot, Caffe Nero*	1 Croissant/104g	286	11.8	273	5.4	37.3	11.3	1.2
Butter, Caffe Nero*	1 Croissant/53g	244	14.6	460	9.1	44.1	27.5	1.7
DANISH PASTRY								
Apple, Caffe Nero*	1 Pastry/75g	255	12.2	340	5.7	42.5	16.3	2.3
Pear & Chocolate, Caffe Nero*	1 Pastry/90g	238	11.5	264	4.7	36.9	12.8	0.0
DRIED FRUIT MIX								
Caffe Nero*	1 Bag/75g	248	4.1	331	1.6	69.1	5.4	5.0
FARFALLE								
with Roasted Vegetable Sauce, Caffe Nero*	1 Serving/324g	275	8.4	85	2.6	13.4	2.6	1.6
FRUIT & NUT MIX								
Caffe Nero*	1 Serving/75g	322	17.5	430	9.8	44.8	23.4	3.5
FRUIT SALAD								
Classic, Caffe Nero*	1 Serving/170g	75	0.2	44	0.5	10.9	0.1	1.5
Spring, Caffe Nero*	1 Salad/174g	47	0.2	27	0.6	6.2	0.1	0.0
Tropical, Caffe Nero*	1 Serving/170g	70	0.2	41	0.6	11.1	0.1	1.4
GINGERBREAD								
Man, Caffe Nero*	1 Man/54g	235	7.7	435	6.7	70.2	14.2	1.6
HOT CHOCOLATE								
Milano, Caffe Nero*	1 Cup/239.8g	446	24.5	186	3.8	19.4	10.2	2.0
Semi Skimmed Milk, Regular, Caffe Nero*	1 Cup/210.5g	280	4.2	133	4.0	25.1	2.0	1.3
Skimmed Milk, No Cream, Regular, Caffe Nero*	1 Cup/210ml	262	2.1	125	4.0	25.5	1.0	1.3
Whipped Cream, Semi Skimmed Milk, Regular, Caffe Nero*	1 Cup/250ml	432	20.5	173	3.7	21.6	8.2	1.1
JUICE								
Apple, Organic, Caffe Nero*	1 Serving/200ml	94	0.0	47	0.5	11.2	0.0	0.0
Apple, Pressed, 100% Premium Juice, Caffe Nero*	1 Serving/250ml	128	0.0	51	0.1	11.9	0.0	0.0
Orange, 100% Squeezed, Caffe Nero*	1 Bottle/250ml	95	0.3	38	0.5	8.8	0.1	0.0
Orange, Organic, Caffe Nero*	1 Serving/200ml	94	0.0	47	0.5	10.4	0.0	0.0
JUICE DRINK								
Fruit Booster, Mango, Caffe Nero*	1 Drink/644g	219	0.6	34	0.5	8.2	0.1	0.6
Pineapple, Orange & Banana, Fruit Booster, Caffe Nero*	1 Serving/651g	202	0.7	31	0.2	7.9	0.1	0.1
Strawberry & Raspberry, Fruit Booster, Caffe Nero*	1 Drink/638ml	166	0.6	26	0.3	6.4	0.1	0.5
Summer Fruits, Fruit Booster, Caffe Nero*	1 Serving/642g	244	0.0	38	0.3	9.4	0.0	0.4
LASAGNE								
Beef, Al Forno, Caffe Nero*	1 Serving/350g	595	36.1	170	10.2	8.3	10.3	0.5
Spinach & Ricotta, Caffe Nero*	1 Serving/375g	633	35.6	169	8.4	13.3	9.5	0.9

CAFFE NERO

	Measure INFO/WEIGHT	per Measure KCAL	FAT	Nutrition Values per 100g / 100ml KCAL	PROT	CARB	FAT	FIBRE
LASAGNE								
Vegetable, Caffe Nero*	1 Serving/371g	482	24.1	130	5.1	13.9	6.5	0.0
LEMONADE								
Sicilian, Still, Caffe Nero*	1 Serving/250ml	115	0.0	46	0.0	11.2	0.0	0.0
MILKSHAKE								
Banana Frappe, Caffe Nero*	1 Frappe/550ml	472	6.6	86	3.1	16.1	1.2	0.0
Double Chocolate, Semi Skimmed, Frappe, Caffe Nero*	1 Frappe/582ml	483	5.8	83	2.8	16.3	1.0	0.4
Double Chocolate, Skimmed Milk, Frappe, Caffe Nero*	1 Frappe/587g	452	2.3	77	2.8	16.3	0.4	0.4
Mint, Frappe, Caffe Nero*	1 Frappe/543ml	462	6.5	85	3.2	15.6	1.2	0.0
Strawberry, Frappe, Caffe Nero*	1 Frappe/545ml	475	6.6	87	3.2	16.2	1.2	0.0
Vanilla, Frappe, Caffe Nero*	1 Serving/543g	473	6.5	87	3.1	16.2	1.2	0.0
MOUSSE								
Chocolate Brownie, Dessert Pot, Caffe Nero*	1 Pot/89g	335	18.8	375	4.3	42.8	21.0	1.5
Sicillian Lemon, Dessert Pot, Caffe Nero*	1 Pot/125g	423	34.7	338	1.7	20.5	27.7	0.1
MUFFIN								
Apple & Ginger, Caffe Nero*	1 Muffin/120g	402	22.1	335	4.4	37.8	18.4	0.7
Blueberry, Caffe Nero*	1 Muffin/120g	430	22.6	358	4.5	42.7	18.8	1.1
Blueberry, Reduced Fat, Caffe Nero*	1 Muffin/120.1g	287	5.5	239	4.7	44.8	4.6	2.9
Carrot & Sultana, Low Fat, Caffe Nero*	1 Muffin/119g	271	3.6	227	5.0	44.8	3.0	0.0
Chocolate, White & Dark, Caffe Nero*	1 Muffin/100g	393	21.2	393	5.7	45.0	21.2	1.7
Lemon & Raspberry, Reduced Fat, Caffe Nero*	1 Muffin/119.7g	365	15.8	305	4.6	41.7	13.2	1.5
Lemon Poppy Seed, Caffe Nero*	1 Muffin/120g	449	22.3	374	5.7	45.9	18.6	0.9
Raspberry & White Chocolate, Caffe Nero*	1 Muffin/120g	461	24.0	384	5.0	46.0	20.0	0.9
Summer Fruit, Caffe Nero*	1 Muffin/120g	410	21.0	342	4.2	41.8	17.5	1.0
Super Seed, Caffe Nero*	1 Muffin/119g	398	19.5	332	5.9	40.4	16.3	2.1
Triple Belgian Chocolate, Caffe Nero*	1 Muffin/124g	488	26.3	393	5.7	45.0	21.2	1.7
White & Dark Chocolate, Caffe Nero*	1 Muffin/120g	472	25.5	393	5.7	45.0	21.2	1.7
White Chocolate & Raspberry, Caffe Nero*	1 Muffin/120g	453	25.3	378	6.0	41.0	21.1	0.0
NUTS								
Cashew, Roasted & Salted, Caffe Nero*	1 Serving/40g	244	20.3	611	20.5	18.8	50.9	3.2
OLIVES								
Green, Marinated, Caffe Nero*	1 Pack/110g	212	22.6	193	1.0	5.0	20.6	4.1
PAIN AU CHOCOLAT								
Almond, Caffe Nero*	1 Pain/100g	406	22.3	406	7.9	45.9	22.3	2.5
Caffe Nero*	1 Pain/62g	277	15.6	446	8.5	46.2	25.2	1.3
PAIN AU RAISIN								
Caffe Nero*	1 Pain/95g	325	14.8	342	5.4	45.0	15.6	1.4
PANINI								
All Day Breakfast, Caffe Nero*	1 Panini/250g	343	11.5	137	9.0	14.8	4.6	2.0
Bacon, Breakfast, Caffe Nero*	1 Panini/109g	298	11.1	271	10.0	35.0	10.1	1.7
Butternut Squash & Soft Cheese, Caffe Nero*	1 Panini/149.6g	208	6.1	139	8.2	20.2	4.1	1.4
Chicken BLT, Caffe Nero*	1 Panini/249g	513	29.4	206	8.7	16.4	11.8	1.3
Chicken Caesar, Caffe Nero*	1 Panini/237g	473	26.0	200	8.9	16.3	11.0	0.9
Chicken, & Creme Fraiche, Spicy, Caffe Nero*	1 Panini/200g	294	6.8	147	9.5	19.4	3.4	1.0
Chicken, Bacon & Arrabbiata Sauce, Caffe Nero*	1 Panini/244g	352	10.3	144	8.8	17.6	4.2	0.9
Chicken, with Herb Creme Fraiche, Caffe Nero*	1 Panini/190g	299	8.6	157	9.2	20.1	4.5	1.2
Club, Italian, Caffe Nero*	1 Panini/212g	454	21.4	214	12.8	17.9	10.1	1.3
Egg Florentine, Breakfast, Caffe Nero*	1 Panini/135g	288	10.5	212	8.6	27.0	7.7	1.7
Egg, Mushroom, & Tomato, Breakfast, Caffe Nero*	1 Panini/145g	297	9.9	205	8.6	27.4	6.8	1.7
Ham, & Brie, Caffe Nero*	1 Panini/229g	392	15.6	171	11.0	16.5	6.8	0.9
Ham, & Egg, Breakfast, Caffe Nero*	1 Panini/145g	334	12.8	230	12.1	25.6	8.8	1.3
Ham, & Smoked Mozzarella, Caffe Nero*	1 Panini/229g	460	20.6	201	13.1	17.0	9.0	0.8
Lemon Chicken, Caffe Nero*	1 Panini/212g	478	17.4	225	9.1	28.8	8.2	0.0

CAFFE NERO

	Measure INFO/WEIGHT	per Measure KCAL	per Measure FAT	Nutrition Values per 100g / 100ml KCAL	PROT	CARB	FAT	FIBRE
PANINI								
Meatball, with Tomato Sauce, Italian, Caffe Nero*	1 Panini/245g	449	20.1	183	8.9	18.5	8.2	0.9
Mediterranean Vegetable & Red Pesto, Caffe Nero*	1 Panini/209g	375	17.6	179	5.9	20.0	8.4	1.6
Mozzarella, & Plum Tomato, Caffe Nero*	1 Panini/216.1g	415	21.2	192	7.9	17.9	9.8	1.1
Mozzarella, & Roasted Mushroom, Caffe Nero*	1 Panini/214g	351	12.0	164	8.1	20.1	5.6	1.2
Parma Ham, & Mascarpone, Caffe Nero*	1 Panini/195g	536	23.2	275	11.3	30.6	11.9	0.0
Prosciutto Ham, & Mascarpone, Caffe Nero*	1 Panini/195g	430	22.4	221	10.0	19.2	11.5	0.9
Roasted Mediterranean Vegetable, Caffe Nero*	1 Panini/204g	255	5.1	125	5.2	20.2	2.5	3.6
Salami Tomato & Mozzarella, Caffe Nero*	1 Panini/214.9g	417	18.5	194	8.9	20.5	8.6	0.0
Soft Cheese & Sweet Chilli Vegetable, Caffe Nero*	1 Panini/223.2g	308	6.9	138	5.1	22.5	3.1	1.5
Tricolore, Caffe Nero*	1 Panini/239g	435	23.2	182	7.2	16.4	9.7	1.3
Tuna, Italian, Melt, Caffe Nero*	1 Panini/224g	440	19.5	196	12.1	17.3	8.7	1.0
Turkey & Cranberry, Caffe Nero*	1 Panini/224.9g	443	14.8	197	9.9	24.4	6.6	1.2
PANNA COTTA								
Raspberry, Caffe Nero*	1 Pot/130g	384	32.0	295	1.2	17.2	24.6	0.0
PASTA SALAD								
Basil Pesto, Caffe Nero*	1 Serving/200g	510	30.2	255	5.9	24.1	15.1	0.4
Red Pepper & Pine Nuts, Caffe Nero*	1 Salad/270g	506	25.4	187	5.7	19.7	9.4	1.9
Sunkissed Tomato, Caffe Nero*	1 Salad/285g	755	44.2	265	6.7	24.6	15.5	0.0
Tomato & Mozzarella, Caffe Nero*	1 Pack/298.47	391	26.0	131	2.9	10.3	8.7	1.1
PASTRY								
Almond Torta, Caffe Nero*	1 Pastry/126g	439	18.3	346	2.7	51.6	14.4	0.5
Creamed Spinach, Savoury, Caffe Nero*	1 Pastry/120g	372	23.4	310	5.7	27.8	19.5	0.0
Frutt Di Bosco, Torta, Caffe Nero*	1 Torta/97g	227	8.0	234	2.9	37.1	8.2	1.5
Ham & Cheese, Puff Pastry, Savoury, Caffe Nero*	1 Pastry/110g	394	25.0	358	11.5	26.9	22.7	0.0
PENNE								
with Roasted Red Pepper Sauce, Caffe Nero*	1 Serving/340g	317	8.2	93	3.0	14.7	2.4	0.6
PIZZA								
Cheese & Tomato, Caffe Nero*	1 Serving/194g	444	13.4	229	10.4	37.9	6.9	3.3
Milano Salami & Peppers, Caffe Nero*	1 Serving/357g	768	23.9	215	9.7	33.7	6.7	2.9
RAVIOLI								
Mushroom, with Chestnut Mushroom Sauce, Caffe Nero*	1 Serving/310g	565	32.0	182	6.9	15.3	10.3	0.0
SALAD								
Cous Cous & Roasted Vegetable, Caffe Nero*	1 Salad/249g	452	14.5	181	4.3	27.5	5.8	1.4
Cous Cous, Mediterranean Style, Caffe Nero*	1 Pack/275g	352	18.7	128	2.8	14.0	6.8	2.1
Crayfish, Caffe Nero*	1 Salad/205g	279	11.1	136	5.2	17.0	5.4	0.0
Prosciutto & Pecorino, Caffe Nero*	1 Salad/217g	369	27.6	170	3.5	10.1	12.7	0.3
Roast Summer Vegetables, & Feta Cheese, Caffe Nero*	1 Serving/263g	460	40.2	175	3.6	4.1	15.3	0.5
Sun Kissed Tomato & Mozzarella, Caffe Nero*	1 Salad/265g	446	17.0	168	6.3	21.4	6.4	1.5
Tuna Nicoise, Caffe Nero*	1 Pack/277.6g	236	11.7	85	6.0	5.9	4.2	0.8
SANDWICH								
BLT, Caffe Nero*	1 Sandwich/167g	375	21.4	224	7.1	20.1	12.8	1.7
Cheese, Simply, Caffe Nero*	1 Serving/161g	506	25.8	314	16.1	26.4	16.0	3.1
Chicken, Italian, Caffe Nero*	1 Serving/174g	361	16.4	207	9.6	21.0	9.4	0.0
Chicken, Oven Roasted Tomatoes, & Spinach, Caffe Nero*	1 Sandwich/169g	289	7.6	171	10.7	22.0	4.5	2.0
Crayfish, with Lemon Mayonnaise, Caffe Nero*	1 Serving/156g	370	19.8	237	8.3	22.4	12.7	0.0
Egg Mayonnaise, & Cress, Caffe Nero*	1 Serving/168g	349	15.0	207	10.7	21.0	8.9	3.3
Feta Cheese & Rocket, Sundried Tom Bread, Caffe Nero*	1 Serving/186g	424	23.6	228	8.2	20.2	12.7	1.2
Focaccia, Goats Cheese & Roasted Pepper, Caffe Nero*	1 Focaccia/182g	344	9.8	189	8.5	26.6	5.4	1.6
Focaccia, Ham, Mozzarella & Mushroom, Caffe Nero*	1 Focaccia/217g	421	10.2	194	10.7	27.3	4.7	1.3
Ham, & Egg, Caffe Nero*	1 Sandwich/204g	371	15.8	181	12.3	15.6	7.7	1.1
Ham, & Mature Cheddar, Caffe Nero*	1 Sandwich/183g	493	26.1	268	15.3	19.6	14.2	1.4
Mozzarella, & Tomato, Caffe Nero*	1 Sandwich/204g	456	24.7	223	10.2	18.2	12.1	1.2

CAFFE NERO

	Measure INFO/WEIGHT	per Measure KCAL	FAT	Nutrition Values per 100g / 100ml KCAL	PROT	CARB	FAT	FIBRE
SANDWICH								
Prawn, Lemon Dressing & Rocket, Caffe Nero*	1 Pack/169g	342	13.0	202	12.4	20.9	7.7	3.2
Salmon, Smoked, & Lemon Mayonnaise, Caffe Nero*	1 Serving/159g	497	32.2	313	10.6	21.8	20.3	0.0
Tuna Mayonnaise, & Salad, Caffe Nero*	1 Sandwich/183g	353	15.4	192	8.8	20.4	8.4	1.3
SCONE								
Luxury Fruit, Caffe Nero*	1 Scone/100g	330	10.2	330	5.9	52.6	10.2	2.0
SHORTBREAD								
Chocolate Chip, Organic, Sharing, Caffe Nero*	1 Serving/105g	502	29.1	478	5.3	51.8	27.7	1.7
Organic, Caffe Nero*	1 Serving/50g	239	13.9	477	5.4	51.3	27.7	1.5
SLICES								
Caramel, Digestive Biscuit, Caffe Nero*	1 Serving/80g	418	23.6	523	4.1	59.2	29.5	1.1
Caramel, Shortcake, Caffe Nero*	1 Slice/98g	514	30.5	524	2.7	49.6	31.1	0.0
SMOOTHIE								
Mango & Passionfruit, Caffe Nero*	1 Smoothie/250ml	154	0.2	62	0.6	14.3	0.1	0.3
Peach & Apricot, Caffe Nero*	1 Smoothie/250ml	132	0.0	53	0.6	12.1	0.0	0.5
Peach & Raspberry, Organic, Bio, Caffe Nero*	1 Smoothie/250ml	188	4.5	75	3.2	11.4	1.8	0.0
Red Berry, Caffe Nero*	1 Smoothie/250ml	130	0.5	52	0.7	11.9	0.2	1.9
Strawberry & Banana, Caffe Nero*	1 Smoothie/250ml	115	0.8	46	0.8	10.4	0.3	5.0
Strawberry, Organic, Bio, Caffe Nero*	1 Smoothie/250ml	188	4.3	75	2.9	11.9	1.7	0.0
SNACK								
Chocolate Coated Coffee Beans, Caffe Nero*	1 Serving/25g	117	6.5	469	8.5	50.0	26.2	11.9
Chocolate Crunch, Caffe Nero*	1 Serving/80g	434	33.7	543	4.1	39.4	42.2	4.4
SOUP								
Broccoli & Blue Cheese, Less Than 5% Fat, Caffe Nero*	1 Serving/331g	205	15.9	62	1.8	3.0	4.8	0.0
Butternut Squash & Roasted Garlic, Caffe Nero*	1 Serving/300g	114	6.3	38	0.7	4.2	2.1	0.9
Carrot & Coriander, Caffe Nero*	1 Serving/300g	186	9.9	62	1.5	6.5	3.3	1.4
Cream of Tomato & Basil, Caffe Nero*	1 Serving/330g	234	16.8	71	1.0	5.8	5.1	0.0
Creamy Mushroom, Caffe Nero*	1 Serving/331g	185	13.5	56	1.0	4.1	4.1	0.0
Mediterranean Vegetable, Caffe Nero*	1 Serving/300g	93	5.7	31	0.7	2.8	1.9	1.0
Potato & Leek, Caffe Nero*	1 Serving/300g	195	14.4	65	1.1	4.3	4.8	0.7
Roast Vegetable, Caffe Nero*	1 Serving/332g	73	4.3	22	0.6	2.2	1.3	0.0
Roasted Tomato, Caffe Nero*	1 Serving/329g	112	3.6	34	0.8	5.1	1.1	0.0
Sun Dried Tomato & Basil, Caffe Nero*	1 Serving/300g	144	6.9	48	2.2	4.7	2.3	0.5
TAGLIATELLE								
Carbonara, Caffe Nero*	1 Serving/349g	856	60.8	245	6.3	15.6	17.4	0.6
TART								
Blueberry, Caffe Nero*	1 Serving/111g	311	18.0	280	3.2	30.3	16.2	1.2
Lemon & Lime, Caffe Nero*	1 Serving/109g	375	24.1	344	4.9	12.7	22.1	0.0
Winter Fruit, Caffe Nero*	1 Serving/145g	434	16.3	299	2.9	46.6	11.2	0.0
TEA								
Chai Latte, Semi Skimmed Milk, Caffe Nero*	1 Grande/405g	284	10.5	70	3.8	8.3	2.6	0.0
Chai Latte, Skimmed Milk, Caffe Nero*	1 Grande/405g	239	5.3	59	3.8	8.4	1.3	0.0
Chia Latte, Iced, Caffe Nero*	1 Latte/548g	466	11.0	85	3.6	13.7	2.0	0.0
TIRAMISU								
Caffe Nero*	1 Serving/112g	386	24.0	342	4.0	33.5	21.3	0.9
WATER								
Spring, Orange & Passion Fruit, Fruity, Caffe Nero*	1 Bottle/500ml	190	0.0	38	0.0	9.3	0.0	0.0
WRAP								
Chicken, & Salsa, Caffe Nero*	1 Wrap/198g	343	8.5	173	11.2	22.3	4.3	1.1
Chicken, Caesar, Caffe Nero*	1 Serving/209.4g	356	11.7	170	11.1	18.8	5.6	0.9
Chicken, Spicy, Caffe Nero*	1 Serving/176g	300	6.0	170	11.4	23.7	3.4	1.2
Chicken, with Yoghurt & Mint, Caffe Nero*	1 Sandwich/180g	418	20.0	232	11.8	21.3	11.1	1.0
Cream Cheese, Grilled Vegetable, & Tomato, Caffe Nero*	1 Serving/216g	344	11.5	159	4.8	22.9	5.3	0.0

	Measure INFO/WEIGHT	per Measure KCAL	FAT	Nutrition Values per 100g / 100ml KCAL	PROT	CARB	FAT	FIBRE
CAFFE NERO								
WRAP								
Ham, Leek, & Cheese, Hot, Caffe Nero*	1 Pack/165g	357	13.9	216	11.9	23.3	8.4	1.2
Ham, Mushroom, & Mozzarella, Caffe Nero*	1 Serving/166g	345	13.4	208	12.2	21.4	8.1	1.0
Houmous, & Red Pepper, Caffe Nero*	1 Serving/202g	303	8.9	150	4.6	23.0	4.4	2.0
Roast Vegetable, Bean & Tomato, Caffe Nero*	1 Serving/200g	332	8.2	166	5.0	27.9	4.1	0.0
Three Bean, Caffe Nero*	1 Wrap/178g	416	20.0	233	9.3	23.7	11.2	1.8
Tuna Nicoise, Caffe Nero*	1 Serving/236.4g	331	11.6	140	8.1	15.9	4.9	0.8
YOGHURT								
Bio, Caffe Nero*	1 Pot/150g	230	14.7	153	6.1	10.4	9.8	0.0
Blackcurrant, Bio, Caffe Nero*	1 Pot/150g	235	12.9	157	5.3	14.2	8.6	0.2
Blueberry, Brunch Pot, Caffe Nero*	1 Pot/126g	165	6.1	130	1.3	19.8	4.8	1.0
Fig & Honey, Brunch Pot, Caffe Nero*	1 Pot/135.3g	203	6.6	150	6.2	19.2	4.9	1.0
Forest Fruits, Muesli Topped, Brunch Pot, Caffe Nero*	1 Pot/150g	228	11.0	152	5.1	13.3	7.3	0.0
Mango & Passion Fruit, Brunch Pot, Caffe Nero*	1 Pot/134.6g	183	6.3	136	5.6	20.7	4.7	1.0
Strawberry, Brunch Pot, Caffe Nero*	1 Pot/125g	150	6.0	120	1.3	17.6	4.8	1.1
Strawberry, Muesli Topped, Brunch Pot, Caffe Nero*	1 Pot/150g	300	12.2	200	5.1	11.5	8.1	0.0
YOGHURT DRINK								
Strawberry, Probiotic, Organic, Caffe Nero*	1 Bottle/250ml	188	4.3	75	2.9	11.9	1.7	0.0
COFFEE REPUBLIC								
FLAPJACK								
Chewy Nutty, Coffee Republic*	1 Flapjack/33g	145	7.7	440	7.1	50.9	23.2	2.0
PANINI								
Ham & Swiss Cheese, Coffee Republic*	1 Panini/223g	558	26.1	250	15.7	20.5	11.7	0.0
Mozzarella & Tomato, Coffee Republic*	1 Panini/255g	566	25.5	222	11.1	23.6	10.0	0.0
SALAD								
Chicken Caesar, Bacon, Grana Padano, Coffee Republic*	1 Pack/139g	201	15.4	145	10.3	1.0	11.1	0.0
SANDWICH								
Cheese, & Ham, Toasted, Coffee Republic*	1 Pack/160g	429	20.3	268	15.7	24.4	12.7	0.0
Ham, & Salad, Coffee Republic*	1 Pack/224g	309	6.0	138	8.6	19.9	2.7	0.0
Mozzarella, & Salad, Coffee Republic*	1 Pack/242g	477	28.6	197	8.6	14.4	11.8	0.0
Salmon, Poached, Coffee Republic*	1 Pack/191g	350	14.5	183	10.3	18.4	7.6	0.0
Turkey, & Sun Dried Tomato, Coffee Republic*	1 Pack/215g	445	14.0	207	11.8	25.3	6.5	0.0
TOASTIE								
Cheese & Ham, Coffee Republic*	1 Serving/164g	436	16.6	266	13.7	30.1	10.1	0.0
COSTA								
BAKE								
Raspberry & Almond, Costa*	1 Slice/100g	451	28.2	451	8.5	40.8	28.2	1.0
BISCUITS								
Almond, Mini, Costa*	1 Serving/25g	124	6.0	494	6.2	63.0	24.1	0.0
Chocolate, Costa*	1 Serving/16g	76	5.0	448	4.9	41.1	29.3	0.0
Garibaldi, Costa*	2 Biscuits/68.1g	316	16.2	464	5.3	57.3	23.8	2.9
Linzer, Raspberry, Costa*	1 Biscuit/75g	312	14.0	416	4.1	56.2	18.6	0.0
Raisin, Cranberry & Hazelnut, Costa*	1 Serving/23g	84	4.2	364	2.7	47.5	18.2	0.0
BROWNIE								
Double Chocolate, Costa*	1 Brownie/80g	372	21.0	465	5.3	51.6	26.3	0.0
CAKE								
Carrot, Costa*	1 Serving/140g	500	25.3	357	5.1	43.4	18.1	0.0
Chocolate, Costa*	1 Serving/171g	667	25.4	388	4.8	58.9	14.8	0.0
Coffee & Walnut, Costa*	1 Serving/70g	334	19.7	472	4.9	50.3	27.9	0.0
Lemon, Costa*	1 Serving/144g	582	26.6	404	4.3	55.0	18.5	0.0
CIABATTA								
Ham, with Plum Tomato & Rocket, Italian, Costa*	1 Serving/50g	115	2.2	231	23.1	24.9	4.4	0.0

COSTA

	Measure INFO/WEIGHT	per Measure KCAL	per Measure FAT	Nutrition Values per 100g / 100ml KCAL	PROT	CARB	FAT	FIBRE
COFFEE								
Caffe Latte, Caramel, Full Fat, Massimo, Costa*	1 Massimo/408ml	282	9.8	69	2.4	9.4	2.4	0.0
Caffe Latte, Caramel, Full Fat, Medio, Costa*	1 Medio/294ml	221	7.1	75	2.3	11.2	2.4	0.0
Caffe Latte, Caramel, Full Fat, Primo, Costa*	1 Primo/220ml	187	5.3	85	1.2	14.7	2.4	0.0
Caffe Latte, Caramel, Skimmed, Massimo, Costa*	1 Massimo/404ml	194	0.4	48	2.3	9.3	0.1	0.0
Caffe Latte, Caramel, Skimmed, Medio, Costa*	1 Medio/291ml	163	0.3	56	2.3	11.3	0.1	0.0
Caffe Latte, Caramel, Skimmed, Primo, Costa*	1 Primo/220ml	143	0.2	65	1.9	14.1	0.1	0.0
Caffe Latte, Full Fat, Massimo, Costa*	1 Massimo/380ml	190	9.9	50	2.6	4.1	2.6	0.0
Caffe Latte, Full Fat, Medio, Costa*	1 Latte/264g	129	6.9	49	2.5	3.8	2.6	0.0
Caffe Latte, Full Fat, Primo, Costa*	1 Cup/190ml	95	5.1	50	1.4	5.0	2.7	0.0
Caffe Latte, Skimmed, Massimo, Costa*	1 Massimo/377ml	102	0.4	27	2.5	4.0	0.1	0.0
Caffe Latte, Skimmed, Medio, Costa*	1 Latte/264ml	71	0.3	27	2.6	3.9	0.1	0.0
Caffe Latte, Skimmed, Primo, Costa*	1 Primo/188g	51	0.2	27	2.2	4.3	0.1	0.0
Caffe Latte, Soya, Massimo, Costa*	1 Massimo/377ml	185	9.8	49	2.3	4.1	2.6	0.0
Caffe Latte, Soya, Medio, Costa*	1 Medio/260ml	86	3.9	33	2.4	2.4	1.5	0.0
Caffe Latte, Soya, Primo, Costa*	1 Primo/187ml	62	2.6	33	2.5	2.5	1.4	0.0
Caffe Latte, Vanilla, Full Fat, Massimo, Costa*	1 Massimo/408ml	290	9.8	71	2.4	9.9	2.4	0.0
Caffe Latte, Vanilla, Full Fat, Medio, Costa*	1 Latte/294g	229	7.1	78	2.3	11.9	2.4	0.0
Caffe Latte, Vanilla, Full Fat, Primo, Costa*	1 Primo/219ml	195	5.3	89	1.2	15.6	2.4	0.0
Caffe Latte, Vanilla, Skimmed, Massimo, Costa*	1 Massimo/404ml	202	0.4	50	2.3	9.8	0.1	0.0
Caffe Latte, Vanilla, Skimmed, Medio, Costa*	1 Medio/294ml	171	0.3	58	2.3	11.9	0.1	0.0
Caffe Latte, Vanilla, Skimmed, Primo, Costa*	1 Latte/220ml	151	0.3	69	1.9	15.0	0.1	0.0
Cappucino, Full Fat, Massimo, Costa*	1 Massimo/279g	123	6.7	44	2.3	3.3	2.4	0.0
Cappucino, Full Fat, Medio, Costa*	1 Medio/246g	101	4.7	41	2.2	3.8	1.9	0.0
Cappucino, Full Fat, Primo, Costa*	1 Cup/183ml	71	3.5	39	2.0	3.4	1.9	0.0
Cappucino, Skimmed, Massimo, Costa*	1 Mug/280ml	73	0.8	26	2.3	3.5	0.3	0.0
Cappucino, Skimmed, Medio, Costa*	1 Medio/241g	58	0.2	24	2.2	3.5	0.1	0.0
Cappucino, Skimmed, Primo, Costa*	1 Primo Cup/183ml	40	0.4	22	1.9	3.1	0.2	0.0
Cappucino, Soya, Massimo, Costa*	1 Massimo/275g	88	4.1	32	2.3	2.2	1.5	0.0
Cappucino, Soya, Medio, Costa*	1 Medio/248g	77	3.2	31	2.3	2.6	1.3	0.0
Cappucino, Soya, Primo, Costa*	1 Primo/180g	47	2.0	26	2.0	1.9	1.1	0.0
Mocha Flake, Full Fat, Massimo, Costa*	1 Massimo/332ml	369	23.6	111	2.9	8.7	7.1	0.0
Mocha Flake, Full Fat, Medio, Costa*	1 Medio/288ml	297	19.3	103	2.7	8.1	6.7	0.0
Mocha Flake, Full Fat, Primo, Costa*	1 Primo/233ml	257	17.3	110	2.6	8.1	7.4	0.0
Mocha Flake, Skimmed, Massimo, Costa*	1 Massimo/334ml	338	17.7	101	3.0	10.3	5.3	0.0
Mocha Flake, Skimmed, Medio, Costa*	1 Medio/287ml	262	14.1	91	2.6	9.0	4.9	0.0
Mocha Flake, Skimmed, Primo, Costa*	1 Primo/234ml	227	13.8	97	2.7	8.3	5.9	0.0
Mocha, Full Fat, Massimo, Costa*	1 Massimo/288ml	170	8.1	59	2.6	5.8	2.8	0.0
Mocha, Full Fat, Medio, Costa*	1 Mocha/253ml	153	6.6	60	2.6	6.7	2.6	0.0
Mocha, Full Fat, Primo, Costa*	1 Primo/188ml	113	4.7	60	2.6	6.7	2.5	0.0
Mocha, Skimmed, Massimo, Costa*	1 Massimo/287ml	138	2.0	48	2.8	7.6	0.7	0.0
Mocha, Skimmed, Medio, Costa*	1 Mocha/253ml	119	1.5	47	2.5	7.8	0.6	0.0
Mocha, Skimmed, Primo, Costa*	1 Primo/190ml	84	1.1	44	2.7	7.0	0.6	0.0
CRISPS								
Sea Salt Flavour, Costa*	1 Pack/50g	252	14.0	503	7.1	55.9	27.9	4.2
CROISSANT								
Almond, Costa*	1 Croissant/104g	432	25.1	415	8.9	40.6	24.1	0.0
Butter, Costa*	1 Croissant/68g	254	8.0	373	9.5	44.5	11.8	0.0
CRUMBLE								
Apple, Costa*	1 Slice/100g	469	30.1	469	5.6	46.7	30.1	0.0
FLAPJACK								
Fruity, Costa*	1 Bar/80g	423	29.0	529	6.5	43.9	36.3	12.5

COSTA

FLATBREAD

	Measure INFO/WEIGHT	per Measure KCAL	FAT	KCAL	PROT	CARB	FAT	FIBRE
Cajun Chicken, Costa*	1 Pack/145g	267	8.2	183	12.8	22.6	5.6	0.0
Cheddar & Caramelised Onion Chutney, Costa*	1 Pack/118g	340	13.3	288	11.9	34.8	11.3	0.0

FRUIT SALAD

Costa*	1 Serving/100g	75	0.3	75	0.9	18.0	0.3	0.0

HOT CHOCOLATE

with Frothed Milk, Full Fat, Massimo, Costa*	1 Massimo/376ml	259	10.9	69	3.1	7.6	2.9	0.0
with Frothed Milk, Full Fat, Medio, Costa*	1 Medio/266ml	157	5.9	59	3.0	6.9	2.2	0.0
with Frothed Milk, Full Fat, Primo, Costa*	1 Primo/192ml	121	4.8	63	3.1	6.9	2.5	0.0
with Frothed Milk, Skimmed, Medio, Costa*	1 Medio/265ml	130	1.3	49	3.4	7.7	0.5	0.0
with Frothed Milk, Skimmed, Primo, Costa*	1 Primo/192ml	98	1.2	51	3.4	7.9	0.6	0.0
with Frothed Milk, Skimmmed, Massimo, Costa*	1 Massimo/380ml	175	1.5	46	3.1	7.6	0.4	0.0
with Marshmallows & Cream, Full Fat, Massimo, Costa*	1 Massimo/419ml	423	20.5	101	3.1	11.2	4.9	0.0
with Marshmallows & Cream, Full Fat, Medio, Costa*	1 Medio/308ml	321	15.4	104	3.0	11.7	5.0	0.0
with Marshmallows & Cream, Full Fat, Primo, Costa*	1 Primo/237ml	285	14.5	120	3.0	13.2	6.1	0.0
with Marshmallows & Cream, Skimmed, Massimo, Costa*	1 Serving/418ml	339	11.3	81	3.1	11.2	2.7	0.0
with Marshmallows & Cream, Skimmed, Medio, Costa*	1 Medio/309ml	294	10.8	95	3.3	12.4	3.5	0.0
with Marshmallows & Cream, Skimmed, Primo, Costa*	1 Primo/238ml	262	10.7	110	3.3	14.0	4.5	0.0

MUFFIN

Banana & Toffee, Costa*	1 Muffin/117g	703	36.1	395	4.4	49.1	20.3	0.0
Blueberry, Costa*	1 Muffin/136g	505	29.7	371	4.7	40.5	21.8	0.0
Chocolate, Mini, Costa*	1 Muffin/19g	81	4.2	425	6.2	53.0	22.3	0.0
Lemon & Orange, Low Fat, Costa*	1 Muffin/135g	328	4.5	243	5.1	48.3	3.3	1.1
Lemon & White Chocolate, Costa*	1 Muffin/129g	472	20.4	366	5.4	52.3	15.8	0.0
Raspberry & White Chocolate, Costa*	1 Muffin/135g	511	26.0	376	4.8	46.4	19.1	0.0
Raspberry & White Chocolate, Mini, Costa*	1 Muffin/19g	71	3.7	371	4.8	44.7	19.4	0.0
Red Berry, Low Fat, Costa*	1 Muffin/124g	381	4.2	307	6.2	63.0	3.4	0.0
Triple Chocolate, Costa*	1 Muffin/133g	525	29.1	392	5.7	47.3	21.7	0.0
Very Berry, Costa*	1 Muffin/140g	354	6.4	253	4.4	48.6	4.6	0.0

PAIN AU RAISIN

Costa*	1 Pastry/99g	289	12.7	292	6.0	38.2	12.8	0.0

PANINI

Chicken & Baby Spinach, Costa*	1 Serving/440g	832	11.0	189	9.8	32.5	2.5	0.0
Chicken Arrabiata, Costa*	1 Pack/204.9g	377	5.5	184	13.7	26.1	2.7	0.0
Ham & Three Cheese, Costa*	1 Panini/174g	460	21.2	263	12.5	26.2	12.1	0.0
Mozzarella, Tomato & Basil, Costa*	1 Panini/190g	460	18.4	242	9.4	29.3	9.7	0.0
Mozzarella, Tomato & Pesto, Costa*	1 Panini/209g	487	14.6	233	9.0	35.0	7.0	5.0
Mushroom & Emmental, Costa*	1 Panini/186g	456	18.3	244	10.9	28.0	9.8	0.0
Spicy Meatball, Costa*	1 Panini/180g	515	17.8	286	11.9	37.1	9.9	0.0
Tuna Melt, Costa*	1 Pack/194g	580	27.8	298	13.8	28.6	14.3	0.0

PASTRY

Pecan Slice, Costa*	1 Pastry/105g	465	29.9	443	5.6	42.1	28.5	3.0

SANDWICH

BLT, Costa*	1 Sandwich/178g	458	24.7	256	8.8	23.9	13.8	0.0
Bacon & Tomato Sauce, Tostato, Costa*	1 Tostato/132.2g	316	6.6	239	8.5	40.2	5.0	0.0
Brie, Apple & Grape, Costa*	1 Serving/225g	536	24.5	238	8.3	28.7	10.9	0.0
Chicken, Roast, Costa*	1 Pack/176.6g	325	7.1	184	13.0	23.8	4.0	0.0
Club, All Day Breakfast, Costa*	1 Sandwich/271g	643	24.1	237	10.1	29.0	8.9	0.0
Club, Chicken & Bacon, Costa*	1 Sandwich/239g	606	18.2	253	14.0	31.6	7.6	0.0
Egg Mayonnaise & Tomato, Free Range, Costa*	1 Pack/174.4g	389	24.1	223	8.6	18.3	13.8	0.0
Egg, Free Range, Costa*	1 Pack/172g	315	8.3	183	10.6	24.3	4.8	0.0
Ham & Three Cheese, Tostato, Costa*	1 Pack/159.1g	409	16.7	257	10.5	30.0	10.5	0.0
Houmous, Costa*	1 Pack/165g	263	4.7	160	6.4	25.9	2.8	0.0

	Measure	per Measure		Nutrition Values per 100g / 100ml				
	INFO/WEIGHT	KCAL	FAT	KCAL	PROT	CARB	FAT	FIBRE

COSTA

SANDWICH

	Measure	per Measure		Nutrition Values per 100g / 100ml				
Prawn, Tiger, with Lime & Chilli Dressing, Costa*	1 Pack/185.4g	366	18.9	198	8.2	21.2	10.2	0.0
Salmon, & Salad, Poached, Oatmeal, Costa*	1 Pack/151g	224	4.2	148	7.7	22.9	2.8	0.0
Sausage, Chorizo, & Vine Ripened Tomato, Costa*	1 Pack/181.0g	315	3.8	174	15.5	26.1	2.1	0.0
Tuna, & Salad, Costa*	1 Pack/206g	363	8.9	176	11.9	22.6	4.3	0.0

SHORTBREAD
Caramel, Costa*	1 Slice/77g	426	26.5	553	4.7	55.9	34.4	0.0

SHORTCAKE
Raspberry, Costa*	1 Shortcake/45g	215	10.7	477	2.4	63.5	23.7	0.0

SOUP
Fish, Bouillabaisse, Costa*	1 Serving/400g	180	5.6	45	5.8	2.2	1.4	0.0

TEA
Iced, Lemon, Costa*	1 Bottle/275ml	91	0.0	33	0.0	8.0	0.0	0.0

WRAP
Sweet Chilli Chicken, Costa*	1 Wrap/192g	365	8.3	190	10.7	27.1	4.3	0.0

CRUSSH JUICE BARS

BAGEL
Salmon, Cream Cheese, Low Fat, Crussh Juice Bars*	1 Pack/191g	365	5.9	190	14.2	28.5	3.1	0.0

BREAKFAST CEREAL
Museli, Berry, Crussh Juice Bars*	1 Serving/225g	295	13.7	131	5.1	13.9	6.1	1.3
Porridge, Cinnamon, Crussh Juice Bars*	1 Serving/300g	285	6.3	95	3.1	15.7	2.1	1.8
Porridge, Summer, Crussh Juice Bars*	1 Serving/330g	495	13.2	150	1.5	27.0	4.0	0.0
Porridge, Traditional, Organic, Crussh Juice Bars*	1 Serving/330g	314	6.9	95	3.1	15.7	2.1	1.8
Porridge, with Soy Milk, Organic, Crussh Juice Bars*	1 Serving/331g	330	11.6	100	3.5	16.5	3.5	1.9

CHOCOLATE
Shot, Fairtrade, Crussh Juice Bars*	1 Shot/100g	210	17.2	210	2.3	12.0	17.2	0.6

COOKIE
Chocolate Chip & Hazelnut, Organic, Crussh Juice Bars*	1 Cookie/50g	228	12.9	457	5.8	50.3	25.8	2.3
Double Chocolate, Crussh Juice Bars*	1 Cookie/50g	210	8.8	421	5.0	60.8	17.6	2.7
Oat & Raisin, Organic, Crussh Juice Bars*	1 Cookie/50g	203	9.1	406	4.8	55.8	18.2	2.7

JUICE
Apple, Crussh Juice Bars*	1 Glass/340ml	119	0.3	35	0.3	8.1	0.1	1.4
Carrot, Crussh Juice Bars*	1 Glass/338ml	122	1.0	36	0.6	7.7	0.3	3.0
Clean & Lean, Crussh Juice Bars*	1 Glass/340ml	146	0.3	43	0.4	10.0	0.1	2.4
Combo, Superjuice, Crussh Juice Bars*	1 Glass/330ml	87	1.3	26	1.3	4.5	0.4	2.0
Energiser, Crussh Juice Bars*	1 Glass/339ml	139	0.7	41	0.5	9.2	0.2	2.9
Green Goddess, Crussh Juice Bars*	1 Glass/341ml	133	0.7	39	0.7	8.5	0.2	2.4
Liquid Lunch, Crussh Juice Bars*	1 Glass/340ml	153	0.7	45	0.4	10.5	0.2	2.1
Love Juice, Crussh Juice Bars*	1 Glass/340ml	143	0.3	42	0.7	9.6	0.1	0.6
Orange, Crussh Juice Bars*	1 Glass/340ml	92	0.3	27	0.8	5.6	0.1	1.7
Purifier, Crussh Juice Bars*	1 Glass/338ml	122	0.7	36	0.6	7.9	0.2	2.7
Super Juice, Crussh Juice Bars*	1 Glass/342ml	113	1.0	33	1.0	6.5	0.3	2.7
Zinger, Crussh Juice Bars*	1 Glass/341ml	133	0.3	39	0.5	9.0	0.1	1.4

SALAD
Chicken Caesar, Free Range, Crussh Juice Bars*	1 Salad/279g	333	16.0	119	8.8	8.8	5.7	1.4
Chicken, Bang Bang, Crussh Juice Bars*	1 Salad/460g	341	26.3	74	3.8	4.0	5.7	2.2
Crayfish & Sweet Chilli Noodle, Crussh Juice Bars*	1 Serving/110.5g	169	3.4	153	6.5	24.5	3.1	0.0
Falafel, Crussh Juice Bars*	1 Salad/300g	321	23.4	107	3.8	5.3	7.8	1.4
Greek, Crussh Juice Bars*	1 Salad/196g	137	8.6	70	2.9	4.4	4.4	0.0
Health Pot, Full O'Beans, Crussh Juice Bars*	1 Salad/159g	243	10.9	152	5.3	17.4	6.8	0.1
Health Pot, Goats Cheese & Sweet Potato, Crussh Bars*	1 Salad/159g	203	9.8	127	7.1	11.6	6.1	1.9
Health Pot, O-Me-Good, Crussh Juice Bars*	1 Pack/290.1g	705	30.8	243	9.7	28.6	10.6	0.9
Health Pot, Puy Lentil, Crussh Juice Bars*	1 Salad/100g	274	13.2	274	12.5	26.4	13.2	6.8

CRUSSH JUICE BARS

	Measure INFO/WEIGHT	per Measure KCAL	FAT	Nutrition Values per 100g / 100ml KCAL	PROT	CARB	FAT	FIBRE
SALAD								
Health Pot, Superfoods, Crussh Juice Bars*	1 Salad/160g	440	24.2	275	10.7	23.9	15.1	4.3
Health Pot, Tuna Lean Bean, Crussh Juice Bars*	1 Pot/159g	213	9.7	134	8.0	11.6	6.1	2.0
Health Pot, Tuscan Chicken & Barley, Crussh Juice Bars*	1 Salad/160g	442	6.6	276	12.2	48.3	4.1	14.3
Super 7, Crussh Juice Bars*	1 Pack/330g	297	12.5	90	7.3	6.7	3.8	2.0
Tuna Nicoise, Crussh Juice Bars*	1 Salad/300g	207	7.5	69	4.5	6.9	2.5	1.3
SANDWICH								
5-A-Day, Wheat Free, Crussh Juice Bars*	1 Sandwich/230g	391	18.9	170	4.2	22.1	8.2	1.3
Chicken, & Salad, Crussh Juice Bars*	1 Pack/171.7g	330	10.8	192	13.6	20.0	6.3	3.0
Egg Mayo & Mustard Cress, Crussh Juice Bars*	1 Pack/421.6g	489	5.5	116	5.6	20.6	1.3	3.7
Ham, Smokey, Swiss, Crussh Juice Bars*	1 Pack/243g	490	19.3	201	12.1	20.2	7.9	3.0
Mature Cheddar & Friars Chutney, Crussh Juice Bars*	1 Pack/152g	390	15.7	255	12.1	28.8	10.3	3.9
Tuna, Cucumber & Mayo, Crussh Juice Bars*	1 Pack/226.7g	340	7.0	150	12.5	18.1	3.1	2.8
SMOOTHIE								
Bananarama, Crussh Juice Bars*	1 Med/339ml	326	1.4	96	3.0	20.1	0.4	1.0
Berry Blast, Crussh Juice Bars*	1 Med/339ml	241	0.7	71	2.0	10.5	0.2	0.6
Berry Breakfast, Crussh Juice Bars*	1 Med/330ml	396	8.9	120	4.5	19.5	2.7	1.5
Bliss Blend, Crussh Juice Bars*	1 Med/339ml	950	0.7	280	1.6	13.9	0.2	0.8
Brainstorm, Crussh Juice Bars*	1 Med/340ml	235	0.7	69	1.8	10.6	0.2	0.9
Brazillian, Crussh Juice Bars*	1 Med/339ml	224	2.0	66	1.8	10.1	0.6	0.9
Breakfast, Crussh Juice Bars*	1 Med/340ml	507	12.6	149	5.0	23.8	3.7	1.8
Energy Explosion, Crussh Juice Bars*	1 Med/344ml	241	0.7	70	1.8	11.5	0.2	0.7
Fat Burner, Crussh Juice Bars*	1 Med/339ml	231	0.7	68	1.9	10.3	0.2	0.7
Mango Madness, Crussh Juice Bars*	1 Med/339ml	248	1.0	73	1.7	15.5	0.3	0.7
Peach Passion, Crussh Juice Bars*	1 Med/340ml	228	0.7	67	1.8	13.9	0.2	0.7
Pineapple Pleasure, Crussh Juice Bars*	1 Med/339g	241	0.7	71	1.8	15.3	0.2	0.5
Strawberry Cool, Crussh Juice Bars*	1 Med/340ml	229	0.7	67	1.7	13.9	0.2	0.7
SOUP								
Beef Chilli, Crussh Juice Bars*	1 Serving/300g	135	3.9	45	4.8	3.4	1.3	0.0
Bengali Tomato, Crussh Juice Bars*	1 Lrg/400g	156	7.6	39	1.2	4.1	1.9	0.0
Boston Clam Chowder, Crussh Juice Bars*	1 Serving/331g	212	9.3	64	2.7	7.0	2.8	0.8
Cauliflower & Brie, Gourmet, Crussh Juice Bars*	1 Lrg/400g	264	15.6	66	3.4	4.3	3.9	1.0
Chicken Chowder, Boston, Gourmet, Crussh Juice Bars*	1 Lrg/400g	312	14.0	78	4.4	7.2	3.5	0.0
Chicken Provencale, Gourmet, Crussh Juice Bars*	1 Med/330g	90	3.3	27	2.6	1.9	1.0	0.0
Chicken Tikka, Organic, Crussh Juice Bars*	1 Med/330ml	330	17.2	100	4.6	8.7	5.2	0.0
Egyptian Lentil, Crussh Juice Bars*	1 Med/331g	288	1.2	87	7.0	15.0	0.4	0.0
Farmhouse Chicken, Crussh Juice Bars*	1 Med/330g	191	8.6	58	3.4	5.2	2.6	0.0
Goats Cheese & Red Pepper, Crussh Juice Bars*	1 Med/330g	139	6.3	42	1.3	4.2	1.9	0.8
Hong Kong, Borscht, Crussh Juice Bars*	1 Med/328g	138	4.6	42	2.8	4.5	1.4	0.0
Lamb Stew, Irish, Crussh Juice Bars*	1 Med/340g	122	4.8	36	2.0	4.2	1.4	1.0
Lentil & Herbs, Crussh Juice Bars*	1 Med/300g	162	1.2	54	4.0	8.6	0.4	10.0
Lentil & Tomato, Crussh Juice Bars*	1 Med Soup/300g	330	3.0	110	4.8	21.4	1.0	0.0
Mediterranean Vegetable, Crussh Juice Bars*	1 Lge/400g	140	4.4	35	2.0	4.4	1.1	1.7
Minestrone, Classic, Italian, Crussh Juice Bars*	1 Med/300g	135	2.4	45	2.3	7.1	0.8	2.1
Mixed Vegetable, Organic, Crussh Juice Bars*	1 Lge /400g	112	2.0	28	2.1	4.0	0.5	0.0
Mulligatawny, Organic, Crussh Juice Bars*	1 Lge/400g	328	18.8	82	3.0	6.9	4.7	0.0
Potato & Leek, Organic, Crussh Juice Bars*	1 Med/330ml	162	7.9	49	1.5	6.0	2.4	0.6
Roasted Tomato & Thyme, Organic, Crussh Juice Bars*	1 Med/330g	99	3.6	30	0.9	4.0	1.1	0.9
Sun Ripened Tomato & Basil, Crussh Juice Bars*	1 Serving/330g	132	6.6	40	0.7	4.8	2.0	1.0
Thai Chicken & Sweet Potato, Crussh Juice Bars*	1 Lge/400g	280	8.8	70	4.8	7.7	2.2	2.0
Thai Tomato, Crussh Juice Bars*	1 Med/329g	313	10.5	95	2.5	15.3	3.2	0.0
Tomato & Basil, Crussh Juice Bars*	1 Large/400g	68	2.0	17	0.6	2.4	0.5	0.8
Tuscan Vegetable, Organic, Crussh Juice Bars*	1 Med/330ml	215	8.6	65	2.4	8.1	2.6	0.0

	Measure INFO/WEIGHT	per Measure		Nutrition Values per 100g / 100ml				
		KCAL	FAT	KCAL	PROT	CARB	FAT	FIBRE
CRUSSH JUICE BARS								
SOUP								
Vegetable, Autumn Garden, Crussh Juice Bars*	1 Med/330g	185	9.3	56	0.9	6.7	2.8	1.0
Vegetable, Chilli Stew, Crussh Juice Bars*	1 Medium/332.1g	93	1.7	28	2.1	4.0	0.5	1.3
Vegetable, Garden, Crussh Juice Bars*	1 Med/336g	168	1.3	50	2.7	8.9	0.4	0.0
Vegetable, Moroccan, Organic, Crussh Juice Bars*	1 Large/400g	104	3.0	26	1.0	4.2	0.7	0.0
Wild Mushroom, Organic, Crussh Juice Bars*	1 Medium/300g	120	7.2	40	0.7	3.9	2.4	1.3
SUSHI								
Salmon, Crussh Juice Bars*	1 Box/280g	344	5.6	123	4.3	21.9	2.0	0.0
Veggie, Crussh Juice Bars*	1 Box/380g	490	18.6	129	2.8	18.3	4.9	0.0
TOASTIE								
Cheddar Cheese, Tasty, Crussh Juice Bars*	1 Toastie/106g	310	10.0	295	14.5	37.9	9.5	0.0
Edam & Ham, Skinny, Crussh Juice Bars*	1 Pack/130g	329	8.7	253	15.4	32.9	6.7	0.0
Jalapeno & Spinach, Crussh Juice Bars*	1 Toastie/150g	404	16.1	269	13.9	29.3	10.7	0.3
Spinach & Chorizo, Crussh Juice Bars*	1 Toastie/150g	333	11.0	222	11.3	28.3	7.3	0.4
Tuna, Swiss, Crussh Juice Bars*	1 Toastie/169g	379	11.6	223	16.3	24.0	6.8	0.1
WRAP								
Caesar, Simply, Crussh Juice Bars*	1 Wrap/190g	538	16.7	283	10.3	40.4	8.8	1.5
Houmous & Falafel, Crussh Juice Bars*	1 Wrap/150g	318	14.4	212	7.5	23.9	9.6	1.0
Salmon Salad & Sushi, Miso Dressing, Crussh Juice Bars*	1 Wrap/301g	379	2.7	126	5.2	24.2	0.9	0.0
Mushroom & Sushi, Soy Vinegar, Crussh Juice Bars*	1 Wrap/298g	310	1.8	104	1.9	22.7	0.6	0.0
Tuna & Salad, Crussh Juice Bars*	1 Wrap/209.8g	365	10.3	174	12.0	20.4	4.9	0.4
Tuna Salad & Sushi, Soy & Vinegar Dressing, Crussh Bars*	1 Wrap/275g	388	7.7	141	4.5	24.4	2.8	0.0
YOGHURT								
with Honey, Low Fat, Greek, Crussh Juice Bars*	1 Pot/140g	209	12.7	150	5.1	12.5	9.1	0.0
CUISINE DE FRANCE								
BREAD								
Baguette, Demi, Cuisine De France*	1 Serving/140g	360	2.0	257	6.7	56.0	1.4	1.7
Baguette, Parisien, Cuisine De France*	1 Serving/70g	172	0.6	245	8.5	51.0	0.8	1.9
Baguette, la Premier, Cuisine De France*	1 Serving/70g	180	0.7	257	7.6	54.3	1.0	1.8
Baps, Brown, Soft, Cuisine De France*	1 Bap/99g	236	0.9	238	11.5	46.0	0.9	7.3
Ciabattina, Cuisine De France*	1 Roll/120g	299	1.9	249	8.3	50.3	1.6	1.5
French, Cuisine De France*	½ Stick/200g	490	1.6	245	8.5	51.0	0.8	1.9
MUFFIN								
Cappuccion, Iced, Luxury, Iced, Cuisine De France*	1 Muffin/105g	457	22.6	435	5.6	54.8	21.5	0.0
Carrot Cake, Cuisine De France*	1 Muffin/105g	373	12.6	355	4.7	56.9	12.0	0.0
DEBENHAMS								
PRAWNS WITH								
Noodles, King, Debenhams*	1 Serving/370g	537	17.8	145	5.4	20.2	4.8	0.0
SANDWICH								
Chicken, with Salad, Chargrilled, Debenhams*	1 Pack/250g	325	9.0	130	7.6	18.0	3.6	0.0
Mozzarella, & Tomato, & Basil, Debenhams*	1 Pack/152.5g	339	14.0	223	10.0	25.0	9.2	0.0
Tuna, & Salad, Debenhams*	1 Pack/249g	309	8.5	124	7.7	16.9	3.4	0.0
DOMINO'S PIZZA								
BREAD								
Garlic, Pizza, Domino's Pizza*	4 Slices/214g	145	5.0	68	4.1	7.6	2.3	0.1
BROWNIES								
Chocolate, Squares, Domino's Pizza*	1 Portion/100g	481	28.0	481	6.7	50.5	28.0	3.6
CHEESECAKE								
Domino's Pizza*	1 Serving/132g	396	24.6	300	5.0	28.5	18.6	0.5
CHICKEN								
Kickers, Domino's Pizza*	7 Kickers/175g	328	10.5	187	19.2	14.1	6.0	0.8
Strippers, Domino's Pizza*	7 Strippers/172g	64	3.7	37	2.8	1.7	2.2	0.1

DOMINO'S PIZZA

	Measure INFO/WEIGHT	per Measure KCAL	per Measure FAT	Nutrition Values per 100g / 100ml KCAL	PROT	CARB	FAT	FIBRE
COLESLAW								
Domino's Pizza*	1 Tub/200g	254	21.4	127	1.1	6.3	10.7	0.0
DESSERT								
Chocolate Indulgence, Domino's Pizza*	1 Pot/125g	449	24.4	359	5.0	40.9	19.5	2.9
Hanky Panky, Domino's Pizza*	1 Serving/125g	463	30.0	370	4.8	34.5	24.0	0.8
Temptation, Domino's Pizza*	1 Serving/125g	404	24.5	323	4.1	32.9	19.6	0.5
Toffee Delight, Domino's Pizza*	1 Pot/125g	401	22.6	321	5.0	34.4	18.1	0.8
DIP								
BBQ, Domino's Pizza*	1 Pot/28g	46	0.0	164	1.0	40.0	0.0	0.0
Chocolate, Domino's Pizza*	1 Pot/28g	90	0.3	320	0.6	77.3	0.9	1.4
Garlic & Herb, Domino's Pizza*	1 Pot/28g	199	21.7	711	1.2	2.1	77.5	0.0
Honey & Mustard, Domino's Pizza*	1 Pot/28g	129	13.2	459	2.1	7.9	47.1	0.0
Sweet Chilli, Domino's Pizza*	1 Pot/28g	56	0.1	200	0.7	48.9	0.2	0.4
PIZZA								
American Hot, Medium, Domino's Pizza*	1 Slice/70g	169	5.9	241	13.1	28.3	8.4	4.0
Americano, Medium, Domino's Pizza*	1 Slice/71g	182	5.0	253	15.6	32.0	7.0	2.6
Ay Carumba Fajita, Domino's Pizza*	1 Slice/56.8g	158	7.0	279	24.5	25.1	12.4	1.8
Bacon Double Cheese Burger, Medium, Domino's Pizza*	1 Slice/94g	207	6.8	221	15.2	23.7	7.3	1.5
Bacon Double Cheese, Medium, Domino's Pizza*	1 Slice/93g	191	6.0	206	13.7	23.2	6.5	3.0
Beef & Onion Pie, Medium, Domino's Pizza*	1 Slice/74g	147	2.6	200	11.9	29.9	3.6	3.3
Beef on the Barbie, Medium, Domino's Pizza*	1 Slice/74g	167	4.1	226	12.8	31.3	5.5	1.9
Calypso, Medium, Domino's Pizza*	1 Slice/73g	152	3.1	209	12.8	30.0	4.2	2.1
Cheese & Tomato, Chicago Thin Crust, Domino's Pizza*	1 Slice/92g	320	14.6	348	16.1	35.1	15.9	3.0
Cheese & Tomato, Double Decadence, Domino's Pizza*	1 Slice/92g	272	11.9	296	17.1	25.6	12.9	2.2
Cheese & Tomato, Medium, Domino's Pizza*	1 Slice/54g	136	2.7	253	13.2	38.6	5.1	3.1
Cheese Steak Melt, Medium, Domino's Pizza*	1 Slice Med/81g	195	5.6	241	15.0	29.8	6.9	1.5
Chicago, Thin Crust, Medium, Domino's Pizza*	1 Slice/44g	151	6.9	348	16.1	35.1	15.9	3.0
Chicken Feast, Medium, Domino's Pizza*	1 Med Slice/73g	145	2.4	199	13.5	28.8	3.3	2.9
Deluxe, Medium, Domino's Pizza*	1 Slice/77g	178	6.3	230	12.8	26.2	8.2	2.2
Dominator, Domino's Pizza*	1 Slice/86g	242	8.1	281	10.6	38.4	9.4	2.9
Double Decadence, Medium, Domino's Pizza*	1 Slice/93g	273	11.9	296	17.1	25.6	12.9	2.2
Extravaganzza, Medium, Domino's Pizza*	1 Slice/96g	201	6.9	209	14.3	21.8	7.2	2.0
Farmhouse, Medium, Domino's Pizza*	1 Slice/71g	147	2.9	205	13.1	29.2	4.0	2.6
Football Fanatic, Domino's Pizza*	1 Slice/73g	215	9.6	295	14.2	29.9	13.2	1.6
Full House, Medium, Domino's Pizza*	1 Slice/84g	190	7.1	226	13.2	24.1	8.5	1.5
Ham & Pineapple, Medium, Domino's Pizza*	1 Slice/70g	148	2.8	211	17.4	26.3	4.0	2.0
Hawaiian, Medium, Domino's Pizza*	1 Slice/72.8g	147	3.0	202	12.9	28.4	4.1	1.7
Hot & Spicy, Medium, Domino's Pizza*	1 Slice/76	146	4.0	192	12.4	23.9	5.2	4.7
Hot Dog, Medium, Domino's Pizza*	1 Slice/91g	237	10.0	260	16.9	23.3	11.0	2.6
Hot Stuff, Domino's Pizza*	1 Slice/78.6g	210	9.0	267	12.2	29.0	11.4	1.6
House Special, Medium, Domino's Pizza*	1 Slice/98g	224	8.5	229	17.1	20.5	8.7	1.8
Jamaican Bombastic, Domino's Pizza*	1 Slice/85.4g	184	4.4	215	11.7	30.4	5.2	1.8
Meat Lovers, Medium, Domino's Pizza*	1 Slice/78g	189	6.6	243	16.0	25.5	8.5	2.3
Meat Packer, Medium, Domino's Pizza*	1 Slice/84g	218	9.0	260	17.1	24.3	10.7	2.1
Meatzza Pizza, Medium, Domino's Pizza*	1 Slice/77g	191	7.0	248	14.3	27.2	9.1	2.5
Mediterranean Spice, Medium, Domino's Pizza*	1 Slice/82g	147	3.4	179	9.6	25.8	4.2	3.1
Mexican Hot, Medium, Domino's Pizza*	1 Slice/84g	186	6.1	220	13.6	25.3	7.2	2.2
Mighty Meaty, Medium, Domino's Pizza*	1 Slice/83g	192	6.6	232	14.7	25.2	8.0	1.9
Mixed Grill, Medium, Domino's Pizza*	1 Slice/88g	203	7.4	229	13.2	25.1	8.4	1.3
New Yorker, Medium, Domino's Pizza*	1 Slice/73.4g	184	6.8	250	16.4	25.3	9.2	2.3
Pepperoni Passion, Medium, Domino's Pizza*	1 Slice/81.8g	199	6.8	243	15.8	26.2	8.3	2.6
Tandoori Hot, Medium, Domino's Pizza*	1 Slice/79.1	154	3.3	195	12.7	26.5	4.2	1.8
Tex Mex, Domino's Pizza*	1 Slice/75.9g	200	8.7	263	12.7	27.5	11.4	2.1

DOMINO'S PIZZA

	Measure INFO/WEIGHT	per Measure KCAL	FAT	Nutrition Values per 100g / 100ml KCAL	PROT	CARB	FAT	FIBRE
PIZZA								
Texas BBQ, Medium, Domino's Pizza*	1 Slice/76g	173	3.6	227	12.1	34.1	4.7	2.8
The Sizzler, Medium, Domino's Pizza*	1 Slice/75g	180	6.2	240	13.6	27.8	8.3	4.8
The Steak Special, Domino's Pizza*	1 Slice/59g	152	4.1	255	15.2	33.3	6.8	2.2
Tuna Delight, Domino's Pizza*	1 Slice/66g	142	2.6	216	13.4	31.6	4.0	3.8
Veg-A-Roma, Medium, Domino's Pizza*	1 Slice/65.6	158	4.0	241	12.2	34.2	6.1	3.3
Vegetarian Supreme, Medium, Domino's Pizza*	1 Slice/80g	138	2.2	172	10.5	26.1	2.8	2.1
Vegi Delight, Medium, Domino's Pizza*	1 Slice/92g	177	4.1	192	13.6	24.3	4.5	1.8
Vegi Lite, Domino's Pizza*	1 Slice/66g	134	2.8	204	11.8	29.8	4.2	3.9
Vegi Volcano, Medium, Domino's Pizza*	1 Slice/94g	155	3.8	166	14.6	17.6	4.1	4.7
POTATO WEDGES								
Domino's Pizza*	1 Serving/165g	316	11.2	192	2.7	29.9	6.8	3.4
STICKY DIPPERS								
Domino's Pizza*	1 Dipper/20.5g	69	1.9	339	10.4	53.3	9.3	3.2
WAFFLES								
Domino's Pizza*	1 Serving/49g	225	12.0	459	5.9	54.3	24.5	3.1
EAT								
ANTIPASTO								
Italian, EAT*	1 Serving/100g	353	29.3	353	19.9	2.4	29.3	1.5
BAGUETTE								
BLT, EAT*	1 Baguette/259g	549	23.0	212	8.9	24.3	8.9	0.9
Brie, Tomato & Basil, EAT*	1 Baguette/120g	578	25.8	482	20.7	51.5	21.5	1.8
Cheese, & Ham, EAT*	1 Serving/132g	652	26.8	494	32.1	45.9	20.3	1.4
Chicken, Tikka, EAT*	1 Baguette/150g	440	10.1	293	20.7	37.5	6.7	2.8
Chorizo, Chargrilled Peppers & Rocket, EAT*	1 Baguette/250g	637	29.7	255	10.6	26.4	11.9	1.3
Ham & Brie, Festive, EAT*	1 Baguette/200g	798	40.1	399	17.9	36.8	20.1	2.4
Ham & Jarlsberg, EAT*	1 Baguette/137g	617	24.1	450	28.9	44.2	17.6	1.3
Ham, Tomato, & English Mustard, Wood Smoked, EAT*	1 Pack/132g	509	20.0	386	19.2	42.7	15.2	2.9
Roast Beef & Rocket, EAT*	1 Pack/250g	682	33.1	273	14.2	24.4	13.2	0.8
Tuna & Cucumber, EAT*	1 Baguette/135g	675	34.7	500	21.6	45.7	25.7	1.6
BARS								
Cereal, Zesty Citrus, EAT*	1 Bar/25g	84	1.3	336	5.6	66.4	5.2	3.6
Oat, Fruit & Nut, EAT*	1 Bar/65g	396	22.2	609	8.6	66.9	34.2	5.2
BREAD								
Wholemeal, Chunk, EAT*	1 Serving/67g	138	1.6	206	9.0	37.2	2.4	7.9
BREAKFAST CEREAL								
Muesli, Swiss Bircher, EAT*	1 Pot/250g	372	6.0	149	5.8	26.3	2.4	1.4
Museli, Mango & Coconut, EAT*	1 Pot/220g	485	26.5	220	4.9	23.2	12.1	3.0
Porridge, Plain, EAT*	1 Serving/340g	226	3.9	66	3.7	10.3	1.2	0.8
Porridge, with Banana & Maple Syrup, EAT*	1 Sm Pot/227g	181	2.6	80	3.7	13.7	1.2	0.9
BROWNIE								
Chocolate, EAT*	1 Brownie/50g	341	18.2	682	8.4	80.0	36.4	2.6
EAT*	1 Slice/70g	345	17.8	493	5.9	61.3	25.4	2.9
CAKE								
Banana & Walnut, EAT*	1 Pack/150g	366	21.7	244	3.2	28.3	14.5	0.7
Chocolate, EAT*	1 Slice/100g	293	15.8	293	4.4	33.3	15.8	0.6
COFFEE								
Cappuccino, Skimmed Milk, EAT*	1 Tall/12oz	118	4.0	33	2.4	3.4	1.1	0.0
Cappuccino, Soya Milk, EAT*	1 Tall/12oz	131	4.9	37	3.2	3.5	1.4	0.9
Cappuccino, Whole Milk, EAT*	1 Tall/12oz	168	9.1	47	2.4	3.4	2.6	0.0
Espresso, Macchiato, Skimmed Milk, EAT*	1 Espresso/4oz	8	0.3	7	0.5	0.7	0.3	0.0
Espresso, Macchiato, Soya Milk, EAT*	1 Espresso/4oz	9	0.4	8	0.6	0.7	0.3	0.2
Espresso, Macchiato, Whole Milk, EAT*	1 Espresso/4oz	11	0.6	9	0.5	0.7	0.5	0.0

EAT

	Measure INFO/WEIGHT	per Measure KCAL	FAT	Nutrition Values per 100g / 100ml KCAL	PROT	CARB	FAT	FIBRE
COFFEE								
Latte, Chai, Skimmed Milk, EAT*	1 Tall/12oz	305	1.0	86	3.2	17.7	0.3	0.0
Latte, Chai, Soya Milk, EAT*	1 Tall/12oz	279	5.3	79	2.5	13.9	1.5	0.5
Latte, Chai, Whole Milk, EAT*	1 Tall/12oz	408	12.9	115	3.1	17.5	3.6	0.0
Latte, Chiller, Skimmed Milk, EAT*	1 Tall/12oz	241	3.3	68	3.1	11.9	0.9	0.0
Latte, Chiller, Soya Milk, EAT*	1 Tall/12oz	251	4.0	71	3.7	12.0	1.1	0.7
Latte, Chiller, Whole Milk, EAT*	1 Tall/12oz	281	7.5	79	3.1	11.9	2.1	0.0
Latte, Iced, Skimmed Milk, EAT*	1 Tall/12oz	95	3.2	27	1.9	2.7	0.9	0.0
Latte, Iced, Soya Milk, EAT*	1 Tall/12oz	105	3.9	30	2.5	2.8	1.1	0.7
Latte, Matcha, Skimmed Milk, EAT*	1 Tall/12oz	204	1.0	57	3.0	10.6	0.3	0.3
Latte, Matcha, Soya Milk, EAT*	1 Tall/12oz	201	5.8	57	3.0	7.4	1.6	0.3
Latte, Matcha, Whole Milk, EAT*	1 Tall/12oz	297	11.8	84	3.0	10.5	3.3	0.3
Latte, Skimmed Milk, EAT*	1 Tall/12oz	142	4.8	40	2.9	4.1	1.4	0.0
Latte, Soya Milk, EAT*	1 Tall/12oz	157	5.9	44	3.8	4.2	1.7	1.1
Latte, Whole Milk, EAT*	1 Tall/12oz	202	11.0	57	2.9	4.1	3.1	0.0
Mocha, Chiller, Skimmed Milk, EAT*	1 Tall/12oz	243	3.4	68	2.5	12.6	1.0	0.0
Mocha, Chiller, Soya Milk, EAT*	1 Tall/12oz	253	4.1	71	3.1	12.7	1.2	0.7
Mocha, Chiller, Whole Milk, EAT*	1 Tall/12oz	283	7.5	80	2.5	12.6	2.1	0.0
Mocha, Skimmed Milk, EAT*	1 Tall/12oz	157	5.0	44	3.1	4.9	1.4	0.0
Mocha, Soya Milk, EAT*	1 Tall/12oz	173	6.1	49	4.0	5.0	1.7	1.2
Mocha, Whole Milk, EAT*	1 Tall/12oz	219	11.4	62	3.0	4.9	3.2	0.0
COOKIES								
Chocolate, EAT*	1 Pack/150g	455	23.0	303	3.6	37.9	15.3	0.4
Muesli, EAT*	1 Cookie/100g	376	12.8	376	4.5	60.8	12.8	1.8
CROISSANT								
Almond, EAT*	1 Croissant/200g	467	26.5	234	4.8	23.8	13.3	1.5
Chocolate, EAT*	1 Croissant/100g	407	23.1	407	6.7	45.9	23.1	3.0
Plain, EAT*	1 Croissant/100g	249	14.0	249	5.4	25.9	14.0	0.0
CUPCAKES								
Chocolate, EAT*	1 Cake/100g	262	13.1	262	2.6	31.5	13.1	0.3
DESSERT								
Chunky Chocolate Fudge, EAT*	1 Pot/200g	447	25.2	224	1.9	25.4	12.6	1.0
Dark Chocolate, Pot, EAT*	1 Pot/50g	211	17.5	422	2.2	27.0	35.0	2.0
DRIED FRUIT & SEED MIX								
EAT*	1 Pack/50g	224	8.9	448	10.0	61.3	17.8	0.0
FRUIT & NUT MIX								
EAT*	1 Pack/70g	253	17.5	361	7.1	27.7	24.9	0.0
FRUIT SALAD								
Big Fruit, EAT*	1 Pot/200g	140	0.3	70	0.9	16.8	0.2	1.3
Fresh, EAT*	1 Std Pack/150g	66	0.0	44	0.5	10.9	0.0	0.0
Mango, Pineapple & Lime, EAT*	1 Pack/100g	64	0.3	64	0.7	15.7	0.3	2.5
Seasonal, EAT*	1 Pack/100g	59	0.1	59	0.7	13.8	0.1	3.5
Tropical, EAT*	1 Pack/150g	64	0.3	43	0.5	10.5	0.2	1.7
FUDGE								
Vanilla, EAT*	1 Pack/100g	405	12.0	405	1.2	73.0	12.0	0.0
HOT CHOCOLATE								
Chiller, EAT*	1 Tall/335ml	533	22.4	159	2.3	24.6	6.7	0.6
Chiller, Whole Milk, EAT*	1 Tall/12oz	19	0.8	158	2.3	23.2	6.3	0.5
Skimmed Milk, EAT*	1 Tall/12oz	171	5.5	48	3.3	5.3	1.5	0.0
Soya Milk, EAT*	1 Tall/12oz	188	6.6	53	4.3	5.4	1.9	1.3
Whole Milk, EAT*	1 Tall/12oz	239	12.4	67	3.3	5.3	3.5	0.0
JUICE DRINK								
Mango & Lime, Blast, EAT*	1 Tall/12oz	253	0.3	71	0.3	17.7	0.1	0.1

EAT

	Measure INFO/WEIGHT	per Measure KCAL	FAT	Nutrition Values per 100g / 100ml KCAL	PROT	CARB	FAT	FIBRE
JUICE DRNK								
Peach & Mint, Blast, EAT*	1 Tall/12oz	216	0.2	61	0.2	15.1	0.1	0.0
Wild Berry, Blast, EAT*	1 Tall/12oz	330	0.2	93	0.2	23.5	0.1	0.5
MILK								
Skimmed, Steamed, EAT*	1 Tall/12oz	169	5.6	48	3.5	4.9	1.6	0.0
Soya, Steamed, EAT*	1 Tall/12oz	187	6.9	53	4.5	5.0	2.0	1.3
Whole, Steamed, EAT*	1 Tall/12oz	241	13.0	68	3.5	4.9	3.7	0.0
MUFFIN								
Blueberry, Low Fat, EAT*	1 Muffin/100g	280	2.7	280	5.7	58.1	2.7	2.3
NOUGAT								
EAT*	1 Pack/30g	132	2.7	440	3.7	86.3	9.0	0.7
PAIN AU CHOCOLAT								
EAT*	1 Pain/120g	368	19.7	307	5.4	34.7	16.4	1.7
PEAS								
Wasabi, EAT*	1 Pack/92.1g	136	5.4	148	1.3	22.4	5.9	7.9
PIE								
Banoffee, EAT*	1 Pie/100g	395	22.7	395	4.8	43.1	22.7	2.2
Beef & Red Pepper Goulash, EAT*	1 Pie/400g	626	29.4	157	7.5	15.1	7.4	0.0
Ratatouille, with Cheesy Crumble, EAT*	1 Pie/400g	563	33.4	141	2.8	13.6	8.4	0.0
SALAD								
Baby Plum Tomato & Mozzarella, Side, EAT*	1 Pack/250g	221	18.9	88	3.8	1.3	7.6	0.4
Chef's, EAT*	1 Serving/200g	414	36.9	207	8.5	1.8	18.4	0.9
Chicken Caesar, EAT*	1oz/28g	105	8.0	374	17.8	11.6	28.6	1.8
Chicken Noodles, Spicy, EAT*	1 Pack/325g	466	18.7	143	8.7	14.2	5.8	0.7
Chicken, & Oriental Vegetable, EAT*	1 Portion/150g	222	9.9	148	11.7	10.1	6.6	2.2
Chicken, Morrocan & Cous Cous, EAT*	1 Pack/100g	688	30.5	688	26.9	75.4	30.5	5.8
Courgette, Feta & Lemon, Side, EAT*	1 Pack/200g	266	12.9	133	4.9	13.8	6.5	1.4
Crayfish & Avocado, EAT*	1oz/28g	108	10.3	387	12.1	2.7	36.7	2.8
Crayfish Noodles, Spicy, EAT*	1 Pack/295.1g	422	9.4	143	6.6	21.8	3.2	0.3
Feta, Lentil & Rice, Side, EAT*	1 Pack	525	20.5	525	21.1	64.0	20.5	8.1
Goats Cheese & Pine Nuts, Superfood, EAT*	1 Pack/250g	348	26.8	139	5.5	5.0	10.7	2.1
Horiatiki Greek, Side, EAT*	1 Pack/250g	298	28.0	119	3.3	1.3	11.2	0.4
Mackerel, Smoked, Super, EAT*	1 Pack/175g	683	53.5	390	15.1	13.7	30.6	2.5
Mezze, Side, EAT*	1 Serving/300g	420	27.0	140	3.0	11.8	9.0	1.7
Moroccan Chicken Couscous, EAT*	1 Pack/100g	688	30.0	688	26.0	75.0	30.0	6.0
Nicoise, EAT*	1 Pack/200g	260	15.9	130	8.0	6.5	8.0	0.7
Noodle, Thai, EAT*	1 Pack/100g	443	20.1	443	12.4	53.9	20.1	3.3
Potato, Spring, EAT*	1 Pack/250g	220	11.2	88	1.2	10.7	4.5	1.0
Satsuma, Carrot & Watercress, Side, EAT*	1 Pack/100g	147	10.3	147	3.2	10.3	10.3	2.9
Smoked Mackerel, Superfood, EAT*	1 Pack/300g	683	53.5	228	8.8	8.0	17.8	1.5
Smoked Salmon, Potato & Horseradish, Side, EAT*	1 Pack/400g	400	29.4	100	3.6	5.0	7.4	0.6
Superfood, EAT*	1 Pack/250g	340	25.5	136	5.6	5.2	10.2	2.0
Supergreens, Side, EAT*	1 Pack/200g	144	3.9	72	4.3	9.6	2.0	1.4
Sushi, Side, EAT*	1 Pack/100g	196	4.5	196	9.5	29.5	4.5	2.1
Tuna, & Bean, Side, EAT*	1 Pack/200g	212	9.5	106	7.5	8.3	4.8	3.4
SANDWICHES								
Avocado, Houmous, & Red Pepper, EAT*	1 Pack/250g	485	24.7	194	5.8	20.6	9.9	3.3
BLT, EAT*	1 Pack/500g	534	30.9	107	4.8	8.0	6.2	0.8
Bacon Butty, EAT*	1 Butty/120g	220	7.8	183	11.8	19.4	6.5	1.0
Beef, & Horseradish, Rare Roast, EAT*	1 Pack/245g	475	18.1	194	13.8	17.9	7.4	1.4
Carrot, & Houmous, EAT*	1 Pack/250g	436	17.4	174	6.2	21.8	7.0	2.0
Cheddar, & Branston Pickle, EAT*	1 Pack/235g	562	27.6	239	10.9	22.5	11.7	1.8
Chicken, & Bacon, EAT*	1 Pack/200g	547	26.0	274	16.0	23.5	13.0	2.0

EAT

SANDWICHES

	Measure INFO/WEIGHT	per Measure KCAL	FAT	KCAL	PROT	CARB	FAT	FIBRE
Chicken, & Mediterranean Vegetables, EAT*	1 Pack/350g	434	14.8	124	7.6	13.9	4.2	1.5
Chicken, & Salad, EAT*	1 Pack/250g	436	16.6	174	9.3	19.3	6.6	2.1
Chicken, & Salad, Less Than 5% Fat, EAT*	1 Pack/242g	337	7.0	139	11.9	16.3	2.9	1.6
Chicken, Aioli, EAT*	1 Pack/250g	424	17.3	170	12.8	14.0	6.9	2.6
Chicken, Caesar, EAT*	1 Pack/250g	605	32.7	242	16.0	15.1	13.1	1.3
Chicken, Thai Citrus, EAT*	1 Pack/250g	479	17.6	192	10.8	21.3	7.1	1.6
Club, EAT*	1 Pack/200g	861	42.3	431	23.1	37.1	21.2	1.7
Crayfish & Rocket, Less Than 5 % Fat, EAT*	1 Pack/200g	292	6.6	146	10.4	18.7	3.3	1.6
Crayfish, Lime & Coriander, Less Than 5% Fat, EAT*	1 Pack/200g	286	6.6	143	9.0	19.5	3.3	1.7
Cumberland Sausage, on a Toasted Muffin, Breakfast, EAT*	1 Sandwich/160g	350	13.2	219	8.2	27.8	8.3	1.3
Egg, & Cress, EAT*	1 Pack/200g	530	28.5	265	11.0	23.2	14.3	2.9
Egg, Spinach & Chargrilled Peppers, EAT*	1 Pack/200g	585	34.9	293	12.2	21.1	17.5	2.4
Eggs Benedict, on a Toasted Muffin, Breakfast, EAT*	1 Muffin/180g	234	9.9	130	6.8	13.3	5.5	0.8
Ham, & Brie, with Honey Mustard, EAT*	1 Pack/250g	618	32.2	247	12.7	20.1	12.9	1.4
Ham, & Mustard Salad, EAT*	1 Pack/85g	363	9.5	427	26.8	54.9	11.2	6.1
Houmous, & Red Pepper, EAT*	1 Pack/250g	402	11.8	161	6.0	23.8	4.7	2.5
Houmous, & Roast Vegetables, EAT*	1 Pack/176g	243	5.6	138	4.9	22.2	3.2	6.0
Prawn Cocktail, EAT*	1 Pack/200g	553	29.5	277	14.0	22.0	14.8	1.9
Salmon, Smoked, EAT*	1 Pack/250g	431	16.6	172	11.3	16.9	6.6	1.3
Steak, Onion, & Cheese, EAT*	1 Pack/300g	789	31.7	263	15.5	26.5	10.6	1.8
Tuna & Sweetcorn, Less Than 5% Fat, EAT*	1 Pack/248.4g	400	9.9	161	9.7	21.5	4.0	1.9
Tuna, & Red Onion, Less Than 5% Fat, Malted, EAT*	1 Pack/225.6g	361	11.1	160	11.4	17.8	4.9	1.8
Tuna, Crunch, EAT*	1 Pack/200g	377	10.5	189	12.2	23.1	5.3	2.3
Tuna, Tuscan, EAT*	1 Sandwich/250g	515	28.8	206	8.8	16.2	11.5	2.0
Turkey & Cranberry, Less Than 5% Fat, EAT*	1 Pack/213.2g	403	9.4	189	15.9	21.4	4.4	1.6

SLICES

Coconut, EAT*	1 Slice/50g	344	21.1	688	9.2	67.8	42.2	6.6

SOUP

Asparagus, Cream & Thyme, EAT*	1 Sm/350ml	90	2.4	26	1.2	3.9	0.7	0.6
Beef Noodle, EAT*	1 Sm/350ml	114	5.7	33	3.2	1.3	1.6	0.4
Beetroot Borscht, EAT*	1 Sm/340ml	98	5.0	29	0.7	3.3	1.5	0.4
Black Bean Chilli Con Carne, EAT*	1 Serving/450ml	358	11.7	80	7.1	7.1	2.6	1.3
Black Bean, Cuban, EAT*	1 Sm/350g	182	6.9	52	2.1	6.4	2.0	0.8
Butter Bean, Chicken & Mint, EAT*	1 Sm/350g	206	4.1	59	5.8	6.4	1.2	2.7
Carrot & Coriander, EAT*	1 Small/12oz	110	7.4	32	0.5	2.7	2.2	1.2
Carrot, Honey & Ginger, EAT*	1 Serving/474ml	178	8.4	38	0.7	5.0	1.8	1.0
Celeriac & Leek, EAT*	1 Small/340ml	171	14.1	50	0.9	2.4	4.2	1.5
Chicken & Egg Noodle, Old Fashioned, EAT*	1 Serving/340g	116	1.5	34	4.1	3.3	0.5	0.5
Chicken Laksa, EAT*	1 Sml/340g	158	5.7	46	3.2	4.7	1.7	0.8
Chicken Pot Pie, No Pastry, EAT*	1 Sm/350ml	171	3.5	49	4.5	5.6	1.0	0.9
Chicken, & Egg Noodle, Old Fashioned, EAT*	1 Small/12oz	95	1.2	28	4.8	1.8	0.4	0.5
Chicken, Tom Kha Gai, EAT*	1 Small/12oz	295	20.3	87	5.0	3.3	6.0	0.9
Chilli Con Carne, EAT*	1 Small/12oz	224	10.6	66	5.4	4.1	3.1	1.4
Chowder, Clam, Boston, EAT*	1 Small/340ml	378	20.0	111	6.1	8.6	5.9	0.7
Chowder, Clam, New England, EAT*	1 Small/12oz	326	19.2	96	4.0	7.0	5.7	1.0
Chowder, Corn, EAT*	1 Serving/340g	383	25.9	113	3.4	7.6	7.6	0.7
Courgette & Coriander, EAT*	1 Lge/454g	164	4.9	36	1.6	4.6	1.1	1.0
Courgette & Green Chilli, EAT*	1 Sml/340g	140	6.1	41	1.3	4.9	1.8	0.9
Cream of Corn, EAT*	1 Sml/340g	303	25.8	89	1.5	3.8	7.6	0.9
Creamy Mushroom, with Truffle Oil, EAT*	1 Small/340g	155	11.4	46	2.0	1.9	3.4	0.5
Fish Bouillabaisse with Rouille, Small, EAT*	1 Small Pot/340g	236	9.0	69	5.8	3.2	2.6	1.5
French Onion, EAT*	1 Small/12oz	164	5.8	48	1.6	6.2	1.7	0.5

EAT

	Measure INFO/WEIGHT	per Measure		Nutrition Values per 100g / 100ml				
		KCAL	FAT	KCAL	PROT	CARB	FAT	FIBRE
SOUP								
Gazpacho, EAT*	1 Sm/350ml	78	2.1	22	0.6	3.6	0.6	0.9
Goulash, Hungarian, EAT*	1 Sm/350g	226	5.8	65	6.5	6.2	1.7	0.6
Gujarati Red Dal, with Riata, EAT*	1 Small/340g	112	3.2	33	1.9	4.3	0.9	0.7
Hungarian Goulash, EAT*	1 Small/12oz	220	5.7	65	6.5	6.2	1.7	0.6
Leek & Potato, EAT*	1 Serving/355ml	156	9.4	44	0.9	4.4	2.7	0.7
Minestrone, with Pesto, EAT*	1 Pack/400ml	276	9.6	69	2.8	9.2	2.4	2.2
Moroccan Chicken & Root Vegetable, EAT*	1 Small/12oz	220	7.8	65	3.9	7.0	2.3	2.2
Mushroom, Tom Yam, EAT*	1 Big/440ml	106	4.8	24	1.1	2.4	1.1	0.4
Pea & Mint, EAT*	1 Lge/480ml	236	7.2	49	1.9	7.3	1.5	1.5
Prawn, Tom Yum, EAT*	1 Big Soup/440ml	70	2.4	16	1.9	0.9	0.6	2.4
Pumpkin, EAT*	1 Small/340ml	155	8.7	46	0.9	5.0	2.6	0.7
Pumpkin, Thai, EAT*	1 Sm/340g	81	2.2	24	0.7	3.8	0.7	1.0
Roast Pumpkin, EAT*	1 Small/12oz	155	8.7	46	0.9	5.0	2.6	0.7
Roast Tomato & Basil, EAT*	1 Small/340.2g	110	3.7	32	1.3	4.4	1.1	1.0
Roasted Red Pepper & Tomato, EAT*	1 Large/454g	98	2.2	22	0.8	3.5	0.5	0.9
Sausage, & 3 Bean, EAT*	1 Sm/340g	310	17.1	91	4.5	6.6	5.0	1.4
Smoked Haddock, EAT*	1 Small/343g	184	6.8	54	3.1	5.8	2.0	0.6
Smokey Bacon & Lentils, EAT*	1 Small/12oz	120	3.6	35	2.7	3.8	1.1	0.6
Spicy Carrot & Coconut, EAT*	1 Sm/350ml	198	15.0	57	0.7	4.0	4.3	1.0
Spicy Cauliflower & Potato, EAT*	1 Small/12oz	69	1.5	20	0.8	3.4	0.4	0.7
Spicy Tomato & Basil, EAT*	1 Small/12oz	71	1.5	21	0.8	3.4	0.4	1.0
Spicy Tomato, EAT*	1 Bowl/354ml	114	5.6	32	0.7	3.5	1.6	0.8
Spinach & Ricotta, EAT*	1 Pack/400ml	224	16.0	56	2.1	3.0	4.0	0.7
Sweet Pepper & Tomato, EAT*	1 Serving/473ml	107	1.3	23	0.7	4.3	0.3	0.8
Sweet Potato, Curried, EAT*	1 Serving/470ml	213	2.5	45	0.7	9.2	0.5	1.7
Sweet Red Pepper, EAT*	1 Small/340g	75	1.1	22	0.8	4.0	0.3	0.7
Thai Butternut Squash, EAT*	1 Big/454g	182	8.9	40	0.7	4.9	2.0	1.4
Tomato & Basil, EAT*	1 Serving/455g	92	2.0	20	0.8	3.4	0.4	0.7
Tomato & Creme Fraiche, EAT*	1 Sm/350g	188	14.0	54	1.0	3.4	4.0	0.8
Tomato & Lentil Rasam, EAT*	1 Large/454g	114	1.9	25	1.5	3.9	0.4	0.5
Tomato Rasam, EAT*	1 Small/12oz	66	1.6	19	1.1	2.7	0.5	0.7
Turkey, & Green Chilli, EAT*	1 Big/473ml	196	5.9	41	4.1	3.5	1.2	0.6
Vegetarian Chilli, EAT*	1 Serving/450ml	205	3.3	46	2.5	7.3	0.7	2.8
Wild Mushroom, EAT*	1 Serving/500ml	192	13.4	38	1.5	2.2	2.7	0.6
Winter Vegetable, EAT*	1 Serving/340g	164	8.7	48	0.9	5.8	2.6	1.1
SUSHI								
Vegetarian, EAT*	1 Pack/150g	240	1.7	160	3.9	33.5	1.1	1.3
TEA								
Chai Latte, Soya, EAT*	1 Cup/355ml	208	6.4	59	4.2	7.1	1.8	0.0
TOASTIE								
Cheese, Mushroom & Roast Tomato, EAT*	1 Pack/300g	519	21.9	173	7.5	19.5	7.3	2.4
Chicken, & Basil, Smoked, EAT*	1 Pack/350g	744	43.0	213	8.9	16.7	12.3	1.3
Ham, Cheese & Mustard, EAT*	1 Pack/250g	593	27.8	237	12.5	21.9	11.1	1.9
Three Cheese, & Caramelised Balsamic Onion, EAT*	1 Pack/100g	477	26.7	477	18.6	40.5	26.7	2.5
WATER								
Lemon & Lime, V, EAT*	1 Bottle/500ml	50	0.0	10	0.0	2.5	0.0	0.0
Pomegranate & Blueberry, V, EAT*	1 Bottle/500ml	50	0.0	10	0.0	2.5	0.0	0.0
WRAP								
Houmous, EAT*	1 Pack/100g	424	22.9	424	10.7	43.9	22.9	2.9
Mexican Chicken, EAT*	1 Pack/200g	386	10.7	193	12.0	24.5	5.4	2.2
Peking Duck, EAT*	1 Pack/250g	475	17.9	190	10.0	21.3	7.2	1.8

	Measure INFO/WEIGHT	per Measure		Nutrition Values per 100g / 100ml				
		KCAL	FAT	KCAL	PROT	CARB	FAT	FIBRE
EAT								
YOGHURT								
Greek, Fruits of the Forest, EAT*	1 Pot/125g	94	1.0	75	5.0	12.3	0.8	0.2
Greek, with Mango, EAT*	1 Tub/100g	100	1.0	100	6.6	16.6	1.0	0.1
Greek, with Muesli & Mixed Berries, Low Fat, EAT*	1oz/28g	45	0.6	161	8.1	27.5	2.2	2.7
FRESH & WILD								
SALAD								
Nicoise, Fresh & Wild*	1 Pack/450g	387	14.4	86	8.0	6.4	3.2	1.2
ITSU								
BEANS								
Edamame, Raw, Cold, Itsu*	1 Pack/80g	100	3.2	125	10.7	12.0	4.0	5.3
DESSERT								
If Bounty Went to Heaven, Itsu*	1 Pot/80g	347	22.6	434	5.9	24.3	28.3	3.8
Valrhona Chocolate Shot, Itsu*	1 Serving/44g	134	1.7	305	7.7	21.1	3.9	0.0
FROZEN YOGHURT								
Skinny, Original, Itsu*	1 Pot/166g	180	0.0	108	3.6	24.1	0.0	0.0
Yo Cream, Itsu*	1 Pot/166g	166	0.0	100	3.0	20.0	0.0	0.0
NUTS								
Squirrel's Dream, Itsu*	1 Pack/70g	210	23.8	300	9.1	40.3	34.0	0.0
PEAS								
Wasabi, Itsu*	1 Pack/70g	301	21.5	430	13.9	15.4	30.7	0.0
RICE CRACKERS								
Peanut, Itsu*	1 Pack/70g	232	9.6	331	12.6	39.6	13.7	0.0
SALAD								
Chicken, Chilli, with Greens, Itsu*	1 Pack/210g	270	8.3	129	10.2	13.0	4.0	2.6
Chicken, Sesame, Itsu*	1 Box/297g	482	24.6	162	9.7	12.1	8.3	2.5
Graze & Dazzle, Itsu*	1 Pack/125g	264	11.0	211	5.9	26.6	8.8	2.2
Gulfstream, Itsu*	1 Pack/356g	402	6.3	113	14.8	9.6	1.8	1.1
Hip, Humble & Healthy, Itsu*	1 Box/314g	336	16.5	107	4.3	11.2	5.3	5.6
Salmon, Skinny, Itsu*	1 Salad/182g	272	13.1	149	11.4	9.7	7.2	1.5
Salmon, Special, Itsu*	1 Box/473g	514	16.6	109	5.8	13.4	3.5	1.5
Sirloin Steak & Noodles, Itsu*	1 Box/397g	367	14.7	92	7.4	8.8	3.7	1.6
SOUP								
Superfood, Itsu*	1 Box/314g	336	16.5	107	4.2	11.1	5.3	5.6
Tuna, Asian Seared, Itsu*	1 Box/100g	212	0.5	212	34.0	18.0	0.5	1.0
Tuna, Yellow Fin, Line Caught, Itsu*	1 Box/328g	401	15.7	122	9.0	10.6	4.8	1.9
Chicken Teriyaki Noodles, Itsu*	1 Serving/805g	453	3.1	56	3.8	9.2	0.4	1.2
Dynamite, Detox, Itsu*	1 Pot/425g	153	0.6	36	0.6	8.1	0.1	0.6
Dynamite, Duck, Itsu*	1 Pot/474g	263	4.0	55	2.1	7.7	0.8	0.6
Dynamite, Itsu*	1 Serving/425g	133	0.4	31	0.3	7.4	0.1	0.5
Dynamite, Salmon, Sense, Itsu*	1 Pot/482g	179	6.3	37	2.6	3.8	1.3	0.7
Miso, Forever Young, Itsu*	1 Serving/395g	86	3.3	22	2.5	1.1	0.8	1.5
Miso, Skinny, Itsu*	1 Serving/500ml	19	0.5	4	0.0	0.0	0.1	0.0
Spicy Dumpling Noodles, Itsu*	1 Serving/782g	589	17.7	75	2.8	10.7	2.3	1.4
SUSHI								
Caviar, Sashimi & Salmon, Itsu*	1 Pack/362g	398	18.1	110	15.1	0.8	5.0	7.5
Health & Happiness, Itsu*	1 Pack/384g	453	21.1	118	8.1	8.9	5.5	3.7
Maki Roll, Chicken, Free Range, Itsu*	1 Pack/221g	241	10.1	109	6.0	11.2	4.6	1.2
Maki Roll, Duck Hoi Sin, Itsu*	1 Box/162g	171	4.0	106	5.4	14.4	2.5	0.8
Maki Roll, Salmon & Avocado, Itsu*	1 Box/211g	239	13.3	113	4.6	9.3	6.3	1.5
Maki Roll, Spicy Crab, Itsu*	1 Box/202g	238	13.5	118	4.3	9.8	6.7	0.8
Maki Roll, Tuna, Itsu*	1 Serving/98g	152	3.5	155	5.1	24.0	3.6	0.0
Maki Roll, Vegetarian Sunrise, Itsu*	1 Box/222g	213	10.9	96	1.9	10.9	4.9	1.9
Prawn, Itsu*	1 Portion/98g	151	1.8	154	6.0	28.5	1.8	0.0

	Measure INFO/WEIGHT	per Measure KCAL	FAT	Nutrition Values per 100g / 100ml KCAL	PROT	CARB	FAT	FIBRE
ITSU								
SUSHI								
Salmon Rushdie, Itsu*	1 Box/400g	488	15.6	122	5.2	16.5	3.9	0.0
Salmon Sashimi, Itsu*	1 Portion/48g	53	2.4	110	15.5	0.8	5.0	0.0
Salmon Supreme, Omega 3, Itsu*	1 Pack/340g	509	24.5	150	7.4	13.6	7.2	1.1
Salmon, Itsu*	1 Portion/64g	129	4.4	202	8.3	26.4	6.9	0.0
Salmon, Super, 3 Ways, Itsu*	1 Pack/391g	451	21.2	115	8.0	8.7	5.4	4.4
Tuna & Salmon, Itsu*	1 Pack/282g	315	7.4	112	7.5	14.2	2.6	0.3
Tuna & Salmon, Junior, Itsu*	1 Pack/175g	181	5.6	103	9.5	9.0	3.2	8.1
Tuna, Avocado & Chives, Itsu*	1 Pack/210g	234	10.0	111	6.4	11.5	4.8	1.5
YOGHURT								
Fruit & Goji Berries, Itsu*	1 Pack/70g	320	11.2	457	44.0	0.0	16.0	0.0
IXXY'S								
BAGEL								
Chicken & Bacon, Ixxy's*	1 Serving/215g	589	26.9	274	12.8	29.3	12.5	0.0
Chicken, Caesar, Ixxy's*	1 Pack/200g	530	25.4	265	12.9	24.7	12.7	1.7
Cranberry & Honey, Multigrain, Mini, Ixxy's*	1 Bagel/34.2g	95	1.3	278	9.2	49.7	3.8	5.3
Ham & Rosemary Ricotta Cheese, Ixxy's*	1 Pack/215g	372	6.9	173	11.1	25.0	3.2	0.3
Plain, Mini, Ixxy's*	1 Bagel/45g	120	0.7	266	9.6	53.6	1.5	3.0
Salt Beef & Dill Pickle, Ixxy's*	1 Bagel/213g	403	10.0	189	11.1	25.5	4.7	1.8
Sesame, Mini, Ixxy's*	1 Bagel/49g	133	1.6	271	9.6	51.0	3.2	3.6
Smoked Salmon & Soft Cheese, Ixxy's*	1 Pack/191.9g	474	18.4	247	11.3	28.8	9.6	1.6
Soft Cheese & Tomato, Low Fat, Ixxy's*	1 Serving/191g	332	2.7	174	7.3	33.1	1.4	0.0
Tuna & Cucumber, Ixxy's*	1 Bagel/260g	390	3.6	150	11.3	23.1	1.4	0.0
Tuna Mayonnaise, Ixxy's*	1 Serving/220g	462	14.9	210	11.1	26.1	6.8	1.4
J & B								
BAGUETTE								
BBQ Chicken & Bacon Melt, Malted Grain, J & B*	1 Baguette/342g	749	25.0	219	11.3	23.0	7.3	1.6
JD WETHERSPOONS								
BAGUETTE								
BLT, Malted Grain, JDW*	1 Baguette/399g	823	45.5	206	8.3	17.8	11.4	1.3
Chicken, BBQ & Bacon, Melt, Malted Grain, JDW*	1 Baguette/342g	1271	49.3	371	20.6	37.4	14.4	2.9
Chicken, Southern Fried, Creole Mayo, JDW*	1 Meal/250g	817	35.7	327	12.6	37.7	14.3	2.0
Club, Malted Grain, JDW*	1 Baguette/387g	768	36.8	198	9.8	18.5	9.5	1.4
Crayfish, Malted Grain, JDW*	1 Baguette/314g	594	25.5	189	6.1	23.2	8.1	1.7
Hot Sausage & Tomato Chutney, JDW*	1 Meal/250g	839	33.4	336	14.1	40.7	13.4	3.8
Mature Cheddar Cheese & Pickle, Malted Grain, JDW*	1 Baguette/360g	696	29.9	193	7.9	21.9	8.3	1.6
Ploughmans, Lloyds, JDW*	1 Baguette/346g	779	34.3	225	8.6	25.5	9.9	2.2
Tuna Mayonnaise, Malted Grain, JDW*	1 Baguette/401g	710	31.3	177	8.9	18.1	7.8	1.3
Wiltshire Ham, JDW*	1 Baguette/346g	536	13.1	155	9.9	20.4	3.8	1.5
BALTI								
Chicken, with Rice, Naan, Chutney & Poppadoms, JDW*	1 Meal/650g	927	27.1	143	6.0	21.1	4.2	1.3
BEEF DINNER								
Roast, with Roast Potatoes, Yorkshire Pud & Veg, JDW*	Portion/836.5g	1305	62.7	156	6.1	17.7	7.5	2.3
BHAJI								
Onion, JDW*	1 Bhaji/30g	43	2.2	143	5.3	18.7	7.3	5.7
BIRYANI								
Chicken, Meal with Naan Bread, Curry Club Dinner, JDW*	1 Meal/706g	897	26.8	127	5.1	18.1	3.8	1.3
Chicken, without Naan, JDW*	1 Meal/614g	700	24.6	114	4.7	14.8	4.0	1.3
BREAD								
Garlic, Ciabatta, JDW*	1 Serving/142g	406	17.9	286	8.0	1.0	12.6	1.5
Naan, JDW*	1 Naan/90g	197	2.5	219	7.6	41.0	2.8	1.4
BREAKFAST								
Baguette, Quorn Sausage, JDW*	1 Baguette/285g	622	18.3	218	10.5	29.4	6.4	3.4

JD WETHERSPOONS

	Measure INFO/WEIGHT	per Measure KCAL	FAT	Nutrition Values per 100g / 100ml KCAL	PROT	CARB	FAT	FIBRE
BREAKFAST								
Blueberry Muffin, JDW*	1 Muffin/124g	467	25.8	374	4.7	43.2	20.7	0.4
Bran, Fruit & Nut Muffin, JDW*	1 Serving/144g	571	31.7	394	7.2	43.0	21.9	1.1
Children's, JDW*	1 Breakfast/340g	613	37.1	180	10.4	10.8	10.9	2.3
Chocolate Muffin, JDW*	1 Muffin/125g	490	28.4	392	5.0	43.6	22.7	4.8
Farmhouse, with Toast, JDW*	1 Serving/795g	1647	101.8	207	9.4	14.0	12.8	1.9
Morning Roll, with Bacon, JDW*	1 Roll/183g	546	34.6	298	11.1	21.7	18.9	1.1
Morning Roll, with Fried Egg, JDW*	1 Roll/143g	400	21.3	280	9.7	27.8	14.9	1.4
Morning Roll, with Quorn Sausage, JDW*	1 Roll/142g	367	16.1	257	10.1	29.5	11.3	2.6
Morning Roll, with Sausage, JDW*	1 Roll/158g	517	28.0	327	13.8	30.1	17.7	2.3
Sandwich, Filled with Sausage, Bacon & Egg, JDW*	1 Sandwich/357g	840	55.8	235	12.6	11.3	15.6	1.5
Scrambled Egg, on Toast, JDW*	1 Serving/264g	503	24.9	190	8.4	17.4	9.4	1.1
Toast & Preserves, JDW*	1 Serving/147g	420	15.2	284	5.7	41.8	10.3	3.2
Traditional, JDW*	1 Breakfast/522g	904	60.1	173	8.4	9.4	11.5	1.8
Vegetarian, JDW*	1 Breakfast/562g	804	47.2	143	6.7	10.2	8.4	2.1
BROWNIES								
Chocolate, Fudge, Warm, with Vanilla Ice Cream, JDW*	1 Portion/108.1g	334	17.5	309	4.5	35.6	16.2	1.5
BURGERS								
Beef, Double, & Chips, JDW*	1 Serving/598g	1382	81.6	231	16.8	11.4	13.6	0.5
Beef, Double, Bacon, Cheese, & Chips, JDW*	1 Serving/729g	1891	119.3	259	18.1	9.4	16.4	0.4
Beef, Double, Cheese, & Chips, JDW*	1 Serving/654g	1565	91.4	239	17.2	10.7	14.0	0.5
Beef, with Bacon, Cheese & Chips, JDW*	1 Serving/531g	1295	78.9	244	15.2	12.6	14.9	0.5
Beef, with Cheese, & Chips, JDW*	1 Serving/456g	966	53.8	212	13.7	13.8	11.8	0.5
Beef, with Chips, JDW*	1 Serving/428g	881	46.4	206	12.8	15.7	10.8	0.7
Chicken, Fillet, with Chips, JDW*	1 Serving/465g	727	17.1	156	10.9	16.7	3.7	0.8
Lamb, Double, Minted, with Chips, JDW*	1 Serving/598g	1077	47.2	180	14.6	14.1	7.9	0.9
Lamb, Minted, with Chips, JDW*	1 Serving/428g	712	27.8	166	11.3	17.2	6.5	0.9
Vegetable, with Chips, JDW*	1 Meal/487g	839	25.9	172	4.7	27.2	5.3	2.0
BUTTY								
Bacon & Egg, Brown Bloomer, JDW*	1 Serving/269g	702	31.1	261	18.3	21.0	11.6	1.4
Bacon & Egg, White Bloomer, JDW*	1 Serving/269g	689	32.7	256	16.7	20.9	12.2	1.2
Bacon, Brown Bloomer, JDW*	1 Serving/309g	869	39.6	281	23.3	18.3	12.8	1.2
Chip & Cheese, Brown Bloomer, JDW*	1 Serving/232g	593	24.4	256	9.7	31.4	10.5	1.6
Chip & Cheese, White Bloomer, JDW*	1 Serving/232g	580	26.0	250	7.9	31.3	11.2	1.4
Chip, Brown Bloomer, JDW*	1 Serving/204g	478	14.7	234	7.6	35.7	7.2	1.9
Chip, White Bloomer, JDW*	1 Serving/204g	465	16.3	228	5.6	35.6	8.0	1.6
Sausage & Egg, Brown Bloomer, JDW*	1 Serving/331g	885	49.0	268	16.8	20.8	14.8	1.3
Sausage & Egg, White Bloomer, JDW*	1 Serving/331g	872	50.6	264	11.4	20.7	15.3	1.1
CAKE								
Chocolate Fudge, & Ice Cream, JDW*	1 Serving/239g	822	47.3	344	4.0	37.6	19.8	0.4
CAULIFLOWER CHEESE								
JDW*	1 Portion/220g	275	151.8	125	4.1	3.6	69.0	0.8
CHEESECAKE								
Chocolate Chip, JDW*	1 Serving/100g	270	11.5	270	4.9	36.8	11.5	0.5
White Chocolate & Raspberry, JDW*	1 Serving/175g	656	36.9	375	5.6	40.8	21.1	0.9
CHICKEN								
Wings, Buffalo, JDW*	1 Portion/328g	636	42.9	194	15.2	4.0	13.1	0.5
CHICKEN ALFREDO								
Pasta, with Dressed Side Salad, JDW*	1 Meal/576g	950	52.4	165	8.7	12.0	9.1	0.3
Pasta, with Garlic Bread, JDW*	1 Meal/501g	1007	47.6	201	10.8	13.0	9.5	0.3
Pasta, without Garlic Bread, JDW*	1 Meal/430g	804	38.7	187	11.3	15.0	9.0	0.1
CHICKEN DINNER								
Roast, Roast Potatoes, Yorkshire Pud & Vegetables, JDW*	1 Meal/993g	1529	63.5	154	10.8	14.6	6.4	2.1

JD WETHERSPOONS

	Measure INFO/WEIGHT	per Measure KCAL	FAT	Nutrition Values per 100g / 100ml KCAL	PROT	CARB	FAT	FIBRE
CHICKEN FORESTIERRE								
JDW*	1 Serving/684g	626	26.0	92	7.7	8.7	3.8	1.0
CHICKEN PHAAL								
Meal, JDW*	1 Serving/720g	1234	46.1	171	7.5	21.0	6.4	1.6
CHICKEN ROAST								
& Chips, Peas, Tomatoes, Mushrooms, JDW*	1 Meal/742g	904	38.6	122	13.0	5.6	5.2	1.2
with BBQ Sauce, JDW*	1 Meal/742g	948	37.5	128	11.3	9.2	5.1	0.6
with Chips & BBQ Sauce, JDW*	1 Meal/768g	1183	53.0	154	11.5	12.2	6.9	0.9
with Chips & Salad, JDW*	1 Meal/695g	983	52.1	141	13.1	5.9	7.5	0.6
with Dressed Side Salad & BBQ Sauce, JDW*	1 Meal/666g	913	46.0	137	12.2	6.0	6.9	0.9
with Jacket Potato, Salad, & Salsa, JDW*	1 Meal/785g	1193	57.3	152	12.2	10.2	7.3	1.3
with Piri Piri Sauce, JDW*	1 Serving/994g	994	47.1	100	8.5	5.8	4.7	0.8
CHICKEN VINDALOO								
JDW*	1 Meal/500g	704	19.0	141	6.4	21.0	3.8	1.3
CHILLI								
Con Carne, with Rice, & Tortilla Chips, JDW*	1 Serving/585g	744	20.0	127	6.5	17.8	3.4	1.6
Five Bean, with Yellow Basmati Rice & Tortilla Chips, JDW*	1 Portion/390.1g	511	9.0	131	3.6	24.0	2.3	1.7
CHIPS								
Bowl, JDW*	1 Serving/300g	363	11.4	121	2.6	21.7	3.8	0.0
with Cheese, JDW*	1 Serving/501g	1002	51.6	200	5.2	21.9	10.3	1.8
with Roast Gravy, JDW*	1 Serving/400g	392	12.4	98	2.5	17.6	3.1	0.0
CHUTNEY								
Mango, JDW*	1 Serving/25g	47	0.2	188	0.4	44.8	0.8	0.4
CIABATTA								
BBQ Chicken & Bacon Melt, JDW*	1 Ciabatta/333g	716	33.6	215	11.3	20.4	10.1	1.8
BLT, JDW*	1 Ciabatta/390g	789	47.3	202	8.2	15.4	12.1	1.5
Club, JDW*	1 Ciabatta/378g	734	38.6	194	9.7	16.1	10.2	1.6
Crayfish, JDW*	1 Ciabatta/304g	561	27.4	184	5.8	20.3	9.0	1.9
Mature Cheddar Cheese & Pickle, JDW*	1 Ciabatta/350g	662	31.5	189	7.8	19.4	9.0	1.7
Tuna Mayonnaise, JDW*	1 Ciabatta/390g	676	32.8	173	8.8	15.8	8.4	1.5
Wiltshire Ham, JDW*	1 Ciabatta/335g	503	14.8	150	9.8	17.7	4.4	1.7
CRUMBLE								
Bramley Apple, Pear, & Raspberry with Custard, JDW*	1 Serving/372g	648	23.8	174	2.5	26.3	6.4	0.0
Bramley Apple, Pear, & Raspberry with Ice Cream, JDW*	1 Serving/300g	579	24.3	193	2.6	27.0	8.1	2.1
CURRY								
Beef, Malaysian, Rendang, with Naan, JDW*	1 Meal/706g	1144	41.0	162	6.8	20.1	5.8	1.1
Beef, Malaysian, Rendang, without Naan, JDW*	1 Meal/615g	947	38.1	154	6.7	17.0	6.2	1.0
Goan, Vegetable, without Naan, JDW*	1 Meal/748g	1017	41.9	136	3.1	18.3	5.6	1.3
Kashmiri, Lamb, with Naan, JDW*	1 Meal/704g	1021	33.1	145	7.2	19.5	4.7	1.2
Kashmiri, Lamb, without Naan, JDW*	1 Meal/615g	824	30.7	134	7.1	16.3	5.0	1.1
Kerala, Fish, with Naan, JDW*	1 Meal/706g	1066	36.0	151	7.0	20.0	5.1	1.0
Kerala, Fish, without Naan, JDW*	1 Meal/616g	869	33.3	141	6.9	16.9	5.4	0.9
Mushroom Dopiaza, with Naan Bread, JDW*	1 Serving/719.2g	899	24.5	125	3.5	21.5	3.4	1.5
Mushroom Dopiaza, without Naan Bread, JDW*	1 Meal/617g	580	14.2	94	2.6	16.7	2.3	1.4
Royal Thali, with Naan, JDW*	1 Meal/948g	1336	48.3	141	7.1	16.8	5.1	1.3
Thai, Green Chicken, without Naan, JDW*	1 Meal/617g	1037	46.9	168	7.5	17.6	7.6	0.5
Vegetable, Goan, with Naan Bread, JDW*	1 Meal/706.8g	1032	36.8	146	3.6	21.2	5.2	1.3
Vegetarian, Thali, with Naan, JDW*	1 Meal/950g	1320	42.7	139	5.3	20.3	4.5	2.4
DHANSAK								
Lamb, Meal, JDW*	1 Serving/720g	983	26.1	137	7.2	19.6	3.6	0.8
FISH & CHIPS								
Haddock, JDW*	1 Meal/496g	806	40.7	162	7.2	14.4	8.2	2.4
Plaice, Breaded, & Peas, JDW*	1 Serving/460g	550	15.6	120	6.8	15.0	3.4	1.7

JD WETHERSPOONS

	Measure INFO/WEIGHT	per Measure		Nutrition Values per 100g / 100ml				
		KCAL	FAT	KCAL	PROT	CARB	FAT	FIBRE
FISH & CHIPS								
Traditional, JDW*	1 Serving/495g	804	40.6	162	7.2	14.4	8.2	2.4
FISH CAKES								
Salmon & Lime, with Tartare Sauce, JDW*	1 Serving/355g	569	31.3	160	5.8	14.5	8.8	1.0
GAMMON								
Steak, 8oz, Eggs, Chips & Pineapple, JDW*	1 Meal/609g	1036	51.8	170	13.4	10.2	8.5	0.8
Steak, Egg, Chips & Side Salad, JDW*	1 Meal/593g	801	41.5	135	10.2	9.0	7.0	0.3
Steak, Egg, Jacket Potato & Dressed Side Salad, JDW*	1 Meal/707g	1040	45.3	147	10.1	13.1	6.4	1.3
Steak, Egg, Jacket Potato, Peas, Tomato, Mushroom, JDW*	1 Meal/660g	963	38.9	146	10.8	13.5	5.9	1.3
GAMMON &								
Chips, Peas, Tomato, & Egg, JDW*	1 Meal/564g	844	41.2	150	15.0	6.7	7.3	1.3
Chips, Peas, Tomato, & Pineapple, JDW*	1 Meal/575g	799	36.2	139	13.6	7.8	6.3	1.4
HAGGIS								
with Neeps & Tatties, JDW*	1 Meal/682g	982	52.5	144	4.6	15.0	7.7	1.9
HAM								
& Eggs, JDW*	1 Serving/396g	253	12.7	64	4.9	3.5	3.2	0.0
ICE CREAM								
Bombe, Mint Chocolate, JDW*	1 Portion/135.1g	300	13.4	222	2.6	30.6	9.9	0.8
Chocolate, Bomb, JDW*	1 Portion/100g	259	13.4	259	5.9	34.3	13.4	5.4
Neopolitan, Movenpick, JDW*	1 Bowl/100g	181	9.6	181	3.0	20.0	9.6	0.0
JALFREZI								
Chicken, Meal, with Naan Bread, JDW*	1 Meal/705g	916	19.7	130	6.8	19.9	2.8	1.3
Chicken, without Naan Bread, JDW*	1 Meal/614.5g	719	17.2	117	6.7	16.9	2.8	1.3
KORMA								
Chicken, Meal, without Naan, JDW*	1 Meal/617g	944	38.2	153	6.4	17.0	6.2	0.8
Chicken, with Naan, JDW*	1 Meal/704g	1141	40.8	162	6.6	20.1	5.8	0.9
LAMB								
Shoulder, Braised, with Mashed Potato & Vegetables, JDW*	1 Meal/843.9g	1114	66.7	132	8.9	6.8	7.9	1.0
LASAGNE								
Al Forno, Wth Dressed Side Salad, JDW*	1 Meal/658g	823	40.8	125	5.5	11.4	6.2	0.8
MASALA								
Chicken, Hot, with Naan, JDW*	1 Meal/707g	1033	31.1	146	6.9	20.1	4.4	1.2
Chicken, Hot, without Naan, JDW*	1 Meal/614g	835	28.2	136	6.8	17.1	4.6	1.1
Prawn, Sri Lankan, with Naan, JDW*	1 Meal/708g	1027	36.1	145	5.7	19.7	5.1	0.8
Prawn, Sri Lankan, without Naan, JDW*	1 Meal/617g	827	33.3	134	5.4	16.6	5.4	1.0
Vegetable, Tandoori, Meal, JDW*	1 Serving/720g	1020	36.0	142	3.4	20.7	5.0	2.3
MEATBALLS								
with Linguine Pasta, JDW*	1 Serving/511.7g	614	24.0	120	6.3	13.1	4.7	1.9
MELT								
BBQ Chicken, & Chips, & Salad, JDW*	1 Serving/643g	849	42.4	132	10.4	8.2	6.6	0.4
MIXED GRILL								
with Chips, & Dressed Side Salad, JDW*	1 Serving/784g	1324	87.0	169	12.0	5.6	11.1	0.3
MOUSSAKA								
Vegetarian, JDW*	1 Serving/555g	582	38.9	105	2.7	7.6	7.0	2.7
NACHOS								
JDW*	1 Serving/366g	1139	67.3	311	7.0	29.2	18.4	3.2
with Chilli Con Carne, JDW*	1 Meal/570g	1505	88.9	264	8.6	22.2	15.6	1.8
with Fajita Chicken, JDW*	1 Serving/486g	1225	70.5	252	5.7	24.7	14.5	2.9
with Five Bean Chilli, JDW*	1 Serving/571g	1399	81.1	245	7.3	21.8	14.2	2.7
PANINI								
BBQ Chicken & Bacon, Melt, JDW*	1 Panini/336.8g	650	27.6	193	9.9	19.9	8.2	1.7
Cheese & Tuna, JDW*	1 Panini/221g	551	22.3	249	15.5	24.9	10.1	0.7
Cheese, Tomato, & Bacon, JDW*	1 Panini/261g	630	29.0	241	14.3	21.6	11.1	0.8

JD WETHERSPOONS

PANINI

	Measure INFO/WEIGHT	per Measure KCAL	FAT	KCAL	PROT	CARB	FAT	FIBRE
Club, JDW*	1 Panini/378g	734	38.6	194	9.7	16.1	10.2	1.6
Fajita Chicken, JDW*	1 Panini/235g	359	6.1	153	4.4	28.8	2.6	1.7
Mature, Cheddar Cheese & Tomato, JDW*	1 Panini/330g	750	27.1	227	10.4	18.0	8.2	1.7
Pepperoni & Mozzarella, JDW*	1 Panini/205g	617	33.4	301	11.6	27.5	16.3	1.0
Tomato, Mozzarella & Green Pesto, JDW*	1 Panini/245g	502	22.9	205	7.3	23.0	9.4	1.4
Wiltshire Ham & Mature, Cheddar Cheese, JDW*	1 Panini/354g	868	49.9	245	12.7	16.7	14.1	1.5

PASTA

Five Cheese & Bacon, with Dressed Side Salad, JDW*	1 Meal/544g	506	28.8	93	2.3	9.1	5.3	1.3
Five Cheese & Bacon, with Garlic Ciabatta, JDW*	1 Meal/469g	563	23.5	120	3.6	9.7	5.0	1.5
Spirale, Vegetable, Chargrilled & Sundried Tomato, JDW*	1 Meal/500g	600	2.5	120	3.6	15.2	0.5	0.7

PASTA BAKE

Mediterranean, JDW*	1 Serving/450g	577	22.1	128	4.3	16.4	4.9	0.9

PEAS

& Ham, with White Poppy Seed Bloomer, JDW*	1 Portion/456g	474	17.8	104	4.4	12.5	3.9	2.0

PIE

Aberdeen Angus, Chips, & Vegetables, JDW*	1 Serving/780g	1356	86.6	174	5.5	15.7	11.1	0.9
British Beef & Abbot Ale, Chips, Vegetables & Gravy, JDW*	1 Meal/850g	1258	68.0	148	4.0	14.9	8.0	1.0
Cottage, with Chips & Peas, JDW*	1 Meal/682g	846	33.4	124	3.7	15.6	4.9	1.9
Fish, Carrot & Broccoli, in Herb Butter, JDW*	1 Serving/550g	612	38.0	111	4.6	9.7	6.9	2.4
Scotch, JDW*	1 Serving/145g	302	15.4	208	13.1	7.8	10.6	0.9
Scotch, with Chips & Beans, JDW*	1 Serving/435g	603	22.2	139	6.8	14.9	5.1	1.5

PLATTER

Italian Style, JDW*	1 Platter/1020g	1985	75.5	195	10.4	22.9	7.4	0.6
Mexican, Chilli, Sour Cream, JDW*	1 Platter/1062g	2560	141.2	241	7.5	22.6	13.3	2.8
Mexican, with Five Bean Chilli, JDW*	1 Platter/1002g	2358	123.2	235	6.2	25.6	12.3	3.6
Western, JDW*	1 Platter/1454g	2973	168.7	205	16.9	9.1	11.6	0.4

POPPADOMS

& Dips, JDW*	1 Serving/134g	425	10.9	317	4.6	28.4	8.1	2.5
JDW*	1 Poppadom/12.4g	35	0.2	281	6.7	45.0	1.9	10.0

POTATO BOMBAY

JDW*	1 Serving/300g	285	14.7	95	1.8	10.8	4.9	2.5

POTATO SKINS

Cheese & Bacon, Loaded, JDW*	1 Serving/439g	949	58.4	216	8.9	15.2	13.3	1.5
Cheese & Red Onion, Loaded, JDW*	1 Serving/414g	835	51.3	202	6.0	16.5	12.4	1.6
Chilli Con Carne, Loaded, JDW*	1 Serving/503g	735	35.7	146	5.0	15.7	7.1	1.9

POTATO WEDGES

Spicy, JDW*	1 Serving/270g	434	15.7	161	2.2	27.7	5.8	1.8
Spicy, with Sour Cream, JDW*	1 Serving/330g	558	27.4	169	2.3	23.4	8.3	1.5

POTATOES

Baked, Jacket, Chill, Sour Cream & Dressed Salad, JDW	*1 Meal/615g	775	30.1	126	4.4	17.0	4.9	1.9
Baked, Jacket, Coleslaw, JDW*	1 Meal/596g	918	48.9	154	2.3	17.1	8.2	1.8
Baked, Jacket, Crayfish, with Marie Rose Dressing, JDW*	1 Meal/524g	796	40.8	152	3.5	18.2	7.8	1.7
Baked, Jacket, Mature, Cheddar Cheese, JDW*	1 Meal/496g	858	44.6	173	5.6	18.7	9.0	1.8
Baked, Jacket, with Baked Beans, & Dressed Salad, JDW*	1 Meal/575g	725	24.7	126	3.3	19.6	4.3	2.4
Baked, Jacket, 5 Bean Chilli, & Dressed Side Salad, JDW*	1 Meal/597g	705	25.7	118	3.0	17.9	4.3	2.4
Baked, Jacket, with Tuna Mayo & Dressed Side Salad, JDW*	1 Meal/645g	1051	57.4	163	7.1	14.7	8.9	1.3
Mashed, Creamy, JDW*	1 Portion/279g	349	21.2	125	1.5	15.0	7.6	1.1
Roast, JDW*	1 Portion/200g	290	9.4	145	2.5	23.0	4.7	2.3

RIBS

Double, JDW*	1 Serving/350g	767	41.0	219	16.7	11.9	11.7	0.4
Double, with Chips, JDW*	1 Serving/500g	949	46.5	190	12.5	14.9	9.3	0.3
Double, with Jacket Potato, JDW*	1 Serving/590g	1159	50.7	196	11.4	19.2	8.6	1.3

JD WETHERSPOONS

	Measure INFO/WEIGHT	per Measure KCAL	FAT	Nutrition Values per 100g / 100ml KCAL	PROT	CARB	FAT	FIBRE
RICE								
Basmati, Yellow, JDW*	1 Portion/200g	286	1.2	143	3.4	31.1	0.6	0.2
JDW*	1 Serving/200g	274	0.4	137	2.9	30.9	0.2	0.2
ROGAN JOSH								
Lamb, Meal, without Naan, JDW*	1 Meal/617g	820	27.7	133	7.1	17.0	4.5	1.0
Lamb, with Naan, JDW*	1 Meal/706g	1017	30.4	144	7.2	20.1	4.3	1.1
SALAD								
Caesar, Chicken, JDW*	1 Meal/230g	507	36.4	220	14.3	5.1	15.8	0.8
Caesar, JDW*	1 Meal/211g	448	38.0	212	6.8	5.8	18.0	1.1
Chicken & Bacon, Warm, JDW*	1 Meal/426g	600	41.3	141	9.8	3.8	9.7	0.6
Chicken, BBQ, Croutons & Dressing, JDW*	1 Portion/350g	315	8.4	90	9.4	7.5	2.4	0.8
Crayfish, JDW*	1 Meal/317g	247	18.0	78	4.4	2.7	5.7	0.6
Side, No Dressing, JDW*	1 Salad/195g	125	4.5	64	2.0	8.9	2.3	1.1
Side, with Dressing & Croutons, JDW*	1 Portion/140g	221	18.3	158	2.1	8.6	13.1	1.1
Side, with Dressing & No Croutons, JDW*	1 Portion/129g	145	14.0	112	1.0	3.2	10.8	0.9
Side, with Dressing, JDW*	1 Salad/215g	263	19.6	122	2.2	8.1	9.1	1.0
Side, without Croutons, JDW*	1 Portion/111g	157	10.8	141	9.8	3.8	9.7	0.6
Thai Noodle, JDW*	1 Portion/393.6g	433	21.3	110	2.7	12.7	5.4	1.4
Thai Noodle, with Chicken, JDW*	1 Meal/554g	637	27.7	115	9.2	9.6	5.0	1.4
Tiger Prawn, Dressing, & Chilli Jam, JDW*	1 Portion/340g	500	33.0	147	4.7	10.1	9.7	0.9
Tuna, with Eggs, Olives, & Croutons, JDW*	1 Portion/395g	679	51.7	172	10.3	3.2	13.1	0.7
SAMOSAS								
Lamb, JDW*	1 Samosa/90g	160	3.8	178	7.9	29.9	4.2	3.9
Vegetable, JDW*	1 Samosa/50g	92	3.1	184	5.4	28.4	6.2	2.2
SANDWICH								
BLT, Brown Bloomer, JDW*	1 Sandwich/404g	885	39.6	219	18.0	14.6	9.8	1.2
BLT, White Bloomer, JDW*	1 Sandwich/404g	872	32.7	216	17.0	14.6	8.1	1.0
Beef, Hot, Brown Bloomer, JDW*	1 Sandwich/299g	618	27.2	207	11.4	19.9	9.1	1.3
Beef, Hot, White Poppy Seed Bloomer, JDW*	1 Sandwich/299g	605	28.7	202	10.0	19.8	9.6	1.1
Cheddar, & Pickle, Brown Bloomer, JDW*	1 Sandwich/260g	665	31.9	256	11.0	25.4	12.3	1.9
Cheddar, & Pickle, White Bloomer, JDW*	1 Sandwich/260g	638	32.8	245	9.2	0.0	12.6	1.5
Chicken, Cheese, Bacon, Mayo, White, JDW*	1 Sandwich/312g	710	39.6	228	13.5	18.8	12.7	1.2
Chicken, Half Fat Mayo, Brown, Hot, JDW*	1 Sandwich/289g	628	28.3	217	11.8	20.7	9.8	1.7
Chicken, Half Fat Mayo, White, Hot, JDW*	1 Sandwich/289g	615	29.8	213	11.3	20.6	10.3	1.5
Egg Mayonnaise, Brown Bloomer, JDW*	1 Sandwich/295g	704	39.5	239	10.1	19.7	13.4	1.3
Egg Mayonnaise, White Bloomer, JDW*	1 Sandwich/295g	692	41.0	235	8.7	19.6	13.9	1.1
Ham, & Tomato, Brown Bloomer, JDW*	1 Sandwich/239g	514	17.2	215	11.4	24.4	7.2	1.8
Ham, & Tomato, White Bloomer, JDW*	1 Sandwich/239g	501	18.6	210	9.7	24.4	7.8	1.5
Prawn Mayonnaise, Brown Bloomer, JDW*	1 Sandwich/244g	579	26.6	237	11.0	23.8	10.9	1.6
Prawn Mayonnaise, White Bloomer, JDW*	1 Sandwich/244g	567	28.3	232	9.3	23.7	11.6	1.4
Salmon, Lemon Mayo, Brown Bloomer, JDW*	1 Sandwich/229g	637	33.7	278	11.4	25.4	14.7	1.7
Salmon, Lemon Mayo, White Bloomer, JDW*	1 Sandwich/229g	625	35.3	273	9.6	25.2	15.4	1.4
Tuna Mayonnaise, Half Fat Mayo, White, JDW*	1 Sandwich/389g	828	47.1	213	11.2	15.6	12.1	1.0
SAUSAGE & MASH								
with Red Wine Gravy, JDW*	Portion/677.1g	887	50.8	131	6.0	10.2	7.5	1.8
SAUSAGES WITH								
Bacon & Egg, JDW*	1 Serving/582g	1040	57.6	179	11.7	11.3	9.9	1.0
SAUSAGES WITH								
Chips & Beans, JDW*	1 Meal/554g	897	42.6	162	7.3	16.4	7.7	2.3
SCAMPI								
Breaded, Chips, Peas, Tartare Sauce, JDW*	1 Meal/560g	987	43.7	176	5.2	19.9	7.8	2.3
SORBET								
Mango & Passionfruit, JDW*	1 Serving/135g	115	0.1	85	0.2	20.0	0.1	0.2

JD WETHERSPOONS

	Measure INFO/WEIGHT	per Measure KCAL	FAT	Nutrition Values per 100g / 100ml KCAL	PROT	CARB	FAT	FIBRE
SOUP								
Leek & Potato, with Malted Grain Baguette, JDW*	1 Bowl/490g	490	8.8	100	3.2	17.9	1.8	1.7
Leek & Potato, without Bread & Butter, JDW*	1 Bowl/420	105	0.8	25	0.9	5.1	0.2	1.0
Mushroom, No Bread, JDW*	1 Serving/305g	500	32.7	83	2.8	5.5	5.4	0.4
Mushroom, with Brown Bloomer, JDW*	1 Serving/429g	561	23.7	131	3.4	16.0	5.5	1.2
Mushroom, with White Bloomer, JDW*	1 Serving/429g	549	25.2	128	3.4	15.9	5.9	1.1
Tomato & Basil, Organic, JDW*	1 Serving/491g	584	23.1	119	2.9	15.8	4.7	1.2
Tomato & Basil, Organic, with Bread, Farmhouse, JDW*	1 Bowl/450g	396	8.6	88	1.0	6.0	1.9	1.1
Tomato & Basil, Organic, with Malted Grain Baguette, JDW*	1 Bowl/491g	584	23.1	119	2.9	15.8	4.7	1.2
Tomato & Basil, Organic, without Bread, JDW*	1 Bowl/350g	200	15.1	57	0.7	3.0	4.3	0.6
Tomato, No Bread, JDW*	1 Serving/305g	393	27.8	65	0.9	3.9	4.6	0.6
Tomato, with Brown Bloomer, JDW*	1 Serving/429g	576	25.8	134	3.7	15.7	6.0	1.3
Tomato, with White Bloomer, JDW*	1 Serving/429g	563	27.3	131	2.8	15.7	6.4	1.2
SPONGE PUDDING								
Treacle, with Hot Custard, JDW*	1 Serving/515g	1267	71.1	246	2.3	41.8	13.8	0.3
SQUASH								
Butternut, Roast Dinner, JDW*	1 Meal/847g	1211	55.9	143	4.9	17.5	6.6	2.9
STEAK								
Ribeye, 8oz, Chips & Side Salad, JDW*	1 Meal/562g	1006	71.9	179	8.0	8.9	12.8	0.3
Ribeye, 8oz, Chips, Peas, Tomato & Mushroom, JDW*	1 Portion/530.9g	945	63.7	178	9.3	9.3	12.0	0.3
Ribeye, 8oz, Jacket & Dressed Side Salad, JDW*	1 Meal/620g	850	43.4	137	8.2	10.1	7.0	1.1
Ribeye, 8oz, Jacket, Peas, Tomato, Mushroom, JDW*	1 Meal/674g	1253	153.6	186	7.8	11.5	22.8	1.9
Ribeye, 10oz, Prawns, Chips, & Side Salad, JDW*	1 Meal/714g	1093	56.4	153	11.0	7.7	7.9	0.3
Ribeye, 10oz, Prawns, Jacket & Side Salad, JDW*	1 Meal/727g	1178	57.4	162	10.8	7.7	7.9	0.3
Rump, 16oz, with Chips & Dressed Side Salad, JDW*	1 Meal/787g	1283	71.6	163	14.3	6.3	9.1	0.2
Rump, 16oz, with Chips, Peas, Tomato & Mushroom, JDW*	1 Meal/759g	1268	70.6	167	14.9	6.5	9.3	0.2
T-Bone, 12oz, with Chips, & Dressed Side Salad, JDW*	1 Meal/673g	1313	97.6	195	9.4	7.4	14.5	0.2
T-Bone, 12oz, with Jacket Potato & Side Salad, JDW*	1 Meal/756g	1496	96.7	198	9.1	12.3	12.8	1.2
STEAK &								
Breaded Scampi, Chips, & Peas, JDW*	1 Serving/816g	1369	72.6	168	10.1	11.3	8.9	1.2
STEAK WITH								
Chips, & Dressed Side Salad, Rump, JDW*	1 Meal/634g	922	60.2	145	9.5	6.3	9.5	0.3
Chips, & Dressed Side Salad, Sirloin, JDW*	1 Meal/577g	979	73.3	170	7.6	6.9	12.7	0.3
Jacket Potato, Salad, & Salsa, Rump, JDW*	1 Meal/724g	1132	64.4	156	9.0	10.9	8.9	1.1
Jacket Potato, Salad, & Salsa, Sirloin, JDW*	1 Meal/667g	1189	77.4	178	7.3	11.8	11.6	1.2
STEW								
Irish, JDW*	1 Serving/600g	516	23.4	86	7.3	5.6	3.9	0.9
STUFFING BALLS								
Sage & Onion, JDW*	1 Portion/70g	137	1.1	196	6.6	32.3	1.6	3.6
TART								
Apple, with Ice Cream, JDW*	1 Serving/235g	464	20.0	197	1.6	29.8	8.5	0.4
TIKKA								
Mixed Grill, Starter, JDW*	1 Portion/374g	460	23.9	123	13.4	3.2	6.4	0.9
TIKKA MASALA								
Chicken, with Rice & No Naan Bread, JDW*	1 Meal/614g	872	33.2	142	6.9	16.9	5.4	1.2
WAFFLES								
Belgian, Ice Cream & Maple Syrup, JDW*	1 Serving/395g	934	33.6	237	13.8	28.4	8.5	0.8
WRAP								
Caesar Wetherwrap & Potato Wedges, JDW*	1 Serving/289g	687	40.2	238	5.0	25.2	13.9	1.6
Caesar Wetherwrap, JDW*	1 Wrap/159g	478	32.6	301	7.0	23.1	20.5	1.5
Caesar Wetherwrap, Tortillas & Salsa, JDW*	1 Serving/244g	624	38.8	256	5.7	23.4	15.9	1.6
Chicken & Cheese, JDW*	1 Wrap/271g	553	26.3	204	10.7	19.6	9.7	1.4
Chicken, Cheese, & Potato Wedges, JDW*	1 Serving/401g	762	34.1	190	8.0	22.2	8.5	1.5

JD WETHERSPOONS

	Measure INFO/WEIGHT	per Measure KCAL	FAT	Nutrition Values per 100g / 100ml KCAL	PROT	CARB	FAT	FIBRE
WRAP								
Chicken, Cheese, Tortilla Chips, Salsa, JDW*	1 Serving/356g	699	32.4	196	8.8	20.6	9.1	1.5
Chicken, Guacamole, Potato Wedges, JDW*	1 Serving/318g	537	18.4	169	7.2	23.7	5.8	2.0
Chicken, Guacamole, Tortillas, Salsa, JDW*	1 Serving/273g	474	16.9	174	8.2	21.9	6.2	2.0
Chicken, Southern Fried, with Creole Mayo, JDW*	1 Wrap/320g	553	30.0	173	7.1	16.3	9.4	1.4
Chicken, with Chicken Breast, JDW*	1 Wrap/292g	450	21.6	154	9.4	14.5	7.4	1.5
Chicken, with Potato Wedges, JDW*	1 Serving/373g	647	24.2	174	6.7	23.9	6.5	1.7
Chicken, with Tortilla Chips & Salsa, JDW*	1 Serving/328g	584	23.0	178	7.5	22.3	7.0	1.6
Club Wetherwrap, Tortilla Chips, Salsa, JDW*	1 Serving/336g	759	42.0	226	12.2	17.1	12.5	1.1
Club Wetherwrap, with Potato Wedges, JDW*	1 Serving/381g	822	43.1	216	10.9	19.2	11.3	1.2
Club, JDW*	1 Wrap/286g	711	40.3	249	12.1	19.2	14.1	1.0
Fajita Chicken, JDW*	1 Wrap/228g	345	14.1	151	3.8	21.2	6.2	1.9
Fajita Chicken, Tortilla Chips, Salsa, JDW*	1 Serving/313g	491	20.3	157	3.5	21.9	6.5	1.9
Fajita Chicken, with Potato Wedges, JDW*	1 Serving/358g	554	21.8	155	3.2	23.5	6.1	1.9
Poached Salmon & Prawn Salad, JDW*	1 Wrap/355g	512	34.1	144	9.8	4.5	9.6	0.5
Poached Salmon, Tortilla Chips, Salsa, JDW*	1 Serving/203g	573	32.9	282	9.9	25.8	16.2	1.6
Poached Salmon, with Potato Wedges, JDW*	1 Serving/298g	656	34.3	220	7.1	24.2	11.5	1.5
YORKSHIRE PUDDING								
JDW*	2 Yorkshires/60g	132	4.6	236	8.2	32.9	8.2	1.1
KFC								
BEANS								
BBQ, Large, KFC*	1 Serving/188g	158	1.4	84	5.3	15.1	0.7	0.0
BBQ, Regular, KFC*	1 Reg Serving/99g	83	0.7	84	5.3	15.1	0.7	0.0
BURGERS								
Fillet, KFC*	1 Burger/245g	441	15.6	180	12.2	18.7	6.4	0.0
Fillet, Mini, KFC*	1 Burger/114g	275	11.2	241	14.8	24.0	9.8	0.0
Tower, KFC*	1 Burger/210g	628	20.8	299	15.9	30.0	9.9	0.0
Tower, Zinger, KFC*	1 Burger/269g	668	33.3	248	11.2	24.4	12.4	0.0
Zinger, Fillet, KFC*	1 Serving/185g	445	19.6	241	13.9	22.4	10.6	1.4
Zinger, KFC*	1 Burger/219g	481	20.8	220	12.2	22.1	9.5	0.0
CHEESECAKE								
Boysenberry, Chateau, KFC*	1 Serving/85g	196	9.4	230	4.0	30.0	11.0	0.0
Cookies & Cream, KFC*	1 Serving/80g	261	17.1	326	4.3	29.1	21.4	0.0
CHICKEN								
Breast, Original Recipe, KFC*	1 Breast/129g	267	12.5	207	24.9	5.6	9.7	0.0
Drumsticks, Original Recipe, KFC*	1 Drumstick/90g	153	9.0	170	11.9	9.1	10.0	0.0
Popcorn, Large, KFC*	1 Serving/182g	477	28.8	262	17.5	13.5	15.8	0.0
Popcorn, Regular, KFC*	1 Reg Serving/117g	294	17.8	251	16.8	12.9	15.2	0.0
Ribs, Original Recipe, KFC*	1 Rib/123g	231	13.0	188	19.8	4.2	10.6	0.0
Strips, Crispy, KFC*	1 Strip/46g	112	5.4	243	15.4	20.4	11.7	0.0
Thighs, Original Recipe, KFC*	1 Thigh/117g	190	12.4	162	12.6	4.4	10.6	0.0
Wings, Hot, KFC*	1 Wing/53g	93	6.4	175	9.4	7.6	12.1	0.0
Wings, Original Recipe, KFC*	1 Wing/13g	112	5.9	862	78.5	39.2	45.4	0.0
COLESLAW								
Large, KFC*	1 Serving/200g	268	22.4	134	0.8	9.5	11.2	0.0
Regular, KFC*	1 Serving/100g	134	11.2	134	0.8	9.5	11.2	0.0
CORN								
Cobs, KFC*	1 Serving/72g	145	8.7	201	4.3	20.1	12.1	0.0
DRESSING								
Caesar, KFC*	1 Sachet/37g	109	11.5	295	19.2	2.7	31.1	0.0
French, KFC*	1 Sachet/45g	30	1.3	66	0.2	2.9	2.9	0.0
Vinaigrette, Low Fat, KFC*	1 Sachet/37g	22	0.8	59	0.5	8.9	2.2	0.0
Yoghurt, Coriander & Chilli, KFC*	1 Sachet/45g	166	16.2	369	2.2	9.3	36.0	0.0

	Measure INFO/WEIGHT	per Measure KCAL	FAT	Nutrition Values per 100g / 100ml KCAL	PROT	CARB	FAT	FIBRE

KFC
FRIES
Large, KFC*	1 Serving/163g	377	19.4	232	3.1	32.4	11.9	0.0
Regular, KFC*	1 Serving/111g	257	13.2	232	3.1	32.4	11.9	0.0

GRAVY
Large, KFC*	1 Serving/242g	171	9.5	71	2.4	7.4	3.9	0.0
Regular, KFC*	1 Serving/102g	72	4.0	71	2.4	7.4	3.9	0.0

ICE CREAM
Avalanche, KFC*	1 Pot/28g	114	5.1	407	10.4	51.4	18.2	0.0
Soft, KFC*	1 Serving/110g	171	7.0	155	3.7	20.6	6.4	0.0

PIE
Apple Slice, Colonel's Pies, KFC*	1 Slice/113g	310	13.9	274	1.7	38.9	12.3	0.0
Strawberry Creme, Slice, KFC*	1 Slice/78g	279	15.0	358	5.4	41.0	19.2	2.5

SALAD
Chicken, Original Recipe, No Dressing, KFC*	1 Salad/266g	246	8.7	92	9.0	7.0	3.3	0.0
Chicken, Zinger, No Dressing, KFC*	1 Salad/266g	287	13.8	108	7.8	8.0	5.2	0.0
Potato, KFC*	1 Portion/160g	229	13.9	143	2.5	14.3	8.7	1.8

WRAP
Twister, Salsa, Toasted, KFC*	1 Wrap/235g	546	26.4	232	8.7	24.6	11.2	0.0
Twister, Toasted, KFC*	1 Wrap/231g	543	26.5	235	8.9	24.6	11.5	0.0
Wrapstar, KFC*	1 Wrapstar/239g	642	36.6	269	11.4	25.9	15.3	0.0

KRISPY KREME
CAKE
Chocolate, Glazed, Krispy Kreme*	1 Doughnut/80g	309	13.6	387	4.0	55.0	17.0	3.0
Vanilla, Krispy Kreme*	1 Doughnut/80g	315	13.7	391	4.0	57.0	17.0	2.0

DOUGHNUTS
Blueberry, Powdered, Filled, Krispy Kreme*	1 Doughnut/86g	307	17.2	357	7.0	36.0	20.0	5.0
Chocolate Iced, Creme Filled, Krispy Kreme*	1 Doughnut/87g	339	17.4	390	6.0	47.0	20.0	4.0
Chocolate Iced, Custard Filled, Krispy Kreme*	1 Doughnut/87g	307	14.8	353	6.0	43.0	17.0	2.0
Chocolate Iced, Glazed, Krispy Kreme*	1 Doughnut/66g	270	13.2	410	5.0	51.0	20.0	3.0
Chocolate Iced, with Creme Filling, Krispy Kreme*	1 Doughnut/87g	350	20.9	402	3.0	42.0	24.0	1.0
Chocolate Iced, with Sprinkles, Krispy Kreme*	1 Doughnut/71g	293	13.5	413	5.0	56.0	19.0	3.0
Cinnamon Apple, Filled, Krispy Kreme*	1 Doughnut/81g	269	14.6	332	7.0	37.0	18.0	5.0
Cruller, Glazed, Krispy Kreme*	1 Doughnut/54g	254	15.6	471	4.0	49.0	29.0	3.0
Glazed, with a Creme Filling, Krispy Kreme*	1 Doughnut/86g	309	15.5	359	5.0	44.0	18.0	4.0
Lemon Filled, Glazed, Krispy Kreme*	1 Doughnut/65g	218	10.5	331	5.0	41.0	16.0	4.0
Maple Iced, Krispy Kreme*	1 Doughnut/66g	279	15.2	422	5.0	49.0	23.0	3.0
Sour Cream, Krispy Kreme*	1 Doughnut/80g	340	18.4	425	4.0	53.0	23.0	1.0
Strawberry Filled, Powdered, Krispy Kreme*	1 Doughnut/74g	248	13.3	335	7.0	36.0	18.0	5.0

LONGLEY FARM
YOGHURT
Lemon, Longley Farm*	1 Pot/150g	159	5.6	106	5.0	13.4	3.7	0.0

MARKS & SPENCER
SANDWICH
Toasted, Mushroom & Gruyere, M & S*	1 Toastie/206.4g	485	22.7	235	10.1	23.9	11.0	2.3

MCDONALD'S
APPLES
McDonald's*	1 Apple/140g	59	0.0	42	0.3	10.0	0.0	2.2

BAGEL
Plain, McDonald's*	1 Bagel/84g	231	1.7	274	8.0	55.0	2.0	2.0
with Bacon, Egg & Cheese, McDonald's*	1 Bagel/177g	481	21.3	271	13.0	28.0	12.0	1.0
with Butter & Jam, McDonald's*	1 Bagel/122g	399	10.2	326	5.9	58.8	8.3	2.2
with Flora & Jam, McDonald's*	1 Bagel/120g	369	6.9	305	6.0	59.4	5.7	2.2
with Philadelphia, McDonald's*	1 Bagel/125g	318	5.9	254	7.7	47.5	4.7	2.1

MCDONALD'S

	Measure INFO/WEIGHT	per Measure KCAL	FAT	Nutrition Values per 100g / 100ml KCAL	PROT	CARB	FAT	FIBRE
BAGEL								
with Sausage & Egg, McDonald's*	1 Bagel/208g	551	26.5	266	13.3	23.3	12.8	1.6
with Sausage, Egg & Cheese, McDonald's*	1 Bagel/207g	561	29.0	271	14.0	25.0	14.0	1.0
BREAKFAST								
Big Breakfast Bun, McDonald's*	1 Bun/242g	571	32.2	236	13.0	15.1	13.3	0.9
Big Breakfast, McDonald's*	1 Breakfast/275g	625	35.8	227	11.0	16.0	13.0	2.0
BREAKFAST CEREAL								
Porridge, Oatso Simple, & Jam, McDonald's*	1 Serving/232g	246	5.3	106	4.0	17.0	2.3	0.9
Porridge, Oatso Simple, & Sugar, McDonald's*	1 Serving/215g	205	5.4	95	4.3	13.7	2.5	0.9
Porridge, Oatso Simple, Plain, McDonald's*	1 Serving/233g	246	4.7	105	4.0	17.0	2.0	1.0
BROWNIE								
Belgian Bliss, McDonald's*	1 Serving/85g	370	20.4	435	6.0	52.0	24.0	2.0
Chocolate Chip, McMini, McDonald's*	1 Brownie/18.9g	68	2.4	360	4.9	58.8	12.7	1.9
BURGERS								
Arizona, Grande, McDonald's*	1 Burger/251.3g	655	40.2	261	16.0	15.0	16.0	2.0
Bacon Cheeseburger, McDonald's*	1 Burger/136.4g	367	16.6	270	16.0	23.6	12.2	2.3
Bacon McDouble, with Cheese, McDonald's*	1 Burger/141g	372	19.0	264	16.1	19.6	13.5	2.2
Beef, Deluxe, McDonald's*	1 Burger/265.3g	650	34.5	245	14.0	18.0	13.0	2.0
Beef, Deluxe, with Bacon, McDonald's*	1 Burger/274g	689	38.4	252	15.0	18.0	14.0	2.0
Big Mac, McDonald's*	1 Burger/216g	496	23.8	229	13.0	19.0	11.0	2.0
Big Mac, No Sauce, No Cheese, McDonald's*	1 Sandwich/181g	400	16.0	221	12.2	23.8	8.8	1.1
Big Tasty, McDonald's*	1 Burger/348g	804	50.5	231	11.7	14.6	14.5	1.6
Big Tasty, with Bacon, McDonald's*	1 Burger/360g	886	57.6	246	13.0	14.0	16.0	2.0
Bigger Big Mac, McDonald's*	1 Burger/324.5g	714	34.0	220	12.9	18.5	10.5	1.6
Cheeseburger, Bacon, McDonald's*	1 Burger/127g	336	15.3	264	16.0	24.0	12.0	2.0
Cheeseburger, Double, McDonald's*	1 Burger/169g	446	22.0	263	17.0	19.0	13.0	1.0
Cheeseburger, McDonald's*	1 Burger/118g	300	12.0	253	14.4	26.2	10.1	2.5
Chicken Deluxe, with Bacon, McDonald's*	1 Burger/255.6g	570	23.0	223	13.0	24.0	9.0	2.0
Chicken Legend, with Cool Mayo, McDonald's*	1 Burger/218g	550	21.8	252	14.0	28.0	10.0	2.0
Chicken Legend, with Spicy Tomato Salsa, McDonald's*	1 Burger/224g	516	13.5	230	13.0	30.0	6.0	2.0
Filet-O-Fish, McDonald's*	1 Burger/146.9g	360	16.2	245	11.0	26.0	11.0	2.0
Filet-O-Fish, No Tartar Sauce, McDonald's*	1 Burger/124g	290	9.0	234	12.1	30.7	7.3	0.8
Grilled Chicken Caprese, McDonald's*	1 Burger/275g	470	21.2	171	12.5	15.0	7.7	2.1
Hamburger, McDonald's*	1 Burger/104g	249	8.3	240	13.0	29.0	8.0	3.0
McChicken Grill with BBQ Sauce, McDonald's*	1 Sandwich/215g	309	5.5	144	12.1	18.1	2.6	2.2
McChicken Premiere, McDonald's*	1 Burger/221g	464	17.0	210	10.4	24.4	7.7	1.4
McChicken Sandwich, McDonald's*	1 Sandwich/170g	380	16.0	224	9.4	25.3	9.4	2.3
Quarter Pounder, Bacon with Cheese, McDonald's*	1 Burger/230g	592	33.2	259	16.5	15.4	14.5	1.3
Quarter Pounder, Deluxe, McDonald's*	1 Burger/253g	521	26.8	206	11.4	16.1	10.6	1.7
Quarter Pounder, Deluxe, Bacon & Cheese, McDonald's*	1 Burger/228.9g	592	33.2	259	16.5	15.4	14.5	1.3
Quarter Pounder, Double, with Cheese, McDonald's*	1 Burger/275g	710	40.3	259	19.5	12.2	14.7	1.1
Quarter Pounder, McDonald's*	1 Burger/178g	424	19.0	238	14.5	20.9	10.7	2.1
Quarter Pounder, with Cheese, McDonald's*	1 Burger/194g	500	25.3	257	17.0	19.0	13.0	2.0
Steak Premiere, McDonald's*	1 Burger/229g	453	14.2	198	14.9	19.4	6.2	1.6
BURGERS VEGETARIAN								
Vegetable, Deluxe, McDonald's*	1 Burger/181g	411	16.3	227	6.0	30.0	9.0	6.0
BUTTER								
McDonald's*	1 Pack/11g	85	9.0	752	0.0	0.0	80.0	0.0
CADBURY BYTE								
McMini, McDonald's*	1 Byte/14.0g	67	2.9	478	6.5	64.7	20.7	1.7
CAKE								
Birthday, McDonald's*	1 Portion/158g	640	22.6	405	2.7	65.4	14.3	1.0

MCDONALD'S

	Measure INFO/WEIGHT	per Measure KCAL	FAT	Nutrition Values per 100g / 100ml KCAL	PROT	CARB	FAT	FIBRE
CARROTS								
Sticks, McDonald's*	1 Bag/80g	25	0.0	31	1.3	6.3	0.0	2.5
CHEESE								
Soft, Philadelphia, Light, McDonald's*	1 Serving/35g	55	4.9	157	6.0	3.0	14.0	0.0
CHICKEN								
McNuggets, 4 Pieces, McDonald's*	4 Pieces/71g	175	9.3	245	14.0	18.0	13.0	1.0
McNuggets, 6 Pieces, McDonald's*	6 Pieces/106g	260	13.8	245	14.0	18.0	13.0	1.0
McNuggets, 9 Pieces, McDonald's*	9 Pieces/159g	390	20.7	245	14.0	18.0	13.0	1.0
Selects, 3 Pieces, McDonald's*	3 Pieces/130g	366	19.6	280	16.0	20.0	15.0	1.0
Selects, 5 Pieces, McDonald's*	5 Pieces/218g	612	32.8	280	16.0	20.0	15.0	1.0
COFFEE								
Cappuccino, Regular, McDonald's*	1 Serving/320ml	128	3.2	40	3.0	4.0	1.0	0.0
Latte, Regular, McDonald's*	1 Serving/368ml	142	3.7	39	3.0	4.0	1.0	0.0
White, Regular, McDonald's*	1 Serving/342ml	24	0.0	7	1.0	1.0	0.0	0.0
COLA								
Coke, Diet, McDonald's*	1 Med/400ml	2	0.0	0	0.0	0.0	0.0	0.0
Coke, McDonald's*	1 Med/400ml	172	0.0	43	0.0	10.5	0.0	0.0
CREAMER								
Uht, McDonald's*	1 Cup/14ml	17	1.4	123	4.2	4.2	10.0	0.0
CROUTONS								
McDonald's*	1 Sachet/14g	60	2.0	426	11.8	63.4	14.0	2.7
DIP								
Caramelised Onion, McDonald's*	1 Dip/31.3g	45	1.9	144	3.0	19.0	6.0	3.0
Sour Cream & Chive, McDonald's*	1 Pot/50g	150	16.0	300	2.0	2.0	32.0	4.0
Sweet Chilli, McDonald's*	1 Pot/31g	80	0.9	256	0.0	58.0	3.0	0.0
DOUGHNUTS								
Chocolate Donut, McDonald's*	1 Donut/79g	345	16.2	437	5.7	43.8	20.5	1.0
Chocolate Donut, McMini, McDonald's*	1 Donut/17.1g	64	3.0	375	6.8	46.9	17.8	1.6
Cinnamon Donut, McDonald's*	1 Donut/72g	302	18.1	419	5.1	43.1	25.1	3.8
Sugared Donut, McDonald's*	1 Donut/49g	175	8.8	357	6.0	45.0	18.0	2.0
DRESSING								
Balsamic, Low Fat, McDonald's*	1 Sachet/33g	20	1.0	60	0.0	9.0	3.0	0.0
Caesar, Low Fat, McDonald's*	1 Sachet/80g	55	1.6	68	2.0	10.0	2.0	0.0
French, Low Fat, McDonald's*	1 Serving/22g	13	0.6	58	0.5	7.1	2.6	1.0
Ranch, Salad, McDonald's*	1 Sachet/78ml	107	6.5	136	3.1	12.3	8.3	0.8
FANTA								
Orange, McDonald's*	1 Reg/250ml	108	0.0	43	0.0	10.4	0.0	0.0
FISH FINGERS								
McDonald's*	3 Fingers/84g	231	11.8	274	14.0	20.0	14.0	2.0
FLATBREAD								
Chicken Salsa, McDonald's*	1 Serving/100g	480	15.5	480	27.3	57.6	15.5	0.0
Greek, McDonald's*	1 Flatbread/100g	433	20.7	433	21.2	47.3	20.7	3.8
FRIES								
French, Large, McDonald's*	1 Lge/160g	456	22.4	284	3.0	35.0	14.0	1.0
French, Medium, McDonald's*	1 Med/114g	325	16.0	284	3.0	35.0	14.0	1.0
French, Small, McDonald's*	1 Sml/79g	225	11.1	284	3.0	35.0	14.0	4.0
FRUIT								
& Yoghurt, McDonald's*	1 Serving/144g	138	2.7	96	2.8	15.9	1.9	1.1
Bag, Apple & Grape, McDonald's*	1 Bag/80g	43	0.1	54	0.3	13.0	0.1	2.3
Bag, McDonald's*	1 Pack/80g	40	0.0	50	0.0	13.0	0.0	3.0
Bag, Pineapple & Grape, McDonald's*	1 Pack/80g	38	0.2	47	0.4	11.1	0.2	1.2
HASH BROWNS								
McDonald's*	1 Hash Brown/57g	140	8.0	246	2.0	28.0	14.0	4.0

MCDONALD'S

	Measure INFO/WEIGHT	per Measure KCAL	FAT	Nutrition Values per 100g / 100ml KCAL	PROT	CARB	FAT	FIBRE
HOT CHOCOLATE								
McDonald's*	1 Serving/330ml	165	3.7	50	0.7	8.8	1.1	0.0
HOT DOG								
& Ketchup, McDonald's*	1 Serving/116g	296	14.6	255	9.6	25.8	12.6	1.3
ICE CREAM								
Smartie, McDonald's*	1 Pot/120g	260	9.5	216	3.4	33.3	7.9	1.0
ICE CREAM CONE								
McDonald's*	1 Cone/90g	141	4.5	156	4.5	24.4	5.0	0.0
with Flake, McDonald's*	1 Cone/107g	204	7.7	191	4.8	27.0	7.2	0.0
JAM								
McDonald's*	1 Serving/21g	55	0.0	261	0.0	64.4	0.0	0.6
Strawberry, McDonald's*	1 Pack/20g	50	0.0	250	0.0	65.0	0.0	0.0
JUICE								
Tropicana, McDonald's*	1 Bottle/250ml	122	0.0	43	1.0	9.0	0.0	0.0
KETCHUP								
Tomato, McDonald's*	1 Portion/23g	25	0.0	109	0.0	26.0	0.0	0.0
LEMONADE								
Sprite, McDonald's*	1 Regular/251ml	108	0.0	43	0.0	10.5	0.0	0.0
MARGARINE								
Flora, Original, McDonald's*	1 Pack/10g	53	5.9	531	0.0	0.0	59.0	0.0
MCFLURRY								
After Eight, McDonald's*	1 McFlurry/203.7g	381	11.0	187	2.8	31.4	5.4	0.5
Cadbury, Shortcake, Limited Edition, McDonald's*	1 McFlurry/205.9g	385	14.4	187	3.0	28.0	7.0	1.0
Cornetto, Mint Choc, McDonald's*	1 Serving/212.9g	430	17.0	202	3.0	30.0	8.0	1.0
Creme Egg, Cadbury's, McDonald's*	1 McFlurry/203g	381	12.9	188	2.9	29.8	6.3	0.5
Crunchie, McDonald's*	1 McFlurry/185g	311	11.1	168	3.0	26.0	6.0	1.0
Dairy Milk, Deluxe, McDonald's*	1 McFlurry/205g	391	14.3	191	3.2	28.6	7.0	0.1
Dairy Milk, McDonald's*	1 McFlurry/181g	314	10.8	173	2.7	26.0	6.0	0.5
Dairy Milk, with Caramel, McDonald's*	1 McFlurry/206g	385	13.0	187	2.9	29.1	6.3	0.0
Jammie Dodger, McDonald's*	1 McFlurry/128g	256	8.2	200	3.9	33.6	6.4	0.3
Rolo, McDonald's*	1 McFlurry/205g	390	13.3	190	4.0	29.2	6.5	0.1
Smarties, McDonald's*	1 McFlurry/185g	310	11.0	168	2.7	26.0	6.0	1.1
Strawberry, Cornetto, McDonald's*	1 McFlurry/211.8g	395	12.7	186	2.0	29.0	6.0	0.0
Toffee Swirl, Oreo Cookie, McDonald's*	1 McFlurry/206ml	400	12.4	194	3.0	31.0	6.0	1.0
Yorkie, McDonald's*	1 McFlurry/204g	379	14.9	186	3.4	27.0	7.3	0.8
MCMUFFIN								
Bacon & Egg, Double, McDonald's*	1 McMuffin/167g	430	25.1	257	15.0	16.0	15.0	1.0
Bacon & Egg, McDonald's*	1 McMuffin/148g	375	20.8	252	13.0	17.0	14.0	1.0
Egg, McDonald's*	1 McMuffin/127g	281	12.8	221	12.2	20.4	10.1	3.2
Sausage & Egg, Double, McDonald's*	1 McMuffin/227g	587	38.7	258	16.0	12.0	17.0	1.0
Sausage & Egg, McDonald's*	1 McMuffin/177g	451	26.6	254	14.0	15.0	15.0	2.0
Scrambled Egg, McDonald's*	1 McMuffin/147g	294	14.1	200	10.9	17.5	9.6	1.3
MELT								
Toasted Ham & Cheese, McDonald's*	1 Serving/100g	239	8.0	239	11.2	30.6	8.0	1.8
MILK								
Fresh, Portion, McDonald's*	1 Portion/14.4ml	10	0.0	69	0.0	7.0	0.0	0.0
MILK SHAKE								
Banana, Large, McDonald's*	1 Lg/432g	510	13.0	118	3.0	20.0	3.0	0.0
Banana, Medium, McDonald's*	1 Med/337g	399	10.1	118	3.0	20.0	3.0	0.0
Banana, Small, McDonald's*	1 Sm/177g	210	5.3	118	3.0	20.0	3.0	0.0
Chocolate, Large, McDonald's*	1 Large/434g	504	13.0	116	3.0	19.0	3.0	0.0
Chocolate, Medium, McDonald's*	1 Med/334g	388	10.0	116	3.0	19.0	3.0	0.0
Chocolate, Small, McDonald's*	1 Sm/178g	207	5.3	116	9.0	19.0	3.0	0.0

MCDONALD'S

	Measure INFO/WEIGHT	per Measure KCAL	FAT	Nutrition Values per 100g / 100ml KCAL	PROT	CARB	FAT	FIBRE
MUFFIN								
Strawberry, Large, McDonald's*	1 Lge/435g	509	13.1	117	3.0	20.0	3.0	0.0
Strawberry, Medium, McDonald's*	1 Med/336g	393	10.1	117	3.0	20.0	3.0	0.0
Strawberry, Small, McDonald's*	1 Sm/178g	208	5.3	117	3.0	20.0	3.0	0.0
Vanilla, Large, McDonald's*	1 Lg/434g	504	13.0	116	3.0	20.0	3.0	0.0
Vanilla, Medium, McDonald's*	1 Med/339g	393	10.2	116	3.0	20.0	3.0	0.0
Vanilla, Small, McDonald's*	1 Sm/178g	207	5.3	116	3.0	20.0	3.0	0.0
MUFFIN								
Blueberry, McDonald's*	1 Muffin/126g	305	2.5	242	4.0	51.0	2.0	2.0
Buttered, McDonald's*	1 Muffin/63g	158	3.7	250	8.6	40.7	5.9	2.9
Buttered, with Preserve, McDonald's*	1 Muffin/93g	234	3.7	252	5.9	48.1	4.0	2.0
Carrot, McDonald's*	1 Muffin/134.8g	360	3.9	267	4.8	55.4	2.9	1.6
Double Chocolate, McDonald's*	1 Muffin/126g	531	30.3	421	6.0	46.0	24.0	2.0
Triple Chocolate, McDonald's*	1 Muffin/138.4g	580	33.5	420	4.7	45.7	24.3	0.9
ONION RINGS								
McDonald's*	1 Serving/80g	180	10.4	225	4.0	26.0	13.0	1.0
PANCAKE								
& Sausage, McDonald's*	1 Serving/169g	431	18.6	254	11.0	28.0	11.0	2.0
& Syrup, McDonald's*	1 Pack/175g	515	12.3	294	4.0	52.0	7.0	2.0
PIE								
Apple, McDonald's*	1 Pie/83g	240	13.3	289	2.0	35.0	16.0	0.0
POTATO WEDGES								
McDonald's*	1 Portion/176g	349	17.7	197	3.3	23.3	10.0	2.8
QUORN*								
Burger, Premiere, McDonald's*	1 Burger/210g	311	6.1	148	9.1	24.2	2.9	2.7
ROLL								
Bacon, McBacon, McDonald's*	1 Roll/122g	349	14.0	286	13.5	30.5	11.5	1.7
Bacon, with Brown Sauce, McDonald's*	1 Roll/126g	351	8.8	278	15.0	37.0	7.0	2.0
Bacon, with Tomato Ketchup, McDonald's*	1 Roll/126g	346	8.8	273	15.0	36.0	7.0	2.0
SALAD								
Caesar, Crispy Chicken, Croutons, McDonald's*	1 Salad/295g	385	18.2	131	9.4	8.8	6.2	1.3
Caesar, Crispy Chicken, Dressing, Croutons, McDonald's*	1 Salad/371g	530	30.0	143	8.0	9.1	8.1	1.2
Caesar, Crispy Chicken, Dressing, McDonald's*	1 Salad/316g	472	28.9	149	8.8	7.5	9.2	1.2
Caesar, Crispy Chicken, McDonald's*	1 Salad/279g	327	17.6	117	9.3	5.8	6.3	1.2
Caesar, Grilled Chicken, Croutons, McDonald's*	1 Salad/294g	280	9.6	95	11.5	4.2	3.3	1.3
Caesar, Grilled Chicken, Dressing & Croutons, McDonald's*	1 Salad/370g	425	21.4	115	9.6	5.4	5.8	1.1
Caesar, Grilled Chicken, Dressing, McDonald's*	1 Salad/305g	367	20.3	120	11.1	3.3	6.7	1.2
Caesar, Grilled Chicken, Plain, McDonald's*	1 Salad/281g	287	13.5	102	8.4	6.4	4.8	1.4
Chicken, No Bacon, Grilled, McDonald's*	1 Salad/261g	117	2.6	45	7.0	2.0	1.0	1.0
Chicken, with Bacon, Grilled, McDonald's*	1 Salad/270g	167	5.4	62	9.0	2.0	2.0	1.0
Crispy Chicken, No Bacon, McDonald's*	1 Salad/281g	271	11.3	96	8.0	6.0	4.0	1.0
Crispy Chicken, with Bacon, McDonald's*	1 Serving/292g	326	14.6	111	10.0	7.0	5.0	1.0
Garden, Side, No Dressing, McDonald's*	1 Salad/90g	10	0.0	11	1.0	1.0	0.0	1.0
Garden, Side, with Balsamic Dressing, McDonald's*	1 Salad/128g	32	0.8	25	1.1	4.2	0.6	1.4
Ranch, Crispy Chicken, Dressing, McDonald's*	1 Salad/401g	501	28.9	125	8.3	6.6	7.2	1.1
Ranch, Crispy Chicken, No Dressing, McDonald's*	1 Salad/320g	394	22.1	123	9.5	5.1	6.9	1.1
Ranch, Grilled Chicken, Dressing, McDonald's*	1 Salad/400g	396	20.0	99	9.8	3.1	5.0	1.1
Ranch, Grilled Chicken, No Dressing, McDonald's*	1 Salad/298g	268	12.5	90	11.4	1.4	4.2	1.0
SANDWICH								
Arizona Grande, McDonald's*	1 Sandwich/251g	657	40.3	261	16.0	15.0	16.0	2.0
California Classic, McDonald's*	1 Sandwich/253g	617	32.9	244	16.0	15.0	13.0	2.0
Chicken, Grilled, McDonald's*	1 Serving/211g	367	14.0	174	11.9	16.9	6.6	0.0
Deli, BBQ Pork, No Cheese or Salad, Brown, McDonald's*	1 Sandwich/166g	382	6.7	229	10.0	39.0	4.0	2.0

MCDONALD'S

	Measure INFO/WEIGHT	per Measure KCAL	per Measure FAT	Nutrition Values per 100g / 100ml KCAL	PROT	CARB	FAT	FIBRE
SANDWICH								
Deli, BBQ Pork, No Cheese or Salad, White, McDonald's*	1 Sandwich/166g	382	6.7	229	11.0	38.0	4.0	2.0
Deli, BBQ Pork, Cheese & Salad, Brown, McDonald's*	1 Sandwich/218g	431	8.7	197	10.0	30.0	4.0	1.0
Deli, BBQ Pork, Cheese & Salad, White, McDonald's*	1 Sandwich/218g	431	8.7	197	11.0	29.0	4.0	1.0
Deli, BBQ Pork, Cheese, No Salad, White Roll, McDonald's*	1 Sandwich/184g	427	9.2	231	13.0	34.0	5.0	2.
Deli, BBQ Pork & Salad, No Cheese, Brown, McDonald's*	1 Sandwich/200g	386	6.0	193	9.0	33.0	3.0	2.0
Deli, BBQ Pork & Salad, No Cheese, White, McDonald's*	1 Sandwich/200g	386	6.0	193	10.0	32.0	3.0	2.0
Deli, Cheese, Ham & Pepperoni, Brown, McDonald's*	1 Sandwich/300g	616	32.0	208	10.4	18.5	10.8	1.6
Deli, Cheese, Ham & Pepperoni, White, McDonald's*	1 Sandwich/300g	601	30.8	203	10.4	17.9	10.4	1.2
Deli, Chicken Salad & Mayo, Brown, McDonald's*	1 Sandwich/292g	390	7.9	134	8.6	20.3	2.7	1.7
Deli, Chicken Salad & Mayo, White, McDonald's*	1 Sandwich/293g	375	6.7	128	8.5	19.5	2.3	1.5
Deli, Chicken Salad, Plain, Brown, McDonald's*	1 Serving/170g	356	5.1	209	12.0	33.0	3.0	2.0
Deli, Chicken Salad, Plain, White, McDonald's*	1 Sandwich/170g	356	5.1	209	13.0	32.0	3.0	2.0
Deli, Chicken Salad, No Cheese, Brown, McDonald's*	1 Sandwich/222g	366	6.7	164	9.0	26.0	3.0	2.0
Deli, Chicken Salad, No Cheese, White, McDonald's*	1 Sandwich/222g	360	4.4	162	10.0	25.0	2.0	1.0
Deli, Chicken Salad, Brown Roll, McDonald's*	1 Sandwich/191g	426	9.6	223	14.0	30.0	5.0	2.0
Deli, Chicken Salad, with Cheese, White, McDonald's*	1 Sandwich/191g	422	9.6	220	14.0	29.0	5.0	2.0
Deli, Chicken Salad, Cheese, Brown, McDonald's*	1 Sandwich/244g	432	9.8	177	11.0	24.0	4.0	2.0
Deli, Chicken Salad, Cheese, White, McDonald's*	1 Sandwich/244g	432	9.8	177	12.0	23.0	4.0	2.0
Deli, Chicken Tikka, Brown, McDonald's*	1 Sandwich/267g	355	5.9	133	9.7	21.0	2.2	1.9
Deli, Chicken Tikka, White, McDonald's*	1 Sandwich/266g	341	4.8	128	9.6	20.3	1.8	1.5
Deli, Ham & Cheddar, Brown, McDonald's*	1 Sandwich/222g	438	15.7	198	10.2	25.0	7.1	1.9
Deli, Ham & Cheddar, White, McDonald's*	1 Sandwich/222g	423	14.6	191	10.2	24.1	6.6	1.5
Deli, Ham Salad, Brown, McDonald's*	1 Sandwich/209g	346	8.0	166	9.1	25.0	3.8	1.4
Deli, Ham Salad, White, McDonald's*	1 Sandwich/207g	344	5.0	166	9.2	27.5	2.4	1.9
Deli, Meatball Melt, with Cheese, Brown, McDonald's*	1 Sandwich/218g	462	17.1	212	10.6	25.8	7.8	1.8
Deli, Meatball Melt, with Cheese, White, McDonald's*	1 Sandwich/216g	455	14.0	211	11.1	27.8	6.5	2.3
Deli, Roast Beef & Mature Cheddar, White, McDonald's*	1 Sandwich/280g	464	16.5	166	9.8	19.5	5.9	1.3
Deli, Roast Beef, Mature Cheddar, Brown, McDonald's*	1 Sandwich/280g	479	17.6	171	9.9	20.2	6.3	1.7
Deli, Spicy Veggie, Plain, Brown, McDonald's*	1 Serving/214g	536	12.8	250	6.0	43.0	6.0	4.0
Deli, Spicy Veggie, Plain, White, McDonald's*	1 Sandwich/214g	536	12.8	250	7.0	42.0	6.0	6.0
Deli, Spicy Veggie, No Cheese, Brown, McDonald's*	1 Sandwich/228g	542	13.7	237	6.0	40.0	6.0	4.0
Deli, Spicy Veggie, No Cheese, White Roll, McDonald's*	1 Sandwich/229g	537	13.8	234	7.0	40.0	6.0	4.0
Deli, Spicy Veggie, with Cheese, Brown, McDonald's*	1 Sandwich/235g	607	16.5	258	8.0	40.0	7.0	4.0
Deli, Spicy Veggie, Cheese, No Salad, White, McDonald's*	1 Sandwich/235g	602	16.5	256	9.0	39.0	7.0	4.0
Deli, Spicy Veggie, Cheese, Brown, McDonald's*	1 Sandwich/248g	606	17.4	243	8.0	37.0	7.0	4.0
Deli, Spicy Veggie, Cheese, White, McDonald's*	1 Serving/248g	606	17.4	243	8.0	37.0	7.0	4.0
Deli, Chilli Chicken, Plain, Brown, McDonald's*	1 Sandwich/239g	600	16.7	251	13.0	35.0	7.0	2.0
Deli, Chilli Chicken, Plain, White, McDonald's*	1 Sandwich/239g	600	16.7	251	13.0	35.0	7.0	2.0
Deli, Chilli Chicken, No Cheese, Brown, McDonald's*	1 Sandwich/271g	606	16.3	223	11.0	31.0	6.0	1.0
Deli, Chilli Chicken, No Cheese, White, McDonald's*	1oz/28g	62	1.7	221	11.0	31.0	6.0	1.0
Deli, Chilli Chicken, with Cheese, Brown, McDonald's*	1 Sandwich/260g	667	20.9	256	13.0	33.0	8.0	2.0
Deli, Chilli Chicken, with Cheese, White, McDonald's*	1 Sandwich/260g	667	20.9	256	14.0	32.0	8.0	2.0
Deli, Chilli Chicken, Cheese, Brown, McDonald's*	1 Sandwich/292g	678	20.7	229	12.0	29.0	7.0	2.0
Deli, Chilli Chicken, Cheese, White, McDonald's*	1 Sandwich/292g	671	20.5	229	13.0	29.0	7.0	1.0
Deli, Veggie Melt, Grilled, Brown Roll, McDonald's*	1 Sandwich/249g	458	17.2	184	8.4	23.6	6.9	2.1
Deli, Veggie Melt, Grilled, White Roll, McDonald's*	1 Sandwich/250g	445	16.0	178	8.4	22.8	6.4	1.7
The Miami Melt, McDonald's*	1 Sandwich/252g	677	40.4	268	16.0	15.0	16.0	2.0
The New York Supreme, McDonald's*	1 Sandwich/252g	657	40.5	260	16.0	14.0	16.0	2.0
SAUCE								
Barbeque, McDonald's*	1 Portion/50g	85	1.0	170	0.0	38.0	2.0	0.0
Curry, Sweet, McDonald's*	1 Portion/29g	50	0.9	171	0.0	38.0	3.0	3.0
Mustard, Mild, McDonald's*	1 Portion/30g	64	3.6	212	1.0	24.8	12.1	0.0

	Measure INFO/WEIGHT	per Measure		Nutrition Values per 100g / 100ml				
		KCAL	FAT	KCAL	PROT	CARB	FAT	FIBRE

MCDONALD'S
SAUCE
Sweet & Sour, McDonald's*	1 Portion/29g	50	0.0	172	0.0	38.0	0.0	0.0

SPRITE*
Z, McDonald's*	1 Med/200ml	1	0.0	1	0.0	0.0	0.0	0.0

SUNDAE
Hot Caramel, McDonald's*	1 Sundae/189g	357	8.3	189	3.8	33.9	4.4	0.0
Hot Fudge, McDonald's*	1 Sundae/187g	352	10.7	188	4.5	30.0	5.7	0.0
No Topping, McDonald's*	1 Sundae/149g	219	7.6	147	4.2	21.6	5.1	0.0
Strawberry, McDonald's*	1 Sundae/214g	346	6.4	161	2.0	31.0	3.0	0.0
Toffee, McDonald's*	1 Sundae/182g	335	9.1	184	3.0	32.0	5.0	1.0

TOASTIE
Ham & Cheese, McDonald's*	1 Serving/91.8g	214	7.7	233	11.5	28.0	8.4	2.2

WRAP
Chicken Fajita, McDonald's*	1 Wrap/259g	647	31.1	250	8.9	26.7	12.0	1.2
Chicken, Cajun, McDonald's*	1 Wrap/222.4g	585	33.4	263	9.0	22.0	15.0	2.0
Chicken, Snack, McDonald's*	1 Wrap/112g	266	11.2	237	10.0	29.0	10.0	2.0

YOGHURT
Berry Crunch, McDonald's*	1 Serving/194.8g	224	5.1	115	3.5	18.9	2.6	1.2
Burst, Strawberry, McDonald's*	1 Yoghurt/40g	21	0.0	52	2.9	11.0	0.0	0.9

MORRISONS
BAGEL
Plain, Morrisons*	1 Bagel/84.7g	216	1.6	255	9.1	50.4	1.9	2.9

PIZZA HUT
BACON BITS
Pizza Hut*	1 Serving/12g	60	3.6	496	8.3	48.7	29.8	0.0

BEANS
Chocolate Coated, Pizza Hut*	1 Serving/30g	143	5.4	475	5.5	72.2	18.1	0.0

BEETROOT
Pizza Hut*	1 Portion/25g	14	0.0	55	0.9	12.0	0.1	0.0

BREAD
Garlic, Ciabatta, Pizza Hut*	2 Ciabattas/253g	820	32.1	324	9.1	43.4	12.7	1.0
Garlic, Dipsters, Pizza Hut*	1 Piece/90g	308	14.2	342	6.8	43.1	15.8	0.0
Garlic, Pizza Hut*	4 Pieces/119g	380	16.5	317	7.3	40.9	13.8	0.0
Garlic, with Cheese, Pizza Hut*	4 Pieces/187g	567	32.6	303	16.2	20.5	17.4	0.0

BREADSTICKS
Garlic, Pizza Hut*	1 Stick/50g	174	6.7	347	9.8	46.9	13.4	1.0

CAKE
Chocolate Fudge, Pizza Hut*	1 Piece/154g	588	33.3	382	4.7	44.8	21.6	0.0

CARROTS
Grated, Pizza Hut*	1 Serving/17g	5	0.1	30	0.7	6.0	0.5	0.0

CHEESECAKE
New York Style, Baked, Pizza Hut*	1 Slice/113g	442	16.2	391	6.6	62.3	14.3	0.0
Vanilla, Madagasca, Pizza Hut*	1 Serving/133g	397	18.1	298	4.8	39.2	13.6	0.0

CHICKEN
Dippin, Pizza Hut*	1 Serving/155g	332	14.4	214	15.7	17.1	9.3	0.0
Goujons, Pizza Hut*	5 Pieces/169.2g	340	14.2	201	17.5	13.8	8.4	1.5
Wings, BBQ, Pizza Hut*	6 Pieces/183.9g	412	24.8	224	21.0	4.5	13.5	0.0
Wings, BBQ, Saucy, Pizza Hut*	6 Wings/159g	355	21.8	223	21.4	3.6	13.7	0.0
Wings, Buffalo, Saucy, Pizza Hut*	6 Wings/181g	380	22.2	209	21.0	3.7	12.2	0.0

CHICKEN
Wings, with Sour Cream & Chive Dip, Pizza Hut*	1 Pack/178g	680	56.1	382	22.8	1.9	31.5	1.3

COLESLAW
Pizza Hut*	1 Pot/38g	54	4.6	143	0.9	7.1	12.3	0.0

PIZZA HUT

	Measure INFO/WEIGHT	per Measure KCAL	per Measure FAT	Nutrition Values per 100g / 100ml KCAL	PROT	CARB	FAT	FIBRE
COLESLAW								
Pizza Flavoured, Pizza Hut*	1 Serving/12g	23	3.1	196	10.1	55.2	26.1	0.0
CHICKEN								
Slices, Pizza Hut*	1 Serving/53g	8	0.0	15	1.0	3.0	0.0	0.0
DIP								
BBQ, Pizza Hut*	1 Pot/28g	38	0.0	135	1.0	31.0	0.0	0.0
Garlic & Herb, Pizza Hut*	1 Pot/28g	144	15.4	513	1.0	2.4	55.0	0.0
Sour Cream & Chive, Pizza Hut*	1 Pot/28g	99	9.2	354	1.0	14.0	33.0	0.0
Sweet Chilli, Pizza Hut*	1 Pot/28g	46	0.3	164	1.0	40.0	1.0	0.0
DRESSING								
1000 Island, Pizza Hut*	1 Serving/38g	107	9.7	279	0.3	12.0	25.4	0.0
Blue Cheese, Pizza Hut*	1 Serving/35g	161	15.3	458	3.5	12.6	43.4	0.0
Caesar, Pizza Hut*	1 Serving/40g	125	10.7	311	0.3	16.8	26.6	0.0
Ranch, Pizza Hut*	1 Serving/30g	163	18.0	510	1.2	1.5	56.4	0.0
Vinaigrette, Low Fat, Pizza Hut*	1 Serving/30ml	21	0.1	71	0.4	15.0	0.4	0.0
FRIES								
Seasoned, Pizza Hut*	1 Portion/145g	247	11.1	171	2.3	23.0	7.7	0.0
ICE CREAM								
Dairy, Pizza Hut*	1 Portion/141.7g	273	12.6	192	4.6	23.3	8.9	0.2
Factory, Pizza Hut*	1 Serving/100g	202	9.5	202	3.9	24.6	9.5	0.0
KETCHUP								
Tomato, Pizza Hut*	1 Pot/28g	39	0.0	141	1.4	34.1	0.1	0.0
MACARONI CHEESE								
Pizza Hut*	1 Serving/40g	57	2.4	140	4.9	16.6	6.0	0.0
MARSHMALLOWS								
Mini, Pizza Hut*	1 Serving/30g	96	0.0	320	5.4	74.3	0.0	0.0
MAYONNAISE								
Sachet, Pizza Hut*	1 Sachet/12g	88	9.8	731	1.3	1.8	81.2	0.0
MUFFIN								
Double Choc Chip, Pizza Hut*	1 Muffin/108g	442	22.7	409	6.4	48.7	21.0	0.0
Mixed Berry, Pizza Hut*	1 Muffin/108g	402	22.6	372	4.4	41.6	20.9	0.0
Strawberry & White Chocolate, Pizza Hut*	1 Muffin/108g	402	22.6	372	4.4	41.6	20.9	0.0
MUSHROOMS								
Breaded, Pizza Hut*	6 Mushrooms/179g	410	14.4	228	4.5	26.1	8.0	0.0
Garlic, Crispy Coated, Pizza Hut*	1 Portion/135g	240	10.1	178	4.1	23.4	7.5	0.0
Garlic, with BBQ Dip, Pizza Hut*	1 Portion/112.2g	264	11.3	234	6.2	30.5	10.0	3.4
Garlic, with Sour Cream & Chive Dip, Pizza Hut*	1 Portion/112.2g	429	34.8	380	6.4	20.0	30.8	3.4
NACHOS								
Pizza Hut*	1 Serving/153g	448	30.9	293	7.6	20.7	20.2	0.0
ONIONS								
White, Pizza Hut*	1 Serving/24g	10	0.0	42	1.0	10.0	0.0	0.0
PASTA								
Ham & Mushroom, Pizza Hut*	1 Serving/450g	473	10.4	105	4.2	17.0	2.3	0.0
PASTA SALAD								
Sweetcorn & Pepper, Pizza Hut*	1 Serving/50g	75	2.5	159	4.6	23.1	5.3	0.0
Tomato & Basil, Pizza Hut*	1 Serving/50g	50	0.8	100	3.7	17.8	1.5	0.0
PENNE								
Mediterranean Vegetable, Pizza Hut*	1 Portion/450g	592	19.7	132	3.7	18.3	4.4	0.0
PEPPERS								
Red & Green Wedges, Pizza Hut*	1 Serving/40g	6	0.1	15	0.8	2.6	0.3	0.0
PIE								
Banoffee, Pizza Hut*	1 Serving/125g	428	25.3	340	2.5	37.3	20.1	0.0

PIZZA HUT

PIZZA

INFO/WEIGHT	Measure	per Measure		Nutrition Values per 100g / 100ml				
		KCAL	FAT	KCAL	PROT	CARB	FAT	FIBRE
BBQ Deluxe, Cheesy Bites, Pizza Hut*	1 Slice/155g	400	13.8	258	13.0	31.4	8.9	0.0
BBQ Deluxe, Italian, Individual, Pizza Hut*	1 Slice/79g	179	2.8	225	11.4	37.0	3.5	0.0
BBQ Deluxe, Italian, Large, Pizza Hut*	1 Slice/94g	239	8.0	252	14.3	29.7	8.4	0.0
BBQ Deluxe, Italian, Medium, Pizza Hut*	1 Slice/104g	253	8.0	241	12.0	31.1	7.6	0.0
BBQ Deluxe, Pan, Individual, Pizza Hut*	1 Slice/79g	200	7.9	253	12.7	28.0	10.0	0.0
BBQ Deluxe, Pan, Large, Pizza Hut*	1 Slice/121g	306	14.8	251	11.8	28.6	12.1	0.0
BBQ Deluxe, Pan, Medium, Pizza Hut*	1 Slice/107g	276	11.3	257	11.7	28.8	10.5	0.0
BBQ Deluxe, Stuffed Crust, Pizza Hut*	1 Slice/151g	365	13.0	241	14.7	26.1	8.6	0.0
Cajun Chicken, Hot One, Italian, Medium, Pizza Hut*	1 Slice/100g	250	9.3	250	12.5	29.1	9.3	0.0
Cajun Chicken, Hot One, Pan, Large, Pizza Hut*	1 Slice/125g	321	14.7	257	12.9	24.7	11.8	0.0
Cajun Chicken, Hot One, Pan, Medium, Pizza Hut*	1 Slice/105g	273	12.3	259	12.7	25.6	11.7	0.0
Cajun Chicken, Hot One, Stuffed Crust, Pizza Hut*	1 Slice/135g	331	10.8	245	13.3	30.0	8.0	0.0
Cheese Feast, Italian, Medium, Pizza Hut*	1 Slice/96g	260	11.3	272	12.3	29.1	11.8	0.0
Cheese Feast, Pan, Medium, Pizza Hut*	1 Slice/106g	299	15.0	283	14.6	24.2	14.2	0.0
Cheese Feast, Stuffed Crust, Pizza Hut*	1 Slice/132g	361	13.8	273	14.3	30.5	10.4	0.0
Chicken Feast, Italian, Medium, Pizza Hut*	1 Slice/100g	249	8.6	248	14.1	28.6	8.6	0.0
Chicken Feast, Pan, Medium, Pizza Hut*	1 Slice/110g	283	12.0	259	15.5	24.6	11.0	0.0
Chicken Feast, Stuffed Crust, Pizza Hut*	1 Slice/133g	337	12.6	254	14.8	27.3	9.5	0.0
Chicken Supreme, Cheesy Bites, Pizza Hut*	1 Slice/155g	370	12.6	238	11.4	29.9	8.1	0.0
Chicken Supreme, Italian, Individual, Pizza Hut*	1 Slice/77g	169	3.6	218	10.9	33.2	4.6	0.0
Chicken Supreme, Italian, Large, Pizza Hut*	1 Slice/99g	216	7.4	217	10.5	27.1	7.4	0.0
Chicken Supreme, Italian, Medium, Pizza Hut*	1 Slice/110g	232	7.2	210	10.9	26.9	6.5	0.0
Chicken Supreme, Pan, Individual, Pizza Hut*	1 Slice/79g	190	7.4	240	11.5	27.4	9.4	0.0
Chicken Supreme, Pan, Large, Pizza Hut*	1 Slice/129g	288	11.6	223	10.5	24.9	9.0	0.0
Chicken Supreme, Pan, Medium, Pizza Hut*	1 Slice/108g	247	10.2	227	11.0	24.6	9.4	0.0
Chicken Supreme, Stuffed Crust, Pizza Hut*	1 Slice/153g	337	18.0	219	11.4	26.3	11.7	0.0
Chicken, Hi Light, Medium, Pizza Hut*	1 Slice/83g	189	5.5	230	13.2	29.2	6.7	0.0
Country Feast, Italian, Medium, Pizza Hut*	1 Slice/109g	252	9.6	232	9.7	28.6	8.8	0.0
Country Feast, Pan, Medium, Pizza Hut*	1 Slice/114.8g	279	12.1	243	11.4	25.8	10.5	0.0
Country Feast, Stuffed Crust, Pizza Hut*	1 Slice/144g	326	10.8	227	11.5	28.4	7.5	0.0
Farmhouse, Cheesy Bites, Pizza Hut*	1 Slice/139g	374	13.5	269	16.5	28.9	9.7	0.0
Farmhouse, Hi Light, Medium, Pizza Hut*	1 Slice/82g	184	5.5	225	12.1	29.1	6.7	0.0
Farmhouse, Italian, Individual, Pizza Hut*	1 Slice/74g	188	6.0	253	11.0	33.1	8.1	0.0
Farmhouse, Italian, Large, Pizza Hut*	1 Slice/100g	243	7.5	244	12.9	31.2	7.5	0.0
Farmhouse, Italian, Medium, Pizza Hut*	1 Slice/97g	239	8.0	248	12.0	31.4	8.3	0.0
Farmhouse, Pan, Individual, Pizza Hut*	1 Slice/76g	184	7.2	241	12.1	27.1	9.4	0.0
Farmhouse, Pan, Large, Pizza Hut*	1 Slice/115g	261	9.2	226	13.0	25.4	8.0	0.0
Farmhouse, Pan, Medium, Pizza Hut*	1 Slice/98g	240	9.6	243	11.2	27.7	9.7	0.0
Farmhouse, Stuffed Crust, Pizza Hut*	1 Slice/139g	335	10.8	241	11.1	31.7	7.8	0.0
Ham, Hi Light, Medium, Pizza Hut*	1 Slice/82g	184	5.5	225	12.1	29.1	6.7	0.0
Hawaiian, Cheesy Bites, Pizza Hut*	1 Slice/143g	348	10.8	242	11.3	32.2	7.5	0.0
Hawaiian, Italian, Individual, Pizza Hut*	1 Slice/76g	193	6.5	251	13.1	30.8	8.4	0.0
Hawaiian, Italian, Large, Pizza Hut*	1 Slice/102g	250	8.2	245	12.2	31.1	8.0	0.0
Hawaiian, Italian, Medium, Pizza Hut*	1 Slice/99g	245	7.8	248	11.9	32.3	7.9	0.0
Hawaiian, Pan, Individual, Pizza Hut*	1 Slice/76g	184	7.2	241	12.1	27.1	9.4	0.0
Hawaiian, Pan, Large, Pizza Hut*	1 Slice/121g	276	11.0	228	12.0	24.4	9.1	0.0
Hawaiian, Pan, Medium, Pizza Hut*	1 Slice/96g	223	9.4	232	11.6	24.4	9.8	0.0
Hawaiian, Stuffed Crust, Pizza Hut*	1 Slice/149g	348	11.5	233	12.8	28.2	7.7	0.0
Hot 'n' Spicy, Cheesy Bites, Pizza Hut*	1 Slice/139g	392	15.3	282	10.7	35.0	11.0	0.0
Hot 'n' Spicy, Italian, Individual, Pizza Hut*	1 Slice/67g	186	7.1	277	11.9	33.4	10.6	0.0
Hot 'n' Spicy, Italian, Large, Pizza Hut*	1 Slice/94g	265	10.8	280	17.5	26.9	11.4	0.0
Hot 'n' Spicy, Italian, Medium, Pizza Hut*	1 Slice/88g	239	9.2	270	9.7	34.3	10.4	0.0

PIZZA HUT

PIZZA

	Measure INFO/WEIGHT	per Measure KCAL	FAT	Nutrition Values per 100g / 100ml KCAL	PROT	CARB	FAT	FIBRE
Hot 'n' Spicy, Pan, Individual, Pizza Hut*	1 Slice/65g	189	9.0	289	12.2	29.3	13.7	0.0
Hot 'n' Spicy, Pan, Large, Pizza Hut*	1 Slice/108g	291	13.1	269	11.1	28.9	12.1	0.0
Hot 'n' Spicy, Pan, Medium, Pizza Hut*	1 Slice/93g	255	10.7	274	10.8	31.7	11.5	0.0
Hot 'n' Spicy, Stuffed Crust, Pizza Hut*	1 Slice/139g	367	13.0	263	11.6	33.3	9.3	0.0
Margherita, Cheesy Bites, Pizza Hut*	1 Slice/133g	364	13.7	273	12.0	33.0	10.3	0.0
Margherita, Italian, Individual, Pizza Hut*	1 Slice/76g	217	7.9	284	13.0	34.7	10.4	0.0
Margherita, Italian, Large, Pizza Hut*	1 Slice/98g	274	9.8	280	15.1	32.3	10.0	0.0
Margherita, Italian, Medium, Pizza Hut*	1 Slice/95g	257	9.6	270	11.7	33.0	10.1	0.0
Margherita, Pan, Individual, Pizza Hut*	1 Slice/76g	202	8.4	265	13.2	28.4	11.0	0.0
Margherita, Pan, Medium, Pizza Hut*	1 Slice/85g	243	12.1	286	14.6	25.0	14.2	0.0
Margherita, Stuffed Crust, Pizza Hut*	1 Slice/140g	355	14.4	252	12.2	27.9	10.2	0.0
Meat Feast, Cheesy Bites, Pizza Hut*	1 Slice/155g	404	17.2	260	12.9	27.0	11.1	0.0
Meat Feast, Italian, Individual, Pizza Hut*	1 Slice/89g	247	10.5	279	13.8	29.1	11.9	0.0
Meat Feast, Italian, Large, Pizza Hut*	1 Slice/124g	334	15.1	269	12.8	26.9	12.2	0.0
Meat Feast, Italian, Medium, Pizza Hut*	1 Slice/104g	301	13.1	290	12.3	31.9	12.6	0.0
Meat Feast, Pan, Individual, Pizza Hut*	1 Slice/82g	233	11.8	281	14.3	24.0	14.2	0.0
Meat Feast, Pan, Large, Pizza Hut*	1 Slice/143.3g	384	20.5	268	15.6	19.1	14.3	0.0
Meat Feast, Pan, Medium, Pizza Hut*	1 Slice/114g	327	17.2	287	15.0	22.7	15.1	0.0
Meat Feast, Stuffed Crust, Pizza Hut*	1 Slice/159g	377	18.6	237	12.3	30.3	11.7	0.0
Meaty, The Edge, Medium, Pizza Hut*	1 Slice/36g	110	5.8	308	17.0	20.4	16.1	0.0
Mediterranean Meat Feast, Cheesy Bites, Pizza Hut*	1 Slice/147g	417	17.2	282	13.3	31.2	11.6	0.0
Mediterranean Meat Feast, Italian, Individual, Pizza Hut*	1 Slice/77g	226	10.1	291	15.2	28.3	13.0	0.0
Mediterranean Meat Feast, Italian, Large, Pizza Hut*	1 Slice/104g	291	13.0	279	11.1	30.6	12.5	0.0
Mediterranean Meat Feast, Italian, Medium, Pizza Hut*	1 Slice/100g	295	12.8	294	12.5	32.2	12.8	0.0
Mediterranean Meat Feast, Pan, Individual, Pizza Hut*	1 Slice/79g	238	12.0	299	18.2	22.5	15.1	0.0
Mediterranean Meat Feast, Pan, Large, Pizza Hut*	1 Slice/117g	506	20.9	285	13.1	31.6	11.8	0.0
Mediterranean Meat Feast, Pan, Medium, Pizza Hut*	1 Slice/104g	297	13.9	284	13.1	27.9	13.3	0.0
Meditterranean Meat Feast, Stuffed Crust, Pizza Hut*	1 Slice/146g	397	16.4	271	13.6	28.9	11.2	0.0
Mountain Fantastico, Cheesy Bites, Pizza Hut*	1 Slice/135g	339	10.8	250	14.6	29.9	8.0	0.0
Mountain Fantastico, Italian, Individual, Pizza Hut*	1 Slice/74g	174	6.5	234	12.8	26.2	8.7	0.0
Mountain Fantastico, Italian, Large, Pizza Hut*	1 Slice/98g	231	7.1	234	13.5	28.9	7.2	0.0
Mountain Fantastico, Italian, Medium, Pizza Hut*	1 Slice/93g	227	7.2	242	8.0	35.2	7.7	0.0
Mountain Fantastico, Pan, Individual, Pizza Hut*	1 Slice/78g	197	8.7	250	13.3	24.3	11.1	0.0
Mountain Fantastico, Pan, Large, Pizza Hut*	1 Slice/116g	294	12.8	252	13.9	24.4	11.0	0.0
Mountain Fantastico, Pan, Medium, Pizza Hut*	1 Slice/99g	234	10.2	235	12.8	23.0	10.2	0.0
Mountain Fantastico, Stuffed Crust, Pizza Hut*	1 Slice/143g	338	12.2	236	9.5	30.3	8.5	0.0
Pepperoni Feast, Cheesy Bites, Pizza Hut*	1 Slice/144g	407	16.8	281	14.4	29.8	11.6	0.0
Pepperoni Feast, Italian, Individual, Pizza Hut*	1 Slice/85.8g	259	12.5	302	15.3	27.4	14.6	0.0
Pepperoni Feast, Italian, Large, Pizza Hut*	1 Slice/115g	327	15.8	284	14.0	26.2	13.7	0.0
Pepperoni Feast, Italian, Medium, Pizza Hut*	1 Slice/105g	306	15.0	293	15.2	25.7	14.4	0.0
Pepperoni Feast, Pan, Individual, Pizza Hut*	1 Slice/81g	235	11.8	290	16.5	23.1	14.6	0.0
Pepperoni Feast, Pan, Large, Pizza Hut*	1 Pizza/800g	2336	120.8	292	13.5	25.4	15.1	0.0
Pepperoni Feast, Pan, Medium, Pizza Hut*	1 Slice/117g	352	19.5	302	14.4	23.4	16.7	0.0
Pepperoni Feast, Stuffed Crust, Pizza Hut*	1 Slice/154g	432	18.4	279	11.1	31.8	11.9	0.0
Seafood Fantastico, Italian, Individual, Pizza Hut*	1 Slice/81g	173	4.6	213	15.3	25.1	5.7	0.0
Seafood Fantastico, Italian, Large, Pizza Hut*	1 Slice/106g	228	6.6	215	15.1	24.6	6.2	0.0
Seafood Lovers, Cheesy Bites, Pizza Hut*	1 Slice/141g	388	14.3	275	11.9	34.2	10.1	0.0
Seafood Lovers, Italian, Individual, Pizza Hut*	1 Slice/68g	164	3.6	241	9.3	38.9	5.3	1.0
Seafood Lovers, Italian, Large, Pizza Hut*	1 Slice/95g	239	8.6	249	10.9	31.0	9.0	0.0
Seafood Lovers, Italian, Medium, Pizza Hut*	1 Slice/91g	233	8.1	254	9.9	33.9	8.8	0.0
Seafood Lovers, Pan, Individual, Pizza Hut*	1 Slice/73g	198	8.6	268	9.8	31.1	11.6	0.0
Seafood Lovers, Pan, Large, Pizza Hut*	1 Slice/108g	286	11.9	263	11.8	29.4	10.9	0.0

PIZZA HUT

	Measure INFO/WEIGHT	per Measure KCAL	FAT	Nutrition Values per 100g / 100ml KCAL	PROT	CARB	FAT	FIBRE
PIZZA								
Seafood Lovers, Pan, Medium, Pizza Hut*	1 Slice/93g	243	10.7	261	9.3	30.0	11.5	0.0
Seafood Lovers, Stuffed Crust, Pizza Hut*	1 Slice/136g	337	11.1	246	11.8	31.4	8.1	0.0
Spicy, Hot One, Italian, Individual, Pizza Hut*	1 Slice/88g	213	8.1	243	11.3	28.7	9.2	0.0
Spicy, Hot One, Italian, Large, Pizza Hut*	1 Slice/114g	270	10.1	236	10.1	29.2	8.8	0.0
Spicy, Hot One, Italian, Medium, Pizza Hut*	1 Slice/116g	299	11.4	258	11.3	31.1	9.8	0.0
Spicy, Hot One, Pan, Medium, Pizza Hut*	1 Slice/115g	274	13.0	239	11.2	23.1	11.3	0.0
Spicy, Hot One, Stuffed Crust, Pizza Hut*	1 Slice/141g	352	13.6	249	13.0	27.6	9.6	0.0
Super Supreme, Cheesy Bites, Pizza Hut*	1 Slice/167g	438	16.1	261	12.2	31.5	9.6	0.0
Super Supreme, Italian, Individual, Pizza Hut*	1 Slice/97g	260	11.0	267	13.9	27.3	11.3	0.0
Super Supreme, Italian, Large, Pizza Hut*	1 Slice/132g	339	16.6	256	12.4	23.5	12.5	0.0
Super Supreme, Italian, Medium, Pizza Hut*	1 Slice/129g	327	14.5	254	14.8	23.3	11.3	0.0
Super Supreme, Pan, Individual, Pizza Hut*	1 Slice/94g	234	11.1	250	12.4	23.2	11.9	0.0
Super Supreme, Pan, Medium, Pizza Hut*	1 Slice/130g	331	16.5	253	13.0	21.8	12.6	0.0
Super Supreme, Stuffed Crust, Pizza Hut*	1 Slice/178g	430	15.5	241	11.7	29.0	8.7	0.0
Supreme, Cheesy Bites, Pizza Hut*	1 Slice/150g	368	14.5	244	11.1	28.4	9.6	0.0
Supreme, Italian, Individual, Pizza Hut*	1 Slice/87g	221	9.4	253	11.2	27.7	10.8	0.0
Supreme, Italian, Large, Pizza Hut*	1 Slice/114g	297	13.2	259	13.2	25.6	11.5	0.0
Supreme, Italian, Medium, Pizza Hut*	1 Slice/106g	277	11.3	261	12.2	28.9	10.7	0.0
Supreme, Pan, Individual, Pizza Hut*	1 Slice/83g	222	10.0	265	12.9	25.9	11.9	0.0
Supreme, Pan, Large, Pizza Hut*	1 Slice/131g	365	19.2	277	12.4	24.0	14.6	0.0
Supreme, Pan, Medium, Pizza Hut*	1 Slice/105.7g	282	14.0	266	12.5	24.4	13.2	0.0
Supreme, Stuffed Crust, Pizza Hut*	1 Slice/156g	389	14.9	248	10.1	30.4	9.5	0.0
The Works, The Edge, Medium, Pizza Hut*	1 Slice/64g	150	6.7	235	12.7	19.5	10.4	0.0
Vegetable Supreme, Cheesy Bites, Pizza Hut*	1 Slice/137g	348	11.8	254	10.8	33.4	8.6	0.0
Vegetable Supreme, Italian, Individual, Pizza Hut*	1 Slice/81g	188	5.6	233	9.5	33.0	7.0	0.0
Vegetable Supreme, Italian, Large, Pizza Hut*	1 Slice/102g	232	8.2	227	12.0	26.8	8.0	0.0
Vegetable Supreme, Italian, Medium, Pizza Hut*	1 Slice/102.6g	236	7.9	230	10.3	29.9	7.7	0.0
Vegetable Supreme, Pan, Individual, Pizza Hut*	1 Slice/77.6g	191	7.8	246	10.7	28.2	10.0	0.0
Vegetable Supreme, Pan, Large, Pizza Hut*	1 Slice/122g	297	13.3	242	10.9	25.2	10.8	0.0
Vegetable Supreme, Pan, Medium, Pizza Hut*	1 Slice/105g	266	12.0	254	11.5	26.0	11.5	0.0
Vegetable Supreme, Stuffed Crust, Pizza Hut*	1 Slice/163g	337	10.8	206	9.0	27.6	6.6	0.0
Vegetarian Hot One, Cheesy Bites, Pizza Hut*	1 Slice/145g	352	12.5	242	13.0	28.1	8.6	0.0
Vegetarian Hot One, Italian, Individual, Pizza Hut*	1 Slice/82g	193	7.4	236	10.2	28.3	9.1	0.0
Vegetarian Hot One, Italian, Large, Pizza Hut*	1 Slice/107g	238	8.1	222	10.9	27.6	7.6	0.0
Vegetarian Hot One, Italian, Medium, Pizza Hut*	1 Slice/104g	248	8.2	238	10.3	31.5	7.9	0.0
Vegetarian Hot One, Pan, Individual, Pizza Hut*	1 Slice/79g	191	7.8	241	10.6	27.7	9.8	0.0
Vegetarian Hot One, Pan, Large, Pizza Hut*	1 Slice/124g	282	11.9	227	10.3	24.8	9.6	0.0
Vegetarian Hot One, Pan, Medium, Pizza Hut*	1 Slice/110g	265	11.4	242	11.0	26.0	10.4	0.0
Vegetarian Hot One, Stuffed Crust, Pizza Hut*	1 Slice/157g	333	11.2	211	10.1	26.6	7.1	0.0
Vegetarian, Hi Light, Medium, Pizza Hut*	1 Slice/80g	170	5.1	221	10.3	30.0	6.6	0.0
Veggie, The Edge, Medium, Pizza Hut*	1 Slice/60g	136	5.4	227	11.2	22.2	9.0	0.0
POTATO SKINS								
Jacket, Loaded, with Cheese, Pizza Hut*	1 Portion/267g	571	34.2	214	13.6	11.2	12.8	0.0
Jacket, Pizza Hut*	1 Portion/ 223.5g	571	37.2	255	3.4	23.0	16.6	2.1
Jacket, with Sour Cream & Chive Dip, Pizza Hut*	1 Portion/223.5g	311	24.2	139	1.4	9.3	10.8	0.8
POTATO WEDGES								
Pizza Hut*	1 Portion/224g	329	13.9	147	2.1	20.8	6.2	0.0
PROFITEROLES								
Pizza Hut*	1 Serving/100g	381	31.3	381	4.6	20.1	31.3	0.0
PUDDING								
Sticky Toffee, Pizza Hut*	1 Serving/105.3g	400	18.2	380	5.5	50.6	17.3	0.0

	Measure INFO/WEIGHT	per Measure KCAL	per Measure FAT	Nutrition Values per 100g / 100ml KCAL	PROT	CARB	FAT	FIBRE
PIZZA HUT								
RAISINS								
Chocolate, Pizza Hut*	1 Serving/30g	122	4.3	405	5.4	63.3	14.2	0.0
SALAD								
4 Leaf Mix, Pizza Hut*	1 Serving/100g	14	0.5	14	0.8	1.7	0.5	0.0
Caesar, Pizza Hut*	1 Salad/195g	344	20.2	177	6.0	14.8	10.4	0.0
Chicken & Bacon, Pizza Hut*	1 Serving/323g	514	32.0	159	10.3	6.9	9.9	0.0
Chicken Caesar, Pizza Hut*	1 Salad/174g	296	14.8	170	11.5	11.7	8.5	0.0
Leaf Mix, Pizza Hut*	1 Serving/40g	7	0.5	17	2.9	6.3	1.1	0.0
Potato, Whole, Pizza Hut*	1 Serving/100g	154	10.1	154	1.6	13.5	10.1	0.0
Tuna, Pizza Hut*	1 Portion/461g	378	8.8	82	10.4	5.9	1.9	2.0
Warm Chicken, Pizza Hut*	1 Salad/341g	403	17.4	118	11.0	6.8	5.1	0.0
SAUCE								
Caramel, Pizza Hut*	1 Serving/25g	77	1.0	307	0.7	67.2	3.9	0.0
Chocolate, Pizza Hut*	1 Serving/25g	75	0.6	298	2.0	66.8	2.5	0.0
Lemon, Pizza Hut*	1 Serving/25g	70	0.0	280	0.1	69.0	0.0	0.0
Strawberry, Pizza Hut*	1 Serving/25g	70	0.0	280	0.0	69.5	0.0	0.0
SPAGHETTI BOLOGNAISE								
Pizza Hut*	1 Portion/475g	745	31.3	157	6.2	17.8	6.6	0.0
SUNDAE								
Double Chocolate, Pizza Hut*	1 Sundae/145g	307	16.2	212	3.1	27.0	11.2	0.0
SWEETCORN								
Pizza Hut*	1 Serving/30g	24	0.2	79	1.8	16.8	0.8	0.0
TAGLIATELLE								
Carbonara, Pizza Hut*	1 Potion/475g	908	51.8	191	5.7	17.6	10.9	0.0
PRET A MANGER								
BAGUETTE								
Beef & Rocket, Artisan, Pret a Manger*	1 Roll/247.6g	619	22.0	250	14.8	27.6	8.9	2.1
Brie, Tomato & Basil, Pret a Manger*	1 Pack/200g	407	15.6	203	9.3	23.9	7.8	0.3
Cheddar & Pickle, Artisan, Posh, Pret a Manger*	1 Baguette/295.5g	779	38.9	264	10.1	25.9	13.2	1.8
Cheddar, & Baby Plum Tomato, Pret a Manger*	1 Pack/300g	625	35.8	208	6.7	18.5	11.9	1.0
Cheese, Kids, Pret a Manger*	1 Pack/105g	329	15.9	313	11.1	29.9	15.1	0.5
Egg Mayo & Bacon, Breakfast, Pret a Manger*	1 Baguette/137g	372	19.9	270	11.9	22.8	14.5	0.2
Egg Mayo & Roasted Tomato, Breakfast, Pret a Manger*	1 Pack/151.6g	352	18.0	232	8.1	23.1	11.9	0.1
Egg, & Salmon, Pret a Manger*	1 Pack/230g	527	24.0	229	10.9	23.0	10.4	2.2
Egg, & Tomato, Pret a Manger*	1 Pack/157g	291	10.7	185	8.1	22.8	6.8	0.7
Ham, Dry Cured & Greve, Pret a Manger*	1 Baguette/225.1g	543	24.5	241	12.3	21.9	10.9	0.3
Ham, Kids, Pret a Manger*	1 Pack/118g	308	13.7	261	12.4	26.8	11.6	0.0
Italian Prosciutti Artisan, Pret a Manger*	1 Baguette/288g	636	28.5	221	9.3	23.5	9.9	2.0
Prosciutto Capreze, Pret a Manger*	1 Pack/255.2g	699	32.9	274	12.6	27.0	12.9	1.9
Salmon, Egg Mayo & Cress, Breakfast, Pret a Manger*	1 Baguette/152g	349	17.7	229	10.6	20.5	11.6	1.2
Tuna Mayonnaise, Pret a Manger*	1 Pack/230g	535	22.9	233	10.8	25.0	10.0	1.7
Tuna, & Salad, Pret a Manger*	1 Pack/227g	506	24.3	223	10.0	21.7	10.7	0.9
Tuna, Dolphin Friendly, Pret a Manger*	1 Baguette/209.7g	474	21.6	226	9.7	22.7	10.3	1.3
BARS								
Choc, Pret a Manger*	1 Bar/105g	555	38.6	529	5.0	44.3	36.8	2.6
Fruit Goodness, Pret a Manger*	1 Bar/70g	286	16.8	408	6.8	41.3	24.0	0.0
Love, Pret a Manger*	1 Bar/72g	324	18.3	450	5.9	49.2	25.4	0.0
Power, Pret a Manger*	1 Bar/65g	265	15.6	408	6.8	41.4	24.0	6.2
BREAKFAST								
Bowl, All Day Breakfast, Pret a Manger*	1 Bowl/220.2g	363	15.1	165	5.2	19.4	6.9	1.2
Bowl, Gooseberry, Pret a Manger*	1 Bowl/216.6g	386	12.1	178	6.6	25.2	5.6	1.7
Bowl, Scottish Raspberry, Pret a Manger*	1 Pack/214g	372	12.2	174	6.7	24.1	5.7	1.7
Bowl, Strawberry, Wild, Pret a Manger*	1 Bowl/214g	364	12.2	170	6.6	23.1	5.7	1.6

PRET A MANGER

	Measure INFO/WEIGHT	per Measure KCAL	FAT	Nutrition Values per 100g / 100ml KCAL	PROT	CARB	FAT	FIBRE
BREAKFAST								
Bowl, Very Berry, Pret a Manger*	1 Bowl/218g	368	15.1	169	5.2	20.3	6.9	1.4
BREAKFAST CEREAL								
Granola, Hot & Warming, Pret a Manger*	1 Pack/226g	579	19.9	256	6.4	38.4	8.8	3.5
BROWNIE								
Chocolate, Pret a Manger*	1 Brownie/60g	267	15.7	445	4.7	47.7	26.2	1.5

PRET A MANGER

	Measure INFO/WEIGHT	per Measure KCAL	FAT	Nutrition Values per 100g / 100ml KCAL	PROT	CARB	FAT	FIBRE
CAKE								
Apple, Card Box, Pret a Manger*	1 Pack/116g	356	17.1	307	3.9	39.6	14.7	1.8
Apple, Pret a Manger*	1 Pack/120g	432	26.3	360	5.3	38.8	21.9	2.1
Banana, Card Box, Pret a Manger*	1 Pack/103g	345	18.3	335	4.6	39.0	17.8	1.9
Carrot, Card Box, Pret a Manger*	1 Pack/112g	402	22.3	359	4.0	41.0	19.9	2.3
Carrot, Pret a Manger*	1 Pack/120g	288	8.3	240	2.9	41.6	6.9	0.2
Chocolate, Card Box, Pret a Manger*	1 Cake/88g	354	20.9	402	5.3	41.7	23.8	1.4
Fudge, Pret a Manger*	1 Pack/140g	537	28.4	384	4.1	46.1	20.3	1.3
Lemon, Card Box, Pret a Manger*	1 Cake/97g	318	14.7	328	5.0	42.8	15.2	0.9
Lemon, Card Cake, Pret a Manger*	1 Pack/97g	318	14.7	328	5.0	42.8	15.2	0.9
Nut Munch, Pret a Manger*	1 Pack/100g	497	34.6	497	8.0	38.5	34.6	7.9
Orange, The Amazing Wheatfree, Pret a Manger*	1 Pack/90g	326	16.0	362	10.2	40.9	17.8	3.8
CHEESECAKE								
Caramel Crunch, Pret a Manger*	1 Serving/105g	395	31.6	376	5.3	21.1	30.1	1.2
Lemon, Pret a Manger*	1 Serving/95g	376	28.8	396	4.3	26.4	30.3	0.6
CHERRIES								
Summer, Pret a Manger*	1 Pot/150g	60	0.2	40	0.8	9.0	0.1	1.8
CHOCOLATE								
Milk, Organic, Pret a Manger*	1 Bar/40g	216	12.8	540	9.5	54.0	32.0	0.0
Plain, Organic, Pret a Manger*	1 Bar/40g	230	16.2	575	7.5	45.5	40.5	0.0
White, Organic, Pret a Manger*	1 Bar/40g	230	15.0	575	7.5	52.5	37.5	0.0
COFFEE								
Cappuccino, Chocolate, Pret a Manger*	1 Serving/340g	106	5.8	31	1.7	2.2	1.7	0.0
Cappuccino, Chocolate, Tall, Pret a Manger*	1 Serving/355ml	106	5.8	30	1.7	2.1	1.6	0.0
Cappuccino, Full-Fat Milk, No Chocolate, Pret a Manger*	1 Serving/355ml	102	5.8	29	1.7	1.9	1.6	0.0
Cappuccino, Toffee, Pret a Manger*	1 Serving/355ml	187	6.9	53	1.6	7.2	1.9	0.0
Latte, Pret a Manger*	1 Serving/340ml	194	11.2	57	3.1	3.9	3.3	0.0
Latte, Toffee, Pret a Manger*	1 Latte/247g	205	8.1	83	2.6	10.9	3.3	0.0
Mocha, Pret a Manger*	1 Serving/340g	233	10.9	68	2.7	7.3	3.2	0.0
Mocha, Skimmed Milk, Pret a Manger*	1 Serving/340ml	91	0.8	27	2.6	3.6	0.2	0.0
CRISP								
Spicy Piri Chilli, Pret a Manger*	1 Pack/40g	190	10.1	475	5.3	56.8	25.3	5.3
Cheddar & Chive, Pret a Manger*	1 Bag/40g	187	9.9	468	7.0	53.8	24.8	6.0
Cheddar & Red Onion, Croxton Manor, Pret a Manger*	1 Bag/40g	181	9.9	453	6.5	50.5	24.8	7.0
Cider Vinegar & Sea Salt, Organic, Pret a Manger*	1 Bag/40g	178	9.6	445	5.3	51.9	24.1	0.0
Crispy Seaweed & Miso, Pret a Manger*	1 Bag/40g	179	9.8	448	6.5	50.5	24.5	5.8
Lightly Salted, Pret a Manger*	1 Bag/40g	198	11.4	495	5.8	58.0	28.5	4.3
Maldon Sea Salt, Pret a Manger*	1 Pack/40g	184	10.2	460	5.5	51.1	25.4	0.0
Mature Cheddar, & Red Onion, Pret a Manger*	1 Bag/40g	196	10.0	490	6.0	60.0	25.0	5.0
Mediterranean Sea Salt, Pret a Manger*	1 Bag/40g	198	11.4	495	5.8	58.0	28.5	4.3
Parsnip, Pret a Manger*	1 Pack/50g	238	14.9	476	5.8	35.4	29.8	12.8
Pickled Onion, Pret a Manger*	1 Bag/40g	177	9.1	443	7.5	52.0	22.8	7.3
Salt & Vinegar, Pret a Manger*	1 Bag/40g	186	10.1	465	6.8	55.0	25.3	6.0
Sea Salt & Balsamic Vinegar, Pret a Manger*	1 Bag/40g	186	10.0	465	6.8	55.0	25.0	6.0
Sea Salt & Black Pepper, Pret a Manger*	1 Bag/40g	186	10.0	465	6.8	55.0	25.0	6.0
Sea Salt & Mixed Peppercorns, Pret a Manger*	1 Pack/40g	178	9.7	445	5.5	51.0	24.3	4.1

PRET A MANGER

	Measure INFO/WEIGHT	per Measure KCAL	FAT	Nutrition Values per 100g / 100ml KCAL	PROT	CARB	FAT	FIBRE
CRISPS								
Sweet Chilli, Pret a Manger*	1 Pack/40g	190	9.4	475	5.5	60.5	23.5	6.3
Vegetable, Pret a Manger*	1 Bag/25g	123	8.7	493	5.5	51.2	34.6	11.4
All Butter, Pret a Manger*	1 Croissant/80g	340	19.9	425	7.6	42.5	24.9	2.4
Almond, Pret a Manger*	1 Croissant/100g	365	21.1	365	8.8	34.9	21.1	1.1
CROISSANT								
Cheese & Tomato, Pret a Manger*	1 Croissant/111g	376	25.1	339	11.4	22.5	22.6	0.0
Chocolate, Pret a Manger*	1 Croissant/95g	364	20.4	383	5.4	42.3	21.5	0.8
Egg & Bacon, Pret a Manger*	1 Croissant/167g	483	20.1	289	11.3	20.6	12.0	1.8
Ham & Cheese, Pret a Manger*	1 Croissant/134g	441	26.8	329	13.3	21.4	20.0	2.2
Ham, Cheese & Smoked Bacon, Pret a Manger*	1 Croissant/100g	359	24.3	359	12.1	22.9	24.3	1.8
Ham, Cheese & Tomato, Pret a Manger*	1 Croissant/115g	337	21.1	293	11.7	19.6	18.4	0.0
Mozzarella & Tomato, Pret a Manger*	1 Croissant/110g	371	24.0	337	12.7	22.7	21.8	1.8
Plain, All Butter, Pret a Manger*	1 Croissant/80g	340	19.9	425	7.6	42.5	24.9	0.0
CRUMBLE								
Mincemeat Crumble, Pret a Manger*	1 Serving/70g	275	12.5	393	3.9	53.0	17.9	2.1
DANDELION & BURDOCK								
Pret a Manger*	1 Serving/100ml	27	0.0	27	0.0	7.1	0.0	0.0
DANISH PASTRY								
Cinnamon & Raisin, Pret a Manger*	1 Danish/85g	408	27.6	480	6.5	40.4	32.5	1.4
DESSERT								
Brownie, Pret Pot, Pret a Manger*	1 Pot/121g	201	10.0	166	5.7	17.7	8.3	0.7
DOUGHNUTS								
Mixed Berry, Pret a Manger*	1 Doughnut/47.5g	160	5.3	337	7.6	51.8	11.2	1.5
DRESSING								
French, Dijon, Pret a Manger*	1 Pot/48g	202	20.2	421	2.3	9.2	42.1	1.0
Sweet Chilli, Pret a Manger*	1 Pot/48g	87	5.5	182	3.8	16.9	11.5	0.2
DRIED FRUIT								
Nuts & Bolts, Pret a Manger*	1 Pack/120g	571	39.0	476	15.5	35.7	32.5	4.4
FALAFEL								
No Bread, Pret a Manger*	1 Pack/255.8g	369	28.4	144	3.8	7.3	11.1	1.5
FOOL								
Raspberry, Pret a Manger*	1 Pot/140g	188	12.4	134	1.7	12.4	8.9	0.4
FRUIT								
Berries & Cherries, Bag, Pret a Manger*	1 Bag/120g	334	0.9	278	2.2	70.4	0.8	3.8
Pot, British Berries, Pret a Manger*	1 Pot/130g	146	0.1	112	0.9	5.4	0.1	1.6
FRUIT BOWL								
British Berries, Pret a Manger*	1 Pack/130g	34	0.1	26	0.9	5.4	0.1	1.6
FRUIT SALAD								
Fresh, Pret a Manger*	1 Pack/250g	98	0.5	39	0.6	8.8	0.2	0.0
GINGER BEER								
Pure Pret, Pret a Manger*	1 Can/330ml	152	0.0	46	0.0	11.4	0.0	0.0
GOULASH								
Hungarian, Pret a Manger*	1 Serving/455g	240	7.6	53	3.2	6.7	1.7	1.2
GRAPES								
Pret a Manger*	1 Pack/130g	78	0.1	60	0.4	15.4	0.1	0.7
ICE CREAM								
Chocolate, Organic, Pret a Manger*	1 Serving/100ml	192	10.8	192	3.9	19.5	10.8	0.9
Vanilla, Organic, Pret a Manger*	1 Serving/100ml	156	9.5	156	3.3	14.3	9.5	0.1
White Chocolate & Caramel, Organic, Pret a Manger*	1 Serving/100ml	223	13.5	100	1.4	10.0	6.1	0.0
JUICE								
Apple, 100% Premium, Pret a Manger*	1 Serving/250ml	128	0.0	51	0.1	11.9	0.0	0.0

PRET A MANGER

INFO/WEIGHT	Measure KCAL	FAT	per Measure KCAL	PROT	CARB	FAT	FIBRE
JUICE							
Blue Bionic, Pret a Manger*	1 Serving/250g	170	3.5	68	2.9	11.3	1.4	1.8
Carrot, Freshly Pressed, Pret a Manger*	1 Serving/250ml	60	0.3	24	0.5	5.7	0.1	0.0
Orange, & Raspberry, Pret a Manger*	1 Serving/250g	110	0.0	44	0.7	10.0	0.0	0.0
Orange, Pret a Manger*	1 Serving/250ml	114	0.0	46	0.6	11.4	0.0	0.1
JUICE DRINK							
Mandarin & Lychee, Pret a Manger*	1 Bottle/250ml	103	0.0	41	0.7	9.5	0.0	0.1
Red Defence, Pure Pret, Pret a Manger*	1 Can/330ml	140	0.0	42	0.0	10.3	0.0	0.0
MANGO							
Dried, Pret a Manger*	1 Pack/60g	200	0.2	333	1.5	84.5	0.4	4.5
MELON							
Fruit Sticks, Pret a Manger*	1 Pack/200g	52	0.4	26	0.5	5.6	0.2	0.0
MILK							
Kids, Pret a Manger*	1 Serving/250g	170	10.0	68	3.4	4.7	4.0	0.0
MOUSSE							
Chocolate, Pret a Manger*	1 Pot/90g	338	26.3	376	3.3	24.6	29.2	1.2
MUFFIN							
Double Berry, Pret a Manger*	1 Muffin/140g	470	23.8	336	4.5	41.4	17.0	1.3
Morning Glory, Pret a Manger*	1 Muffin/140g	521	31.6	372	7.4	35.2	22.6	3.2
Orange, & Lemon, Pret a Manger*	1 Muffin/160g	603	28.2	377	4.9	38.1	17.6	1.1
Yoghurt & Pecan, Pret a Manger*	1 Muffin/140g	521	31.6	372	7.4	35.2	22.6	3.2
PANNACOTTA							
Mango & Passion Fruit, Pret a Manger*	1 Pot/110g	330	26.4	300	2.1	18.8	24.0	0.5
PIE							
Pecan, Pret a Manger*	1 Pie/80g	376	25.8	470	5.9	39.1	32.3	0.3
POPCORN							
Honey, Organic, Pret a Manger*	1 Bag/35g	157	6.1	449	4.0	75.7	17.4	6.3
Sea Salt, Organic, Pret a Manger*	1 Pack/35g	138	5.5	394	11.1	52.0	15.7	13.1
PRETZELS							
Plain, Sesame Or Poppy, Pret a Manger*	1 Pretzel/120g	371	7.8	309	10.9	51.6	6.5	2.5
SALAD							
Chicken Avocado, Pret a Manger*	1 Salad/311g	342	23.9	110	7.8	2.6	7.7	2.6
Chicken Provencal, No Bread, Pret a Manger*	1 Pack/288.4g	234	13.8	81	6.5	3.1	4.8	1.0
SALAD							
Chicken, Al Fresco, Pret a Manger*	1 Pack/287g	439	34.4	153	6.9	4.8	12.0	1.6
Crayfish, & Smoked Salmon, Pret a Manger*	1 Pack/230.40g	134	3.9	58	9.4	1.4	1.7	0.9
Crayfish, Pret a Manger*	1 Pack/320g	200	16.7	63	3.0	0.8	5.2	0.3
Houmous & Pitta Bread, Pot, Pret a Manger*	1 Pot/200g	393	28.8	197	4.8	12.0	14.4	3.4
Humous, Chunky, Pret a Manger*	1 Salad/268g	539	31.1	201	6.0	18.5	11.6	2.8
Pesto Pasta, Pret a Manger*	1 Pot/320g	425	34.1	133	2.7	6.9	10.7	0.9
Salmon, Smoked, with Wild Crayfish, Pret a Manger*	1 Pack 226.5g	125	3.9	55	8.6	1.2	1.7	1.0
Super Club, Pret a Manger*	1 Pack/200g	213	12.6	107	10.8	1.6	6.3	0.6
Tuna Nicoise, Pret a Manger*	1 Pack/300g	381	27.2	127	7.9	3.7	9.1	1.2
Tuna, Tricolore, No Dressing, Pret a Manger*	1 Serving/320.5g	240	11.5	75	9.2	1.5	3.6	1.3
SALAD BOWL							
Crayfish, with Sweet Chilli Dressing, Pret a Manger*	1 Bowl/243.5g	149	6.3	61	4.8	4.6	2.6	0.5
Houmous & Feta Salad, Pret a Manger*	1 Bowl/252g	399	26.2	158	6.1	10.2	10.4	1.6
Houmous & Feta, Pret a Manger*	1 Bowl/200g	422	34.0	211	5.8	9.1	17.0	1.5
Pasta, Basil, Pret a Manger*	1 Bowl/334.20g	629	36.8	188	4.4	17.7	11.0	0.8
Tuna, No Dressing, Dolphin Friendly, Pret a Manger*	1 Bowl/261.1g	178	6.8	68	9.2	2.3	2.6	1.4
SANDWICH							
All Day Breakfast, Pret a Manger*	1 Sandwich/306g	560	27.5	183	9.6	16.0	9.0	1.5
All Day Breakfast, Slim Pret, Pret a Manger*	1 Pack/148.9g	306	17.9	206	8.6	15.7	12.0	1.5

PRET A MANGER
SANDWICH

	INFO/WEIGHT	KCAL	FAT	KCAL	PROT	CARB	FAT	FIBRE
Avocado, & Alfalfa Sprout, Pret a Manger*	1 Pack/250g	329	20.0	132	3.4	11.6	8.0	2.4
Avocado, & Bacon, Pret a Manger*	1 Pack/286g	543	35.5	190	5.8	13.4	12.4	2.6
Avocado, & Italian Cheese Salad, Pret a Manger*	1 Pack/290g	552	36.6	190	5.7	13.4	12.6	2.7
Avocado, & Roasted Tomatoes, Pret a Manger*	1 Pack/300g	560	34.1	187	5.2	14.4	11.4	2.6
BLT, Beech Smoked, Slim Pret, Pret a Manger*	1 Sandwich/123g	248	14.4	200	8.5	15.4	11.6	1.7
BLT, Big, Pret a Manger*	1 Pack/200g	398	23.2	199	8.5	15.4	11.6	1.6
BLT, Slim, Pret a Manger*	1 Pack/123.9g	248	14.4	200	8.5	15.4	11.6	1.7
Beef, & Horseradish, Pret a Manger*	1 Pack/250g	382	10.9	153	11.2	17.7	4.4	2.5
Big Prawn, Pret a Manger*	1 Pack/208.6g	445	24.9	213	10.6	16.5	11.9	1.5
Brie & Roasted Tomato, Pret a Manger*	1 Pack/234.6g	530	30.0	226	8.3	17.2	12.8	1.5
Cheddar, Christmas, Pret a Manger*	1 Pack/270g	671	41.9	249	8.8	18.3	15.5	2.0
Cheddar, Roasted Tomatoes & Pickle, Pret a Manger*	1 Pack/301.4g	648	24.1	215	9.0	20.0	8.0	1.8
Cheese, Three, & Roasted Tomato, Pret a Manger*	1 Pack/350g	417	21.8	119	3.8	11.5	6.2	1.5
Chicken & Pepper Sauce, Special, Pret a Manger*	1 Pack/215.4g	397	17.9	184	10.1	17.5	8.3	1.9
Chicken & Whole-Leaf Basil, with Salad, Pret a Manger*	1 Pack/275.8g	480	22.6	174	10.1	15.1	8.2	1.8
Chicken Avocado, Pret a Manger*	1 Pack/250.7g	456	23.7	182	8.7	15.8	9.5	3.0
Chicken Caesar, Slim Pret, Pret a Manger*	1 Pack/135.4g	239	12.6	177	8.4	14.2	9.3	1.7
Chicken Ceaser, No Bread, Pret a Manger*	1 Pack/226.2g	360	27.1	159	8.6	2.6	12.0	1.0
Chicken Valentino, Pret a Manger*	1 Pack/271g	516	25.2	190	9.8	14.8	9.3	1.7
Chicken, & Basil Salad, Pret a Manger*	1 Pack/284.3g	576	34.9	203	9.7	13.6	12.3	1.8
Chicken, & Coriander, on Rye, Pret a Manger*	1 Pack/200g	500	27.8	250	10.8	22.1	13.9	2.0
Chicken, & Mango, Summer, Pret a Manger*	1 Pack/242g	486	20.1	201	10.7	20.9	8.3	2.1
Chicken, Black Pepper, Bloomer, Pret a Manger*	1 Pack/250g	642	24.2	257	13.0	29.5	9.7	1.8
Chicken, Caesar, Pret a Manger*	1 Pack/261.4g	429	20.4	164	8.5	14.5	7.8	1.7
Chicken, Charred Pepper, Yoghurt Dressing, Pret a Manger*	1 Pack/221.8g	466	21.3	210	13.0	17.9	9.6	2.5
Chicken, Coronation, Pret a Manger*	1 Pack/250g	415	13.6	166	7.9	21.2	5.4	0.2
Chicken, Devonshire Red, Free Range, Pret a Manger*	1 Sandwich/192g	504	27.5	262	14.2	19.2	14.3	1.5
Club, Caesar's, Pret a Manger*	1 Pack/284g	558	27.9	196	11.3	13.9	9.8	1.5
Club, Cheddar, Pret a Manger*	1 Pack/298g	641	41.4	215	8.9	13.7	13.9	1.6
Club, Pret a Manger*	1 Pack/250g	542	25.2	217	12.8	18.7	10.1	2.3
Club, Super, Pret a Manger*	1 Sandwich/226.9g	445	25.6	196	10.4	13.6	11.3	1.5
Club, Super, Slim Pret, Pret a Manger*	1 Pack/143.40g	290	17.4	202	10.3	13.6	12.1	1.6
Crayfish & Roacket, Wild, Slim Pret, Pret a Manger*	1 Sandwich/97g	185	8.6	190	8.3	19.4	8.8	1.6
Crayfish & Rocket, Pret a Manger*	1 Pack/194.9g	370	17.2	190	8.3	19.4	8.8	1.6
Crayfish & Rocket, Wild, Pret a Manger*	1 Sandwich/194g	370	17.2	190	8.3	19.4	8.8	1.6
Crayfish, & Avocado, No Bread, Pret a Manger*	1 Pack/241g	258	22.2	107	4.2	1.8	9.2	2.0
Crayfish, & White Crab, Pret a Manger*	1 Pack/250g	391	19.3	156	5.0	16.8	7.7	2.2
Duck & Mango, Special, Pret a Manger*	1 Pack/249g	376	20.2	151	7.8	15.8	8.1	1.7
Egg Florentine, Pret a Manger*	1 Sandwich/284g	504	27.6	177	8.1	14.1	9.7	1.5
Egg Mayonnaise, Pret a Manger*	1 Pack/250g	360	15.8	144	6.8	14.9	6.3	1.4
Egg, Bacon & Tomato, Free Range, Pret a Manger*	1 Sandwich/219g	522	28.8	238	11.8	18.1	13.1	1.5
Egg, Florentine, No Bread, Pret a Manger*	1 Pack/232g	263	18.4	113	5.7	4.9	7.9	0.7
Egg, Sunny, & Salad, Pret a Manger*	1 Sandwich/289g	488	27.2	169	7.0	14.1	9.4	1.4
Falafel, Spinach & Tomato, Pret a Manger*	1 Pack/271g	360	9.2	133	5.2	20.5	3.4	1.6
Grilled Peppers & Salad, Pret a Manger*	1 Pack/275.2g	421	21.7	153	5.1	15.5	7.9	2.3
Ham, & Egg Salad, Pret a Manger*	1 Pack/287.60	426	15.7	148	9.2	15.6	5.5	1.3
Ham, & Egg, Bloomer, Pret a Manger*	1 Pack/290g	476	26.1	164	6.0	19.0	9.0	0.0
Ham, & Salad, Summer, Pret a Manger*	1 Pack/285.5g	454	19.4	159	10.5	14.1	6.8	1.5
Ham, Cheese, & Pickle, Pret a Manger*	1 Pack/250g	592	27.6	237	11.9	25.0	11.0	2.4
Ham, Egg & Greve, Pret a Manger*	1 Pack/324.8g	552	26.6	170	11.5	12.7	8.2	1.4
Houmous Salad, Slim Pret, Pret a Manger*	1 Pack/128.30g	201	9.1	157	5.1	18.4	7.1	2.6
Houmous, & Oven Roasted Tomato, Pret a Manger*	1 Pack/350g	404	18.2	115	3.5	13.6	5.2	3.1

PRET A MANGER

	Measure INFO/WEIGHT	per Measure KCAL	FAT	Nutrition Values per 100g / 100ml KCAL	PROT	CARB	FAT	FIBRE
SANDWICH								
Houmous, & Roasted Peppers, Pret a Manger*	1 Pack/268.1g	477	24.9	178	5.5	18.4	9.3	3.1
Humous, & Roasted Peppers, Pret a Manger*	1 Sandwich/268g	477	24.9	178	5.5	18.4	9.3	3.1
Humous, & Roasted Tomatoes, Wheat Free, Pret a Manger*	1 Sandwich/280g	613	33.0	219	5.6	22.9	11.8	5.2
Lamb, Pea & Mint Relish, Roast, Pret a Manger*	1 Pack/250g	938	31.8	375	21.8	44.1	12.7	7.4
Mature Cheddar, & Pret Pickle, Pret a Manger*	1 Sandwich/281g	547	30.3	195	8.1	16.5	10.8	1.6
More Than Mozzarella, No Bread, Pret a Manger*	1 Pack/285.4g	377	31.4	132	5.7	2.7	11.0	1.9
More Than Mozzarella, Pret a Manger*	1 Sandwich/250g	508	29.5	203	9.3	15.0	11.8	1.6
New Tuna Salad, Slim Pret, Pret a Manger*	1 Pack/115g	234	12.7	202	1.0	16.2	11.0	2.3
Pastrami, Bloomer, Pret a Manger*	1 Pack/301g	434	14.8	144	7.1	18.1	4.9	2.5
Pastrami, on Rye, Pret a Manger*	1 Pack/200g	391	15.3	196	10.3	22.6	7.7	1.9
Prawn, & Rocket, Pret a Manger*	1 Pack/280g	435	19.4	155	8.4	14.9	6.9	1.3
Prawn, Gourmet, Pret a Manger*	1 Pack/250g	454	25.4	182	7.8	15.2	10.2	1.8
Prawn, with Yummy Yoghurt, Pret a Manger*	1 Pack/277g	282	5.8	102	7.5	13.6	2.1	1.4
Salmon, & Horseradish, Pret a Manger*	1 Pack/300g	462	20.2	154	9.0	14.2	6.7	1.8
Salmon, Really Wild, Pret a Manger*	1 Sandwich/265.5g	440	16.2	166	11.8	16.0	6.1	1.6
Salmon, Really Wild, Summer, Pret a Manger*	1 Sandwich/221g	473	24.3	214	12.0	17.0	11.0	1.6
Salmon, Smoked & Free Range Egg, Pret a Manger*	1 Pack/231.8g	438	18.3	189	13.0	16.3	7.9	1.6
Smoked Salmon, Pret a Manger*	1 Pack/157.9g	348	11.5	220	16.5	21.8	7.3	1.7
Soft Cheese, & Spicy Aubergine, Pret a Manger*	1 Pack/250g	319	6.8	128	4.6	21.2	2.7	2.8
Tabbouleh, No Bread, Pret a Manger*	1 Pack/342g	250	17.4	73	2.1	4.8	5.1	2.2
Tuna Mayonnaise, No Bread, Pret a Manger*	1 Pack/233g	193	8.8	83	10.8	1.9	3.8	0.5
Tuna Nicoise, on Whole Grain, Pret a Manger*	1 Pack/295g	486	26.5	165	7.9	13.4	9.0	1.9
Tuna, Dolphin Friendly, Pret a Manger*	1 Sandwich/227g	442	22.7	195	8.8	16.8	10.0	1.5
Tuna, Dolphin Friendly, Slim Pret, Pret a Manger*	1 Pack/115.8g	234	12.7	202	9.7	16.2	11.0	2.3
Tuna, Nicoise, Pret a Manger*	1 Sandwich/305g	467	23.8	153	8.1	12.4	7.8	2.0
Tuna, St Tropez, Pret a Manger*	1 Pack/250g	387	19.0	155	7.4	14.7	7.6	2.0
Turkey Club, Pret a Manger*	1 Pack/295.7g	593	31.3	200	10.0	15.1	10.6	1.8
SHORTBREAD								
Fingers, Pret a Manger*	1 Pack/28.40g	148	10.0	521	5.6	58.5	35.2	2.8
SLICES								
Oat & Fruit, Pret a Manger*	1 Slice/80g	342	16.2	427	5.3	56.0	20.3	5.1
SMOOTHIE								
Mango, Pret a Manger*	1 Serving/250g	130	0.5	52	0.6	12.4	0.2	1.2
SMOOTHIE								
Strawberry, Pret a Manger*	1 Serving/250g	105	0.3	42	0.3	9.6	0.1	0.9
Vitamin Volcano, Pret a Manger*	1 Serving/250ml	103	0.3	41	0.4	10.1	0.1	0.9
SNACK POT								
Banoffee, Pret a Manger*	1 Pot/198g	273	6.7	138	5.9	21.5	3.4	0.5
SOUP								
Bacon, Tomato & Creme Fraiche, Pret a Manger*	1 Pack/334g	220	14.9	66	1.7	4.7	4.5	0.8
Bean & Herb, Summer, Pret a Manger*	1 Serving/335g	191	12.7	57	1.8	3.8	3.8	1.3
Carrot & Roast Cumin, Pret a Manger*	1 Serving/282g	167	9.5	59	1.4	5.6	3.4	1.3
Carrot, Arabian Spiced, Pret a Manger*	1 Serving/334g	194	9.1	58	2.5	5.8	2.7	0.7
Celeriac & Mash, Pret a Manger*	1 Serving/297g	125	10.1	42	0.8	2.2	3.4	1.0
Chicken Curry, Pret a Manger*	1 Serving/275g	283	14.6	103	5.1	8.7	5.3	1.6
Chicken Salsa, Verde, Pret a Manger*	1 Serving/345g	197	9.3	57	4.5	3.6	2.7	4.6
Chicken, Malaysian, Pret a Manger*	1 Serving/347g	243	11.8	70	5.1	4.8	3.4	0.9
Chilli & Rice, Pret a Manger*	1 Serving/334g	244	8.4	73	5.4	7.3	2.5	2.8
Classic Tomato, Pret a Manger*	1 Serving/336g	179	7.1	53	0.9	7.5	2.1	0.7
Five Bean Cassoulet, Pret a Manger*	1 Serving/294g	174	5.9	59	3.6	6.6	2.0	4.9
Fresh Tomato, & Herb, Pret a Manger*	1 Serving/307g	123	6.8	40	0.6	3.3	2.2	0.9
Italian Meatball, Pret a Manger*	1 Serving/340g	221	13.9	65	1.8	5.1	4.1	1.2

PRET A MANGER

	Measure INFO/WEIGHT	per Measure KCAL	FAT	Nutrition Values per 100g / 100ml KCAL	PROT	CARB	FAT	FIBRE
SOUP								
Kedgeree, Chowder, Pret a Manger*	1 Serving/334g	197	12.0	59	1.9	4.8	3.6	1.2
Lentil & Bacon, Hotpot, Pret a Manger*	1 Serving/296g	219	9.2	74	5.9	6.3	3.1	1.2
Lentil, Tomato & Tumeric, Pret a Manger*	1 Pack/345g	248	7.2	72	4.5	8.7	2.1	5.0
Minestrone, Pret a Manger*	1 Serving/455g	187	6.3	41	1.7	5.6	1.4	1.5
Mushroom Risotto, Pret a Manger*	1 Serving/347g	202	9.3	58	1.5	7.0	2.7	1.2
Pea & Pancetta Risotta, Pret a Manger*	1 Pot/335g	214	14.4	64	2.4	3.9	4.3	3.6
Porcini Musroom, Pret a Manger*	1 Serving/455g	210	8.2	46	1.4	5.6	1.8	0.9
Red Pepper & Goats Cheese, Pret a Manger*	1 Serving/335g	208	15.9	62	1.8	2.9	4.8	0.9
Spinach, Nutmeg & Sage, Pret a Manger*	1 Serving/334g	248	19.1	74	1.2	4.4	5.7	1.0
Tomato & Basil, Pret a Manger*	1 Serving/453.6g	147	6.4	32	0.6	4.7	1.4	0.7
Tomato & Mountain Wheat, Pret a Manger*	1 Serving/455g	220	6.0	48	1.3	8.1	1.3	0.7
Tuscan Bean & Sausage, Pret a Manger*	1 Serving/340g	267	11.2	79	4.8	8.1	3.3	3.8
Yoghurt, Cumin & Carrot, Spicy, Pret a Manger*	1 Serving/100g	191	8.9	191	8.3	19.1	8.9	2.3
STRUDEL								
Cinnamon, Pret a Manger*	1 Serving/92g	363	17.7	392	6.1	49.0	19.1	4.7
SUSHI								
Deluxe, Pret a Manger*	1 Pack/258g	364	3.6	141	6.0	25.1	1.4	1.2
Salmon, Nigiri, Pret a Manger*	1 Pack/200g	314	8.4	157	5.4	23.4	4.2	0.0
Vegetarian, Pret a Manger*	1 Pack/193g	277	5.4	144	3.4	25.9	2.8	5.6
VEGETABLE CHIPS								
Parsnip, Beetroot & Carrot, Pret a Manger*	1 Bag/25g	126	9.2	504	5.6	37.2	36.8	10.0
WATER								
Blackcurrant, Pure Still, Pret a Manger*	1 Serving/500ml	80	0.0	16	0.0	3.6	0.0	0.0
Cranberry, Pure Pret, Pret a Manger*	1 Can/330ml	119	0.0	36	0.0	8.6	0.0	0.0
Grape & Elderflower, Pure Pret, Pret a Manger*	1 Can/330ml	146	0.0	44	0.0	10.6	0.0	0.0
Lemon Barley, Pure Pret, Pret a Manger*	1 Serving/500ml	80	0.0	16	0.0	3.7	0.0	0.0
Lemon, Pure Pret, Pret a Manger*	1 Can/330ml	175	0.0	53	0.0	12.6	0.0	0.0
Orange, Pure Pret, Pret a Manger*	1 Can/330ml	158	0.0	48	0.0	11.3	0.0	0.0
Orange, Still, Pure Pret, Pret a Manger*	1 Serving/500ml	85	0.0	17	0.0	3.8	0.0	0.0
Yoga Bunny, Pret a Manger*	1 Can/330ml	132	0.0	40	0.0	9.7	0.0	0.0
WRAP								
All Day Breakfast, Hot, Pret a Manger*	1 Pack/255g	512	24.2	201	10.0	18.9	9.5	1.9
Avocado & Herb Salad, Pret a Manger*	1 Pack/251.8g	461	30.2	183	4.8	14.1	12.0	2.7
Beef, with Salt, Hot, Pret a Manger*	1 Pack/233g	476	21.9	204	14.1	16.3	9.4	2.0
WRAP								
Chicken Salad, Pret a Manger*	1 Pack/230g	378	17.6	164	8.3	15.6	7.7	1.3
Chicken, Jalapeno, Hot, Pret a Manger*	1 Pack/261g	433	14.6	166	12.7	16.4	5.6	1.8
Falafel, Spicy, Melt, Hot, Pret a Manger*	1 Pack/226.5g	460	19.3	203	8.9	22.7	8.5	2.4
Houmous Salad, Pret a Manger*	1 Pack/230g	351	15.6	153	5.0	17.9	6.8	3.4
Lamb, Pret a Manger*	1 Pack/271.4g	421	20.9	155	7.9	13.7	7.7	1.7
Meatball Ragu, Swedish, Hot, Pret a Manger*	1 Pack/218.5g	566	26.0	259	13.3	24.9	11.9	2.2
Salmon Fish Cake, Hot, Pret a Manger*	1 Pack/250g	460	25.0	184	10.9	12.7	10.0	0.7
Tuna Nicoise & Salad, Pret a Manger*	1 Pack/287g	430	20.6	150	7.7	13.9	7.2	1.6
Tuna Nicoise, Pret a Manger*	1 Pack/200g	338	18.2	169	7.0	15.1	9.1	2.1
YOGHURT								
Goosberry, Pret Pot, Pret a Manger*	1 Pot/151g	161	4.7	107	5.9	13.7	3.1	0.3
Honey & Granola, Pret Pot, Pret a Manger*	1 Pot/135g	255	8.4	189	7.6	25.8	6.2	1.7
Red Berry, Blender, Pret a Manger*	1 Pot/125g	175	3.8	140	5.6	23.0	3.0	2.4
Vanilla, Blender, Pret a Manger*	1 Pot/250ml	230	6.8	92	4.5	12.8	2.7	0.0
Very Berry, Pret Pot, Pret a Manger*	1 Pot/148g	151	4.7	102	6.0	12.5	3.2	0.3
YOGHURT DRINK								
Blueberry Blender, Pret a Manger*	1 Drink/250g	170	3.5	68	2.9	11.3	1.4	1.8

	Measure INFO/WEIGHT	per Measure KCAL	per Measure FAT	Nutrition Values per 100g / 100ml KCAL	PROT	CARB	FAT	FIBRE
PRET A MANGER								
YOGHURT DRINK								
Mango's & Minerals, Pret a Manger*	1 Drink/250g	203	3.5	81	2.6	14.4	1.4	0.1
Vanilla, Pret a Manger*	1 Drink/250ml	230	6.8	92	4.5	12.8	2.7	0.0
SPARKY								
COFFEE								
Iced, Latte, Vanilla, Tall, Skimmed Milk, Sparky*	1 Tall Cup/335ml	114	0.0	34	1.7	6.8	0.0	0.0
STARBUCKS								
BAGEL								
Cheese, & Jalapeno, Starbucks*	1 Bagel/115g	292	3.6	254	10.8	45.8	3.1	1.5
Cheesy, Starbucks*	1 Bagel/90g	253	6.6	281	11.9	41.7	7.3	2.2
Cinamon & Raisin, Starbucks*	1 Bagel/83g	190	1.2	229	44.8	9.4	1.4	1.3
Fruity, Starbucks*	1 Bagel/90g	338	16.1	376	9.7	44.5	17.9	3.4
BARS								
Almond, Cranberry & Yoghurt, Starbucks*	1 Bar/50g	220	12.8	440	6.6	46.0	25.5	10.2
Chocolate, Milk, Starbucks*	1 Bar/45g	252	16.5	559	8.4	48.8	36.7	0.0
Granola, Starbucks*	1 Bar/90g	392	22.1	435	7.3	46.4	24.6	4.4
Mango, Pistachio & Cashew, Fruit & Nut, Starbucks*	1 Bar/50g	201	10.6	401	7.7	45.0	21.1	16.9
Rocky Road, Starbucks*	1 Bar/90g	459	30.0	510	4.8	47.1	33.3	2.5
BISCOTTI								
Almond, Starbucks*	1 Biscuit/55g	219	9.1	399	8.0	54.4	16.6	2.5
Starbucks*	1 Biscuit/27g	100	4.0	370	7.4	55.6	14.8	0.0
BISCUITS								
Ginger Snaps, Organic, Starbucks*	3 Biscuits/60g	267	9.2	445	4.8	71.9	15.4	1.5
Golden Crunch, Starbucks*	1 Biscuit/29.9g	144	6.6	481	5.1	65.4	22.1	2.0
Oat & Fruit, Starbucks*	1 Biscuit/60g	258	10.5	430	4.2	64.0	17.5	2.2
BREAD								
Fruit, Luxury, Starbucks*	2 Slices/160g	477	8.6	298	6.3	56.2	5.4	2.2
BROWNIE								
Chocolate, Fudge, Classic, Starbucks*	1 Brownie/72g	301	15.2	418	4.9	52.3	21.1	0.5
CAKE								
Banana & Date, Skinny, Starbucks*	1 Slice/120g	300	3.5	250	3.9	52.1	2.9	2.5
Banana Date & Raisin, Wholemeal, Low Fat, Starbucks*	1 Slice/70g	169	2.0	242	5.0	49.1	2.9	3.4
Butterfly, Starbucks*	1 Slice/80g	361	18.2	451	3.4	58.2	22.7	0.5
Carrot & Valencia Orange, Low Fat, Starbucks*	1 Slice/79.7g	169	2.2	212	3.9	43.3	2.7	3.7
Carrot Loaf, Starbucks*	1 Slice/100g	352	19.9	352	4.7	38.4	19.9	2.3
Carrot, Passion, Starbucks*	1 Slice/128g	465	28.1	364	4.3	37.2	22.0	1.8
Carrot, Skinny, Starbucks*	1 Slice/75g	192	2.5	256	4.0	54.1	3.3	2.1
Chocolate Decadence, Starbucks*	1 Slice/187g	755	42.9	405	4.5	44.8	23.0	0.6
Chocolate Orange, Starbucks*	1 Slice/70g	276	14.8	395	5.7	45.4	21.2	1.9
Chocolate, Cornflake, Starbucks*	1 Serving/70g	320	16.4	460	4.2	57.5	23.6	2.3
Chocolate, Fairtrade, Starbucks*	1 Serving/70g	300	19.1	430	7.9	37.8	27.4	4.6
Fruit, Starbucks*	1 Slice/80g	236	7.0	295	3.6	50.1	8.7	2.8
Iced Fancies, Starbucks*	1 Cake/81g	307	10.5	379	2.3	63.7	13.0	0.6
Marshmallow Twizzle, Starbucks*	1 Serving/35g	145	4.9	410	4.0	67.1	13.9	0.6
Orange, Summer Valencia, Wheat & Dairy Free, Starbucks*	1 Slice/70g	190	9.8	271	7.6	28.9	14.0	2.9
Orange, Wheat & Gluten Free, Starbucks*	1 Serving/55g	138	7.3	251	7.4	25.8	13.2	3.3
Victoria Sponge, Classic, Starbucks*	1 Slice/127g	490	25.1	385	3.2	48.4	19.7	0.8
Victoria Sponge, Mini, Starbucks*	1 Cake/64.8g	243	12.2	375	3.7	47.5	18.8	0.9
Yoghurt & Berry Loaf, Low Fat, Starbucks*	1 Slice/94g	254	4.8	270	5.3	50.8	5.1	1.7
CHEESECAKE								
Blueberry Swirl, Starbucks*	1 Slice/155g	555	36.7	360	6.7	29.1	23.8	1.1
CHOCOLATE								
Chocolate, Starbucks*	1 Serving/185g	723	49.6	391	6.9	30.5	26.8	0.8

	Measure INFO/WEIGHT	per Measure KCAL	FAT	Nutrition Values per 100g / 100ml KCAL	PROT	CARB	FAT	FIBRE
STARBUCKS								
CHOCOLATE								
Dark, Organic, Fairtrade, 70% Cocoa Solids, Starbucks*	1 Square/5g	28	2.3	554	6.7	27.6	46.3	0.0
Caramel Macchiato, Venti, Soy, Starbucks*	1 Venti/591ml	256	6.5	43	1.9	6.3	1.1	0.2
Brewed, Grande, Starbucks*	1 Grande/473ml	5	0.1	1	0.1	0.0	0.0	0.0
Brewed, Short, Starbucks*	1 Short/236ml	2	0.1	1	0.1	0.0	0.0	0.0
Brewed, Tall, Starbucks*	1 Tall/335mls	4	0.1	1	0.2	0.0	0.0	0.0
COFFEE								
Brewed, Venti, Starbucks*	1 Venti/591ml	6	0.0	1	0.1	0.0	0.0	0.0
Caffe Americano, Grande, Starbucks*	1 Grande/473ml	17	0.0	4	0.2	0.6	0.0	0.0
Caffe Americano, Short, Starbucks*	1 Short/236ml	6	0.0	3	0.2	0.4	0.0	0.0
Caffe Americano, Tall, Starbucks*	1 Tall/335mls	11	0.0	3	0.1	0.3	0.0	0.0
Caffe Americano, Venti, Starbucks*	1 Venti/591ml	23	0.0	4	0.2	0.7	0.0	0.0
Caffe Latte, Grande, Semi Skimmed Milk, Starbucks*	1 Grande/473ml	188	7.0	40	2.6	4.0	1.5	0.0
Caffe Latte, Grande, Skimmed Milk, Starbucks*	1 Grande/473ml	131	0.3	28	2.7	4.0	0.1	0.0
Caffe Latte, Grande, Soy, Starbucks*	1 Grande/473ml	148	5.3	31	2.2	2.8	1.1	0.3
Caffe Latte, Grande, Whole Milk, Starbucks*	1 Grande/473ml	223	11.5	47	2.6	3.8	2.4	0.0
Caffe Latte, Short, Semi Skimmed Milk, Starbucks*	1 Short/236ml	67	0.1	28	2.7	4.2	0.0	0.0
Caffe Latte, Short, Skimmed Milk, Starbucks*	1 Short/236ml	67	0.1	28	2.7	4.2	0.0	0.0
Caffe Latte, Short, Soy, Starbucks*	1 Short/236ml	75	2.7	32	2.3	3.0	1.1	0.3
Caffe Latte, Short, Whole Milk, Starbucks*	1 Short/236ml	113	5.8	48	2.6	3.8	2.5	0.0
Caffe Latte, Tall, Semi Skimmed Milk, Starbucks*	1 Tall/335ml	148	5.6	44	2.9	4.2	1.7	0.0
Caffe Latte, Tall, Skimmed Milk, Starbucks*	1 Tall/335ml	102	0.2	30	3.0	4.5	0.1	0.0
Caffe Latte, Tall, Soy, Starbucks*	1 Tall/335ml	116	4.3	35	2.4	3.0	1.3	0.3
Caffe Latte, Tall, Whole Milk, Starbucks*	1 Tall/335ml	176	9.2	53	2.8	4.2	2.8	0.0
Caffe Latte, Venti, Semi Skimmed Milk, Starbucks*	1 Venti/591ml	242	9.1	41	2.7	4.1	1.5	0.0
Caffe Latte, Venti, Skimmed Milk, Starbucks*	1 Venti/591ml	210	0.5	36	3.5	5.3	0.1	0.0
Caffe Latte, Venti, Soy, Starbucks*	1 Venti/591ml	190	7.0	32	2.3	2.7	1.2	0.3
Caffe Latte, Venti, Whole Milk, Starbucks*	1 Venti/591ml	289	15.0	49	2.6	3.9	2.5	0.0
Caffe Misto, Cafe Au Lait, Semi Skimmed Milk, Starbucks*	1 Grande/473ml	106	4.1	22	1.5	2.1	0.9	0.0
Caffe Misto, Cafe Au Lait, Skimmed Milk, Starbucks*	1 Grande/473ml	73	0.2	15	1.5	2.1	0.0	0.0
Caffe Misto, Cafe Au Lait, Soy, Starbucks*	1 Grande/473ml	82	3.2	17	1.3	1.3	0.7	0.2
Caffe Misto, Cafe Au Lait, Whole Milk, Starbucks*	1 Grande/473ml	126	6.8	27	1.5	1.9	1.4	0.0
Caffe Misto, Cafe Au Lait, Semi Skimmed Milk, Starbucks*	1 Short/236ml	54	2.1	23	1.5	2.1	0.9	0.0
Caffe Misto, Cafe Au Lait, Skimmed Milk, Starbucks*	1 Short/236ml	37	0.1	16	1.6	2.1	0.0	0.0
Caffe Misto, Cafe Au Lait, Soy, Starbucks*	1 Short/236ml	42	1.6	18	1.3	1.3	0.7	0.2
Caffe Misto, Cafe Au Lait, Whole Milk, Starbucks*	1 Short/236ml	65	3.5	28	1.5	2.1	1.5	0.0
Caffe Misto, Cafe Au Lait, Semi Skimmed Milk, Starbucks*	1 Tall/335ml	81	3.2	24	1.6	2.1	1.0	0.0
Caffe Misto, Cafe Au Lait, Skimmed Milk, Starbucks*	1 Tall/335ml	56	0.2	17	1.7	2.4	0.1	0.0
Caffe Misto, Cafe Au Lait, Soy, Starbucks*	1 Tall/335ml	63	2.4	19	1.3	1.5	0.7	0.2
Caffe Misto, Cafe Au Lait, Whole Milk, Starbucks*	1 Tall/335ml	97	5.2	29	1.6	2.1	1.6	0.0
Caffe Misto, Cafe Au Lait, Semi Skimmed Milk, Starbucks*	1 Venti/591ml	134	5.2	23	1.5	2.0	0.9	0.0
Caffe Misto, Cafe Au Lait, Skimmed Milk, Starbucks*	1 Venti/591ml	92	0.3	16	1.6	2.2	0.1	0.0
Caffe Misto, Cafe Au Lait, Soy, Starbucks*	1 Venti/591ml	104	4.0	18	1.3	1.4	0.7	0.2
Caffe Misto, Cafe Au Lait, Whole Milk, Starbucks*	1 Venti/591ml	160	8.6	27	1.5	2.0	1.5	0.0
Caffe Misto, Skimmed Milk, Starbucks*	1 Tall/354ml	64	0.0	18	1.8	2.5	0.0	0.0
Caffe Misto, Whole Milk, Starbucks*	1 Grande/442ml	143	7.5	30	1.6	2.3	1.6	0.0
Caffe Mocha, Skimmed Milk, Starbucks*	1 Tall/354ml	175	1.3	49	0.3	9.3	0.4	0.4
Caffe Mocha, Skimmed Milk, with Whip, Starbucks*	1 Grande/473ml	324	11.6	69	3.0	9.3	2.5	0.4
Caffe Mocha, Whole Milk, Starbucks*	1 Tall/354ml	233	9.3	66	2.9	8.8	2.6	0.4
Caffe Mocha, Whole Milk, with Whip, Starbucks*	1 Tall/354ml	313	17.3	88	2.9	9.0	4.9	0.4
Caffe Mocha, with Whip, Semi Skimmed Milk, Starbucks*	1 Grande/473ml	335	15.0	71	2.8	9.1	3.2	0.4
Caffe Mocha, with Whip, Skimmed Milk, Starbucks*	1 Grande/473ml	288	9.5	61	2.8	9.3	2.0	0.4
Caffe Mocha, with Whip, Soy, Starbucks*	1 Grande/473ml	302	13.7	64	2.5	8.0	2.9	0.6

STARBUCKS
COFFEE

	Measure INFO/WEIGHT	per Measure KCAL	FAT	KCAL	PROT	CARB	FAT	FIBRE
Caffe Mocha, with Whip, Whole Milk, Starbucks*	1 Grande/473ml	364	18.7	77	2.8	8.9	4.0	0.4
Caffe Mocha, with Whip, Semi Skimmed Milk, Starbucks*	1 Short/236ml	184	9.1	78	2.8	9.3	3.9	0.4
Caffe Mocha, with Whip, Skimmed Milk, Starbucks*	1 Short/236ml	160	6.4	68	2.9	9.3	2.7	0.4
Caffe Mocha, with Whip, Soy, Starbucks*	1 Short/236ml	167	8.5	71	2.5	8.5	3.6	0.6
Caffe Mocha, with Whip, Whole Milk, Starbucks*	1 Short/236ml	198	11.0	84	2.8	9.3	4.7	0.4
Caffe Mocha, with Whip, Semi Skimmed, Starbucks*	1 Short/236ml	228	8.0	97	4.5	14.4	3.4	0.6
Caffe Mocha, with Whip, Skimmed Milk, Starbucks*	1 Tall/335ml	228	8.0	68	3.2	10.2	2.4	0.4
Caffe Mocha, with Whip, Soy, Starbucks*	1 Tall/335ml	24	1.1	7	0.3	0.9	0.3	0.1
Caffe Mocha, with Whip, Whole Milk, Starbucks*	1 Tall/335ml	290	15.5	87	3.0	9.9	4.6	0.4
Caffe Mocha, with Whip, Semi Skimmed Milk, Starbucks*	1 Venti/591ml	409	17.5	69	2.9	9.1	3.0	0.4
Caffe Mocha, with Whip, Skimmed Milk, Starbucks*	1 Venti/591ml	347	10.2	59	2.9	9.3	1.7	0.4
Caffe Mocha, with Whip, Soy, Starbucks*	1 Venti/591ml	366	15.7	62	2.5	8.1	2.7	0.6
Caffe Mocha, with Whip, Whole Milk, Starbucks*	1 Venti/591ml	448	22.5	76	2.8	9.0	3.8	0.4
Cappuccino, Semi Skimmed Milk, Starbucks*	1 Grande/473ml	115	4.1	24	1.6	2.5	0.9	0.0
Cappuccino, Skimmed Milk, Starbucks*	1 Grande/473ml	116	0.3	24	2.3	3.6	0.1	0.0
Cappuccino, Grande, Soy, Starbucks*	1 Grande/473ml	92	3.2	19	1.4	1.7	0.7	0.2
Cappuccino, Grande, Whole Milk, Starbucks*	1 Grande/473ml	136	6.8	29	1.6	2.3	1.4	0.0
Cappuccino, Semi Skimmed Milk, Starbucks*	1 Short/236ml	78	2.8	33	2.2	3.4	1.2	0.0
Cappuccino, Skimmed Milk, Starbucks*	1 Short/236ml	55	0.1	23	2.2	3.4	0.0	0.0
Cappuccino, Soy, Starbucks*	1 Short/236ml	62	2.2	26	1.8	2.5	0.9	0.3
Cappuccino, Whole Milk, Starbucks*	1 Short/236ml	92	4.7	39	2.1	3.4	2.0	0.0
Cappuccino, Semi Skimmed Milk, Starbucks*	1 Tall/335ml	91	3.4	27	1.8	2.7	1.0	0.0
Cappuccino, Skimmed Milk, Starbucks*	1 Tall/335mls	64	0.1	19	1.8	2.7	0.0	0.0
Cappuccino, Soy, Starbucks*	1 Tall/335ml	72	2.6	21	1.5	1.8	0.8	0.2
Cappuccino, Whole Milk, Starbucks*	1 Tall/335ml	108	5.6	32	1.8	2.7	1.7	0.0
Cappuccino, Semi Skimmed Milk, Starbucks*	1 Venti/591ml	155	5.7	26	1.7	2.5	1.0	0.0
Cappuccino, Skimmed Milk, Starbucks*	1 Venti/591ml	109	0.2	18	1.8	2.7	0.0	0.0
Cappuccino, Soy, Starbucks*	1 Venti/591ml	123	4.4	21	1.5	1.9	0.7	0.2
Cappuccino, Whole Milk, Starbucks*	1 Venti/591ml	184	9.3	31	1.7	2.5	1.6	0.0
Caramel Macchiato, Semi Skimmed Milk, Starbucks*	1 Grande/473ml	240	6.7	51	2.2	7.2	1.4	0.0
Caramel Macchiato, Skimmed Milk, Starbucks*	1 Grande/473ml	193	1.1	41	2.3	7.4	0.2	0.0
Caramel Macchiato, Soy, Starbucks*	1 Grande/473ml	207	5.3	44	1.9	6.1	1.1	0.2
Caramel Macchiato, Whole Milk, Starbucks*	1 Grande/473ml	269	10.5	57	2.2	7.2	2.2	0.0
Caramel Macchiato, Semi Skimmed Milk, Starbucks*	1 Short/236ml	122	3.8	52	2.3	6.8	1.6	0.0
Caramel Macchiato, Skimmed Milk, Starbucks*	1 Short/236ml	97	0.9	41	2.4	7.2	0.4	0.0
Caramel Macchiato, Soy, Starbucks*	1 Short/236ml	104	3.0	44	1.9	5.9	1.3	0.3
Caramel Macchiato, Whole Milk, Starbucks*	1 Short/236ml	137	5.7	58	2.3	6.8	2.4	0.0
Caramel Macchiato, Skimmed Milk, Starbucks*	1 Tall/354ml	173	0.8	49	3.1	8.5	0.2	0.0
Caramel Macchiato, Tall, Semi Skimmed Milk, Starbucks*	1 Tall/335ml	178	5.3	53	2.4	7.5	1.6	0.0
Caramel Macchiato, Tall, Skimmed Milk, Starbucks*	1 Tall/335ml	142	0.9	42	2.4	7.5	0.3	0.0
Caramel Macchiato, Tall, Soy, Starbucks*	1 Tall/335ml	153	4.2	46	2.0	6.3	1.3	0.3
Caramel Macchiato, Tall, Whole Milk, Starbucks*	1 Tall/335ml	201	8.2	60	2.3	7.2	2.5	0.0
Caramel Macchiato, Venti, Semi Skimmed Milk, Starbucks*	1 fl oz/30ml	15	0.4	51	2.2	7.3	1.4	0.0
Caramel Macchiato, Venti, Skimmed Milk, Starbucks*	1 Venti/591ml	239	1.2	40	2.3	7.5	0.2	0.0
Caramel Macchiato, Venti, Whole Milk, Starbucks*	1 Venti/591ml	337	13.1	57	2.2	7.1	2.2	0.0
Caramel Macchiato, Whole Milk, Starbucks*	1 Tall/354ml	244	10.4	69	2.8	7.9	2.9	0.0
Espresso Con Panna, Doppio, Starbucks*	1 Doppio/60ml	36	2.5	60	1.5	5.0	4.2	0.0
Espresso Con Panna, Solo, Starbucks*	1 Solo/30ml	31	2.5	103	1.7	6.7	8.3	0.0
Espresso Macchiato, Doppio, Semi Skimmed, Starbucks*	1 Doppio/60ml	14	0.1	23	1.5	3.3	0.2	0.0
Espresso Macchiato, Doppio, Skimmed Milk, Starbucks*	1 Doppio/60ml	13	0.0	22	1.7	3.3	0.0	0.0
Espresso Macchiato, Doppio, Soy, Starbucks*	1 Doppio/60ml	13	0.1	22	1.5	3.3	0.2	0.0
Espresso Macchiato, Doppio, Whole Milk, Starbucks*	1 Doppio/60ml	15	0.2	25	1.5	3.3	0.3	0.0

STARBUCKS

	Measure INFO/WEIGHT	per Measure KCAL	FAT	Nutrition Values per 100g / 100ml KCAL	PROT	CARB	FAT	FIBRE
COFFEE								
Espresso Macchiato, Solo, Semi Skimmed Milk, Starbucks*	1 Solo/30ml	8	0.1	27	1.7	3.3	0.3	0.0
Espresso Macchiato, Solo, Skimmed Milk, Starbucks*	1 Solo/30ml	7	0.0	23	1.7	3.3	0.0	0.0
Espresso Macchiato, Solo, Soy, Starbucks*	1 Solo/30ml	7	0.1	23	1.7	3.3	0.3	0.0
Espresso Macchiato, Solo, Whole Milk, Starbucks*	1 Solo/30ml	8	0.2	27	1.7	3.3	0.7	0.0
Espresso, Con Panna, Doppio, Starbucks*	1 Doppio/60ml	111	9.3	185	1.2	6.7	15.5	0.0
Espresso, Con Panna, Solo, Starbucks*	1 Solo/30ml	105	9.3	350	1.3	10.0	31.0	0.0
Espresso, Doppio, Starbucks*	1 Doppio/60ml	11	0.0	18	1.2	3.3	0.0	0.0
Espresso, Solo, Starbucks*	1 Solo/30ml	6	0.0	20	1.3	3.3	0.0	0.0
Hazelnut Mocha, & Whip, Semi Skimmed Milk, Starbucks*	1 Grande/473ml	399	14.5	84	2.6	12.9	3.1	0.4
Hazelnut Mocha, & Whip, Skimmed Milk, Starbucks*	1 Tall/335ml	252	6.7	75	2.7	13.1	2.0	0.4
Hazelnut Mocha, & Whip, Soy, Starbucks*	1 Grande/473ml	369	13.3	78	2.3	12.1	2.8	0.6
Hazelnut Mocha, & Whip, Whole Milk, Starbucks*	1 Grande/473ml	425	17.9	90	2.6	12.7	3.8	0.4
Hazelnut Mocha, & Whip, Semi Skimmed Milk, Starbucks*	1 Short/236ml	216	8.9	92	2.7	13.1	3.8	0.4
Hazelnut Mocha, & Whip, Skimmed Milk, Starbucks*	1 Short/236ml	197	6.2	83	2.8	13.6	2.6	0.4
Hazelnut Mocha, & Whip, Soy, Starbucks*	1 Short/236ml	201	8.3	85	2.3	12.3	3.5	0.6
Hazelnut Mocha, & Whip, Whole Milk, Starbucks*	1 Short/236ml	229	10.6	97	2.6	13.1	4.5	0.4
Hazelnut Mocha, & Whip, Semi Skimmed Milk, Starbucks*	1 Tall/335ml	312	12.0	93	2.9	13.7	3.6	0.4
Hazelnut Mocha, & Whip, Skimmed Milk, Starbucks*	1 Tall/335ml	277	7.9	83	3.0	13.7	2.4	0.4
Hazelnut Mocha, & Whip, Soy, Starbucks*	1 Tall/335ml	288	11.1	86	2.6	12.5	3.3	0.7
Hazelnut Mocha, & Whip, Whole Milk, Starbucks*	1 Tall/335ml	334	14.8	100	2.9	13.4	4.4	0.4
Hazelnut Mocha, & Whip, Semi Skimmed Milk, Starbucks*	1 Venti/591ml	487	16.8	82	2.7	12.9	2.8	0.4
Hazelnut Mocha, & Whip, Skimmed Milk, Starbucks*	1 Venti/591ml	430	10.1	73	2.7	13.0	1.7	0.4
Hazelnut Mocha, & Whip, Soy, Starbucks*	1 Venti/591ml	448	15.2	76	2.4	11.8	2.6	0.6
Hazelnut Mocha, & Whip, Whole Milk, Starbucks*	1 Venti/591ml	523	21.4	88	2.6	12.7	3.6	0.4
Iced, Caffe Americano, Grande, Starbucks*	1 Grande/473ml	17	0.0	4	0.2	0.6	0.0	0.0
Iced, Caffe Americano, Tall, Starbucks*	1 Tall/335ml	11	0.0	3	0.2	0.6	0.0	0.0
Iced, Caffe Americano, Venti, Starbucks*	1 Venti/591ml	23	0.0	4	0.2	0.7	0.0	0.0
Iced, Caffe Latte, Grande, Semi Skimmed Milk, Starbucks*	1 Grande/473ml	126	4.5	27	1.8	2.8	1.0	0.0
Iced, Caffe Latte, Grande, Skimmed Milk, Starbucks*	1 Grande/473ml	90	0.2	19	1.8	2.8	0.0	0.0
Iced, Caffe Latte, Grande, Soy, Starbucks*	1 Grande/473ml	104	3.6	22	1.5	1.9	0.8	0.2
Iced, Caffe Latte, Grande, Whole Milk, Starbucks*	1 Grande/473ml	149	7.5	32	1.7	2.5	1.6	0.0
Iced, Caffe Latte, Tall, Semi Skimmed Milk, Starbucks*	1 Tall/335ml	97	3.6	29	1.9	3.0	1.1	0.0
Iced, Caffe Latte, Tall, Skimmed Milk, Starbucks*	1 Tall/335ml	68	0.2	20	1.9	3.0	0.1	0.0
Iced, Caffe Latte, Tall, Soy, Starbucks*	1 Tall/335ml	80	2.9	24	1.7	2.1	0.9	0.2
Iced, Caffe Latte, Tall, Whole Milk, Starbucks*	1 Tall/335ml	115	5.9	34	1.9	2.7	1.8	0.0
Iced, Caffe Latte, Venti, Semi Skimmed Milk, Starbucks*	1 Venti/591ml	142	5.1	24	1.6	2.4	0.9	0.0
Iced, Caffe Latte, Venti, Skimmed Milk, Starbucks*	1 Venti/591ml	100	0.2	17	1.6	2.5	0.0	0.0
Iced, Caffe Latte, Venti, Soy, Starbucks*	1 Venti/591ml	118	4.2	20	1.4	1.9	0.7	0.2
Iced, Caffe Latte, Venti, Whole Milk, Starbucks*	1 Venti/591ml	168	8.5	28	1.5	2.4	1.4	0.0
Iced, Caffe Mocha, & Whip, Semi Skimmed Milk, Starbucks*	1 Grande/473ml	316	16.8	67	2.0	8.0	3.6	0.4
Iced, Caffe Mocha, & Whip, Skimmed Milk, Starbucks*	1 Grande/473ml	289	13.6	61	2.0	8.3	2.9	0.4
Iced, Caffe Mocha, & Whip, Soy, Starbucks*	1 Grande/473ml	300	16.1	63	1.8	7.6	3.4	0.6
Iced, Caffe Mocha, & Whip, Whole Milk, Starbucks*	1 Grande/473ml	333	18.9	70	2.0	8.0	4.0	0.4
Iced, Caffe Mocha, & Whip, Semi Skimmed, Starbucks*	1 Tall/335ml	234	12.4	70	2.1	8.7	3.7	0.4
Iced, Caffe Mocha, & Whip, Skimmed Milk, Starbucks*	1 Tall/335ml	212	9.8	63	2.2	8.7	2.9	0.4
Iced, Caffe Mocha, & Whip, Soy, Starbucks*	1 Tall/335ml	221	11.8	66	2.0	8.1	3.5	0.6
Iced, Caffe Mocha, & Whip, Whole Milk, Starbucks*	1 Tall/335ml	248	14.1	74	2.1	8.4	4.2	0.4
Iced, Caffe Mocha, & Whip, Semi Skimmed, Starbucks*	1 Venti/591ml	340	16.7	58	1.8	7.6	2.8	0.4
Iced, Caffe Mocha, & Whip, Skimmed Milk, Starbucks*	1 Venti/591ml	310	13.2	52	1.8	7.8	2.2	0.4
Iced, Caffe Mocha & Whip, Soy, Starbucks*	1 Venti/591ml	322	16.0	54	1.6	7.1	2.7	0.5
Iced, Caffe Mocha, & Whip, Whole Milk, Starbucks*	1 Venti/591ml	358	19.0	61	1.7	7.6	3.2	0.4
Iced, Caramel Macchiato, Semi Skimmed Milk, Starbucks*	1 Grande/473ml	231	6.3	49	2.0	7.0	1.3	0.0

STARBUCKS
COFFEE

	INFO/WEIGHT	KCAL	FAT	KCAL	PROT	CARB	FAT	FIBRE
Iced, Caramel Macchiato, Skimmed Milk, Starbucks*	1 Grande/473ml	188	1.3	40	2.1	7.2	0.3	0.0
Iced, Caramel Macchiato, Soy, Starbucks*	1 Grande/473ml	206	5.3	44	1.8	6.3	1.1	0.2
Iced, Caramel Macchiato, Whole Milk, Starbucks*	1 Grande/473ml	257	9.8	54	2.0	7.0	2.1	0.0
Iced, Caramel Macchiato, Semi Skimmed Milk, Starbucks*	1 Tall/335ml	171	4.9	51	2.1	7.2	1.5	0.0
Iced, Caramel Macchiato, Skimmed Milk, Starbucks*	1 Tall/335ml	139	1.2	41	2.1	7.5	0.4	0.0
Iced, Caramel Macchiato, Soy, Starbucks*	1 Tall/335ml	152	4.2	45	1.8	6.6	1.3	0.2
Iced, Caramel Macchiato, Whole Milk, Starbucks*	1 Tall/335ml	191	7.5	57	2.0	7.2	2.2	0.0
Iced, Caramel Macchiato, Semi Skimmed Milk, Starbucks*	1 Venti/591ml	262	6.8	44	1.8	6.6	1.2	0.0
Iced, Caramel Macchiato, Skimmed Milk, Starbucks*	1 Venti/591ml	215	1.3	36	1.8	6.8	0.2	0.0
Iced, Caramel Macchiato, Soy, Starbucks*	1 Venti/591ml	234	5.7	40	1.6	5.9	1.0	0.2
Iced, Caramel Macchiato, Whole Milk, Starbucks*	1 Venti/591ml	291	10.5	49	1.7	6.6	1.8	0.0
Iced, Grande, Starbucks*	1 Grande/473ml	4	0.1	1	0.1	0.0	0.0	0.0
Iced, Hazelnut Mocha & Whip, Semi Skimmed, Starbucks*	1 Grande/473ml	452	20.1	96	2.4	12.3	4.3	0.0
Iced, Hazelnut Mocha & Whip, Skimmed Milk, Starbucks*	1 Grande/473ml	425	16.9	90	2.4	12.5	3.6	0.0
Iced, Hazelnut Mocha & Whip, Soy, Starbucks*	1 Grande/473ml	437	19.4	92	2.2	11.8	4.1	0.2
Iced, Hazelnut Mocha & Whip, Whole Milk, Starbucks*	1 Grande/473ml	469	22.2	99	2.3	12.3	4.7	0.0
Iced, Hazelnut Mocha & Whip, Semi Skimmed Starbucks*	1 Tall/335ml	318	14.1	95	2.4	12.1	4.2	0.0
Iced, Hazelnut Mocha, with Whip, Tall, Skimmed, Starbucks*	1 Tall/335ml	297	11.6	89	2.4	12.4	3.5	0.0
Iced, Hazelnut Mocha & Whip, Soy, Starbucks*	1 Tall/335ml	325	14.3	97	2.4	12.5	4.3	0.2
Iced, Hazelnut Mocha & Whip, Whole Milk, Starbucks*	1 Tall/335ml	351	16.6	105	2.5	12.8	5.0	0.0
Iced, Hazelnut Mocha & Whip, Semi Skimmed, Starbucks*	1 Venti/591ml	599	23.1	101	2.6	14.2	3.9	0.0
Iced, Hazelnut Mocha, & Whip & Skimmed Milk, Starbucks*	1 Venti/591ml	563	18.8	95	2.7	14.4	3.2	0.0
Iced, Hazelnut Mocha & Whip, Soy, Starbucks*	1 Venti/591ml	578	22.2	98	2.5	13.7	3.8	0.2
Iced, Latte, Vanilla, Semi Skimmed Milk, Starbucks*	1 Grande/473ml	187	3.9	40	1.5	6.3	0.8	0.0
Iced, Latte, Vanilla, Skimmed Milk, Starbucks*	1 Grande/473ml	155	0.2	33	1.6	6.6	0.0	0.0
Iced, Latte, Vanilla, Soy, Starbucks*	1 Grande/473ml	168	3.2	36	1.4	5.7	0.7	0.2
Iced, Latte, Vanilla, Whole Milk, Starbucks*	1 Grande/473ml	207	6.5	44	1.5	6.3	1.4	0.0
Iced, Latte, Vanilla, Semi Skimmed Milk, Starbucks*	1 Tall/335ml	134	2.9	40	1.6	6.5	0.9	0.0
Iced, Latte, Vanilla, Soy, Starbucks*	1 Tall/335ml	120	2.3	36	1.4	5.6	0.7	0.2
Iced, Latte, Vanilla, Whole Milk, Starbucks*	1 Tall/335ml	149	4.9	45	1.6	6.2	1.5	0.0
Iced, Latte, Vanilla, Venti, Semi Skimmed Milk, Starbucks*	1 Venti/591ml	182	0.2	31	1.4	6.3	0.0	0.0
Iced, Latte, Vanilla, Venti, Skimmed Milk, Starbucks*	1 Venti/591ml	182	0.2	31	1.4	6.3	0.0	0.0
Iced, Latte, Vanilla, Venti, Soy, Starbucks*	1 Venti/591ml	197	3.5	33	1.2	5.6	0.6	0.2
Iced, Latte, Vanilla, Venti, Whole Milk, Starbucks*	1 Venti/591ml	240	7.2	41	1.3	6.1	1.2	0.0
Iced, Tall, Starbucks*	1 Tall/335ml	3	0.1	1	0.1	0.0	0.0	0.0
Iced, Venti, Starbucks*	1 Venti/591ml	5	0.1	1	0.1	0.0	0.0	0.0
Mocha, Peppermint, Skimmed, Grande, Starbucks*	1 Grande/473ml	304	2.3	64	2.9	13.3	0.5	0.4
Mocha, Peppermint, Skimmed, Tall, Starbucks*	1 Tall/354ml	237	1.4	67	3.1	13.6	0.4	0.4
Mocha, Peppermint, Skimmed, Venti, Starbucks*	1 Venti/591ml	385	2.9	65	3.0	13.4	0.5	0.4
Mocha, Peppermint, Skimmed, Whip, Grande, Starbucks*	1 Grande/473ml	405	20.8	86	2.9	13.7	4.4	0.4
Mocha, Peppermint, Skimmed, Whip, Tall, Starbucks*	1 Tall/354ml	317	9.4	90	3.1	13.8	2.7	0.4
Mocha, Peppermint, Skimmed, Whip, Venti, Starbucks*	1 Venti/591ml	486	12.3	82	3.0	13.7	2.1	0.4
Mocha, Peppermint, Whole, Grande, Starbucks*	1 Grande/473ml	372	11.4	79	2.7	12.9	2.4	0.4
Mocha, Peppermint, Whole, Tall, Starbucks*	1 Tall/354ml	293	9.0	83	2.9	13.3	2.5	0.4
Mocha, Peppermint, Whole, Venti, Starbucks*	1 Venti/591ml	475	15.2	80	2.8	12.9	2.6	0.4
Mocha, Peppermint, Whole, Whip, Grande, Starbucks*	1 Grande/473ml	473	20.8	100	2.7	13.3	4.4	0.4
Mocha, Peppermint, Whole, Whip, Tall, Starbucks*	1 Tall/354ml	373	17.0	105	2.9	13.6	4.8	0.4
Mocha, Peppermint, Whole, Whip, Venti, Starbucks*	1 Venti/591ml	576	24.6	97	2.8	13.2	4.2	0.4
Vanilla Latte, Grande, Semi Skimmed Milk, Starbucks*	1 Grande/473ml	251	6.4	53	2.4	7.6	1.4	0.0
Vanilla Latte, Grande, Skimmed Milk, Starbucks*	1 Grande/473ml	199	0.3	42	2.5	7.8	0.1	0.0
Vanilla Latte, Grande, Soy, Starbucks*	1 Grande/473ml	214	4.9	45	2.1	6.6	1.0	0.3
Vanilla Latte, Grande, Whole Milk, Starbucks*	1 Grande/473ml	284	10.6	60	2.4	7.6	2.2	0.0

STARBUCKS

	Measure INFO/WEIGHT	per Measure KCAL	FAT	Nutrition Values per 100g / 100ml KCAL	PROT	CARB	FAT	FIBRE
COFFEE								
Vanilla Latte, Short, Semi Skimmed Milk, Starbucks*	1 Short/236ml	127	3.3	54	2.5	7.6	1.4	0.0
Vanilla Latte, Short, Skimmed Milk, Starbucks*	1 Short/236ml	101	0.1	43	2.5	8.1	0.0	0.0
Vanilla Latte, Short, Soy, Starbucks*	1 Short/236ml	108	2.5	46	2.1	6.8	1.1	0.3
Vanilla Latte, Short, Whole Milk, Starbucks*	1 Short/236ml	144	5.4	61	2.4	7.6	2.3	0.0
Vanilla Latte, Tall, Semi Skimmed Milk, Starbucks*	1 Tall/335ml	195	5.2	58	2.7	8.1	1.6	0.0
Vanilla Latte, Tall, Skimmed Milk, Starbucks*	1 Tall/335ml	152	0.2	45	2.8	8.4	0.1	0.0
Vanilla Latte, Tall, Soy, Starbucks*	1 Tall/335ml	165	4.0	49	2.3	6.9	1.2	0.3
Vanilla Latte, Tall, Whole Milk, Starbucks*	1 Tall/335ml	221	8.6	66	2.7	8.1	2.6	0.0
Vanilla Latte, Venti, Semi Skimmed Milk, Starbucks*	1 Venti/591ml	321	8.5	54	2.5	7.8	1.4	0.0
Vanilla Latte, Venti, Skimmed Milk, Starbucks*	1 Venti/591ml	252	0.4	43	2.6	8.0	0.1	0.0
Vanilla Latte, Venti, Soy, Starbucks*	1 Venti/591ml	272	6.5	46	2.1	6.6	1.1	0.3
Vanilla Latte, Venti, Whole Milk, Starbucks*	1 Venti/591ml	364	14.0	62	2.5	7.6	2.4	0.0
Vanilla, with Whip, Grande, Starbucks*	1 Grande/473ml	364	14.2	77	1.2	11.4	3.0	0.0
Vanilla, with Whip, Tall, Starbucks*	1 Tall/335ml	284	10.4	85	1.3	13.1	3.1	0.0
Vanilla, with Whip, Venti, Starbucks*	1 Venti/591ml	412	13.8	70	1.1	11.2	2.3	0.0
White Chocolate Mocha & Whip, Semi Skimmed, Starbucks*	1 Grande/473ml	471	18.4	100	3.2	13.3	3.9	0.0
White Chocolate Mocha & Whip, Skimmed Milk, Starbucks*	1 Grande/473ml	425	12.9	90	3.2	13.5	2.7	0.0
White Chocolate Mocha & Whip, Soy, Starbucks*	1 Grande/473ml	439	17.0	93	2.8	12.3	3.6	0.2
White Chocolate Mocha & Whip, Whole Milk, Starbucks*	1 Grande/473ml	500	22.1	106	3.1	13.1	4.7	0.0
White Chocolate Mocha & Whip, Skimmed Milk, Starbucks*	1 Short/236ml	229	8.0	97	3.3	13.6	3.4	0.0
White Chocolate Mocha & Whip, Soy, Starbucks*	1 Short/236ml	236	10.1	100	2.9	12.7	4.3	0.3
White Chocolate Mocha & Whip, Whole Milk, Starbucks*	1 Short/236ml	267	12.7	113	3.2	13.6	5.4	0.0
White Chocolate Mocha, & Whip, Semi Skimmed, Starbucks*	1 Tall/335ml	369	15.0	110	3.5	14.3	4.5	0.0
White Chocolate Mocha & Whip, Skimmed Milk, Starbucks*	1 Tall/335ml	331	10.5	99	3.6	14.3	3.1	0.0
White Chocolate Mocha & Whip, Soy, Starbucks*	1 Tall/335ml	342	13.9	102	3.1	13.1	4.2	0.3
White Chocolate Mocha & Whip, Whole Milk, Starbucks*	1 Tall/335ml	392	18.0	117	3.4	14.0	5.4	0.0
White Chocolate Mocha & Whip, Semi Skimmed, Starbucks*	1 Venti/591ml	581	21.7	98	3.3	13.4	3.7	0.0
White Chocolate Mocha & Whip, Skimmed Milk, Starbucks*	1 Venti/591ml	518	14.3	88	3.3	13.5	2.4	0.0
White Chocolate Mocha & Whip, Soy, Starbucks*	1 Venti/591ml	537	19.9	91	2.9	12.4	3.4	0.3
White Chocolate Mocha & Whip, Whole Milk, Starbucks*	1 Venti/591ml	619	26.6	105	3.2	13.2	4.5	0.0
COOKIES								
Chocolate Chip, Giant, Starbucks*	1 Cookie/110g	539	25.1	490	6.1	62.7	22.8	0.8
Fruit & Oat, Starbucks*	1 Cookie/80g	344	14.0	430	4.2	64.0	17.5	2.2
CRISPS								
Strong Cheese & Onion, Starbucks*	1 Bag/50g	228	11.3	455	7.1	56.2	22.6	4.0
CROISSANT								
Almond Filled, Starbucks*	1 Croissant/92g	360	22.8	391	7.7	34.3	24.8	2.0
Butter, Starbucks*	1 Croissant/82g	289	17.3	352	5.9	34.9	21.1	1.6
Cheese, & Ham, Starbucks*	1 Pack/114g	359	20.6	315	13.2	24.9	18.1	0.8
CUPCAKES								
Banana & Chocolate Chip, Starbucks*	1cake/80g	342	14.9	428	4.7	57.8	18.6	0.5
Lemon, Sicilian, Starbucks*	1 Cake/80g	350	18.0	437	3.3	55.3	22.5	0.5
DOUGHNUT								
Chocolate & Custard, Starbucks*	1 Doughnut/25g	55	4.1	218	1.2	16.3	16.4	0.3
Jam, Starbucks*	1 Donut/24g	57	3.1	237	0.9	24.5	13.1	0.9
FLAPJACK								
Banana & Caramel, Starbucks*	1 Serving/70g	301	15.4	430	3.3	54.4	22.0	2.5
FRAPPUCCINO								
Caramel Cream, Grande, Starbucks*	1 Grande/473ml	339	5.2	72	2.8	12.7	1.1	0.0
Caramel Cream, Tall, Starbucks*	1 Tall/354ml	261	3.9	74	2.8	13.0	1.1	0.0
Caramel Cream, Venti, Starbucks*	1 Venti/591ml	409	6.0	69	2.6	12.4	1.0	0.0
Caramel Cream, with Whip, Grande, Starbucks*	1 Grande/473ml	470	17.4	99	2.8	13.1	3.7	0.0

STARBUCKS
FRAPPUCCINO

	Measure INFO/WEIGHT	per Measure KCAL	FAT	Nutrition Values per 100g / 100ml KCAL	PROT	CARB	FAT	FIBRE
Caramel Cream, with Whip, Tall, Starbucks*	1 Tall/354ml	355	12.6	100	2.8	13.6	3.6	0.0
Caramel Cream, with Whip, Venti, Starbucks*	1 Venti/591ml	540	18.2	91	2.6	12.7	3.1	0.0
Caramel, Grande, Starbucks*	1 Grande/473ml	294	3.9	62	0.0	12.5	0.8	0.0
Caramel, Light, Grande, Starbucks*	1 Grande/473ml	158	1.6	33	1.3	6.3	0.3	0.5
Caramel, Light, Tall, Starbucks*	1 Tall/335ml	129	1.4	39	1.4	7.5	0.4	0.6
Caramel, Light, Venti, Starbucks*	1 Venti/591ml	192	1.7	32	1.2	6.4	0.3	0.5
Caramel, Tall, Starbucks*	1 Tall/354ml	228	3.1	64	0.0	12.7	0.9	0.0
Caramel, Venti, Starbucks*	1 Venti/591ml	370	4.7	63	0.0	12.7	0.8	0.0
Caramel, with Whip, Grande, Starbucks*	1 Grande/473ml	382	14.9	81	1.2	12.1	3.2	0.0
Caramel, with Whip, Tall, Starbucks*	1 Tall/335ml	302	11.0	90	1.3	13.7	3.3	0.0
Caramel, with Whip, Venti, Starbucks*	1 Venti/591ml	431	14.4	73	1.1	11.7	2.4	0.0
Chocolate, Grande, Starbucks*	1 Grande/473ml	338	5.7	71	3.0	12.7	1.2	0.0
Chocolate, Tall, Starbucks*	1 Tall/354ml	260	4.5	73	3.0	13.0	1.3	0.0
Chocolate, Venti, Starbucks*	1 Venti/591ml	413	7.1	70	2.8	12.7	1.2	0.0
Chocolate, with Whip, Grande, Starbucks*	1 Grande/473ml	469	17.9	99	3.0	13.1	3.8	0.1
Chocolate, with Whip, Tall, Starbucks*	1 Tall/354ml	354	13.2	100	3.0	13.6	3.7	0.2
Chocolate, with Whip, Venti, Starbucks*	1 Venti/591ml	544	19.3	92	2.8	13.0	3.3	0.2
Coffee, Grande, Starbucks*	1 Grande/473ml	261	9.4	55	1.2	11.0	2.0	0.0
Coffee, Light, Grande, Starbucks*	1 Grande/473ml	128	1.0	27	1.3	5.3	0.2	0.6
Coffee, Light, Tall, Starbucks*	1 Tall/335ml	91	0.7	27	1.3	5.4	0.2	0.5
Coffee, Light, Venti, Starbucks*	1 Venti/591ml	151	1.2	26	1.2	4.9	0.2	0.5
Coffee, Tall, Starbucks*	1 Tall/335ml	184	2.4	55	1.2	11.0	0.7	0.0
Coffee, Venti, Starbucks*	1 Venti/591ml	278	3.6	47	1.0	9.5	0.6	0.0
Cream, Caramel, with Whip, Tall, Starbucks*	1 Tall/335ml	329	10.4	98	2.7	14.9	3.1	0.0
Cream, Chocolate Chip, with Whip, Grande, Starbucks*	1 Grande/473ml	498	18.0	105	2.9	15.6	3.8	0.3
Cream, Chocolate Chip, with Whip, Tall, Starbucks*	1 Tall/335ml	368	12.9	110	3.0	16.7	3.9	0.4
Cream, Chocolate Chip, with Whip, Venti, Starbucks*	1 Venti/591ml	562	18.9	95	2.6	14.9	3.2	0.4
Cream, Chocolate, with Whip, Grande, Starbucks*	1 Grande/473ml	425	14.2	90	2.7	13.5	3.0	0.1
Cream, Chocolate, with Whip, Tall, Starbucks*	1 Tall/335ml	322	10.4	96	2.9	14.6	3.1	0.2
Cream, Chocolate, with Whip, Venti, Starbucks*	1 Venti/591ml	480	14.1	81	2.5	13.0	2.4	0.2
Cream, Vanilla, with Whip, Grande, Starbucks*	1 Grande/473ml	431	14.2	91	2.6	13.5	3.0	0.0
Cream, Vanilla, with Whip, Tall, Starbucks*	1 Tall/335ml	310	9.8	93	2.7	14.0	2.9	0.0
Cream, Vanilla, with Whip, Venti, Starbucks*	1 Venti/591ml	470	13.0	80	2.4	12.7	2.2	0.0
Espresso, Grande, Starbucks*	1 Grande/473ml	209	2.7	44	1.0	8.9	0.6	0.0
Espresso, Tall, Starbucks*	1 Tall/335ml	146	1.9	44	1.0	8.7	0.6	0.0
Espresso, Venti, Starbucks*	1 Venti/591ml	243	3.1	41	0.9	8.1	0.5	0.0
Grande, Starbucks*	1 Grande/473ml	239	3.1	51	1.1	10.2	0.7	0.0
Java Chip, with Whip, Grande, Starbucks*	1 Grande/473ml	456	18.6	96	1.5	14.6	3.9	0.3
Java Chip, with Whip, Tall, Starbucks*	1 Tall/335ml	345	13.6	103	1.7	16.1	4.1	0.4
Java Chip, with Whip, Venti, Starbucks*	1 Venti/591ml	650	24.5	110	1.8	17.6	4.1	0.5
Mango Passion, Grande, Starbucks*	1 Grande/473ml	191	0.3	40	0.2	9.7	0.1	0.3
Mango Passion, Tall, Starbucks*	1 Tall/335ml	157	0.2	47	0.2	11.3	0.1	0.3
Mango Passion, Venti, Starbucks*	1 Venti/591ml	228	0.3	39	0.2	9.3	0.1	0.3
Mocha, Light, Grande, Starbucks*	1 Grande/473ml	144	1.4	30	1.4	6.1	0.3	0.6
Mocha, Light, Tall, Starbucks*	1 Tall/335ml	113	1.1	34	1.5	6.9	0.3	0.7
Mocha, Light, Venti, Starbucks*	1 Venti/591ml	184	2.0	31	1.3	6.3	0.3	0.6
Mocha, White Chocolate, with Whip, Grande, Starbucks*	1 Grande/473ml	408	15.6	86	1.4	12.9	3.3	0.0
Mocha, White Chocolate, with Whip, Venti, Starbucks*	1 Venti/591ml	481	16.2	81	1.4	13.0	2.7	0.0
Mocha, with Whip, Grande, Starbucks*	1 Grande/473ml	378	14.8	80	1.3	12.1	3.1	0.1
Mocha, with Whip, Venti, Starbucks*	1 Venti/591ml	428	14.9	72	1.3	11.7	2.5	0.1
Raspberry Tea, Grande, Starbucks*	1 Grande/473ml	200	0.2	42	0.1	11.0	0.0	0.2
Raspberry Tea, Tall, Starbucks*	1 Tall/354ml	144	0.1	41	0.1	10.5	0.0	0.2

	INFO/WEIGHT	KCAL	FAT	KCAL	PROT	CARB	FAT	FIBRE
STARBUCKS								
FRAPPUCCINO								
Raspberry Tea, Venti, Starbucks*	1 Venti/591ml	261	0.2	44	0.1	11.3	0.0	0.2
Raspberry, Black Currant, with Zen Tea, Grande, Starbucks*	1 Grande/473ml	192	0.1	41	0.1	9.9	0.0	0.2
Raspberry, Black Currant, with Zen Tea, Tall, Starbucks*	1 Tall/335ml	158	0.1	47	0.1	11.6	0.0	0.2
Raspberry, Black Currant, with Zen Tea, Venti, Starbucks*	1 Venti/591ml	229	0.1	39	0.1	9.5	0.0	0.1
Strawberries & Cream, Grande, Starbucks*	1 Grande/473ml	424	5.2	90	2.9	17.3	1.1	0.0
Strawberries & Cream, Tall, Starbucks*	1 Tall/354ml	299	3.6	84	2.7	16.4	1.0	0.0
Strawberries & Cream, Venti, Starbucks*	1 Venti/591ml	543	6.7	92	3.0	17.6	1.1	0.0
Strawberries & Cream, with Whip, Grande, Starbucks*	1 Grande/473ml	555	17.4	117	2.9	17.8	3.7	0.1
Strawberries & Cream, with Whip, Tall, Starbucks*	1 Tall/354ml	393	12.3	111	2.7	17.0	3.5	0.1
Strawberries & Cream, with Whip, Venti, Starbucks*	1 Venti/591ml	674	18.9	114	3.0	17.9	3.2	0.1
Tazo Chai, Grande, Starbucks*	1 Grande/473ml	405	5.1	86	2.9	16.5	1.1	0.0
Tazo Chai, Tall, Starbucks*	1 Tall/354ml	294	3.8	83	2.9	15.8	1.1	0.0
Tazo Chai, Venti, Starbucks*	1 Venti/591ml	487	5.9	82	2.7	16.1	1.0	0.0
Tazo Chai, with Whip, Grande, Starbucks*	1 Grande/473ml	536	17.3	113	2.9	16.9	3.7	0.0
Tazo Chai, with Whip, Tall, Starbucks*	1 Tall/354ml	388	12.5	110	2.9	16.4	3.5	0.0
Tazo Chai, with Whip, Venti, Starbucks*	1 Venti/591ml	618	18.1	105	2.7	16.4	3.1	0.0
Tropical Citrus Tea, Grande, Starbucks*	1 Grande/473ml	178	0.3	38	0.3	9.3	0.1	0.3
Tropical Citrus Tea, Tall, Starbucks*	1 Tall/354ml	128	0.2	36	0.3	9.0	0.1	0.3
Tropical Citrus Tea, Venti, Starbucks*	1 Venti/591ml	232	0.4	39	0.3	9.8	0.1	0.3
Vanilla, with Whip, Grande, Starbucks*	1 Grande/473ml	460	17.2	97	2.8	12.7	3.6	0.0
Vanilla, with Whip, Tall, Starbucks*	1 Tall/354ml	344	12.5	97	2.8	13.0	3.5	0.0
Vanilla, with Whip, Venti, Starbucks*	1 Venti/591ml	530	18.0	90	2.6	12.4	3.1	0.0
White Chocolate Mocha, with Whip, Tall, Starbucks*	1 Tall/335ml	319	11.7	95	1.6	14.6	3.5	0.0
FRUIT SALAD								
Starbucks*	1 Salad/300g	126	0.6	42	0.5	9.7	0.2	1.0
HOT CHOCOLATE								
Signature & Whip, Grande, Semi Skimmed Milk, Starbucks*	1 Grande/473ml	537	30.7	114	3.2	12.5	6.5	6.5
Signature & Whip, Grande, Skimmed Milk, Starbucks*	1 Grande/473ml	505	27.0	107	3.3	12.5	5.7	1.4
Signature & Whip, Grande, Soy, Starbucks*	1 Grande/473ml	515	29.8	109	3.0	11.8	6.3	1.6
Signature, with Whip, Grande, Whole Milk, Starbucks*	1 Grande/473ml	556	33.5	118	3.2	12.5	7.1	1.4
Signature & Whip, Short, Semi Skimmed Milk, Starbucks*	1 Short/236ml	283	16.9	120	3.3	12.7	7.2	1.4
Signature & Whip, Short, Skimmed Milk, Starbucks*	1 Short/236ml	267	15.0	113	3.3	12.7	6.4	1.4
Signature & Whip, Short, Soy, Starbucks*	1 Short/236ml	272	16.4	115	3.1	11.9	7.0	1.6
Signature & Whip, Short, Whole Milk, Starbucks*	1 Short/236ml	293	18.1	124	3.2	12.7	7.7	1.4
Signature & Whip, Tall, Semi Skimmed Milk, Starbucks*	1 Tall/335ml	418	24.2	125	3.5	13.4	7.2	1.5
Signature & Whip, Tall, Skimmed Milk, Starbucks*	1 Tall/335ml	393	21.3	117	3.6	13.7	6.4	1.5
Signature & Whip, Tall, Soy, Starbucks*	1 Tall/335ml	401	23.5	120	3.3	12.8	7.0	1.7
Signature & Whip, Tall, Whole Milk, Starbucks*	1 Tall/335ml	433	26.1	129	3.5	13.4	7.8	1.5
Signature & Whip, Venti, Semi Skimmed Milk, Starbucks*	1 Venti/591ml	665	37.2	113	3.3	12.7	6.3	1.4
Signature & Whip, Venti, Skimmed Milk, Starbucks*	1 Venti/591ml	624	32.4	106	3.3	12.7	5.5	1.4
Signature & Whip, Venti, Soy, Starbucks*	1 Venti/591ml	637	36.0	108	3.1	12.0	6.1	1.6
Signature & Whip, Venti, Whole Milk, Starbucks*	1 Venti/591ml	690	40.4	117	3.3	12.5	6.8	1.4
Skimmed Milk, Grande, Starbucks*	1 Grande/473ml	261	2.4	55	3.3	10.6	0.5	0.4
Skimmed Milk, Tall, Starbucks*	1 Tall/354ml	209	1.5	59	3.5	11.3	0.4	0.4
Skimmed Milk, Venti, Starbucks*	1 Venti/591ml	340	2.9	58	3.3	11.2	0.5	0.4
White, Skimmed Milk, Grande, Starbucks*	1 Grande/442ml	361	16.6	82	3.9	14.0	3.8	0.0
White, Skimmed Milk, Tall, Starbucks*	1 Tall/354ml	301	3.9	85	4.1	14.4	1.1	0.0
White, Skimmed Milk, Venti, Starbucks*	1 Venti/591ml	493	7.1	83	4.0	14.2	1.2	0.0
White, Skimmed Milk, with Whip, Grande, Starbucks*	1 Grande/443ml	456	14.1	103	3.9	14.4	3.2	0.0
White, Skimmed Milk, with Whip, Tall, Starbucks*	1 Tall/354ml	381	11.9	108	4.1	14.7	3.4	0.0
White, Skimmed Milk, with Whip, Venti, Starbucks*	1 Venti/553ml	556	15.4	101	4.0	14.6	2.8	0.0
White, Whole Milk, Grande, Starbucks*	1 Grande/443ml	449	16.7	101	3.6	13.3	3.8	0.0

STARBUCKS

INFO/WEIGHT	Measure	KCAL	FAT	KCAL	PROT	CARB	FAT	FIBRE
HOT CHOCOLATE								
White, Whole Milk, Tall, Starbucks*	1 Tall/354ml	377	14.2	107	3.8	13.8	4.0	0.0
White, Whole Milk, Venti, Starbucks*	1 Venti/591ml	618	24.0	105	3.7	13.5	4.1	0.0
White, Whole Milk, with Whip, Grande, Starbucks*	1 Grande/443ml	543	25.5	123	3.6	13.7	5.8	0.0
White, Whole Milk, with Whip, Tall, Starbucks*	1 Tall/354ml	457	22.2	129	3.8	14.1	6.3	0.0
White, Whole Milk, with Whip, Venti, Starbucks*	1 Venti/553	673	31.2	122	3.7	13.9	5.7	0.0
Whole Milk, Grande, Starbucks*	1 Grande4/473ml	347	14.1	73	3.0	9.9	3.0	0.4
Whole Milk, Tall, Starbucks*	1 Tall/354ml	277	10.7	78	3.1	10.7	3.0	0.4
Whole Milk, Venti, Starbucks*	1 Venti/591ml	448	17.6	76	3.0	10.7	3.0	0.4
Whole Milk, with Whip, Grande, Starbucks*	1 Grande/443ml	420	22.0	95	3.0	10.4	5.0	0.4
Whole Milk, with Whip, Tall, Starbucks*	1 Tall/354ml	357	18.7	101	3.1	11.0	5.3	0.4
Whole Milk, with Whip, Venti, Starbucks*	1 Venti/553ml	514	25.3	93	3.0	11.0	4.6	0.4
HOUMOUS								
with Crunchy Vegetables, Starbucks*	1 Pot/219g	359	9.6	164	4.7	26.4	4.4	2.9
with Tomato, Vegetables, Red Pepper, Starbucks*	1 Pack/217.7g	405	14.4	186	5.4	26.2	6.6	2.0
MUFFIN								
Apple & Cinnamon, Starbucks*	1 Muffin/100g	377	20.2	377	4.7	45.1	20.2	0.4
Banana & Caramel, Starbucks*	1 Muffin/100g	585	30.6	585	6.7	66.8	30.6	1.4
Banana & Nut, Starbucks*	1 Muffin/140g	476	22.3	340	5.0	44.2	15.9	1.1
Bran, Honey Raisin, Starbucks*	1 Muffin/100g	315	15.2	315	5.9	38.9	15.2	4.5
Classic Blueberry, Starbucks*	1 Muffin/129g	548	30.9	422	5.5	47.5	23.8	0.6
Golden Syrup Filled, Starbucks*	1 Muffin/130g	499	23.0	384	4.8	57.4	17.7	1.3
Orange & Lemon, Starbucks*	1 Muffin/140g	552	28.0	394	5.5	48.1	20.0	0.8
Skinny Blackcurrant & Redcurrant, Starbucks*	1 Muffin/125g	341	4.0	273	5.4	55.6	3.2	1.1
Skinny Blueberry, Starbucks*	1 Muffin/129g	342	5.4	264	5.5	51.4	4.2	0.9
Skinny Lemon Poppy Seed, Starbucks*	1 Muffin/130g	390	5.2	300	5.7	63.6	4.0	3.2
Skinny Peach & Raspberry, Starbucks*	1 Muffin/120.2g	286	4.4	238	5.1	46.5	3.7	1.4
Skinny Sunrise, Starbucks*	1 Muffin/130g	255	3.9	194	4.6	36.7	3.0	1.3
Sunrise, Starbucks*	1 Muffin/150g	592	34.6	395	5.5	40.8	23.1	1.9
MUFFIN								
White Chocolate & Strawberry, Starbucks*	1 Muffin/142g	583	33.5	411	5.7	49.0	23.6	2.3
PAIN AU CHOCOLAT								
Starbucks*	1 Pastry/64.9g	241	14.0	371	5.8	38.7	21.5	1.5
PAIN AU RAISIN								
Starbucks*	1 Pastry/130g	360	16.8	275	3.9	36.3	12.8	1.3
PANINI								
Beef Pastrami, New York Style, Starbucks*	1 Panini/220g	528	21.6	240	12.3	25.0	9.8	1.3
Cheese & Marmite, Breakfast, Starbucks*	1 Panini/105g	305	13.1	290	15.1	31.1	12.5	1.9
Chicken, Mediterranean Style, with Green Pesto, Starbucks*	1 Panini/224g	387	9.2	173	11.4	22.6	4.1	1.3
Croque Monsieur, Starbucks*	1 Panini/200g	460	19.0	230	13.6	22.9	9.5	1.1
Egg & Bacon, Breakfast, Starbucks*	1 Panini/165g	305	10.5	185	10.0	22.0	6.4	1.5
Egg Mayo, Breakfast, Starbucks*	1 Panini/146g	327	11.8	224	12.3	25.4	8.1	1.7
Falafel, Starbucks*	1 Pack/213.3g	384	7.0	180	6.8	30.9	3.3	2.7
Grilled Chicken Salsa, Lightly Spiced, Starbucks*	1 Panini/237.7g	386	8.1	162	7.9	25.0	3.4	2.0
Grilled Chicken Salsa, with Creme Fraiche, Starbucks*	1 Panini/180g	385	8.1	214	10.4	32.9	4.5	0.0
Ham, Cheese & Roasted Vegetable, Starbucks*	1 Panini/216.8g	388	8.0	179	11.0	25.4	3.7	1.4
Mozzarella with Sun Dried Tomatoes, Starbucks*	1 Panini/192g	530	25.1	275	13.5	25.8	13.0	2.4
Pesto Chicken, with Sunblush Tomato, Starbucks*	1 Panini/207g	399	10.0	192	13.1	24.1	4.8	3.0
Roasted Vegetable & Taw Valley Cheddar, Starbucks*	1 Panini/225.6g	485	19.9	215	9.2	25.1	8.8	1.7
Roasted Vegetables & Cheese, Starbucks*	1 Panini/215g	542	32.5	252	8.7	20.6	15.1	0.0
Sausage, Egg & Baked Bean, Starbucks*	1 Panini/100g	395	9.8	395	16.9	59.8	9.8	1.5
Steak, & Cheese, New York Style, Starbucks*	1 Panini/200g	486	16.9	243	15.4	26.4	8.5	2.9
Steak, New York Style, Starbucks*	1 Panini/227g	490	17.5	215	12.7	23.2	7.7	1.2

STARBUCKS

INFO/WEIGHT	KCAL	FAT	KCAL	PROT	CARB	FAT	FIBRE

PANINI

	INFO/WEIGHT	KCAL	FAT	KCAL	PROT	CARB	FAT	FIBRE
Tuna Melt, Toasted, Starbucks*	1 Panini/198g	485	20.6	245	13.7	24.2	10.4	1.6

PASTA SALAD

	INFO/WEIGHT	KCAL	FAT	KCAL	PROT	CARB	FAT	FIBRE
Salmon & Dill, Starbucks*	1 Pack/260g	614	34.8	236	7.8	21.0	13.4	1.0

PASTRY

	INFO/WEIGHT	KCAL	FAT	KCAL	PROT	CARB	FAT	FIBRE
Apricot, Starbucks*	1 Pastry/115g	279	15.3	243	4.7	26.1	13.3	1.1
Belgian Chocolate & Orange, Swirl, Starbucks*	1 Pastry/140g	525	18.5	375	7.5	57.4	13.2	2.6
Cheese, Savoury, Starbucks*	1 Pastry/126g	417	26.1	331	8.4	27.9	20.7	1.2
Cinnamon Swirl, Starbucks*	1 Pastry/116g	553	15.3	333	6.2	51.6	9.2	1.5

SALAD

	INFO/WEIGHT	KCAL	FAT	KCAL	PROT	CARB	FAT	FIBRE
Chicken Caesar, Starbucks*	1 Pack/233g	403	18.4	173	8.7	18.0	7.9	1.2
Chicken, Roasted, Starbucks*	1 Pack/157g	165	10.2	105	7.1	5.1	6.5	1.2
Mozarella & Cherry Tomato, Starbucks*	1 Pack/172g	322	29.2	187	5.5	2.9	17.0	17.0
Salmon Nicoise, Starbucks*	1 Pack/260g	291	18.2	112	6.9	7.2	7.0	1.0
Tuna Nicoise, Starbucks*	1 Pack/184.2g	175	9.8	95	7.8	4.6	5.3	1.2

SANDWICH

	INFO/WEIGHT	KCAL	FAT	KCAL	PROT	CARB	FAT	FIBRE
Atlantic Prawn, Starbucks*	1 Pack/185g	348	12.4	188	10.1	22.0	6.7	2.7
BLT, Starbucks*	1 Pack/203.5g	524	25.4	257	10.1	26.1	12.5	2.3
Beef, & Horseradish, Roast, Starbucks*	1 Pack/200g	546	22.2	273	18.7	23.1	11.1	1.0
Beef, Scottish, Roast, Mustard Mayonnaise, Starbucks*	1 Pack/157.8g	303	8.4	192	16.3	19.7	5.3	3.6
Cheddar Cheese & Pickle, Starbucks*	1 Pack/190.1g	504	29.8	265	10.2	20.5	15.7	1.6
Cheddar, & Italian Style Roasted Vegetables, Starbucks*	1 Pack/223g	553	30.6	248	5.3	25.8	13.7	0.0
Cheese, & Tomato, & Apple Chutney, Half Fat, Starbucks*	1 Pack/200g	318	8.4	159	8.8	21.3	4.2	0.0
Chicken, & Bacon, Club, Starbucks*	1 Pack/252g	590	38.6	234	11.5	12.8	15.3	0.0
Chicken, Club, Starbucks*	1 Pack/206g	422	19.4	205	12.6	17.8	9.4	1.7
Chicken, Lightly Spiced, Starbucks*	1 Pack/200g	286	4.8	143	11.2	18.2	2.4	0.0
Chicken, in Lemon Pepper Dressing, Starbucks*	1 Pack/198.1g	307	6.9	155	11.8	19.4	3.5	1.6
Egg Mayonnaise, & Cress, Starbucks*	1 Pack/200g	410	20.4	205	10.5	17.4	10.2	1.9
Egg Mayonnaise, on Gluten Free Bread, Starbucks*	1 Pack/226g	340	11.6	150	6.2	20.3	5.1	2.9
Falafel & Houmous, in Flatbread, Starbucks*	1 Pack/250g	468	9.5	187	7.0	34.8	3.8	3.6
Ham, & Tomato, Smoked, Starbucks*	1 Pack/206g	297	8.0	144	5.2	22.0	3.9	0.0
Ham, Yorkshire, Starbucks*	1 Pack/208g	374	11.0	180	10.0	23.0	5.3	2.3
Houmous, with Crunchy Vegetables, Starbucks*	1 Pack/218.9g	359	9.6	164	4.7	26.4	4.4	2.9
Prawn, Mayo, Starbucks*	1 Sandwich/189g	496	30.7	262	10.2	19.0	16.2	1.0
Salmon, Oaked Smoked, Starbucks*	1 Pack/180g	405	16.3	224	12.1	23.6	9.0	2.0
Salmon, Smoked & Edamane Bean Flatbread, Starbucks*	1 Sandwich/218g	461	15.7	211	9.6	27.1	7.2	2.1
Soft Cheese, & Tomato, Extra Light, Starbucks*	1 Pack/186g	283	5.0	152	8.0	24.0	2.7	3.1
Tuna Mayonnaise, & Spring Onion, Starbucks*	1 Pack/209g	318	8.4	152	9.0	19.9	4.0	1.5
Tuna Mayonnaise, Cucumber & Mixed Salad, Starbucks*	1 Pack/190.3g	295	8.4	155	10.1	18.6	4.4	1.5
Turkey, & Salad, Smoked, Starbucks*	1 Pack/198g	303	4.8	153	10.8	22.3	2.4	1.5
Turkey, Pork & Herb, Starbucks*	1 Pack/198g	465	21.4	235	11.7	22.6	10.8	2.1

SCONE

	INFO/WEIGHT	KCAL	FAT	KCAL	PROT	CARB	FAT	FIBRE
Berry, Starbucks*	1 Scone/90g	302	14.7	335	5.6	40.3	16.3	2.1
Blueberry, Starbucks*	1 Scone/128g	460	18.0	359	3.9	53.1	14.1	2.3
Raisin, Jumbo, Starbucks*	1 Scone/150g	564	22.2	376	5.9	54.9	14.8	2.1

SHORTBREAD

	INFO/WEIGHT	KCAL	FAT	KCAL	PROT	CARB	FAT	FIBRE
Chocolate Caramel, Starbucks*	1 Bar/64.9g	305	17.6	470	2.7	53.9	27.1	1.1
Bar Mocha, 1 Pump, Starbucks*	1 Pump/17g	26	0.6	153	3.5	35.3	3.5	5.9
Flavoured, 1 Pump, Starbucks*	1 Pump/10g	20	0.0	200	0.0	50.0	0.0	0.0

SYRUP

	INFO/WEIGHT	KCAL	FAT	KCAL	PROT	CARB	FAT	FIBRE
Flavoured, Sugar Free, 1 Pump, Starbucks*	1 Pump/10g	0	0.0	0	0.0	0.0	0.0	0.0
Hazelnut Flavoured, Starbucks*	1 Pump/10g	20	0.0	200	0.0	50.0	0.0	0.0

STARBUCKS

	Measure INFO/WEIGHT	per Measure KCAL	FAT	Nutrition Values per 100g / 100ml KCAL	PROT	CARB	FAT	FIBRE
TEA								
Brewed, Grande, Starbucks*	1 Grande Cup/473ml	0	0.0	0	0.0	0.0	0.0	0.0
Brewed, Short, Starbucks*	1 Short Cup/236ml	0	0.0	0	0.0	0.0	0.0	0.0
Brewed, Tall, Starbucks*	1 Tall Cup/335ml	0	0.0	0	0.0	0.0	0.0	0.0
Brewed, Venti, Starbucks*	1 Venti Cup/591ml	0	0.0	0	0.0	0.0	0.0	0.0
Chai, Latte, Tazo, Grande, Semi Skimmed Milk, Starbucks*	1 Grande/473ml	236	4.0	50	1.6	9.3	0.9	0.0
Chai, Latte, Tazo, Grande, Skimmed Milk, Starbucks*	1 Grande/473ml	204	0.2	43	1.6	9.3	0.0	0.0
Chai, Latte, Tazo, Grande, Soy, Starbucks*	1 Grande/473ml	213	3.2	45	1.3	8.7	0.7	0.2
Chai, Latte, Tazo, Grande, Whole Milk, Starbucks*	1 Grande/473ml	255	6.5	54	1.5	9.1	1.4	0.0
Chai, Latte, Tazo, Short, Semi Skimmed Milk, Starbucks*	1 Short/236ml	119	2.0	50	1.6	9.3	0.9	0.0
Chai, Latte, Tazo, Short, Skimmed Milk, Starbucks*	1 Short/236ml	103	0.1	44	1.7	9.3	0.0	0.0
Chai, Latte, Tazo, Short, Soy, Starbucks*	1 Short/236ml	108	1.6	46	1.4	8.5	0.7	0.2
Chai, Latte, Tazo, Short, Whole Milk, Starbucks*	1 Short/236ml	129	3.3	55	1.6	9.3	1.4	0.0
Chai, Latte, Tazo, Tall, Semi Skimmed Milk, Starbucks*	1 Tall/335ml	179	3.0	53	1.7	9.9	0.9	0.0
Chai, Latte, Tazo, Tall, Skimmed Milk, Starbucks*	1 Tall/335ml	154	0.2	46	1.7	9.9	0.1	0.0
Chai, Latte, Tazo, Tall, Soy, Starbucks*	1 Tall/335ml	162	2.4	48	1.4	9.3	0.7	0.2
Chai, Latte, Tazo, Tall, Whole Milk, Starbucks*	1 Tall/335ml	194	5.0	58	1.6	9.9	1.5	0.0
Chai, Latte, Tazo, Venti, Semi Skimmed Milk, Starbucks*	1 VentiCup/591ml	297	5.0	50	1.6	9.3	0.9	0.0
Chai, Latte, Tazo, Venti, Skimmed Milk, Starbucks*	1 Venti/591ml	256	0.3	43	1.6	9.5	0.1	0.0
Chai, Latte, Tazo, Venti, Soy, Starbucks*	1 Venti/591ml	268	4.0	45	1.3	8.6	0.7	0.2
Chai, Latte, Tazo, Venti, Whole Milk, Starbucks*	1 Venti/591ml	322	8.3	54	1.5	9.3	1.4	0.0
Iced, Chai, Latte, Tazo, Semi Skimmed Milk, Starbucks*	1 Grande/473ml	238	4.2	50	1.6	9.3	0.9	0.0
Iced, Chai, Latte, Tazo, Grande, Skimmed Milk, Starbucks*	1 Grande/473ml	205	0.2	43	1.6	9.3	0.0	0.0
Iced, Chai, Latte, Tazo, Grande, Soy, Starbucks*	1 Grande/473ml	219	3.4	46	1.4	8.7	0.7	0.2
Iced, Chai, Latte, Tazo, Grande, Whole Milk, Starbucks*	1 Grande/473ml	259	6.9	55	1.5	9.3	1.5	0.0
Iced, Chai, Latte, Tazo, Tall, Semi Skimmed, Starbucks*	1 Tall/335ml	176	3.0	53	1.6	9.9	0.9	0.0
Iced, Chai, Latte, Tazo, Tall, Skimmed Milk, Starbucks*	1 Tall/335ml	152	0.2	45	1.6	9.9	0.1	0.0
Iced, Chai, Latte, Tazo, Tall, Soy, Starbucks*	1 Tall/335ml	153	2.3	46	1.4	8.7	0.7	0.2
Iced, Chai, Latte, Tazo, Tall, Whole Milk, Starbucks*	1 Tall/335ml	191	5.0	57	1.6	9.6	1.5	0.0
Iced, Chai, Latte, Tazo, Venti, Semi Skimmed Milk, Starbucks*	1/591ml	277	4.4	47	1.3	9.0	0.7	0.0
Iced, Chai, Latte, Tazo, Venti, Skimmed Milk, Starbucks*	1 Venti/591ml	242	0.3	41	1.4	9.0	0.1	0.0
Iced, Chai, Latte, Tazo, Venti, Soy, Starbucks*	1 Venti/591ml	256	3.5	43	1.2	8.5	0.6	0.2
Iced, Chai, Latte, Tazo, Venti, Whole Milk, Starbucks*	1 Venti/591ml	299	7.2	51	1.3	9.0	1.2	0.0
TOPPING								
Caramel, Starbucks*	1 Serving/4g	15	0.6	375	0.0	50.0	15.0	0.0
Chocolate, Starbucks*	1 Serving/4g	6	0.1	150	2.5	25.0	2.5	2.5
Sprinkles, Starbucks*	1 Sprinkle/1g	4	0.0	400	0.0	100.0	0.0	0.0
Whipped Cream, Cold, Grande Beverage, Starbucks*	1 Serving/35g	114	11.2	326	1.7	8.6	32.0	0.0
Whipped Cream, Cold, Tall Beverage, Starbucks*	1 Serving/25g	81	8.0	324	1.6	8.0	32.0	0.0
Whipped Cream, Cold, Venti Beverage, Starbucks*	1 Serving/32g	104	10.2	325	1.9	9.4	31.9	0.0
Whipped Cream, Hot, Grande/venti, Starbucks*	1 Serving/22g	72	7.0	327	1.8	9.1	31.8	0.0
Whipped Cream, Hot, Short Beverage, Starbucks*	1 Serving/16g	52	5.1	325	1.9	6.3	31.9	0.0
Whipped Cream, Hot, Tall Beverage, Starbucks*	1 Serving/19g	62	6.1	326	1.6	10.5	32.1	0.0
WAFFLES								
Caramel, Starbucks*	1 Waffle/30g	140	6.1	467	4.3	66.7	20.3	1.3
WRAP								
Chicken, Breast, in Honey Mustard, Starbucks*	1 Pack/200g	332	7.8	166	7.3	25.8	3.9	1.4
Chicken, Chargrilled, Tomato & Pepper Salsa, Starbucks*	1 Pack/187.1g	320	8.2	171	10.4	22.5	4.4	1.6
Chicken, Roasted, Starbucks*	1 Pack/197g	374	13.0	190	11.6	21.2	6.6	2.2
Chicken, with Lightly Spiced Salsa, Starbucks*	1 Pack/187g	320	8.2	171	10.4	22.5	4.4	1.6
Emmental Cheese, & Roasted Aubergines, Starbucks*	1 Pack/225g	517	25.7	230	8.9	22.3	11.4	0.0
Greek Salad, Starbucks*	1 Pack/181.5g	265	7.3	146	6.1	21.5	4.0	2.0
Houmous & Falafel, Starbucks*	1 Wrap/213g	383	8.5	180	6.4	30.0	4.0	2.8

	Measure INFO/WEIGHT	per Measure KCAL	FAT	Nutrition Values per 100g / 100ml KCAL	PROT	CARB	FAT	FIBRE

STARBUCKS
WRAP
Prawn Caesar, Starbucks*	1 Pack/173.1g	464	27.2	268	11.4	20.2	15.7	1.1
Roasted Chicken Salad, with Mange Tout, Starbucks*	1 Pack/184g	294	3.7	160	12.2	23.5	2.0	1.7
Three Bean, Starbucks*	1 Pack/200g	350	11.8	175	5.9	24.5	5.9	2.0

YOGHURT
Blueberry with Mixed Seeds, Organic, Starbucks*	1 Pot/180g	194	6.5	108	3.6	15.1	3.6	0.6
Blueberry, Starbucks*	1 Pot/130g	116	0.0	89	4.4	17.8	0.0	0.0
Greek, with Crunchy Granola, Starbucks*	1 Pot/150g	267	15.0	178	1.7	20.5	10.0	1.1
Strawberry with Mixed Seeds, Organic, Starbucks*	1 Pot/179.8g	178	6.5	99	3.6	12.6	3.6	1.1

SUBWAY
BACON
Strips, Subway*	2 Strips/9g	40	2.9	444	33.3	0.2	32.2	0.0

BREAD
Roll, Hearty Italian, 6", Subway*	1 Roll/79g	189	2.3	239	8.9	46.8	2.9	3.2
Roll, Honey Oat, 6", Subway*	1 Roll/91g	224	3.0	246	9.9	45.1	3.3	3.6
Roll, Italian, Herbs & Cheese, Subway*	1 Roll/86g	220	5.2	256	10.5	41.9	6.1	0.5
Roll, Parmesan & Oregano, 6", Subway*	1 Roll/79g	190	2.7	241	8.9	45.6	3.4	3.5
Roll, Wheat, 6", Subway*	1 Roll/80g	183	2.3	229	10.0	43.8	2.9	3.5
Roll, Wheat, Mini, Subway*	1 Roll/53g	122	1.6	230	8.1	49.1	3.0	3.4
Roll, White, Italian, 6", Subway*	1 Roll/75g	178	2.1	237	9.3	46.7	2.8	2.7
Roll, White, Italian, Mini, Subway*	1 Roll/50g	117	1.2	234	9.6	46.0	2.4	2.6

CHEESE
Cheddar, Sliced, Processed, Subway*	1 Serving/24g	88	7.2	367	16.7	0.0	30.0	0.0

COOKIES
Chocolate Chip & Candy, Subway*	1 Cookie/45g	218	9.7	484	4.4	68.9	21.6	2.2
Chocolate Chip, Subway*	1 Cookie/45g	214	10.3	476	4.4	68.9	22.9	2.7
Chocolate Chunk, Subway*	1 Cookie/45g	226	10.1	502	4.4	68.9	22.4	2.2
Double Chocolate Chip, Subway*	1 Cookie/45g	212	9.5	471	4.4	66.7	21.1	2.2
Oatmeal & Raisin, Subway*	1 Cookie/45g	206	8.2	458	6.7	68.9	18.2	3.1
Sugar, Subway*	1 Cookie/45g	231	11.8	513	4.4	64.4	26.2	1.3
White Chip Macadamia Nut, Subway*	1 Cookie/45g	222	10.8	493	4.4	64.4	24.0	1.6

DOUGHNUTS
Chocolate, Subway*	1 Doughnut/55g	243	15.5	442	7.3	38.2	28.2	2.2
Sugared, Subway*	1 Doughnut/49g	207	11.6	422	6.1	42.9	23.7	1.0

DRESSING
Ranch, Subway*	1 Serving/21g	42	4.3	200	0.0	0.0	20.5	0.0

MAYONNAISE
Light, Subway*	1 Serving/15g	56	6.0	373	0.0	6.7	40.0	0.0
Subway*	1 Serving/15g	108	11.9	720	0.0	0.0	79.3	0.0

MUFFIN
Blueberry, Subway*	1 Muffin/111g	352	20.6	317	4.5	36.0	18.6	2.7
Chocolate Chunk, Subway*	1 Muffin/111g	394	22.9	355	5.4	39.6	20.6	2.6
Double Chocolate Chip, Subway*	1 Muffin/111g	389	22.0	350	5.1	40.5	19.8	2.8

OIL
Olive, Blend, Subway*	1 Serving/5g	44	5.0	880	0.0	0.0	100.0	0.0

SALAD
Beef, No Dressing, Subway*	1 Salad/371g	127	2.5	34	4.9	1.9	0.7	1.2
Chicken, Breast, No Dressing, Subway*	1 Salad/385g	152	3.3	39	5.7	2.1	0.9	1.1
Club, No Dressing, Subway*	1 Salad/404g	153	3.4	38	5.7	2.0	0.8	1.1
Ham, No Dressing, Subway*	1 Salad/371g	113	3.0	30	3.5	2.2	0.8	1.2
Sweet Onion Chicken Teriyaki, No Dressing, Subway*	1 Serving/427g	206	3.7	48	5.4	4.7	0.9	1.1
Turkey Breast & Ham, No Dressing, Subway*	1 Serving/380g	121	3.0	32	4.0	2.1	0.8	1.2
Turkey, Breast, No Dressing, Subway*	1 Salad/371g	111	2.5	30	3.8	1.9	0.7	1.2

SUBWAY

SANDWICH

	Measure INFO/WEIGHT	per Measure KCAL	FAT	Nutrition Values per 100g / 100ml KCAL	PROT	CARB	FAT	FIBRE
Veggie Delite, No Dressing, Subway*	1 Salad/314g	58	1.1	18	1.0	2.2	0.4	1.4
Italian Bmt, & Cheese, White Bread, 6", Subway*	1 Sub/240g	424	21.0	177	9.6	16.3	8.8	1.3
Sub, Bacon, Breakfast, Wheat Bread, 6", Subway*	1 Sub/98g	264	8.1	269	15.3	36.7	8.3	2.9
Sub, Bacon, Breakfast, White Bread, 6", Subway*	1 Sub/93g	259	7.9	278	15.1	38.7	8.5	2.2
Sub, Bacon, Egg & Cheese, 6", Subway*	1 Sub/184g	437	23.1	238	12.0	20.1	12.6	1.7
Sub, Bacon, Egg & Cheese, White, 6", Subway*	1 Sub/179g	432	22.9	241	11.7	20.7	12.8	1.3
Sub, Beef, Wheat Bread, Lite, 6, Subway*	1 Sub/226g	272	4.1	120	10.6	17.3	1.8	1.8
Sub, Beef, Wheat Bread, Mini, Subway*	1 Sub/148g	181	2.7	122	10.8	17.6	1.8	1.8
Sub, Beef, White Bread, Lite, 6, Subway*	1 Sub/221g	267	3.9	121	10.4	17.7	1.8	1.5
Sub, Beef, White Bread, Mini, Subway*	1 Sub/145g	176	2.3	121	11.4	15.9	1.6	1.5
Sub, Chicken & Bacon Ranch, Cheese, Wheat, 6", Subway*	1 Sub/299g	489	20.9	164	13.0	13.7	7.0	1.3
Sub, Chicken & Bacon Ranch, Cheese, White, 6", Subway*	1 Sub/294g	484	20.7	165	12.9	14.0	7.0	1.1
Sub, Chicken Breast, Wheat Bread, Lite, 6", Subway*	1 Sub/240g	298	4.8	124	11.7	16.7	2.0	1.7
Sub, Chicken Breast, White Bread, Lite, 6", Subway*	1 Sub/235g	293	4.6	125	11.5	17.0	2.0	1.4
Sub, Chicken Teriyaki & Onion, Wheat, Lite, 6", Subway*	1 Sub/283g	352	5.3	124	10.3	18.0	1.9	1.6
Sub, Chicken Teriyaki & Onion, White, Lite, 6", Subway*	1 Sub/278g	347	5.1	125	10.1	18.4	1.8	1.3
Sub, Chicken, Reggae Reggae, 6", Subway*	1 Sub/100g	380	9.3	380	29.7	47.8	9.3	3.9
Sub, Club, Wheat Bread, Lite, 6", Subway*	1 Sub/259g	299	5.0	115	11.2	15.1	1.9	1.5
Sub, Club, White Bread, Lite, 6", Subway*	1 Sub/254g	294	4.8	116	11.0	15.4	1.9	1.3
Sub, Egg & Cheese, Breakfast, Wheat Bread, 6", Subway*	1 Sub/162g	352	16.5	217	10.5	22.8	10.2	1.9
Sub, Egg & Cheese, Breakfast, White Bread, 6", Subway*	1 Sub/157g	347	16.3	221	10.2	23.6	10.4	1.5
Sub, Ham, & Salad, Subway*	1 Sub/222g	290	5.0	131	8.1	20.7	2.3	1.8
Sub, Ham, Wheat Bread, Lite, 6", Subway*	1 Sub/226g	259	4.5	115	8.4	17.3	2.0	1.8
Sub, Ham, Wheat Bread, Mini, Subway*	1 Sub/138g	162	2.7	117	8.0	18.8	2.0	1.9
Sub, Ham, White Bread, Lite, 6", Subway*	1 Sub/221g	254	4.3	115	8.1	17.7	2.0	1.5
Sub, Ham, White Bread, Mini, Subway*	1 Sub/135g	157	2.3	116	8.5	17.0	1.7	1.6
Sub, Italian, Bmt, & Cheese, Wheat Bread, 6", Subway*	1 Sub/245g	429	21.2	175	9.8	15.9	8.7	1.6
Sub, Meatball Marinara, & Cheese, Wheat, 6", Subway*	1 Sub/382g	520	22.4	136	7.3	14.9	5.9	1.8
Sub, Meatball Marinara, & Cheese, White, 6", Subway*	1 Sub/377g	515	22.2	137	7.2	15.1	5.9	1.6
Sub, Mega Breakfast & Cheese, White Bread, 6, Subway*	1 Sub/242g	569	31.6	235	12.4	17.8	13.1	1.6
Sub, Mega Breakfast, Wheat Bread, 6, Subway*	1 Sub/247g	574	31.8	232	12.6	17.4	12.9	1.9
Sub, Melt, & Cheese, Wheat Bread, 6, Subway*	1 Sub/257g	351	11.1	137	10.5	15.6	4.3	1.6
Sub, Melt, & Cheese, White Bread, 6", Subway*	1 Sub/252g	346	10.9	137	10.3	15.9	4.3	1.3
Sub, Sausage, Breakfast, Wheat Bread, 6", Subway*	1 Sub/156g	364	14.6	233	12.2	26.9	9.4	2.7
Sub, Sausage, Breakfast, White Bread, 6", Subway*	1 Sub/151g	359	14.4	238	11.9	27.8	9.5	2.3
Sub, Sausage, Egg & Cheese, Breakfast, Wheat, 6", Subway*	1 Sub/238g	533	28.9	224	11.8	18.1	12.1	1.9
Sub, Sausage, Egg & Cheese, Breakfast, White, 6", Subway*	1 Sub/233g	528	28.7	227	11.6	18.5	12.3	1.6
Sub, Spicy Italian, & Cheese, Wheat Bread, 6", Subway*	1 Sub/229g	461	26.1	201	9.6	17.0	11.4	1.8
Sub, Spicy Italian, & Cheese, White Bread, 6", Subway*	1 Sub/224g	456	25.9	204	9.4	17.4	11.6	1.4
Sub, Steak & Cheese, Wheat Bread, 6", Subway*	1 Sub/253g	336	9.8	133	9.9	16.2	3.9	1.6
Sub, Steak & Cheese, White Bread, 6, Subway*	1 Sub/248g	331	9.6	133	9.7	16.5	3.9	1.3
Sub, Tuna & Cheese, White Bread, Mini, Subway*	1 Sub/155g	251	11.1	162	8.7	15.5	7.2	1.4
Sub, Tuna, & Cheese, Wheat Bread, 6", Subway*	1 Sub/253g	402	18.6	159	8.7	16.2	7.4	1.6
Sub, Tuna, & Cheese, Wheat Bread, Mini, Subway*	1 Sub/158g	256	11.5	162	8.2	17.1	7.3	1.7
Sub, Tuna, & Cheese, White Bread, 6", Subway*	1 Sub/248g	397	18.4	160	8.5	16.5	7.4	1.3
Sub, Turkey Breast & Ham, Wheat Bread, Lite, 6", Subway*	1 Sub/236g	267	4.5	113	8.9	16.5	1.9	1.7
Sub, Turkey Breast & Ham, White Bread, Lite, 6", Subway*	1 Sub/231g	262	4.3	113	8.7	16.9	1.9	1.4
Sub, Turkey Breast, Subway*	1 Sub/235g	264	3.4	112	8.1	16.6	1.5	1.7
Sub, Turkey Breast, Wheat Bread, Lite, 6", Subway*	1 Sub/226g	256	4.1	113	8.9	17.3	1.8	1.8
Sub, Turkey Breast, Wheat Bread, Mini, Subway*	1 Sub/148g	170	2.7	115	8.8	17.6	1.8	1.8
Sub, Turkey Breast, White Bread, Lite, 6", Subway*	1 Sub/221g	251	3.9	114	8.6	17.7	1.8	1.5
Sub, Turkey Breast, White Bread, Mini, Subway*	1 Sub/145g	165	2.3	114	9.3	15.9	1.6	1.5

	Measure INFO/WEIGHT	per Measure		Nutrition Values per 100g / 100ml				
		KCAL	FAT	KCAL	PROT	CARB	FAT	FIBRE

SUBWAY
SANDWICH

	Measure INFO/WEIGHT	KCAL	FAT	KCAL	PROT	CARB	FAT	FIBRE
Sub, Turkey, & Ham, 6", Subway*	1 Sub/244g	271	3.8	111	7.8	16.0	1.6	1.6
Sub, Veggie Delite, Wheat Bread, Lite, 6", Subway*	1 Sub/169g	203	2.6	120	5.3	22.5	1.5	2.4
Sub, Veggie Delite, White Bread, Lite, 6", Subway*	1 Sub/164g	198	2.4	121	4.9	23.2	1.5	2.0
Sub, Veggie Patty, & Cheese, Wheat Bread, 6", Subway*	1 Sub/267g	414	13.3	155	8.6	17.6	5.0	1.5
Sub, Veggie Patty, & Cheese, White Bread, 6, Subway*	1 Sub/262g	409	13.1	156	8.4	17.9	5.0	1.2

SAUCE

		KCAL	FAT	KCAL	PROT	CARB	FAT	FIBRE
Chipotle Southwest, Subway*	1 Serving/21g	88	9.0	419	0.0	9.5	42.9	1.0
Honey & Mustard, Subway*	1 Serving/21g	32	0.2	152	0.0	33.3	1.0	0.5
Sweet Onion, Subway*	1 Serving/21g	38	0.2	181	0.0	42.9	1.0	0.5

WRAP

		KCAL	FAT	KCAL	PROT	CARB	FAT	FIBRE
Chicken, & Bacon Ranch, Subway*	1 Wrap/256g	374	20.0	146	13.3	3.9	7.8	5.0
Tuna, & Cheese, Subway*	1 Wrap/210g	406	31.0	193	10.0	3.8	14.8	6.1
Tuna, Subway*	1 Wrap/210g	310	19.0	148	10.0	3.8	9.1	6.2
Turkey & Bacon, with Chipotle Sauce, Melt, Subway*	1 Wrap/242g	386	23.0	160	12.0	5.0	9.5	5.3
Turkey Breast & Bacon Melt, Subway*	1 Wrap/242g	386	24.0	160	12.0	5.0	9.9	5.4
Turkey, Subway*	1 Wrap/184g	157	3.7	85	10.9	4.4	2.0	7.1

WIMPY
BAGUETTE

		KCAL	FAT	KCAL	PROT	CARB	FAT	FIBRE
BLT, Best, Wimpy*	1 Serving/177g	320	6.9	181	9.9	25.1	3.9	1.6
Beef, Big, Wimpy*	1 Serving/240g	578	29.5	241	13.2	19.3	12.3	1.2
Cheese, Big, Wimpy*	1 Serving/185g	474	23.1	256	11.8	24.0	12.5	1.5
Chicken, Hot 'n' Spicy, Wimpy*	1 Serving/230g	522	22.8	227	9.5	24.9	9.9	1.8
Sausage, Sizzler, Wimpy*	1 Serving/193g	519	23.9	269	10.8	28.6	12.4	1.7
Spicy Beanburger, Wimpy*	1 Serving/254g	597	26.7	235	5.9	29.3	10.5	2.5

BEANS

		KCAL	FAT	KCAL	PROT	CARB	FAT	FIBRE
Baked, Wimpy*	1 Portion/110g	83	0.2	75	4.7	13.6	0.2	3.7

BREAKFAST

		KCAL	FAT	KCAL	PROT	CARB	FAT	FIBRE
All Day, Wimpy*	1 Serving/410g	730	39.8	178	8.3	14.5	9.7	2.0
Big Breakfast, Wimpy*	1 Serving/216g	404	26.4	187	12.7	5.6	12.2	0.5
The Country Breakfast, Wimpy*	1 Serving/265g	339	17.0	128	8.5	8.8	6.4	1.8
The Great, Wimpy*	1 Breakfast/443g	793	41.2	179	9.7	14.2	9.3	1.3
Wimpy*	1 Serving/301g	452	25.0	150	10.6	7.7	8.3	1.6

BURGERS

		KCAL	FAT	KCAL	PROT	CARB	FAT	FIBRE
Cheeseburger, Bacon, Wimpy*	1 Burger/145g	345	15.3	238	13.2	22.3	10.6	0.0
Cheeseburger, Wimpy*	1 Burger/118g	317	14.8	269	14.7	24.7	12.5	1.3
Chicken & Bacon, Melt, Wimpy*	1 Burger/174g	447	21.8	257	13.9	21.0	12.5	1.3
Chicken, Fillet, Gourmet, Wimpy*	1 Burger/327g	513	13.7	157	14.8	15.3	4.2	0.8
Chicken, Hot 'n' Spicy, in a Bun, Wimpy*	1 Burger/188g	414	20.5	220	9.7	20.7	10.9	1.6
Chicken, in a Bun, Wimpy*	1 Burger/154g	411	22.3	267	11.3	22.0	14.5	1.5
Double Decker, Wimpy*	1 Burger/270g	830	51.4	307	19.0	15.7	19.0	2.5
Gourmet, Wimpy*	1 Burger/291g	675	32.6	232	14.4	18.8	11.2	1.0
Half Pounder, Wimpy*	1 Burger/299g	852	53.5	285	18.5	12.8	17.9	1.6
Hamburger, Wimpy*	1 Burger/104g	277	11.5	266	14.2	27.3	11.1	1.4
Leanburger, Wimpy*	1 Burger/191g	315	12.2	165	12.4	14.6	6.4	0.9
Quarter Pounder, Wimpy*	1 Burger/200g	548	31.2	274	15.3	18.9	15.6	2.4
Quarter Pounder, with Cheese, Wimpy*	1 Burger/214g	589	34.2	275	15.4	17.9	16.0	2.2
Spicy Bean, Wimpy*	1 Burger/221g	526	24.3	238	6.3	29.1	11.0	3.8
Spicy Bean, with Cheese, Wimpy*	1 Burger/205g	520	22.0	254	7.9	33.5	10.7	7.8
The Classic, Kingsize, Wimpy*	1 Burger/229g	559	32.1	244	16.4	13.1	14.0	0.8
The Classic, Wimpy*	1 Burger/159g	343	16.1	216	12.8	18.4	10.1	1.1
The Classic, with Cheese & Bacon, Wimpy*	1 Burger/194g	411	20.0	212	14.0	15.5	10.3	0.9
The Classic, with Cheese, Wimpy*	1 Burger/173g	386	19.4	223	13.2	17.3	11.2	1.0

	Measure INFO/WEIGHT	per Measure KCAL	FAT	Nutrition Values per 100g / 100ml KCAL	PROT	CARB	FAT	FIBRE

WIMPY

BURGERS VEGETARIAN

	Measure INFO/WEIGHT	KCAL	FAT	KCAL	PROT	CARB	FAT	FIBRE
Quorn, in a Bun, Wimpy*	1 Burger/170g	380	18.2	224	9.8	22.1	10.7	0.0
CHICKEN &								
Chips, Chunks, Wimpy*	1 Serving/317g	713	41.8	225	7.9	19.5	13.2	1.9
CHIPS								
Large, Wimpy*	1 Serving/143g	335	17.2	234	3.0	30.4	12.0	3.0
Standard, Wimpy*	1 Serving/114g	267	13.7	234	3.0	30.5	12.0	3.0
COOKIES								
Chocolate, Triple, Wimpy*	1 Serving/80g	377	17.4	471	7.9	60.9	21.8	2.3
Milk Chocolate, Wimpy*	1 Serving/70g	311	10.5	444	6.9	69.6	15.0	1.4
White Chocolate, Wimpy*	1 Serving/80g	383	17.4	479	10.5	60.3	21.8	1.0
DESSERT								
Apple Pie, with Ice Cream, Wimpy*	1 Serving/194g	483	25.2	249	3.2	31.7	13.0	1.4
Apple Pie. with Cream, Wimpy*	1 Dessert/174g	459	25.1	264	3.0	32.4	14.4	1.6
Chocolate Fudge Cake, with Cream, Wimpy*	1 Dessert/95g	315	5.9	332	3.6	65.5	6.2	0.4
Chocolate Fudge Cake, with Ice Cream, Wimpy*	1 Dessert/115g	340	6.0	296	3.7	58.6	5.2	0.3
Spotted Dick, with Cream, Wimpy*	1 Dessert/140g	466	19.2	333	4.1	48.9	13.7	0.6
Spotted Dick, with Custard, Wimpy*	1 Dessert/280g	602	21.0	215	3.6	33.6	7.5	0.3
Spotted Dick, with Ice Cream, Wimpy*	1 Dessert/160g	490	19.4	306	4.2	46.1	12.1	0.6
Treacle Sponge Pudding, with Cream, Wimpy*	1 Dessert/140g	533	24.1	381	3.8	52.6	17.2	0.4
Treacle Sponge Pudding, with Custard, Wimpy*	1 Dessert/280g	669	26.0	239	3.4	35.4	9.3	0.2
Treacle Sponge Pudding, with Ice Cream, Wimpy*	1 Pudding/160g	558	24.3	349	3.9	49.3	15.2	0.3
FISH								
in a Bun, Wimpy*	1 Serving/245g	515	13.5	210	14.0	26.1	5.5	1.5
FISH & CHIPS								
Wimpy*	1 Serving/266g	519	28.2	195	7.6	18.2	10.6	2.4
GRILL								
Bacon, Classic, Wimpy*	1 Grill/306g	719	45.3	235	12.0	14.6	14.8	1.3
Classic, Wimpy*	1 Grill/314g	754	50.9	240	11.1	14.1	16.2	1.2
Double Egg & Chips, Wimpy*	1 Grill/214g	445	27.6	208	7.9	16.3	12.9	1.6
Frankfurter, Wimpy*	1 Grill/308g	684	45.3	222	8.8	14.4	14.7	1.2
Quarterpounder, Wimpy*	1 Grill/395g	955	63.5	242	12.8	11.8	16.1	0.0
The International, Wimpy*	1 Grill/400g	896	58.8	224	12.8	11.2	14.7	1.0
HASH BROWNS								
Wimpy*	1 Serving/55g	93	7.8	169	2.2	19.6	14.2	1.8
HOT DOG								
Frankfurter, in a Bun, with Cheese, Wimpy*	1 Hotdog/172g	432	24.3	251	10.3	20.6	14.1	1.1
Frankfurter, in a Bun, with Chips, Wimpy*	1 Meal/158g	389	21.0	246	9.7	22.0	13.3	1.2
Wimpy*	1 Hot Dog/146g	412	21.0	282	11.0	27.1	14.4	1.4
ICE CREAM								
Banana Longboat, with Dairy Ice Cream, Wimpy*	1 Serving/199g	285	9.2	143	2.4	24.0	4.6	0.7
Banana Longboat, with Soft Ice Cream, Wimpy*	1 Serving/209g	259	6.1	124	2.3	23.9	2.9	0.7
Brown Derby, with Dairy Ice Cream, Wimpy*	1 Serving/125g	399	20.8	319	5.4	36.9	16.6	1.5
Brown Derby, with Soft Ice Cream, Wimpy*	1 Serving/138g	397	19.7	288	5.1	35.2	14.3	1.4
Chocolate, Wimpy*	1 Serving/67g	177	7.1	264	7.0	32.1	10.6	0.0
Ice Mountain, Wimpy*	1 Serving/230g	531	27.1	231	3.9	27.7	11.8	0.4
Knickerbockerglory, with Dairy Ice Cream, Wimpy*	1 Serving/194g	386	15.1	199	2.5	30.3	7.8	0.3
Knickerbockerglory, with Soft Ice Cream, Wimpy*	1 Serving/136g	196	6.0	144	2.7	25.1	4.4	4.4
Mint, Choc Chip, Wimpy*	1 Serving/67g	187	13.0	279	4.0	24.9	19.4	0.0
Strawberry, Wimpy*	1 Serving/67g	148	6.4	221	4.0	29.6	9.6	0.0
Sundae, Mint Chocolate, Wimpy*	1 Serving/113g	325	15.6	288	4.1	36.6	13.8	0.4
Sundae, Neopolitan, Wimpy*	1 Sundae/135g	329	13.9	244	4.1	33.0	10.3	0.2
Sundae, Strawberry, Triple, with Dairy Ice Cream, Wimpy*	1 Serving/170g	394	17.7	232	3.4	31.6	10.4	0.5

WIMPY

ICE CREAM

Sundea, Strawberry, with Soft Ice Cream, Wimpy*	1 Serving/78g	123	3.3	158	2.9	28.5	4.2	0.3
Vanilla, Wimpy*	1 Serving/67g	150	7.8	224	4.6	25.2	11.6	0.0

MUSHROOMS

Wimpy*	1 Serving/114g	179	18.5	157	2.4	0.3	16.2	1.5

NUGGETS

Veg & Cheese, with Chips, Wimpy*	1 Meal/234g	571	34.0	244	3.9	25.4	14.5	2.1

ONION RINGS

12, Wimpy*	1 Portion/180g	401	23.2	223	3.2	23.6	12.9	3.0
6, Wimpy*	1 Serving/90g	201	11.6	223	3.2	23.6	12.9	3.0

POTATO JACKET

Plain, with Butter, Wimpy*	1 Serving/356g	491	7.8	138	3.5	28.0	2.2	2.4
with Baked Beans, Wimpy*	1 Serving/481g	587	7.7	122	3.8	24.3	1.6	2.8
with Coleslaw, Wimpy*	1 Serving/481g	818	40.9	170	2.9	21.8	8.5	2.2

RIBS

Pork, Wimpy*	1 Rib/189g	455	21.9	241	12.9	21.1	11.6	1.4

ROLL

Bacon & Egg, Breakfast, Wimpy*	1 Roll/194g	369	12.0	190	13.4	18.3	6.2	1.1
Bacon & Egg, in a Bun, Wimpy*	1 Roll/155g	308	11.5	199	13.3	18.2	7.4	1.0
Bacon, Breakfast, Wimpy*	1 Roll/144g	278	5.0	193	13.3	24.7	3.5	1.5
Bacon, in a Bun, Wimpy*	1 Roll/105g	218	4.6	208	13.1	26.9	4.4	1.5
Quorn, in a Bun, Wimpy*	1 Roll/165g	380	18.2	230	10.1	22.8	11.0	3.5
Sausage & Egg, Breakfast, Wimpy*	1 Roll/211g	528	28.5	250	11.8	20.3	13.5	1.2
Sausage, Breakfast, Wimpy*	1 Roll/161g	436	21.6	271	11.3	26.6	13.4	1.6

SALAD

Chicken, Gourmet, Wimpy*	1 Serving/383g	253	4.2	66	11.1	2.7	1.1	0.4
Chicken, Hot 'n' Spicy, Wimpy*	1 Salad/310g	267	13.3	86	4.9	7.3	4.3	1.0
Fish, Wimpy*	1 Serving/320g	262	11.8	82	5.8	6.5	3.7	1.4
Side, Wimpy*	1 Salad/155g	143	13.3	92	0.9	2.7	8.6	0.9
Spicy Beanburger, Wimpy*	1 Serving/320g	330	18.6	103	1.8	11.3	5.8	1.7

TEACAKE

with Butter, Wimpy*	1 Serving/62g	239	9.1	385	8.1	56.7	14.6	2.6

TOAST

Butter & Jam, Wimpy*	1 Serving/89g	278	8.4	312	7.3	52.8	9.4	1.7

Useful Resources

Beating Bowel Cancer
Beating Bowel Cancer is a leading UK charity for bowel cancer patients, working to raise awareness of symptoms, promote early diagnosis and encourage open access to treatment choice for those affected by bowel cancer.
Tel: 020 8892 5256   Email: info@beatingbowelcancer.org
Website: http://www.bowelcancer.org

Cancer Research
Cancer Research UK is the leading UK charity dedicated to research, education and fundraising for all forms of cancer.
Tel: 0207 242 0200 Email: via their website
Website: www.cancerresearchuk.org

Diabetes Advice
Diabetes UK is the leading charity working for people with diabetes. Their mission is to improve the lives of people with diabetes and to work towards a future without diabetes
Tel : 0845 120 2960 Email: info@diabetes.org.uk
Website: www.diabetes.org.uk

Dietary Advice
The British Dietetic Association has helpful food fact leaflets and information on how to contact a registered dietitian.
Tel: 0121 200 8080 Email: webmaster@bda.uk.com
Website: : www.bda.uk.com

Exercise Equipment for Home
Diet and Fitness Resources has a range of equipment for exercise at home, from pedometers to treadmills and fitballs to weights. As well as diet tools such as food diaries, a weight loss kit and diet plates.
Tel: 01733 345592   Email: helpteam@dietandfitnessresources.co.uk
Website: www.dietandfitnessresources.co.uk

Healthy Eating
The British Nutrition Foundation has lots of in depth scientifically based nutritional information, knowledge and advice on healthy eating for all ages.
Tel: 0207 404 6504 Email: postbox@nutrition.org.uk
Website: www.nutrition.org.uk

Healthy Heart

The British Heart Foundation provides advice and information for all on all heart aspects from being healthy, to living with heart conditions, research and fundraising.
Tel: 0845 070 8070 Email: via their website
Website: www.bhf.org.uk

Safety and Standards

The Food Standards Agency is an independent watchdog, set up to protect the public's health and consumer interests in relation to food.
Tel: 0207 276 8000 Email: helpline@foodstandards.gsi.gov.uk
Website: www.foodstandards.gov.uk

Weight Loss

Weight Loss Resources is home to the UK's largest calorie and nutrition database along with diaries, tools and expert advice for weight loss and health.
Tel: 01733 345592 Email: helpteam@weightlossresources.co.uk
Website: www.weightlossresources.co.uk

Feedback

If you have any comments or suggestions about The Calorie, Carb & Fat Bible, or would like further information on Weight Loss Resources, please call, email, or write to us:

Tel: 01733 345592
Email: helpteam@weightlossresources.co.uk
Address: Pat Wilson,
          Weight Loss Resources Ltd,
          29 Metro Centre,
          Woodston,
          Peterborough,
          PE2 7UH.

Reviews for The Calorie Carb & Fat Bible

'What a brilliant book. I know I'll be sinking my teeth into it.'
GMTV Nutritionist Amanda Ursell, BSc RD

'To help you make low-cal choices everyday, invest in a copy.'
ZEST magazine

'There is no doubt that the food listings are extremely helpful
for anyone wishing to control their calorie intake in order to lose
pounds or maintain a healthy weight.'
Women's Fitness magazine

'Useful if you don't want to exclude any overall food groups.'
Easy Living magazine

'Quite simply an astonishing achievement by the authors.'
Evening Post, Nottingham

'The book gives you all the basic information so you can work out
your daily calorie needs.'
Woman magazine

'This is a welcome resource in view of the 'national epidemic of obesity.'

Bryony Philip, Bowel Cancer UK

'The authors seem to understand the problems of slimming.'

Dr John Campion

'Jam-packed with info on dieting, and full to bursting point with the calorie, carbohydrate and fat values of thousands of different foods, it's the perfect weight loss tool.'

Evening Express, Aberdeen

'Excellent resource tool - used by myself in my role as a Practice Nurse.'

Pam Boal, Sunderland

'I recently bought your book called the Calorie, Carb & Fat Bible and would love to tell you what a brilliant book it is. I have recently started a weight management programme and I honestly don't know where I'd be without your book. It has helped me a lot and given me some really good advice.'

Rachel Mitchell

About Weight Loss Resources

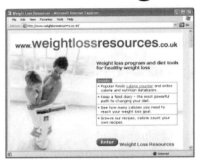

"What this does is put you in control with no guilt, no awful groups and no negativity! Fill in your food diary, get support on the boards and watch it fall off!"

LINDAB, Weight Loss Resources Member

How Does It Work?

Weight Loss Resources is home to the UK's biggest online calorie and nutrition database. You simply tap in your height, weight, age and basic activity level - set a weight loss goal, and the programme does all the necessary calculations.

What Does It Do?

The site enables you to keep a food diary which keeps running totals of calories, fat, fibre, carbs, proteins and portions of fruit and veg. You can also keep an exercise diary which adds the calories you use during exercise. At the end of a week, you update your weight and get reports and graphs on your progress.

How Will It Help?

You'll learn a great deal about how your eating and drinking habits affect your weight and how healthy they are. Using the diaries and other tools you'll be able to make changes that suit your tastes and your lifestyle. The result is weight loss totally tailored to your needs and preferences. A method you can stick with that will help you learn how to eat well for life!

Try It Free!

Go to **www.weightlossresources.co.uk** and take a completely free, no obligation, 24 hour trial. If you like what you see you can sign up for membership from £7.95 per month.